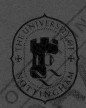

Encyclopedia of Pharmaceutical Technology

Second Edition

Volume 2
E–Pat
Pages 1033–2044

edited by

James Swarbrick

President
PharmaceuTech, Inc., Pinehurst, North Carolina
and
Vice President for Scientific Affairs, aaiPharma, Inc.
Wilmington, North Carolina, U.S.A.

and

James C. Boylan

Pharmaceutical Consultant
Gurnee, Illinois, U.S.A.

MARCEL DEKKER, INC.   NEW YORK • BASEL

Cover Art: Leigh A. Rondano, Boehringer angelheim Pharmaceuticals, Inc.

ISBN: Volume 1:   0-8247-2822-X
        Volume 2:   0-8247-2823-8
        Volume 3:   0-8247-2824-6
        Prepack: 0-8247-2825-4

ISBN: Online: 0-8247-2820-3

This book is printed on acid-free paper.

Headquarters
Marcel Dekker, Inc.
270 Madison Avenue, New York, NY 10016
tel: 212-696-9000; fax: 212-685-4540

Eastern Hemisphere distribution
Marcel Dekker AG
Hutgasse 4, Postfach 812, CH-4001 Basel, Switzerland
tel: 41-61-261-8482; fax: 41-61-261-8896

World Wide Web
http://www.dekker.com

Current printing (last digit)

10 9 8 7 6 5 4 3 2 1

PRINTED IN THE UNITED STATES OF AMERICA

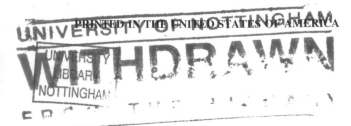

List of Contributors

Phillip M. Achey/*University of Florida, Gainesville, Florida, U.S.A.*

James P. Agalloco/*Agalloco & Associates, Belle Mead, New Jersey, U.S.A.*

Jean-Marc Aiache/*Faculty of Pharmacy, University of Clermont-Ferrand, Clermont-Ferrand, France*

James E. Akers/*Akers Kennedy & Associates, Kansas City, Missouri, U.S.A.*

Michael J. Akers/*Cook Pharmaceutical Solutions, Bloomington, Indiana, U.S.A.*

Loyd V. Allen, Jr./*International Journal of Pharmaceutical Compounding, Edmond, Oklahoma, U.S.A.*

David G. Allison/*University of Manchester, Manchester, United Kingdom*

Hemant H. Alur/*University of Missouri–Kansas City, Kansas City, Missouri, U.S.A.*

Norman Anthony Armstrong/*Cardiff University, Cardiff, United Kingdom*

Agnès Artiges/*European Directorate for the Quality of Medicines (EDQM), Council of Europe, Strasbourg, France*

Carolyn H. Asbury/*University of Pennsylvania, Philadelphia, Pennsylvania, U.S.A.*

Larry L. Augsburger/*University of Maryland School of Pharmacy, Baltimore, Maryland, U.S.A.*

J. Desmond Baggot/*Monash University, Parkville, Victoria, Australia*

Paul Baldrick/*Regulatory Affairs-Pharmaceuticals, Covance Laboratories Ltd., Harrogate, England*

Debra Barnes/*Hoffmann-LaRoche, Palo Alto, California, U.S.A.*

Onkaram Basavapathruni/*Pharmacia Corporation, Peapack, New Jersey, U.S.A.*

G. J. P. J. Beernink/*University of Florida, Gainesville, Florida, U.S.A.*

Leslie Z. Benet/*University of California San Francisco, San Francisco, California, U.S.A.*

David H. Bergstrom/*Cardinal Health Pharmaceutical Technologies & Services Center, Somerset, New Jersey, U.S.A.*

Ira R. Berry/*International Regulatory Business Consultants, L.L.C., Somerset, New Jersey, U.S.A.*

Guru Betageri/*Western University of Health Sciences, Pomona, California, U.S.A.*

Erick Beyssac/*Faculty of Pharmacy, University of Clermont-Ferrand, Clermont-Ferrand, France*

Haresh Bhagat/*Alcon Research Ltd., Fort Worth, Texas, U.S.A.*

Hridaya Bhargava/*Massachusetts College of Pharmacy and Health Sciences, Boston, Massachusetts, U.S.A.*

M.J. Blanco-Príeto/*Universidad de Navarra, Pamplona, Spain*

Daniel Blankschtein/*Massachusetts Institute of Technology, Cambridge, Massachusetts, U.S.A.*

Roland A. Bodmeier/*Freie Universität Berlin, Berlin, Germany*

Michael J. Bogda/*Barr Laboratories, Inc., Pomona, New York, U.S.A.*

iii

René Bommer/*E. Pfeiffer GmbH, Radolfzell, Germany*

Charles Bon/*AAI International, Wilmington, North Carolina, U.S.A.*

Carol A. Borynec/*University Hospital, Edmonton, Alberta, Canada*

David W.A. Bourne/*University of Oklahoma, Oklahoma City, Oklahoma, U.S.A.*

J. Phillip Bowen/*University of Georgia, Athens, Georgia, U.S.A.*

Gayle A. Brazeau/*University of Florida, Gainesville, Florida, U.S.A.*

Ron J. Brendel/*Mallinckrodt, Inc., St. Louis, Missouri, U.S.A.*

Harry G. Brittain/*Center for Pharmaceutical Physics, Milford, New Jersey, U.S.A.*

Albert W. Brzeczko/*Atlantic Pharmaceutical Services, Owings Mills, Maryland, U.S.A.*

Robert A. Buerki/*The Ohio State University College of Pharmacy, Columbus, Ohio, U.S.A.*

Diane J. Burgess/*University of Connecticut, Storrs, Connecticut, U.S.A.*

John B. Cannon/*Abbott Laboratories, Abbott Park, Illinois, U.S.A.*

Allen Cato III/*Cato Research Ltd., San Diego, California, U.S.A.*

Allen Cato/*Cato Research Ltd., Durham, North Carolina, U.S.A.*

Hak-Kim Chan/*University of Sydney, Sydney, New South Wales, Australia*

L.F. Chasseaud/*Huntingdon Life Sciences, Huntingdon, United Kingdom*

Xiu Xiu Cheng/*Andrx Pharmaceuticals, Inc., Fort Lauderdale, Florida, U.S.A.*

Nora Y.K. Chew/*University of Sydney, Sydney, New South Wales, Australia*

Yie W. Chien/*Kaohsiung Medical University, Kaohsiung, Taiwan*

Masood Chowhan/*Alcon Laboratories, Fort Worth, Texas, U.S.A.*

Sebastian G. Ciancio/*State University of New York at Buffalo, Buffalo, New York, U.S.A.*

Emil W. Ciurczak/*Purdue Pharma LP, Ardsley, New York, U.S.A.*

Bradley A. Clark/*Pharmacia, Skokie, Illinois, U.S.A.*

C. Randall Clark/*Auburn University, Auburn, Alabama, U.S.A.*

Sophie-Dorothée Clas/*Merck Frosst Canada & Co., Pointe Claire-Dorval, Quebec City, Canada*

Sarah M.E. Cockbill/*University of Wales College, Cardiff, United Kingdom*

Douglas L. Cocks/*Indiana University, Bloomington, Indiana, U.S.A.*

James J. Conners/*Dura Pharmaceuticals, San Diego, California, U.S.A.*

Kenneth A. Connors/*University of Wisconsin-Madison, Madison, Wisconsin, U.S.A.*

Chyung S. Cook/*Pharmacia Corporation, Skokie, Illinois, U.S.A.*

James F. Cooper/*Charles River Endosafe, Charleston, South Carolina, U.S.A.*

Geoffrey A. Cordell/*University of Illinois at Chicago, Chicago, Illinois, U.S.A.*

Owen I. Corrigan/*University of Dublin, Trinity College, Dublin, Ireland*

Michael Cory/*GlaxoSmithKline, Research Triangle Park, North Carolina, U.S.A.*

Diane D. Cousins/*United States Pharmacopeia, Rockville, Maryland, U.S.A.*

Alan L. Cripps/*GlaxoSmithKline, Ware, Hertfordshire, United Kingdom*

Patrick J. Crowley/*GlaxoSmithKline, H'arlow, United Kingdom*

Anthony M. Cundell/*Wyeth-Ayerst Pharmaceuticals, Pearl River, New York, U.S.A.*

Chad R. Dalton/*Merck Frosst Canada & Co., Pointe Claire-Dorval, Quebec City, Canada*

James T. Dalton/*The Ohio State University, Columbus, Ohio, U.S.A.*

Ira Das/*St. Louis, Missouri, U.S.A.*

Judith A. Davis/*University of Florida, Gainesville, Florida, U.S.A.*

Jack DeRuiter/*Auburn University, Auburn, Alabama, U.S.A.*

M. Begoña Delgado-Charro/*Centre Interuniversitaire de Recherche et d'Enseignement, Archamps, France University of Geneva, Switzerland*

Nigel J. Dent/*Country Consultancy Ltd., Northamptonshire, United Kingdom*

Jeffrey Ding/*Battelle Pulmonary Therapeutics, Inc., Columbus, Ohio, U.S.A.*

Marilyn D. Duerst/*University of Wisconsin-River Falls, River Falls, Wisconsin, U.S.A.*

Gillian M. Eccleston/*University of Strathclyde, Glasgow, United Kingdom*

Ronald P. Evens/*Clinical Research, Amgen Inc., Thousand Oaks, California, U.S.A.*

Kevin L. Facchine/*GlaxoSmithKline, Research Triangle Park, North California, U.S.A.*

Gordon J. Farquharson/*Bovis Lend Lease Pharmaceutical, United Kingdom*

Elias Fattal/*University of Paris XI, Châtenay-Malabry, France*

J.C. Ferdinando/*R.P. Scherer Limited, Swindon, United Kingdom*

Charles W. Fetrow/*St. Francis Medical Center, Pittsburgh, Pennsylvania, U.S.A.*

John W.A. Findlay/*Pharmacia, Skokie, Illinois, U.S.A.*

Joseph A. Fix/*Yamanouchi Pharma Technologies, Inc., Palo Alto, California, U.S.A.*

James L. Ford/*Liverpool John Moores University, Liverpool, United Kingdom*

Farrel L. Fort/*TAP Pharmaceutical Products, Inc., Lake Forest, Illinois, U.S.A.*

Cara R. Frosch/*Covance Central Laboratory Services, Inc., Indianapolis, Indiana, U.S.A.*

Kumar G. Gadamasetti/*ChemRx Advanced Technologies, Inc., San Francisco, California, U.S.A.*

Bruno Gander/*Institute of Pharmaceutical Sciences, Zürich, Switzerland*

David Ganderton/*The University of North Carolina at Chapel Hill, Chapel Hill, North Carolina, U.S.A.*

Isaac Ghebre-Sellassie/*Pfizer Global Research and Development, Morris Plains, New Jersey, U.S.A.*

Peter J. Giddings/*SmithKline Beecham plc, Brentford, United Kingdom*

Peter Gilbert/*University of Manchester, Manchester, United Kingdom*

Danièlle Giron/*Novartis Pharma AG, Basel, Switzerland*

Samuel Givens/*Hoffmann-LaRoche, Nutley, New Jersey, U.S.A.*

Igor Gonda/*Aradigm Corporation, Hayward, California, U.S.A.*

Lee T. Grady/*United States Pharmacopoeia, Rockville, Maryland, U.S.A.*

Jerry J. Groen/*Abbott Laboratories, Abbott Park, Illinois, U.S.A.*

Richard A. Guarino/*Oxford Pharmaceutical Resources, Inc., Totowa, New Jersey, U.S.A.*

Pramod K. Gupta/*TAP Pharmaceuticals, Deerfield, Illinois, U.S.A.*

Richard H. Guy/*Centre Interuniversitaire de Recherche et d'Enseignement, Archamps,
France University of Geneva, Switzerland*

J. Richard Gyory/*ALZA Corporation, Mountain View, California, U.S.A.*

Huijeong A. Hahm/*University of Maryland School of Pharmacy, Baltimore, Maryland, U.S.A.*

Nigel A. Halls/*GlaxoSmithkline Global Manufacturing and Supply, Uxbridge, United Kingdom*

Jerome A. Halperin/*United States Pharmacopeia, Rockville, Maryland, U.S.A.*

Bruno C. Hancock/*Pfizer Inc., Groton, Connecticut, U.S.A.*

Henri Hansson/*Galenica AB, Meleon, Malmö, Sweden*

D.R. Hawkins/*Huntingdon Life Sciences, Huntingdon, United Kingdom*

Leslie C. Hawley/*Pharmacia Corporation, Kalamazoo, Michigan, U.S.A.*

Anne Marie Healy/*University of Dublin, Trinity College, Dublin, Ireland*

Herbert Michael Heise/*Institute of Spectrochemistry and Applied Spectroscopy, Dortmund, Germany*

Jeffrey M. Herz/*Applied Receptor Sciences, Mill Creek, Washington, U.S.A.*

Anthony J. Hickey/*The University of North Carolina, Chapel Hill, North Carolina, U.S.A.*

Gregory J. Higby/*American Institute of the History of Pharmacy, Madison, Wisconsin, U.S.A.*

Anthony J. Hlinak/*Pharmacia, Skokie, Illinois, U.S.A.*

Harm HogenEsch/*Purdue University, West Lafayette, Indiana, U.S.A.*

R. Gary Hollenbeck/*University of Maryland School of Pharmacy, Baltimore, Maryland, U.S.A.*

Stephen A. Howard/*Purdue Pharma L.P., Ardsley, New York, U.S.A.*

Carmel M. Hughes/*The Queen's University of Belfast, Belfast, United Kingdom*

Jeffrey A. Hughes/*University of Florida, Gainesville, Florida, U.S.A.*

Ho-Wah Hui/*Abbott Laboratories, Abbott Park, Illinois, U.S.A.*

D. Hunkeler/*Laboratoire des Polyélectrolytes et BioMacromolécules, Lausanne, Switzerland*

Anwar A. Hussain/*University of Kentucky, Lexington, Kentucky, U.S.A.*

Daniel A. Hussar/*University of the Sciences in Philadelphia, Philadelphia, Pennsylvania, U.S.A.*

Juhana E. Idänpään-Heikkilä/*Council for International Organizations of Medical Sciences,
WHO, Geneva, Switzerland*

Victoria Imber/*CastleRock Technologies, Inc., Sausalito, California, U.S.A.*

David M. Jacobs/*David M. Jacobs Consulting, Basel, Switzerland*

Thomas P. Johnston/*University of Missouri–Kansas City, Kansas City, Missouri, U.S.A.*

Brian E. Jones/*Shionogi Qualicaps, Alcobendas, Spain*

Deborah J. Jones/*Norton Steripak, Cheshire, United Kingdom*

Maik W. Jornitz/*Sartorius Group, Germany*

Jose C. Joseph/*Abbott Laboratories, Abbott Park, Illinois, U.S.A.*

Hans E. Junginger/*Leiden/Amsterdam Center for Drug Research, Leiden University, The Netherlands*

Galina N. Kalinkova/*Medical University, Sofia, Bulgaria*

Isadore Kanfer/*Rhodes University, Grahamstown, South Africa*

Aziz Karim/*Pharmacia Corporation, Skokie, Illinois, U.S.A.*

Brian H. Kaye/*Laurentian University, Sudbury, Ontario, Canada*

David P. Kessler/*Purdue University, West Lafayette, Indiana, U.S.A.*

Ban-An Khaw/*Northeastern University, Boston, Massachusetts, U.S.A.*

Arthur H. Kibbe/*Wilkes University, Wilkes-Barre, Pennsylvania, U.S.A.*

Chris C. Kiesnowski/*Bristol-Myers Squibb Pharmaceutical Research Institute, New Brunswick, New Jersey, U.S.A.*

Kwon H. Kim/*St. John's University, Jamaica, New York, U.S.A.*

Florence K. Kinoshita/*Hercules Incorporated, Arlington, Virginia, U.S.A.*

Cathy M. Klech-Gelotte/*McNeil Consumer Healthcare, Fort Washington, Pennsylvania, U.S.A.*

Axel Knoch/*Pfizer Global Research and Development, Freiburg, Germany*

John J. Koleng, Jr./*The University of Texas at Austin, Austin, Texas, U.S.A.*

Sheldon X. Kong/*Merck & Co. Inc., Whitehouse Station, New Jersey, U.S.A.*

Mark J. Kontny/*Pharmacia, Kalamazoo, Michigan, U.S.A.*

Sylvie Laganière/*Origenix Technologies, Inc., Quebec, Canada*

Duane B. Lakings/*Drug Safety Evaluation Consulting, Inc., Birmingham, Alabama, U.S.A.*

Robert Langer/*Massachusetts Institute of Technology, Cambridge, Massachusetts, U.S.A.*

Destin A. LeBlanc/*Cleaning Validation Technologies, San Antonio, Texas, U.S.A.*

Jason M. LePree/*Boehringer Ingelheim Pharmaceuticals, Ridgefield, Connecticut, U.S.A.*

Chi H. Lee/*The University of Missouri-Kansas City, Kansas City, Missouri, U.S.A.*

Kyung Hee Lee/*University of Illinois at Chicago, Chicago, Illinois, U.S.A.*

Mike S. Lee/*Milestone Development Services, Newtown, Pennsylvania, U.S.A.*

Vincent H.L. Lee/*University of Southern California, Los Angeles, California, U.S.A.*

Yong-Hee Lee/*Trega Biosciences, Inc., San Diego, California, U.S.A.*

Gareth A. Lewis/*Sanofi-Synthelabo, Chilly Mazarin, France*

Luk Chiu Li/*Abbott Laboratories, Abbott Park, Illinois, U.S.A.*

Eric J. Lien/*University of Southern California, Los Angeles, California, U.S.A.*

Senshang Lin/*St. John's University, Jamaica, New York, U.S.A.*

Nils-Olof Lindberg/*Pharamacia AB, Helsingborg, Sweden*

B. Lindsay/*University of Strathclyde, Glasgow, United Kingdom*

John M. Lipari/*Abbott Laboratories, Abbott Park, Illinois, U.S.A.*

Robert L. Maher, Jr./*Duquesne University, Pittsburgh, Pennsylvania, U.S.A.*

Henri R. Manasse, Jr./*American Society of Health-System Pharmacists, Bethesda, Maryland, U.S.A.*

Laviero Mancinelli/*University of California San Francisco, San Francisco, California, U.S.A.*

Peter Markland/*Southern Research Institute, Birmingham, Alabama, U.S.A.*

Diego Marro/*Centre Interuniversitaire de Recherche et d'Enseignement, Archamps, France University of Geneva, Switzerland*

Luigi G. Martini/*GlaxoSmithKline, Harlow, United Kingdom*

Michael B. Maurin/*DuPont Pharmaceuticals Company, Wilmington, Delaware, U.S.A.*

Joachim Mayer/*University of Lausanne, Lausanne, Switzerland*

Orla McCallion/*Vandsons Research, Islington, London, United Kingdom*

James C. McElnay/*The Queen's University of Belfast, Belfast, United Kingdom*

Iain J. McGilveray/*McGilveray Pharmacon, Inc., Ottawa, Ontario, Canada*

Jim W. McGinity/*The University of Texas at Austin, Austin, Texas, U.S.A.*

Michael McKenna/*Pfizer, Inc., New York, New York, U.S.A.*

Marghi R. McKeon/*Lab Safety Corp., Des Plaines, Illinois, U.S.A.*

Eugene J. McNally/*Boehringer Ingelheim Pharmaceuticals, Inc., Ridgefield, Connecticut, U.S.A.*

Duncan E. McVean/*Consultant, Solon, Ohio, U.S.A.*

Robert W. Mendes/*Massachusetts College of Pharmacy and Health Sciences (Retired), Dedham, Massachusetts, U.S.A.*

Marvin C. Meyer/*University of Tennessee, Memphis, Tennessee, U.S.A.*

Ashim K. Mitra/*University of Missouri–Kansas City, Kansas City, Missouri, U.S.A.*

Samir S. Mitragotri/*University of California, Santa Barbara, California, U.S.A.*

Suresh K. Mittal/*Purdue University, West Lafayette, Indiana, U.S.A.*

Lorie Ann Morgan/*GlaxoSmith Kline, Research Triangle Park, North Carolina, U.S.A.*

Karen Morisseau/*University of Rhode Island, Kingston, Rhode Island, U.S.A.*

Gerold Mosher/*CyDex, Inc., Overland Park, Kansas, U.S.A.*

Christel C. Mueller-Goymann/*Universität Braunschweig Mendelssohnstr, Braunschweig, Germany*

Ronald L. Mueller/*GlaxoSmithKline, King of Prussia, Pennsylvania, U.S.A.*

Suman K. Mukherjee/*University of Southern California, Los Angeles, California, U.S.A.*

Sandy J.M. Munro/*GlaxoSmithKline, Ware, Hertfordshire, United Kingdom*

Fernando J. Muzzio/*Rutgers University, Piscataway, New Jersey, U.S.A.*

Paul B. Myrdal/*The University of Arizona, Tucson, Arizona, U.S.A.*

Venkatesh Naini/*Barr Laboratories, Inc., Pomona, New York, U.S.A.*

Jintana M. Napaporn/*University of Florida, Gainesville, Florida, U.S.A.*

Robert A. Nash/*Consultant, Mahwah, New Jersey, U.S.A.*

Deanna J. Nelson/*BioLink Technologies, Inc., Cary, North Carolina, U.S.A.*

Sandeep Nema/*Pharmacia Corporation, Skokie, Illinois, U.S.A.*

Michael T. Newhouse/*Inhale Therapeutic Systems, Inc., San Carlos, California, U.S.A.*

Ann W. Newman/*SSCI, Inc., West Lafayette, Indiana, U.S.A.*

J.M. Newton/*University of London, London, United Kingdom*

Thomas M. Nowak/*Abbott Laboratories, Abbott Park, Illinois, U.S.A.*

Thomas M. O'Connell/*GlaxoSmithKline, Research Triangle Park, North California, U.S.A.*

Christine K. O'Neil/*Duquesne University, Pittsburgh, Pennsylvania, U.S.A.*

B. O'Mahony/*University of Strathclyde, Glasgow, United Kingdom*

John P. Oberdier/*Abbott Laboratories, Abbott Park, Illinois, U.S.A.*

Clyde M. Ofner III/*University of the Sciences in Philadelphia, Philadelphia, Pennsylvania, U.S.A.*

Claudia C. Okeke/*United States Pharmacopeia, Rockville, Maryland, U.S.A.*

Wayne P. Olson/*Consultant, Beecher, Illinois, U.S.A.*

Rama V. Padmanabhan/*ALZA Corporation, Mountain View, California, U.S.A.*

Jagdish Parasrampuria/*Galderma R&D, Cranbury, New Jersey, U.S.A.*

Eun Jung Park/*University of Illinois at Chicago, Chicago, Illinois, U.S.A.*

Jung Y. Park/*Boehringer Ingelheim Pharmaceuticals, Inc., Ridgefield, Connecticut, U.S.A.*

Kinam Park/*Purdue University, West Lafayette, Indiana, U.S.A.*

Barbara Perry/*Hoffmann-LaRoche, Welwyn, United Kingdom*

Adam Persky/*University of Florida, Gainesville, Florida, U.S.A.*

Gregory F. Peters/*Lab Safety Corporation, Des Plaines, Illinois, U.S.A.*

John M. Pezzuto/*University of Illinois at Chicago, Chicago, Illinois, U.S.A.*

J. Bradley Phipps/*ALZA Corporation, Mountain View, California, U.S.A.*

Michael J. Pikal/*University of Connecticut, Storrs, Connecticut, U.S.A.*

Wayne L. Pines/_Pharmaceutical Consultant, Washington, D.C., U.S.A._

Dario Pistolesi/_Fedegari Autoclavi S.p.A., Albuzzano, PV, Italy_

Michael E. Placke/_Battelle Pulmonary Therapeutics, Inc., Columbus, Ohio, U.S.A._

Therese I. Poirier/_Duquesne University, Pittsburgh, Pennsylvania, U.S.A._

Jacques H. Poupaert/_Université Catholique de Louvain, Brussels, Belgium_

Sunil Prabhu/_Western University of Health Sciences, Pomona, California, U.S.A._

Neil Purdie/_Oklahoma State University, Stillwater, Oklahoma, U.S.A._

R. Raghavan/_Abbott Laboratories, Abbott Park, Illinois, U.S.A._

M.S. Rahman/_Cardinal Health Pharmaceutical Technologies & Services Center, Somerset, New Jersey, U.S.A._

Ali R. Rajabi-Siahboomi/_Colorcon Limited, Kent, United Kingdom_

Suneel Rastogi/_Forest Laboratories, Inc., Inwood, New York, U.S.A._

William R. Ravis/_Auburn University, Auburn, Alabama, U.S.A._

Thomas L. Reiland/_Abbott Laboratories, Abbott Park, Illinois, U.S.A._

Jean Paul Remon/_Ghent University, Ghent, Belgium_

Shijun Ren/_University of Southern California, Los Angeles, California, U.S.A._

Michael Repka/_The University of Mississippi, University, Mississippi, U.S.A._

Christopher T. Rhodes/_University of Rhode Island, Kingston, Rhode Island, U.S.A._

Martin M. Rieger/_M&A Rieger, Morris Plains, New Jersey, U.S.A._

Jean G. Riess/_University of California at San Diego, San Diego, California, U.S.A._

Thomas N. Riley/_Auburn University, Auburn, Alabama, U.S.A._

Ronald J. Roberts/_AstraZeneca, Macclesfield, Cheshire, United Kingdom_

Naír Rodríguez-Hornedo/_University of Michigan, Ann Arbor, Michigan, U.S.A._

Raymond C. Rowe/_AstraZeneca, Macclesfield, Cheshire, United Kingdom_

Joseph T. Rubino/_Wyeth-Ayerst Research, Pearl River, New York, U.S.A._

J. Howard Rytting/_The University of Kansas, Lawrence, Kansas, U.S.A._

Rosalie Sagraves/_University of Illinois at Chicago, Chicago, Illinois, U.S.A._

Peter C. Schmidt/_University of Tübingen, Tübingen, Germany_

David R. Schoneker/_Colorcon, West Point, Pennsylvania, U.S.A._

Stephen G. Schulman/_University of Florida, Gainesville, Florida, U.S.A._

Erik R. Scott/_ALZA Corporation, Mountain View, California, U.S.A._

Gerald Scucci/_Rutgers University, Piscataway, New Jersey, U.S.A._

Richard B. Seymour/_Haight Ashbury Free Clinics, San Francisco, California, U.S.A._

Jaymin C. Shah/_Pfizer Inc., Groton, Connecticut, U.S.A._

Umang Shah/_Parke-Davis Division, Warner Lambert, Morris Plains, New Jersey, U.S.A._

Shalaby W. Shalaby/_Poly-Med, Inc., Pendleton, South Carolina, U.S.A._

Leon Shargel/_Eon Labs Manufacturing, Inc., Laurelton, New York, U.S.A._

Joseph Sherma/_Lafayette College, Easton, Pennsylvania, U.S.A._

Troy Shinbrot/_Rutgers University, Piscataway, New Jersey, U.S.A._

Brent D. Sinclair/_University of Michigan, Ann Arbor, Michigan, U.S.A._

Ambarish K. Singh/_The Bristol-Myers Squibb Pharmaceutical Research Institute, New Brunswick, New Jersey, U.S.A._

Brahma N. Singh/_St. John's University, Jamaica, New York, U.S.A._

Shailesh K. Singh/_Wyeth–Ayerst Research, Pearl River, New York, U.S.A._

Patrick J. Sinko/_Rutgers University, Piscataway, New Jersey, U.S.A._

Jerome P. Skelly/_Consultant, Alexandria, Virginia, U.S.A._

Michael F. Skinner/_Rhodes University, Grahamstown, South Africa_

William H. Slattery III/_House Ear Institute, Los Angeles, California, U.S.A._

David E. Smith/_Haight Ashbury Free Clinics, San Francisco, California, U.S.A._

Edward J. Smith/_Packaging Science Resources, King of Prussia, Pennsylvania, U.S.A._

Marshall Steinberg/*International Pharmaceutical Excipients Council-Americas, Arlington, Virginia, U.S.A.*

Ralph Stone/*Alcon Laboratories, Fort Worth, Texas, U.S.A.*

Raj Suryanarayanan/*University of Minnesota, Minneapolis, Minnesota, U.S.A.*

Stuart R. Suter/*Suter Associates, Glenside, Pennsylvania, U.S.A.*

Lynda Sutton/*Cato Research Ltd., Durham, North Carolina, U.S.A.*

Hanne Hjorth Tønnesen/*University of Oslo, Oslo, Norway*

Hua Tang/*Massachusetts Institute of Technology, Cambridge, Massachusetts, U.S.A.*

Kevin M.G. Taylor/*University of London, London, United Kingdom*

Bernard Testa/*University of Lausanne, Lausanne, Switzerland*

Maya Thanou/*Leiden/Amsterdam Center for Drug Research, Leiden University, The Netherlands*

C. Thomasin/*The R.W. Johnson Pharmaceutical Research Institute, Schaffhausen, Switzerland*

Diane O. Thompson/*CyDex, Inc., Overland Park, Kansas, U.S.A.*

William J. Thomsen/*Arena Pharmaceuticals, San Diego, California, U.S.A.*

Youqin Tian/*Alcon Research, Ltd., Fort Worth, Texas, U.S.A.*

Jeffrey Tidwell/*University of North Carolina, Chapel Hill, North Carolina, U.S.A.*

James E. Tingstad/*Tingstad Associates, Green Valley, Arizona, U.S.A.*

Richard Turton/*West Virginia University, Morgantown, West Virginia, U.S.A.*

Mitsuru Uchiyama/*Japan Pharmacists Education Center, Tokyo, Japan*

Madhu K. Vadnere/*NJ Pharma LLC, Chatham, New Jersey, U.S.A.*

Lynn Van Campen/*Inhale Therapeutic Systems, Inc., San Carlos, California, U.S.A.*

Koen Van Deun/*Janssen Pharmaceutica N.V., Beerse, Belgium*

Mark D. VanArendonk/*Pharmacia Corporation, Kalamazoo, Michigan, U.S.A.*

Christine Vauthier/*University of Paris XI, Châtenay-Malabry, France*

Geraldine Venthoye/*Inhale Therapeutic Systems, Inc., San Carlos, California, U.S.A.*

J. Coos Verhoef/*Leiden/Amsterdam Center for Drug Research, Leiden University, The Netherlands*

Vesa Virtanen/*Orion Pharma, Kuopio, Finland*

Imre M. Vitez/*Bristol-Myers Squibb Pharmaceutical Research Institute, New Brunswick, New Jersey, U.S.A.*

Karel Vytras/*University of Pardubice, Pardubice, Czech Republic*

Roderick B. Walker/*Rhodes University, Grahamstown, South Africa*

Kenneth A. Walters/*An-eX Analytical Services Ltd, Cardiff, United Kingdom*

Ch. Wandrey/*Laboratoire des Polyélectrolytes et BioMacromolécules, Lausanne, Switzerland*

R.P. Waranis/*Cardinal Health Pharmaceutical Technologies & Services Center, Somerset, New Jersey, U.S.A.*

Richard J. Washkuhn/*Lexington, Kentucky, U.S.A.*

Alan L. Weiner/*Alcon Research, Ltd., Fort Worth, Texas, U.S.A.*

Peter G. Welling/*University of Strathclyde, Glasgow, Scotland*

Albert I. Wertheimer/*Temple University, Philadelphia, Pennsylvania, U.S.A.*

Cheryl A. Wiens/*University of Alberta, Edmonton, Alberta, Canada*

Ellen M. Williams/*Pfizer, Inc., New York, New York, U.S.A.*

Roger L. Williams/*U.S. Pharmacopeia, Rockville, Marryland, U.S.A.*

C. G. Wilson/*University of Strathclyde, Glasgow, United Kingdom*

A. David Woolfson/*The Queen's University of Belfast, Belfast, United Kingdom*

Samuel H. Yalkowsky/*The University of Arizona, Tucson, Arizona, U.S.A.*

Victor C. Yang/*The University of Michigan, Ann Arbor, Michigan, U.S.A.*

Andrew B.C. Yu/*U.S. Food and Drug Administration, Rockville, Maryland, U.S.A.*

Mark J. Zellhofer/*University Pharmaceuticals of Maryland, Inc., Baltimore, Maryland, U.S.A.*

Feng Zhang/*The University of Texas at Austin, Austin, Texas, U.S.A.*

William C. Zimlich, Jr./*Battelle Pulmonary Therapeutics, Inc., Columbus, Ohio, U.S.A.*

Preface to the Second Edition

Pharmaceutical science and technology have progressed enormously in recent years. Significant advances in therapeutics and a greater understanding of the need to optimize drug delivery in the body have brought about an increased awareness of the valuable role played by the dosage form in therapy. This, in turn, has resulted in an increased sophistication and level of expertise in the design, development, manufacture, testing, and regulation of drugs and dosage forms.

The *Encyclopedia of Pharmaceutical Technology* is a unique, comprehensive compilation that brings together knowledge from every specialty encompassed by pharmaceutical technology. It is the ideal place for initiation of research projects or for becoming acquainted with or updating oneself in a specific topic.

It has been 17 years since we first began organizing topics and contacting potential authors for the first edition of the *Encyclopedia of Pharmaceutical Technology*. The first volume appeared in 1988. The last volume of the first edition, Volume 20, appeared in 2001. As the usefulness of the encyclopedia became evident, a second edition was launched. The constant progress in the many fields comprising pharmaceutical technology has resulted in a second edition that will be available in print and online, which will allow for quarterly updates and expansions.

The print version of the encyclopedia consists of three volumes totaling over 3,000 pages and over 200 articles arranged alphabetically by subject. Each article is written by an expert in a particular specialty and represents the latest advances in the field.

The online version includes everything in the print version and also offers the convenience of a keyword search engine as well as the inclusion of color illustrations. New articles and revised articles will be digitally posted quarterly and available to all subscribers of the electronic version.

The production and publishing of a work of this nature is not possible without the dedication and talent of numerous individuals. In particular, we gratefully acknowledge the efforts of the authors, several of whom have contributed multiple articles. Clearly, without this talented and responsive cadre of world class scientists, there would be no *Encyclopedia of Pharmaceutical Technology*.

Our publisher, Marcel Dekker, Inc., has always been supportive of our efforts and receptive to our editorial needs. We are especially indebted to Carolyn Hall, Managing Editor of the Encyclopedia Department, for her marvelous assistance in working with us to bring this work to fruition.

Finally, we would be remiss if we did not thank you, our readers, for your numerous comments and continuing support. We hope the second edition meets and exceeds your expectations. As always, we welcome your comments.

James Swarbrick
James C. Boylan
Editors

Aims and Scope

The need for a comprehensive, authoritative, contemporary, and relevant collection of articles detailing that area of the pharmaceutical sciences embraced by the term "pharmaceutical technology" has been amply confirmed by the success of the First Edition of the *Encyclopedia of Pharmaceutical Technology*.

With the first volume published in 1988 and the last in 2000, this 20 volume set contained over 300 articles covering a wide range of topics described in over 9000 pages of text, illustrations, tables, references, and indices.

As with the First Edition, the new, Second Edition focuses on a list of topics relevant to the discovery, development, regulation, manufacture, and commercialization of drugs and dosage forms. Consistent with the phrase "pharmaceutical technology," it emphasizes contributions in such areas as pharmaceutics, pharmacokinetics, analytical chemistry, quality assurance, drug safety, and the manufacturing process—not solely on discussion of the chemical and/or pharmacological profiles of individual drugs or classes of drugs.

The aim of the Second Edition is to essentially match the breadth of coverage found in the First Edition but with a more consistent format and style for the approximately 200 topics. At the same time, the number of volumes is being reduced to three, each of approximately 1000 pages, which will be published simultaneously. This more condensed, but consistent, three-volume presentation will appeal to institutional libraries and organizations, as well as individual pharmaceutical scientists.

All First Edition entries selected for inclusion in the Second Edition have been updated. New topics have been included, and some topics reorganized from multiple headings in the First Edition to single entries in the Second Edition, and vice versa, to reflect the current significance of a particular area. As before, the authors are recognized experts in their respective fields of activity.

The online version of the *Encyclopedia* has a powerful search engine, user-friendly interface, and customer-focused features. The database that is *EPT Online* is dynamic, with a number of articles added each quarter. Users can browse the Table of Contents and search the full text in query-based and menu-driven modes. Search features ensure the return of a limited number of useful search results quickly.

EPT Online will be marketed as a subscription product updated quarterly. Purchase of the print *Encyclopedia* will not be a prerequisite for purchase of *EPT Online*. We plan to track the activities of users and broaden our business plan.

Contents

Volume 2

Volume 3

ECONOMIC CHARACTERISTICS OF THE R&D-INTENSIVE PHARMACEUTICAL INDUSTRY

Douglas L. Cocks
Indiana University, Bloomington, Indiana

INTRODUCTION

This article presents a brief sketch of the economics of the R&D-intensive ethical pharmaceutical industry, highlighting its dynamic characteristics. The approach taken here minimizes the use of static analysis, and thus avoids the use of pure or perfect competition as an analytical tool. In this theoretical discussion, certain empirical studies will be cited as support for aspects of the theory being developed.

The theory discussed here will concentrate on allocative efficiency, but as with all discussions of allocative efficiency, elements of technical efficiency will automatically be involved and at least implicit recognition of these elements will be evident. The allocative efficiency concerns will be placed in a dynamic framework; we will be attempting to establish a notion of "dynamic pure competition" that has analytical and public policy implications. The concept of dynamic pure competition will describe a hybrid form of workable competition as the term is used by industrial organization economists.

AN OUTLINE OF A COMPETITIVE PROCESS

Before we get into an outline of the theory of pharmaceutical economics, we need to establish pure competition as a *competitive process*. Traditional microeconomics has assumed implicitly that the "natural state" is one that is depicted by pure competition. Deviations from the natural state occur as a disequilibrium, by the establishment of monopoly power, or through other often cited market failures. In cases of disequilibrium, the tatonnement will bring us to the equilibrium ideal of pure competition. Interestingly, the model of pure competition never really describes the process of the tatonnement (equilibration) but only the conditions necessary for the process to operate and the final equilibrium to result when the process has worked itself out.

The monopoly power deviation arises because the nature of "economic man" causes him or her to attempt to break out of a pure competitive equilibrium, or the equilibrating tatonnement process, and maximize his or her own economic situation relative to the rest of the world. The economic man will attempt to establish a monopoly power position through "entry barrier" meansemp (1a, 1b).

According to traditional microeconomics, then, the natural economic process is one that proceeds from the natural state of pure competitive equilibrium, or from where the necessary conditions exist for the pure competitive tatonnement process to take place, to conditions of monopoly.

The competitive process that is relevant here is one in which a naturally occurring monopoly is systematically faced with a pressure that erodes this position. It is a process that occurs on a continuum and which must be considered on the basis of changes through time. Reverting to the static sense, the economic concept of deadweight welfare loss is a representation of the social opportunity cost that is associated with having entrepreneurs, singular and corporate, invading previously held monopoly positions by providing new and improved products and services. This in turn represents the economic progress that generates welfare gains, in the technically economic context and not in the sense of providing public funds to needy populations. Through time, economic life is characterized as a continual process of monopoly establishment and systematic erosion via entrepreneurial activity. This entrepreneurial activity constitutes the observation of, and action upon, profit opportunities as evidenced by static monopoly rents.

We can think of dynamic pure competition as a process where naturally occurring monopoly is systematically eroded. It represents a kind of entropy that properly allocates resources in the production of current and future goods and services. The underlying characteristics of the competitive process are that it recognizes that economic imperfections are inherent; that economic man realizes this as a matter of course; and he or she is willing to compensate economic agents who act to ameliorate these imperfections.

EMPIRICAL EVIDENCE OF COMPETITION IN THE PHARMACEUTICAL INDUSTRY

The issue of competition in the pharmaceutical industry is implicitly addressed in the works of Cocks and Virts (2, 3), who show a significant lack of price rigidity in various drug markets and among individual drug products. But its clearest discussion is given by Brozen (4):

> The Cocks data also destroy the common fiction of rigid prices for drugs and the fiction of inelastic demands for each of these patented products. Prices are remarkably flexible, thus producing large effects on market position. Leading products in the anti-infective market, for example, suffered price declines from 1962 to 1971 ranging from 7% (for product number 8) to 67% (for product number 3). The average price decline in this inflationary period for these products was 32%, while the consumer price index rose 34%. The price of leading anti-infectives fell by 51% in constant dollars. This is a remarkable record.

Sales of these products also demonstrate what a complete fiction is the story that the average physician pays no attention to prices in writing prescriptions. Product 11 among the anti-infectives languished at 0.1% of the market for 5 years until it had cut its price by 47%. At that point, its market share rose to 0.7%, a sixfold increase. Another 14% price cut raised its market share another 170%. Still further cuts over the next three years amounting to 12% raised its market share by still another 68%. This would seem to demonstrate a remarkably high price elasticity of demand for a branded patented product; particularly in view of the price cuts of competitive products.

Product number 3 had a fading market position from 1962 through 1969 "despite its price cuts, but then a 16% price cut in 1970 stopped the decline and added 14% to its market share. A further 27% cut in 1971 jumped its market share by another 40%. The market for ethical drugs responds remarkably vigorously to price changes, the myth of the price-insensitive prescribing physician to the contrary nothwithstanding.

There appears to be competition among products within each class despite whatever unique features each possesses. A product only singular enough to win 0.1% of the market over a five-year span won a 310% increase in market share when it cut its price relative to most of the other products in its market. A fading product turned itself around and reclaimed a major portion of its market position as it undertook similar price action."

One area that has been emphasized in economic theory is that price competition does not exist if a firm or group of firms can charge different prices to different segments of the market. In the pharmaceutical industry, this "market failure" has been emphasized relative to the prices charged to the elderly. It has been claimed that the elderly pay higher prices than the rest of the population. A recent study by Berndt et al. provides statistical evidence that the elderly do not.

A study by Reekie provides a more systematic analysis of pricing behavior regarding pharmaceutical products (5). This study provides a statistically strong inference that physicians are indeed sensitive to drug prices. The paper provides statistical evidence on pharmaceutical product price elasticity in which the coefficient of elasticity is determined to be greater than 1. Schwartzman also provides significant evidence on the amount of price competition in the pharmaceutical industry, especially in the area of antibiotics (6). The elderly generally pay higher prices than the rest of the population, and in some drug categories they pay lower prices (7).

INTERNAL ORGANIZATION CHARACTERISTICS OF THE PHARMACEUTICAL FIRM

The model of the pharmaceutical firm that we have constructed so far leaves us with a fundamental dichotomization of the firm. The dichotomy is between the firm consisting of the production of existing, marketed products, and the production of new products through research and development. The existence of this naturally leads us to question why the firm has to consist of these seemingly different activities. In other words, why could there not be firms who engage in research and development and only produce new products? They could sell these new products on the open market to firms whose specialized function it is to produce and sell the products developed by research firms. In addressing this issue, it is hoped that greater insight into the subtleties of the theory of the pharmaceutical firm can be garnered.

There are two basic elements as to why it is economically efficient to have both characteristics—current product production and new production—present in one firm. The first element relates to corporate finance and the sources and uses of cash flows in the firm. The second element relates to the efficiencies that can be gained by resorting to markets within the firm (as opposed to external markets that are thought of in conventional microeconomic theory) (8a, 8b, 8c). It should be obvious from the discussion that follows there is an inherent interaction between these elements. This discussion also points out the entrepreneurial function in the firm and its implications for considering the efficiency of the firm.

A characteristic of the pharmaceutical industry, and very likely other R&D-intensive industries, is the interrelationship among new products, the cash flows of the firm, profit expectations, and the utility-enhancing characteristics of new drugs. This flow of economic events can be depicted in the following:

→ Portfolio of products composed of past R&D induced competitive products contributes to forming, maintaining, or raising expected present values of portfolio of current products and portfolio of research products. → Increasing cash flows (this relates to high accounting profits, discussed elsewhere in this article), → Increasing real R&D investment. → A portfolio of products that contains the previous products plus the newly developed products. →

→ Determination of number of new drug products.

This is a series of events that occurs on a continuum, and the main characteristic is the internally generated cash flows that provide the wherewithal for R&D investment to come from the portfolio of existing products. To provide the necessary cash flows, this portfolio must contain products that have a range of price-marginal manufacturing cost differentials.

The relevance of the two elements, just discussed, can be elaborated on by considering the employment relation that is the primary aspect of the R&D process described above. Pharmaceutical R&D is really an investment in and accumulation of human capital through the employment of scientists and technicians. Like all human capital its "producing" aspects are necessarily embodied in individuals. Unlike normal labor (6) and any associated human capital characteristics that go with it (learning by doing), the human capital associated with pharmaceutical R&D creates

complexities of monitoring and metering work effort. These difficulties exacerbate the contingent claims contracts, bounded rationality, opportunism, and information impactedness problems that would prevail if external markets were used. The use of a hierarchical system clearly presents a less costly alternative. In addition, it is evident from the previous description of the R&D process that the internal market organization allows the combining of the R&D inputs and yields output that is larger than the sum of the products if inputs are used separately.

We can now address the significance of a third element—what can be described as the entrepreneurial, combined element. The six stages of the R&D system process are really the steps that characterize going from invention to innovation, as discussed in the economics of innovation literature. The role of the concept of the entrepreneur is very crucial here. If we view the entrepreneur as the economic visionary, the importance of his or her role is especially apparent in stage 1 of our stage process. At this stage something more than mere "scientific" ability is required. It is also necessary to have the vision to convert "science" or knowledge into a useful product. However, each step of the system process requires entrepreneurial input.

The pharmaceutical firm amalgamates the diverse entrepreneurial activities that make up the complex process from invention through getting a marketable pharmaceutical product. In essence, we are making a distinction between the R&D inputs: scientist and scientist-entrepreneur. In many cases, the scientist does not have the full extent of entrepreneurial ability, and the firm provides the mechanism to achieve this. In addition, when dealing with both the scientist and scientist-entrepreneur, the problems with the Williamson (9) concepts are attenuated; resources are economized because the elements of complexity of contingent claims contracts, bounded rationality, information impactedness, and opportunism are separately prevalent in both the scientists' and scientist-entrepreneurs' activities. It is likely that there are distinctive aspects of the Williamson characteristics that are interactive, and this compounds the difficulties and thus makes the internal organization alternative less resource-costly.

In summary, the pharmaceutical R&D process lends itself to the efficiency gains that come from internally organizing these activities. These efficiencies are derived from the existence of the complex technological environment that surrounds the R&D process.

The essence of the theory that we are attempting to apply to the pharmaceutical industry has clearly been outlined by Demsetz. The crucial point is that there are efficiency gains that are apparent not by comparing them with some ideal, but by comparing them with "real world" alternatives (10).

CONCLUSIONS

The model of the economics of the pharmaceutical industry that is developed here has four basic assumptions:

1. There is price sensitivity on the part of pharmaceutical consumers or, in particular, their agents-physicians, for new products as well as for existing products.
2. Research and development (R&D) serves as the primary catalyst for change among drug firms and is the focal point of entrepreneurial activity that ensures dynamic welfare gains (a continuum of static welfare losses being offset by concomitant higher utility, yielding benefits from new products and systematic erosion of monopoly power through price pressures for older products). As an institutional consideration, there will be a substantial number of firms intensively engaged in R&D activity. In the late 1990s there have been attempts at mega mergers in the industry that would create firms approaching the $100 billion or more sales amount. These mergers seem to be due to the significant rise in the R&D cost of developing new drugs—possibly exceeding $500 million.
3. The utility benefits from even small improvements in therapy can theoretically offset substantial differences in the prices of the new improvement relative to existing drug therapies. (This is basically a corollary to assumption 2).
4. The economic profitability of the industry will reflect all dynamic opportunity costs and will through time tend toward normal returns. As such, economic profitability serves as the ultimate guide to the proper allocation of resources as it does with the pure competitive model.

It has been the purpose of this article to apply certain aspects of economic analysis to the pharmaceutical industry. In doing this, we have described a dynamic competitive process that generates new products and serves as a mechanism that pushes us toward the optimal allocation of resources for the production of existing products. A model of the pharmaceutical firm was also presented. Finally, the welfare implications of the competitive process and the model of the firm were discussed.

REFERENCES

1a. Schumpeter, J.A. *Capitalism, Socialism, and Democracy*; Harper & Row, Publishers, Inc.: New York, 1947.
1b. Winston, A.P. The Chimera of Monopoly. *The Competitive Economy: Selected Readings*; Brozen, Y., Ed.
2. Cocks, D.L.; Virts, J.R. Pricing Behavior in the Ethical Pharmaceutical Industry. J. Bus. **1977**, *47*, 349–362.
3. Cocks, D.L. Product Innovation and the Dynamic Elements of Competition in the Ethical Pharmaceutical Industry. *Drug Development and Marketing*; Helms, R.B., Ed.; American Enterprise Institute: Washington, D.C., 1975; 225–254.
4. Cocks, D.L. Product Innovation and the Dynamic Elements of Competition in the Ethical Pharmaceutical Industry. *Drug Development and Marketing*; Helms, R.B., Ed.; American Enterprise Institute: Washington, D.C., 1975; 225–254.
5. Reekie, W.D. Price and Quality Competition in the United States Drug Industry (Mimeographed). *Pricing New Pharmaceutical Products*; Croom Helm: London, 1977.
6. Schwartzman, D. *Innovation in the Pharmaceutical Industry*; The Johns Hopkins University Press: Baltimore, 1976; 251–299.
7. Berndt is Price Inflation for the Elderly? An Empirical Analysis of Prescription Drugs. *Frontiers of Health Policy Research*; Garber, A., Ed.; National Bureau of Economic Research: Cambridge, MA, 1998.
8a. Coase, R.H. The Nature of the Firm. Economica N. S. **1937 November**, *4*, 386–405.
8b. Alchian, A.; Demsetz, H. Production, Information Costs, and Economic Organization. Am. Eco. Rev. **1972**, *62*, 777–795.
8c. Williamson, O.E. *Markets and Hierarchies: Analysis and Antitrust Implications*; The Free Press: New York, 1975; 183–192.
9. Williamson, O.E. *Markets and Hierarchies: Analysis and Antitrust Implications*; The Free Press: New York, 1975; 183–192.
10. Demsetz, H. Information and Efficiency: Another Viewpoint. J. Law Eco. **April 1969**, 1–2.

EFFERVESCENT PHARMACEUTICALS

Nils-Olof Lindberg
Pharamacia AB, Helsingborg, Sweden

Henri Hansson
Galenica AB, Meleon, Malmö, Sweden

INTRODUCTION

Effervescent tablets are uncoated tablets that generally contain acid substances and carbonates or bicarbonates, and that react rapidly in the presence of water by releasing carbon dioxide. They are usually dissolved or dispersed in water before administration (1).

Effervescent mixtures have been known for over 250 years. During the 1930s, the success of Alka Seltzer created a vogue for effervescent products, including tablets (2). Effervescent tablets have been reviewed (3–5).

Effervescent reactions have also been employed in other dosage forms, such as suppositories (laxative effect), vaginal suppositories (mainly contraceptive effect), and drug delivery systems (e.g., floating systems and tablets rapidly dissolving in the saliva).

Effervescent products should be stored in tightly closed containers. Desiccants are usually added to the containers.

PHARMACOPEIAL MONOGRAPHS

Soluble, effervescent tablets are prepared by compression. In addition to active ingredients, they contain mixtures of acids (citric acid, tartaric acid) and sodium bicarbonate ($NaHCO_3$) that release carbon dioxide when dissolved in water (6). The *United States Pharmacopeia* (USP) 24 includes the following seven monographs: Acetaminophen for Effervescent Oral Solution; Aspirin Effervescent Tablets for Oral Solution; Potassium Bicarbonate Effervescent Tablets for Oral Solution; Potassium Bicarbonate and Potassium Chloride for Effervescent Oral Solution; Potassium Bicarbonate and Potassium Chloride Effervescent Tablets for Oral Solution; Potassium and Sodium Bicarbonates and Citric Acid for Oral Solution; and Potassium Chloride, Potassium Bicarbonate, and Potassium Citrate Effervescent Tablets for Oral Solution (7).

Effervescent tablets as well as effervescent granules and powders are mentioned in the *European Pharmacopoeia* (Ph. Eur.), although it does not contain any monographs regarding specific drugs (1, 8).

THE EFFERVESCENT REACTION

Acid–base reactions between alkali metal bicarbonate and citric or tartaric acid have been used for many years to produce pharmaceutical preparations that effervesce as soon as water is added. In such systems, it is practically impossible to achieve much more than an atmospheric saturation of the solution with respect to the released carbon dioxide. If the acid dissolves first, then the bulk of the reaction takes place in the saturated solution in close proximity to the undissolved bicarbonate particles. If the bicarbonate dissolves faster, the reaction essentially takes place near the surface of the undissolved acid. Such suspension systems do not favor supersaturation with respect to carbon dioxide because the particulate solids act as nuclei for bubble formations (9).

RAW MATERIALS

General Characteristics

With regard to compressibility and compactibility, the considerations pertaining to raw materials in effervescent products are similar to the ones that prevail in evaluating raw materials intended for conventional tablets. However, poor compactibility cannot usually be compensated for by the use of binders, as this will prevent a rapid dissolution of the effervescent tablet. Addition of a binder is generally not as critical for the dissolution of effervescent granules or powders.

The general tablet compaction process normally is described by a number of sequential phases: rearrangement, deformation (elastic, plastic) of initial particles, fragmentation, and deformation of fragments. Particle surfaces are brought into close proximity and interparticulate attraction or bonds will be formed (10). Similar conditions will prevail with the effervescent tablets.

A very important property for effervescent products is the adsorption/desorption isotherm of the raw material and, consequently, its moisture content. To avoid a premature effervescent reaction in the tablets, substances with low moisture contents will have to be used. The aqueous solubility is another important property of the substances used in effervescent products. It is also important to use raw materials that are easily wetted. Of course, the taste of the employed substances is important.

Acid Materials

The acidity for the effervescent reaction can be obtained from three main sources: acids, acid anhydrides, and acid salts. Traditional sources of acid materials are the organic acids, citric and tartaric acid; however, some acid salts also are used.

Acids

Citric acid: Citric acid is obtained as a monohydrate or an anhydrate. A variety of particle-size grades are available—colorless, translucent crystals, or white, granular-to-crystalline powder. Citric acid is odorless and has a strong acidic taste. It is soluble in less than 1 part of water and 1 in 1.5 parts of ethanol (11).

Citric acid monohydrate melts at 100°C. It loses water at 75°C, becomes anhydrous at 135°C, and fuses at 153°C. At relative humidities (RH) lower than approximately 65%, it effloresces at 25°C; the anhydrous acid is formed at humidities below approximately 40%. At RH between approximately 65 and 75%, it sorbs insignificant amounts of moisture, but above this, substantial amounts are absorbed (Fig. 1) (11).

Figure 1 also includes the sorption curve of the anhydrate. The anhydrous form melts at 135°C during decomposition (12). At RH approaching 75%, the monohydrate is formed (11).

Information from Heckel plots indicates that anhydrous citric acid is predominantly fragmented during compression (13). The elastic deformation and consequently the elastic recovery during decompression are low (14).

Tartaric acid: Tartaric acid is soluble 1 in 0.75 parts of water, and 1 in 2.5 parts of alcohol (15). It sorbs insignificant amounts of moisture at RH up to approximately 65%, but at RH above approximately 75%, substantial amounts are absorbed (Fig. 1).

Studies indicate that tartaric acid behaves in a manner similar to that of anhydrous citric acid. During compression, the acid fragments predominantly, and the

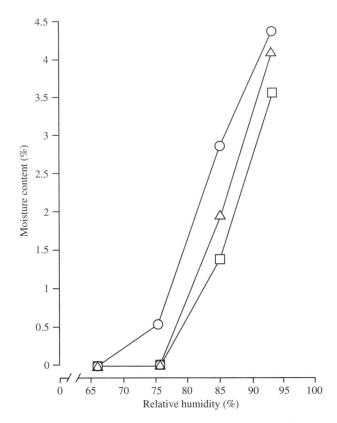

Fig. 1   Sorption isotherms of some hygroscopic acids. *Key*: *x* axis = relative humidity, %; *y* axis = moisture content, %; ○ = citric acid monohydrate; △ = anhydrous citric acid; □ = tartaric acid. (Adapted from Ref. 16.)

elastic deformation and consequently the elastic recovery were low (14).

A comparison of the formation of carbon dioxide from effervescent tablets based on anhydrous citric acid, ascorbic acid or tartaric acid, and $NaHCO_3$ in stoichiometric proportions indicated that ascorbic acid and anhydrous citric acid behaved similarly. However, tartaric acid formed the most carbon dioxide, but the disintegration time was longer (16).

Ascorbic acid: Ascorbic acid occurs as white to light yellow crystalline powder or colorless crystals with a sharp, acidic taste and no odor. It is not hygroscopic. Upon exposure to light, it gradually darkens. Ascorbic acid is soluble 1 in 3.5 parts of water and 1 in 50 parts of ethanol (17).

Ascorbic acid particles show an intermediate fragmentation during compaction. The relatively low tablet strength indicates that the attraction forces are relatively weak and not very resistant to stress relaxation and elastic recovery (18).

Ascorbic acid can be used as the acid source. The speed of release of carbon dioxide from a mixture of ascorbic acid and

$NaHCO_3$ is comparable with that produced by citric or tartaric acid–$NaHCO_3$ combinations. Since ascorbic acid is less hygroscopic than citric and tartaric acid, using ascorbic acid as the only acid source makes it possible to produce effervescent tablets in a nonairconditional area (19).

Fumaric acid: Fumaric acid is a white, odorless or nearly odorless crystalline powder. It is soluble 1 in 222 parts of water and 1 in 28 parts of ethanol (20). The sorption isotherm indicates that fumaric acid is not a hygroscopic substance (16).

Acetylsalicylic acid (aspirin): Although acetylsalicylic acid is a drug frequently used in effervescent form, it cannot be used as the acid source because of its low water solubility. Additional acid is necessary to decrease the reaction time.

Other acids: Malic acid is hygroscopic and readily soluble in water. It has been suggested for effervescent products (3).

Other acids have been mentioned in connection with effervescent products (3, 5).

Acid anhydrides: The use of acid anhydrides as the acid precursor has been investigated. However, their use in commercial products is limited.

Acid salts: Amino acid hydrochlorides readily release acid when in solution. However, these materials have the disadvantage of being expensive and rather hygroscopic (4). Other suggested acid sources include: sodium dihydrogen citrate (21), a nonhygroscopic substance (16); disodium hydrogen citrate, which is nonhygroscopic below approximately 93% RH/20°C (16); and sodium acid phosphate, which is very soluble in water.

Sources of Carbon Dioxide

Both carbonates and bicarbonates are used as carbonate sources, but the latter is most often used.

Sodium bicarbonate ($NaHCO_3$)

$NaHCO_3$ is an odorless, white crystalline powder with a saline, slightly alkaline taste. A variety of particle-size grades of powders and granules are available. The carbon dioxide yield is approximately 52% by weight. At RH below approximately 80% (at room temperature), the moisture content is less than 1%. Above 85% RH, it rapidly absorbs an excessive amount of water and may start to decompose. Its solubility in water is 1 part in 11 parts at 20°C, and it is practically insoluble in 95% ethanol at 20°C. When heated to 250–300°C, $NaHCO_3$ decomposes and is converted into anhydrous sodium carbonate. However, this process is both time- and temperature-dependent, commencing at about 50°C. The reaction proceeds via surface-controlled kinetics, and when $NaHCO_3$ crystals are heated for a short period of time, very fine needle-shaped crystals of anhydrous sodium carbonate appear on the surface (22).

In humid air, there is a slow decarboxylation of $NaHCO_3$, where as sodium sesquicarbonate $Na_2CO_3 \cdot NaHCO_3 \cdot 2H_2O$ is formed (23).

$NaHCO_3$ mainly consolidates by plastic deformation and not by fragmentation (18). It is a nonelastic substance (13).

In order to overcome the poor flowability and low compressibility of $NaHCO_3$, a spray-drying technique was used. Additives such as polyvinylpyrrolidone and silicon oil were found to be essential to obtain direct compressible spray-dried $NaHCO_3$. The product showed good compression characteristics without being transformed into sodium carbonate (24).

Sodium carbonate: Sodium carbonate is commercially available as an anhydrous form and as a monohydrate or a decahydrate. All forms are very soluble in water. The anhydrate is hygroscopic (25).

Potassium bicarbonate: Potassium bicarbonate ($KHCO_3$) is very soluble in water. When heated to approximately 200°C, it is decomposed, and potassium carbonate, water, and carbon dioxide are formed (26). Consequently, $KHCO_3$, is less sensitive to heat in connection with drying than is $NaHCO_3$. Above approximately 80% RH at 20°C, substantial amounts of water are adsorbed by $KHCO_3$.

Potassium carbonate: The moisture scavenging effect of potassium carbonate in effervescent tablets has been investigated (27).

Calcium carbonate: Precipitated calcium carbonate occurs as fine, white, odorless, and tasteless powder or crystals. It is practically insoluble in water and ethanol (95%). Precipitated calcium carbonate is nonhygroscopic (28). Calcium carbonate is a high-density, not very compressible material (29). It is known to consolidate by fragmentation (30).

Other sources: Amino acid–alkali metal carbonate derivatives, such as sodium glycine carbonate, have been suggested as sources of carbon dioxide.

Sodium glycine carbonate is a nonhygroscopic, heat-resistant, stable substance (31). However, the carbon dioxide yield—approximately 18% by weight—is only about one-third of $NaHCO_3$.

PRODUCTS

Dosage Forms

Effervescent tablets (1, 6), granules, and powders (8) are mentioned in the pharmacopoeias and exist as products

E

on the market. The effervescent tablet provides several advantages over conventional oral solid dosage forms. It is administered as a reasonably palatable, sparkling solution. Consequently, it can be given to patients who have difficulties swallowing capsules or tablets. Since the drug is administered as a solution, problems associated with dissolution, that is, absorption rate and extent of bioavailability, are avoided. Drugs that are unstable when stored in aqueous solutions are more often stable in the effervescent tablet.

Effervescent dosage forms have several drawbacks when compared with aqueous solutions and plain tablets. For example, they are relatively expensive to produce due to the use of large amounts of more or less expensive excipients and the necessary special production facilities, as well as high Na+ and/or K+ concentrations. In addition, when compared with plain tablets, effervescent tablets are bulky, even though small packages that are easy to carry in a pocket or handbag are available. Finally, it is sometimes difficult to make unpleasant tasting drugs sufficiently palatable in an effervescent form.

When an effervescent product is dropped into a glass of water, the reaction between the acid and the $NaHCO_3$ is quite rapid, usually completed within 1 minute or less (32). The effervescent reaction is also used in other pharmaceutical dosage forms than the traditional effervescent products. Effervescent laxative suppositories that release carbon dioxide have been thoroughly studied (33). One product has been on the Swedish market for many years. Effervescent vaginal suppositories are described (34). Pulsatile and gastric floating drug delivery systems for oral administration based on a reservoir system consisting of a drug-containing effervescent core and a polymeric coating also have been investigated (35).

Drugs (Product Categories)

Many drugs and drug compositions have been used for effervescent products. Some of these are listed below.

Acetylsalicylic acid (aspirin) is a common drug in many different effervescent products (36, 37).

Paracetamol (acetaminophen) is another analgesic used in effervescent preparations (38).

Effervescent compositions of ibuprofen, another analgesic, are marketed.

Among effervescent antacid preparations, Alka-Seltzer, an effervescent antacid analgesic product, has been available since the 1930s. Pure effervescent antacid products are marketed in many countries.

Effervescent tablets of ascorbic acid, 0.5–1 g, are well known. Other vitamins as well as calcium and some minerals have also been included.

Acetylcysteine, a mycolytic agent that also is used as an antidote for paracetamol overdose, is available as an effervescent tablet.

Effervescent products of water-insoluble drugs have been manufactured. A successful example is the effervescent activated charcoal preparation suggested in the management of theophylline poisoning (39).

Electrolyte Balance Considerations

Effervescent tablets normally have a high sodium content. In most of the effervescent analgesic products in Sweden, the sodium content is approximately 15 mmol. This sodium content may be contraindicated in some patients (e.g., in patients with active sodium-retaining status such as congestive heart failure or renal insufficiency). Otherwise, there are no restrictions concerning the sodium content of effervescent tablets.

Biopharmaceutical Aspects

Drugs are most rapidly absorbed from the gastrointestinal (GI) tract when administered as aqueous solutions. Although dilution of the drug solution in the gastric fluids sometimes results in precipitation, the extremely fine nature of the precipitate permits rapid redissolution (40). The rapid absorption of the aqueous solution is the idea behind effervescent analgesic products, for example. Furthermore, consistent absorption is expected with the solution, as disintegration and dissolution in the GI tract are bypassed.

Effervescence may produce physiological changes within the body. Carbon dioxide bubbling directly onto the intestinal epithelium induced enhanced drug permeability due to an alteration of the paracellular pathway. This, in addition to fluid flow and membrane hydrophobicity concepts, may account for observed increases in drug flux (41).

Buffered effervescent aspirin tablets are generally believed to have a less irritant effect on the gastric mucosa and cause less GI blood loss than conventional tablets. This view has been questioned.

The bioavailability of acetylsalicylic acid from three different dosage forms—two types of effervescent tablets with different buffering properties and tablets of a conventional type—was studied in healthy volunteers. Complete absorption was found for all the preparations studied. Both effervescent tablets were rapidly absorbed. The buffering properties did not influence the rate of absorption (36).

Effervescent aspirin, soluble aspirin, and soluble aspirin to which sufficient $NaHCO_3$ had been added to give it the same buffering capacity as the effervescent preparation, were compared in healthy volunteers. There were no significant differences in plasma salicylate levels at any time after taking these preparations (37).

The absorption of the effervescent formulation of paracetamol was compared with that of a plain tablet in normal volunteers. As to the rate of absorption, this was more rapid and consistent from the effervescent preparation than from the plain tablet. This may have important therapeutic implications where a rapid and predictable analgesic effect may be desired (38).

The bioavailability of an effervescent ibuprofen tablet was compared to a sugar-coated tablet. Ibuprofen was absorbed more rapidly from the effervescent tablet but both formulations were bioequivalent in respect to peak plasma concentrations and area under the plasma concentration curves (42).

PROCESSING

Environment

The manufacturing of effervescent tablets requires careful control of environmental factors. As early as the 1930s, it was clear that it was essential to maintain RH throughout the plant of no more than 20%. In addition, a uniform temperature of 21°C also was desirable (2).

A maximum of 25% RH at a controlled room temperature of 25°C or less is usually sufficient to avoid problems caused by atmospheric moisture (3).

Equipment

Conventional processing equipment (mixers, granulators, roller compactors, drying equipment, and mills) can be used to produce effervescent preparations if the influence of atmospheric moisture is considered. As a rule, tablet presses have to be adapted to handle effervescent products, except for tablets with a sufficient proportion of a self-lubricating substance, such as acetylsalicylic acid.

Wet Granulation Methods

The acid and carbonate parts of the effervescent formulation can be granulated either separately or as a mixture with water (crystal water of citric acid, liquid water, or water vapor), ethanol (possibly diluted with water), isopropanol, or other solvents.

When granulating with solvents without any moisture, no effervescent reaction will occur provided the raw materials are dry and the process is performed in a low humidity atmosphere. However, citric acid will partly dissolve in ethanol or isopropanol, and function as a binder when the solvent is evaporated.

When granulating either with solvents containing water or pure water, the effervescent reaction will start. Care must be taken to maintain adequate control of the process. Vacuum processing is often beneficial due to the ability to control the effervescent reaction and the drying process.

In the fusion method of granulation, the effervescent mixture is heated to approximately 100°C (the melting point of the monohydrate) so that the water of crystallization from hydrous citric acid is released. This process is sporadic and difficult to control, especially in a static bed (3).

By means of high-shear mixers and the heat generated during mixing, it was possible to prepare granular effervescent products in batch sizes of 60–300 kg using the fusion method (43).

Citric acid is moistened and added to the $NaHCO_3$. Partial wet fusion occurs, and granules are formed by kneading in a suitable mixer. The granules are tableted while still damp, with the moist citric acid acting as a lubricant. The compressed tablets are transferred immediately and continuously to ovens where they are dried at 70–75°C. Drying also hardens them. As soon as they leave the dryer, the tablets are packed in aluminum foil lined with polyethylene (44).

X-ray diffractometry and infrared (IR) spectrophotometry were used to study the reaction between citric acid and $NaHCO_3$ when granulating the mixture with water in a high-shear mixer and vacuum drying the wet mass. The contact time before drying varied as did the water content. At low water levels, varying the contact times did not change the citric acid. However, with higher levels of water content, the presence of monocitrates, dicitrates, and tricitrates was verified. The loss of carbon dioxide during granulation occurred in the presence of, especially, dicitrates and tricitrates (45).

Effervescent granules were prepared in a fluid bed granulator/dryer (46).

The drug can be mixed with the effervescent granulate and other excipients or be a part of the granulation. When mixing low proportions of drug with granulate, the risk of segregation must be taken into account.

Dry Granulation

Granulation by slugging (slugs or large tablets that are compressed using heavy-duty tableting equipment) or roller compaction is suitable for materials that cannot be wet granulated. The slugs and the material from the roller compactor are reduced to the proper size. Lubrication is often necessary during slugging but not always with roller compaction. The acidic and basic components may be dry granulated separately or together.

Direct Compression

Some effervescent tablet products are successfully produced by direct compression (e.g., acetylsalicylic acid products). Direct compression normally requires careful selection of raw materials to achieve a free-flowing, nonsegregating, compressible mixture. Effervescent products present the same problems as conventional products in direct compression.

Tableting

The adaptation of a single-punch tablet press for compressing effervescent tablets via external lubrication has been described (5, 47). Only rotary presses are normally used in connection with the commercial production of effervescent tablets. Tablet machine manufacturers have applied various adaptations to their existing equipment to avoid problems due to internal lubrication and punch adhesion. Consequently, many effervescent tablets are produced on rotary presses with external lubrication. Liquid or solid lubricants can be used.

FORMULATION

Excipients (Including Sweeteners and Flavors)

Lubricants

A perfect lubricant (or auxiliary agent, in general) for effervescent products must be nontoxic, tasteless, and water-soluble. Very few traditional lubricants fulfill these requirements.

Intrinsic lubricants are added to the powder mixture and consequently included in the formulation. When added in solid form, the lubricant will have to be finely divided.

Metal stearates, such as magnesium or calcium stearate that serve as lubricants in conventional tablets, are seldom used as intrinsic lubricants in connection with effervescent tablets due to their insolubility in water. Use of stearates results in an undissolved, foamy, soapy-tasting layer on the surface of the cloudy solution. In addition, normal lubricant concentrations of metal stearates make the tablets hydrophobic, which entails a slow dissolution of the effervescent tablet in the water. However, very low concentrations of metal stearates can be used to improve the rate of solution of effervescent tablets as the tablet will remain immersed in the water during dissolution and not float to the surface the way a tablet without metal stearate would. A floating tablet presents a smaller surface area to the water than a tablet immersed in the liquid.

Sodium stearate and sodium oleate are water-soluble in low concentrations. They have the characteristic soapy taste, which virtually precludes their use in effervescent products.

A combination of 4% polyethylene glycol (PEG) 6000 and 0.1% sodium stearyl fumarate proved to be a good lubricant for ascorbic acid tablets made by direct compression on a small scale (48). Sodium chloride, sodium acetate, and D,L-leucine (water-soluble lubricants) also have been suggested for effervescent tablets (44).

Twenty lubricants for effervescent tablets were tested for lubrication efficiency in direct compression of a standard effervescent formulation. The lubricant concentration was high as compared to traditional tablet lubricants. By increasing the lubricant concentration and the compression force, most lubricants became more effective. The lubricant used in effervescent formulations should combine hydrophobic and hydrophilic properties in order to achieve both good lubrication and a short disintegration time. A medium polar lubricant was the best compromise. Fumaric acid was chosen and its concentration optimized (49). Other research that studied the lubrication of effervescent products indicated optimal concentrations of spray-dried L-leucine and PEG 6000 at levels of 2 and 3%, respectively (50).

Surfactants such as sodium lauryl sulfate and magnesium lauryl sulfate also act as lubricants.

Extrinsic lubrication is provided via mechanisms that apply a lubricating substance, normally paraffin oil, to the tableting tool surface during processing. One method makes use of an oiled felt washer attached to the lower punch below the tip. This washer wipes the die cavity with each tablet ejection. To avoid having tablets stick to the punch faces, materials such as polytetrafluorethylene or polyurethane have been applied to the faces. Another lubrication method sprays a thin layer of lubricant (either liquid or solid lubricant) onto the tool surfaces after one tablet is ejected and before the granulate of the next tablet enters the die cavity.

Products containing acetylsalicylic acid do not usually require additional lubrication.

Glidants

Glidants are usually not necessary. Free-flowing granulates, ingredients of appropriate physical form for direct compression, and the large tablet diameters make it possible to exclude the use of glidants.

Antiadherents

The adherence of the granulate or powder mixture to the punch surfaces, so-called picking, can be eliminated by using discs, such as polytetrafluorethylene or polyurethane, cemented to the punch surfaces.

Binders

Binders are commonly used when making conventional tablets. The binders are either added in dry form or dissolved in a suitable solvent and then added in connection with a wet-granulation process. Most binders are polymers and increase the plastic deformation of the formulation.

The use of binders will normally prevent a rapid dissolution of the effervescent tablet. Therefore, many effervescent tablets are formulated without any binder. However, effervescent granules may be formulated with binders since their large surface area, when compared with that of the conventional or the effervescent tablet, will result in rapid dissolution. An effervescent granulation composed of anhydrous citric acid and $NaHCO_3$ was made with dehydrated alcohol as the granulating liquid. A portion of the citric acid dissolved during the massing and functioned as a binder (51).

In order to compress ascorbic acid from a combination with $NaHCO_3$, granulation was required. Common water-soluble binders, such as polyvinylpyrrolidone (polyvidone) or polyvinylpyrrolidone–poly(vinyl acetate)-copolymer, led to a change of color on the part of the ascorbic acid granules. Hydrogenated maltodextrins containing high amounts of maltitol were chosen from a wide range of dextrins and maltodextrins as possible binders. Maltitol was a suitable binder for ascorbic acid effervescent tablets. Formation of crystal bridges of maltitol was the assumed binding mechanism (19). PEG 6000 functions both as a binder and as a lubricant.

Disintegrants or dissolution aids

Disintegrants, which are used in conventional tablets, are not normally used in effervescent tablets because one of the marketing demands is that a clear solution should be obtained within a few minutes after adding the tablet to a glass of cold water.

Diluents

Effervescent products generally do not require diluents. The effervescent materials themselves will have to be added in large quantities.

Sweeteners

Sucrose and other natural sweeteners, such as sorbitol, can be used in effervescent products, although artificial sweetening agents are customary. However, the application of artificial sweeteners is restricted by health regulations. Therefore, the use of such sweeteners will vary from one country to the next based on national standards.

Saccharin or its sodium and calcium salts are used as sweeteners. Aspartame is also employed as a sweetener in effervescent tablets. Earlier, cyclamates and cyclamic acid were the artificial sweeteners of choice, but their use has now been restricted.

Flavors

The simple use of sweetening agents may not be sufficient to render palatable a product containing a drug with an unpleasant taste. Therefore, a flavoring agent can be included. Various dry flavors are available from suppliers. The flavors used must be water-soluble or water-dispersible.

Colors

Water-soluble colors may be added; however, some dyes change color according to pH variations, a consideration that must be noted before a dye is selected.

Surfactants

This type of excipient is sometimes used to increase the wetting and dissolution rate of drugs. Attention must be paid to the formation of foam.

Antifoaming agents

To reduce the formation of foam, and consequently the tendency of drugs to stick to the wall of the glass above the water level, an antifoaming agent, such as polydimethylsiloxane, can be used. However, antifoaming agents do not normally form constituents of effervescent products.

Formulations (Including Optimization)

Literature on formulations of effervescent products it relatively sparse. Table 1 presents some examples of effervescent products on the Nordic market.

A fractional factorial design was employed in the preparation of effervescent aspirin tablets. The optimum conditions for preparing the tablets were determined following the path of steepest ascent (53).

Table 1 Some compositions of effervescent tablets on the Nordic market: Components and weight per tablet

	Product A		Product B		Product C	
	Component	mg	Component	mg	Component	mg
Drugs	Ascorbic acid	1000	Acetylsalicylic acid	500	Paracetamol	500
			Caffeine	50		
Excipients	Citric acid, anhydrous	700	Citric acid, anhydrous	500	Citric acid, anhydrous	1200
	Sodium bicarbonate	490	Sodium bicarbonate	1250	Sodium bicarbonate	1550
	Polyethylene glycol 6000	45	Docusate sodium	0.85	Polyvidone	25
			Sodium benzoate	0.15	Sodium cyclamate	45
	Sorbitol	25			Saccharin sodium	5
	Saccharin sodium	12			Lemon flavor	25
	Riboflavin sodium phosphate (for color)	1			Magnesium stearate	1.4
	Orange flavor	2				

(Adapted from Ref. 52.)

An experiment investigating the effects of tablet manufacturing conditions, tablet formulations, tablet compression pressures, storage conditions, and storage times was performed on five different formulations (54). The effects of two formulation factors (the ratio of citric acid/$NaHCO_3$ and the polyvidone content) and two process factors (the temperature and the velocity of the fluidizing air) on granule size, powder content, and dissolution rate of the tablets were studied using factorial design. In addition, the levels of the significant factors were optimized with the path of steepest ascent (46).

Solid dispersions of poorly water-soluble drugs were made by the fusion method. Citric acid was employed in various ratios with $NaHCO_3$ as the carrier for these drugs (55).

Stability

The greatest problem with effervescent products is the loss of reactivity with time if exposed prematurely to moisture (i.e., the stability of the effervescent system). In addition, the stability of the drug and some excipients, such as flavors, also must be considered.

Effervescent products are not stable in the presence of moisture. Most effervescent products are hygroscopic and can therefore adsorb enough moisture to initiate degradation if they are not suitably packaged.

Tablets made with equivalent amounts of $NaHCO_3$ and tartaric acid were stored at 70°C. In a closed system, a reaction between the $NaHCO_3$ and the tartaric acid occurred. When the tablets were stored as an open system,

the weight loss was concluded to be a decarboxylation of the $NaHCO_3$ (56).

Effervescent compositions may be markedly stabilized if the $NaHCO_3$ is partly converted to the corresponding carbonate. Usually, the desired degree of stability is attained if approximately 2–10% of the weight of the bicarbonate is converted to the carbonate (57). The addition of sodium carbonate did not by itself improve stability. One explanation for the stabilizing effect caused by heating of the bicarbonate could be that heating causes a uniform distribution of the carbonate on the surface of the bicarbonate so that the water-scavenging efficiency is greater. Another explanation is that the carbonate formed by the rupture of the bicarbonate crystals would be much finer than added crystalline sodium carbonate, however finely ground. A third explanation is the possibility that double salts might be present and that they could be better scavengers than the carbonate itself (56). The moisture scavenging effect of potassium carbonate was determined and the concentration optimized for a specific formulation (27).

The stability of three commercial effervescent and one dispersible aspirin tablet were evaluated by factorially designed experiments. Temperature affected the hydrolysis of all tablets, whereas humidity influenced one product in a plastic tube and one in an aluminum tube (58).

Mercury-intrusion porosimetry and a cantilever beam-proximity transducer balance were used to monitor the stability of selected effervescent tablet systems. An index of reactivity was obtained from the balance measurements. The porosity measurements proved to be useful in elucidating tablet-pore structure changes over time.

Compression pressure and manufacturing conditions were not significant factors in the stability of an effervescent system when nonhygroscopic materials were used (54).

Codeine phosphate in a paracetamol-codeine effervescent tablet was found to react at room temperature with the citric acid constituents to form citrate esters of codeine. The esterification was confirmed in a solid-state reaction at an elevated temperature. Tartaric acid also yielded an ester with codeine phosphate in a similar nonsolvolytic reaction (59).

PRODUCTION

Granulation

At the Pharmacia plant in Helsingborg, Sweden, approximately 1200 kg of effervescent granulate is produced daily. Anhydrous citric acid and $NaHCO_3$ are massed with ethanol in a planetary mixer and the wet mass is dried on trays. Additional effervescent granulates are produced with vacuum equipment (Topo granulator) where water is the main component of the granulation liquid. The Topo granulator, developed for preparation of granules and coated particles in a vacuum, handles the mixing, granulation, drying, and milling/sieving as a closed system.

The fusion method, which employs heat to liberate water of crystallization from hydrous citric acid in order to effect moistening, was applied by using a high-shear mixer to generate heat (43). Batch sizes of 60 and 300 kg were granulated.

Anhydrous citric acid and $NaHCO_3$ were granulated with ethanol in a twin-screw extruder at powder flow rates of 60–90 kg/h in a continuous process (51).

The air suspension coating–reacting technique also is used in the production of effervescent granulates.

Tableting

Effervescent tablets are normally produced by machines with external lubrication systems. Most tablet machine manufacturers can add this type of equipment to their rotary machines. Products with a high proportion of acetylsalicylic acid can be manufactured without any traditional lubricants. Consequently, conventional rotary tablet presses can be used. Effervescent acetylsalicylic acid tablets are produced on ordinary high-speed rotary presses at the Pharmacia plant in Helsingborg, Sweden.

Effervescent granules can be tableted while still damp since moist citric acid acts as a lubricant. The compressed tablets are transferred immediately and continuously to ovens where they are dried. Drying also hardens them (44).

Several types of steel are normally used in the manufacture of compression tooling. Material rich in nickel was found to have the best resistance to rusting induced by a hydrochloride salt, although other factors, such as humidity, temperature, and contact time, also were responsible for the rusting of tooling material (60). This information may be useful when ordering and managing tooling materials for effervescent tablets.

The compression of effervescent mixtures usually results in severe picking and sticking. By means of flat-faced punches with discs of polytetrafluorethylene, the sticking to tablet-punch surfaces is overcome (61). Other nonadherent materials, such as Vulkollan® (a polyethane), Hostalit® (polyvinyl chloride), and Resopal® (a melamine), have been used (62). The disc of the plastic material is attached to the recess of the punch surface by glue or adhesive tape. It should be noted that fragments of the polymer can rub off during compression.

Effervescent tablets were produced using four different formulations that contained citric and/or tartaric acid and $NaHCO_3$ with polyvidone and PEG 6000. The adhesion of each formulation to the metal faces of the punch tips was determined by means of electron microscopy, surface-roughness measurements, and quantification of punch-weight variations during tablet production. The basic formulations were inherently adhesive and produced tablets with a weak, porous structure; the tablets were rougher than conventional, noneffervescent compressed tablets. Both formulations that contained tartaric acid produced tablets with a lower surface roughness and had less of a tendency to stick to tablet-punch faces than the two formulations that contained citric acid alone. The addition of a water-soluble sucrose ester had a beneficial effect, especially on formulations with inherently high adhesive tendencies (63).

In-Process Quality Control

For a rapid determination of loss on drying, an IR drying balance may be used. In the matter of size distribution, effervescent granulations are controlled by sieve analysis.

During the compression of effervescent tablets, in-process tests are routinely run to monitor the process. These tests include controls of tablet weight, weight variation, thickness, crushing strength, disintegration, and appearance of the tablet. Friability and pH of the solution may be additionally tested. Electronic devices that monitor tablet weight are normally used.

Inspection of the punches is carried out during the manufacturing of the tablets when plastic insertions are used. Inspections ensure that the plastic insertions are intact, i.e., that no loss or damage to the discs has occurred.

Product Evaluations

Both chemical and physical properties have to be considered when evaluating effervescent products. In this review, only the physical properties will be discussed, except where the chemical characteristics are especially influenced by the effervescent base. For more detail, Ph. Eur. includes a special disintegration test for effervescent tablets (1) and granules (8).

Many tests (e.g., titrimetric, gravimetric, colorimetric, and volumetric tests as well as loss-of-weight measurements and pressure measurements) have been proposed in order to determine carbon dioxide content (16, 48, 64). Methods based on monitoring carbon dioxide pressure generation and weight loss have been applied (16, 65).

Results from weight-loss measurements were modeled (65). Research indicates that the determination of water content by Karl Fischer analysis in effervescent tablets was possible after extraction with dioxane (66). $NaHCO_3$, which reacts with the Karl Fischer reagent, is insoluble in dioxane and does not interfere during the determination.

Near IR (NIR) is a quick and nondestructive method for the determination of water in effervescent products. In addition, it is suitable for in-process quality control. Measurement of pH of the solution is often performed. The conditions are important for congruent results.

Tablets

The disintegration and dissolution times are very important characteristics of effervescent products. A well-formulated effervescent tablet will disintegrate and dissolve within 1–2 min to form a clear solution. Consequently, the residue of undissolved drug must be minimal. The temperature of the water influences the dissolution time. It is, therefore, important to choose a water temperature that is actually used by consumers (e.g., cold tap water). Ph. Eur. includes a general requirement on disintegration time of 5 min in water 15–25°C (1).

Factors such as crushing strength and friability will influence the possibility of packaging the tablets on packaging lines, as effervescent tablets chip easily at the edges during handling. When the tablets are filled in tubes, the tablet height is of the utmost importance since the looseness or tightness of the packaging depends on the tablet height. When small or fairly small amounts of drug form part of the formulation, it is essential that content uniformity be carefully supervised.

Powders and Granules

Disintegration and dissolution time is an important characteristic, as is powder weight variation. The Ph. Eur. requirement time for disintegration of granules is 5 min (8).

Production Area

As the mass of an effervescent tablet is, as a rule, many times larger than that of a conventional tablet, larger amounts of raw material will have to be handled when packaging the same number of tablets. Therefore, the production area will be larger, too, unless a compact continuous line has been constructed.

At the Pharmacia plant in Helsingborg, Sweden, all steps during the production of effervescent tablets (i.e., mixing, granulating, drying, milling, final mixing of granulate and other constituents, tableting, and packaging) are performed in dehumidified areas of <25% RH and <25°C. Other companies perform mixing, granulating, drying, and milling at normal humidities but store the final mixture in dehumidified areas while slowly bubbling dehumidified air through the mixture. The mixture is then tableted and packaged in a small, dehumidified area around the tablet and packaging machine.

In direct compression, the mixing can be performed at normal humidities; however, in that case, the mixture is dried (to prevent a premature effervescent reaction) by means of causing dehumidified air to flow through the bed in a suitable container. Tableting and packaging are also performed in the dehumidified area. Thus, the number of manufacturing stages in the low humidity zone is reduced.

PACKAGING

Effervescent tablets should be stored in tightly closed containers or moisture-proof packs (6).

Even the moisture in the air may be enough to initiate the effervescent reaction of an effervescent product if it is not properly protected. When the consumer opens the container, the effervescent product will again be exposed to the moisture in the air. Consequently, the packaging of all effervescent products is very important. The time between tablet production and start of packaging operation should be kept as short as possible.

Ph. Eur. recommends that effervescent granules and powders be stored in airtight containers (8). In the past, acidic and alkaline components were wrapped separately to prevent effervescent reactions during the storage of powders and granules.

Materials

Effervescent products are usually packed in individual aluminum foil pouches and effervescent tablets are often packed in metal tubes. To avoid excessive laminate stress, the dimensions of the sachets should be adapted to the dimensions of the tablet or the amount of granulate. These pouches are arranged in conveniently sized strips and stacked in a paperboard box.

The metal tube is a multiple-use container sealed with a moisture-proof closure. The tablets are stacked on top of one another. Consequently, a minimum of air surrounds them. The tubes are seamless, extruded aluminum packages. They are closed by tightly fitting plastic snap caps that contain a desiccant chamber. Tubes of plastic materials, such as polyvinyl chloride or polypropene, have been tested with effervescent tablets. Acceptable stability was obtained with some of these products. Plastic tubes are used more often due to their lower cost and lower noise level during the packaging operation.

Aluminum-foil blisters can provide hermetic packs. Similar protection can be achieved by using a foil-bearing laminate or a strip pack. A special strip pack for effervescent tablets, where each tablet is connected to a desiccant via a channel, has been suggested (67).

The effect of environmental moisture on the physical stability of effervescent tablets in foil-laminate packages containing microscopic imperfections was examined. Physical stability, after storing at different RH and temperature conditions, was assessed by noting whether the tablet components reacted prematurely. A penetrating dye-solution test was used in order to determine whether the foil packages permitted any transmission of moisture. High humidity accelerated the physical deterioration of effervescent tablets when stored in packets of poor integrity (68).

Filling

Packaging operations must be conducted in a low humidity environment if the long-term stability of the product is to be maintained. The tablets must be hard enough so as not to break during packaging.

Quality Control

Individual foil packets are tested for proper sealing. Several methods of rapid seal integrity testing have been devised, such as the vacuum underwater method, detection of tracer material sealed within the pouch, purging with detectable gas, IR seal inspection, and electronic air-tightness testers (3).

CONCLUSION

The traditional effervescent product is dissolved prior to oral intake. This requires the drug to have an acceptable taste. Since the drug is given as a solution, the absorption is normally rapid and the bioavailability is usually good.

The commercial manufacturing of effervescent products involves controlling air humidity in the production area. Special tablet machines are generally required, and the package is a very important part of the effervescent product. Over-the-counter analgesics have been very successful as effervescent tablets on certain markets.

ACKNOWLEDGMENT

We are indebted to Ms. Margareta Duberg, Diabact AB, Uppsala for her valuable contribution.

REFERENCES

1. *European Pharmacopoiea*, 3rd Ed.; Council of Europe: Strasbourg, France, 1999; 1347, Suppl. 2000.
2. Chilson, F. Effervescent Tablets. Drug Cosm. Ind. **1936**, *39*, 738–740.
3. Mohrle, R. Effervescent Tablets. *Pharmaceutical Dosage Forms*, 2nd Ed.; Lieberman, H.A., Lachman, L., Schwartz, J.B., Eds.; Marcel Dekker, Inc.: New York, 1989; 1, 285–328.
4. Sendall, F.E.J.; Staniforth, J.N.; Rees, J.E.; Leatham, M.J. Effervescent Tablets. Pharm. J. **1983**, *230*, 289–294.
5. Schmidt, P.C.; Christin, I. Brausetabletten—Eine Fast Vergessene Arzneiform. Pharmazie **1990**, *45*, 89–101.
6. *The United States Pharmacopeia USP 24*, United States Pharmacopeial Convention: Rockville, MD, 1999, 2117.
7. *The United States Pharmacopeia USP 24*; United States Pharmacopeial Convention: Rockville, MD, 1999; 18, 167, 1354, 1355, 1356, 1360.

8. *European Pharmacopoeia,* 3rd Ed.; Council of Europe: Strasbourg, France, 1996; 1749, 1752.

9. Higuchi, T.; Perrin, J.; Robinson, J.; Repta, A.J. Carbonation of Aqueous Solutions with Acid Anhydrides. J. Pharm. Sci. **1965,** *54,* 1273–1276.

10. Nyström, C.; Karehill, P.-G. The Importance of Intermolecular Bonding Forces and the Concept of Bonding Surface Area. *Pharmaceutical Powder Compaction Technology*; Alderborn, G., Nyström, C., Eds.; Marcel Dekker, Inc.: New York, 1996; 17–53.

11. Wade, A., Weller, P.J., Eds. *Handbook of Pharmaceutical Excipients,* 2nd Ed.; The American Pharmaceutical Association and the Pharmaceutical Society of Great Britain: Washington and London, 1994; 123–125.

12. Kommentar, Böhme, H., Hartke, K., Eds.; Acidum citricum. *Europäisches Arzneibuch*; Wissenschaftliche Verlagsgesellschaft mbH: Stuttgart, and Govi-Verlag GmbH: Frankfurt, 1979; III, 215–219.

13. Duberg, M.; Nyström, C. Studies on Direct Compression of Tablets. XVII. Porosity—Pressure Curves for the Characterization of Volume Reduction Mechanisms in Powder Pompression. Powder Technol. **1986,** *46,* 67–75.

14. Duberg, M.; Diabact, A.B. Personal Communications. Box 303, S-751 05, Uppsala, Sweden.

15. Wade, A., Weller, P.J., Eds.; *Handbook of Pharmaceutical Excipients,* 2nd Ed.; The American Pharmaceutical Association and the Pharmaceutical Society of Great Britain: Washington and London, 1994; 522–523.

16. Schmidt, P.C.; Brögmann, B. Brausetabletten. Welche Säurekomponenten Sind Die Geeignesten. Dtsch. Apoth.-Ztg. **1987,** *127,* 991–997.

17. Wade, A., Weller, P.J., Eds.; *Handbook of Pharmaceutical Excipients,* 2nd Ed.; The American Pharmaceutical Association and the Pharmaceutical Society of Great Britain: Washington and London, 1994; 15–18.

18. Nyström, C.; Glazer, M. Studies on Direct Compression of Tablets. XIII. The Effect of Some Dry Binders on the Tablet Strength of Compounds with Different Fragmentation Propensity. Int. J. Pharm. **1985,** *23,* 255–263.

19. Schmidt, P.C.; Brögmann, B. Effervescent Tablets: Choice of a New Binder for Ascorbic Acid. Acta Pharm. Technol. **1988,** *34,* 22–26.

20. Wade, A., Weller, P.J., Eds.; *Handbook of Pharmaceutical Excipients,* 2nd Ed.; The American Pharmaceutical Association and the Pharmaceutical Society of Great Britain: Washington and London, 1994; 197–198.

21. Rothe W.; Groppenbächer G.; Heinemann H. Brausetabletten, Brausepulver und Verfahren zur Herstellung Derselben. German Patent Application No. 1,962,791.

22. Wade, A., Weller, P.J., Eds. *Handbook of Pharmaceutical Excipients,* 2nd Ed.; The American Pharmaceutical Association and the Pharmaceutical Society of Great Britain: Washington and London, 1994; 436–438.

23. Neumüller, O.A. *Römpps Chemie-Lexicon,* 7th Ed.; Franckh'sche Verlagshandlung: Stuttgart, 1974; 2277.

24. Saleh, S.I.; Boymond, C.; Stamm, A. Preparation of Direct Compressible Effervescent Components: Spray-Dried Sodium Bicarbonate. Int. J. Pharm. **1988,** *45,* 19–26.

25. Parfitt, K., Ed. *Martindale: The Complete Drug Reference,* 32nd Ed.; The Pharmaceutical Press: London, 1999; 1630.

26. Neumüller, O.A. *Römpps Chemie-Lexicon,* 7th Ed.; Franchkh'sche Verlagshandlung: Stuttgart, 1974; 1697.

27. Wells, M.L.; Wood, D.L.; Sanftleben, R.; Shaw, K.; Hottovy, J.; Weber, T.; Geoffroy, J.-M.; Alkire, T.G.; Emptage, M.R.; Sarabia, R. Potassium Carbonate as a Desiccant in Effervescent Tablets. Int. J. Pharm. **1997,** *152,* 227–235.

28. Wade, A., Weller, P.J., Eds.; *Handbook of Pharmaceutical Excipients,* 2nd Ed.; The American Pharmaceutical Association and the Pharmaceutical Society of Great Britain: Washington and London, 1994;, 52–55.

29. Ejifor, O.; Esezobo, S.; Pilpel, N. The Plasto-Elasticity and Compressibility of Coated Powders and the Tensile Strengths of their Tablets. J. Pharm. Pharmacol. **1986,** *38,* 1–7.

30. Roberts, R.J.; Rowe, R.C. The Effect of Punch Velocity on the Compaction of a Variety of Materials. J. Pharm. Pharmacol. **1985,** *37,* 377–384.

31. Fiedler, H.P. *Lexikon der Hilfsstoffe für Pharmazie, Kosmetik und Angrenzende Gebiete,* 2nd Ed.; Editio Cantor: Aulendorf, Germany, 1981; 647.

32. Banker, G.S.; Anderson, N.R. *Tablets: The Theory and Practice of Industrial Pharmacy,* 3rd Ed.; Lachman, L., Lieberman, H.A., Kanig, J.L., Eds.; Lea & Febiger: Philadelphia, 1986; 293–345.

33. Hakata, T.; Ijima, M.; Kimura, S.; Sato, H.; Watanabe, Y.; Matsumoto, M. Effects of Bases and Additives on Release of Carbon Dioxide from Effervescent Suppositories. Chem. Pharm. Bull. **1993,** *41,* 351–356.

34. Kurobe, T.; Kasai, M.; Kayano M. Stable Effervescent Vaginal Suppositories, US Patent 4,853,211.

35. Krögel, I.; Bodmeier, R. Floating or Pulsatile Drug Delivery Systems Based on Coated Effervescent Cores. Int. J. Pharm. **1999,** *187,* 175–184.

36. Ekenved, G.; Elofsson, R.; Sölvell, L. Bioavailability Studies on a Buffered Acetylsalicylic Acid Preparation. Acta Pharm. Suec. **1975,** *12,* 323–332.

37. Orton, K.; Treharne; Jones, R.; Kaspi, T.; Richardson, R. Plasma Salicylate Levels after Soluble and Effervescent Aspirin. Br. J. Clin. Pharmacol. **1979,** *7,* 410–412.

38. Hedges, A.; Clive, M.K.; Maclay, W.P.; Turner, P. A Comparison of the Absorption of Effervescent Preparations of Paracetamol and Penicillin V (Phenoxymethylpenicillin) with Solid Dosage Forms of these Drugs. J. Clin. Pharmacol. **1974,** *14,* 363–368.

39. Helliwell, M.; Berry, D. Theophylline Absorption by Effervescent Activated Charcoal (Medicoal®). J. Int. Med. Res. **1981,** *9,* 222–225.

40. Gibaldi, M. Biopharmaceutics. *The Theory and Practice of Industrial Pharmacy,* 2nd Ed.; Lachman, L., Lieberman, H.A., Kanig, J.L. Eds.; Lea & Febiger: Philadelphia, 1976; 78–140.

41. Eichman, J.D.; Robinson, J.R. Mechanistic Studies on Effervescent-Induced Permeability Enhancement. Pharm. Res. **1998,** *15,* 925–930.

42. Altomare, E.; Wendemiale, G.; Benvenuti, C.; Andreatta, P. Bioavailability of a New Effervescent Tablet of Ibuprofen in Healthy Volunteers. Eur. J. Clin. Pharmacol. **1997,** *52,* 505–506.

43. Murray, R.B. New Approach to the Fusion Method for Preparing Granular Effervescent Products. J. Pharm. Sci. **1968,** *57,* 1776–1779.

44. Gunsel, W.C.; Kanig, J.L. Tablets. *The Theory and Practice of Industrial Pharmacy,* 2nd Ed.; Lachman, L.,

Lieberman, H.A., Kanig, J.L. Eds.; Lea & Febiger: Philadelphia, 1976; 321–358.

45. Joachim, J.; Kalantzis, G.; Jacob, M.; Mention, J.; Maury, L.; Rambaud, J. Tehnologie d'un Granule Effervescent. Etudes Physico-Chimiques. J. Pharm. Belg. **1986**, *41*, 197–208.

46. Devay, A.; Uderszky, J.; Racz, I. Optimization of Operational Parameters in Fluidized Bed Granulation of Effervescent Pharmaceutical Preparations. Acta Pharm. Technol. **1984**, *30*, 239–242.

47. Lindberg, N.-O. Preparation of Effervescent Tablets Containing Nicotinic Acid and Sodium Bicarbonate. Acta Pharm. Suec. **1970**, *7*, 23–28.

48. Saleh, S.I.; Aboutaleb, A.; Kassem, A.A.; Stamm, A. A Contribution to the Formulation of Effervescent Tablets by Direct Compression. Labo-Pharma Probl. Tech. **1984**, *32*, 763–766.

49. Röscheisen, G.; Schmidt, P.C. The Combination of Factorial Design and Simplex Method in the Optimization of Lubricants for Effervescent Tablets. Eur. J. Pharm. Sci. **1995**, *41*, 302–308.

50. Rotthäuser, B.; Kraus, G.; Schmidt, P.C. Optimization of an Effervescent Tablet Formulation Containing Spray Dried L-leucine and Polyethylene Glycol 6000 as Lubricants Using a Central Composite Design. Sur. J. Pharm. Sci. **1998**, *46*, 85–94.

51. Lindberg, N.-O.; Tufvesson, C.; Olbjer, L. Extrusion of an Effervescent Granulation with a Twin Screw Xxtruder, Baker Perkins MPF 50 D. Drug Dev. Ind. Pharm. **1987**, *13*, 1891–1913.

52. SWEDIS, Medical Products Agency, Box 26, S-751 03. Uppsala, Sweden.

53. El-Banna, H.M.; Minina, S.A. The Construction and Uses of Factorial Designs in the Preparation of Solid Dosage Forms. Part 1: Effervescent Acetylosalicylic Acid Tablets. Pharmazie **1981**, *36*, 417–420.

54. Anderson, N.R.; Banker, G.S.; Peck, G.E. Quantitative Evaluation of Pharmaceutical Effervescent Systems II: Stability Monitoring by Reactivity and Porosity Measurements. J. Pharm. Sci. **1982**, *71*, 7–13.

55. Desai, S.R.; Allen, L.V.; Greenwood, R.B.; Stiles, M.L.; Parker, D. Effervescent Solid Dispersions of Prednisone, Griseofulvin and Primidone. Drug Dev. Ind. Pharm. **1989**, *15*, 671–689.

56. Usui, F.; Carstensen, J.T. Interactions in the Solid State I: Interactions of Sodium Bicarbonate and Tartaric Acid under Compressed Conditions. J. Pharm. Sci. **1985**, *74*, 1293–1297.

57. White, B. Stable Effervescent Compositions and Method of Preparing Same. US Patent 3,105,792.

58. Bulut, P.; Özer, A.Y.; Sumnu, M.; Hincal, A.A. Evaluation of the Stability of Commercial Effervescent and Dispersible Aspirin Tablets by Factorial Analysis. S.T.P. Pharm. Sci. **1991**, *1*, 357–361.

59. Silver, B.; Sundholm, G. Solid-State Esterification of Codeine Phosphate by the Acid Constituent of Effervescent Tablets. J. Pharm. Sci. **1987**, *76*, 53–55.

60. Narurkar, A.N.; Purkaystha, A.R.; Sheen, P.-C. Effect of Various Factors on the Corrosion and Rusting of Tooling Material Used for Tablet Manufacturing. Drug Dev. Ind. Pharm. **1985**, *11*, 1487–1495.

61. Siegel, S.; Hanus, E.J.; Carr, J.W. Polytetrafluoorethylene Tipped Tablet Punches. J. Pharm. Sci. **1963**, *52*, 604–605.

62. Stammberger, W. Entwicklung von Brausezubereitungen. Acta Pharm. Technol. **1975**, *21*, 177–184.

63. Sendall, F.E.J.; Staniforth, J.N. A Study of Powder Adhesion to Metal Surfaces During Compression of Effervescent Pharmaceutical Tablets. J. Pharm. Pharmacol. **1986**, *38*, 489–493.

64. Amela, J.; Salazar, R.; Cemeli, J. Methods for the Determination of the Carbon Dioxide Evolved from Effervescent Systems. Drug Dev. Ind. Pharm. **1993**, *19*, 1019–1036.

65. Anderson, N.R.; Banker, G.S.; Peck, G.E. Quantitative Evaluation of Pharmaceutical Effervescent Systems I: Design of Testing Apparatus. J. Pharm. Sci. **1982**, *71*, 3–6.

66. Spitz, H.D. Determination of Water in Aluminum Chlorohydrate and Effervescent Tablets by Karl Fischer analysis. J. Pharm. Sci. **1979**, *68*, 122–123.

67. Ritschel, W.A. Die Tablette. *Grundlagen und Praxis Des Tablettierens, Granulierens und Dragierens*; Editio Cantor KG: Aulendorf Germany, 1966; 116.

68. David, S.T.; Gallian, C.E. The Effect of Environmental Moisture and Temperature on the Physical Stability of Effervescent Tablets in Foil Laminate Package Containing Minute Imperfections. Drug Dev. Ind. Pharm. **1986**, *12*, 2541–2550.

FURTHER READING

Mohrle, R. Effervescent Tablets. *Pharmaceutical Dosage Forms*, 2nd Ed.; Lieberman, H.-A., Lachman, L., Schwartz, J.B. Eds.; Marcel Dekker, Inc.: New York, 1989; 1.

Schmidt, P.C.; Christin, I. Brausetabletten —eine fast vergessene Arzneiform. Pharmazie **1990**, *45*, 89–101.

Sendall, F.-E.-J.; Staniforth, J.-N.; Rees, J.-E.; Leatham, M.J. Effervescent Tablets. Pharm. J. **1983**, *230*, 289–294.

ELASTOMERIC COMPONENTS FOR THE PHARMACEUTICAL INDUSTRY

Edward J. Smith

Packaging Science Resources, King of Prussia, Pennsylvania

INTRODUCTION

The primary function of elastomeric components used by the pharmaceutical industry, which includes both drugs and medical devices, is to protect and deliver. Elastomeric components are typically primary packaging components; that is, they are or may be in direct contact with the dosage form. They must neither interact with the dosage form nor allow the ingress or egress of materials. Elastomeric or rubber components typically provide the means for sealing parenteral containers of varying size and shape because of their unique physical properties. Elasticity particularly permits intimate contact between the closure and the relatively rigid surfaces of container openings. No other material known today has this same unique property. This property is primarily responsible for the ability of the closure to be pierced with a sharp device, such as a hypodermic needle, and then to reseal. This is an example of the delivery function of elastomeric components. Rubber closures are an essential component of the primary package for most parenteral or injectable products. Typical rubber components are pictured in Figs. 1 and 2.

In order to understand how rubber performs its unique "protect and deliver" function, it is necessary to know how rubber is compounded and manufactured.

RUBBER COMPOUNDS

Rubber, like all other primary packaging materials, is not inert. Any material used in the compounding of the rubber component may be leached into and/or chemically react with the dosage form. The basic materials used in the compounding of rubber components used by the drug and medical device industries are listed in Table 1. These materials, and the amounts used, are significantly different from those that may be used in industrial rubber belts, tires, and hoses where heat, abrasion, and solvent resistance are typically the main concern. More than one type of each material may be used in a rubber compound. For example, compounds containing two elastomers, such as isoprene and chlorobutyl rubber, and two pigments, such as titanium dioxide and carbon black, are very common. Compounds used for parenteral closures consist of an elastomer as the base material combined chemically and physically with other necessary rubber chemicals.

The elastomer determines most of the physical and chemical characteristics of a rubber compound. Typical elastomers are natural elastomers such as natural rubber (NR), sometimes called crepe, and synthetic elastomers such as butyl (including chlorobutyl and bromobutyl), ethylene propylene diene monomer (EPDM), and styrene butadiene rubber (SBR). A list of commonly used elastomers is shown in Table 2.

In the pharmaceutical industry, natural rubber and its synthetic analog, isoprene rubber, are normally used in products that require good physical strength or that must be able to withstand multiple punctures while maintaining seal integrity. Due the "latex sensitivity" issue, the use of natural rubber is declining. This issue is discussed in a later section. Neoprene, a halogenated form of polyisoprene, is typically used for oil-based pharmaceutical products, such as mineral oil or vegetable oil. SBR and nitrile rubber (NBR), which is used primarily for oil-based products, are specialty elastomers that are not as commonly used. Butyls and halobutyls comprise the largest segment of pharmaceutical rubber compounds, having properties that make them applicable for the packaging of many products, especially those requiring protection from moisture vapor or oxygen. Most lyophilized and powdered products require this protection, and some liquid products require protection from oxygen. EPDMs are less commonly used, though they have been selected for large intravenous (IV) stoppers. Silicones also are not often used due to their permeability to moisture vapor and oxygen as well as their relatively high cost. A list of common elastomers and their chemical structures is found in Table 3.

Curing (or vulcanizing/cross-linking) agents are chemicals used to cross-link elastomer chains into the three-dimensional (3D) network required to give a rubber component the desired elasticity. The term "vulcanization" indicates that heat is employed in the manufacturing or molding process. Common curing agents are sulfur,

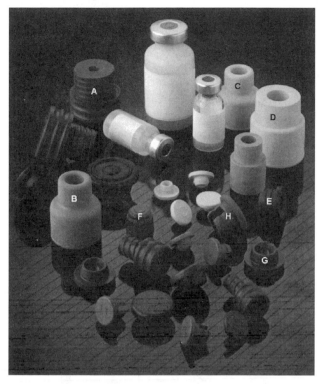

Fig. 1 Typical rubber components. A) Syringe plunger. B,C,D) Sleeve stoppers. E) Abbott ADDVantage vial stopper. F) IV bag injection site. G) Serum vial stopper. H) Lyophilization vial stopper. (Photograph provided by Abbott Laboratories.)

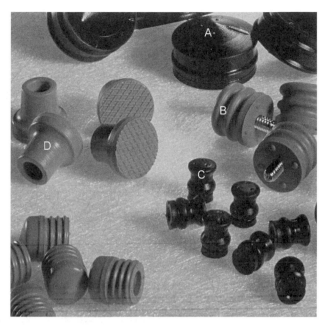

Fig. 2 Typical rubber syringe plungers. A) Plunger for 10-mL sterile-empty syringe. B) Plunger for sterile-prefilled dental cartridge. C) Plunger for 1mL sterile-empty syringe. D) Tip cap for Luer Tip syringe. (Photograph provided by West Pharmaceutical Services, Inc.)

thiurams, zinc oxide, peroxides, resins, and amines. A desirable property of pharmaceutical rubber formulations is "cleanliness," that is, that they contain materials that neither leach nor volatilize into the packaged pharmaceutical. Sulfur-cured rubber, because it requires other chemicals to effect an efficient cure, is not usually as clean as resin-, metal oxide-, or peroxide-cured formulations. The demands of the pharmaceutical industry and regulatory agencies are such that these relatively clean cure systems are becoming more common.

Accelerators reduce the cure time considerably by increasing the cure rate. They are not catalysts because they are chemically altered and, in many cases, also react as curing agents. Common sulfur-cure accelerators are amines, dithiocarbamates, sulfenamides, thiazoles, and thiurams. Some accelerators, because of their reactivity, may form toxic compounds, such as 2-(2-hydroxyethylmercapto)benzothiazole from mercaptobenzothiazole (2-MCBT), residues of which may be extractable. Accelerators that are secondary amines may form toxic nitrosamines.

Activators, which affect the efficiency of accelerators, are commonly added. Normally these are metal oxides, such as zinc oxide or stearic acid.

Antioxidants are classified as antidegradants or age resistors. Chemically, antioxidants protect the reactive (sensitive) sites of the rubber chains against oxygen attack. Typical antioxidants are chemicals such as hindered phenols and amines. Unsaturated elastomers, such as natural rubber, require antioxidants for protection against oxidation, which causes surface cracking and loss of elasticity. Saturated elastomers, such as silicones and fluoroelastomers, are resistant to oxidation and usually require no added antioxidants. Some antioxidants are classified as antiozonants, which are designed to provide protection when high levels of reactive ozone are likely to be in the environment. A list of saturated and unsaturated elastomers is found in Table 4.

Table 1 Rubber compounding materials and their function

Material	Function
Elastomer	Base material
Curing agent	Forms cross-links
Accelerator	Affects type and rate of cross-links
Activator	Alters efficiency of accelerator
Antioxidant	Antidegradant
Plasticizer	Processing aid
Filler	Affects physical properties
Pigment	Color

Table 2   Common elastomers used in parenteral packaging components

Elastomer	% Use	Reason
Butyl/halobutyls	~80	Excellent O_2 and moisture barrier
Natural/isoprene	~10	Excellent physical properties such as reseal
EPDM	~5	Good heat resistance and surface lubricity
Nitrile and neoprene	~3	Resistance to vegetable and mineral oils
SBR	~1	Blended with isoprene/NR or halobutyls to improve physical properties
Silicone	≪1	Excellent heat resistance; poor O_2 and moisture barrier; high cost

Table 3   Chemical structures of common elastomers

Common name	Chemical name	Structure
Butyl rubber	Poly(isobutylene-isoprene)	$+(CH_2-\underset{CH_3}{\overset{CH_3}{C}})_{50}(CH_2-\underset{CH_3}{C}=CH-CH_2)_n+$
Halobutyl rubber[a]	Halogenated poly(isobutylene-isoprene)	$+(CH_2-\underset{CH_3}{\overset{CH_3}{C}})_{65}(CH=\underset{CH_3}{C}-\overset{X}{CH}-CH_2)_n+$
Ethylene-propylene rubber	Poly(ethylene-propylene)	$+(CH_2-CH_2)_3(CH_2-\underset{CH_3}{CH})]_n$
Ethylene-propylene-diene rubber	Poly(ethylene-propylene-diene)	$+(CH_2-CH_2)_{15}(CH_2-\underset{CH_3}{CH})_5(diene)_n+$
Silicone rubber	Polydimethylsiloxane	$+\underset{CH_3}{\overset{CH_3}{Si}}-O-]_n$
Urethane rubber	Adipic acid-ethylene glycol polyester	$HO+(CH_2)_2+O-\overset{O}{\overset{\|}{C}}-(CH_2)_4-\overset{O}{\overset{\|}{C}}-O-(CH_2)_2+_n OH$
Fluoroelastomers	Polytetrafluorethylene	$+\underset{F}{\overset{F}{C}}-\underset{F}{\overset{F}{C}}-]_n$
Natural rubber	cis-(1.4-Polyisoprene)	$+(CH_2-\underset{CH_3}{C}=CH-CH_2)_n+$
Polyisoprene rubber	cis-(1.4-Polyisoprene)	$+(CH_2-\underset{CH_3}{C}=CH-CH_2)_n+$
Neoprene rubber	Polychloroprene	$+(CH_2-\underset{Cl}{C}=CH-CH_2)_n+$
Styrene-butadiene rubber	Poly(butadiene-styrene)	$+(CH_2-CH=CH-CH_2)_4(CH_2-\underset{C_6H_5}{CH})_n+$
Nitrile rubber	Poly(butadiene-acrylonitrile)	$+(CH_2-CH=CH-CH_2)_5(CH_2-\underset{CN}{CH})_2)_n+$
Polybutadiene	Polybutadiene	$+(CH_2-CH=CH-CH_2)_n+$

(From Ref. 22.)

[a] X = Cl or Br.

Table 4 Saturated and unsaturated elastomers

Saturated	ASTM abbreviation	Unsaturated	ASTM abbreviation
Butyl	IIR	Natural	NR
Halobutyls (chlorobutyl and bromobutyl)	CIIR, BIIR	Isoprene	IR
Ethylene-propylene-diene monomer rubber	EPDM	Styrene butadiene	SBR
Silicone	Q	Nitrile	NBR
Urethane	U	Neoprene	CR
Fluoroelastomers	FKM	Polybutadiene	BR

Plasticizers are used in rubber compounds to assist in the mixing or molding of the rubber, to soften the final vulcanized rubber, or to add surface lubricity to the surface of the rubber component. Examples are paraffinic wax, silicone oil, paraffinic and naphthenic oils, phthalates, and organic phosphates. Silicone oil is commonly used in syringe pistons that must slide freely within a glass or plastic barrel; it also reduces the coring or fragmentation tendency of vial stoppers.

Fillers are materials that modify rubber characteristics (e.g., hardness) and improve its physical characteristics (e.g., tensile strength), in addition to reducing costs. Rubber is sometimes compounded without the use of fillers; the resultant product is called "gum rubber." Typical fillers are calcined and hydrated clays, magnesium silicate (talc), magnesium oxide, and silicas. Carbon black, a common filler used to increase the heat resistance in industrial components such as tires, is not used as a filler in pharmaceutical components but it is used in smaller amounts as a black pigment. Polynuclear aromatic (PNA) hydrocarbons are a concern with carbon blacks but the grades used by manufacturers of pharmaceutical components contain very low concentrations.

The pigments used are inorganic salts and oxides, carbon black, or organic dyes that are used for aesthetic or functional purposes (e.g., identification, designating a dosage, etc.). Typical pigments are carbon black, titanium dioxide, and iron oxide. With these three pigments white, black, red, and many shades of gray and pink can be produced. These pigments are chemically pure and stable, nontoxic, and relatively inexpensive. Other pigments such as phthalocyanines and ultramarine blue can be used for blues and greens, but their color fastness in not as good as the aforementioned pigments.

A typical thermoset rubber compound is shown in Table 5. In terms of percentage by weight, the elastomer and filler are the chief materials used, accounting typically for over 90% of a compound. However, the other "minor" materials are quite necessary in order for the compound to have the necessary chemical, physical, and toxicological properties required for a functional packaging component. For example, without the curing agent the compound would remain a physical mixture of materials that would have the consistency of chewing gum. On the other hand, materials such as pigments may be omitted from the compound with only minor consequences — i.e., the loss of the desired color.

SELECTION OF COMPOUND MATERIALS

Many materials may be used in a rubber compound; however, only a fraction of materials are acceptable in components used for the drug industry. A source of

Table 5 Typical thermoset rubber compound

Material	Percent by weight
Chlorobutyl rubber (elastomer)	52.7
Calcined clay (filler)	39.4
Paraffinic oil (plasticizer)	4.4
Titanium dioxide (pigment)	1.1
Carbon black (pigment)	0.13
Thiuram (curing agent/accelerator)	0.14
Zinc oxide (activator)	1.6
2,6-Di-tert-butyl-4-sec-butyl phenol (antioxidant)	0.53

acceptable materials is the U.S. Code of Federal Regulations (CFR). Since the CFR has no list for drug contact, the drug industry uses the CFR list designated for foods. Applicable sections of 21 CFR are as follows:

Section 175—Indirect Food Additives
Sections 177 and 178—Indirect Food Additives Polymers
Sections 182, 184, 185—Generally Regarded as Safe (GRAS) Lists
Section 177.2600—Rubber Articles Intended for Repeated Use (The primary section containing a list of materials used in rubber formulations for pharmaceutical items.)

There are some cautions with the CFR lists. First, manufacturers may not always submit materials to the Food and Drug Administration (FDA) for listing in the CFR. They may not want to take the time or incur the costs if they see only a limited market for their material in the pharmaceutical or food market. Second, some materials, such as 2-MCBT, which is not permitted by the FDA, are listed but are strongly discouraged. Finally, some materials listed in the CFR, such as food, drug, and cosmetic dyes, are really not applicable for rubber compounds used for pharmaceuticals. Many of these dyes are water-soluble and are not applicable for rubber formulations that come in contact with aqueous solutions, since the dyes could be extracted from the rubber and discolor the drug.

Component manufacturers may use materials not listed in the CFR provided that acceptable toxicity data is available to the reviewing health authority.

TYPES OF RUBBER AND THE MANUFACTURING PROCESS

Elastomeric closures for parenteral products are made from two types of elastomers or rubbers. Thermoset rubber, the most common, undergoes a chemical reaction during the molding or component-forming processing. In this chemical reaction cross-links, or bonds are inserted between the long polymer chains to form a resilient 3D network. Without these cross-links elastomeric closures would have properties resembling those of chewing gum, which is an uncross-linked rubber blended with sugar, flavors, and food coloring. The cross-linking process is not reversible. Once a closure is molded it cannot be remolded into another shape or size. Addition of heat only causes degradation or reversion of the rubber.

Another type of rubber that is used frequently is thermoplastic rubber (1, 2). Components are fabricated in a process that is similar to that used for common hard plastics, such as polyethylene or polystyrene, but the final product is an elastic material with properties otherwise equivalent to those of thermoset rubbers. No chemical reactions are involved in the processing of a thermoplastic rubber. The fabrication process consists of heating the rubber compound until it liquefies, injecting the liquid into a mold, cooling the mold, and finally removing the closure from the mold. The process is reversible. Closures can be remelted and remolded into different shapes or sizes as desired. Cross-linking in this case is not a chemical process but a physical intertwining of polymeric chains. The resulting intertwined 3D network gives thermoplastic elastomers their elasticity and resiliency.

Currently, thermoplastics account for less than 5% of the elastomeric closures for parenterals. Their limited resistance to heat deformation under stress during autoclave sterilization is the main reason for this limited use. However, thermoplastics have two advantages over thermosets. First, they are chemically less complex and therefore less prone to interact with parenteral medications, and second, they may be manufactured by a simpler and more automated process. Thermoplastic elastomers have found use in baby bottle nipples and dropper bulbs that are not typically heat sterilized under compression.

The manufacturing of rubber components for pharmaceutical applications is a multistep process with controls on each step. Fully validated processes are now common. The process is outlined in Table 6.

There are generally three molding processes used for manufacturing pharmaceutical closures: compression molding, injection molding, and transfer molding. The choice of molding method usually depends on the necessary final dimensional tolerances of the item being molded. Injection molding gives the best dimensional tolerances; however, it is usually the most expensive technique, especially as compared to compression molding. Thermoset rubbers are commonly compression or transfer molded, while thermoplastic rubbers are typically injection molded. The compression molding cycle is illustrated in Fig. 3. Sheets of molded components vary in shape from round to rectangular, and in size from 12 in. in diameter to 36 × 36 inches square, and may contain 50–10,000 components.

A recent trend in rubber component manufacturing is the production of "preprocessed" components. Components are prepared for shipment in either one of two states:

1. *Ready to Sterilize (RtS):* Typically components are washed, then rinsed with Water For Injection (WFI) to reduce bioburden and endotoxin levels, lubricated with

Table 6　Manufacturing process for rubber components for pharmaceutical use

Process step	Comment
1. Raw material specifications and testing	Tests for identity and purity
2. Weighing of batch ingredients according to DMF-filed "recipe"	Weighted to ±0.2% of nominal batch weight
3. Mixing to get homogeneous batch of material	Mixed either in an internal mixer or on an open mill
4. Testing representative samples of the mixed batch of rubber	Blend of ingredients is tested for cure characteristics; molded test piece is tested for common attributes such as durometer hardness, specific gravity, percentage ash, IR spectrum of pyrolizate, and UV spectrum of an aqueous extract.
5. Preform material by extrusion, calendering or pelletizing	Material is formed into blocks, trips, sheets or pellets for ease of handling
6. Preformed material is placed on mold or into mold feeder mechanism	
7. Molding by compression, transfer, or injection techniques	Unvulcanized mixtures of materials are shaped into the desired component by heat and pressure; chemical reaction causes cross-links to form between polymer chains
8. Trimming	Convert molded sheets of connected components into individual components
9. Washing	Remove particulate matter, and mold and trim lubricants
10. Rinsing	Reduce surface endotoxins and bioburden when WFI water is used
11. Sterilization	Only done when presterilized components are produced
12. Final QC testing	Tests for identity, dimensional measurements, and physical, chemical and biological tests
13. Packing	A counted number of components are placed in containers, usually bags made of polyethylene or Tyvek®, then sealed in cardboard cartons for shipping
14. Shipping	Cartons are grouped by lot number, palletized and shipped by truck, ship or air

silicone oil, and finally packaged in a classified area (Classes 100–10,000) in Tyvek® bags that can be steam sterilized by the drug or device manufacturer

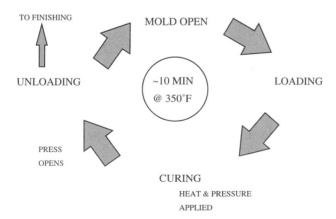

Fig. 3　Compression molding cycle.

before use. Alternately polyethylene bags may be used if the end user is utilizing gamma radiation for sterilization.

2. *Ready to Use (RtU):* The process is identical to that used for RtS components except that the component manufacturer takes responsibility for component sterilization and the sterilized components are received by the drug or device manufacturer. No additional component processing is required before use.

Both processes typically require extensive validation by the component manufacturer, a description of the process in a Drug Master File (DMF), quality audits by customers, and perhaps FDA approval before RtS or RtU components are utilized. Nevertheless, RtS and RtU are trends that are moving rapidly; most major rubber component manufacturers now market RtS components (3). A list of pharmaceutical rubber manufacturers is shown in Table 7.

STERILIZATION OF RUBBER COMPONENTS

Heat, radiation, and sterilizing gases may be used to sterilize rubber components. However, components, especially vial stoppers, are most frequently sterilized by pressurized steam (autoclaving), a highly effective method and probably the most reliable of available methods when an F_0 value of at least 8 min is reached (4). However, the poor thermal conductivity of rubber and the relatively large mass of wet stoppers placed in a stainless steel container for sterilization require a careful validation of the process. Assurance must be obtained that the moist heat penetrates throughout the mass of stoppers so that every stopper receives a dose equivalent to a minimal F_0 of 8 min. However, rubber closures subjected to elevated temperatures or extended heating even at moderate temperatures degrade or revert, which is most frequently evidenced by stickiness. Therefore, the application of moist heat must be controlled because this degradation is most likely to be greatest at the outer layers of the mass of stoppers. This undesirable effect can be markedly reduced by distributing the stoppers in a shallow tray or otherwise reducing the mass, thus making it possible to reduce the thermal cycle time and the applied heat. Cycle times of 121°C for 30–60 min are usually well tolerated by rubber components made from butyl or halobutyl rubbers. Natural and isoprene rubbers are less tolerant. Increasing the sterilization temperature above 121°C or the time above 60 min is not recommended unless components have been tested to assure that no significant degradation will take place. Dry heat sterilization or drying of components above 105°C is also not recommended without prior testing. Testing may include inspection of the surface for cracks or tackiness, swelling studies to determine state of cure, functional tests such as coring and reseal, and chemical tests such as the United States Pharmacopoeia (USP) protocol or extraction studies performed before and after the sterilization cycle.

Under the usual autoclaving conditions, moist heat does not destroy pyrogens. For closures to be pyrogen-free, a final rinse with WFI before sterilization is necessary.

Ethylene oxide, a sterilizing gas, may be used to sterilize rubber components when they are part of a medical device; however, the gas is readily absorbed by the rubber and sufficient time must be allowed after sterilization for the concentration of residual ethylene oxide to dissipate to acceptable levels (5, 6).

Radiation sterilization, by either gamma or e-beam, also may be utilized to sterilize rubber components. However, some elastomers, such as butyl, chlorobutyl, and bromobutyl, do not tolerate high doses of radiation, while others, such as natural, isoprene, neoprene, and nitrile rubbers are readily radiation-sterilized without degradation (7, 8). The challenge with radiation sterilization of rubber components in bulk (i.e., cartons or bags) is to obtain a uniform dose of radiation throughout the entire package—enough of a dose to assure the desired sterility assurance level (SAL), usually 10^{-6}, without degrading the components, especially those nearest the radiation source. There are generally two approaches that can be followed. One is to target a uniform dose of 25 kGy, which is generally accepted to assure sterility, while the other is to follow the ANSI/AAMI/ISO 11137:1994 standard and target a dose of radiation that is dependent on the bioburden of the components (9). The first approach is usually overkill but may be acceptable for radiation-resistant rubbers. The second approach usually results in lower doses applied, which may be critical with butyl and other rubbers that are not so radiation resistant. There are several necessary steps if the ANSI/AAMI/ISO standard is used. These are:

- Selection of the SAL, usually 10^{-6}
- Determination of the average bioburden from samples taken from three consecutive production lots
- Establishment of the Verification Dose. This is the dose in kGy found in Table B.1 of the standard that will give a SAL of 10^{-2}
- Confirmation of the Verification Dose by irradiating 100 components and testing each for sterility. No more than two positives are permitted
- Establishment of the Sterilizing Dose from Table B.1 of the standard
- Dose mapping, using dosimeters, on a shipping container filled with components. Irradiate and determine the maximum and minimum doses (D_{max} and D_{min}) received in the container
- Calculation of the Target Dose by multiplying the Sterilizing Dose by the ratio, D_{max}/D_{min}. The Target Dose is typically increased 6% or more to account for dosimeter error and to add additional sterility assurance.

TESTS AND STANDARDS

In-Process Tests

Several tests may be performed on unvulcanized rubber or on standard-shaped test specimens to measure the properties of a rubber compound (10). These include the following:

1. *Rheometer measurements* measure cure and cure rate characteristics of the rubber. The component

Table 7 Pharmaceutical rubber packaging component manufacturers

Name	Symbol[a]	Address	Phone	Website or e-mail address
Abbott Laboratories	AB	268 E. Fourth Street, Ashland, OH 44805, USA	+419-282-5378	www.abbott.com
AL group Wheaton	AL	618 Beam St., Salisbury, MD 21801, USA	+410-546-6441	www.alcanpackaging.com
Bryant Rubber Corp.	BR	1112 Lomita Blvd., Harbor City, CA 90710, USA	+310-530-2530	www.bryantrubber.com
Daikyo Seiko, Ltd.	DS	38-2, Sumida 3-Chome, Sumida-Ku, Tokyo 131, Japan	+81-3-3614-5461	
Helvoet Pharma	HP	Industrieterrein Kolmen 1519, B-3570 Alken, Belgium	+32-11-59-08-00	www.helvoetpharma.com
Itran-Tompkins Rubber Corp.	IT	375 Metuchen Rd., South Plainfield, NJ 07080, USA	+908-754-8100	www.itranrubber.com
Kokoku Rubber Inc.	KO	1450 E. American Lane, Zurich Towers, #1545, Schaumburg, IL 60173, USA	+847-517-6770 Ext 12	www.kokokurubber.com
Lexington Medical	LR	663 Bryant Blvd. Rock Hill, SC 29732, USA	+803-366-7036	
The Plasticoid Company	PL	249 High Street, Elkton, MD 21921, USA	+410-398-2800	www.plasticoid.com
Samsung Medical Rubber Co., Ltd.	SA	474-4, Mokae-Dong, Ansan-City, Kyunggi Province, Korea	+82-345-491-8071	www.smrco.co.kr
Seal Line S.p.A.	SL	Via Bernarde, 7, 36040 Montegaldella (VI), Italy	+39-0444/737221	Sealline@keycomm.it
Stelmi Trading International	ST	121, avenue Jean Mermoz, BP-93, F-93127 La Courneuve Cedex, France	+(33)-1-49-92-64-00	www.stelmi.com
West Pharmaceutical Services	WP	101 Gordon Drive, Lionville, PA 19341, USA	1-800-231-3000	www.westpharma.com

[a] Abbreviation for reference use in this chapter only.

manufacturer performs this test on unvulcanized rubber. The rheometer measures the viscosity of the rubber as a function of time at a constant temperature. As time increases, the degree of cure or cross-linking increases and thus the viscosity increases.

2. *Durometer hardness is* measured on tests specimens that meet specific standards for shape and thickness (11). Durometer hardness is usually measured using the Shore A scale, which measures relative hardness on a scale of 0 to 100 units. Most rubber components for medical use are found in the 35–60 range with 40–50 typical for rubber vial stoppers. Durometer Hardness may be measured on some actual components if they have a sufficiently large flat surface and thickness, i.e., 28–32 mm IV stoppers.

3. *Compression set is* commonly used as a measure of the dimensional recovery of a rubber compound after compression at a defined level, usually 25%, at a specified time and temperature, usually 24 h at 70°C (12). High compression set values are associated with rubber that "takes a set" or loses its ability to spring back after compression. Low compression set is important for rubber closures and syringe plungers that are heat sterilized while under compression and remain under compression for long periods of time before use but must remain elastic and resilient to maintain seal integrity. Compression Set is measured on dimensionally defined test specimens.

4. *Tensile, modulus, and elongation* are measures of the strength of a rubber compound (13). They are measured on bow tie-shaped specimens that are clamped in a tensile measuring apparatus and stretched.

5. *Water vapor and oxygen transmission (WVT and O$_2$T)* are commonly measured on thin-film specimens. Butyl and halobutyl compounds have very low WVT and O$_2$T rates, while rates for natural and isoprene rubbers are higher and for silicone even higher.

Finished Component Tests

Finished component tests may be divided into three categories: those used as routine identity and/or quality control tests, those tests recommended or mandated by government, standards, and compendial groups, and those test that are part of the larger rubber component acceptance and drug/device approval process. In many instances, a test may fall into more than one category.

Identity and quality control tests (14, 15)

Percentage ash is a measure of the nonvolatile materials in a rubber formulation, such as clays and other fillers.

Specific gravity is a measure of the type and quantity of fillers in a formulation.

An *infrared spectrum* of a compound pyrolysate identifies the elastomer qualitatively (natural, butyl, etc.).

An *ultraviolet (UV) spectrum* of an aqueous rubber extract identifies and quantifies the antioxidants, curing agents, accelerators, and other UV-absorbing species extracted from the compound.

Percentage swelling in an organic solvent is a measure of the degree and consistency of cure or cross-linking that determines the physical and functional properties of a component.

These five tests may be used to characterize a rubber formulation or serve, either individually or in combinations, as quality control tests.

Compendial, standard, and government tests

The most influential of these test protocols are the USP (16), the *European Pharmacopoeia* (EP) (17), the *Pharmacopoeia of Japan* (JP) (18), the Organization for International Standardization (ISO) (19), and the Parenteral Drug Association (PDA) (15, 20). USP<381>, Elastomeric Closures for Injections, contains five chemical tests and two biological tests. Closures must meet the biological requirements but there are no current specifications for the chemical tests. All USP chemical tests are commonly performed on aqueous extracts but isopropyl alcohol and the drug product vehicle are also permitted. A brief description of the USP<381> tests follows (21).

Turbidity. The clarity of the closure extract is measured with a nephelometer with appropriate standards. Turbidity is a measure of the insoluble extractables from a closure and is affected by the type and amounts of ingredients in a formulation, pretreatments such as washing, extractions, sterilizations, and degree of cure.
Reducing agents. Organic extractables oxidizable by iodine are determined in this procedure. It is affected by the same variables as turbidity.
Heavy metals. Extractable lead as well as other metals, such as zinc and cadmium, are determined colorimetrically or by atomic absorption.
pH change. The pH of the extract is a measure of the acidic and alkaline water-soluble extractables from a compound.
Total extractables. The sum of the inorganic, organic (nonvolatile), soluble, and insoluble extractables is measured in this test. The weight of total extractables is an indication of the "cleanliness" of a formulation.
Biological tests. USP 24 lists two levels of biological tests—the in vitro tissue culture test and the in vivo systemic injection and intracutaneous tests. A parenteral

closure must pass either type of test to meet USP requirements.

The application of numerical specifications to the USP <381> chemical tests is under discussion and probably will become effective in USP 24 via a supplement. The JP, EP, and ISO have specifications for rubber closures and these test protocols are compared with the USP in Table 8. Not all pharmacopeias and standards groups designate the same tests; therefore, it is important to consult a wide spectrum of references to design a test protocol for specific applications and geographical submissions. Of the four protocols compared, the JP is the most stringent in terms of limits for extractables. The USP, EP, and ISO test protocols are based on a specific closure "area" per volume of water in the extraction step. The JP test protocols, on the other hand, are based on a specific "weight" of closures per volume of water. This difference makes it more difficult for smaller closures than for larger closures in the same rubber compound to meet JP specifications; i.e., 13-mm closures will be less likely to meet JP specifications than 20-mm closures, and 20-mm closures are less likely than 28-mm closures to meet JP specifications.

Although packaging components, such as vial closures, syringe plungers, and needle shields, may meet all compendial and accepted standards, this does not mean that they will be acceptable for use with any specific drug or device. Specific evaluation tests must be performed for that purpose. Compendial and standard tests should be regarded as the first necessary but not sufficient hurdle in the race to gain approval of a component for use with a drug or device.

Specific tests for component evaluation and regulatory approval

There are three requirements for a rubber component:

1. Compatible with the drug
2. Meets functional requirements
3. Provides closure-container seal integrity

Many factors influence the choice of a rubber compound for a particular drug, the most important of which is the solvent vehicle. If the solvent vehicle is an aqueous material, then a butyl, natural, or EPDM may be used. If the solvent vehicle is an oil, then a neoprene or nitrile is utilized.

Configuration is also important and is determined by the required function. A lyophilization stopper, designed to keep out moisture, almost certainly requires a butyl formulation, while a vial stopper for aqueous-based solutions could be formulated from isoprene rubber.

Some preservatives are especially reactive with rubber. Bromobutyl rubbers, but not chlorobutyls, are recommended for drug formulations that contain chlorobutanol. A pH that is either very low or very high affects rubber formulations more than a pH in the range of 5–8. Buffer systems may also affect the choice of rubber formulations. Materials such as phosphates not only attack the rubber at high pHs but also may attack glass as well.

Metallic sensitivities affect compatibility, as drug formulations that are sensitive to divalent cations, such as calcium, zinc, or iron, may not be able to use certain rubber compounds that are cured or pigmented with these materials.

An obvious factor is the need for oxygen or moisture vapor protection. A butyl-based compound is normally chosen whenever protection from materials transmitted either into or from a drug product is required.

When it comes to color preference, most rubber manufacturers of closures used for drugs prefer to use three pigments: iron oxide to produce reds, carbon black for blacks, and titanium dioxide for whites; combinations of these are used for pinks and grays. Organic materials used as pigments are not generally acceptable since they are not very heat stable and are generally more toxic than the three pigments mentioned.

Choice of sterilization method is extremely important in choosing a rubber formulation. Many heat-sensitive drugs, such as proteins, are packaged aseptically; that is, the rubber closure, the vial, and drug are sterilized separately, and then all three items are brought together in a sterile environment to form the final package. The FDA, however, encourages terminal sterilization. In this method, the three materials are brought together and then the entire package, the drug in contact with the vial and closure, is sterilized by heat. This method is much more demanding on the closure than aseptic processing.

Radiation (Co-60) is used to sterilize many rubber items, especially those used in devices. The effect of gamma radiation on rubber closures is a function of the elastomer, dose, and postirradiation time. NR and isoprene are much more resistant to irradiation effects than butyl.

To give the drug manufacturer a high degree of assurance that the closures being investigated for a possible package will be acceptable, a prescreening procedure is commonly used by component suppliers. In this procedure, information and a sample of the drug are obtained from the drug manufacturer. Then three to five possible closures, along with an inert control stopper (a Teflon® plug or coated closure), are used to package vials of the drug. The closures are put onto the drug-containing vials using an exaggerated closure area-to-volume ratio (2× to 3× the normal ratio). Vials are stored at higher and/or lower temperatures than

Table 8 Comparison of USP, EP, JP, and ISO test protocols for rubber closures

	USP[a]	EP[b]	JP[c]	ISO[d]
Test types and limits				
Chemical tests	Y	Y	Y	Y
Biological tests	Y	N	Y	N
Functional tests	N	N	N	Y
Test limits	Y, only on Biological Tests	Y	Y	Y
Specific tests				
Alkalinity/pH	Y	Y	Y	Y
Ammonia	N	Y	N	Y
Appearance/turbidity	Y	Y	Y	Y
Ash, total	N	Y	N	Y
Conductivity	N	N	N	Y
Container-closure integrity	N	N	N	Y
Design/dimensional specifications	N	N	N	Y
Elasticity	N	Y	N	Y
Extractable zinc	N	Y	Y	Y
Foam	N	N	Y	N
Fragmentation/coring	N	N	N	Y
Halides	N	N	N	Y
Hardness	N	N	N	Y
Heavy metals	Y	Y	N	Y
Hemolysis	N	N	Y	N
Intracutaneous injection	Y	N	N	N
IR of pyrolysate	N	Y	N	Y
Particulate matter	N	N	N	Y
Penetrability	N	N	N	Y
Pyrogens	N	N	Y	N
Reducing substances	Y	Y	Y	Y
Residue on evaporation	Y	Y	Y	Y
Resistance to steam	N	N	N	Y
Self sealing	N	N	N	Y
Storage	N	N	N	Y
Systemic injection	Y	N	Y	N
Tissue culture	Y	N	N	N
Total Cd and Pb	N	N	Y	N
UV absorbance	N	Y	Y	Y
Volatile sulfides	N	Y	N	Y

[a]From Ref. 16, Section <381>.
[b]From Ref. 17, Section 3.1.12.
[c]From Ref. 18, Section 49.
[d]From Ref. 19, ISO 8871, ISO 8362-2 & 8362-5, ISO 8536-2 & 8536-6.

the drug package will normally experience in the upright, inverted and on-side positions.

An inert control stopper should be used since a drug may be stable against glass but not against uncoated rubber. Only when an inert control is used will it be possible to determine whether the rubber and/or glass vial is the cause of the drug instability. Ampoules do not make good controls for the prescreening of drugs in vials since the glass for vials may be different from that used for ampoules.

Table 9 summarizes the important drug compatibility factors that must be considered when choosing a rubber component for a specific drug/device application. These factors along with the functional and seal integrity requirements can be used to write specifications for components. The packaging engineer, as with the rubber compounder, faces the challenge of choosing a compound that best meets the overall requirements but, only at best, provides a balance of all the actual chemical and functional needs. For example, an engineer may choose an isoprene vial closure because multiple punctures with a large cannula are required. Isoprene will provide the low coring and excellent reseal required. But the engineer may give up some shelf life since isoprene is a poor oxygen barrier. Choosing a butyl closure would give additional shelf life due to its better barrier properties, but coring and reseal would not be acceptable. Closure compound choice is always a give-and-take proposition where drug/device requirements must be prioritized before the choice of a rubber compound can be made. Table 10 lists important physical and chemical properties of elastomers (22).

There are four general types of closure–drug interactions:

1. Adsorption occurs when a drug is concentrated at the surface of a closure or vial.
2. Absorption occurs when a drug material is dispersed in the closure matrix.
3. Permeation is the transmission of a drug ingredient through a closure into the atmosphere or transmission of an outside material into the container.
4. Leaching is the process by which closure ingredients are extracted into the drug product.

All four of these interactions commonly occur. No rubber compound is absolutely inert to a drug. In many cases, the extent of the particular interaction is extremely small and may not be measurable, but generally all four are occurring, albeit at a low rate. With proteins, adsorption can be a problem. Many proteinaceous materials made by the biotechnology industry are highly adsorbent onto rubber surfaces and their potency may be readily lost. Other drugs products, especially ones that are very acidic or basic, may attack the stopper and cause the extraction of rubber compound ingredients. Common leachables from rubber closures include low molecular weight elastomer fragments, metal ions, antioxidants, plasticizers, lubricants, curing agents, and accelerators. The rate and relative importance of these four interactions determines the degree of compatibility or incompatibility of a stopper with a drug product.

In May 1999, the FDA issued an updated guidance entitled "Container Closure Systems for Packaging Human Drugs and Biologics—Chemistry, Manufacturing and Controls Documentation," that listed in tables the packaging information that should be submitted in an application (23). The guidance divides the information into four sections:

1. *Description*—Overall general description of the container-closure system plus specific information on suppliers, materials of construction, and postmanufacturing treatments.

Table 9 Drug compatibility factors affecting the choice of rubber component

Liquid or solid?
  Liquid
    1. Aqueous—pH, preservative, buffer cosolvent?
    2. Oil—Vegetable or Mineral?
  Solid
    1. Lyophilized or powder fill?
Configuration?
Need for O_2, H_2O, CO_2 protection?
Drug type?
Metallic sensitivities?
Method of closure and package sterilization?
Color preference?

2. *Suitability*—This section prescribes that tests must be done to assure protection of the drug product, safety of the packaging component material, compatibility of the component with the drug product, and performance of the component.
3. *Quality control*—The rubber component manufacturer's release criteria and drug packager's acceptance are found in this section. Also recommended is a method to monitor the consistency in composition of elastomeric components such as periodic extraction profiles.
4. *Stability*—Testing of the drug product using the packaging component is required. Unlike compendial tests that utilize water for extraction studies of the packaging component, the complete drug product is utilized in these stability studies.

This guideline advocates more information on rubber extractables and the proper use of DMFs.

Knowledge of extraction data from elastomeric components refers not only to the broad (and usually nonspecific) type of extractable data generated in USP<381> testing, but also to the identification and quantification, where necessary, of specific extractable species. Example of nonspecific extractables include turbidity, reducing agents, heavy metals, pH change, and total extractables-; They all measure broad types of extractables. Specific extractables include inorganics, such as zinc or lead and organics, such as PNA, stearic acid, nitrosamines, tetramethylthiuram disulfide, or 2,6-di-*tert*-butyl-4-*sec*-butyl phenol. Both liquid (HPLC) and gas chromatography (GC) are well suited for this purpose (24). Drug/device producers who utilize elastomeric packaging components require information from their suppliers on extractables (extractable profiles), including test methods, that are generated in water at various pH values (i.e., 3, 7, and 10) and in organic solvents such as isopropanol.

Table 10 Physical and chemical properties of elastomers[a,b]

				Common name of elastomer (chemical name)					
Property	Butyl/halobutyl (Isobutylene-isoprene copolymer)	Natural/Isoprene (cis-1,4-polyisoprene)	Neoprene (polychloroprene)	Nitrile (butadiene-acrylonitrile copolymer)	Silicone (polydimethylsiloxane)	Fluoro-elastomers (fluoro-rubber)	Urethane (polyester isocyanate)	EPDM (ethylene propylene diene monomer)	Butadiene (cis-Polybutadiene)
Abrasion resistance	Fair	Good	Fair	Good	Fair	Good	Excellent	Good	Fair
Compression set	Poor	Excellent	Good	Good	Poor	Good	Excellent	Good	Good
Coring	Fair	Excellent	Good	Fair	Poor	N.D.[c]	Excellent	Fair	Fair
Gas transmission resistance	Excellent	Good	Fair	Good	Poor	Good	Poor	Fair	Fair
Heat resistance	Excellent	Good	Good	Good	Excellent	Excellent	Poor	Very Good	Good
Machine-ability	Poor	Good	Fair	Good	Fair	N.D.	Fair	Fair	Good
Moisture vapor resistance	Excellent	Good	Fair	Fair	Poor	Good	Poor	Fair	Fair
Ozone resistance	Excellent	Poor	Good	Fair	Excellent	Excellent	Good	Good	Fair
Radiation resistance	Fair to Poor	Good	Good	Good	Fair to Good	Fair to Good	Fair	Fair	Poor
Resilience	Poor	Excellent	Good	Good	Good	Fair	Good	Good	Good
Shelf-life	Good	Fair	Good	Fair	Excellent	Excellent	Excellent	Excellent	Fair
Solvent resistance									
Acid, dilute	Good	Good	Good	Good	Fair	Fair	Poor	Good	Fair
Aliphatic solvents	Poor	Poor	Good	Poor	Poor	Excellent	Excellent	Good	Poor
Alkali, dilute	Good	Good	Good	Good	Good	Good	Poor	Good	Fair
Animal oil	Excellent	Poor	Good	Excellent	Good	Excellent	Excellent	Fair	Fair to poor
Aromatic solvents	Good	Good	Poor	Good	Poor	Excellent	Poor	Fair	Poor
Chlorinated solvents	Poor	Poor	Poor	Poor	Poor	Excellent	Good	Poor	Poor
Mineral oil	Poor	Poor	Good	Excellent	Fair	Excellent	Excellent	Poor	Poor
Vegetable oil	Excellent	Poor	Good	Excellent	Excellent	Excellent	Excellent	Fair	Fair to poor
Water	Excellent	Good	Fair	Good	Excellent	Good	Poor	Good	Good

[a]Ratings adapted from Ref. 22.
[b]Ratings expressed are typical for rubber compounds made from the elastomers; they can vary significantly from compound to compound.
[c]ND, not determined.

Armed with this information, they can look for extractables in their drug products.

Confidential packaging component information, such as the compound recipe, may be placed in a Type III DMF so that the FDA can review the information when it reviews the drug application (IND, NDA, ANDA, or BLA) (25). Most elastomeric compounds are filed at the request of a pharmaceutical manufacturer who has chosen to use the rubber closure in one or more drug packages or devices applications. The name of a rubber compound is associated with a precise recipe that designates specific ingredients and quantities. Once a rubber compound is filed in a DMF, no changes can be made in that compound without changing the DMF and notifying all customers on whose behalf the DMF was accessed and reviewed by the FDA. Since changes in a supplier's DMF may require additional stability studies by the drug manufacturer, changes are infrequent.

RECENT ISSUES AND DEVELOPMENTS

Latex Sensitivity

There are medical and regulatory issues surrounding the use of "latex rubber" due to allergic reactions that have resulted in medical emergencies. Even deaths have been noted (26, 27). There are two broad types of rubber—natural and synthetic. Several synthetic rubbers or elastomers are used for pharmaceutical components. These are listed in Table 10. However, there is only one type of commercial NR, which is derived from the rubber tree *Hevea Brasiliensis*. "Latex sensitivity" is associated only with NR and not with the synthetics, although other types of allergic reactions can result from contact with synthetic rubbers. NR is processed and used in two forms—liquid or latex rubber and solid or dry rubber, often referred to as crepe, SMR, and SIR. Specific proteins that are contained in both the latex and dry types cause the sensitivity to NR. Thus, the medical community and regulatory authorities have used the term "latex" for both forms of NR when "latex sensitivity" is discussed. Latex reactions reported in the literature have thus far been attributed to contact with components made from liquid rubber but not from dry rubber. Components made from liquid rubber are made by a dipping process that is best suited for thin-walled items such as gloves, condoms, and catheters. None of the typical rubber packaging components shown in Figs. 1 and 2 is made from latex rubber; —they are all made from dry rubber via a molding process. Many studies have been published regarding the allergic

properties of latex and dry rubber (28, 29) and further studies are in progress to determine if exposure to these dry rubber components can cause allergic latex reactions (30).

There is a great deal of regulatory activity in an attempt to protect the public from unexpected latex reactions. In 1996, the USP proposed a change in section <381> that would prohibit the use of NR in elastomeric closures (31); however, it rescinded this change in April 1997, stating that closure manufacturers should instead devise latex protein limits. A test for the water-soluble protein content of elastomers, based on an ASTM test (2), was published as USP <836> but no specifications or limits were proposed (33). At the same time, the FDA published a final rule that made it mandatory to provide labeling statements on medical devices and packaging components that contain NR (34). This rule was later amended to exclude combination drug/device and biologic/device products such as rubber stoppers and plungers for prefilled syringes (35). The uncertainty about the allergic risk from dry NR components and pending regulations have significantly reduced the use of NR in packaging for new drugs and in devices. Substitutes such as isoprene and SBR rubbers are finding increased use.

Preprocessed Components

Preprocessed closures, commonly referred to as RtS or Ready for Sterilization and RtU or Ready for Use, are an unstoppable trend in pharmaceutical packaging. Information on the manufacturing of these products was described previously in this review. The purpose of preprocessed closures is to reduce total processing costs and improve closure characteristics. Typical RtS closure characteristics are as follows:

Endotoxin Level: < 1 EU/closure
Bioburden Level: < 2 cfu/closure
Silicone Level: 10–40 μg/closure
Visible Particulate Matter: < 20 particles in 25 to 50-μ range; < 2 particles in 50 to 100-μ range; < 1 particle over 100 μ.

Coating and Surface Treatments

Although the material science of rubber compounds has greatly improved, drug-closure-interactions and surface lubricity are problematic for packaging engineers. Surface modifications of closures are frequently necessary to meet acceptance standards set by the USP, EP, JP, and ISO as well as the expectations of regulatory authorities. In practice, both liquids and solids are applied to closure surfaces to minimize interactions and improve lubricity.

Table 11 Commercially available coated and surface treated components

Product name	Material	Primary use	% Surface coated	Supplier[a]
Abboclad	Fluorinated polymer solid film	Compatibility	Plug surface	AB
B2	Silicone, polymerized liquid	Lubricity	Top, plug or both surfaces	WP
Coated stopper	Parylene deposited solid film	Compatibility	Total	IT
Deposition coated stopper	Vapor deposition coated solid film	Compatibility	Total	AB
Flurotec	ETFE solid film	Compatibility	Top, plug or both surfaces	WP & DS
Omniflex plus	Solid fluoropolymer coating	Compatibility	Total	HP
R2	Polymer, nonsilicone solid	Lubricity	Total	ST
SAF	Silicone, high viscosity liquid	Lubricity	Total	HP
Slipcoat	Plasma deposited polymer solid	Lubricity	Total	AL

[a]See Table 7 for supplier information.

A compilation of commercially available coated and surface treated components is shown in Table 11 (36). Although these coating and surface treatments may add significantly to the purchase price of closures they often reduce the total drug product cost by providing the following benefits:

- Increased lubricity, which allows faster processing speeds
- Decreased drug–closure interactions, which permits the marketing of some products not compatible with uncoated rubber and better quality and longer shelf life for others
- Decreased particulate matter, which reduces the number of units rejected for visible particulate matter

Container-Closure Seal Integrity

The FDA Guidance on Container Closure Systems (Ref. May 1999 Guidance) lists sterility or container integrity as an important parameter to be considered in the section on Protection. Seal integrity tests can be done by both physical and microbial methods, but historically, sterility testing alone has been used. A 1998 FDA draft guidance discusses the replacement of the sterility test with an appropriate container-closure integrity test in the stability protocol, permitting an alternative to sterility testing for proving the continued capability of containers to maintain sterility (37). Kirsch et al. (38–41) published a series of four papers that studied mass spectrometry-based helium leak detection, microbial ingress, and vacuum decay and the correlation between these methods. The PDA also published an updated technical report that provides guidance for evaluating pharmaceutical package integrity (42), and Guazzo has published an excellent review article that outlines the advantages and limitations of current methods (43).

SUMMARY

Rubber packaging and device components are an important part of the overall medical delivery system. Without innovative packaging systems, modern drugs would not be available today. Advances in drug development have initiated research in new packaging and delivery systems while the availability of innovative packaging has led to the introduction of new drug therapies. Innovation, while containing costs and conforming to regulations, is the challenge for the 21st century.

REFERENCES

1. Williams, J.L. Medical Applications for Thermoplastic Elastomers Proceedings of the 1st International Conference on Thermoplastic Elastomer Markets and Technology, Schotland Business Research, Inc.: Princeton, NJ, 1988.
2. Naugle, D.G., Djiauw, L.K., Elastomerics **1989**, *121*, 23–32.
3. Manufacturers HP, ST, and WP, see Table 7 for contact information.
4. Avis, K.E., Smith, E.J., Elastomeric Parenteral Closures. *Encyclopedia of Pharmaceutical Technology*, 1st Ed.; Swarbrick, J., Boylan, J.C., Eds.; Marcel Dekker, Inc. New York, 1992.
5. Anderson, S.R., Ethylene Oxide Residues in Medical Materials. Bull. Parent. Drug Assoc. **1973**, 27 (2), 49–58.
6. Baan, E. Ethylene Oxide Adsorption and Desorption of Elastomers and Plastics, Bull. Parent. Drug Assoc. **1976**, *30* (6), 299–305.
7. Effects of Gamma Irradiation on Elastomeric Closures, Technical Report No. 16. PDA. J. Parent. Sci. Technol. **1992**, *52*, S1–S13.
8. Langlade, V., Le Gall, P.A., *Complying with the EC Note for Guidance for Gamma Irradiation: Validation of Rubber Closure Radiosterilization*; PDA International Congress: Basel, Switzerland, 1994; 261–273.

9. *Sterilization of Health Care Products—Requirements for Validation and Routine Control: Radiation Sterilization*; ANSI/AAMI/ISO 1137:1994, AAMI: Arlington, VA, 1994.

10. Morton, M. Ed. *Rubber Technology*, 2nd Ed.; Van Nostrand Reinhold: New York, 1973.

11. *Standard Test Method for Rubber Properties: Durometer Hardness*, ASTM D2240-97el, ASTM: West Conshohocken PA, 1999.

12. *Standard Test Method for Rubber Properties in Compression*, ASTM D 575-91(1996), ASTM: West Conshohocken, PA, 1999.

13. *Standard Test Method for Vulcanized Rubber and Thermoplastic Rubbers and Thermoplastic Elastomers—Tension*, ASTM D 412-98a, ASTM: West Conshohocken, PA, 1999.

14. *Standard Test Methods for Rubber Products—Chemical Analysis*, ASTM D 297-93(1998), ASTM: West Conshohocken, PA, 1999.

15. *Elastomeric Closures: Evaluation of Significant Performance and Identity Characteristics*, Technical Methods Bulletin No. 2, PDA, Bethesda, MD, 1981.

16. *The United States Pharmacopeia 24/ National Formulary 19,* The United States Pharmacopeial Convention, Inc.: Rockville, MD, 2000.

17. Rubber for Closures for Containers for Aqueous Parenteral Preparations and for Powders for Freeze-Dried Products. *European Pharmacopoeia*, Section 3.1.12 in 1999 Addendum European Pharmacopoeia Commission, Strasbourg, France, 1996.

18. Test for Rubber Closer for Aqueous Infusions, *The Pharmacopoeia of Japan, Yakuji Nippo, Ltd.* Section 49, Society of Japanese Pharmacopoeia, Tokyo, Japan, 1996.

19. International Organization for Standardization (ISO), Geneva, Switzerland. Some Important ISO Standards are 8362, Parts 2 & 5, Closures for Injection Vials; 8536, Parts 2 & 6, Closures for Infusion Bottles; and 8871, Part 1, Extractables from Elastomeric Parts for Parenterals. (ISO Standards are in Continual Revision; Contact ISO for Latest Revision.).

20. Extractables from Elastomeric Closures, Analytical Procedures for Functional Group Characterization/Identification. *Technical Methods Bulletin No. 1*, PDA, Bethesda, MD, 1980.

21. *Elastomeric Closures for Injections*; USP<381>, USP 24 The United States Pharmacopeia Convention, Inc., Rockville, MD, 2000.

22. Smith, E.J., Nash, R.J. Elastomeric Closures for Parenterals. *Pharmaceutical Dosage Forms: Parenteral Medications*; Avis, K.E., Lieberman, H.A., Lachman, L., Eds.; Marcel Dekker, Inc.: New York, 1992; 1.

23. FDA Guidance for Industry, *Container Closure Systems for Packaging Human Drugs and Biologics—Chemistry, Manufacturing, and Controls Documentation*, Food and Drug Administration, Rockville, MD, May 1999.

24. Milano, C.J., Bailey, L.C., Evaluation of Current Compendial Physicochemical Test Procedures for Pharmaceutical Elastomeric Closures and Development of an Improved HPLC Procedure, PDA. J. Pharm. Sci. Tech. **1999**, *53*, 202–210.

25. INDA, Investigational New Drug Application; NDA, New Drug Application; ANDA, Abbreviated New Drug Application; BLA, Biologic License Application.

26. Allergic Reaction to Latex Containing Medical Devices, FDA Medical Alert, MDA 91-1 **1992**, 1–2.

27. Smith, E.J., *Natural Rubber/Latex Closures and Devices: The Issues*; PDA Spring Meeting, San Diego, CA, 1997.

28. Yip, E., Turjanmaa, K., Makinen-Kiljunen, S., The "Non-allergenicity" of NR Dry Rubber Products, with Reference to Type 1 Protein Allergy, Rubber Developments **1995**, *48*, 48–52.

29. Slater, J.E., Latex Allergy, J. Allergy Clin. Immunol. **1994**, *94*, 139–149.

30. Hamilton, R.G., Allergenic Content of Elastomeric Closures, Private Communication. The Johns Hopkins University School of Medicine, Baltimore, MD, 1999.

31. Elastomeric Closures for Injections, Pharmaceutical Forum **1996**, *22* (5), 2886–2887, USP<381>.

32. *Standard Test Method for Analysis of Protein in Natural Rubber and Its Products*, ASTM D 5712-95, ASTM, West Conshohocken, PA, 1999.

33. Natural Rubber—Water-Soluble Protein Content, Pharmacopoeial Forum **1997**, *23* (5), 4681–4683, USP<836>.

34. 21 CFR Part 801 Natural Rubber-Containing Medical Devices, User Labeling, Fed. Reg. **1997**, *62* (189), 51021–51030.

35. 21 CFR Part 8021, Amended Economic Analysis of Final Rule Requiring Use of Labeling on Natural Rubber Containing Devices, Fed. Reg. **1998**, *63* (104), 29552–29590.

36. Smith, E.J. Coatings and Surface Treatments for Rubber Closures for Parenterals, PDA Annual Meeting: Washington, DC, 1999.

37. FDA Draft Guidance for Industry, *Container and Closure Integrity Testing in Lieu of Sterility Testing as a Component of the Stability Protocol for Sterile Products*, Food and Drug Administration: Rockville, MD, 1998.

38. Kirsch, L.E., Nguyen, L., Moeckly, C.S., Pharmaceutical Container/Closure Integrity I: Mass Spectrometry-Based Helium Leak Rate Detection for Rubber-Stoppered Glass Vials, PDA J. Pharm. Sci. Technol. **1997**, *51*, 187–195.

39. Kirsch, L.E., Nguyen, L., Moeckly, C.S., Gerth, R. Pharmaceutical Container/Closure Integrity II: The Relationship Between Microbial Ingress and Helium Leak Rates in Rubber-Stoppered Glass Vials. PDA J. Pharm. Sci. Technol. **1997**, *51*, 195–202.

40. Kirsch, L.E., Nguyen, L., Gerth, R. Pharmaceutical Container/Closure Integrity III: Validation of the Helium Leak Rate Method for Rigid Pharmaceutical Containers. PDA J. Pharm. Sci. Technol. **1997**, *51*, 203–207.

41. Nguyen, L.T., Muangsiri, W., Schiere, R., Guazzo, D.M., Kirsch, L.E., Pharmaceutical Container/Closure Integrity IV: Development of an Indirect Correlation Between Vacuum Decay Leak Measurement and Microbial Ingress, PDA J. Pharm. Sci. Technol. **1999**, *53*, 211–218.

42. Pharmaceutical Package Integrity, Technical Report No. 27. PDA J. Parent. Sci. Technol. **1998**, *52* (S2), 1–48.

43. Guazzo, D.M., Current Approaches in Leak Testing Pharmaceutical Packages. PDA J. Pharm. Sci. Technol. **1996**, *50*, 378–385.

EMULSIONS AND MICROEMULSIONS

Gillian M. Eccleston
University of Strathclyde, Glasgow, United Kingdom

EMULSIONS

An emulsion is a heterogeneous preparation composed of two immiscible liquids (by convention described as oil and water), one of which is dispersed as fine droplets uniformly throughout the other. Emulsions are thermodynamically unstable and revert back to separate oil and water phases by fusion or coalescence of droplets unless kinetically stabilized by a third component, the emulsifying agent. The phase present as small droplets is called the disperse, dispersed, or internal phase and the supporting liquid is known as the continuous or external phase. Droplet diameters vary enormously, but in pharmaceutical emulsions they are typically polydispersed with diameters ranging from approximately 0.1 to 50 μm. Emulsions are conveniently classified as oil-in-water (o/w) or water-in-oil (w/o), depending on whether the continuous phase is aqueous or oily. Fig. 1a shows a photomicrograph of a simple o/w system. Practical pharmaceutical emulsions, however, are rarely simple two-phase oil and water preparations; many are multicomponent systems containing additional solid or liquid crystalline (e.g. lamellar) phases (Fig. 1b). Multiple emulsions, which are prepared from oil and water by the reemulsification of an existing emulsion so as to provide two dispersed phases, are also of pharmaceutical interest. Multiple emulsions of the oil-in-water-in-oil (o/w/o) type are w/o emulsions in which the water globules themselves contain dispersed oil globules; conversely, water-in-oil-in-water (w/o/w) emulsions are those where the internal and external aqueous phases are separated by the oil (Fig. 1c). These more complex emulsions are covered by the broader International Union of Pure and Applied Chemistry (IUPAC) definition of emulsions, which extends the classical definition to include "liquid droplets and/or liquid crystals dispersed in a liquid" (1).

Emulsions are formulated for virtually all the major routes of administration, and there are a number of dermatological, oral and, parenteral preparations available commercially. The internal phase may contain water-soluble drugs, preservatives, and flavoring agents whilst the oil phase may itself be therapeutically active or may act as a carrier for an oil-soluble drug. Such preparations provide an effective approach to many of the problems in drug delivery, often showing distinct advantages over other dosage forms by way of improved bioavailability and/or reduced side effects. However, despite such advantages, emulsions are not used as extensively as other oral or parenteral dosage forms due to the fundamental problems of emulsion instability that result in unpredictable drug release profiles and possible toxicity. The full potential of emulsions will not be realized until stable systems are developed with predictable in vitro and in vivo release patterns. Much of the emulsion research over the past decade is based on attempts to understand the relationships between emulsion stability, physicochemical properties, and biological fate. Multiple emulsions are even more difficult to stabilize, and characterize and although there is an increasing interest in their potential applications for drug delivery, at present there are no commercial preparations available (2).

PHARMACEUTICAL APPLICATIONS

The current and potential pharmaceutical applications of emulsions have been the subject of a number of general reviews (3–6). Traditionally the term "emulsion" is restricted to mobile emulsions for internal use; emulsions for external use are described by their pharmaceutical types as liniments, lotions, and creams. This tends to conceal the fact that by far the largest group of emulsions currently used in pharmacy and medicine are dermatological emulsions for external use (7, 8). Both oil-in-water and water-in-oil emulsions are extensively used for their therapeutic properties and/or as vehicles to deliver drugs and cosmetic agents to the skin. The emulsion facilitates drug permeation into and through the skin by its occlusive effects and/or by the incorporation of penetration-enhancing components. Particular attention is paid to patient acceptance of such formulations, which range in consistency from mobile liniments and lotions to semisolid ointments and creams. In the past, the development of dermatological emulsions was essentially empirical with only a limited understanding of the

(a)   (b)   (c)

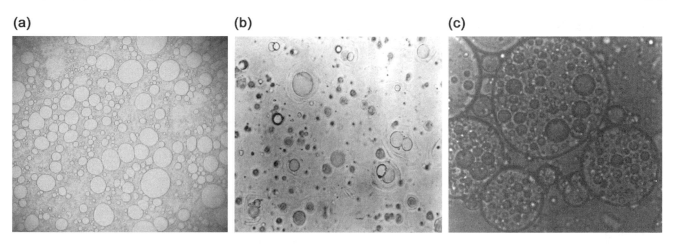

Fig. 1 Photomicrographs of typical emulsions. (a) A liquid paraffin-in-water emulsion stabilized by 1.89% Span 40 and 1.62% Tween 80. The polydispersity of the oil droplets before homogenization is clearly seen. (b) A liquid paraffin–water cream stabilized by a cationic emulsifying wax. Note the lamellar structures surrounding the oil droplets. (c) A multiple w/o/w emulsion. Water droplets can clearly be seen within the larger oil droplets.

underlying principles. Today, although the microstructure of many of these complex formulations is now better understood (9, 10), the mechanisms by which the structure of an emulsion can influence drug bioavailability are far from clear and much of the literature on the role of emulsions in drug release to the skin is contradictory. Confusion arises because the majority of investigations concerning in vitro vehicle effects on drug release are only on bulk formulation. As most emulsions are applied to the skin as a thin film, the drug delivery system is not one of bulk emulsion, but rather a dynamic evaporating system in which phase changes can occur as the preparation is rubbed into the skin and the relative concentrations of volatile ingredients alter. Droplet size appears to influence drug delivery to the skin, with submicron lipid emulsions enhancing the transcutaneous permeation and efficiency of a number of lipophilic drugs (11).

Oral emulsions are almost exclusively of the oil-in-water type. They provide a degree of taste masking as the aqueous external phase effectively isolates the oil from the tongue. Mineral and castor oils have been emulsified in water and administered orally for the local treatment of constipation for many years (cf. Mineral Oil Emulsion USP) as have various nutritional oils from fish liver (generally halibut or cod) or vegetable origin to produce oral liquid food supplements. It has long been established that the use of o/w emulsions as carriers for lipophilic drugs may improve oral bioavailability and efficacy (3–6). For example, griseofulvin formulated as an o/w emulsion has enhanced gastrointestinal absorption when compared with suspensions, tablets, or capsule dosage forms (12). The mechanisms by which emulsions modify and improve

absorption processes are complex and not fully understood, although the oil itself influences gastric motility. Fats and oils are solubilized by the bile salts so that the administration of already emulsified oil droplets containing a high concentration of drug may increase the likelihood of further droplet and drug solubilization and transport across the GI tract by the fat absorption pathways.

The type of emulsion used parenterally depends on the route of injection and the intended use (13–15). Oil-in-water emulsions are administered by all the major parenteral routes whereas water-in-oil emulsions are generally reserved for intramuscular or subcutaneous administration where sustained release is required. Drug action is prolonged in such oily emulsions because the drug has to diffuse from the aqueous dispersed phase through the oil-continuous environment to reach the tissue fluids. Water-in-oil emulsions are used to disperse water-soluble immunizing antigens in mineral oil for injection via subcutaneous or intramuscular routes as adjuvant preparations where they prolong and enhance the antigenic stimulus and increase the antibody titer. Oily emulsion formulations also show promise in cancer chemotherapy as vehicles for prolonging drug release after intramuscular or intratumoral injection, and as a means of enhancing the transport of anticancer agents via the lymphatic system (16). Water-in-oil emulsions for sustained release are often difficult to inject because of the high viscosities of the oily continuous phases. Although these problems can be overcome by reemulsification of the primary w/o emulsion to produce a less viscous multiple w/o/w emulsion, a study using

Table 1 Some commercial lipid emulsions for parenteral nutrition

Trade name	Oil phase (%)	Emulsifier (%)	Other components (%)
Intralipid® (Fresenius Kabi)	Soybean (10 and 20)	Egg lecithin (1.2)	Glycerol (2.2), phosphate (15mm/l)
Lipovenos® (Fresenius Kabi)	Soybean (10 and 20)	Egg lecithin (1.2)	Glycerol (2.5)
Liposyn® (Abbott)	Safflower and soybean, 1:1 (10 and 20)	Egg lecithin (1.2)	Glycerol (2.5)
Lipofundin® (Braun)	Cottonseed (15)	Soybean lecithin (0.75)	Sorbitol (5.0), DL-α-Tocopherol
Lipofundin N® (Braun)	Soybean (10 and 20)	Egg lecithin (0.75 and 1.2)	Glycerol (2.5)
Lipofundin MCT/LCT® (Braun)	Soybean and MCT, 1:1 (10 and 20)	Egg lecithin (0.75 and 1.2)	Glycerol (2.5)

5-fluorouracil implied that sustained release was actually less marked with multiple emulsions (17).

Sterile parenteral oil-in-water emulsions have been used extensively for over 40 years for the intravenous administration of fats, carbohydrates, and vitamins to debilitated patients. Several vegetable oil-in-water emulsions are now available commercially with droplet sizes similar to that of chylomicrons (approximately 0.5–2 μm), the natural fat droplets in the blood that transport ingested fats to the lymphatic and circulatory systems (Table 1). More recently, such emulsions have been employed as intravenous carriers for poorly water-soluble lipophilic drugs such as vitamin K (e.g., Sterile Phytonadione Injection U.S.P.) diazepam (e.g., Diemuls®), vitamin A (Vitlipid N®), and profonol (Diprovan®) as alternatives to the traditionally used cosolvent, surfactant solubilized, or pH controlled parenteral solutions. The drug dissolved in the oil phase of the emulsion is unlikely to precipitate and cause pain when diluted by blood on injection, and if susceptible to hydrolysis or oxidation, it will be protected by the nonaqueous environment. Emulsion formulations of diazepam and more recently clarithromycin have been clinically shown to be less painful than solubilized preparations (18, 19) while emulsions containing amphoteracin B are less toxic (20). This emulsion was also shown to be an equally effective, cheaper, and more elegant alternative to a liposomal system. The enormous literature on the potential of lipid emulsions for drug delivery and targeting is discussed in a recent book (21).

Radiopaque emulsions, which have long been used as contrast media in conventional X-ray examinations of body organs, are finding further application with more sophisticated techniques including computed tomography, ultrasound, and nuclear magnetic resonance. Perfluorochemical emulsions are used as artificial blood substitutes. The potential advantages of such systems over donated blood are enormous with the elimination of major donor associated problems such as blood group incompatibilities and blood disease. The first commercial product, Fluosol-DA® (Green Cross Corporation, Osaka, Japan) was licensed several years ago in a number of countries to reduce myocardial ischaemia in patients undergoing angioplasty; however, Fluosol-DA was not a commercial success due to its slow excretion rate and to its marked instability, which meant that it had to be stored in the frozen state. In addition, some patients were sensitive to one of the emulsifiers, pluronic F68®. Currently, a second generation of emulsions is being evaluated to resolve the problems encountered with Fluosol (22) and these are discussed in another chapter of this encyclopedia.

There are only a few studies on the ocular and nasal applications of emulsions. Lipid (submicron) emulsions exhibited a long-lasting antidepressant effect on the intraocular pressure of rabbits after a single application when used as carriers for lipophilic antiglaucoma drugs (23). Medium-chain triglyceride emulsions formulated at pH 8 show potential as controlled release formulations for nasal delivery (24, 25) for they give prolonged drug residence in the nasal cavity (Fig. 2). Enhanced nasal delivery of insulin was observed when insulin was incorporated into the continuous phase of an o/w emulsion, but not when incorporated into the aqueous phase of a w/o emulsion (26).

FORMULATION CONSIDERATIONS

The choice of oil, emulsifier, and emulsion type (o/w, w/o, or multiple) is limited by its ultimate use and route of

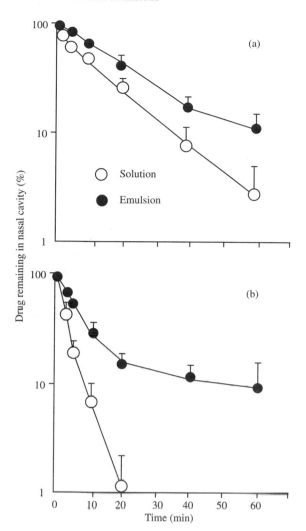

Fig. 2 Disappearance profiles of (a) tetrahydrozoline hydrochloride and (b) chlorpheniramine maleate from rat nasal cavity after nasal administration of an o/w emulsion and an aqueous solution at pH 8. (From Ref. 25.)

administration. Potential toxicity and chemical incompatibilities in the final formulation must be taken into account as must processing details for these also affect the variables that control emulsion stability and therapeutic response such as droplet size distributions and rheology. The design of stable emulsions with the correct pharmacokinetic characteristics and tissue distribution is currently an area of enormous interest, particularly for parenteral IV emulsions. Immediately after injection, the surface of the parenteral emulsion droplets is altered by adsorption of blood components (optosonation) and they are then distributed rapidly through the circulation. Their subsequent fate depends on whether they are treated by the body in the same manner as chylomicrons, or whether they

are recognized as foreign particles and cleared by the RES. Many factors, including droplet size and charge, the type of lipid, and the emulsifier composition influence their fate. A major factor to be considered in the formulation of oral preparations is the low pH and high ionic strength of stomach fluids, which may destabilize the emulsion by its effect on the emulsifier.

Pharmaceutical Oils

Oils used in the preparation of pharmaceutical emulsions are of various chemical types, including simple esters, fixed and volatile oils, hydrocarbons, and turpenoid derivatives. The oil itself may be the medicament, it may function as a carrier for a drug, or even form part of a mixed emulsifier system as in the case of some fixed oils that contain sufficient free fatty acids. Many oils, particularly those of vegetable origin, are liable to autooxidation with subsequent rancidity, and it is frequently necessary to add an antioxidant and/or preservative to inhibit this degradation process. For externally applied emulsions, mineral oils, either alone or combined with soft or hard paraffins, are widely used both as the vehicle for the drug and for their occlusive and sensory characteristics. The most widely used oils in oral preparations are nonbiodegradable mineral and castor oils that provide a local laxative effect, and fish liver oils or various fixed oils of vegetable origin (e.g., arachis, cottonseed, and maize oils) as nutritional supplements.

The choice of oil is severely limited in emulsions for parenteral administration for reasons of toxicity. Purified soybean, sesame, safflower, and cottonseed oils composed mainly of long-chain triglycerides have been used for many years as they are resistant to rancidity and show few clinical side effects. More recently, it has been recognized that the structure of the oil will influence the fate of emulsion droplets after injection. Mixtures containing both long- and medium-chain triglycerides are not only better energy sources for nutritional purposes but they are also cleared more rapidly from the circulation (27); such mixtures are now used in commercial preparations (c.f. Table 1). Structured triglycerides, formed by modifying the oil enzymatically to produce 1,3-specific triglycerides are an area of increasing interest because of their influence on the in vivo circulation time of an emulsion (28). Purified mineral oil is used in some water-in-oil depot preparations where mineral toxicity (e.g., abscess formation at the injection site) must be carefully balanced against efficiency. Emulsified perfluorochemicals are considered acceptable for IV use provided that they are excreted relatively fast. A major problem in the formulation of the early perfluorocarbon emulsions was that the oils that form the most stable emulsions were not cleared rapidly from the body.

Pharmaceutical Emulsifiers

Emulsifying agents are used both to promote emulsification at the time of manufacture and to control stability during a shelf life that can very from days for extemporaneously prepared emulsions to months or years for commercial preparations. In practice, combinations of emulsifiers rather than single agents are used. The emulsifier also influences the in vivo fate of lipid parenteral emulsions by its influence on the surface properties of the droplets and on the droplet size distributions. For convenience, most pharmacy texts classify emulsifiers into three groups: i) surface active agents, ii) natural (macromolecular) polymers, and iii) finely divided solids.

Surface Active Agents

The range of surfactant emulsifiers used in pharmaceutical preparations is illustrated in Table 2. Surfactants are manufactured from a variety of natural and synthetic sources and consequently they show considerable batch-to-batch variations in their homologue compositions and in trace impurities from the starting material. For example, batch variations in the number of neutral phospholipids occur in lecithin surfactants and nonionic polyethylene surfactants show variations in the number of moles of ethylene oxide. The mechanisms by which such batch variations lead to differences in emulsifying properties are now better understood (29).

Although synthetic and semisynthetic surfactants form by far the largest group of emulsifiers studied in the scientific literature and many of them are available commercially, their use in pharmaceutical emulsions is limited by the fact that the majority are toxic (i.e., haemolytic) and irritant to the skin and mucous

Table 2 Synthetic surface active emulsifying agents

Class	Example	Type	Compatibility
Anionic			Efficient to various degrees above pH 7; incompatible with cationic surfactants and polyvalent cations
Alkali and ammonium soaps	Sodium stearate	o/w	
Divalent and trivalent metallic soaps	Calcium oleate	w/o	
Organic sulfates	Sodium lauryl sulfate	o/w	
Cationic			Efficient below pH 7; incompatible with anionic surfactants and polyvalent anions
Quaternary ammonium compounds	Cetrimonium bromide	o/w	
Pyridium compounds	Hexadecyl pyridinium chloride	o/w	
Nonionic			Efficient to various degrees over pH range 4–8; good tolerance to ionic surfactants and polyvalent ions
Alcohol polyethylene glycol ethers	Ceteth 20	o/w	
Fatty acid polyethylene glycol esters	Polyethylene glycol 40 stearate	o/w	
Ethoxylated fatty acid polyethylene glycol esters	Sorbitan mono-oleate (Span 80)	w/o	
	Polyoxyethylene sorbitan monooleate (Tween 80)	o/w	
Polymeric			
Polyoxyethylene-polyoxypropylene block co-polymers	Poloxomers, Pluronic F-68®	o/w	
Amphiphiles			Generally used combined with a surfactant to form a o/w emulsion
Fatty alcohols	Cetyl alcohol	w/o	
Fatty acids	Stearic acid	w/o	

membranes of the gastrointestinal tract. In general, cationic surfactants are the most toxic and irritant and nonionic surfactants the least. Surfactants are therefore used mainly at relatively low concentrations in topical preparations. The quaternary ammonium compounds constitute an important group of cationic emulsifiers in dermatological preparations because they have antimicrobial properties in addition to their o/w emulsifying action. There are many nonionic surfactants with different oil and water solubilities available commercially because for each fatty starting material the polyoxyethylene chain length can be modified by the systematic addition of ethylene oxide groups. However, a limited number of polysorbate surfactants are used in oral emulsions, and parenteral preparations appear to be based only on the lecithins from plant or animal sources and the nonionic polyoxyethylene oxide/polyoxypropylene oxide block copolymer poloxomer 188 (Poloxamer F68®), although some patients using the first generation of perfluorochemical emulsions were sensitive to this poloxomer. The emulsifier influences both emulsion stability and in vivo disposition by its influence on droplet surface properties.

Natural macromolecular materials and finely divided solids

Materials derived from natural sources (Table 3) may originate from animal or vegetable sources and many of these products are susceptible to degradation. For example, depolymerization (the polysaccharides) or hydrolysis (the steroids) usually lead to loss in emulsifying power. Some of these materials, polysaccharides and proteins in particular, provide good culture medium for microorganisms, and therefore preservation of emulsions containing them is imperative. To overcome

these problems, a number of purified and semisynthetic derivatives are available, including various purified wool fat derivatives and semisynthetic celluloses such as methylcellulose and sodium carboxymethylcellulose. These are generally more stable than the unmodified materials. These celluloses are used in oral preparations; they are less suitable for topicals because of their unpleasant feel. Finely divided solids such as clays are used in dermatological preparations as structuring agents.

Preservatives

It is essential that emulsions are formulated to resist microbial attack, as this not only can affect the physicochemical properties of the formulation, causing color, odor, or pH changes and even phase separation, but may also constitute a health hazard. The potential sources of contamination can be from raw materials (especially if these are natural products), water, manufacturing and packaging equipment, or patients themselves. W/o emulsions are less susceptible to attack than o/w emulsions because the aqueous continuous external phase can produce ideal conditions for the growth of bacteria, moulds, and fungi. Preservatives are not used in parenteral emulsions, which are sterilized, generally by autoclaving, but sometimes by using sterile components and aseptically assembling the final emulsion.

There is no simple way of predicting the ideal preservative for a particular emulsion. In addition to requiring a wide spectrum of activity against bacteria, yeasts, and molds, the preservative should be free from toxic, irritant, or sensitizing activity. Some commonly used preservatives in oral and topical preparations include phenoxyethanol, benzoic acid, parabenzoates, and chlorcresol. Emulsions are heterogeneous products, and the

Table 3 Emulsifying agents derived from natural products and finely divided solids

Class	Example	Emulsion type, route of administration	Comments
Polysaccharide	Acacia	o/w; oral	Stable over a wide pH range
	Carageen	o/w; oral	As above
	Methylcellulose	o/w; oral, parenteral	As above, less prone to hydrolysis
Protein	Gelatin	o/w; oral,	Emulsifying properties pH dependent
Glycoside	Saponin	o/w; topical	
Phospholipid	Lecithin	o/w; oral, parenteral	Emulsifying properties dependent on number of negative lipids
Sterol	Wool fat	w/o; topical	Poor emulsifiers alone
	Cholesterol and its esters	w/o; topical	As above
Finely divided solids	Bentonite	o/w and w/o; topical	Gelation dependent on processing conditions
	Veegum	o/w; oral, topical	As above
	Aluminium hydroxide	o/w; oral	

preservative partitions between the oil and aqueous phases. As a sufficient aqueous concentration of the active (usually unionized) form must be present to ensure proper preservation, pH is an additional factor to be considered. Problems often arise because many of the materials used in emulsion formulation, for example hydrocolloids or polyoxyethylene surfactants, can interact with the preservatives, thus depleting their activity. The use of a single preservative is often considered unrealistic, and attention is being increasingly focused on the use of mixtures for a wider spectrum of activity, although this may introduce additional compatibility problems.

Antioxidants and Humectants

Antioxidants are added to many pharmaceutical preparations to prevent oxidative deterioration on storage of the oil, emulsifier, or the drug itself. Such deterioration, as well as destabilizing the formulation, imparts an unpleasant odor or taste. Some oils are supplied containing antioxidants already. Those commonly used in pharmacy include butylated hydroxyanisole (BHA) and butylated hydroxytoluene (BHT) at concentrations up to 0.2%, and the alkyl gallates. Humectants such as propylene glycol, glycerol, and sorbitol (5%) are often added to dermatological preparations to reduce the evaporation of water from the emulsion during storage and use. They are sometimes claimed to prevent evaporation of water from the surface of the skin, although their use at high concentrations would be expected to have the opposite effect (i.e., remove moisture and dehydrate the skin).

EMULSION FORMATION

There are essentially two major considerations in emulsification: first, the formation of emulsions of the correct type, oil-in-water, water-in-oil, or multiple emulsion with the required droplet size distributions and second, the stabilization of the dispersed droplets so formed. When given amounts of two immiscible liquids are mixed or mechanically agitated in the absence of other additives, both phases tend to form droplets of various sizes. The size distributions are related to the forces involved during the agitation process, and the number of droplets of each liquid depends on its relative volume. The surface free energy of the system, which is dependent on both total surface area and interfacial tension is raised by the increase in surface area produced during dispersion, and the system is thermodynamically unstable. To reduce this, high-energy droplets first assume a spherical shape, as this gives the

minimum surface area for a given volume, and then on collision the droplets will coalesce (fuse) to reduce the interfacial area, the interfacial tension remaining constant.

The type of emulsion that forms, either o/w or w/o, depends on the relative rates of coalescence of each type of droplet, with the more rapidly coalescing droplets forming the continuous phase. Generally, this is the liquid present in the larger amount because higher number of droplets increase the probability of collision and coalescence. With phase volumes of oil and water close to 50%, other factors such as the order and rate of addition of each liquid are important. If agitation ceases, coalescence will continue until complete phase separation—the state of minimum free energy—is reached. Thus, emulsification can be considered as the result of two competing processes, namely the disruption of bulk liquids to produce fine droplets and the recombination of the droplets to give back the original bulk liquids. With the inclusion of surfactants or other classes of emulsifiers, the type of emulsion that forms is no longer simply a function of the phase volume and the order of mixing, but also the relative solubilities of the emulsifier in oil and water. In general, the phase in which the emulsifier is most soluble becomes the continuous phase (Bancroft's Rule); thus, hydrophilic polymers and surfactants promote o/w emulsions whereas lipophilic surfactants promote w/o emulsions. Preferential coalescence of the phase in which the emulsifier is most soluble occurs because when droplets collide, the emulsifier is easily displaced from the interface into the droplet, thus providing little protection against coalescence. Theoretically, the disperse phase of an emulsion can occupy up to 74% of the phase volume, and such high internal phase o/w emulsions have been produced with suitable surfactants. It is more difficult to formulate w/o emulsions with greater than 50% disperse phase because of the steric mechanisms involved in their stabilization (discussed later), and the addition of extra water sometimes causes inversion to an o/w emulsion.

Emulsion Characteristics

In general, an emulsion exhibits the characteristics of its external phase. Several methods are available for identifying the emulsion type. Dilution tests are based on the fact that the emulsion is only miscible with the liquid that forms its continuous phase. Conductivity measurements rely on the poor conductivity of oil compared with water, and give low values in w/o emulsions where oil is the continuous phase. Staining tests in which a water-soluble dye is sprinkled onto the surface of the emulsion also indicate the nature of the continuous phase. With an o/w emulsion there is rapid incorporation of the dye into the system whereas with the w/o emulsion the dye forms microscopically visible clumps. The reverse happens on addition of an oil-soluble dye. These tests essentially identify the continuous phase and do not indicate whether a multiple emulsion has been produced. This can be resolved by microscopy.

Rheology

The rheological properties of emulsions are influenced by a number of interacting factors, including the nature of the continuous phase, the phase volume ratio, and to a lesser extent, particle size distributions. A variety of products ranging from mobile liquids to thick semisolids can be formulated by altering the dispersed phase volume and/or the nature and concentration of the emulsifiers. For low internal phase volume emulsions, the consistency of the emulsion is generally similar to that of the continuous phase; thus, w/o emulsions are generally thicker than o/w emulsions, and the consistency of an o/w system is increased by the addition of gums, clays, and other thickening agents that import plastic or pseudoplastic flow properties. Some mixed emulsifiers interact in water to form a viscoelastic continuous phase to give a semisolid o/w cream (7).

Droplet Size Distributions

Droplet size distributions in pharmaceutical emulsions are important from both stability and biopharmaceutical considerations. The larger the particle size, the greater the tendency to coalesce and further increase droplet size. Thus, fine particles generally promote better stability. Size distributions are influenced by the characteristics of the emulsifier and the method of manufacture. From a biological point of view, fine emulsification enhances gastrointestinal absorption and whilst this is desirable with oral formulations of nutrient oils alone or with drugs dissolved in them, it may give adverse clinical effects with mineral oils that are used for a local effect and are toxic if absorbed. Droplets in emulsions used as contrast media in computed tomography are approximately 1–3 μm. Parenteral emulsions should be formulated so that the dispersed droplet sizes range from approximately 100 nm to 1 μm. In any event, sizes should never be greater than 5 μm in diameter because of the danger of pulmonary emboli. There is clear evidence that, as with other colloidal preparations, droplet size distributions influence the clearance kinetics of parenteral emulsions. Larger droplets are treated as foreign bodies and rapidly cleared by elements of the RES while smaller droplets may be treated

as natural fat sorting lipoproteins, with a different in vivo fate (30). Drug delivery from dermatological preparations also appears to be improved in lipid emulsions containing submicron droplets (11).

EMULSION STABILITY

A stable emulsion is considered to be one in which the dispersed droplets retain their initial character and remain uniformly distributed throughout the continuous phase for the desired shelf life. There should be no phase changes or microbial contamination on storage, and the emulsion should maintain elegance with respect to odor, color, and consistency. Instabilities of both chemical and physical origins can occur in emulsion formulations. Chemical instabilities, such as the development of rancidity in natural oils due to oxidation by atmospheric oxygen, the depolymerization of macromolecular emulsifiers by hydrolysis, or microbial degradation can be minimized by the addition of suitable antioxidants and preservatives. More general chemical instabilities involving interactions between the drug and emulsion excipients or between the excipients themselves may lead to physical instabilities. If these interactions involve the emulsifying agent, they may destroy its emulsifying properties, causing the emulsion to break. For example, interactions between phenolic preservatives and polyoxyethylene nonionic emulsifiers may lead to loss of emulsifying power as well as poor preservation.

Physical Instability

As emulsions are inherently unstable, they eventually revert to the original state of two separate liquids, that is, will break or crack. In the presence of an emulsifier and other additives, this state is approached via several distinct processes, some of which are reversible such as creaming and flocculation and others irreversible such as coalescence and Ostwald ripening. Phase inversion when an oil-in-water emulsion inverts to form a water-in-oil emulsion or visa versa is a special case of irreversible instability that occurs only under well-defined conditions such as a change in emulsifier solubility due to specific interactions with additives or to a change in temperature (Fig. 3).

Flocculation describes a weak reversible association between emulsion globules separated by thin films of continuous phase. The individual droplets retain their separate identities, but each floccule or cluster of droplets behaves physically as a single unit. The association arises from the interaction of attractive and repulsive forces between droplets and is reversible in the sense that the original dispersion can generally be regained by mild agitation. Flocculation is generally regarded as a precursor to the irreversible process of coalescence, although sometimes the time scale between flocculation and coalescence can be extended almost indefinitely by the adsorbed emulsifier, giving a kinetically stable emulsion.

Coalescence, where dispersed phase droplets merge to form larger droplets, takes place in two distinct stages. It begins with the drainage of liquid films of continuous phase from between the oil droplets as they approach one another and ends with the rupture of the film when a critical thickness is reached. The approaching droplets may deform as the opposing surfaces distort to either flatten (small droplets) or dimple (larger droplets) under the hydrodynamic pressures generated by viscous flow of the continuous phase.

Coalescence is not the only mechanism by which dispersed phase droplets increase in size. If the emulsion is polydispersed and there is significant miscibility between the oil and water phases, then Ostwald ripening, where droplet sizes increase due to large droplets growing at the expense of smaller ones, may also occur. This destabilizing process is a result of the Kelvin effect and occurs when small emulsion droplets (less than 1 μm) have higher solubilities (and vapor pressures) than do larger droplets (i.e. the bulk material) and consequently are thermodynamically unstable. To reach the state of equilibrium, molecules from these droplets dissolve and diffuse through the continuous phase to enlarge the larger droplets. As the small droplets lose their oil, they become even smaller, the vapor pressure difference increases, and Ostwald ripening is further enhanced.

Creaming or sedimentation occurs when the dispersed droplets or floccules separate under the influence of gravity to form a layer of more concentrated emulsion, the cream. Generally a creamed emulsion can be restored to its original state by gentle agitation. This process, which

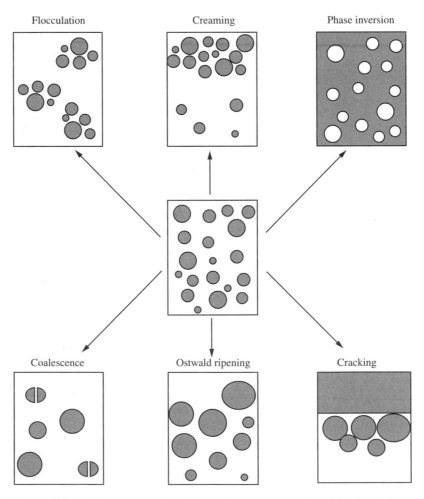

Fig. 3 Schematic representation of the various processes of emulsion breakdown.

inevitably occurs in any dilute emulsion if there is a density difference between the phases as a consequence of Stokes law, should not be confused with flocculation which is due to particle interactions resulting from the balance of attractive and repulsive forces. Most oils are less dense than water so that the oil droplets in o/w emulsions rise to the surface to form an upper layer of cream. In w/o emulsions, the cream results from sedimentation of water droplets and forms the lower layer. According to Stokes Law, the rate of creaming can be minimized by reducing droplet sizes and/or thickening the continuous phase. Adjustment of the densities of the two phases has received little attention.

The destabilization processes are not independent and each may influence or be influenced by the others. For example, the increased droplet sizes after coalescence or Ostwald ripening will enhance the rate of creaming, as will the formation of large floccules which behave as single entities. In practice, creaming, flocculation, and Ostwald ripening may proceed simultaneously or in any order followed by coalescence.

Coalescence and Ostwald ripening are obviously the most serious types of instability as they result in the formation of progressively larger droplets and ultimately lead to phase separation. Creaming and flocculation, on the other hand, are more subtle forms of instability, for although they represent potential steps towards coalescence and breaking due to the close proximity of the droplets, many practical emulsions remain in this state for long periods of time without significant coalescence and can be redispersed simply by shaking the container.

EMULSION STABILIZATION

Emulsifiers stabilize emulsions in a number of different ways, all of which act to prevent or delay the various destabilization processes described previously. The emulsifier may form an interfacial film at the oil–water interface and/or structure (i.e., thicken) the continuous phase. The interfacial film introduces additional repulsive (e.g., electrostatic, steric, or hydrational) forces between droplets to counteract attractive van der Waals forces and inhibit the close approach of droplets. It may also provide a barrier to the coalescence of droplets in close proximity, particularly if the film is close-packed and elastic. Surfactant interfacial films also lower the interfacial tension between oil and water. Although this effect is important during the emulsification process where it facilitates the breakup of droplets, it is not a major factor in maintaining the long-term stability of emulsions. In emulsions that are thickened

by the emulsifier, the interfacial film does not play the dominant role in maintaining stability; rather, it is the structured continuous phase that forms a rheological barrier to prevent the movement and hence the close approach of droplets and also inhibits Ostwald ripening.

Classical (Interfacial) Theories

Classical theories of emulsion stability focus on the manner in which the adsorbed emulsifier film influences the processes of flocculation and coalescence by modifying the forces between dispersed emulsion droplets. They do not consider the possibility of Ostwald ripening or creaming nor the influence that the emulsifier may have on continuous phase rheology. As two droplets approach one another, they experience strong van der Waals forces of attraction, which tend to pull them even closer together. The adsorbed emulsifier stabilizes the system by the introduction of additional repulsive forces (e.g., electrostatic or steric) that counteract the attractive van der Waals forces and prevent the close approach of droplets. Electrostatic effects are particularly important with ionic emulsifiers whereas steric effects dominate with nonionic polymers and surfactants, and in w/o emulsions. The applications of colloid theory to emulsions stabilized by ionic and nonionic surfactants have been reviewed as have more general aspects of the polymeric stabilization of dispersions (4, 31, 32).

The DLVO theory, which was developed independently by Derjaguin and Landau and by Verwey and Overbeek to analyze quantitatively the influence of electrostatic forces on the stability of lyophobic colloidal particles, has been adapted to describe the influence of similar forces on the flocculation and stability of simple model emulsions stabilized by ionic emulsifiers. The charge on the surface of emulsion droplets arises from ionization of the hydrophilic part of the adsorbed surfactant and gives rise to electrical double layers. Theoretical equations, which were originally developed to deal with monodispersed inorganic solids of diameters less than 1 μm, have to be extensively modified when applied to even the simplest of emulsions, because the adsorbed emulsifier is of finite thickness and droplets, unlike solids, can deform and coalesce. Washington (33) has pointed out that in lipid emulsions, an additional repulsive force not considered by the theory due to the solvent at close distances is also important.

The theory states that the forces between droplets can be considered as the sum of an attractive van der Waals part V_A and a repulsive electrostatic part V_R when identical electrical double layers overlap. As the origin of each force is independent of the other, each is evaluated separately, and the total potential of interaction V_T between the two droplets as a function of their surface-to-surface separation is obtained by summation

$$V_T = V_A + V_R$$

A schematic potential energy of interaction with distance plot is shown in Fig. 4a. It can be seen that a weak attraction occurs at large droplet separations represented by the secondary energy minimum, and a very strong attraction at small droplet separations hence the very deep primary minimum. At intermediate distances, double-layer repulsion dominates and there is

a maximum in the curve. Flocculation occurs in the secondary minimum, where the attractive forces are relatively weak and floccules are easily separated by low energy agitation. Once flocculated, droplets are prevented from approaching closer by the potential energy barrier. If they have sufficient energy to overcome the barrier, the process of coalescence commences as the droplets move closer together. Once in the primary minimum the aggregates formed are separated by only a small distance so that stability against coalescence is determined by the resistance of the interfacial film to rupture.

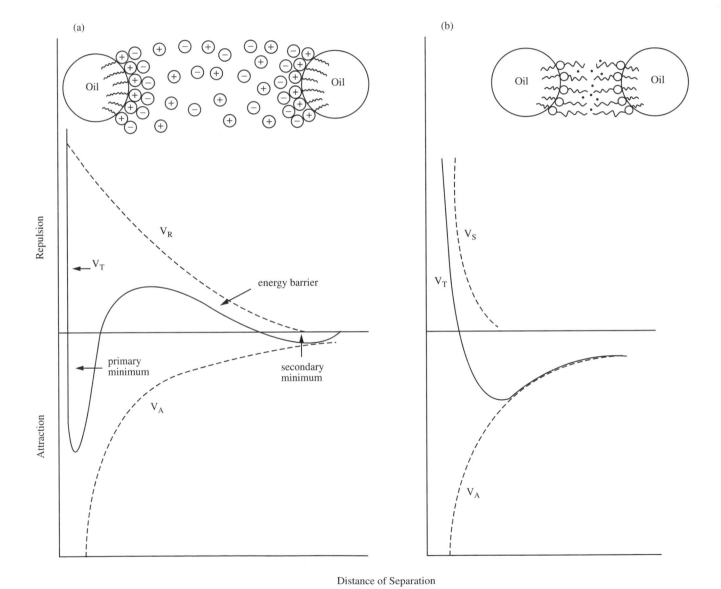

Fig. 4   The total potential energy of interaction V_T as a function of distance of surface separation H for two similar oil droplets in an oil-in-water emulsion. (a) Electrostatic stabilization by a monolayer of ionic surfactant. (b) Steric stabilization by a monolayer of nonionic surfactant. V_A: van der Waals attractive force; V_R: electrostatic repulsive force; V_S: steric repulsive force.

The height of the energy barrier, which is crucial to emulsion stabilization, depends on the state of ionization of the emulsifying agent. Most surfactants are used at pH values where they are totally ionized so that the surface potential is high, giving a correspondingly high energy barrier. The surface potential cannot be measured directly, but can be estimated from the experimentally derived zeta potential. In lipid emulsions for parenteral nutrition, the electrostatic barrier is provided by the ionization of the negatively charged phospholipids in the emulsifier film at the oil droplet–water interface. At physiological pH, a typical fat emulsion carries a negative charge with the zeta potential between 30 and 60 mV. This is sufficient to ensure stability because of the high potential energy barrier. The addition of electrolytes or a change in pH can have a devastating effect on emulsion stability by compressing the double layers, thus reducing the zeta potential and energy barrier and allowing droplets to move into the primary minimum. Thus, great care must be exercised when electrolytes are added nutritional emulsions. With emulsifiers such as proteins and gums, ionization, and hence emulsifying activity, is also pH dependent (c.f. Table 3).

The DLVO theory does not explain either the stability of water-in-oil emulsions or the stability of oil-in-water emulsions stabilized by adsorbed nonionic surfactants and polymers where the electrical contributions are often of secondary importance. In these, steric and hydrational forces, which arise from the loss of entropy when adsorbed polymer layers or hydrated chains of nonionic polyether surfactant intermingle on close approach of two similar droplets, are more important (Fig. 4b). In emulsions stabilized by polyether surfactants, these interactions assume importance at very close distances of approach and are influenced markedly by temperature and degree of hydration of the polyoxyethylene chains. With block copolymers of the ethylene oxide–propylene oxide type, such as the poloxamers, the hydrated polyoxyethylene chains extend into the continuous phase to provide steric stabilization and the hydrophobic propylene oxide portion is anchored onto the droplet surface to form a strong protecting layer against coalescence. Stability is optimized when the droplet surfaces are completely coated by polymer chains so that desorption and lateral movement of the polymer is inhibited. With w/o emulsions, steric hindrance of the adsorbed chains of emulsifier can also result in entropic repulsion effects at small distances of separation.

Some natural polymeric emulsifiers such as the gums, in addition to forming steric and electrostatic barriers form thick multilayered films that are very resistant to film rupture. They may also thicken the continuous phases

of o/w emulsions, thereby reducing the rate of film drainage in the initial stages of coalescence. Small solid particles may stabilize emulsions if they are wetted by both phases and possess sufficient adhesion for one another to form a coherent interfacial film. The film serves as a mechanical barrier to prevent the coalescence of droplets, and if charged, electrostatic mechanisms further assist in the stabilization of the emulsion. Although solids are not generally sufficient to stabilize emulsions on their own, they often reinforce the effectiveness of other emulsifiers.

Stabilization by Mixtures of Emulsifiers

Most pharmaceutical emulsions, whether dilute mobile systems for internal use or thick semisolid creams for application to the skin, contain mixtures of emulsifiers, as these provide more stable preparations. For example, traditional oral preparations are sometimes stabilized by mixtures of gums such as acacia and tragacanth and mixtures of nonionic surfactants of high and low hydrophile–lipophile balance (HLB) generally form more stable emulsions than a single surfactant. The lecithins used to stabilize parenteral emulsions are usually mixtures of neutral and charged lipids as are the partially neutralized glyceryl esters such as self-emulsifying glyceryl monostearate. Combinations of sparingly soluble long-chain acids, alcohols, or glyceryl esters with more soluble ionic and non-ionic surfactants are widely used in dermatological o/w lotions and creams, where they are sometimes added in the form of a preblended emulsifying wax (Table 4). Surfactant/fatty acid combinations are also present in traditional liniment and lotion emulsion formulations prepared by the nascent soap method and in preparations where triethanolamine soaps are formed in situ from the interaction of triethanolamine and excess fatty acid.

Equations from the DLVO theory even if modified to allow for the steric repulsive forces cannot cope with mixtures of emulsifiers. Increased stability in model emulsions (c.f. Fig. 1a) is attributed not so much to the control of flocculation (although this does occur), but rather to the prevention or retardation of coalescence by closer packing of the molecules in the adsorbed monolayer to form a more rigid and condensed film. There is now substantial evidence that interactions between emulsifier components to form specific lamellar phases, either liquid crystalline or gel, that are capable of incorporating large volumes of water are important for the stability of many parenteral and dermatological emulsions. Mobile parenteral injections stabilized by

Table 4 Typical emulsifying waxes and their component surfactants

Emulsifying wax	Components
Emulsifying wax USNF	Cetearyl alcohol, polysorbate
Cationic emulsifying wax BP	Cetearyl alcohol, cetrimonium bromide
Cetomacrogol emulsifying wax BP	Cetearyl alcohol, ceteth 20
Glyceryl stearate, SE	Glyceryl stearate, soap

phospholipid mixtures usually contain swollen lamellar liquid crystals (34) whereas a swollen gel phase which generally provides better stability as well as a means of controlling rheological properties dominates in semisolid dermatological emulsions prepared with emulsifying waxes. The relevance of bilayer gel and liquid crystalline phases in dermatological and parenteral emulsions have been discussed in reviews (10, 29). Much of the information about their structures was obtained from investigations of the phase behaviour of emulsifiers and their components in water over the ranges of concentration and temperature relevant to the manufacture, storage, and use of the formulations. It is interesting to note that the same electrostatic, hydrational, and steric forces that operate in simple emulsions also dominate the stability and properties of the lamellar phases (35).

Ostwald Ripening

Ostwald ripening has not been studied as extensively in emulsions as has coalescence, although it is a major mechanism for instability in lipid and perfluorochemical emulsions with submicron droplet sizes where a condensed monolayer is not always necessary for emulsion stability (36). Although surfactant interfacial films protect against flocculation and coalescence, Ostwald ripening may in fact be enhanced if the surfactant is above the critical micelle concentration (cmc) because of the diffusion of solubilized oil through the continuous phase. The addition of a third component to the emulsion that has a lower vapor pressure and solubility than the disperse phase has will also inhibit Ostwald ripening. The addition of long-chain alkanes to comparatively unstable oil-in-water emulsions prepared with sodium dodecyl sulfate resulted in marked increases in stability even though the alkanes do not effect the composition or mechanical properties of the oil–water interface (37). The stability of pure perfluorodecalin emulsions used as blood substitutes is enhanced by the addition of a small quantity of perfluorotributylamine, and lipid emulsions containing local anaesthetic/analgesic drugs show enhanced stability

in the presence of hydrophobic excipients of lower solubility than the disperse phase (38). Polymeric emulsifiers possibly stabilize emulsions against Ostwald ripening by increasing the viscosity of the continuous phase. The relative lack of Ostwald ripening in emulsions prepared from oils immiscible with water, such as mineral oil, may partly explain why they are easier to emulsify than are more miscible vegetable oils used in parenteral preparations.

Selection of Emulsifier

Over the years there have been many attempts to find systemic methods for screening potential emulsifiers from the enormous number of surfactants available commercially. Although the mechanisms governing the stability of emulsions, including the complex multiple phase systems of pharmacy are becoming clearer, there are still few scientific guidelines to assist in the proper selection of emulsifiers for a particular emulsion. Semiempirical methods based on both interfacial considerations and the phase behavior of the emulsifiers are considered briefly next.

The hydrophile–lipophile balance (HLB) concept

Griffin devised the concept of hydrophile–lipophile balance (HLB) and its additivity many years ago for selection of nonionic emulsifiers and this rather empirical method is still widely used. The enormous literature on the HLB of surfactants has been reviewed by Becher (39). Each surfactant is allocated an HLB number usually on a scale of 0–20, based on the relative proportions of the hydrophilic and hydrophobic part of a molecule. Water-in-oil emulsions are formed generally from oil-soluble surfactants of low HLB number and oil-in-water emulsions from more hydrophilic surfactants of high HLB number. The method of selection is based on the observation that each type of oil will require an emulsifying agent of a specific HLB number to produce a stable emulsion. Thus, oils are often designated two "required" HLB numbers, one low and one high, for their emulsification to form water-in-oil and oil-in-water emulsions respectively. A series of emulsifiers and their blends with HLB values close to the required HLB of the oil are then examined to see which one forms the most stable emulsion (c.f. Fig. 1a).

Although the HLB concept narrows the range of emulsifiers to select and provides a schematic approach for the formulator, it is limited by its strict relation to molecular structure of the individual surfactants. The concept does not consider the total emulsion and is therefore insensitive to interactions between emulsifier components, the influence of temperature changes, or the presence of additional ingredients in the emulsion. Consequently, not all emulsifier blends of the correct HLB form stable systems. For example, when surfactants of widely different HLB numbers are blended to give the optimum theoretical HLB, the high solubility of the surfactant in the oil and aqueous phases change the balance of the molecules at the interface and unstable emulsions may result. Similarly, if the added surfactants form intermolecular associations at the interface, the association complex is unlikely to have properties that are related in any simple way to the individual properties of the constituent molecules.

The phase inversion temperature (PIT) method (HLB-temperature)

A complementary means of emulsifier selection, the phase inversion temperature (PIT), which employs a characteristic property of the emulsion rather than the properties of the emulsifiers in isolation, was introduced by Shinoda (40). The method uses the fact that the stabilities of oil-in-water emulsions containing nonionic surfactants are closely related to the degree of hydration of the interfacial films. Emulsion stability is reduced by increase in temperature or added salts because these decrease the extent of interfacial film hydration. Phase inversion, due to a change from preferential water solubility of the emulsifier film at low temperature to preferential oil solubility at high temperature, will occur at a specific temperature unique to the particular emulsion and this can be determined experimentally. As a general rule, relatively stable oil-in-water emulsions are obtained when their temperatures during storage and use are between 20 and 65°C below the PIT, presumably because the films are sufficiently hydrated. Mixtures of emulsifiers with identical HLBs produce emulsions with quite different PITs because additives and interactions between the components affect PIT but not HLB.

Microscopic selection for multiple phase emulsions

The better understanding of the mechanisms of stability in complex dermatological emulsions stabilized by surfactants and amphiphiles has enabled the development of a rapid microscopic method for evaluation of potential emulsifiers. The method is based on the observation that good emulsifier blends that stabilize emulsions by the formation of multilayers of stable gel phase also swell spontaneously in water at ambient temperature and this process can be observed microscopically. Mixtures that do not form gel phase or form metastable gels only after a heating and cooling cycle cannot be observed to swell spontaneously at ambient temperature (4).

Emulsification Techniques

Emulsions are usually prepared by the application of mechanical energy produced by a wide range of agitation techniques. These disrupt droplets by the application of either shear forces in laminar flow or inertial forces in turbulent flow. Emulsifying devices ranging from simple hand mixers and stirrers to the use of propeller or turbine mixers, static mixers, colloid mills, homogenizers, and ultrasonic devices have been used.

Emulsifiers also have an important role in the process of emulsification. Surfactant emulsifiers reduce interfacial tensions during emulsification, making droplets easier to break up as well as reducing the tendency for recombination. Other emulsifiers such as the polymer macromolecules alter the hydrodynamic forces during the agitation process by their influence on rheological properties. Scale-up procedures from the laboratory to manufacture can introduce a number of problems due to the difficulties in matching the exact conditions of mixing, and, because of entrapment of air, especially in emulsions of high consistency that have a yield value. Along with being inelegant, even traces of atmospheric air can cause decomposition in drugs or excipients susceptible to oxidation.

There are additional constraints when manufacturing parenteral emulsions that must be sterile and of fine particle size. Perfluorochemical and fat emulsions are usually prepared by homogenization at high temperature and pressure, as a large output of energy is required to produce droplet sizes considerably less than 1 μm. Although heat sterilization is widely used, this places a severe test on the stability, and emulsions are sometimes prepared from sterile components under strict aseptic conditions and further sterilized by filtration (15).

Processing variables

Differences in manufacturing techniques such as the rate of the heating and cooling cycle, the extent and order of mixing can cause variations in the consistency and rheology of the resulting emulsions. The initial particle size of the emulsion depends on the emulsifiers used, the emulsification equipment, the addition speed, and the phase volume. If the surfactant is placed in one of the phases prior to emulsification, it will migrate to the other to establish equilibrium. Thus, emulsification temperatures and cooling rates are important and the time of the mixing should be sufficient to allow the surfactant to migrate to and equilibrate at the interface throughout the process. Oil-in-water emulsions are sometimes prepared by the phase inversion technique, where the aqueous phase is added to the oil phase to form a w/o emulsion that inverts to an o/w emulsion on addition of further amounts of water. This process is claimed to give finer emulsions.

Preparation techniques, in particular cooling rates and mixing procedures, have a marked effect on initial and final consistencies of emulsions prepared with nonionic emulsifying waxes. For example, "shock" cooling and limited mixing initially produces very mobile systems whereas slow cooling with adequate mixing produces semisolid emulsions. Mixing time, when the emulsifiers are in the molten state, influences the distribution of surfactant within the molten masses and bilayers and the relative lamellar order within the system. With ionic emulsifying waxes, different preparation techniques cause comparatively minor variations in the consistency of the final product. It was shown that differences are not due to the gel phase component of cationic ternary systems, but rather due to the variations in size of the crystalline alcohol that precipitates after manufacture. Systems formed by a rapid "shock" cooling method exhibited smaller but greater numbers of cetostearyl alcohol crystals and were thicker than similar ternary systems manufactured by a more lengthy procedure (29).

MICROEMULSIONS

Microemulsions are thermodynamically stable, transparent (or translucent) dispersions of oil and water that are stabilized by an interfacial film of surfactant molecules. The surfactant may be pure, a mixture, or combined with a cosurfactant such as a medium-chain alcohol (e.g., butanol, pentanol). These homogeneous systems, which can be prepared over a wide range of surfactant concentrations and oil to water ratios (20–80%), are all fluids of low viscosity.

The term microemulsion, which implies a close relationship to ordinary emulsions, is misleading because the microemulsion state embraces a number of different microstructures, most of which have little in common with ordinary emulsions. Although microemulsions may be composed of dispersed droplets of either oil or water, it is now accepted that they are essentially stable, single-phase swollen micellar solutions rather than unstable two-phase dispersions. Microemulsions are readily distinguished from normal emulsions by their transparency, their low viscosity, and more fundamentally their thermodynamic stability and ability to form spontaneously. The dividing line, however, between the size of a swollen micelle (~10–140 nm) and a fine emulsion droplet (~100–600 nm) is not well defined, although microemulsions are very labile systems and a microemulsion droplet may disappear within a fraction of a second whilst another droplet forms spontaneously elsewhere in the system. In contrast, ordinary emulsion droplets, however small, exist as individual entities until coalescence or Ostwald ripening occurs.

Figure 5 shows a hypothetical phase diagram with representation of microemulsion structures. At high water concentrations, microemulsions consist of small oil droplets dispersed in water (o/w microemulsion), while at lower water concentrations the situation is reversed and the system consists of water droplets dispersed in oil (w/o microemulsions). In each phase, the oil and water droplets are separated by a surfactant-rich film. In systems containing comparable amounts of oil and water, equilibrium bicontinuous structures in which the oil and the water domains interpenetrate in a more complicated manner are formed. In this region, infinite curved channels of both the oil and the water domains extend over macroscopic distances and the surfactant forms an interface of rapidly fluctuating curvature, but in which the net curvature is near zero.

Pharmaceutical and Biological Applications of Microemulsions

Microemulsions provide ultralow interfacial tensions and large interfacial areas as well as the ability to concentrate and localize significant amounts of both oil- and water-soluble materials within the same isotropic medium. Over the years, attention has been focused on their potential use as novel reaction media for a wide range of chemical, biochemical, and photochemical reactions, and as carriers for chemicals and small particles, reviewed by Eccleston (41). Inverse microemulsions of the w/o type are the subject of particular interest because of the rapidly emerging range of biotechnological applications based on their ability to solubilize enzymes in the water domains without denaturation or loss of activity. The ability of such solubilized hydrophilic enzymes to transform hydrophobic substrates dissolved in the organic

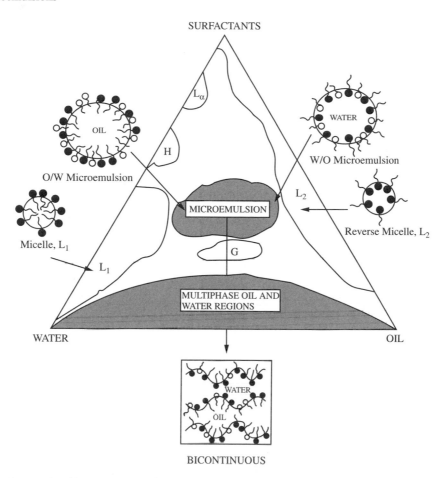

Fig. 5 Ternary phase diagram for oil, water, and surfactant mixtures showing micellar, microemulsion, and multiphase macroemulsion regions with schematic representations of various structures.

phase could lead eventually to the synthesis of new drugs. As with ordinary emulsions, microemulsions show improved gastrointestinal absorption. They also have a number of other advantages over macroemulsions for drug delivery. Microemulsions form spontaneously without the aid of high shear equipment or significant heat input (heat and gentle mixing are required only if it is necessary to melt any of the ingredients) and their microstructures are independent of the order of addition of the excipients. Optical transparency and low viscosity of microemulsions ensure that they are cosmetically elegant and easy to handle and pack, and their indefinite stabilities ensure a long shelf life. Microemulsions have thus attracted much interest in their drug delivery potential. Both o/w and w/o emulsions have been shown to enhance the oral bioavailability of drugs, including various peptides (42). A peroral concentrate of cyclosporine is now available commercially (Sandimmune Neoral® Novartis), which forms a microemulsion in the aqueous fluids of the gastrointestinal tract. In this preparation, the rate of absorption of cyclosporin is more rapid and less variable than it is with the conventional oily dispersion. Calcein administered intraduodenally in the aqueous phase of a w/o microemulsion prepared from medium-chain triglycerides (43) produces significantly higher plasma levels of the drug compared with an aqueous solution.

Microemulsions have also been used for topical delivery where they increase drug absorption. For example, cetyl alcohol, which is commonly used as an emulsifier in lotions and creams, is absorbed faster and deeper into the skin when formulated as a component of a microemulsion (44). Although efficient skin penetration may be desirable for a therapeutic agent, the relatively high concentrations of surfactant (10–25%) and cosurfactant or cosolvent (5–10%) in such formulations could enhance skin absorption of potential irritants or carcinogens. In fact, the main limitations in realizing the full potential of microemulsions as drug delivery systems are the narrow range of surfactants, cosurfactants, solvents, and other materials acceptable pharmaceutically.

Microemulsion Formation

Many approaches have been used to explore the mechanisms of microemulsion formation and stability [summarized by Eccleston (41) and Attwood (45)]. Early theories considered interfacial aspects of microemulsions and did not distinguish between thermodynamically stable systems and very fine kinetically stable emulsions. For microemulsions to form spontaneously, the free energy involved when the interfacial area is increased, ΔG ($\Delta G = \gamma \Delta A$, where ΔA is the increase in interfacial area) must be negative. An essential requirement is that the interfacial tension between the oil and water phases γ, is reduced to a very low value by the interfacial film, giving a small but positive free-energy value. The dispersion of the droplets in the continuous phase increases the entropy of the system. Microemulsions form because the negative free energy changes due to the entropy of the dispersion of droplets in the continuous phase overcomes the positive product of the small interfacial tension and the large interfacial area A.

The curvature of the oil–water interface in microemulsions varies from highly curved towards oil (o/w) or water (w/o) to zero mean curvature in bicontinuous structures. The type of microemulsion that forms depends on the properties of the surfactant, cosurfactant and the oil. Although there are no strict rules for choosing the appropriate microemulsion components, there are a number of general guidelines based on empirical observations. The surfactant(s) chosen for a particular oil must:

1. lower interfacial tension to a very low value to aid dispersion processes during the preparation of the microemulsion.
2. be of the appropriate hydrophile-lipophile character to provide the correct curvature at the interfacial region for the desired microemulsion type, o/w, w/o or bicontinuous.
3. provide a flexible film that can readily deform round small droplets.

The analysis of film curvature for surfactant associations leading to microemulsion formation has been rationalized by Mitchell and Ninham. They used a packing ratio P defined as V/al, where V is the partial molar volume of the surfactant, a the cross sectional area (i.e. size) of the surfactant head group, and l the maximum length of the surfactant chain (46). The packing ratio provides a direct measure of HLB and is influenced by the same factors. Oil-in-water microemulsions are favored if the effective polar part of the surfactant is more bulky than the hydrophobic part, that is, P varies from 0 to 1, and the interface curves spontaneously towards water (positive curvature). Water-in-oil microemulsions form when the interface curves in the opposite direction, that is, P is greater than 1 (negative curvature). At zero curvature, when the HLB is balanced and P is zero, either bicontinuous or lamellar structures may form according to the rigidity of the film. The critical packing parameter P is based purely on geometric considerations. Hydration of the surfactant head group and penetration of the oil and the cosurfactant into the surfactant film also affect the packing and curvature, as summarized in Table 5, which also illustrates how formulation variables may be manipulated to produce a microemulsion of the desired type (47).

Most single-chain surfactants do not lower the oil–water interfacial tension sufficiently to form microemulsions nor are they of the correct molecular structure, and

Table 5 Factors affecting spontaneous curvature of monolayers

Variable	Curvature effect	Cause
Increase oil chain length	More positive	Less penetration of surfactant tail region
Addition of shorter chain cosurfactant	More positive	Alcohol swells head region more than tail region
Addition of longer chain cosurfactant	More negative	Alcohol swells surfactant chain region more than head region
Addition of salt (ionic surfactant)	More negative	Screened repulsion between polar head groups
Addition of salt (nonionic surfactant)	More negative	Headgroup size reduced by dehydration
Branched or double chained surfactant	More negative	Increased tail group area
Reduced surfactant head group size	More negative	
Increased temperature (nonionic surfactant)	More negative	Headgroup size reduced by dehydration
Increased temperature (ionic surfactant)	More positive	Increased surfactant counter-ion dissociation

(Adapted from Ref. 47.)

short- to medium-chain length alcohols are necessary as cosurfactants. The cosurfactant also ensures that the interfacial film is flexible enough to deform readily around each droplet as their intercalation between the primary surfactant molecules decreases both the polar head group interactions and the hydrocarbon chain interactions. Medium-chain alcohols such as pentanol and hexanol have been used by many investigators as they are particularly effective cosurfactants. They are not, however, suitable for pharmaceuticals due to their high irritant potential. Double-chain surfactants such as anionic Aerosol-OT (bis-2-ethylhexyl sulfosuccinate) or cationic DDAB (didodecyldimethylammonium bromide), which have relatively small head groups and bulky hydrophobic portions, are already of the required HLB to form w/o microemulsions spontaneously without a cosurfactant. Unfortunately, these widely investigated surfactants are too toxic for general pharmaceutical or biotechnological applications. Double-chain phospholipids such as the phosphatidylcholines of lecithin are an obvious possibility. Although lecithin is too lipophilic to form microemulsions, pharmaceutically acceptable microemulsions have been prepared from double-chain phospholipids by using acceptable cosurfactants such as ethanol, propanol, or n-butanol with isopropyl myristate (48, 51). Self-emulsifying drug delivery systems are composed of triglyceride oils and surfactant mixtures that undergo spontaneous emulsification when mixed with water (52). This principle is used in the commercial product Sandimmune Neoral®, which forms a microemulsion in situ when diluted by gastric fluid.

Formulation and Preparation of Microemulsions

As microemulsions are thermodynamically stable, they can be prepared simply by blending oil, water, surfactant, and cosurfactant with mild agitation. Once the appropriate microemulsion components have been selected, quaternary phase diagrams or ternary pseudo-phase diagrams may be constructed to define the extent and nature of the microemulsion regions and the surrounding two- and three-phase domains. The microemulsion region can be identified and characterized using the range of light, neutron, and X-ray scattering and other techniques such as NMR and microscopy (45). Problems arise in interpretation of data in systems of high droplet volume fraction due to interdroplet interactions. The normal practice of investigating systems at relatively low concentrations and then extrapolating to zero concentration in order to eliminate interparticle interactions cannot be applied to

microemulsions as it is not possible to dilute the systems without affecting their structure. Hard sphere models, such as those adapted from Percus and Yevick, have been successfully used to analyze scattering data from concentrated w/o microemulsions (53).

REFERENCES

1. International Union of Pure and Applied Chemistry, IUPAC. *Manual of Colloid and Surface Chemistry*; Butterworths: London, 1971.
2. Garti, N.; Aserin, A. Double Emulsions Stabilized by Macromolecular Surfactants. *Micelles Microemulsions and Monolayers*; Shah, D.O. Ed.; Marcel Dekker, Inc.: New York, 1998; 333–362.
3. Davis, S.S.; Washington, C.; West, P.; Illum, L.; Liversidge, G.; Sternson, L.; Kirsh, R. Lipid Emulsions as Drug Delivery Systems. Ann. N. Y. Acad. Sci. **1987**, *507*, 75–88.
4. Eccleston, G.M.; Emulsions. *Encyclopedia of Pharmaceutical Technology*, 1st Ed.; Swarbrick, J., Boylan, J.C. Eds.; Marcel Dekker, Inc.: New York, 1992; 5, 137–188.
5. Block, L.H. Pharmaceutical Emulsions and Microemulsions. *Pharmaceutical Dosage Forms: Disperse Systems*; Lieberman, H.A., Rieger, M.M., Banker, G.S, Eds.; Marcel Dekker, Inc.: New York, 1996; 2, 47–109.
6. Rosoff, M.; Specialised Pharmaceutical Emulsions. *Pharmaceutical Dosage Forms: Disperse Systems*; Lieberman, H.A., Rieger, M.M., Banker, G.S., Eds.; Marcel Dekker, Inc.: New York, 1997; 3, 1–22.
7. Barry, B.W. *Dermatological Formulation. Percutaneous Absorption*; Marcel Dekker, Inc.: New York, 1983; 480.
8. Flynn, G.L.; Cutaneous and Transdermal Delivery: Processes and Systems of Delivery. *Modern Pharmaceutics*, 3rd Ed.; Banker, G.S., Rhodes, C.T. Eds.; Marcel Dekker, Inc.: New York, 1996; 239–298.
9. Eccleston, G.M.; The Microstructure of Semisolid Creams. Pharm. Int. **1986**, *7* (3), 63–70.
10. Eccleston, G.M.; Functions of Mixed Emulsifiers and Emulsifying Waxes in Dermatological Lotions and Creams. Colloids and Surfaces **1997**, 169–182.
11. Amselem, S.; Friedman, D.; Submicron Emulsions as Drug Carriers for Topical Administration. *Submicron Emulsions in Drug Delivery*; Benita, S. Ed.; Harwood Academic: Amsterdam, 1998; 9, 152–173.
12. Carrigan, P.; Bates, T.; Biopharmaceutics of Drug Administered in Lipid-Containing Dosage Forms 1: GI Absorption of Griseofulvin from an Oil-in-Water Emulsion in Rat. J. Pharm. Sci. **1973**, *62*, 1476–1414.
13. Collins Gold, L.C.; Lyons, R.T.; Bartholow, L.C.; Parenteral Emulsions for Drug Delivery. Adv. Drug Del. Rev. **1990**, *5*, 189–208.
14. Prankerd, R.J.; Stella, V.J.; The Use of Oil-In-Water Emulsions as a Vehicle for Parenteral Administration. J. Parent. Sci. Technol. **1990**, *44*, 139–149.
15. Floyd, A.G.; Jain, S. Injectable Emulsions and Suspensions. *Pharmaceutical Dosage Forms: Disperse Systems*; Lieberman, H.A., Rieger, M.M., Banker, G.S., Eds.; Marcel Dekker, Inc.: New York, 1996; 2, 261–318.

16. Nomura, T.; Koreeda, N.; Yamashita, F.; Takakura, Y.; Hashida, M. Effect of Particle Size on the Disposition of Lipid Carriers after Intratumoral Injection into Tissue Isolated Tumors. Pharm. Res. **1998**, *15* (1), 128–132.

17. Omotosho, J.A.; Whateley, T.L.; Florence, A.T. Release of 5-Fluorouracil from Intramuscular W/O/W Multiple Emulsions. Biopharm. and Drug Disposit **1989**, *10*, 257–268.

18. Von Dardel, O.; Mebius, C.; Mossberg, T.; Svensson, B. Fat Emulsion as a Vehicle for Diazepam. A Study of 9492 Patients. Br. J. Anaesth. **1983**, *55*, 41–47.

19. Lovell, M.W.; Johnson, H.W.; Hui, H.W.; Cannon, J.B.; Gupta, P.K.; Hsu, C.C. Less Painful Emulsion Formulations for Intravenous Administration of Clarithromycin. Int. J. Pharm. **1994**, *109*, 45–57.

20. Kirsh, R.; Goldstein, R.; Tarloff, J.; Parris, D.; Hook, J.; Hanna, N.; Bugelski, P.; Poste, G.J. An Emulsion Formulation of Amphoteracin B Improves the Therapeutic Index when Treating Systemic Murine Candidiasis. Infect. Dise. **1988**, *158*, 1065–1070.

21. Submicron Emulsions in Drug Targeting and Delivery. *Drug Targeting and Delivery*; Benita, S., Ed.; Harwood Academic: Amsterdam, 1998; 333.

22. Spahn, D.R. Current Status Of Artificial Oxygen Carriers. Adv. Drug Del. Rev. **2000**, *40*, 143–151.

23. Naveh, N.; Muchtar, S.; Benita, S. Pilocarpine Incorporated into a Submicron Emulsion Vehicle Causes Unexpectedly Prolonged Ocular Hypotensive Effects in Rabbits. J. Ocular Pharmacol. **1994**, *10* (3), 509–520.

24. Kararli, T.T.; Needham, T.E.; Schoenhard, G.; Baron, D.A.; Schmidt, R.E.; Katz, B.; Belonio, B. Enhancement of Nasal Delivery of a Renin Inhibitor in the Rat Using Emulsion Formulations. Pharm. Res. **1992**, *9*, 1024–1028.

25. Aikawa, K.; Matsumoto, K.; Uda, H.; Tanaka, S.; Shimamura, H.; Aramaki, Y.; Ysuchiya, S. Prolonged Release of Drug from O/W Emulsion and Residence in Rat Nasal Cavity. Pharm. Dev. Technol. **1998**, *3* (4), 461–469.

26. Mitra, R.; Pezron, I.; Chu, W.A.; Mitra, A.K. Lipid Emulsions as Vehicles for Enhanced Nasal Delivery of Insulin. Int. J. Pharm. **2000**, *205* (1–2), 127–134.

27. Mascioli, E.A.; Babayan, V.K.; Bistrian, B.R.; Blackburn, G.L. Novel Triglycerides for Special Medical Purposes. J. Parent. Ent. Nut. **1989**, *12* (6), 127S–132S.

28. Hedeman, H.; Brondsted, H.; Mullertz, A.; Frokjaer, S. Fat Emulsions Based on Structured Lipids (1,3 Specific Triglycerides): An Investigation of the In Vivo Fate. Pharm. Res. **1996**, *13* (5), 725–733.

29. Eccleston, G.M. Multiple-Phase Oil-in-Water Emulsions. J. Soc. Cosmet. Chem. **1990**, *41*, 1–22.

30. Nishikawa, M.; Yoshinobu, T.; Hashida, M. Biofate of Fat Emulsions. *Submicron Emulsions in Drug Targeting and Delivery*; Benita, S., Ed.; Harwood Academic: Amsterdam, 1998; 99–118.

31. Eccleston, G.M.; Florence, A.T. Application of Emulsion Theory to Complex and Real Systems. Int. J. Cosmet. Sci. **1985**, *7*, 195–212.

32. Hough, D.B.; Thompson, L. Effect of Nonionic Surfactants on the Stability of Dispersions. *Nonionic Surfactants. Physical Chemistry*; Schick, M.J., Ed.; Marcel Dekker, Inc.: New York, 1987; 601–676.

33. Washington, C. The Electrokinetic Properties of Phospholipid Stabilized Fat Emulsions. III. Interdroplet Potentials and Stability Ratios in Monovalent Electrolytes. Int. J. Pharm. **1990**, *64*, 67–73.

34. Rydhag, L.; Wilton, I. The Function of Phospholipids of Soybean Lecithin in Emulsions. Am. J. Oil Col. Chem. **1981**, *58*, 830–837.

35. Eccleston, G.M.; Behan-Martin, M.K.; Jones, G.R.; Townes-Andrews, E. Synchrotron X-Ray Investigations into the Lamellar Gel Phase Formed in Pharmaceutical Creams Prepared with Cetrimide and Fatty Alcohols. Int. J. Pharm. **2000**, *203*, 127–139.

36. Buscall, R.; Davis, S.S.; Potts, D.C. The Effect of Long-Chain Alkenes on the Stability of Oil-in-Water Emulsions. The Significance of Ostwald Ripening. Colloid Polym. Sci. **1979**, *257*, 636–644.

37. Davis, S.S.; Round, H.P.; Purewal, T.S. Ostwald Ripening and the Stability of Emulsion Systems: An Explanation for the Effect of an Added Third Component. J. Colloid Int. Sci. **1981**, *80* (2), 508–511.

38. Welin-Berger, K.; Bergenstahl, B. Inhibition of Ostwald Ripening in Local Anaesthetic Emulsions by Using Hydrophobic Excipients in the Disperse Phase. Int. J. Pharm. **2000**, *200* (2), 249–260.

39. Becher, P. Hydrophile-Lipophile Balance: An Updated Biography. *Encyclopedia of Emulsion Technology*; Becher, P., Ed.; Marcel Dekker, Inc.: New York, 1985; 2, 425–512.

40. Shinoda, K.; Saito, H. The Stability of O/W Type Emulsions as Functions of Temperature and the HLB of Emulsifiers: The Emulsification by PIT Method. J. Colloid Int. Sci. **1969**, *30*, 258–263.

41. Eccleston, G.M. Microemulsions. *Encyclopedia of Pharmaceutical Technology*, 1st Ed.; Swarbrick, J., Boylan, J.C., Eds.; Marcel Dekker, Inc.: New York, 1995; 9, 375–421.

42. Ritschel, W. Microemulsions for Improved Peptide Absorption from the Gastrointestinal Tract. Meth. Find. Exp. Clin. Pharmacol. **1991**, *13*, 205–220.

43. Constantinides, P.P.; Scalart, J.; Lancaster, C.; Marcello, J.; Marks, G.; Ellens, H.; Smith, P.L. Formulation and Intestinal Absorption Enhancement Evaluation of Water-In-Oil Microemulsions Incorporating Medium Chain Triglycerides. Pharm. Res. **1994**, *11* (10), 1385–1390.

44. Linn, E.E.; Pohland, R.C.; Byrd, T.K. Microemulsions for Intradermal Delivery of Cetyl Alcohol and Octyl Dimethyl PABA. Drug Dev. Ind. Pharm. **1990**, *16* (9), 899–920.

45. Attwood, D. Microemulsions. *Colloidal Drug Delivery Systems*; Kreuter, J., Ed.; Marcel Dekker, Inc.: New York, 1994; 66, 31–71.

46. Mitchell, D.J.; Ninham, B. Micelles Vesicles and Microemulsions. J. Chem Soc. Faraday Trans. **1981**, *2* (677), 601–629.

47. Fletcher, D.I.; Parrott, D. Protein Partitioning between Microemulsion Phases and Conjugate Aqueous Phases. *Structure and Reactivity in Reverse Micelles*; Pileni, M.P., Ed.; Elsevier: New York, 1988; 303–322.

48. Attwood, D.; Mallon, C.; Taylor, C.J. Phase Studies on Oil-in-Water Phospholipid Microemulsions. Int. J. Pharm. **1992**, *84*, R5–R8.

49. Aboofazeli, R.; Lawrence, M.J. Investigations into the Formation and Characterisation of Phospholipid Microemulsions. 1. Pseudo-ternary Phase Diagrams of Systems Containing Water-Lecithin-Alcohol-Isopropyl Myristate. Int. J. Pharm. **1993**, *93*, 161–175.

50. Aboofazeli, R.; Lawrence, M.J. Investigations into the Formation and Characterisation of Phospholipid Microemulsions. II. Pseudo-Ternary Phase Diagrams of Systems Containing Water-Lecithin-Isopropyl Myristate-Alcohol: Influence of Purity. Int. J. Pharm. **1994**, *106* , 51–61.

51. Aboofazeli, R.; Lawrence, M.J. Investigations into the Formation and Characterisation of Phospholipid Microemulsions. II. Pseudo-Ternary Phase Diagrams of Systems Containing Water-Lecithin-Isopropyl Myristate. Int. J. Pharm. **1994**, *111*, 63–72.

52. Pouton, C. Lipid Formulations for Oral Administration of Drugs: Non-Emulsifying, Self-Emulsifying and Self-Microemulsifying Drug Delivery Systems. Eur. J. Pharm. Sci. **2000**, *1* (11), S93–S98.

53. Percus, J.K.; Yevick, G.J. Analysis of Classical Statistical Mechanics by Means of Collective Co-ordinates. Phys. Rev. **1958**, *110*, 1–13.

E

ENZYME IMMUNOASSAY AND RELATED BIOANALYTICAL METHODS

John W.A. Findlay

Pharmacia, Skokie, Illinois

Ira Das

St. Louis, Missouri

INTRODUCTION

Enzyme immunoassay, a bioanalytical method incorporating an antigen–antibody reaction to capture the analyte of interest and an enzyme reporter system to detect the captured analyte, is one of the most widely used immunoassay formats. The method is sometimes applied only qualitatively to indicate the presence of an antigen in a matrix. However, in the more common quantitative implementation, a calibration (standard) curve is incorporated, from which the concentration of the analyte in unknown samples is interpolated. In the decades since the development of a radioimmunoassay for insulin by Yalow and Berson (1), immunoassays have been widely applied in support of medical practice and drug development. However, in recent years, there has been a decline in the application of immunoassays to the quantitation of low-molecular-weight xenobiotics, primarily due to the advent of liquid chromatography–mass spectrometry (LC–MS) methods, which have high sensitivity and specificity. This is particularly so for support of early drug discovery, where assay development times of as little as a day and analytical run times of only a few minutes per sample make LC–MS ideally suited to fast delivery of results to discovery scientists. Nonetheless, the remarkable specificity of antibodies allows their application in well-characterized immunoassays to the support of Phase III and Phase IV clinical trials as a cost-effective alternative to LC–MS methods. In addition, these methods are still widely used for therapeutic drug monitoring and analysis of low-molecular-weight hormones, such as steroids, in support of medical diagnostics. Immunoassays remain the method of choice for the quantitation of protein macromolecules and antibodies in complex matrices. Another major application of immunoassays is in the detection and quantitation of biomarkers, which are evolving to be of pivotal importance in the evaluation of pharmacological, toxicological, and clinical activities of candidate drugs (2).

Immunoassays generally vary in the type of critical antibody binding reagent or the detection and reporter systems used to monitor the end-point of the binding reaction. These different types of immunoassays have many characteristics in common; therefore, this chapter will include discussions of both enzyme immunoassays and other closely related methods. The enzyme immunoassay technique has been the subject of several textbooks, monographs, and review articles, including an excellent, comprehensive discussion in an earlier edition of this series (3). Thus, this chapter does not provide an in-depth review of the mechanistic details for producing and processing antibodies as reagents or on assay conditions for enzyme immunoassay. Rather, the intent is to present this technique in the context of several primary topics, namely the range of bioanalytical applications, the different, and sometimes additional, validation considerations imposed upon an enzyme immunoassay and its fraternal immunoassay methods, and some newer techniques that are complementary to enzyme immunoassay and offer potential performance enhancements. The chapter is written from the perspective of bioanalysis in biological fluids and does not address in any detail other applications of enzyme immunoassay, such as support of process control or product release, although such topics have been addressed elsewhere (4).

FORMAT OF ENZYME IMMUNOASSAYS

The format of an enzyme immunoassay refers to the configuration in which the components of the assay are assembled for routine application. Once this format has been established and assay conditions defined during assay development, they must remain unchanged through validation and subsequent application to sample analysis. Enzyme immunoassay formats fall broadly into two categories, namely heterogeneous and homogeneous. In a heterogeneous assay, at least one key reagent is immobilized on a solid surface and there is at least one "washing" step before the final detection step. In contrast, in a homogeneous assay, all reagents are in solution together and there is no "washing" step prior to signal generation and detection. Both categories of assay include formats described as competitive and noncompetitive. In a competitive assay, there is direct competition between the labeled and the unlabeled antigen (analyte or ligand) in solution or, in some cases, between immobilized and soluble antigen for a limited number of antibody binding sites. In noncompetitive assays, antibody binding sites to capture and detect the antigen are not limiting because the antigen is incubated with excess capture antibody and enzyme-labeled detection antibody. An example of a competitive homogeneous assay format is the enzyme-multiplied immunoassay (EMIT) system (5), in which enzyme-labeled antigen competes directly in solution with unlabeled antigen in the biological sample (or calibration standard and quality control samples) for a limited number of antibody binding sites. The reaction endpoint is detected and quantitated spectrophotometrically without any intervening wash steps. This assay configuration is shown in Fig. 1. Enzyme-linked immunosorbent assay (ELISA) is an example of a heterogenous noncompetitive immunoassay. In this format, the primary antibody against the analyte of interest is immobilized on a solid plastic surface, usually a multiwell (or microtiter) plate. The biological sample is dispensed into the multiwell plate and incubated. The immobilized antibody then captures the analyte of interest, and the excess analyte is removed by washing. The antigen–antibody complex is then detected by two-step incubation with conjugated antibody and its substrate. First, an enzyme-labeled antibody, directed against the captured analyte, sandwiches the immobilized antibody–antigen complex. In a second incubation with an appropriate enzyme-specific substrate solution, a colored (or fluorescent or chemiluminescent) product is generated and quantitated spectrophotometrically. This assay format is depicted in Fig. 2. The ELISA can also be established in a competitive heterogenous format in which the antigen is immobilized on a multiwell plate and competition is established between the immobilized antigen and the antigen in solution for a limited number of binding sites on the primary antibody, also in solution. Following a fixed incubation period, the plates are washed and incubated with excess enzyme-labeled secondary antibody (directed against immunoglobulin from the species in which the primary, anti-antigen antibody was generated). The endpoint of this competition is then detected, following appropriate washing steps, by incubations with a signal-generating substrate. This assay format is depicted in Fig. 3.

It should be noted that the relationship between the final signal output and concentration of the analyte (dose–response) may be one of direct or inverse proportionality, and is dependent on the specific assay format. In addition, a number of different reporter enzymes may be used (e.g., horseradish peroxidase, alkaline phosphatase, β-galactosidase), along with a number of different signaling systems (e.g., substrates that yield chromogenic or fluorescent or chemiluminescent products, activation of signaling enzymes, amplification by biotin–avidin system or polymerase chain reaction).

ENZYME IMMUNOASSAYS FOR LOW-MOLECULAR-WEIGHT ANALYTES

Although the advent of sensitive LC–MS assays with short development times has reduced the need for immunoassays for low-molecular-weight compounds, the sensitivity, high-throughput and relatively low-cost characteristics of these assays still allow them to play an important role in some cases. Immunoassay support at the drug discovery stage may still be viable in such areas as the evaluation of biomarkers or determination of peptides, in which the elimination of sample cleanup prior to assay may constitute a valuable advantage of immunoassay over LC–MS. In addition, for low-molecular-weight therapeutic candidates, immunoassays can be used to support late-stage (Phases III and IV) clinical trials, when the metabolic pathways and the use of concomitant medications have been clearly defined. Critical to the application of immunoassay for analysis of low-molecular-weight compounds is the development of an antibody with clearly defined specificity for the analyte of interest. Low-molecular-weight compounds (less than 1000–2000 Da) are generally nonimmunogenic, or only weakly immunogenic, when administered directly to animals. To elicit an immune response producing antibodies suitable for use as reagents in immunoassays, these compounds must be conjugated to a carrier protein, e.g., bovine serum albumin (BSA), prior to immunization. This subject has been reviewed in depth previously (3). The immune system of the immunized animal responds to the carrier, and then secondarily to the hapten (the analog of the analyte bound to the carrier protein) attached to it. Although antibodies to the carrier protein are often produced in large amounts, they are easily removed by such techniques as affinity chromatography (6). Conversely, the desired antibodies to the analyte may be removed by affinity chromatography, which may also improve their specificity by eliminating or reducing

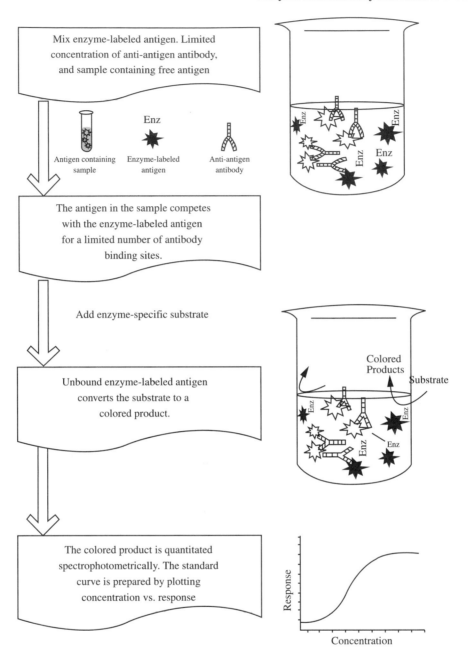

Fig. 1 An illustration of enzyme-multiplied immunoassay.

antibody populations that may cross-react with closely related chemicals, such as metabolites or degradation products. However, in many cases, carrier antibodies do not interfere in the assay to quantitate the analyte of interest and, therefore, anti-antigen antibodies in crude antiserum may be used in immunoassays without further purification. The site of attachment of the hapten to the carrier protein (either directly with the molecule via functional groups that are suitable for chemical coupling, or via a synthetic analog prepared to incorporate chemical

coupling functionality) will determine the specificity profile of the resulting antiserum. As a result, the site of attachment of hapten to carrier protein must be selected judiciously, considering all available knowledge of the metabolism of the compound in the animal system under investigation. Metabolic changes closest to the site of attachment will be poorly discriminated from the parent molecule, whereas metabolic changes distant from the conjugation site will be distinguished most clearly (i.e., will have lowest cross-reactivity). The ultimate

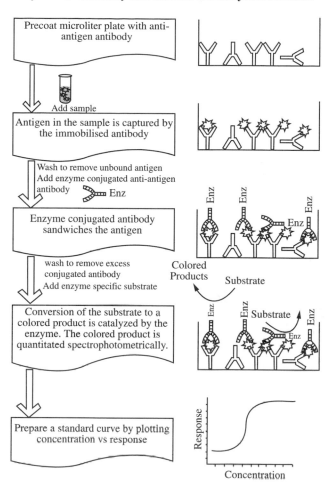

Precoat microliter plate with anti-antigen antibody

Add sample

Antigen in the sample is captured by the immobilised antibody

Wash to remove unbound antigen
Add enzyme conjugated anti-antigen antibody   Enz

Enzyme conjugated antibody sandwiches the antigen

wash to remove excess conjugated antibody
Add enzyme specific substrate

Colored Products

Substrate

Conversion of the substrate to a colored product is catalyzed by the enzyme. The colored product is quantitated spectrophotometrically.

Substrate

Prepare a standard curve by plotting concentration vs response

Response

Concentration

Fig. 2 An illustration of enzyme-linked immunosorbent assay.

result of this strategy is the ability of antibodies, and the resulting assays, to distinguish between enantiomers of chiral drugs (7). Although coupling methods generally have involved condensation reactions of hapten carboxylic or amino groups (or activated derivatives thereof) with amino or carboxylic groups on proteins, newer conjugation methods continue to be developed. These include the use of two-level, heterobifunctional agents such as *N*-(*m*-aminobenzoyloxy) succinimide, first to form a peptide bond to carrier protein and then, following diazotization of the aromatic amino group, to couple to a suitable hapten containing an imidazole, phenol, or indole residue. An example is the coupling of thyroid stimulating hormone to BSA (8). Another example involves interesting steroid chemistry in the preparation of an 11-Alpha-(3-Sulfanylpropyl)oxy hapten analog of the 3-Sulfamate ester of estradiol, and its subsequent coupling to bovine gamma globulin via a heterobifunctional crosslinker (9).

IMMUNOASSAYS FOR MACROMOLECULES

Immunoassays for macromolecules generally fall into one of two categories, namely those for endogenous proteins applied in support of clinical medicine (for example, assays for gonadotrophins or insulin) or those for new, genetically engineered proteins. The advent of genomics, proteomics, and recombinant technology has greatly advanced our understanding of the potential roles of regulatory proteins in the pathogenesis and modulation of diseases, and led to a sharp increase in the number of biological therapeutics under development. Several regulatory proteins are being developed as therapeutic agents and some have reached the market. Fig. 4 indicates the wide distribution of these agents across many different therapeutic categories, with a concentration in the field of cancer treatment. These products are often recombinant analogs of endogenous proteins, with the resulting challenge of developing enzyme immunoassays that are specific enough to distinguish between native and recombinant molecules.

Unlike low-molecular-weight xenobiotics, macromolecules are often immunogenic. An immune response is often elicited against several sites on the molecules called epitopes or antigenic determinants. The number of epitopes per antigen is determined by the size and complexity of the molecule. These epitopes can be linear, consisting of as few as four amino acids in a sequence, or conformational, involving different regions of the molecule in a three-dimensional configuration. Use of antibodies against conformational epitopes can be problematic if the antigen of interest loses its three-dimensional structure in vivo, or during sample analysis. In general, assay formats for macromolecules use at least two antibodies that react with two different regions of the molecule. Use of two antibodies against different regions of the molecule can confer additional specificity and may distinguish the analyte of interest from its metabolites or isoforms.

IMMUNOASSAYS FOR ANTIBODIES

Many of the new biological agents under development are recombinant versions of naturally occurring human proteins, or analogs of human proteins containing minor changes in their primary sequence, or differences in the extent of post-translation modifications. Marketed recombinant proteins include hormones (insulin, erythropoietin and growth hormone), enzymes (DNAase, asparaginase), cytokines (interleukins 1, 2, 11, interferon), growth factors

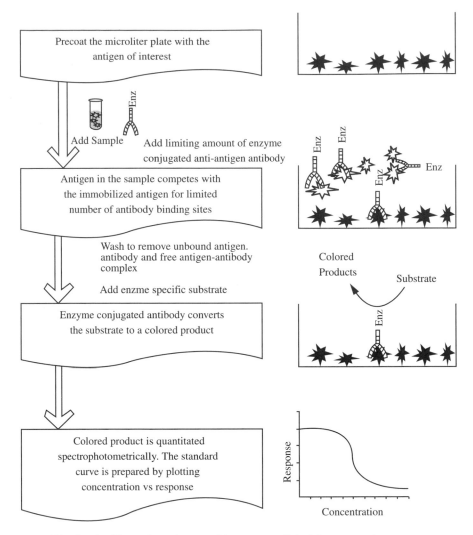

Fig. 3 An illustration of competitive enzyme-linked immunosorbent assay.

(G-CSF, GM-CSF), clotting factors (Factor VIII) and vaccines (hepatitis B). Some other biotechnology products are novel fusion proteins, such as etanercept (Enbrel®), whereas yet others are therapeutic antibodies, for example muromonab (Orthoclone OKT3), abciximab (ReoPro®), and trastuzumab (Herceptin®). Administration of these recombinant proteins to animals and humans may result in their recognition by the host's immune system as "non-self," resulting in an antibody response. Several factors contribute to the potential immunogenicity of these molecules, including the structure of the protein (including post-translation modifications), the presence of protein fragments or protein aggregates in the administered formulation, and the cell substrate or media components that may co-purify with the therapeutic agent. Clinical factors, such as genetic background, disease state or immune status, may also influence the immunogenicity of

a biological product, as well as the route and frequency of dose administration.

In both preclinical and clinical studies, evaluation of immune response to the administered product is necessary to evaluate accurately the safety, pharmacokinetic and pharmacodynamic response as anti-drug antibodies can bind the drug and neutralize the therapeutic effect, or eliminate it by-Fc receptor-mediated uptake and destruction in the reticuloendothelial system. Conversely, the pharmacodynamic response could be enhanced if the distribution or clearance of the drug–antibody complex is altered (10). Antibodies to therapeutic agents may also react with the endogenous analog protein, abrogate its activity, and precipitate a severe adverse event. The presence of such antibodies may also interfere with the immunoassay for the quantitation of the therapeutic agent in biological matrices. In addition, the presence of

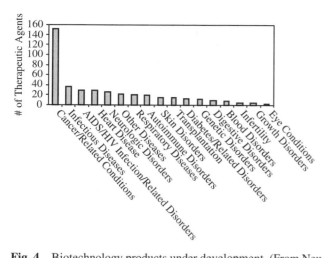

Fig. 4 Biotechnology products under development. (From New Medicines in Development, Biotechnology, PhRMA, April 1998.)

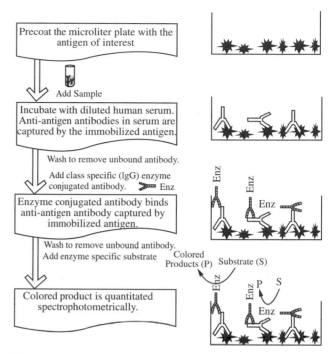

Fig. 5 An illustration of antigen capture antibody detection assay.

pre-existing antibodies (autoantibodies) to endogenous proteins can further complicate the quantitation of the molecule in biological fluids and its safety assessment in preclinical and clinical studies. Anti-drug antibodies may also interfere in imaging and diagnostic procedures utilizing antibodies; for example, human anti-mouse antibodies (HAMA) in the serum of patients treated with a murine antibody-based therapeutic may interfere in diagnostic assays using murine monoclonal antibodies.

Although several immunoassay formats [precipitin reactions, agglutination, radioimmunoassay (RIA), immunoradiometric assay (IRMA), western blot] have been used to detect and quantitate antibodies, enzyme immunoassay is the most commonly applied method. Several factors should be considered when developing an assay to detect the antibody response to a therapeutic agent. It is essential to understand the purpose for the antibody detection assay as it will influence the selection of the assay format. If the aim of the work is to detect only high-affinity antibodies with concomitant high specificity, a competitive assay format would be most appropriate. However, if all antibodies to the administered molecules (regardless of their affinity) are to be detected, best results will be obtained with a noncompetitive ELISA. In addition, random orientation of the antigen to expose all potential epitopes should be confirmed during assay development. These formats are illustrated in Figs. 5, 6. Product characteristics, such as the impurity profile, protein structure, and the presence of fragments and aggregates of the administered protein, need to be understood so that the most appropriate antigen is used in the assay. The potential loss of epitopes when the

protein is directly adsorbed on the surface of the plate, the possibility of circulating antigen–antibody complexes, circulating antigen aggregates, and the source species of antibodies for capture and detection in the assay should also be evaluated. In some instances, cross-reactivity of the detected antibody with subclasses of the macromolecule (e.g., interferon) may need to be evaluated because the binding affinities of each subtype may vary greatly and may influence the interpretation of the results. Pre-existing antibodies can also limit the application of another antibody raised in the same species as that used in the assay configuration (e.g., as the detection antibody). Concomitant medications or high levels of the circulating macromolecular therapeutic agent may also be potential interferents in the assay.

Whether these assays should be established as truly quantitative is controversial. Although a quantitative response seems, from a bioanalytical perspective, desirable, the difficulties in so establishing the assay are significant and the added value is debatable. The primary challenge in developing a quantitative antibody assay is the lack of well-characterized, species-specific, polyclonal anti-drug antibody reference materials to be used as calibration standards (11). Heterologous polyclonal antibody could be used as reference standard (e.g., monkey antibody for human studies), or even nonspecific human IgG. However, although a true quantitative titer

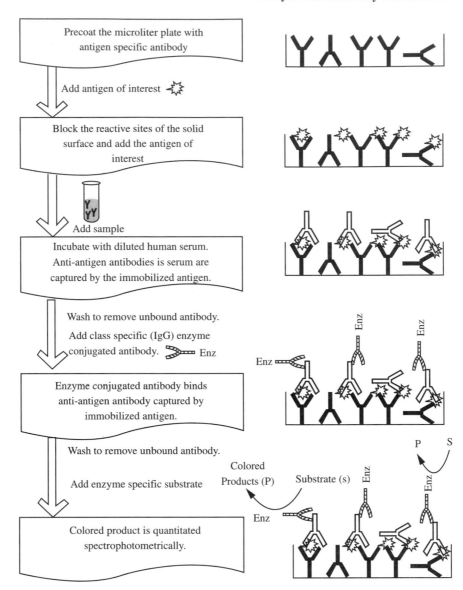

Fig. 6 An illustration of antibody detection method using an antigen–antibody capture configuration.

value may be calculated with reference to a standard of one of these types, the greater value of ELISA assays for antibodies to macromolecules lies in comparative titers determined over time following administration of the candidate therapeutic protein, in conjunction with the assessment of any clinical sequelae.

IMMUNOASSAYS FOR BIOMARKERS

A biomarker is defined as an in vivo biological response to a disease or a toxicological event. Pharmacological markers are a subset of biomarkers that respond to drug intervention, whereas surrogate markers are markers that predict clinical endpoints. In a clinical setting, biomarkers may indicate the response of a disease to therapeutic intervention. In the pharmaceutical industry, correctly chosen biomarkers may help with compound selection, identify mechanism of action, predict dose, demonstrate efficacy and, in cases where sufficiently sensitive assays are unavailable, substitute for direct pharmacokinetic evaluation. Identification of relevant biomarkers at the discovery stage will optimize target selection and validation, facilitate preclinical toxicological evaluation, and markedly shorten the time needed to demonstrate proof of concept in early clinical trials. Rapid and effective implementation of appropriate biomarker assays will result in major resource savings in drug development. A biomarker may be a physiological measurement, such as blood pressure or heart rate, an enzyme activity, or a quantifiable discrete molecule. Biomarkers can be either low-molecular-weight analytes or large macromolecules. Many of these molecules (especially macromolecules) are measured by immunoassay, particularly by enzyme immunoassay.

Many biomarkers are found in blood and urine, where the basal levels may be low or high, depending on the nature of the marker. Thus, one of the additional challenges in establishing enzyme immunoassays for these analytes is obtaining analyte-free matrix for use in preparation of calibration standard and quality control samples. Appropriate analyte-free matrix may sometimes be prepared by extraction of the analyte from matrix by such techniques as affinity chromatography (6) or charcoal adsorption, but care must be taken to ensure that the processed matrix is still representative of the matrix to be analyzed. Alternative solutions to this problem include use of the same matrix type from a different species in which the endogenous biomarker does not occur, pooled baseline samples of low biomarker concentration, or use of a protein-containing buffer. In each case, dilutional linearity of study samples, containing high concentration of the analyte, with the assay matrix should be demonstrated. However, although calibration standards may be prepared in an alternative matrix, whenever possible the quality control samples should be prepared in the matrix to be analyzed so that they reflect the assay performance for the study samples. The concentration range for the calibration standards should attempt to bracket the anticipated concentrations of the biomarkers in both physiological (including such factors as circadian rhythm and intra-individual variability) and pathological states. The concentration levels in the quality controls should also reflect concentration levels in physiological and pathological disease states. Physiological levels may be affected by gender, race, intra-individual variation, circadian rhythm, and seasonal variations, whereas the levels in pathological samples may be affected by stage of the disease, intercurrent disease, current therapies, and overall patient status.

Another challenge in developing assays for biomarkers is the inconsistent availability of well-characterized reference standards. For many macromolecular biomarkers, purified species-specific reference materials are not available. If available, proteins are often not characterized by a standardized method. Different sources of antibodies may also give different results for the same lot of reference standard. It is suggested that crossover studies using standards, quality control pools, and some study samples should be conducted when the source or lot number of reference standard or antibody is changed.

The data from crossover studies will help to normalize study results obtained with different lots of reagents. In addition, biomarkers may exist in multiple forms, such as isoforms, or have homology with other biomarkers in the same class of molecules. Thus, an immunoassay may be developed to measure all forms nonspecifically or target a specific isoform. Cross-reactivity of the antibody selected for use in a biomarker assay should be rigorously tested for potential cross-reactivity with other isoforms and homologous molecules.

VALIDATION OF ENZYME IMMUNOASSAYS

Validation of bioanalytical methods has been a subject of increasing attention over the last 10–15 years. A conference addressing this issue, cosponsored by the US Food and Drug Administration (FDA), the Health Protection Branch (HPB) Canada, the American Association of Pharmaceutical Scientists (AAPS), the European Federation of Pharmaceutical Societies and the United States Pharmacopoeia (USP), was convened in Arlington, Virginia, in December 1990. The proceedings of this meeting, which came to be known as the Crystal City meeting, were published (12) and have subsequently been used as an informal guideline for bioanalytical method validation.

Since 1990, bioanalytical method validation has been a topic of discussion at the International Conference on Harmonization, and was also the topic of a draft guidance document from the FDA (13). Although, many of the validation considerations for chromatographic assays also apply to immunoassay validation, some of the unique considerations for immunoassays were not addressed in the draft guidance. The present authors, along with a number of pharmaceutical industry colleagues, have recently discussed validation issues specific to immunoassays (14). Topics covered in that review included the proper use of quality control (QC) samples for acceptance of assay runs, and statistical aspects of assay validation. Specifically addressed was the issue of how differences in bioanalytical techniques should be considered when developing validation acceptance criteria. In recent years, several publications have reviewed issues related to validation of immunoassays both broadly (15, 16), and specifically for assays for macromolecules (17). In 2000, two conferences were held to "revisit" the issue of bioanalytical methods validation in general (18), as well as specifically for assays for macromolecules, primarily immunoassays and cell-based assays (19).

As for any bioanalytical method, the extent of validation for an immunoassay should be related to the intended application of the assay. Thus, if an immunoassay is intended to support rapid screening in discovery R&D, the characterization of specificity and the accuracy and precision specifications may be less stringent than if the assay is used to support preclinical and clinical development studies. Indeed, an assay for discovery support may be designed to detect active metabolites as well as parent molecule, so that an estimate of total, circulating, pharmacologically active agents may be made. However, at the development stage, such an assay may be applicable only with clear definition of the cross-reactivities of both the parent and the active metabolite in the assay.

DIFFERENTIATING CHARACTERISTICS OF IMMUNOASSAYS AND THEIR IMPACT ON VALIDATION

The key difference between chromatographic assays and immunoassays is the biological nature of the critical binding reagent in an immunoassay, namely the antibody. As antibodies are produced in biological systems, lot-to-lot variability may occur, and this is greatest for polyclonal antibodies because they are produced in whole animals. Monoclonal antibodies, produced from a single cell line in an in vitro biological system, tend to have much lower variability between different production batches. Immunoassays have at least one timed incubation period, which means that variations in binding affinity and avidity between different lots of antibody reagents can result in differences in rates at which equilibrium is reached. Another important difference between immu-noassay and chromatographic assays is the use of analyte–protein and antibody–protein conjugates in immunoassays. During validation, the stability of these critical reagents should be demonstrated to ensure that their degradation does not adversely affect assay performance. The availability of reference standards may also differentiate chromatographic and immunoassay procedures. Thus, although well-characterized reference standards are readily available for low-molecular-weight xenobiotics, it is sometimes much more difficult to obtain similarly well characterized reference materials for macromolecule immunoassays. Macromolecular products are not always available in a highly purified state, and are often characterized in terms of biological activity rather than percentage purity. In some cases, more widely studied proteins are available as reference standards from independent agencies such as the World Health Organization.

Another important difference between immunoassays and most chromatographic assays, with significant implications for validation, is the nonlinear nature of the relationship between concentration and response for immunoassays. For optimum calibration curve fit, it is sometimes appropriate to include calibration points above and below the defined limits of quantitation. The calibration curve fit algorithm should evaluate the overall fit of the experimental data with and without the use of these additional standards in the asymptotic regions of the calibration curve. In general, the authors have observed that the use of additional standards in the asymptotic regions improves the accuracy and precision of the assay at the limits of quantitation. The option to include additional standards is not addressed in the draft FDA guideline for bioanalytical method validation (13), which states that the lowest and highest concentrations on the calibration curve should serve as the limits of quantitation.

Precision, accuracy and specificity also raise some interesting and different considerations for immunoassay methods. The biological nature of the reagents and the antibody–antigen reaction can potentially confer higher imprecision on immunoassays, and a larger number of validation runs may be needed to determine the true precision of the method. This higher imprecision also increases the likelihood that a higher number of assay runs will not meet the so called 4-6-20 rule relating to quality control acceptance criteria for method implementation (20, 21), leading to a recommendation (14, 19) that the 20% limit for accuracy be relaxed to 25% for immunoassays. However, as many immunoassays can also have precision comparable to that of chromatographic methods, the acceptance criteria should be determined based on the demonstrated capability of the method during validation and not set arbitrarily to 4-6-25 for all immunoassays.

Although antibodies can be exquisitely specific, the biological nature of these reagents also poses some new specificity issues for immunoassays when compared to chromatographic assays. In immunoassays, the analyte of interest is usually detected and quantitated directly (i.e., without prior extraction) in complex biological matrices such as serum, plasma, or urine. Furthermore, the specificity of the assay can potentially be compromised if cross-reacting metabolites of the analyte of interest are present in the study sample. Nonspecificity in immunoas-says can arise from a variety of sources, but may be broadly classified as "specific" or "nonspecific" nonspecificity. Specific nonspecificity can arise from interferents that share similar physicochemical characteristics with the analyte of interest, and include metabolites, degraded forms of the analyte, impurities, or concomitant medications. For macromolecules, post-translation modified proteins, protein aggregates or host anti-idiotypic antibodies may affect the specificity of the assay in a "specific" manner. Nonspecific nonspecificity arises from a variety of factors unrelated to the analyte, and is often referred to as "matrix effects." Matrix effects may be due to hemolysis, lipemia, ionic strength differences, pH, serum proteins such as complement or rheumatoid factor, anticoagulants, binding proteins, autoantibodies or heterophilic anti-IgG antibodies. Nonspecific interferences may arise from the matrix chosen for preparation of calibration standards and quality control samples, or the study sample itself. Evaluation of the matrix should include comparison of the concentration–response relationship in spiked (and unspiked) matrix to that in a buffer matrix. Dilution with buffer may adequately decrease the intensity of matrix effects; however, if this approach fails, sample cleanup or full analyte extraction from the matrix may be needed. In these cases, it is important to treat all samples, including calibration standards, quality control or validation samples and study samples, identically, to obviate the need for recovery corrections in the assay.

VALIDATION CONSIDERATIONS FOR IMMUNOASSAYS FOR LOW-MOLECULAR-WEIGHT XENOBIOTICS AND MACROMOLECULES

An essential prerequisite component of small-molecule immunoassay validation is the demonstration of specificity for the analyte of interest. Assay interference (cross-reactivity) due to known metabolites, concomitant medications and, in some cases, endogenous molecules, should be evaluated. These experiments should assess the cross-reactivity of the potential interferents individually and in combination with each other and the analyte of interest to simulate the most likely biological milieu for the analyte. For small molecule immunoassays, the specificity of the assay should be established, whenever possible, by conducting a comparator study over a specified number of analytical runs, using a different, validated and specific bioanalytical method, such as LC–MS. Samples for these comparative analyses should be selected from an earlier study (incurred samples), and should have been collected at two or more time points following drug administration (e.g., approximate time of maximum plasma concentration and a succeeding time corresponding to several elimination half-lives) to allow performance of the immunoassay to be evaluated in an environment of increasing metabolite(s) concentration. If the immunoassay meets the predefined criteria for accuracy and precision

relative to the reference method, the immunoassay may be considered equivalent to the reference method.

The metabolism/catabolism of protein drugs and protein drug candidates is generally much less clearly elucidated than that of conventional small-molecule therapeutics. The dearth of information regarding the metabolism of protein-based drug candidates can hamper efforts to develop a highly specific and accurate enzyme immunoassay. In addition, there are few, sufficiently sensitive, comparator methods available to perform comparative analysis. Approaches to define specificity and, thus, predict reliability of a given assay, include epitope mapping experiments or the use of chromatographic separation prior to immunoassay, although the latter approach can be cumbersome and may result in markedly reduced assay sensitivity. Consequently, complete investigation of assay specificity for a therapeutic protein is more difficult than for a low-molecular-weight xenobiotic. The immunoreactivity of the analyte may be decreased with relatively minor changes in the region of antigenic determinants, such as a change in the amino acid sequence or by oxidation/deamination of an amino acid. On the other hand, proteolytic formation of major fragments of the parent protein may result in retention of the antigenic determinants and preserve the immunoreactivity of the protein metabolite. Such structural changes may or may not result in changes in biological activity, so that immunoreactivity may or may not correlate with biological activity in the study samples collected after administration of the protein. If assay sensitivity permits, methods such as chromatography or electrophoresis, coupled with immunoassay, may shed some light on the structural nature of the compounds in the study samples giving a positive response in the immunoassay. For many recombinant proteins, antigenic determinants of the therapeutic agent are often indistinguishable from those of the endogenous equivalent protein and, therefore, assays for such recombinant proteins are prone to interference from endogenous analog proteins. Such an occurrence poses challenges for the validation analyst in the selection of the preferred homologous matrix for the preparation of calibration standards, validation pools and quality control samples. The problem is accentuated when the administered doses of the exogenous product are so low that circulating concentrations are not increased markedly over the background endogenous concentrations. Clearly, in cases where in vivo concentrations of the exogenous product are very high after dosing, the contribution of low basal levels of the endogenous analyte to the total measured concentration may be small enough to be ignored. An alternative approach to this problem is to remove the endogenous analyte from the matrix by one of a number of methods, as discussed previously (under the heading

"Immunoassays for Biomarkers") or to use a heterologous biological matrix devoid of the specific interfering endogenous substance for the preparation of calibration standards and control samples. In all of these approaches, it is important that the final prepared calibration curve reflects negligible bias due to the presence of endogenous analyte.

VALIDATION CHALLENGES FOR ENDOGENOUS ANALYTE AND BIOMARKER IMMUNOASSAYS

Immunoassays are often developed for the quantitation of endogenous equivalents of therapeutic molecules and biomarkers. Challenges in developing immunoassays for these compounds are similar to those experienced with macromolecules. As the biomarker is normally always present in the matrix of interest, it is difficult to obtain analyte-free matrices. Standard curves and lower limit of quantitation (LLOQ) validation pools may be prepared by choosing and pooling matrix from individuals with low baseline concentrations, diluting baseline samples with a protein-based buffer, or using an alternative species matrix with negligible concentrations of the analyte. The upper limit of quantitation (ULOQ) can be established by fortifying the baseline sample with the analyte of interest. Whenever possible, the appropriate biological matrix should be used for QC sample preparation. This may be a systemic matrix such as whole blood or plasma, or target-specific matrix such as sputum, cerebrospinal fluid, aqueous humor, platelets, T-cells or tissues. Alternatively, if no matrix effects can be demonstrated, quality control pools may be prepared in an "analyte-free" protein-based buffer.

As with macromolecules, obtaining well-characterized reference material can be difficult. Whenever possible, reference materials should also be species-specific. In situations where well-characterized standards are not available, crossover studies should be conducted to permit normalization of data obtained using reference standards from different vendors or different lots.

VALIDATION CONSIDERATIONS FOR IMMUNOASSAYS FOR ANTIBODIES

Anti-drug antibodies are polyclonal in nature and rarely does one have access to species-specific (especially human) anti-drug antibodies to prepare a calibration curve. Despite the problems associated with developing a quantitative anti-drug antibody assay, most validation parameters for immunoassays still apply. Although true accuracy cannot be determined, relative recovery using

quality control samples can be monitored through the life of the assays. Assay specificity evaluation should include assessment of any nonspecific binding of the antibody to the microtiter plate, potential interference of the administered protein, endogenous protein analogs, concomitantly administered drugs, and antigen–antibody complex or cross-reacting antibodies that may be present in the sample under evaluation.

A major issue with anti-drug antibody assays is definition and interpretation of a positive antibody response. During validation, a negative cut-off value, to distinguish antibody negative and positive results, should be determined by evaluating the analytical noise (imprecision) of the assay and the background absorbance readings from individual baseline samples from healthy volunteers and patients from the appropriate disease population. The recommended number of baseline samples is at least 25 (preferably 100) from each of the volunteer and patient groups. If the background responses tend to cluster closely together and the assay is precise, a negative cut-off can be defined as the mean absorbance ± 3 SD at a given dilution factor(s). If, however, there is greater variability in the background absorbance, developing a negative cut-off is more difficult. The cut-off should be based on an acceptable level of false negative and false positive results. The assay validation scheme should include a process to distinguish true responses from false positives. This is particularly important as auto-antibodies against various proteins may be present in otherwise healthy individuals. Several approaches can be taken to elucidate whether an apparent antibody response is truly positive, such as an alternative method for detecting the antibody (e.g., western blotting). In some cases, when antibody response is evaluated against several different antigens, true positives may be distinguished from false positives by cross-reactivity patterns. Finally, examination of the response prior to drug administration, and the change in this response over time, with continued exposure to the agent, will normally distinguish between true and false positives. In addition, results of in vitro neutralizing activity assays and clinical effects (in vivo neutralization) may provide further support for the presence of clinically significant, drug-specific antibodies.

MODERN TECHNOLOGICAL ADVANCES RELATED TO ENZYME IMMUNOASSAY

Immunoassays are inherently sensitive and specific. However, with continued need to develop increasingly sensitive assays to support preclinical and clinical studies, there have been ongoing efforts to enhance the capabilities of these techniques. Advances in critical binding reagents, detection systems, new assay formats and automation have resulted in improved immunoassay technology.

Critical Binding Reagents

Although most immunoassays have used polyclonal antibodies as the critical binding reagents, development of monoclonal antibodies by Kohler and Milstein in 1975 (22), has resulted in their widespread use, particularly in assays for macromolecules. Their unique epitope specificity conveys advantages in double antibody immunoassays for proteins, where one monoclonal antibody may be used to capture the protein by a specific subunit or epitope, and another, directed against a different region or subunit of the protein, may be used to detect it. Use of antibodies against specific regions of the molecule can enhance the specificity of the assay such that one can distinguish the parent molecule from its catabolic products, one isoform from another, or an individual protein from its family members. Although monoclonal antibodies are highly specific, their affinity for the antigen is generally lower than that observed with polyclonal antibodies. Consequently, competitive immunoassays established with monoclonal antibodies as the critical binding reagent are generally less sensitive than those using polyclonal antibodies. For this reason, the application of monoclonal antibodies to competitive immunoassays for low-molecular-weight analytes has been limited.

A nonantibody binding reagent that has received increasing attention recently is the aptamer. Aptamers are oligonucleotide sequences that bind ligands or antigens in a way that is similar in many respects to antibody–ligand interactions (23). Thus, aptamers have been shown to bind with high affinity and selectivity to molecules as diverse as proteins and low-molecular-weight ligands. Aptamer libraries have also been generated, from which members with the desired binding properties may be identified and their concentrations enriched for use in binding assays. The use of these molecules as complements to, or substitutes for, antibodies has been reviewed elsewhere (24). These reagents offer the promise of similar sensitivity and specificity achievable with antibodies, without the need for time-consuming in vivo work to generate them.

Phage display technology provides a source of recombinant antibodies with defined affinity and specificity for use in immunoassay, without the need for extended immunization of animals. This approach involves genetic manipulation of the coat proteins of the filamentous phage, a bacteriophage that lives on *Escherichia coli*. In one approach, the coding sequences of the antibody variable regions (Fv) are first isolated from spleen cells of immunized mice. The coding sequence for a single chain Fv fragment is then fused to the phage coat protein. With the assistance of a series of molecular biology steps, a library containing millions of single-chain antibodies can be displayed on the surface of the phage particles and released into the medium. Through a series of binding and elution steps ("panning"), the mixture of antibodies with the desired affinity and selectivity may be sequentially enriched. To obtain single-chain antibodies of suitable affinity and selectivity against new drug entities, one can repeatedly and rapidly screen the recombinant antibody phage library and avoid the traditional, time-consuming process of antibody production. A detailed discussion of antibody phase display technology is provided in reviews by Hoogenboom (25) or Peterson (26).

Molecularly imprinted polymers (MIPs) also offer some potential as synthetic alternative binding reagents (27) for assay of small molecules. These binding reagents are synthesized by polymerization of functional monomers (e.g., methylacrylic acid, 4-vinyl pyridines) in the presence of the ligand (antigen), which acts as a template. Depending on experimental conditions during polymerization, the template ligand may interact with the monomers by either noncovalent interactions, reversible covalent interactions, or metal-ion-mediated interactions, with the noncovalent approach being most commonly used. Upon completion of the polymerization reaction, the ligand may be washed out to leave its imprint in the polymer. The binding properties of these molecular imprints are characterized by remarkable specificity for the ligand originally imprinted. These MIPs have been applied in place of biologically derived antibodies for the binding assay of a range of low-molecular-weight analytes following extraction of the analyte from the biological matrix. The assays were initially conducted in an organic solvent. Under these conditions, a good correlation was found between the MIP binding assay and an established radioimmunoassay for theophylline (28). Subsequent developments of aqueous assay conditions led to a MIP-based assay for propranolol directly in plasma (29). These high-affinity binding reagents have high chemical and thermal stabilities, resulting in long shelf lives at ambient temperature, an advantage over antibodies. Additionally, although most MIP-based assays have employed radiolabeled analyte as the detection system, some recent studies have successfully used a fluorescence detection system. However, there are currently some limitations with this technology. The MIPs often have lower binding affinities than do antibodies, resulting in lower assay sensitivities than immunoassays have. The use of MIPs is also limited to analytes stable in organic matrices, and further research is necessary to establish them fully in aqueous media, so that they are competitive with conventional immunoassays for the direct analysis of biological fluids.

Detection Systems

The need for greater sensitivity to monitor extremely low concentrations of either highly potent therapeutic agents, endogenous biomarker molecules, or environmental toxicants has been the primary driver in the development of newer detection systems as more sensitive alternatives to the chromogenic substrates normally used in enzyme immunoassay.

There are numerous examples in the literature of fluorescence being used in place of ultraviolet light absorption as the end-point detection system for an immunoassay. In particular, methods using time-resolved fluorescence detection (30) offer high sensitivity while largely avoiding the problem of background fluorescence in complex matrices by allowing this short-lived fluorescence to decay, before fluorescence of the labeled antibody complex is measured. These procedures frequently employ lanthanide chelates as the long-lived fluorophores. An interesting recent example of this method is the time-resolved fluoroimmunoassay for plasma enterolactone, a lignan produced from fiber-rich foods by intestinal bacteria, and thus claimed to be a biomarker of a healthy diet (31). This assay used a derivative of enterolactone coupled with a europium chelate as the fluorophore, and achieved sensitivity of 1.5 nmol/L. Examples from the pharmaceutical field include the assays for enalaprilat in human serum (32) and sampatrilat in human plasma (33), which are characterized by lower limits of quantitation of 200–500 pg/mL. In the technique of fluorescence polarization, detection is based on the change in polarization of light emitted by a fluorophore molecule when bound to an antibody. This change in polarization is correlated with the concentration of unlabeled antigen, and a standard curve is developed to interpolate the analyte concentration in an unknown sample. This method, which has the advantage of being homogeneous and easily automatable, has been widely available commercially for some time for such applications as therapeutic drug monitoring, but more recently has seen new application to high throughput screening in drug discovery (34).

Chemiluminescence (35) offers yet another sensitive detection system, which is easily implemented with simple instrumentation, but suffers to some extent from background interference in complex matrices. A recent example of an enzyme immunoassay with chemiluminescence as the detection system is the assay for 8-oxoguanine in DNA (36), which uses a secondary antibody conjugated with peroxidase–anti-peroxidase complex and a substrate solution containing hydrogen peroxide, luminol and p-Iodophenol.

The utility of chemiluminescence as a detection system has been extended greatly with the development of electrochemiluminescence. Although electrochemiluminescence has been studied since the 1960s, only relatively recently has the system been commercialized by the IGEN Corporation (Rockville, MD). In their system (37), a precursor molecule, tripropylamine (TPA) diffuses to an electrode surface to be activated, resulting in the excitation of a reporter molecule, ruthenium tris-bipyridyl. When the reporter molecule returns to ground state from the excited state, it emits a photon of light at a specific wavelength, which is detected by a sensitive photomultiplier tube. The system includes an electrochemical flow cell and magnetic bead technology to trap the ruthenium-tagged molecules on the electrode and thus allow the electrochemical cycle to proceed. Thus, in a typical immunoassay for a macromolecule, two different anti-analyte antibodies (recognizing different epitopes) may be used. One antibody may be labeled with biotin, which complexes with strepavidin-complexed magnetic beads, whereas the second antibody is labeled with the ruthenium complex. During incubation, the analyte is sandwiched between the two antibodies, after which the mixture is drawn into the flow cell, and the antigen–antibody complex is trapped on the electrode surface by magnetic forces. After washing, the amount of ruthenium complex in the trapped antigen–antibody complex is measured by activating the electrode and quantitating the emitted light. This method has been applied to bioanalysis of many analytes; an example is the biotin–avidin coupled assay for interferon alfa-2b in human serum, with a sensitivity of 4 IU/mL (38).

Detection systems have extended into the area of biosensors and immunosensors, with the application of surface plasmon resonance (SPR) in immunochemistry. SPR is one of a number of optical immunosensor techniques (39) in which a change in the resonance angle of incident light occurs when antigen-antibody binding takes place. In an instrument such as the Biacore, a typical experimental design might involve adsorption of an antibody to the gold or silver surface of a microcell, which is backed by a prism or diffraction grating. When a solution containing the antigen of interest flows through the cell, the formation of the antigen–antibody complex results in a change in the angle of the reflected light (resonance angle) at the metal surface. The shift in the resonance angle has been reported to have a linear relationship to the concentration of antigen added to the system. As no labeled reagents are needed for this method, SPR can be quite simple; however, the technique cannot distinguish between antigen recognition and nonspecific binding, and poor sensitivity can also be a limiting factor. However, recent advances include the incorporation of liposomes linked to a sandwich immunoassay format, resulting in picomolar sensitivity in an assay for interferon (40). In another application for a low-molecular-weight xenobiotic, sulfamethazine, in milk, the analyte was covalently coupled to the gold surface of the sensor chip (41). The final response was the result of competition between covalently bound sulfamethazine and free antigen in calibration solutions and study samples for binding sites on polyclonal antibodies, also in solution. The assay sensitivity was in the range of 1.7–8.0 μg/kg.

Assay Configuration and Automation

When immunoassay specificity has not been inherent in the antibody employed in the assay, separation steps such as high performance liquid chromatography have been applied prior to immunoassay. One of the more promising of such coupled methods is capillary electrophoretic immunoassay (CEIA) (42). This method offers a number of potential advantages, including a smaller sample size and lower reagent consumption, simple and readily automatable process, potential for simultaneous determination of multiple analytes, and a broad range of detection techniques. When coupled with laser-induced fluorescence as the detection method and enzyme amplification, CEIA appears to be competitive with standard immunoassay techniques, with assay sensitivity in the 10-pM range. The resolving capabilities of CEIA can separate antibody-bound from free antigen, followed by application of the detection method. Thus, the technique is configured for on-line application. Although clearly having the potential for high throughput, CEIA has been applied only in a serial mode to date, analyzing one sample at a time. CEIA has been applied widely to the characterization of antibodies, as well as to immunoassay of a number of low-molecular-weight analytes, including digoxin, morphine and cortisol.

Immunoassay has achieved considerable success in the medical diagnostic arena largely due to its facile adaptation to automation, high sample throughput and relatively low per sample cost. Issues and challenges involved in the automation of immunoassays have been addressed recently by Bock (43). An interesting recent application of enzyme immunoassay in an automated mode has been in the support of high throughput screening in drug discovery (44). In this case, the assay reagents are incorporated into a gel matrix rather than in a multiwell format, which permits 1,000–10,000 assays to be run per day, with the assistance of automation, by a single technician. The development of multianalyte immunoassays in miniaturized, microarray formats has also been reported (45).

The move toward automation has also led to development of online and flow injection immunoassays. These methods involve sequential injection of assay reagents and antigen–antibody reactions in flowing systems. One such system with some promise is flow injection renewable surface immunoassay (FIRSI), with fluorescence detection (46). In this flowing system, antibody-coated beads are retained on a flat surface adjacent to the detector; labeled and unlabeled analyte are then injected and flow over the beads, while reaction occurs. The beads are then washed, the final antibody-bound reading occurs at the detector and the flow is reversed to remove the beads in preparation for the next injection. Similar systems, sometimes using magnetic particle-coupled immunoglobulin to facilitate the separation of antibody-bound and free ligand (47), have been used in conjunction with electrochemiluminescence (48) or laser-induced fluorescence (49) as the detection methods.

CONCLUSIONS

Enzyme immunoassay is widely used, both in competitive and noncompetitive formats, for the bioanalysis of a broad range of low-molecular-weight compounds and macromolecules. Through the use of fluorogenic substrates and amplification systems such as avidin–biotin, the sensitivity of enzyme immunoassay has been developed to equal or exceed that of radioimmunoassay (50). The technique has found particularly wide applicability in the determination of new recombinant proteins, in demonstrating antibody responses to macromolecules, and in the measurement of biomarkers of disease, as well as in diagnostic medicine.

As for all bioanalytical methods applied to support of drug development, validation of immunoassays is important. However, several validation issues need special attention for immunoassays. These include stability of the critical reagents, the curvilinear nature of the calibration curve, the greater variability of immunoassays, and, particularly important, the specificity of the assay.

Finally, a number of newer binding reagents, detection methods, assay configurations, and automation applications are being investigated to develop further the potential of immunoassays. These include binding reagents requiring little or no animal immunization for their production, such as phage display antibody libraries, aptamer libraries, and synthetic molecular imprints. Detection methods such as electrochemiluminescence and surface plasmon resonance hold promise of sensitivity equal to, or better than, that of radioimmunoassay without the limitations of radioactivity. Progress has also been made in automation and miniaturization of immunoassays, as well as online techniques, such as CEIA and flow injection methods. These efforts will continue to ensure that improvements in sensitivity and specificity of immunoassays will be widely available through commercialization.

REFERENCES

1. Yalow, R.S.; Berson, S.A. Immunoassay of Endogenous Plasma Insulin in Man. J Clin. Invest. **1960**, *39*, 1157–1175.
2. Colburn, W.A. Selecting and Validating Biologic Markers for Drug Development. J. Clin. Pharmacol. **1997**, *37* (5), 355–362.
3. Tai, H.H. Enzyme Immunoassay, 1st Ed.; *Encyclopedia of Pharmaceutical Technology*, Swarbrick, J., Boylan, J.C., Eds.; Marcel Dekker, Inc.: New York, 1992; 5, 201–233.
4. Mattiasson, B.; Hakanson, H. Immunochemically Based Assays for Process Control. Adv. Biochem. Eng. Biotechnol. **1992**, *46*, 81–102.
5. Rubenstein, K.E.; Schneider, R.S.; Ullman, E.F. "Homogeneous" Enzyme Immunoassay: New Immunochemical Technique. Biochem. Biophys. Res. Commun. **1972**, *47* (4), 846–851.
6. Hage, D.S. Affinity Chromatograpy. Clin. Chem. **1999**, *45* (5), 593–615.
7. Got, P.A.; Scherrmann, J.M. Stereoselectivity of Antibodies for the Bioanalysis of Chiral Drugs. Pharm. Res. **1997**, *14* (11), 1516–1523.
8. Fujiwara, K.; Matsumoto, N.; Masuyama, Y.; Kitagawa, T.; Inoue, Y.; Inouye, K.; Hougaard, D.M. New Hapten-Protein Conjugation Method Using *N*-(*M*-aminobenzoyloxy) Succinimide as a Two-Level Heterobifunctional Agent: Thyrotropin-Releasing Hormone as a Model Peptide without Free Amino or Carboxyl Groups. J. Immunol. Methods **1994**, *175* (1), 123–129.
9. Schwarz, S.; Schumacher, M.; Ring, S.; Nanninga, A.; Weber, G.; Thieme, I.; Undeutsch, B.; Elger, W. 17 β-Hydroxy-11α-(3'-Sulfanylpropyl)oxy-estra-1,3,5(10)-trien-3-yl sulfamate—A Novel Hapten Structure: Toward the Development of a Specific Enzyme Immunoassay (EIA) for Estra-1,3,5(10)-trien-3-yl sulfamates. Steriods **1999**, *64* (7), 460–471.
10. Working, P.K.; Cossum, W.A. Clinical and Preclinical Studies with Recombinant Human Proteins: Effect of Antibody Production. *Pharmacokinetics and Pharmacodynamics: Peptides, Peptoids and Proteins*; Garzone, P.D., Colburn, W.A., Mokotoff, M., Eds.; Ch. 13; Harvey Whitney Books: New York, 1991; 201–233.
11. Food and Drug Administration, Center for Biologics Evaluation and Review. Meeting of the Biological, Response Modifiers Advisory Committee, Bethesda, Maryland, July, 15, 1999.
12. Shah, V.P.; Midha, K.K.; Dighe, S.; McGilveray, I.J.; Skelly, J.P.; Yacobi, A.; Layloff, T.; Viswanathan, C.T.; Cook, C.E.; McDowell, R.D.; Pittman, K.A.; Spector, S. Analytical Methods Validation: Bioavailability, Bioequivalence and Pharmacokinetic Studies. Pharm. Res. **1992**, *9*, 588–592.
13. Food and Drug Administration, Draft Guidance for Industry on Bioanalytical Methods Validation for Human Studies, Docket No 98D-1168, Federal Register *64*, 1999; 517.
14. Findlay, J.W.A.; Smith, W.C.; Lee, J.W.; Nordblom, G.D.; Das, I.; DaSilva, B.S.; Khan, M.N.; Bowsher, R.R. Validation of Immunoassays for Bioanalysis: A Pharmaceutical Industry Perspective. J. Pharm. Biomed. Anal. **2000**, *21*, 1249–1273.
15. Findlay, J.W.A.; Das, I. Some Validation Considerations for Immunoassay. J. Clin. Ligand Assay **1997**, *20* (1), 49–55.
16. Findlay, J.W.A. Validation in Practice–Experience with Immunoassay. *Bio-International 2. Bioavailability, Bioequivalence and Pharmacokinetic Studies*; Blume, H.H., Midha, K.K., Eds.; Medpharm Scientific Publishers: Stuttgart, 1995; 361–370.
17. Findlay, J.W.A.; Das, I. Validation of Immunoassays for Macromolecules from Biotechnology. J. Clin. Ligand Assay **1998**, *21* (2), 249–253.
18. Shah, V.P.; Midha, K.K.; Findlay, J.W.A.; Hill, H.M.; Hulse, J.D.; McGilveray, I.J.; McKay, G.; Miller, K.J.; Patnaik, R.N.; Powell, M.L.; Tonelli, A.; Viswanathan, C.T.; Yacobi, A. Bioanalytical Method Validation: A Revisit with a Decade of Progress. Pharm. Res. **2000**.
19. AAPS Workshop. Bioanalytical Methods Validation for Macromolecules, Arlington, VA, 1–3 March 2000, American Association of Pharmaceutical Scientists: Alexandria, VA.
20. Smith, W.C.; Sittampalam, G.S. Conceptual and Statistical Issues in the Validation of Analytic Dilution Assays for Pharmaceutical Application. J. Biopharm. Stat. **1998**, *8* (4), 509–532.
21. Kringle, R.O. An Assessment of the 4-6-20 Rule for Acceptance of Analytical Runs in Bioavailability, Bioequivalence, and Pharmacokinetic Studies. Pharm. Res. **1994**, *11* (4), 556–560.
22. Kohler, G.; Milstein, C. Continuous Culture of Fused Cells Secreting Specific Antibody of Predefined Specificity. Nature **1975**, *256* (5517), 495–497.
23. Ellington, A.D.; Szostak, J.W. In Vitro Selection of RNA Molecules that Bind Specific Ligands. Nature **1990**, *346* (6287), 818–822.
24. Jaysena, S.D. Aptamers: An Emerging Class of Molecules That Rival Antibodies in Diagnostics. Clin. Chem. **1999**, *45* (9), 1628–1650.
25. Hoogenboom, H.R.; de-Bruine, A.P.; Hufton, S.E.; Hoet, R.M.; Arends, J.W.; Roovers, R.C. Antibody Phage Display

Technology and its Applications. Immunotechnology **1998**, *4* (1), 1–20.

26. Peterson, N.C. Recombinant Antibodies: Alternative Strategies for Developing and Manipulating Murine-Derived Monoclonal Antibodies. Lab. Anim. Sci. **1996**, *46* (1), 8–14.

27. Andersson, L.I. Molecular Imprinting for Drug Bioanalysis: A Review on the Application of Imprinted Polymers to Solid-Phase Extraction and Binding Assay. J. Chromatogr. B **2000**, *739* (1), 163–173.

28. Vlatakis, G.; Andersson, L.I.; Muller, R.; Mosbach, K. Drug Assay Using Antibody Mimics Made by Molecular Imprinting. Nature **1993**, *361* (6413), 645–647.

29. Bengtsson, H.; Roos, U.; Andersson, L.I. Molecular Imprint-Based Radioassay for Direct Determination of S-Propranolol in Human Plasma. Anal. Commun. **1997**, *34* (9), 233–235.

30. Dickson, E.F.; Pollack, A.; Diamandis, E.P. Ultrasensitive Bioanalytical Assays Using Time-Resolved Fluorescence Detection. Pharma. Ther. **1995**, *66* (2), 207–235.

31. Adlercreutz, H.; Wang, G.J.; Lapcik, O.; Hampl, R.; Wahala, K.; Makela, T.; Lusa, K.; Talme, M.; Mikola, H. Time-Resolved Fluoroimmunoassay for Plasma Enterolactone. Anal. Biochem. **1998**, *265* (2), 208–215.

32. Yuan, A.S.; Gilbert, J.D. Time-Resolved Fluoroimmunoassay for the Determination of Lisinopril and Enalaprilat in Human Serum. J. Pharm. Biomed. Anal. **1996**, *14* (7), 773–781.

33. Venn, R.F.; Bernard, G.; Kaye, B.; Macrae, P.V.; Saunders, K.C. Clinical Analysis of Sampatrilat, a Combined Renal Endopeptidase and Angiotensin-Converting Enzyme Inhibitor II: Assay in Plasma and Urine of Human Volunteers by Dissociation Enhanced Lanthanide Fluorescence Immunoassay (DELFIA). J. Pharm. Biomed. Anal. **1998**, *16* (5), 883–792.

34. Nasir, M.S.; Jolley, M.E. Fluorescence Polarization: An Analytical Tool for Immunoassay and Drug Discovery. Comb. Chem. High Throughput Screen **1999**, *2* (4), 177–190.

35. Baeynes, W.R.; Schulman, S.G.; Calokerinos, A.C.; Zhao, Y.; Garcia-Campana, A.M.; Nakashima, K.; De Keukeleire, D. Chemiluminescence-Based Detection: Principles and Analytical Applications in Flowing Streams and in Immunoassays. J. Pharm. Biomed. Anal. **1998**, *17* (6/7), 941–953.

36. Bruskov, V.I.; Masalimov, Z.K.; Usacheva, A.M. Chemiluminescence Enzyme Immunoassay of 8-Oxoguanine in DNA. Biochemistry (Moscow) **1999**, *64* (7), 803–808.

37. Yang, H.; Leland, J.K.; Yost, D.; Massey, R.J. Electrochemiluminescence: A New Diagnostic and Research Tool. Biotechnology **1994**, *12* (2), 193–194.

38. Obenauer-Kutner, L.J.; Jacobs, S.J.; Kolz, K.; Tobias, L.M.; Bordens, R.W.A. A Highly Sensitive Electrochemiluminescence Immunoassay for Interferon Alfa-2b in Human Serum. J. Immunol. Meth. **1997**, *206* (1-2), 25–33.

39. Rabbany, S.Y.; Donner, B.L.; Ligler, F.S. Optical Immunosensors. Crit. Rev. Biomed. Eng. **1994**, *22* (5-6), 307–346.

40. Wink, T.; van Zuilen, S.J.; Bult, A.; van Bennekom, W.P. Liposome-mediated Enhancement of the Sensitivity in Immunoassays of Proteins and Peptides in Surface Plasmon Resonance Spectrometry. Anal. Chem. **1998**, *70* (5), 827–832.

41. Gaudin, V.; Pavy, M-L. Determination of Sulfamethazine in Milk by Biosensor Immunoassay. J. AOAC Int. **1999**, *82* (6), 1316–1320.

42. Bao, J.J. Capillary Electrophoretic Immunoassays. J. Chromatogr. B **1997**, *699* (1/2), 463–480.

43. Bock, J.L. The Era of Automated Immunoassay. Am. J. Clin. Pathol. **2000**, *113* (5), 628–646.

44. Karet, G. More Compound Tested with Less Automation. Drug Dis. Dev. **June-July 2000**, *48–51*.

45. Silzel, J.W.; Cercek, B.; Dodson, C.; Tsay, T.; Obremski, R.J. Mass-Sensing, Multianalyte Microarray Immunoassay with Imaging Detection. Clin. Chem. **1998**, *44* (9), 2036–2043.

46. Pollema, C.H.; Ruzicka, J. Flow Injection Renewable Surface Immunoassay: A New Approach to Immunoanalysis with Fluorescence Detection. Anal. Chem. **1994**, *66* (11), 1825–1831.

47. Sole, S.; Alegret, S.; Cespedes, F.; Fabregas, E.; Diez-Caballero, T. Flow Injection Immunoanalysis Based on a Magnetoimmunosensor System. Anal Chem. **1998**, *70* (8), 1462–1467.

48. Arai, K.; Takahashi, K.; Kusu, F. An Electrochemiluminescence Flow-Through Cell and its Applications to Sensitive Immunoassays Using N-(aminobutyl)-N-ethylisoluminol. Anal. Chem. **1999**, *71* (11), 2237–2240.

49. Tao, L.; Kennedy, R.T. On-line Competitive Immunoassay for Insulin Based on Capillary Electrophoresis with Laser-Induced Fluorescence Detection. Anal Chem. **1996**, *68* (22), 3899–3906.

50. Hashida, S.; Hashinaka, K.; Ishikawa, E. Ultrasensitive Enzyme Immunoassay. Biotechnol. Ann. Rev. **1995**, *1*, 403–451.

EQUIPMENT CLEANING

Destin A. LeBlanc

Cleaning Validation Technologies, San Antonio, Texas

INTRODUCTION

REGULATORY BACKGROUND

GMP Issues

Cleaning of process equipment has been part of the good manufacturing practices (GMPs) for pharmaceutical manufacturing for many years (1, 2). This has included recommendations for written procedures, cleaning logs, and appropriate design of equipment to facilitate cleaning. Good cleaning practices are necessary to preserve the safety and efficacy of the manufactured drugs and drug products. Possible consequences of inadequate cleaning include cross-contamination (the presence of one drug active in another drug product at an unacceptable level), the presence of foreign material (e.g., a cleaning agent, solvent, or excipient from another drug product), the presence of microbial contamination (numbers and/or species of microbes), or the presence of endotoxins (particularly in parenteral or ophthalmic products). The presence of such contaminants in a drug product may pose safety problems depending on the level of the contaminant. Such contaminants may also affect the efficacy of a drug product; effects could include modifying the bioavailability of the active, the dissolution time of tablets, or the stability of the finished drug. Needless to say, failing to follow GMPs relating to cleaning processes also renders the product "adulterated" and subject to regulatory action.

Expectation of Validation

What is new since about 1990 is the regulatory expectation that certain cleaning processes in pharmaceutical manufacturing be validated. Validation of cleaning processes had been discussed in numerous articles prior to that time (3, 4). However, issues with drug product contamination due to poorly controlled cleaning processes (5), culminating in the Barr Laboratories decision (6), brought this issue to the forefront and clearly established the FDA's authority to require the validation of cleaning processes. As cleaning is a process, the principles of process validation apply to the cleaning process. The Barr decision was followed soon by FDA cleaning validation guidance documents in 1992 (7) and 1993 (8). In 1996, the FDA proposed amendments to the GMPs which clearly defined (if approved) validation of cleaning processes as a GMP requirement (9). The U.S. FDA took the lead in requiring validation of cleaning processes, and other agencies also issued similar requirements. This includes the Pharmaceutical Inspection Cooperation Scheme (PIC/S) document PR-1-99 (10), the Draft Annex 15 to the EU GMPs (11), and the Canadian Therapeutic Products Programme "Cleaning Validation Guidelines" (12). Although the initial emphasis was on cleaning validation related to finished drug products, additional guideline documents clarified that cleaning validation should be considered for active pharmaceutical ingredients (13, 14) and for pharmaceutical excipients (15).

Applicability of Cleaning Validation

It should be noted that these cleaning validation requirements apply only to *critical* cleaning processes. Although GMPs require the cleaning of (and cleaning SOPs for) floors, walls, and the outside of process vessels, such processes are not considered critical cleaning processes. The processes that are critical generally include processes for cleaning product-contact surfaces of equipment or utensils. It is these product-contact surfaces that have the possibility of *directly* contaminating the next product made in the same equipment. In addition, the cleaning of nonproduct-contact surfaces that could reasonably *indirectly* contaminate subsequently manufactured products should also be considered for cleaning validation. For example, some companies have, either on their own or because of regulatory requirements, validated the cleaning of internal surfaces of lyophilizers used for production. On the other hand, validation of cleaning between lots of the same product is not necessarily a requirement (16). This is based on the fact that cross-contamination of the active is not an issue. However, other concerns such as contamination with degradation products, with cleaning agent residues, or with microorganisms may suggest that such cleaning is critical, and therefore should be validated.

boilerplate
Encyclopedia of Pharmaceutical Technology
Copyright © 2002 by Marcel Dekker, Inc. All rights reserved.

CLEANING PROCESSES

The overall cleaning process comprises the soiled equipment, a cleaning method with the associated cleaning equipment, a cleaning agent(s), and process parameters (time, temperature, etc.). These factors should all be captured in a cleaning standard operating procedure (SOP).

Equipment Design

As regards the equipment to be cleaned, this depends on both the equipment itself and the residues to be removed. Ideally the equipment to be cleaned has been designed with cleaning in mind. Design characteristics may be different for manual versus automated cleaning. The equipment design may also affect the extent of disassembly of the equipment as part of the cleaning process. Design characteristics that help maximize cleaning include minimizing deadlegs, minimizing cracks and crevices where soils can be trapped, improving accessibility of the cleaning solution to difficult-to-clean portions of the equipment, and providing adequate drainage. Materials of construction should be selected for the equipment based on the expected cleaning process; such materials may affect both chemical (such as acids, alkalis, and solvents) and physical (such as temperature) compatibility. Although it is difficult to cover all the possibilities because of the varieties of equipment to be cleaned, the principle is the same—the selection of the cleaning process will be limited by the original equipment design (except to the extent that such designs can be modified).

Cleaning Methods

Although cleaning methods are sometimes divided into clean-in-place (CIP) and clean-out-of-place (COP) applications, it may be more useful to consider two significant features of cleaning methods to provide broad categorizations of cleaning processes.

Extent of automation

One factor involves the extent of automation. At one extreme of the "automation" continuum is the fully automatic process—no operator intervention is required for preparation of the cleaning solution, for the cleaning cycle, or for any disassembly or reassembly. The only operator requirement might be pushing a button at the beginning of a cycle, recording the cleaning process in the cleaning log book, and perhaps a visual examination as part of the monitoring procedure at the end of cleaning (and/or before the manufacture of the next product). At the other extreme is the fully manual process. The operator is required for preparation of the cleaning solution, for isolating the system to be cleaned, for applying the cleaning solution, perhaps for applying mechanical action through brushes or wipers, for rinsing the system, and for monitoring process parameters (including the timing of all events). It should be clear that in between these two extremes are various semiautomated processes, which could cover a broad continuum.

Extent of disassembly

A second continuum for cleaning processes involves the degree of disassembly (and consequent reassembly). At one extreme is equipment that requires no disassembly at all (true "clean-in-place"). At the other extreme is equipment that requires disassembly of each component part for cleaning. Disassembly (and reassembly) is preferably avoided for several reasons, including the time it adds to the overall cleaning process (equipment downtime), the concern over damage to the equipment because of stresses during the disassembly/reassembly process, and the concern over incorrect reassembly. However, it should be recognized that there are situations in which partial or complete disassembly of equipment might be required. This includes the removal of filters prior to cleaning, or the opening of a process vessel for placement of a spray device of a portable CIP system into the vessel.

Simplification of cleaning processes

Design of a cleaning process must be taken into consideration not only the nature of the process itself but also the engineering design of the equipment to be cleaned, the various products manufactured in the equipment (such products become "soils" to be cleaned at the end of manufacturing), and the cleaning process parameters (discussed in more detail later). In many pharmaceutical facilities, the objective is to make the process as simple and universal as possible so that one cleaning SOP can be used either for all manufactured products made in the same equipment or for all equipment cleaned in the same process. This simplifies documentation and training and may (because of grouping or bracketing strategies) simplify validation.

Cleaning process steps

The general steps or stages of most cleaning processes involve the following:

Disassembly and isolation: This involves preparation of the equipment for application of the cleaning solution(s). Disassembly may involve complete disassembly for washing individual parts elsewhere, or may involve partial disassembly, such as removal of filters for separate cleaning elsewhere. The preferred technique for cleaning is to isolate the equipment (or parts thereof) and then clean the entire isolated portion. In a validated process, it is difficult to clean only one portion of a piece of equipment without isolating it (for example, trying to clean a storage vessel only to the level of product in the vessel; the entire vessel, including the vessel dome, should be cleaned).

Prewashing (or prerinsing): In aqueous cleaning, this involves flushing all parts of the system with water (usually at ambient temperature) to physically remove soils that can be readily removed by a flowing water stream. The purpose of the prewash is to minimize soils on the surface for the cleaning step. In this manner, the action of those cleaning agents in the cleaning step are focused on residues that are more tenaciously bound to the surface. In biotechnology manufacture or any manufacture that involves proteinaceous deposits, a second objective of this prewash is to prevent "setting" of those proteinaceous deposits when they are immediately cleaned with a hot water solution. If the cleaning process uses a CIP system, the prewash step is usually a "once through to drain" rather than a recirculating process. The objective is to immediately remove loosely bound soils and discharge them from the equipment rather than to spread them evenly over all equipment surfaces (which would occur to a certain extent in a recirculating system).

Washing: This involves application of the cleaning solution (which may be plain water, but which usually involves some cleaning agent) to all equipment surfaces to effectively remove those soils not removed by the prewash. The washing step may involve continuous application of fresh cleaning solution (such as in a non-recirculating CIP system or in a manual application using a high pressure spray hose), a recirculating application of the cleaning agent in which partially "depleted" cleaning solution is reapplied to surfaces (as in a recirculating CIP system or an automatic machine parts washer), or a static soak of equipment or utensils. The purpose of the washing step is to either dissolve, solubilize, emulsify, suspend, or chemically affect the soils on the surface so they can be readily removed from the equipment either in the washing step (in a non-recirculating process) and/or the rinse step.

Rinsing: The rinsing step is designed to remove both washing solution and associated soluble, solubilized, emulsified, or suspended soils from the equipment. For solvent cleaning, the rinsing solution is usually a fresh application of the same solvent used for the washing step. In aqueous processing, the rinsing solution is usually water. The rinsing step should usually be a non-recirculating application of the rinsing solution. A general rule of thumb followed for finished product manufacture involving aqueous-based drug products is that the quality of water used in the final rinse should be at least as good as the quality of water used in the manufacture of the next product. The rationale behind this is that any water contaminants in the final rinse left behind on equipment surfaces by the final rinse are identical in quality to water used in manufacturing of the next product. If the drug does not contain water, such as in the manufacture of a synthetic organic active substance, there may be other considerations for the selection of the quality of the final rinse water. A common practice in bulk pharmaceutical manufacture, suitable for most applications where aqueous cleaning is performed, is to use deionized water as a final rinse.

Drying: Drying is an optional step. One factor in whether drying should be done is the time period before the next use of the equipment. Equipment that is to be used immediately (within a few hours) may not have to be dried, particularly if the equipment is effectively drained to minimize any dilution effect of residual rinse water or solvent. However, the effect of residual water on microbial proliferation during extended storage is a significant issue. Options for drying include heated (and optionally filtered) air and the use of a final alcohol/water rinse. The final alcohol/water rinse may also further reduce the bioburden due to the antimicrobial action of the alcohol. This use has to take into consideration the flammability of such a mixture.

Reassembly and storage: These should be part of the cleaning SOP. "Reassembly" may involve removal of temporarily installed cleaning equipment (e.g., the spray device of a portable CIP unit) or reassembly of equipment parts themselves. If the equipment is to be stored for a significant time before reuse, critical elements for storage include whether the equipment is dry, physical protection of equipment from recontamination by use of items such as plastic wrapping, and the room conditions (air quality, temperature, and humidity) where the equipment is stored. Typically it is expected that stored equipment will be tagged as cleaned with an expiration (or "use by") date. Expiration dates for stored equipment are established based on the possible routes and extent of recontamination during storage. For storage, the focus of regulatory agencies is microbial contamination; however, other types of contamination should also be evaluated.

Automated CIP systems

The discussion of CIP processes deserves special comment because of industry trends to use CIP systems. As used in a broad sense, CIP refers to any system in which the equipment is cleaned with no or minimal disassembly. In a more narrow sense (and in this sense it is more commonly used now), CIP is used to refer to systems in which one or more spray devices is placed in the equipment to be cleaned. A control unit, comprising a pump, associated valves, and a PLC (programmable logic controller), pumps a cleaning solution from a storage tank through the spray device(s). The spray device(s) is engineered and placed so that solution is either directly sprayed or else sprayed so that the solution cascades down the equipment sidewalls to cover all surfaces of the equipment for effective cleaning. In a non-recirculating CIP system, the cleaning solution passes once through the process vessel and associated piping, and then goes to drain. In a recirculating system, the cleaning solution passes through the process vessel and associated piping and then back to the cleaning solution storage tank. It is then pumped through the spray device again, for multiple passes.

The spray device may be either permanently mounted in the process vessel, or installed for cleaning and then removed for product manufacture. Spray devices may be stationary. Stationary spherical devices, the most common type, are called "spray balls." Spray balls are usually stainless steel hollow spheres in which holes are drilled. The placement of the holes is designed to provide adequate coverage for the vessel to be cleaned. Stationary spray devices are usually considered "sanitary" because they are self-draining. The other type of spray device is a dynamic (or rotating) spray device. These are similar in principle to a stationary spray device (they are designed to distribute cleaning solution over all surfaces of the process vessel) except that dynamic spray devices will rotate in one or more planes to provide more even distribution of the cleaning solution. Dynamic spray devices also typically operate at high spray pressures, so that the impingement of the cleaning solution on the vessel surfaces provides more mechanical energy to help dislodge residues. Dynamic spray devices are typically not mounted permanently because they are not self-draining (and thus sanitary); however, some newer dynamic devices are claimed to be sanitary.

A key to operation and validation of a spray device is to perform a "coverage" test, such as a "riboflavin test." Riboflavin is readily water soluble, and also fluoresces under an ultraviolet light. Such a test involves spraying the interior surfaces of the equipment with a dilute solution of riboflavin. A short CIP rinse cycle is then performed using just water in a non-recirculating mode. Following this, the interior surfaces are examined using an ultraviolet light source. If any surfaces fluoresce green, it is an indication that solution coverage in those areas may be inadequate. Poor coverage should require a redesign of the spray device system, either by adding additional spray devices,

using a different spray device, or by drilling additional holes in a stationary spray ball. Such a modified spray system should be retested for adequate coverage. Such riboflavin testing is usually part of the operational qualification (OQ) of the equipment.

Cleaning Agents

Aqueous vs. nonaqueous

In addition to the cleaning method used, the cleaning agents used in the washing step are critical. It should be appreciated that selection of the cleaning method and cleaning agent(s) are somewhat interdependent. Selection of a cleaning method may limit the available cleaning agents that can effectively be used in that process. For example, a CIP process requires a low foaming aqueous cleaning agent, while extent of foam may not be critical for manual cleaning. Cleaning agents may be divided into aqueous and nonaqueous cleaning products. Nonaqueous products are typically solvents, and are more common in cleaning in the bulk manufacture of an active pharmaceutical ingredient (API). Typically, the solvent used for cleaning is the same as that used for manufacture. The cleaning effectiveness depends on the solubility of the residue(s) in the solvent at the temperature of cleaning. Particularly for cleaning of distillation columns, refluxing with a volatile solvent is a common practice for effective cleaning. The trend in the manufacture of APIs is to move away from solvent cleaning to aqueous cleaning. However, it should recognized that in many cases this not practical, and even if it is, the aqueous cleaning may be followed by one or more solvent flushes to remove the water from the process vessels.

Types of aqueous cleaning agents

Aqueous processes involve cleaning with water and, optionally, other ingredients to assist in the cleaning process. If aqueous cleaning can be suitably performed, it is preferred over solvent cleaning because of cost issues (including the cost of the solvent as well as the costs of disposal or reclamation of the solvent) and because of environmental issues relating to the use or emissions of solvents. In aqueous processes, the use of water alone should be considered because it eliminates the concerns over having to consider potential contaminants from the cleaning agent during cleaning validation. However, in most cases, the performance characteristics of various aqueous cleaning agents more than overcome the concerns about cleaning agent residues (particularly if the cleaning agents selected are free-rinsing). The successful use of water alone for the washing step depends solely on the solubility of the residues in water at the temperature of cleaning, and may not typically provide other cleaning mechanisms such as emulsification and dispersion. Therefore, use of water alone may not meet other cleaning objectives such as short processing times.

Another option for aqueous cleaning involves the use of commodity chemicals, including alkalis such as sodium or potassium hydroxide, acids such as phosphoric or citric acid, or sodium hypochlorite solution. These are typically diluted in water at levels of 0.05–1% (w/w), and the resultant solution is typically used at elevated temperatures (45–80°C). Commodity chemicals may provide better cleaning than water alone, and they do so at a relatively inexpensive cost. Residue detection of cleaning agents during validation is relatively straightforward because there is usually only one chemical species to detect from the cleaning agent itself.

A third option for aqueous cleaning is to use a formulated cleaning agent. These formulated products usually contain several functional agents including a surfactant(s), an alkalinity or acidity source, water miscible solvents such as glycol ethers, dispersants such as low-molecular-weight polymers, and various builders such as chelants. The main advantage of such formulated cleaning products is that they are multifunctional because of the variety of components; each component broadens the performance in terms of being applicable on a wider variety of soil types. Well-formulated products thus enable a pharmaceutical manufacturer to use one cleaning agent in one cleaning SOP to effectively clean not only the variety of components in a finished drug product, but also a broader range of finished drugs themselves. It should be noted in the former case that for many (if not most) finished drugs, it is the excipients in the finished drug that are more difficult to clean (as compared to the cleaning of the active ingredient). However, the selection of a formulated cleaning product necessitates that the pharmaceutical manufacturer knows the ingredients in the product, both as a check on the consistency of the formulation over time and to effectively establish residue limits for the cleaning agent.

Basis of selection of cleaning agent

The selection of an aqueous cleaning system is simplified if only water alone, or water and a commodity chemical alone, are used. The cleaning performance can be somewhat predicted based on solubility characteristics (at the appropriate pH) or by consideration of the peptizing performance of alkalinity on protein or the oxidizing action of sodium hypochlorite on denatured protein. In the case of formulated multifunctional cleaning agents, the performance is more difficult to predict based on

chemistry alone, and an acceptable cleaning agent is preferably selected based on experience or on laboratory studies. The selection of cleaning agents is also complicated by the fact that sometimes proper cleaning necessitates the use of two cleaning agents at the same time (a primary cleaning agent and a functional additive of some sort), or by the use of two cleaning agents in succession (for example, the use of an alkaline cleaning product followed by an acidic cleaning product).

Cleaning Parameters

While selection of the cleaning method and cleaning agent(s) is important, equally important are the various parameters to consider in the overall cleaning system. These include cleaning process parameters as well as parameters related to the system actually cleaned. Probably the most important cleaning process parameters are the time of cleaning, the temperature of cleaning, the concentration of the cleaning agent, the water quality, the impingement action of the cleaning solution, and any mixing in the cleaning solution.

Time

Three aspects of time are important to the cleaning process. The first is the time from the end of product manufacture to the beginning of the cleaning process. This is important in validated cleaning because the nature of the soil to be cleaned may change over time. Changes may include the drying of the soil residue (thus possibly making it more difficult to clean) or microbial proliferation (thus increasing the bioburden to be cleaned during the cleaning process). A maximum time between the end of manufacture and the beginning of the cleaning process must be specified, and this maximum time must be considered in the selection of worst case conditions for the validation of cleaning processes. A second aspect of time is the times of the cleaning process steps, as well as the time between steps. This includes specifying the time of the prewash, of the washing step, and of rinsing. These are usually established based on laboratory and scale-up trials in the development of a cleaning SOP. The times between these three steps may be critical; if so a maximum time interval should be specified. For example, in the manual cleaning of larger equipment, the time interval between the washing step and the rinse could be significant if the cleaning agent on the washed part is allowed to dry before the rinsing step starts. Drying after the washing step may redeposit soils and prevent effective rinsing. The expectation for validated cleaning is that the times for the various phases are specified. It is generally unacceptable to specify an open-end time frame such as "test until clean" (that is, continue repeating the cleaning process until tests indicate the equipment is clean) in a validated process. Such performance is indicative of an uncontrolled cleaning process. The third aspect of time is the time of storage of cleaned equipment. Although recontamination of equipment is generally known to be event related rather than time related, time is known to affect microbial proliferation. For this reason it is expected for validated cleaning processes that an expiration date (or "use by" date) for cleaned equipment be established.

Temperature

A second important process parameter is the temperature, not only of the cleaning solution, but also of the prewash and rinse solution. The solution temperature can significantly affect cleaning performance, including the rate of solubility and the extent of hydrolysis. Control of temperature during cleaning is preferable. However, it should be recognized that consistency is more important than just constancy of temperature. A consistent decrease in temperature (due to the lack of a heat exchanger in a cleaning circuit) may be acceptable for validated cleaning, provided that the decrease in temperature is consistent from one cleaning event to the next. Temperature of the prewash is generally ambient to prevent setting of certain residues at higher temperatures. The temperature of the rinse is probably least critical. However, it should be recognized that the higher temperature of a rinse might facilitate faster rinsing. In addition, if the temperature of a first rinse is significantly lower than the temperature of the cleaning solution, the temperature "shock" may cause a cleaning solution containing emulsified soils to "break," thus redepositing soils on the equipment surfaces. Temperature should be controlled within reasonable limits, for example, within 5°C of the control point.

Cleaning agent concentration

Cleaning agent concentration should be specified and controlled. Cleaning agent concentration can usually be controlled by diluting based on weight or volume, or by diluting to a known control point, such as to a known conductivity. Within reasonable limits for aqueous cleaning, higher cleaning agent concentrations result in more effective cleaning. Concerns with higher cleaning agent concentration include deleterious effects on equipment and safety issues in manual cleaning.

Water quality

In certain circumstances, water quality can be critical for cleaning performing. If the washing step involves the use of surfactants for cleaning, the presence of hard-water ions (calcium and magnesium) is well known to interfere with effective detergency. Additionally, in the presence of alkalinity sources (which raise the pH), calcium ions will precipitate as calcium carbonate. Such deposits, if not removed from the equipment surfaces, can contribute to the equipment being judged visually dirty. Some formulated cleaners will contain chelants (such as salts of ethylenediamine tetra-acetic acid) to minimize such possibilities. For most cleaning applications, pharmaceutical manufacturers will also use the same quality of water (Purified Water or Water for Injection) that is used for manufacture of the drug product. Lesser quality water, such as tap water, can be used provided the water quality (both chemical and microbiological) is carefully monitored. In addition, if the tap water quality may vary (due to seasonality or source, for example), the worst-case water conditions must be considered for validation purposes.

Impingement

The impingement of the cleaning solution refers to the physical action of a cleaning solution as it hits the surface from a spray application. Such a spray application may include that from a spray device in a CIP system, or may be from a high-pressure hose spray application. Impingement provides mechanical action to help dislodge residues from surfaces. Such impingement can be beneficial if the dislodged residues can then be suspended, emulsified, or otherwise carried away from the equipment surfaces and removed from the cleaning system. Dislodging residues and just displacing them to another location on equipment surfaces may not prove beneficial. In some circumstances, impingement with a solution containing added cleaning agents may be preferred.

Mixing

Mixing refers to the movement within the cleaning solution itself. With a static application of a cleaning solution, as the soils on the surfaces dissolve, emulsify, or otherwise migrate into the cleaning solution, a concentration gradient of saturated or partially saturated cleaning solution is established near the equipment surfaces. This concentration gradient minimizes the chemical cleaning action. Mixing eliminates this concentration gradient and places fresh cleaning solution (or at least a less saturated cleaning solution) in contact with soils on surfaces. This optimizes the cleaning process. It is desirable that mixing be such that the cleaning solution experiences turbulent flow.

The six parameters discussed above are parameters that usually can be controlled by proper design of the cleaning process. Other parameters that are important for cleaning are things that are controlled more by equipment design or by manufacturing process design. Those characteristics include the nature of the equipment surfaces, the physical nature of the soil, and the amount of soil.

Nature of the surface

In removing manufactured product soils from equipment, the nature of the surface may also affect the cleaning process. This includes any special factors in the adhesion of the soil to different surfaces. Different surfaces include differences in type, such as stainless steel, glass, and various plastics. Effective removal of soils from all representative surface types is usually considered in a sampling plan for cleaning validation. Different surfaces also include the roughness or smoothness of the surface itself. Although there is controversy on this, as a general rule for most surfaces involved in pharmaceutical manufacturing, smoother surfaces are more easily cleaned. This may be related to the fact that rougher surfaces have cracks or crevices where soils can more easily "hide." For example, etched glass surfaces are generally more difficult to clean as compared with highly polished glass surfaces. A third factor in considering the nature of the surface is the chemical or physical compatibility of the cleaning solution with the surface itself. The objective in cleaning is to remove the soils and restore the surface to its original condition (or as close to that condition as practical). Two examples of substrate compatibility issues are the repeated use of high levels of hypochlorite on stainless steel (leading to rouge formation) and the use of high levels of aqueous alkalis (sodium or potassium hydroxide) at high temperatures for prolonged periods on glass-lined vessels (leading to etching of the glass surfaces). Other issues might be temperature compatibility of plastics or of gasket materials. Although some deleterious effects may be expected in any cleaning process, the process should be designed to clean effectively and yet keep substrate compatibility issues to a minimum.

Condition of soil

A second factor to consider is the soil condition itself. Three "states" of the soil may be considered—freshly deposited soil, dried soil, and baked-on soils. The difference between the last two is that drying just involves the removal of water without any chemical changes in the soil. Baking usually involves not only the removal of water but also a significant chemical change in the soil. Such chemical changes usually result in the soil being more difficult to remove. For example, drying sugar on a surface may render it slightly more difficult to remove; however, baking it at elevated temperatures will caramelize the sugar and render it extremely difficult to remove. The condition of the soil may change because of manufacturing process conditions, such as product splashing onto a vessel

dome that is steam jacketed and baking onto the surfaces. It also may change because of a time delay after manufacture and before cleaning, allowing the product to dry out. It should be noted that merely drying of certain polymers on surfaces might render them extremely difficult to remove. For example, dried solutions of carboxymethylcellulose (CMC) can be extremely difficult to remove from surfaces.

Although it may be difficult to control the extent of drying or baking in certain processes, these phenomena should be evaluated, and if they do occur, the cleaning process should be designed to remove those soils in the more difficult dried or baked conditions.

Amount of soil

A third factor to consider is the amount of soil on the surface. As a general rule, the greater the amount of soil on the surface, the more difficult the cleaning. For freshly deposited soils, this may not be a serious issue if the bulk of the soil can be readily removed in the prewash. On the other hand, with dried or baked-on soils, the prewash may have little benefit in reducing the amount of soil on the surface. Unfortunately, surfaces that are most likely to have larger amounts of soils (dead legs, cracks, crevices, low flow areas) are also those that are more difficult to clean because of accessibility of the cleaning solution to the surfaces. For cleaning process design purposes, worst cases in soil amounts should be considered.

CLEANING STRATEGIES IN LIGHT OF VALIDATION

Although cleaning processes should be primarily based on what is necessary for good cleaning, they may be modified somewhat based on the regulatory needs for validation. As most pharmaceutical companies will want to validate a cleaning process and not have to do additional significant revalidation work in the near future, this may limit the selection of cleaning agents. As a key part of any validated process is consistency and control, cleaning SOPs for validated processes will also generally have more detail and specificity.

Cleaning for Multiproduct Equipment

Several strategies are possible for cleaning of equipment used to make two or more different products. One option is to optimize a cleaning process for each product made on the equipment. This may mean different cleaning agents for cleaning after each manufactured product, although usually what it means is that the same cleaning agent is used under different process conditions (such as time and/or cleaning agent concentration). Each manufactured product will have its specific cleaning SOP. Another option is to use only one cleaning process for all products manufactured on that individual piece of equipment. One cleaning SOP (with all process conditions the same) is used for all manufactured products. Such a strategy allows for the possibility of "grouping" or "bracketing" for validation protocol purposes. However, it should be recognized that the decision to use one cleaning SOP for all manufactured products has implications for both cleaning and for validation purposes. A strategy of "one SOP for everything" has advantages for cleaning in terms of simplifying documentation and simplifying training. However, such a strategy can be pursued regardless of whether one adopts grouping strategies for validation or not. Clearly, one can also adopt a hybrid strategy, in which several manufactured products are cleaned with one SOP and another group of products (manufactured on the same equipment) is cleaned with a different SOP.

Cleaning in Campaigns

Cleaning between lots of the same product made successively on the same equipment in a campaign may allow for less aggressive cleaning procedures. The reason is that in such cleaning there is no concern about cross-contamination with an active from a different product. However, there are concerns about cleaning. First is the issue of lot integrity—how much of the active or product from one lot can comingle with a different lot and be considered different lots for such purposes as recalls? In addition, while cross-contamination is not an issue, other issues such as contamination from residues of cleaning agents and microbial contamination should also be considered. Another issue in campaigns in which cleaning is minimal is the possibility of degradation product accumulating on the equipment.

VALIDATION ISSUES

IQ/OQ/PQ

Cleaning validation is a type of process validation, and the principles of process validation (17) apply equally to a cleaning process. This includes installation qualification (IQ), operational qualification (OQ), and process or performance qualification (PQ). IQ and OQ should focus on the equipment used for the cleaning process, such as a CIP skid, a spray device, or the monitoring equipment (such as a conductivity probe).

PQ involves performance of the cleaning procedure three consecutive times and evaluating the success of the cleaning procedure, usually by measuring the amount or degree of potential contaminants on the cleaned equipment surfaces. The cleaning SOP should be challenged during the three PQ runs, using (as much as possible) process conditions within the normal ranges that are more likely to induce failure. For example, if the time from the end of manufacture until the beginning of cleaning is specified as a maximum of 12 h, then at least one of the PQ runs should be performed at that maximum time to demonstrate adequate performance.

Cleaning validation is different from other types of process validation in that with cleaning validation both the product cleaned as well as the next product manufactured must be considered. The cleaning SOP is primarily based on what is required to remove the manufactured product. However, the types and acceptable levels of residues following cleaning are also determined by the nature of the next product manufactured in the cleaned equipment. For this reason, cleaning validation is more dependent on what other products are made on the same equipment. Furthermore, the addition of a new product to equipment previously validated for cleaning with multiple manufactured products requires a reevaluation of that previous validation work to determine whether or not the previously validated residue acceptance limits are still applicable in light a new "next product."

Residue Limits

Validating a cleaning process includes selecting target residues and setting limits for those residues following the cleaning process. Target residues are selected based on possible residues that can be left after the cleaning process. This requires an understanding of the cleaning process, and may require an investigation into possible degradation products that may occur during the cleaning process. Acceptable levels of those specific residues are based on what could occur should those residues contaminate the subsequently manufactured product (18, 19). Analytical determinations of residues are usually required. In addition to those measurements, it is expected that the equipment will be visually clean. Examination of equipment for visual cleanness requires training of the observers and may require auxiliary lighting. A visual examination may be supplemented by use of a video camera for recording purposes or by use of a boroscope for pipes. In some cases, equipment may be disassembled for visual examination (and optionally for analytical sampling) to determine cleanness.

Limit in next product

It is important in any discussion of "residue limits" to understand that limits for a cleaning process may be expressed in different ways. This includes the limit of the residue in the subsequently manufactured product, the limit of the residue on the cleaned equipment surfaces, and the limit of the residue in the analyzed sample. These are all related, but they are usually different numbers. For an active ingredient in the cleaning of a finished drug product, the limit in the next product is usually calculated based on application of a safety factor (usually 0.001 or lower) to the minimum daily dose of that active in the maximum daily dose of the subsequently manufactured product. The active or level of active in the subsequently manufactured product is irrelevant unless there is information about unusual deleterious interactions. This calculation is also independent of manufacturing issues such as batch size and equipment surfaces areas, and can be calculated solely on information about the dosing of the two products as follows:

$$L_1 = \frac{\text{MinDA} \times \text{SF}}{\text{MaxDSP}} \qquad (1)$$

where L_1 is the limit of the active in the next product, MinDA is the minimum (daily) dose of the active (the target residue), MaxDSP is the maximum (daily) dose of the subsequently manufactured drug product, and SF represents an appropriate safety factor. Care needs to be paid to selection of units; the L_1 limit is usually expressed in μg/g (or ppm).

Limit per surface area

The next limit calculated is usually the limit per equipment surface area. This is calculated based on the limit in the next product, the batch size of the subsequently manufactured product, and the equipment shared surface area. This is expressed as:

$$L_2 = \frac{L_1 \times \text{BS}}{\text{SSA}} \qquad (2)$$

where L_2 is the limit per surface area, BS is the batch size, and SSA is the shared surface area. Units should be consistent, and the L_2 limit is usually expressed in units of μg/cm^2.

Limit in analytical sample

The next limit is the limit in the analytical sample. If the sampling method involves swabbing, the surface area swabbed and the amount of diluent used for desorbing the swab must be considered. The limit per swab sample is then calculated as:

$$L_3 = \frac{L_2 \times \text{SA}}{\text{AD}} \qquad (3)$$

where L_3 is the limit per analytical sample, SA is the swabbed area, and AD is the amount of diluent for swab elution. Here again units need to be consistent, and the L_3 limit is usually expressed as μg/g or μg/mL. It should be clear that the limit in the analytical sample can be manipulated by changing the area sampled (higher areas result in larger limits per analytical sample) or the amount of diluent used (lower amounts result in larger analytical sample limits). If a sampling rinse is used (in place of swabbing), SA effectively becomes the total surface area of the equipment, and AD becomes the volume of solution used for the sampling rinse.

Nondose limits

For residues (such as cleaning agents) that do not have a defined dose, some measure of toxicity, such as an acceptable daily intake (ADI), is used for residue limit purposes. If the subsequently manufactured product is an in vitro diagnostic (IVD), and has no defined dose, then some evaluation of the effects of target residues on the performance or stability of the IVD product should be performed. These nondose factors are used only for the L_1 limit; there are no changes for calculation of L_2 and L_3 limits.

Limits for multiple subsequent products

When a residue limit is to be calculated for a product where there may be more than one subsequently manufactured product, calculations should be made to compare the surface area residue limits (L_2 limits) by using each subsequent product. If the manufacturing order is not to be restricted, the cleaning validation of the first product should be established using the lowest surface area limit.

Sampling Procedures

Sampling procedures for cleaned surfaces can be divided into four types. Direct surface sampling involves a fiberoptic probe (such as a near infrared probe) that is placed directly on the surface. An output is provided as to the type of residue and the level. Such systems are currently in development (20), but are not commercially practical. Swab sampling involves wiping a fixed area of the surface with a premoistened swab. The swabbing procedure is designed to remove any residues from the surface, and the swab is then placed in diluent to desorb the residue from the swab to the diluent. The residue is then measured in the diluent by a suitable analytical technique.

Such swabbing is commonly called "direct surface sampling," although it clearly is an indirect measure. Rinse sampling involves flushing the equipment surface with a fixed amount of rinse solution (aqueous or solvent), capturing the rinse solution, and then measuring the target residue in the rinse solution. A true sampling rinse is distinct from the final process rinse, and may involve a solution different from that for the process rinse. A fourth sampling procedure is placebo sampling. This involves making a placebo of the subsequently manufactured product in the cleaned equipment. Following manufacture of the placebo, the placebo is sampled and analyzed for the target residue. Any target residue in the placebo would come from the cleaned equipment, and it could be expected that the level present in the placebo would be the level present in any such subsequently manufactured product. Placebo sampling is not widely used because of regulatory concerns related to uniformity of contamination of the placebo from the equipment surfaces and the analytical challenge of finding low levels of residues in placebos.

Analytical Methods

Relationship to target residue

The analytical method selected to measure the target residue must provide a direct measurement of that target residue. When regulatory authorities first began requesting that cleaning be validated, some companies merely tested the rinse water by USP Purified Water specifications to determine if the equipment was clean. The rationale was that the effluent met the same standard as the incoming water. Regulatory authorities (quite rightly) rejected such arguments (because of the possibility of unacceptable levels of potent drugs being present, and because of the possibility that the target residue not being removed in the rinsing procedure), and requested that analytical techniques target the specific residues of concern. However the requirements for analytical methods for residue determination are slightly different from methods for actives level determination in finished product in one important way. For finished product actives determination, a method is required to unequivocally measure the active in the presence of known potential interferences and provide an exact level of the active present. For cleaning validation residue analysis, it is not so as important to know exactly how much residue is present as to know that the amount present is below the acceptance criteria in the validation protocol. For this reason both specific and nonspecific analytical methods can be used for residue detection purposes.

Specificity of methods

Specific methods are preferred because they can more accurately provide information for evaluating potential problems. Because they are designed to eliminate the effects of potential interferences, they can more reliably meet the acceptance criteria. The most common method for residue determination for cleaning validation purposes is the high performance liquid chromatography (HPLC) procedure. In contrast, nonspecific methods such as total organic carbon (TOC) can only provide an upper limit value of the target residue, provided there are no negative interferences (that is, all interferences contribute positively to the analytical response). For TOC, this is usually the case. If the anaytical response is treated as if the response comes only from the target residue, then an upper limit calculation of the target residue can be obtained. If such upper limit calculation is below the acceptance criterion, then it is safe to claim that the residue is within acceptance limits. Nonspecific methods such as TOC are more commonly used in biotech manufacture, where proteinaceous actives are readily degraded by the cleaning procedure. In such cases, the TOC values are treated as if the carbon were due solely to the protein active. Actually, some of the carbon may be due to the cleaning agent, and some may be due to the excipients or processing aids.

Validation of methods

It is expected that any analytical method chosen be validated, including an evaluation of specificity, sensitivity (limit of detection and limit of quantitation), accuracy, precision, range, and linearity (21). The range validated is preferably a range around the expected value in the analytical sample. However, it is wise to also include values up to the acceptance limit in the analytical sample.

Sampling/Analytical Method Recovery

The sampling method chosen must be challenged in combination with the analytical procedure to determine the recovery of the sampling method. This is typically a laboratory study involving spiking a model surface with the target residue and performing the sampling procedure on the surface and measuring the residue with the analytical procedure (22). The amount of residue measured is compared to the amount spiked to give a percent recovery. Recoveries of greater than 80% are considered good, but recoveries of greater than 50% are acceptable. As the analytical values have to be transformed by the recovery values, it is desirable to obtain as high a recovery as consistently possible.

MICROBIAL CONTROL ISSUES

Issues in Cleaning

GMPs require that procedures be in place to limit objectionable microorganisms in both nonsterile and sterile drug products. This should be interpreted to include both the number of organisms as well as the type (species) of organism. Protection of subsequently manufactured product from microbial contamination can be accomplished in part by effective cleaning, by a separate sanitizing step, and/or by storage procedures. In many cases effective microbial control is achieved by a good aqueous cleaning process. The conditions of cleaning can either physically remove microbes, or these conditions (hot alkaline or acidic aqueous conditions) can be conducive to the destruction of microbes. The use of hypochlorite for removal of denatured proteins also serves as an effective oxidizing biocide. If cleaning alone does not achieve adequate microbial reduction, the use of either a chemical sanitizer or elevated temperature (steam or hot air) can be considered. Chemical sanitizers include hydrogen peroxide, peracetic acid, quaternary ammonium chlorides, and alcohols; as a general rule phenolic sanitizers are not used for process equipment because of the difficulty of rinsing from equipment surfaces. If the sanitizer leaves a residue, then a final rinse should be considered to reduce that residue to an acceptable level. Acceptable levels of microbes in the cleaned equipment can be established depending on the nature of the subsequently manufactured product. Limits for nonsterile products can be established based on accepted levels of microorganisms in nonsterile products. Such calculations usually result in acceptance levels that are considerably above what can be routinely achieved with good cleaning procedures. Limits for equipment surfaces used for manufacture of terminally sterilized products are usually related to assumptions of the maximum bioburden for product sterilization purposes. Limits for equipment surfaces used for manufacture of aseptically produced products are usually related to assumptions of the maximum bioburden for equipment sterilization purposes.

Issues in Storage

One major regulatory issue in the cleaning of equipment is the possible microbial proliferation due to improper storage, such as in a wet condition or with pools of water. The preferred method for dealing with such concerns is to effectively dry the equipment before prolonged storage. An alternative (but less desirable option) is to include an additional cleaning and/or sanitizing step after storage and before the next use of the equipment. If this alternative is used, the measurement of both chemical and microbial residues should be performed at the end of this cleaning/sanitizing step.

VALIDATION MAINTENANCE

Once a cleaning process has been appropriately validated, steps should be taken to help insure that the cleaning process remains consistent and in control. Steps that are taken to help assure this include regular monitoring, a change control system, training, and revalidation.

Monitoring

The testing that is done for routine monitoring of the cleaning process should be distinguished from the testing that is part of PQ process qualification. Monitoring tests are usually done on each individual cleaning run. Tests are selected which could be indicative of a cleaning system that is either out of control, or could be trending out of control. Examples of process parameters that could be monitored include the concentration of the diluted cleaning agent, temperature of the cleaning solution, times of various process steps, pressure at a spray device, flow rates, volumes of solutions used, and conductivity of the final rinse water. As these monitoring steps should be part of the cleaning SOP, they should also be performed during the three PQ runs. Some monitoring can give pass/fail information, which clearly indicates the cleaning process is out of control, requiring an investigation and correction of the problem. For example, a higher than specified pressure at a spray device may suggest that spray nozzles were blocked, and that perhaps cleaning coverage was inadequate. This would require an immediate investigation of whether the equipment was adequately cleaned. Such equipment should not be used until a confirmation of adequate cleaning is performed, and the cause of the high pressure corrected. On the other, hand monitoring of the final rinse water conductivity or TOC may show results which do not necessarily suggest that cleaning was inadequate, but rather may display a trend which suggests that cleaning may become inadequate if such a trend continues. This is the value of action and alert limits for monitoring, and of control charts which show trends. It is possible that in certain situations the full range of testing done in the PQ runs would be repeated. However, the value of validation is that consistency has been demonstrated, and the emphasis in monitoring should be tests that might indicate a process change.

Change Control

Validated cleaning processes should be subject to change control. Changes include unplanned and planned changes. Examples of unplanned changes include the failure of a process pump, the clogging of a spray device, and the discontinuance of a cleaning agent by a supplier. The keys to change control are to evaluate the effects of any change, correct the changed item (if possible), implement any increased monitoring as needed, and document the procedure. For example, failure of a pump in a CIP skid may just require a switch of like for like, IQ on the new pump, optionally OQ on the new pump, and proper documentation. Clogging of a spray device may require cleaning of the device and an investigation of the cause of clogging. This should be followed by preventive measures, such as installation of a filter screen to remove material with the potential to clog and some kind of preventive maintenance to regularly clean the screen and inspect the spray device. In both these cases, it may not be necessary to repeat a PQ run. On the other hand, a slight compositional change of the cleaning agent may require laboratory studies to suggest equivalence, followed by one PQ run to confirm equivalence. A change in the manufacturing process itself, and the possible effect of such a change on the cleanability of the equipment, should not be neglected when considering change control for a cleaning process. A change such as increased processing temperature may modify the condition of the soil and, therefore, make it more difficult to clean. In all cases documentation of changes according to a change control SOP is mandatory.

Training

Training operators in the cleaning SOP is an important part of validation maintenance, particularly for manual cleaning methods. Training in a manual method should include a classroom discussion of the method, observation of the SOP being performed by a trained operator, and then demonstration of proficiency by performance of the SOP by the trainee. Training should always follow revision of the SOP, and retraining should follow any deviations that were attributable to operator error.

Revalidation

There are two aspects to revalidation of a previously validated cleaning process. First is revalidation upon any significant change. What is "significant" is a matter of professional judgment. However, a change in cleaning method, such as from manual cleaning to automated cleaning will generally require revalidation even though the cleaning agent and process parameters are the same. In essence this is not really revalidation but rather validation of a new cleaning process. The other aspect of revalidation is based on the evaluation of the consistency and control of a cleaning process on a regular basis to confirm that the process is still under control. The time of this periodic revalidation should be specified in a cleaning validation policy (such as in the cleaning validation master plan), and typically is every one or two years. Such a periodic revalidation involves an evaluation of the monitoring data, change control, cleaning process deviations, and quality records of products manufactured after the cleaning process. If the monitoring data is adequate, the change control is minor, any deviations have had attributable to corrected causes, and there have been no product quality problems possibly related to cleaning, then all this information is suggestive of a cleaning process that is still under control. In such a case it is possible to document such findings in a revalidation report with a conclusion that the cleaning process is still under control and that the original validation work is sill applicable. On the other hand, if the monitoring data show continual trends which require corrections, if numerous individual changes have been made (each of which was acceptable) but the overall cleaning process is now seen as significantly different, if deviations in the cleaning process have either not been attributable to a cause or the cause has not been corrected, and/or if there have been product quality issues related to the cleaning process, then such an investigation may result in a repeat of one or more PQ runs. In such a case, usually there will be some laboratory or pilot scale evaluations before PQ runs are performed.

REFERENCES

1. Current Good Manufacturing Practice in Manufacturing, Processing, Packing, or Holding of Drugs: General, 21 CFR210, 1 April 1997 (revised).
2. Current Good Manufacturing Practice for Finished Pharmaceuticals, 21 CFR 211, 1 April, 1997 (revised).
3. Harder, S.W. The Validation of Cleaning Procedures. Pharm. Technol. **1984**, *8* (5), 29–34.
4. Mendenhall, D.W. Cleaning Validation. Drug Dev. Ind. Pharm. **1989**, *15* (13), 2105–2114.
5. FDA. *Guide to Inspections of Validation of Cleaning Processes*; FDA Office of Regulatory Affairs: Rockville MD, 1993.
6. United States vs. Barr Laboratories,812F, Supp. 458 (DNJ 1993).
7. FDA. *Mid-Atlantic Region Inspection Guide: Cleaning Validation, July 28*; 1992.

8. FDA. *Guide to Inspections of Validation of Cleaning Processes*; FDA Office of Regulatory Affairs: Rockville, MD, 1993.

9. FDA. *Current Good Manufacturing Practice: Proposed Amendment of Certain Requirements for Finished Pharmaceuticals*; Federal Register, 1996; 61, 20103.

10. Recommendations on Cleaning Validation. *Document PR 1/99-2. Pharmaceutical Inspection Cooperation Scheme*; Geneva, Switzerland, 1 April, 2000.

11. Draft 4 of Annex 15 to 1997 EU Guide to Good Manufacturing Practice—Eudralex Volume 4, *Validation Master Plan/Design Qualification/Installation and Operational Qualification/Non-Sterile Process Validation/Cleaning Validation*, European Commission, Working Party on Control of Medicines and Inspections, 17 September 1999. http://dg3.eudra.org/pharmacos/docs/doc99/ GMPanx15.pdf (accessed September 2000).

12. Cleaning Validation Guidelines, Health Canada Therapeutic Products Programme, 1 May, 2000. http://www.hc-sc.gc.ca/hpb-gps/therapeut/zfiles/english/guides/ validate/ validation_guide_e.pdf(accessed September 2000).

13. ICH Steering Committee, Draft Consensus Guideline: Good Manufacturing Practice Guide for Active Pharmaceutical Ingredients, 19 July, 2000.www.ifpma.org/pdfifpma/Q7Astep2.pdf (accessed September 2000).

14. PhRMA Quality Committee, Bulk Pharmaceuticals Working Group. PhRMA Guideline for the Validation of Cleaning Procedures for Bulk Pharmaceutical Chemicals. Pharm. Technol. **1997**, *21* (9), 56–73.

15. Good Manufacturing Practice Guide for Bulk Pharmaceutical Excipients. *International Pharmaceutical Excipient Council*; Arlington VA, 1995.

16. FDA. *Guide to Inspections of Validation of Cleaning Processes*; FDA Office of Regulatory Affairs: Rockville, MD, 1993.

17. FDA, Guideline on General Principles of Process Validation, May 1987. http://www.fda.gov/cder/guidance/pv.htm (accessed September 2000).

18. Fourman, G.L.;Mullen, M.V. Determining Cleaning Validation Acceptance Limits for Pharmaceutical Manufacturing Operations. Pharm.Technol. **1993**, *17* (4), 54–60.

19. LeBlanc, D.A. Establishing Scientifically Justified Acceptance Criteria for Cleaning Validation of Finished Drug Products. Pharm.Technol. **1999**, *23* (10), 136–148.

20. FTIR.com, Cleaning Validation and Coat Weight Analysis., http://.www.ftir.com/remspec/grazing05html. htm(accessed September 2000).

21. Kirsch, R.B. Validation of Analytical Methods Used in Pharmaceutical Cleaning Assessment and Validation. Analytical Validation in the Pharmaceutical Industry (Suppl. to Pharm. Technol.) **1998**, *22* (10), 40–46.

22. Kirsch, R.B. Validation of Analytical Methods Used in Pharmaceutical Cleaning Assessment and Validation. Analytical Validation in the Pharmaceutical Industry (suppl. to Pharm. Technol.) **1998**, *22* (10), 40–46.

FURTHER READING

Bismuth, G.; Neumann, S. *Cleaning Validation: A Practical Approach*; Interpharm Press: Denver, CO, 1999.

Brunkow, R.; Delucia, D.; Haft, S.; Hyde, J.; Lindsay, J.; McEntire, J.; Murphy, R.; Myers, J.; Nichols, K.; Terranova, B.; Voss, J.; White, E. *Cleaning and Cleaning Validation: A Biotechnology Perspective*; PDA: Bethesda, MD, 1996.

LeBlanc, D.A. *Validated Cleaning Technologies for Pharmaceutical Manufacturing*; Intepharm Press: Denver CO, 2000.

Points to Consider for Cleaning Validation; PDA Technical Report No. 29: Bethesda, MD, August 1998.

Verghese, G. Developing a Validatable Cleaning Process. *Proceedings of the 1999 Interphex Conference*; New York, April 20–22, 1999; Reed Exhibition Companies: Norwalk CT, 1999; 461–469.

EUROPEAN AGENCY FOR THE EVALUATION OF MEDICINAL PRODUCTS (EMEA)

David M. Jacobs

David M. Jacobs Consulting, Basel, Switzerland

INTRODUCTION

History of the European Union

After the Second World War, the idea of a "United States of Europe" was promulgated and in 1957, the Treaty of Rome was signed instituting the European Economic Community (EEC) between six countries (Germany, Belgium, France, Italy, Luxembourg, and the Netherlands). In 1973, Ireland, the United Kingdom, (UK) and Denmark joined the EEC. In 1974, heads of state and government decided that a European Parliament should be elected by direct universal suffrage and that it would meet regularly as the European Council (EC) to deal with community affairs and political cooperation. Greece acceded to the EC in 1981, and Spain and Portugal joined in 1986. In 1992, the 12 Foreign Affairs Ministers signed the Maastricht Treaty instituting the European Union (EU), which also included the four freedoms of labor, capital, goods, and services. Finally, Austria, Finland, and Sweden joined the EU in 1995. The Treaty of Amsterdam, which entered into force on May 1, 1999, made further institutional changes such that no draft text can become law without the formal agreement of both the European Parliament and the Council. Thus, the EU now consists of 15 member states, each of which has its own national government and legislative bodies.

The EEC has three important powers:

1. It adopts "European laws" that apply in the 15 countries ("directives" and "regulations").
2. It disposes of a budget to finance certain programs carried out in its member states.
3. It signs international agreements on cooperation or trade.

All these decisions are taken by common institutions sitting in Brussels, Strasbourg, and Luxembourg. Since 1974, the EC has brought together heads of state and government of the 15 member states, as well as the the president of the Commission, to set key guidelines and political goals and to arbitrate on questions for which agreement has not been found within the EU Council of Ministers. Each member country presides over the Council for a six-month period.

EUROPEAN UNION INSTITUTIONS AND LEGISLATIVE INSTRUMENTS

The European Commission, representing the Community's interests, draws up common projects and, after a decision has been taken by the EU Council of Ministers, sees that they are properly implemented. It is directed by 20 commissioners and is assisted in its work by a permanent staff of 17,000, most of who are based in Brussels. It is independent of the governments but is subject to control of the European Parliament. It implements common policies and negotiates international agreements. It may bring an action before the European Court of Justice should Community laws not be respected by the member states. It is here, within the Pharmaceuticals and Cosmetics Unit of the Directorate-General for Enterprise (formerly the Directorate-General for Industry, DG III), that European legislation on medicines is drawn up and implemented.

The European Parliament is made up of 626 deputies who are elected by direct universal suffrage every 5 years. It examines all proposals for European directives and regulations, which it may accept, modify, or refuse. It supervises the work of the European Commission, which it can dismiss with a motion of censure, and it votes the annual Community budget.

The EU Council of Ministers meets in order to adopt proposed European directives and regulations in light of the advice given by the European Parliament. The ministers convene depending on the subject that the Council is dealing with and according to their areas of competency (i.e., the ministers of health of the 15 member states are present for a Council dealing with questions of drug regulation or health.) The country presiding over the EC holds the presidency of the EU Council of Ministers. Due to the principle of subsidiarity, Community legislation is only introduced on points of common interest and in order to further the aim of a balanced and dynamic Europe.

The Council of Ministers can adopt several types of legislation, which are more or less restrictive:

"Regulations" are binding and directly applicable to all citizens.

"Directives" are binding on all citizens but indirectly (i.e., after they have been "transposed" into the laws of each country).

"Decisions" are binding and directly applicable but only to the institutions, bodies, businesses, or citizens specifically named.

"Recommendations," "advisory opinions," and "resolutions" are consultative or guidance texts addressed to the states.

EU LEGISLATION FOR PHARMACEUTICAL AND VETERINARY PRODUCTS

The foundation of European pharmaceutical legislation is Directive 65/65/EEC (1), which when promulgated in 1965, applied only to the initial six member states. In this directive, the definition of a medicinal product is given and the data required to obtain approval is described. This original directive is continually updated, amended, and supplemented with subsequent legislation, but remains the basis of pharmaceutical legislation.

Ten years following the first direction, three new directives sought to further promote public health and the free movement of medicinal products within the community. Directive 75/318/EEC (2) set analytical, pharmaco-toxicological, and clinical standards for testing proprietary medicinal products. Directive 75/319/EEC (3) established the Committee for Proprietary Medicinal Products (CPMP) and its partial mutual recognition procedure, while Directive 75/320/EEC (4) set up a Pharmaceutical Committee to examine problems in implementing the pharmaceutical directives.

In the years that followed, cooperation between national health authorities at EU level was further encouraged. Two Directives, 83/570/EEC (5) and 87/22/EEC (6), set up the Multistate procedure and the Concertation procedure. These procedures provided a mechanism for exchange of information on all aspects of product licensing between member states and made it easier for national licensing authorities to recognize each other's decisions. In the Concertation procedure, the CPMP was charged with forming an opinion on the feasibility of an application, which, however, was not binding on the member states' national authorities. The Multistate procedure was based on the principle of recognition of an approval in one member state by the national health authorities in other member states.

The European Agency for the Evaluation of Medicinal Products (EMEA) was established by Council Regulation (EEC) No 2309/93 (7) of July 22, 1993, with London chosen as its seat by decision of the Council on October 29, 1993. It began operation on February 1, 1995. Regulation 2309/93 also established the legal basis for a single community-wide centralized procedure for the approval of medicinal and veterinary products.

Simultaneously, Directive 93/39/EEC (8) amended Directives 65/65/EEC (1), 75/318/EEC (2), and 75/319/EEC (3) and established the Decentralized Procedure (commonly known as the Mutual Recognition Procedure).

THE EMEA

Mission

The Mission of the EMEA is to contribute to the protection and promotion of public and animal health by:

Mobilizing scientific resources from throughout the EU to provide high quality evaluation of medicinal products, to advise on research and development programs, and to provide useful and clear information to users and health professionals

Developing efficient and transparent procedures to allow timely access by users to innovative medicines through a single European marketing authorization

Controlling the safety of medicines for humans and animals, in particular through a pharmacovigilance network and the establishment of safe limits for residues in food-producing animals

Structure

The European system is based on cooperation between the national health authorities of the member states and the EMEA. The EMEA acts as a focal point of a network that coordinates the scientific resources made available by the member states. This partnership between the EMEA, national health authorities, and the EU institutions is crucial to the functioning of the European authorization procedures.

A Management Board supervises the EMEA, while its scientific activities are largely carried out through its two scientific committees and their working parties. The Board, scientific committees, and their working parties are supported by the EMEA secretariat, headed by an Executive Director.

The Management Board is made up of two representatives from each member state, from the European Parliament and from the European Commission. Representatives of Iceland and Norway, who are members of the European Economic Area (EEA) but not of the EU, also attend meetings of the Board. As of January 1, 2000, these countries formally joined the EMEA. The Management Board appoints the Executive Director, and approves the budget and work program each year. On the recommendation of the European Parliament, it gives discharge to the Executive Director for the implementation of the budget.

The principal scientific bodies of the EMEA are the CPMP and the Committee for Veterinary Medicinal Products (CVMP). They are made up of two members from each member state as well as from Norway and Iceland, and are appointed to give independent scientific advice to the EMEA. The EMEA Secretariat comprises four units: administration, evaluation of medicines for human use, technical coordination, and evaluation of medicines for veterinary use.

The Administration Unit is responsible for carrying out administrative and financial functions to ensure that the Secretariat and staff are able to perform their statutory tasks under satisfactory conditions and thus, has two subsections for personnel, budget and facilities, and for accounting.

The Unit for the Evaluation of Medicines for Human Use is responsible for the following:

- management and follow-up of marketing authorization applications under the centralized procedure;
- postmarketing maintenance of authorized medicinal products;
- management of community referrals and arbitrations arising from the mutual recognition procedure; and
- provision of support to European and international harmonization activities of the CPMP and its working parties.

This unit consists of three subdivisions or sectors: for regulatory affairs and pharmacovigilance, for biotechnology and biologicals, and for new chemical substances.

The Unit for the Evaluation of Medicines for Veterinary Use is responsible for the following:

- management and follow-up of marketing authorization applications under the centralized procedure;
- management of applications for the establishment of maximum limits for residues of veterinary medicinal products that may be permitted in foodstuffs of animal origin;
- postmarketing maintenance of authorized medicinal products;

- management of community referrals and arbitrations arising from the mutual recognition procedure; and
- provision of support to European and international harmonization activities of the CVMP and its working parties.

It has two sectors: for CVMP and veterinary procedures, and for safety of veterinary medicines.

The Technical Coordination Unit is responsible for providing logistical support to both human and veterinary medicine evaluation activities as well as a number of general services to the EMEA, including document management, conference services, and information technology support. It has four sectors: for inspections, for document management and publishing, for conference services, and for information technology. The sector for inspections coordinates the work of inspectors, the implementation of mutual recognition agreements, and the monitoring of medicines authorized in the community. It provides the secretariat of the Quality Working Party and coordinates the Agency's quality management program.

EMEA Scientific Committees

The CPMP and the CVMP are the scientific committees set up to facilitate the adoption of scientific decisions between member states on the authorization of medicinal products on the scientific criteria of quality, safety, and efficacy.

When working for the EMEA, members of the CPMP and CVMP act independently of their nominating member state. The scientific committees are aided by a network of approximately 2300 European experts, nominated by the national competent authorities of the member states on the basis of proven experience in the assessment of medicinal products. Experts may serve on working parties or expert groups of the CPMP or CVMP.

The scientific committee decides the appointment of rapporteurs and corapporteurs, i.e., those members of the CPMP or CVMP who take the lead in reviewing a dossier. The committees are required to ensure that all members undertake the role of rapporteur or corapporteur. Compensation is provided to national competent authorities for the services provided by committee members or European experts at the specific request of the agency.

THE CPMP AND THE EVALUATION OF MEDICINAL PRODUCTS FOR HUMAN USE

A CPMP member acts as rapporteur or corapporteur for centralized procedures and the CPMP gives an official opinion on whether an application for marketing is approvable or not. The EMEA is intimately involved in the management of this procedure up to the issue of the marketing authorization. The EMEA's involvement also includes preparation of the CPMP opinion in all 11 official EU languages. Quality management standards have been implemented for the preparation of scientific advice and opinions, and a tracking system throughout the life cycle of centrally authorized products has been developed. Postauthorization, variations, and extensions to the license may be submitted and rapporteurs play a major role with these maintenance activities. There is also ongoing activity with regard to adverse drug reaction (ADR) reporting, periodic safety update reports (PSURs), and other follow-up measures. Rapporteurs and corapporteurs are particularly involved in urgent safety restriction procedures.

Pharmaceutical sponsors may seek advice on their development programs from the CPMP. The CPMP has set up a scientific advice review group to strengthen and widen CPMP input and to guarantee the availability of proper expertise. A standard operating procedure for the giving of scientific advice by the CPMP for innovator medicinal products has been adopted.

Working Parties

The CPMP and CVMP each have four working parties, as well as a joint CPMP/CVMP Quality Working Party. There is also an EMEA working party on Herbal Medicinal Products.

The CPMP working parties are concerned with biotechnology, efficacy, safety, and pharmacovigilance. The CVMP working parties are concerned with safety of residues, immunological veterinary products, veterinary pharmacovigilance, and efficacy.

These working parties produce position papers, points to consider, notes for guidance, and joint CPMP/CVMP/International Conference on Harmonization (ICH) Guidelines that provide up-to-date scientific opinions on matters of current interest to all member states and pharmaceutical and veterinary manufacturers.

Biotechnology working party

This working party considers aspects of the manufacture and control of biotechnological and biological medicinal products and is also involved in the provision of scientific advice. For example, workshops were held recently on the application of assays for markers of transmissible spongiform encephalopathies (TSE) and on the potential risk of transmitting new variant Creutzfeld–Jakob Disease (nv-CJD) through plasma-derived medicinal products.

Efficacy working party

Clinical trial methodology and guidelines for special disease-related therapeutic fields are discussed in this party. In cooperation with other working parties, guidance on modified release oral and transdermal dosage forms, on pharmacokinetics, and on clinical investigation of new vaccines, gene therapy, and cell-cultured influenza vaccines has been given.

Pharmacovigilance working party

This working party considers safety-related issues at the request of both the CPMP and national authorities, resulting in the harmonization of the summary of product characteristics and package leaflets of marketed products. Regular video conferences are held with the U.S. Food and Drug Administration (U.S. FDA) to discuss issues of mutual interest. A pilot project was started for the electronic transmission of individual case safety reports with a restricted number of participants from national authorities and marketing authorization holders.

Safety working party

Preclinical and safety issues are discussed, and in cooperation with the Biotechnology Working Party, a note for guidance on the quality, preclinical, and clinical aspects of gene transfer products was produced recently.

Ad hoc and other groups

Ad hoc groups on excipients, Lipodystrophy, and antiretroviral medicinal products have been formed. A multidisciplinary group has been set up to evaluate medicinal products containing thiomersal with a view to limiting exposure to mercury and organomercurial compounds.

Cooperation with Competent Authorities

European Monitoring Centre for Drugs and Drug Addiction (EMCDDA)

The EMEA has supported the development of guidelines on risk assessment of new synthetic drugs.

International Conference on Harmonization (ICH and VICH)

The EMEA, as one of the six partners in the ICH process, is intimately involved in production and update of ICH guidelines. The Unit for the Evaluation of Medicinal Products for Human Use supports the Steering Committee, the EU topic leaders, the CPMP, and the various working parties in the preparation, review, and administration of ICH guidelines. Similarly, since establishment of the VICH in 1996, the Unit for Evaluation of Veterinary Medicinal Products supports the Steering Committee and the CVMP as well as the various working parties in this initiative.

Central and Eastern Europe

Many central and eastern European countries (CEEC) are candidates for accession to the EU. The candidates are Bulgaria, Czech Republic, Estonia, Hungary, Latvia, Lithuania, Poland, Romania, Slovakia, Slovenia, and Cyprus. In order to help pharmaceutical registration authorities in these countries prepare for EU membership, a Collaborative Agreement of Drug Regulatory Authorities of European Union Associated Countries (CADREAC) was formed. In addition to this agreement, a simplified procedure for the recognition of centrally authorized medicinal products by the national authorities of CEEC was established. The procedure is optional and is initiated at the request of the marketing authorization holder in the EU.

In addition, under the auspices of a pharmaceutical Pan-European Regulatory Forum (PERF) set up by the European Commission, the EMEA administers and provides executive assistance to CEEC and EU regulators in the conduct of working groups and training sessions in order to facilitate the adoption of common technical requirements. Topics include the implementation of Community legislation, pharmacovigilance, and the assessment of dossiers for marketing authorization for quality safety and efficacy.

Meanwhile, to help eliminate technical barriers to pharmaceutical trade with the CEECs, protocols to permit mutual recognition of good manufacturing practice compliance for medicinal products are being negotiated.

THE CVMP AND THE EVALUATION OF MEDICINAL PRODUCTS FOR VETERINARY USE

The CVMP operates in a similar fashion to the CPMP and is heavily involved in the review of centralized procedures for veterinary products. The CVMP has developed a broad range of new guidelines to assist applicants on topics related to research and development and for which no guidance existed previously.

The Unit for the Evaluation of Medicinal Products for Veterinary Use has also been involved in the PERF initiative as well as other activities related to implementation of Community legislation and the quality of medicinal products.

When the EMEA opened in January 1995, more than 600 "old" substances remained for which maximum residue limits (MRLs) had to be established. The assessment of these products was completed before the January 2000 deadline.

Veterinary Working Parties

Similarly to the CPMP Working Parties, the Efficacy, Safety of Residues, Immunologicals, and Pharmacovigilance Working Parties develop guidelines for the testing and reporting requirements of studies for products for veterinary use.

INSTITUTIONAL PARTNERS

The major contact within the services of the European Commission is the Pharmaceuticals and Cosmetics Unit of the Directorate-General for Enterprise; however, there is also continued exchange of information with the Directorate-General for Health and Consumer Protection. Other contacts include the Directorate-General for Research and the Joint Research Center.

European Technical Office for Medicinal Products (ETOMEP)

The European Commission Joint Research Center has established a technical office at the EMEA responsible for the management of a telecommunications network and other computer technologies to facilitate the dissemination of information on medicinal products. It also manages the EMEA Internet website. A new mechanism for the secure exchange of documents through the Internet has been put in place to facilitate, among other things, the transmission of individual case safety reports within the pilot project on pharmacovigilance between EMEA, national authorities, and the pharmaceutical industry.

The European Union drug regulatory authorities' network (EudraNet) is an internetworking service provided to EU medicinal regulatory authorities in collaboration with the European Commission Directorate-General for Industry. Part of the EudraNet is accessible to industry and the general public.

Joint Interpreting and Conference Service (JICS)

The JICS of the European Commission serves the institutions of the EU, as well as the decentralized agencies and bodies located in EU member states. A representative of the JICS is based at the EMEA to coordinate translation and conference needs. A glossary of specialized and technical EMEA terms to assist interpreters at EMEA meetings is being developed.

The European Department for the Quality of Medicines (EDQM)

European Pharmacopoeia (EP)

The EP was founded by Belgium, France, Germany, Italy, Luxembourg, Netherlands, Switzerland, and the United Kingdom in 1964, under a Council of Europe Convention, to help standardize their national pharmacopoeias. The EP now has 26 signatories (15 member states, the European community, and 10 other European countries). Its monographs have force of law, replacing the old national pharmacopoeias. Directive 75/318/EEC requires EU pharmaceutical manufacturers to use these monographs when compiling marketing authorization applications. The EMEA participates in the work of the EP Commission as part of the EU delegation.

European Network of Official Medicines Control Laboratories (OMCL)

This is a joint project between the EU and the Council of Europe to allow the coordination of laboratory controls between the EU and EFTA members. In 1999, a contract was signed between the EMEA and the EDQM to organize sampling and testing of centrally authorized medicinal products by the OMCL network.

EUROPEAN APPROVAL PROCEDURES

There are two European procedures for obtaining a marketing authorization in more than one country belonging to the EU. These are the Centralized Procedure and the Decentralized or Mutual Recognition Procedure.

Centralized Procedure

The Centralized Procedure must be used for biotechnology products and can be used for so-called high technology products as well as for new active pharmaceutical ingredients (i.e., products that have never before been approved for marketing). The Centralized Procedure is laid down in Council Regulation (EEC) N° 2309/93 (7) and Directive 93/41/EEC (9).

In the Centralized Procedure, one license to market the drug in the entire EU is issued and in principle there is only one evaluation of the dossier. In fact, both a rapporteur and corapporteur are appointed, and each assesses the dossier with its own team. The rapporteur and corapporteur are members of the CPMP who are assigned to a particular

dossier by the CPMP. Each member is obliged to act as rapporteur or corapporteur.

Before submission of the dossier, the Sponsor Company contacts the CPMP or CVMP to announce its intention to make a registration submission and to request appointment of a rapporteur. If, as is usually the case, the Sponsor has had contact with national health authorities, it may request that a particular CPMP or CVMP member be appointed as rapporteur. The CPMP/CVMP is not obliged to follow this request, but in many cases either the rapporteur or the corapporteur is the CPMP/CVMP member requested.

After submission, the rapporteur and corapporteur have 120 days to perform their review and to write a draft assessment report. The two assessments are then discussed by the parties and a list of outstanding issues is sent to the sponsor, at which point the clock is stopped. When the answers have been received, the rapporteur has another 30 days to finalize the assessment report, which is sent to the CPMP or CVMP. CPMP/CVMP members also receive a copy of Part I of the dossier and may request the full dossier. After a total of 210 days, the CPMP or CVMP delivers an opinion: favorable or unfavorable.

If the opinion is favorable, the second stage of the procedure, the decision-making process, begins. During the decision-making process, the Commission Services check that the marketing authorization complies with community law and turn the agency opinion into a binding decision for all the member states. Should the CPMP decision be unfavorable, the sponsor may appeal and a second CPMP opinion must be prepared within 60 days.

The agency sends the Pharmaceutical Unit of the Commission its opinion in all 11 community languages together with the Summary of Product Characteristics (SPC), the particulars of the manufacturing authorization holder responsible for batch release and of the manufacturer of the active substance, as well as the labeling and package leaflet. The commission has 30 days to prepare a draft decision. During this period, various commission directorates-general are consulted and are able to give their opinions.

The draft decision is then sent to the Standing Committee on Medicinal Products or the Standing Committee on Veterinary Products for their opinions. Should there be detailed opposition from a member state to the draft commission decision, the standing committee can refer it back to the CPMP if the opposition is scientific. If the matter is nonscientific, a vote is taken and the council decision is made on the basis of a qualified majority. Each member state has a different number of votes depending on size and importance, and the majority of votes must be in favor. If there is no opposition within 30 days, the draft decision is forwarded to the Commission

Secretariat-General for adoption, enabling the Commissioner for Enterprise and the Information Society to issue the final decision. The final decision is published in the Official Journal of the European Communities.

Decentralized Procedure

The Decentralized Procedure is made on the basis of mutual recognition. Council Directive 93/39/EEC (8) has been implemented in all member states in accordance with Directives 65/65/EEC (1) and 75/319/EEC (3). The sponsor makes a submission to the national health authority of one member state, with a request to assess the dossier for mutual recognition. Within 210 days, the so-called Reference Member State (RMS) must approve the application, prepare an assessment report, and agree on an SPC. The clock may be stopped to obtain further information during this time.

The mutual recognition submission can then be made to any number of the other member states, and the RMS sends a copy of the assessment report to the concerned member states (CMS). Within 90 days, member states must raise serious objections and if there are none, each CMS issues a national marketing authorization with an identical SPC.

To facilitate the mutual recognition procedure, a Mutual Recognition Facilitation Group (MRFG) and a Veterinary Mutual Recognition Facilitation Group have been set up, although this was not foreseen in the original directive. These groups meet one day before each CPMP/CVMP meeting. The objections raised are discussed within the group and the RMS tries to reach agreement on the approval possibilities of the dossier and the most appropriate labeling. If necessary, breakout sessions with the sponsor can be held to finalize labeling details.

Should no agreement be reached within the MRFG/VMRFG, the matter is sent to the CPMP/CVMP for an opinion. Thereafter, the procedure is similar to that during the centralized procedure—the end result being a commission decision after which national licenses must be issued within 30 days.

Referrals and Arbitration

A sponsor company or a national authority may make referrals to the EMEA under Article 10 of Directive 75/319/EEC, in order to harmonize the summary of product characteristics in all member states for products previously approved under national legislation.

Similarly, where there are public health concerns as a result of pharmacovigilance data, nationally authorized products or products authorized by the mutual recognition procedure may be referred under Articles 12 or 15 of Directive 75/319/EEC. The CPMP/CVMP gives an opinion on variation, suspension, or withdrawal of the marketing authorization in such cases.

REFERENCES

1. Official Journal of the European Communities N° 022, **Feb 9, 1965**, 0369–0373.
2. Official Journal of the European Communities N° L 147, **June 9, 1975**, 0001–0002.
3. Official Journal of the European Communities N° L 147, **June 9, 1975**, 0013–0022.
4. Official Journal of the European Communities N° L 147, **June 9, 1975**, 0023–0024.
5. Official Journal of the European Communities N° L 332, **Nov 28, 1983**, 0001–0002.
6. Official Journal of the European Communities N° L 15, **Jan 17, 1997**, 0038–0041.
7. Official Journal of the European Communities N° L 214, **Aug 24, 1993**, 0001–0002.
8. Official Journal of the European Communities N° N L 214, **Aug 24, 1993**, 0022–0030.
9. Official Journal of the European Communities N° L 214, **Aug 24, 1993**, 0040.
10. EUhttp://europa.eu.int, http://europa.eu.int/eur-lex.
11. Pharmaceuticals in the EU. http://pharmacos.eudra.org, http://www.eudraportal.eudra.org, http://emea.eu.int, http://perf.eudra.org.
12. National Agencies. http://heads.medagencies.org, http://hevra.org.
13. ICH. http://www.ifpma.org/ich1.html, http://vich.eudra.org.
14. European Pharmacopoeia. http://www.pheur.org.

EVAPORATION AND EVAPORATORS

David P. Kessler

Purdue University, West Lafayette, Indiana

INTRODUCTION

In the general sense, *evaporation* refers to any change in phase of a component from liquid to gas. *Vaporization*, sometimes used interchangeably with *evaporation*, is at times specifically used to designate the total change of a liquid phase to gas (vapor).

In this article only the term *evaporation* will be used. Evaporation will be defined as processes carried out in process equipment conventionally classified as *evaporators*. This, in turn, implies that nonequipment-contained classes of evaporation, such as solar ponds and oil tanker spills, will be ignored.

Evaporators are used to increase the concentration of relatively nonvolatile dissolved or suspended components in a solution or slurry (the *liquor*) by evaporating portions of the liquid phase using energy supplied by a *medium*, often steam. The dissolved or suspended components do not appear in the vapor phase to a substantial extent. (If they do, the process is referred to as *distillation*.)

Other methods that will not be discussed here, but also can be used to increase concentration (some with and some without concomitant evaporation) are reverse osmosis, ion exchange, dialysis, electrodialysis, osmotic distillation, and applications that involve fluidized beds, cooling towers, or evaporation of aerosols.

In most evaporators, the solvent or suspending phase is primarily or totally one constituent, most frequently water. The important product in evaporation can be either the more concentrated mixture left behind or the overhead vapor (which is often, but not necessarily, subsequently condensed).

The overhead solvent vapor in solvent recovery processes or boiler water vapor in power plant applications typifies vapor products. *Blowdown* refers to the periodic or continuous purging of the bottoms used to control buildup of undesirable material in the liquid phase when producing a vapor product (1).

Some processes of evaporation can be accompanied by crystallization, as the residual liquor grows more and more concentrated. Carried yet further, evaporation evolves to *drying* (or dehydration, if the constituent removed is water), as the bottoms product obtained becomes primarily solid rather than liquid.

TYPICAL APPLICATIONS FOR EVAPORATORS

Historically, a classic example of an evaporation process is the production of table salt. Maple syrup has traditionally been produced by evaporation of sap. Concentration of black liquor from pulp and paper processing constitutes a large-volume present application. Evaporators are also employed in such disparate uses as: desalination of seawater, nuclear fuel reprocessing (1), radioactive waste treatment (2, 3), preparation of boiler feed waters, and production of sodium hydroxide (2). They are used to concentrate stillage waste in fermentation processes, waste brines, inorganic salts in fertilizer production, and rinse liquids used in metal finishing, as well as in the production of sugar, vitamin C, caustic soda, dyes, and juice concentrates, and for solvent recovery in pharmaceutical processes.

TYPES OF EVAPORATORS

Extended discussion of types (including photographs and schematic diagrams), design, and operation of evaporators can be found in the literature (4–6).

Because evaporation of a liquid phase usually requires addition of large amounts of thermal energy, the method of transferring this heat to the liquor tends to dominate evaporator capital cost. The source of heat for evaporators is usually a medium such as hot combustion gases or a condensing vapor, typically steam. Molten salts and electrical resistance heaters are less commonly used sources of thermal energy.

Flash evaporators operate by an adiabatic decrease of the pressure on a liquid that has been previously heated. These were first used for production of potable water on ships; now they are used for more general brackish waters and seawater as well as for processed liquids (7).

Encyclopedia of Pharmaceutical Technology

Disk or *cascade* evaporators use the partial immersion of either disks mounted perpendicular to, or bars mounted parallel to a rotating shaft to carry films of liquid into a hot gas stream (8).

The most efficient method of transferring the energy of a heating medium to the liquor is direct injection of the heating medium. Because of the consequent contamination of the liquor with the heating medium, this method of heat transfer is of relatively less importance in the pharmaceutical industry and will not be discussed here.

The more useful methods for pharmaceutical products maintain purity at the expense of additional resistance to heat transfer by interposing a solid wall of some thermally conductive material between the heating medium and the liquor. The solid wall is usually metallic, but can be coated with materials such as glass, porcelain enamel, or polymers. Glass or ceramic themselves can be used for walls.

The solid wall can be the wall of the evaporator itself, as in *jacketed* evaporators. The area available for heat transfer in jacketed vessels, however, is quite limited. Jacketed vessels frequently incorporate some sort of internal agitator.

Heat transfer can be supplied from within a vessel by a heating coil, but again, the available heat transfer area is not large; however, such coils can be designed in ways that

make their removal for cleaning relatively easy. The alternative is to have the heat exchange external to the main chamber of the evaporator.

Some applications use plate-type exchangers. In plate exchangers, the bounding surface may be in the plate-and-frame form (parallel plates with the heating medium and the liquor flowing in alternate interstitial spaces), or in a spiral-plate configuration that contains a concentric pair of spiral passages (7). Such exchangers can be cleaned easily. They do, however, require a large gasketed area. Fig. 1 shows a typical plate-type evaporator.

The most common geometry for the separating surface between the heating medium and the liquor is probably that of tube bundles, which can be oriented either horizontally or vertically, with the liquor flowing on either the outside or the inside of the tubes. Depending on the application, the tube bundle can be either inside or outside the vessel in which the evaporation takes place.

The heating element of an evaporator is sometimes referred to as a *calandria*. Usually this term is applied to a heating system in which the liquor rises through a vertical tube bundle surrounded by the heating medium and then descends through a central well.

The *short-tube vertical* evaporator is an early type that still sees considerable industrial use. The heating element,

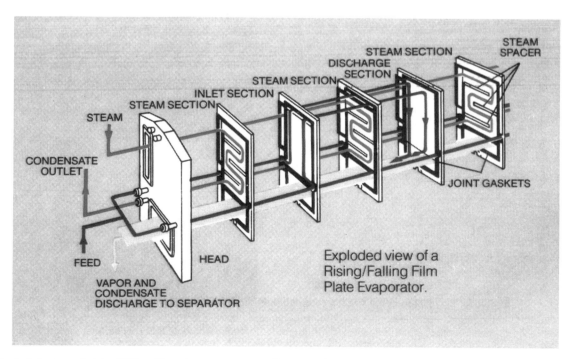

Fig. 1 Exploded view of rising/falling film plate evaporator. (Courtesy of APV Crepaco, Inc., APV Americas, Rosemont, IL—An Invensys Company.)

a vertical bundle of tubes around a center well, is sometimes colloquially referred to as the basket. Circulation is upward through the tubes, the *rising film* mode, and then downward through the central well or *downtake*. Liquid boils in the tubes, which decreases the overall density therein and thus creates the driving force for circulation, since the density of the (nonboiling) fluid in the downtake is greater than that in the tubes.

Mechanical cleaning is fairly easy with such units, and the capital investment is relatively low. Circulation stops, however, if the heat input is interrupted, creating the danger of the settling of any solids suspended in the liquor. This type of unit is not well suited to viscous liquids because of the low heat transfer coefficients associated with the low velocities of natural convection (8). Short-tube vertical evaporators have largely been surpassed by other types, particularly for applications involving liquors that foam, deposit excessive scale, are excessively viscous, or are heat sensitive.

Long-tube vertical evaporators are normally the cheapest per unit of capacity (8). When operated in the rising film mode, temperature variation along the inside of the tubes is both substantial and difficult to predict. The variation in pressure from high at the bottom to low at the top normally means that the liquid enters the bottom of the tubes below its boiling temperature. The liquid is subsequently heated to boiling as it rises, and the boiling temperature simultaneously decreases as the pressure decreases toward the top of the tube (assuming any boiling point rise from increasing concentration is overshadowed by the effect of the reduced pressure on the boiling point).

By operating a long-tube evaporator in the *falling film* mode, the problem of temperature variation induced by pressure differences is mitigated. Here, a film of liquid surrounding a gas core flows down the walls of the tube, so pressure drop is very much less than in the rising film mode. The low residence time of the falling film units makes them useful for heat-sensitive materials, but the necessity of maintaining a film on the walls of the tubes makes feed distribution a problem. They are readily adapted to sanitary processing. Evaporators that combine rising film sections and falling film sections in the same unit are also available.

Forced circulation evaporators have relatively higher heat transfer coefficients, and are somewhat less subject to fouling, salting, and scaling. This advantage is offset by both the cost of external power required for the circulating machinery and a relatively high holdup (8). At times they more frequently experience plugging from deposits detached from the walls of the unit by the force of the circulating fluid. The introduction of a pump may lead to mechanical problems, particularly with liquors that are slurries.

Liquor velocities required to prevent surface deposits are often greater than can be obtained with natural circulation at reasonably low temperature differences (9). In addition to mitigating scale formation, forced circulation also improves the heat transfer coefficient.

For viscous liquids, one way to increase the heat transferred is to improve the heat transfer coefficient by scraping or stirring the fluid adjacent to the wall, as in *agitated film* or *wiped film* evaporators. Accommodation of the mechanical devices used to mix the fluid close to the wall requires a fairly large diameter tube, so these devices tend to consist of only a single tube; thus, heat transfer area is relatively small. The introduction of moving mechanical parts may lead to maintenance problems.

In *horizontal tube* evaporators, the liquor is usually on the outside of the tubes and the heating medium on the inside. Rather than submerging the tubes, the boiling liquid is sometimes sprayed on the outside of the tubes. This gives a performance approaching that of falling film evaporators (8).

Evaporators can be operated at a variety of pressures (9). Reduced pressure, with its concomitant reduction in boiling temperature, offers advantages for heat-sensitive materials and materials that are sensitive to exposure to air.

Evaporation operations are often staged in *multiple effect* systems (1) to achieve better efficiency. Such systems can have a variety of relative directions for flow of liquor and vapor. A typical example of such staging is illustrated in Figs. 2 and 3.

Detailed discussion of the advantages and disadvantages of various types of evaporators is available (8). A table summarizing the advantages and disadvantages of common types of evaporators also is available (10).

Since most evaporators are purchased from outside suppliers either prefabricated or on-site-fabricated, such suppliers can be an excellent source of information on selection of evaporator type. Suppliers and addresses can be found in the literature (11, 12).

DESIGN OF EVAPORATORS

A number of publications have addressed the design of evaporators at both the elementary and complex levels (1, 2, 7–9, 13–18). The reader is referred to these and to their bibliographies for details.

Efficiency of steam-heated evaporators is commonly described in terms of steam economy, defined as the pounds of solvent evaporated per pound of steam consumed (7).

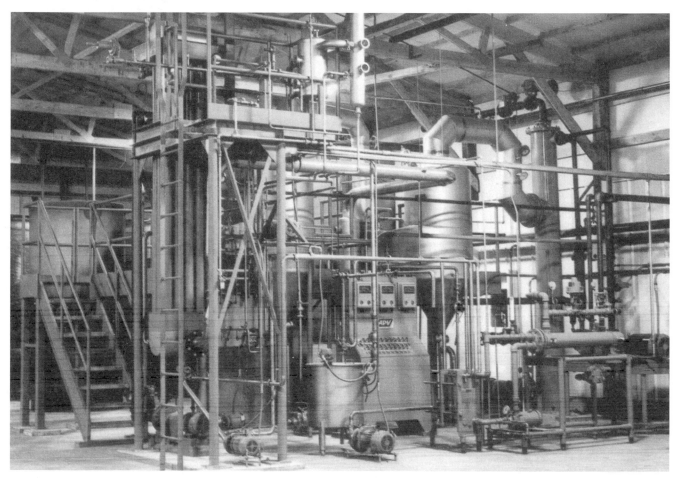

Fig. 2 Two-effect rising/falling film plate evaporator. (Courtesy of APV Crepaco, Inc., APV Americas, Rosemont, IL—An Invensys Company.)

Important to the design of evaporators is the concept of boiling point rise. Boiling point rise, which normally accompanies increasing concentration in a liquor, is defined as the difference between the boiling temperature of the liquor and that of pure water at the same pressure.

A plot of the boiling point of pure water on the abscissa versus the boiling point of the liquor on the ordinate, with lines of constant concentration plotted as a parameter, is known as a Dühring plot. A Dühring plot is unique to the particular chemical species. A monograph summarizing the boiling point rise for a number of inorganic salts, is available (19), as well as information on general equations to predict boiling point rise either empirically or from other thermodynamic properties (9).

During batch operation, the composition of the liquor in the evaporator is continuously changing. For batch operation in the absence of significant potential and kinetic energy changes, an energy balance on the system constituted by the liquor in the evaporator shows that the sum of the rate of enthalpy removed in the overhead stream and the change in internal energy of the liquor in the evaporator must equal the rate of energy addition as heat:

$$\hat{H}_{ov}\dot{w} + \frac{d(\hat{U}M)}{dt} = \dot{Q} \tag{1}$$

where

$\hat{H}_{ov}$ enthalpy of overhead vapor (energy/mass)
$\dot{W}$ mass flow rate of overhead vapor (mass/time)
$\hat{U}$ internal energy of liquor (energy/mass)
M mass of liquor (mass)
$\dot{Q}$ rate of heat input (energy/time)
t time (time)
$(\ )$ units

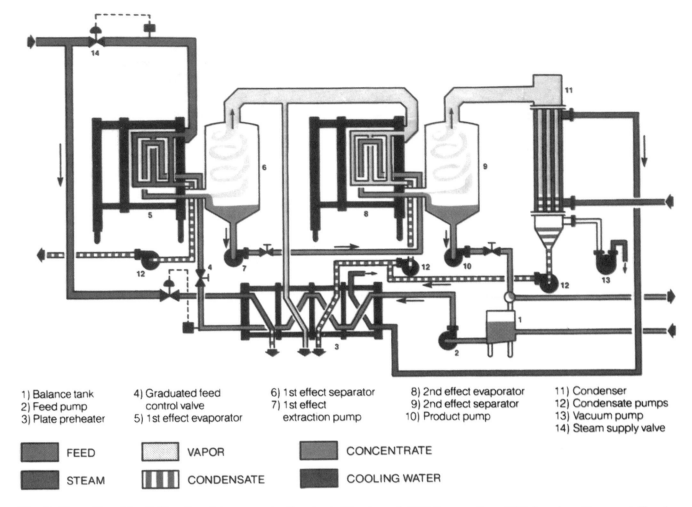

1) Balance tank
2) Feed pump
3) Plate preheater

4) Graduated feed
   control valve
5) 1st effect evaporator

6) 1st effect separator
7) 1st effect
   extraction pump

8) 2nd effect evaporator
9) 2nd effect separator
10) Product pump

11) Condenser
12) Condensate pumps
13) Vacuum pump
14) Steam supply valve

FEED   VAPOR   CONCENTRATE

STEAM   CONDENSATE   COOLING WATER

Fig. 3 Two-effect rising/falling film plate evaporator flowsheet. (Courtesy of APV Crepaco, Inc., APV Americas, Rosemont, IL—An Invensys Company.)

A way to estimate vapor enthalpy and data on the internal energy of the liquor as a function of concentration is required.

Even though both the enthalpy and rate of the overhead vapor are often quite constant in time (except for the small sensible thermal energy contribution from the boiling point rise), the rate of heat addition may vary with time because of changes in the overall heat transfer coefficient from surface changes (see below) and because of significant changes in the temperature difference between the liquor and heating medium induced by the boiling point rise. A simple example calculation of batch evaporation can be found in reference (14). The equations involved are similar to those that govern batch distillation.

Many evaporators are operated at substantially steady-state conditions (although heat transfer coefficients will vary slowly with time because of surface changes from scaling, deposition, etc., as noted above). The design of an evaporator for steady-state operation typically is initiated from the specification of the mass flow rate of material to be processed and its required change in concentration. This information is used in mass balances, which proceed via an energy balance to yield the required rate of heat transfer.

For an evaporator system which has a liquid feed, overhead vapor, and bottoms liquid product, and is used to concentrate species A:

Total mass balance

$$\dot{W}^{(\text{feed})} = \dot{W}^{(\text{overhead vapor})} + \dot{W}^{(\text{bottoms liquid})} \qquad (2)$$

Species mass balance

$$\dot{W}^{(\text{feed})} x_{\text{A}}^{(\text{feed})} = \dot{W}^{(\text{overhead vapor})} x_{\text{A}}^{(\text{overhead vapor})}$$
$$+ \dot{W}^{(\text{bottoms liquid})} x_{\text{A}}^{(\text{bottoms liquid})} \qquad (3)$$

where

$\dot{W}$ mass flow rate (total mass/time)

x mass concentration of species A (mass A/total-mass)

Normally, the feed flow rate and concentration are specified, as are the overhead and bottoms concentrations (the overhead concentration is most often zero). This set of two equations in 2 unknowns can then be solved for the unknown overhead and bottoms mass flow rates.

The required rate of heat transfer can then be calculated from the steady-state energy balance, assuming negligible changes in potential and kinetic energy and no work input (the latter not valid, of course, for vapor recompression evaporators).

$$\dot{Q} = \dot{W}^{(\text{overhead vapor})} \hat{H}^{(\text{overhead vapor})}$$
$$+ \dot{W}^{(\text{bottoms liquid})} \hat{H}^{(\text{bottoms liquid})} - \dot{W}^{(\text{feed})} \hat{H}^{(\text{feed})} \quad (4)$$

where

$\dot{Q}$ heat transfer rate into system (energy/time)

$\dot{W}$ flow rate (mass/time)

$\hat{H}$ enthalpy (energy/mass)

In the above equation, the mass flow rates are known from the mass balance calculation. The enthalpies must be determined from thermodynamic data, which will require specification of the temperature and/or pressure of the stream in combination with the concentrations that were originally specified.

Calculation of the rate of heat transfer required does not of itself determine the heat transfer area required or the configuration thereof. The configuration (tubes, plates, etc.) is typically chosen first, by rules of thumb and experience, depending on the liquor to be processed.

The area is usually calculated, once the configuration is chosen, by using an overall heat transfer coefficient that lumps together all forms of heat transfer in terms of an overall coefficient paired with a characteristic area:

$$\dot{Q} = UAT \quad (5)$$

where

U overall heat transfer coefficient, valid only when paired with a specified area (energy/time $\times$ length^2 $\times$ temperature)

A a specified area normal to heat flow; (e.g., the outside area of the tubes or the inside area of the tubes (length^2),

ΔT Temperature difference between temperature of heating medium and temperature of the liquor

(usually either freestream or bulk temperatures) (temperature).

The overall heat transfer coefficient depends on the properties and flow pattern of the heating medium, the properties and flow pattern of the liquor, the properties of the solid surface that separates the medium and the liquor, and the properties of any deposits at the interface on either side of the separating surface.

In general, heat can be transferred by the three mechanisms of conduction, convection, and radiation (20). In evaporators, the mechanisms of importance are usually convection in the liquor and medium, and conduction through the solid separating them.

In order to calculate the overall heat transfer coefficient in the equation above, the heat transfer properties of the heating medium and the liquor are described in terms of individual heat transfer coefficients, and the heat transfer properties of the separating solid in terms of its thermal conductivity. Deposits at the interface, which one might expect to be described by a thermal conductivity, are usually described instead in terms of either a fouling (heat transfer) coefficient or a "fouling factor" (which is usually defined to have a value of 1000/[fouling coefficient]).

Individual heat transfer coefficients for convection are defined by the equation:

$$\dot{Q} = h A T \quad (6)$$

where

h individual heat transfer coefficient (energy/time $\times$ length^2 $\times$ temperature),

A a characteristic area normal to the flow of heat: typically, the area of the unfouled surface initially in contact with the fluid. In cases where area varies along the heat transfer path, (e.g., tubes), it is necessary to specify on which area the coefficient is based, such as, inside, outside (length^2),

ΔT a specified temperature difference, usually the difference between either the freestream or the bulk temperature and the temperature at the surface.

The rate of heat transfer by conduction can be written in terms of the thermal conductivity:

$$\dot{Q} = k A_{\text{avg}} T x \quad (7)$$

where

k thermal conductivity of solid (energy/time$\times$ length $\times$ temperature),

A_{avg} average area through which heat transfer occurs, e.g., logarithmic mean area for concentric cylinders (length^2),

ΔT temperature drop from one outside surface of the solid to the other outside surface (temperature)

Δx thickness of solid normal to heat flow (length)

One can relate the overall heat transfer coefficient to the individual steps:

$$\frac{1}{U_{ov}A_{ov}} = \frac{1}{h_{medium}A_{medium}}$$

$$+ \frac{1}{h_{fouling,medium}A_{fouling,medium}} + \frac{x}{kA_{avg,solid}}$$

$$+ \frac{1}{h_{fouling,liquor}A_{fouling,liquor}} + \frac{1}{h_{liquor}A_{liquor}}$$

(8)

The overall heat transfer coefficient can be calculated by evaluation of the individual terms in the above equation. Knowledge of the overall temperature drop then permits calculation of the required area. A detailed development of the above is available (5).

The individual heat transfer coefficients for the medium and the liquor can be calculated from general correlations using the properties of the fluid and the velocity fields in the system (20–25). Additional information can be found in the continuing series of the American Society of Mechanical Engineers (26). Detailed studies and bibliographies on prediction of individual heat transfer coefficients for evaporating films on/in horizontal/vertical tubes, can be found in other publications (21, 22, 24–27).

The limiting step in heat transfer is usually the thermal resistance from the liquor itself and/or deposit formation on the liquor side (the last two terms in the previous equation.) On the heating medium side, the heat transfer coefficients are usually for condensation and are therefore substantially larger than those on the liquor side, which are for boiling. The conduction resistance of the tube wall is usually small (but this is not necessarily true of the resistance of deposits that accumulate on the tube wall).

Deposits typically accumulate more on the boiling side than the condensing side. To determine coefficients for systems with substantial surface deposition, experimental data on that particular system is usually necessary.

Heat-sensitive products can break down to insoluble forms that deposit on the surface and inhibit heat transfer. For example, some soluble proteins, when heated, convert to an insoluble form (18). Change in the heat transfer characteristics of the tube surface can also be induced by corrosion.

The liquor can be on either the inside or the outside of the tubes, depending on the physical and chemical characteristics of the materials involved. Considerations include convenience in cleaning deposits from the heat transfer surface, the heat transfer characteristics of the fluids involved, and fluid velocities required for efficient heat transfer or prevention of scale deposition.

A useful table of criteria and data for the rapid design and selection of evaporators is available (10).

Natural circulation evaporators have overall coefficients of the order of 1.1–3.4 kW/(m²°K) = 200–600 Btu/(h ft²°F). Adding forced circulation may raise this to the order of 11 kW/(m²°K) = 2000 Btu/(h ft²°F). In agitated-film units, for Newtonian liquids with viscosity of the order of water, coefficients of the order of 2.3 kW/(m²°K) = 400 Btu/(h ft²°F) may be obtained. As the viscosity increases to 10 Newton sec/m² = 10,000 centiPoise, the coefficient will drop to the order of 0.7 kW/(m²°K) = 120 Btu/(h ft²°F). More extensive listings of overall coefficients for evaporators may be found in the literature (1, 8, 10, 28).

The heating medium must be at a higher temperature than the liquor, and the resultant temperature driving force must be sufficiently large that excessive area for transfer is not required. One means of increasing the temperature driving force for a heating medium at a given temperature is to reduce the pressure of the liquor side to decrease the boiling temperature. This is a common device in evaporation, and is often accomplished with a steam-jet ejector. Design (and cost) of such ejectors is detailed in the literature (29).

If the overhead vapor is water and the heating medium is steam, the vapor generated is usually comparable in amount and quality to the heating steam used, but is at a lower pressure because the heating steam must be at a higher temperature (therefore, pressure) than the liquor in order to furnish an adequate temperature driving force for heat transfer. A logical question is whether or not to attempt to recover the latent heat in the vapor generated.

The condensing temperature of the vapor does not usually furnish an appropriate temperature difference to permit transferring heat to the liquor (except, perhaps, a small part to sensible heat of the incoming liquor). However, compressing the vapor will raise both its temperature and its condensing temperature, permitting the vapor to be used to transfer its heat of vaporization/condensation to the liquor with consequent recovery of thermal energy.

Unfortunately, the work required for such compression is high-quality (and therefore, expensive) mechanical energy that ends up as low-quality thermal energy. Either thermocompression or mechanical compression may supply the required mechanical energy. Thermocompression is accomplished by means of high-pressure steam in an ejector system [for design and cost of ejectors see (29)], while mechanical compression is usually done by a centrifugal compressor (1).

An alternative scheme is to split the evaporation process into stages (in different vessels), commonly referred to as *effects*, where the flow of liquor may be in the same direction, the backward direction, or normal to the flow of vapor (1, 9). In such a scheme, the vapor generated in a given effect is used to boil the liquid in a different effect where a proper temperature driving force exists. In multiple-effect evaporation, one exchanges savings in steam costs for increased capital investment in equipment.

Pennink (30) notes that the optimum is usually 3 or 4 effects in a 50,000 lb/h system and 7 to 8 effects in very large systems. Ramakrishna (31) details a shortcut method to estimate the optimum number of effects for multi-effect evaporation, and Ulrich (10) gives a shortcut algorithm for the design of multiple-effect evaporators. A sample calculation can be found in Schilt (15). Cole (18) gives specific steam consumption and minimum evaporation rates for single and multiple-effect evaporators with and without steam-jet thermocompression, as well as data on mechanical vapor recompression cost per ton of water evaporated.

For those who wish to pursue more detailed design, a good starting point for mechanical design of heat exchange equipment is Azbel (9), who also discusses alternative materials of construction. For general discussion of evaporation as well as insight into safety/environmental considerations, see a report from the U.S. Environmental Protection Agency (32). This document discusses failure analysis as applied to evaporators for treatment of effluent from the metal finishing industry. Other useful references, which have extensive bibliographies, are Rubin et al. (33), Knudsen et al. (34), Chisholm (35), and Taborek et al. (36). The continuing series from the American Society of Mechanical Engineers, as exemplified by Shah (37), contains additional information.

COSTS ASSOCIATED WITH EVAPORATORS

The two major costs associated with evaporators, as with any process equipment, are capital investment and operating costs. The best estimate of the installed cost of evaporation systems is, of course, a firm bid from a vendor. The installed cost, however, can be estimated based on the heat transfer surface area, as in Peters and Timmerhaus (38). Costs taken from published references

must be adjusted for changes subsequent to the time of publication. To do this, one may use an index such as the Marshall and Swift all-industry index. The value of this index is published each month in *Chemical Engineering*, a McGraw-Hill publication. Further information on the use of this and other cost indices as well as their histories are available, for example, in Peters and Timmerhaus (38) and Ulrich (10). Variation of purchased evaporator costs with material of construction and pressure can also be found in Ulrich (10).

A chart to estimate the costs of ejectors for thermocompression has been developed (29). Approximate costs of compressors for mechanical vapor recompression also can be found (38–40). In addition, these publications contain details of cost estimation for heat exchangers. For more detailed estimation of cost of shell-and-tube exchangers, see Purohit (41–43). Plate-and-frame and spiral-plate heat exchanger costs can be estimated using Kumana (44).

Operating expenses can be approximated using published techniques (10, 38. These are mainly useful for preliminary cost estimates only. Such items as raw materials, operating labor, utilities, supervisory expenses, maintenance and repairs, etc., may vary greatly depending on the specific process in question.

OPERATION AND CONTROL OF EVAPORATORS

Many of the problems in operation and control of a given evaporator system will be specific to the application. However, all systems need to answer such questions as how to evaluate performance, how best to schedule periodic *boil outs* (cleaning), how to measure and control variables typified by temperature, pressure, fluid level, fluid flow rate, composition, etc., and how to detect faults in evaporator operation quickly and efficiently (45, 46).

At one time, the American Institute of Chemical Engineers issued a guide to performance testing of evaporators (47). The Instrument Society of America issues a book-length guide for the operation and control of evaporators (2), which covers, among other topics, such operational considerations as the optimum use of boil outs. Instrumentation is covered in detail, including variables, the choice of measurement and measurement method, and both design and implementation of the control system including digital techniques. This work contains both chapter bibliographies and a general bibliography.

Operation of an evaporator for minimum cost of production involves scheduling cleaning cycles to remove scale or deposits. Minimizing costs requires the balancing of increased evaporation rate against out-of-service time. Shutdown involves costs associated not only with cleaning, but emptying and refilling as well. The crux of such optimization is the function used to describe the evolution of scale formation with time.

REFERENCES

1. Gupta, J.P. Evaporators and Vaporizers. *Fundamentals of Heat Exchanger and Pressure Vessel Technology*; Hemisphere: Washington, 1986; 187–211.

2. Nisenfeld, A.E. *Industrial Evaporators: Principles of Operation and Control*; Instrument Society of America: Research Triangle Park, NC, 1985.

3. Anthony, D. Improved Evaporators for Radioactive Waste, Chem. Eng. Progress **1983**, 58–63.

4. Billet, R. VCH Verlagsgesellschaft MbH. *Evaporation Technology—Principles, Applications, Economics*; Weinheim: Germany, 1989.

5. Kakac, S., Ed. *Boilers, Evaporators, and Condensers*; Wiley Interscience: New York, 1991.

6. Cheremisinoff, N.P.; Cheremisinoff, P.N. *Heat Transfer Equipment*; Prentice Hall: Englewood Cliffs, NJ, 1993.

7. Freese, H.L. *Evaporation, Fermentation and Biochemical Engineering Handbook*; Vogel, H.C., Ed.; Noyes Publications: Park Ridge, NJ, 1983; 227–276.

8. Standiford, F.C. Thermal Design of Evaporators. *Perry's Chemical Engineers' Handbook*; Perry, R.H., Green, D.W., Maloney, J.O., Eds.; McGraw-Hill Book Company: New York, 1984; 10–34–10–38.

9. Azbel, D. *Heat Transfer Applications in Process Engineering*; Noyes Publications: Park Ridge, NJ, 1984.

10. Ulrich, G.D. *A Guide to Chemical Engineering Process Design and Economics*; John Wiley Sons: New York, 1984.

11. Evaporators. *Thomas Register of American Manufacturers*; Thomas Publishing Company: New York, 1990; 5, 8584–8595.

12. Chemical Processing Guide and Directory. Chem. Process. **1991**, *53* (15), 118–122.

13. Myers, A.L.; Seider, W.D. *Introduction to Chemical Engineering and Computer Calculations*; Prentice Hall: Englewood Cliffs, NJ, 1976.

14. Blackadder, D.A.; Nedderman, R.M. *A Handbook of Unit Operations*; Academic Press: London, 1971.

15. Schilt, E.A. *Evaporation Transfer Operations in Process Industries*; Bhatia, M.V., Ed.; Technomic Publishing Co., Inc.: Lancaster, PA, 1983; 5, 267–299.

16. Esplugas, S.; Mata, J. Calculator Design of Multistage Evaporators. *The Chemical Engineering Guide to Heat Transfer*; McNaughton, K.J., Ed.; Hemisphere: Washington, 1986; II, 261–265.

17. Krishna, R. Book Review of: Evaporation Technology—Principles, Applications, Economics, by R. Billet. The Chemical Engineer **1989**, (462), 53.

18. Cole, J. A Guide to the Selection of Evaporation Plant. The Chemical Engineer **1984**, (404), 20–23.

19. Luyben, W.L.; Wenzel, L.A. *Chemical Process Analysis: Mass and Energy Balances*; Prentice Hall: Englewood Cliffs, NJ, 1988.

20. Kessler, D.P.; Greenkorn, R.A. *Momentum, Heat, and Mass Transfer Fundamentals*; Marcel Dekker, Inc.: New York, 1999.

21. Sandall, O.C.; Hanna, O.T.; et al. Heating and Evaporation of Turbulent Falling Liquid Films. AIChE J. **1988**, *34* (3), 502–505.

22. Kocamustafaogullari, G.; Chen, I.Y. Falling Film Heat Transfer Analysis on a Bank of Horizontal Tube Evaporator. AIChE J. **1988**, *34* (9), 1539–1549.

23. Han, J.; Fletcher, L.S. Falling Film Evaporation and Boiling in Circumferential and Axial Grooves on Horizontal Tubes. Ind. Eng. Chem. Process Design Dev. **1985**, *24*, 570–575.

24. Palen, J.W. Falling Film Evaporation in Vertical Tubes. *Heat Exchanger Technology*; Chisholm, D., Ed.; Elsevier Applied Science: London, 1988; 189–218.

25. Steiner, D.; Ozawa, M. Flow Boiling Heat Transfer in Horizontal and Vertical Tubes. *Heat Exchangers: Theory and Practice*; Taborek, J., Hewitt, G.F., Afgan, N., Eds.; Hemisphere: Washington, 1983; 19–34.

26. Chen, I.Y.; Kocamustafaogullari, G. An Experimental Study and Practical Correlations for Overall Heat Transfer Performance of Horizontal Tube Evaporator Design. *Heat Transfer Equipment Fundamentals, Design, Applications, and Operating Problems*; Shah, R.K., Ed.; The American Society of Mechanical Engineers: New York, 1989; 108, 23–32.

27. Han, J.; Fletcher, L.S. Falling Film Evaporation and Boiling in Circumferential and Axial Grooves on Horizontal Tubes. Ind. & Eng. Chem. Process Design Dev. **1985**, *24*, 570–575.

28. Evans, F.L., Jr. *Ejectors, Equipment Design Handbook for Refineries and Chemical Plants*; Gulf Publishing Company: Houston, 1979; 1, 105–117.

29. Evans, F.L., Jr. *Ejectors, Equipment Design Handbook for Refineries and Chemical Plants*; Gulf Publishing Company: Houston, 1979; 1, 105–117.

30. Pennink, H. Cost Savings from Evaporator Vapor Compression. Chem. Eng. **1986**, *93*, 79–81.

31. Ramakrishna, P. Estimate Optimum Number of Effects for Multi-Effect Evaporation. Chem. Eng. **1987**, *94*, 82.

32. Evaporation Process, Center for Environmental Research Information, National Risk Management Research Laboratory, Office of Research and Development, U.S. Environmental Protection Agency, Capsule Report EPA/625/R-96/008, Cincinnati, OH, 1996.

33. Rubin, F.L.; Moak, H.A. Heat-Transfer Equipment. *Perry's Chemical Engineers' Handbook*; Perry, R.H., Green, D.W., Maloney, J.O., Eds.; McGraw-Hill Book Company: New York, 1984; 11–3–11–59.

E

34. Knudsen, J.G.; Bell, K.J. Heat Transmission. *Perry's Chemical Engineers' Handbook*; Perry, R.H., Green, D.W., Maloney, J.O., Eds.; McGraw-Hill Book Company: New York, 1984; 11–3–11–59.

35. Chisholm, D. *Heat Exchanger Technology*; Elsevier Applied Science: London, 1988.

36. Taborek, J.; Hewitt, G.F.; *Heat Exchangers: Theory and Practice*; Hemisphere Publishing Corporation: Washington, 1983.

37. Shah, R.K. *Heat Transfer Equipment Fundamentals, Design, Applications, and Operating Problems*; The American Society of Mechanical Engineers: New York, 1989.

38. Peters, M.S.; Timmerhaus, K.D. *Plant Design and Economics for Chemical Engineers*; McGraw-Hill, Inc.: New York, 1991.

39. Hall, R.S.; Matley, J. Current Costs of Process Equipment. *The Chemical Engineering Guide to Heat Transfer*; McNaughton, K.J., Ed.; Hemisphere: Washington, 1986; II, 337–357.

40. Hall, R.S.; Matley, J. Current Costs of Process Equipment. Chem. Eng. **1982**.

41. Purohit, G.P. Estimating Costs of Shell-And-Tube Heat Exchangers. *The Chemical Engineering Guide to Heat Transfer*; McNaughton, K.J., Ed.; Hemisphere: Washington, 1986; II, 319–330.

42. Purohit, G.P. Costs of Double-Pipe and Multitube Heat Exchangers-Part 1. *The Chemical Engineering Guide to Heat Transfer*; McNaughton, K.J., Ed.; Hemisphere: Washington, 1986; II, 331–334.

43. Purohit, G.P. Costs of Double-Pipe and Multitube Heat Exchangers-Part 2. *The Chemical Engineering Guide to Heat Transfer*; McNaughton, K.J., Ed.; Hemisphere: Washington, 1986; II, 335–336.

44. Kumana, J.D. Cost Update on Specialty Heat Exchangers. *The Chemical Engineering Guide to Heat Transfer*; McNaughton, K.J., Ed.; Hemisphere: Washington, 1986; II, 358–360.

45. To, L.C. Robust Nonlinear Control of Industrial Evaporation Systems. World Scientific: River Edge, NJ, 1999.

46. Dukelow, S.G. *The Control of Boilers*; The Instrument Society of America: Research Triangle Park, NC, 1991.

47. Equipment Testing Procedures Committee. *Evaporators: A Guide to Performance Evaluation*; AIChE Equipment Testing Procedure American Institute of Chemical Engineers: New York, 1978.

EXCIPIENTS—POWDERS AND SOLID DOSAGE FORMS

Hak-Kim Chan
Nora Y.K. Chew
University of Sydney, Sydney, New South Wales, Australia

INTRODUCTION

Excipients are the additives used to convert pharmacologically active compounds into pharmaceutical dosage forms suitable for administration to patients (1). Although excipients are the nonactive ingredients, they are essential in the successful production of acceptable solid dosage forms such as tablets and powders. For example, the lack of filling materials would make it exceedingly challenging, if not impossible, to produce a 1 mg dose tablet of a potent drug.

The following general criteria are essential for excipients (2): physiological inertness; physical and chemical stability; conformance to regulatory agency requirements; no interference with drug bioavailability; absence of pathogenic microbial organisms; and commercially available at low cost.

In reality, no single excipient would satisfy all the criteria; therefore, a compromise of the different requirements has to be made. For example, although widely used in pharmaceutical tablet and capsule formulations as a diluent, lactose may not be suitable for patients who lack the intestinal enzyme lactase to break down the sugar, thus leading to the gastrointestinal tract symptoms such as cramps and diarrhea. The role of excipients varies substantially depending on the individual dosage form.

EXCIPIENTS IN TABLETS AND CAPSULES

For tablets and capsules, excipients are needed both for the facilitation of the tableting and capsule-filling process (e.g., glidants) and for the formulation (e.g., disintegrants). Except for diluents, which may be present in large quantity, the level of excipient use is usually limited to only a few percent and some lubricants will be required at <1%. Details of the types, uses, and mechanisms of action of various excipients for tablet and capsule production have been discussed at length in other articles

^aSee *Tablet Compression*, page 000; *Tablet Formulation*, page 000.

in this encyclopedia.^a The types and functions of excipients for tablet production are summarized in Table 1. Although binders, lubricants, and antiadherents are specific for making tablets, other excipients in Table 1 are also used in capsule production for reasons similar to those for tablets.

It is worth noting that some of these tableting excipients may exert effects in opposition to each other. For example, binders and lubricants, because of their respective bonding and waterproofing properties, may hinder the disintegration action of the disintegrants. In addition, some of these tableting excipients may possess >1 function that may be similar (e.g., talc as lubricant and glidant) or opposite (e.g., starch as binder and disintegrant) to each other. Furthermore, the sequence of adding the excipients during tablet production depends on the function of the excipient. Whereas the diluents and the binders are to be mixed with the active ingredient early on for making granules, disintegrants may be added before granulation (i.e., inside the granules), and/or during the lubrication step (i.e., outside the granules) before tablet compression.

EXCIPIENTS IN FREEZE-DRIED (LYOPHILIZED) POWDERS

Freeze-dried (lyophilized) powders are obtained by the process of freeze-drying (lyophilization), which involves freezing of an aqueous-based drug solution in a glass vial followed by sublimation of the ice in a vacuum (3). Because the process is carried out at low temperatures, it is most suitable for heat-sensitive compounds. Antibiotics, such as cephalosporins, are among the preparations commonly prepared by freeze-drying (4). An interesting finding of excipients in freeze-drying is related to breakage of the glass vial (5). This was observed in excipients, such as mannitol, which would undergo mechanical expansion during warming after fast freezing.

Excipients are used in freeze-drying for various purposes. They act as bulking agents to give a pleasing

Table 1 Summary of types and functions of tableting excipients

Excipient	Functions	Examples
Diluent	To act as a bulking agent or filling material	Sugars, lactose, mannitol, sorbitol, sucrose
		Inorganic salts, primarily calcium salts
		Polysaccharides, primarily microcrystalline celluloses
Binders and adhesives	To hold powders together to form granules for tableting	Sugars, glucose, syrup
		Polymers, natural gums, starch, gelatin or synthetic celluloses, polyvinylpyrrol-pyrrolidone (PVP), poly-methycrylate (Eudragit™)
Glidants	To improve the flow of granules from the hopper to the die cavity to ensure uniform fill for each tablet	Fine silica, magnesium stearate, purified talc
Disintegrants	To facilitate the breakup of a tablet in the gastrointestinal tract	Starch and derivatives (polyplasdone XL)
		Microcrystalline cellulose
		Clays, algins, gums, surfactants
Lubricants	To reduce the friction between the granules and the die wall during compression and ejection of the tableting process	Water-insoluble: metal stearates, stearic acid, talc
		Water-soluble: boric acid, sodium chloride, benzoate and acetate, sodium or magnesium lauryl sulfate Carbowax 4000 or 6000
Antiadherents	To minimize the problem of picking, i.e., portion of the tablet face picked out and adhered to the punch face during tableting	Talc, cornstarch, metal stearates, sodium lauryl sulfate
Colorants	For identification purposes and visual marketing values	Natural pigments
		Synthetic dyes
Flavors and sweeteners	To improve the taste of chewable tablets	Natural, e.g., mannitol
		Artificial, e.g., aspartame

appearance to the freeze-dried products. Buffers are present to control the pH of the products that are stable only within a narrow pH range in solution, both during freezing and the subsequent reconstitution. However, it is important to realize that certain buffers, such as the phosphate buffer, in which $Na_2HPO_4 \cdot H_2O$ crystallizes during freezing, cause a pronounced drop in pH (6). This can lead to deleterious effects on the active ingredients, according to the pH dependence of the product stability. Other excipients that may be present in freeze-dried powders include: solubility enhancers (e.g., surfactants or cosolvents), osmotic agents (e.g., saline and sugars), antioxidants (e.g., ascorbic acid), and preservatives for multiple-injection containers (e.g., benzyl alcohol and chlorobutanol). In addition, freeze-dried biological powders may also contain excipients that function to reduce protein adsorption onto the container surface (e.g., surfactants and albumins) (7). A particularly important

use of excipients for therapeutic protein formulations is the stabilization of the protein molecules in the dry state, as discussed later.

Therapeutic Protein Formulations

Therapeutic proteins are usually prepared in liquid formulations or as freeze-dried powders that are to be reconstituted immediately before use. A number of the proteins have been found to be unstable when dried alone, with aggregation being a major problem. It has been found that stability can be greatly improved if the proteins are dried in the presence of certain excipients (8, 9). However, not all excipients that can stabilize protein against aggregation are suitable. Other considerations required of the excipients for use in protein pharmaceuticals include:

Redox reaction potential: reducing sugars such as lactose and sucrose may not be suitable if they react with the protein (e.g., via the lysine residue) resulting in protein glycosylation [e.g., lactosylation of recombinant deoxyribonuclease I by lactose (10)] and other reaction products. However, glycosylation alone may not necessarily be a problem if the glycosylated proteins do not cause toxicity and immunogenicity while maintaining the therapeutic efficacy.

Parenteral use suitability: excipients such as trehalose, which has not been used in any products acceptable by regulatory authorities, may create concerns over toxicity.

Nonparenteral use feasibility: for example, inhalation drug delivery; lactose has been used for marketed aerosol products and hence may be more suitable for inhalation protein formulations.

Table 2 gives some examples of excipients used as stabilizers for proteins in freeze-dried formulations. Among others, saccharides are the most widely used excipients for stabilizing freeze-dried therapeutic proteins. There are exceptions to the need for stabilizing excipients, e.g., recombinant (α-Antitrypsin was stable when freeze-dried alone or with lactose, sucrose, and polyvinylpyrrolidone (11).

The mechanism of the protective effects imparted by the excipients has not been fully elucidated. Empirical observations have pointed to the following contributing factors: formation of a glassy state of the protein–excipient system; crystallinity of the excipients; hydrogen bonding between the excipient and protein molecules; and residual water content.

Glass is an amorphous or noncrystalline solid. It is characterized by the glass transition temperature above which the glassy state softens to the rubbery state. Protein stabilization imparted by excipients can be achieved when the freeze-dried powders are held below the glass transition temperature (T_g) of the protein–excipient systems (i.e., in the glassy state). Of particular relevance to the protein stability is that in the glassy state, the diffusion rate and mobility of the molecules are much less than those in the rubbery state. Thus, any physicochemical reactions leading to protein degradation will be diminished as the protein molecules are "frozen" in the glass formed by the excipients (12).

In contrast to the amorphous excipients, crystalline excipients, such as mannitol, were reported to reduce the stability of proteins (13). Mannitol can be used if the powder is rendered amorphous by the presence of other excipients such as glycine (14). Evidence for protein stabilization by hydrogen bonding has mainly come from the Fourier transformed infrared (FTIR) spectroscopy (15), which provides information on the protein secondary structures. The amide I absorption band (approximately $1600–1700\ cm^{-1}$) of freeze-dried proteins with excipients was found to bear more similarities than the freeze-dried proteins alone to the native proteins in the aqueous environment. This has been explained by sustenance of the native protein structures by protein–excipient hydrogen bonding in the dry powders. However, FTIR measurements were mostly carried out in compressed potassium bromide disks containing the protein. The integrity of the compressed proteins has been largely overlooked (16).

Water affects the stability of proteins by enhancing the mobility of the protein molecules (17). It has been established that an optimal level of water is required to maintain stability of proteins during storage (18). Moisture was known to increase the mobility of the surface groups of protein as measured by solid-state nuclear magnetic resonance spectroscopy (19, 20). The distribution of water between the protein and the excipients in a freeze-dried powder depends on the crystalline or amorphous nature of the excipients (21). For example, if a protein is formulated with an amorphous excipient and stored in a sealed container, water would distribute according to the water affinity of the protein and excipients (21). When the amorphous excipient crystallizes (e.g., because of elevated temperatures), it will expel its sorbed water, which may cause stability problems in the protein (8).

EXCIPIENTS IN POWDER AEROSOL FORMULATIONS

Pharmaceutical inhalation aerosols are widely used for treatment of diseases such as asthma and chronic bronchitis. There are three basic types of aerosol products: the propellant-driven metered-dose inhalers, the dry powder inhalers, and the nebulizers (33). Because of the ozone-depleting and greenhouse effects of the chlorofluorocarbon (CFC) propellants, interest in the dry powder aerosols has risen in recent years.

The main use of excipients in the dry powder inhaler formulations has been to act as carriers for the active ingredients (Table 3). The performance of a dry powder system depends on both the aerosol device and the powder formulation. To generate respirable aerosols, powder formulations must meet two opposing criteria: the particles have to be sufficiently fine (e.g., $<7\ \mu m$) for lung deposition, and yet coarse enough for optimal flow in device (and capsule)-filling and emptying. To achieve this, the drug is blended with coarse inert excipient carriers (34).

Table 2 Some examples of excipients used as protectants for freeze-dried protein and peptide formulations

Protein	Excipients and uses	Reference
Recombinant human growth hormone (rhGH)	Mannitol and glycine as amorphous excipients to prevent human growth hormone (hGH) aggregation. Trehalose as a lyoprotectant, reserves the secondary structure of rhGH.	14
Bovine and human insulins	Dextrin, Emdex™ (spray-dried dextrose) and hydroxypropyl β-cyclodextrin minimized insulin aggregation	22
Recombinant factor IX	Polysorbate 80 as protectant for drying; histidine as pH buffer; glycine for cake appearance	23
Recombinant human interleukin-6	Aggregation prevented by amorphous trehalose, sucrose or a combination of sucrose, and glycine or mannitol	24
Recombinant human interleukin-1 receptor antagonist	Sucrose, sorbitol, trehalose and alanine as protectants against aggregation and deamidation; mannitol and glycine as bulking agent; sodium citrate as buffer	25
FK906 tripeptide	Sugars (sucrose, lactose, trehalose, maltose), polymer (dextran) and salts (NaCl, KCl) to modify the glass transition temperatures of the freeze-dried powders	26
Recombinant human albumin	Organic acid excipient molecules with either a carboxyl group or an amino group present at C-1 position completely stabilized rHA against aggregation	27
Lactate dehydrogenase Phosphofructokinase	Polyethylene glycol as protectant for freezing; sugars (mannitol, lactose, trehalose) as lyoprotectants against loss of bioactivity	28
Alkaline phosphatase	Lactose and trehalose maintain activity longer at elevated temperatures than mannitol	29
Recombinant bovine somatotropin, lysozyme	Both the excipient type (sucrose, sorbitol, glycerol) and moisture content affected protein degradation	30
Hemoglobin	Mannitol protected protein from phase separation induced damage during freeze drying	31
Recombinant human factor XIII	Trehalose and sucrose preserved the native dimeric structure of the protein and prevented aggregates formation	32

Table 3 Some examples of excipients used for dry powder aerosols

Active ingredient	Excipient carrier	Reference
Salbutamol sulfate	Lactose (63–90 μm): regular, spray-dried, and recrystallized	34
Budesonide	Lactose (α-monohydrate (<32 μm, 63–90 μm, 125–180 μm)	39
rhDNase	Lactose (50 wt% < 42 and 115 μm) Mannitol (50 wt% < 43 μm) Sodium chloride (50 wt% < 87 μm)	38
Bovine serum albumin–maltodextrin (50–50)	Lactose (α-monohydrate (63–90 μm) Fine particle lactose (76 wt% < 10 μm) Micronized polyethylene glycol 6000 (97.5 wt% < 10 μm)	40
Recombinant human granulocyte-colony stimulating factor-mannitol	Polyethylene glycol 8000 (38–75 μm, 90–125 μm)	41

Thus, the primary reason of using excipient carrier is to enhance flowability of the drug powder. The excipient carriers are large particles which, because of their sizes (>50 μm), would not be inhaled into the lung. They provide surfaces for the fine drug particles to adhere (Fig. 1), forming an interactive powder mix that would have an improved flowability than the drug alone for handling. On dispersion of the powder by air flow, the fine drug particles are detached from the carriers for inhalation. In an ideal drug–carrier system, the adhesion of the drug to the carriers is strong enough to prevent demixing during filling, handling, and storage, but not so strong as to prevent the generation of fine drug particles by detachment from the carrier during inhalation.

Another reason for using excipient carrier is to improve the availability of fine drug particles in the aerosol cloud. Surface texture of excipients appears to play a prominent role. The fine particle fraction of the antiasthmatic drug salbutamol sulfate was significantly higher with the recrystalline lactose as carrier than with regular or spray-dried lactose. The difference was attributed to the lower surface rugosity (roughness) of the recrystalline lactose (35). With another antiasthmatic compound, salmeterol xinofoate, a formulation using lactose carrier produced a higher fine particle fraction than formulations containing sucrose or spray-dried sorbitol (36). The implication is that using a suitable excipient as carrier it is possible to generate the desirable amount of fine drug particles in an aerosol with a minimal inspiratory effort. Recombinant human deoxyribonuclease I (rhDNase), the first therapeutic protein approved by the Food and Drug Administration (FDA) in the United States for inhalation use in the treatment of cystic fibrosis (37), generated a twofold increase in the fine particle fraction in the aerosol when blended with excipients lactose, mannitol, or sodium chloride (38). In this case, the increase was independent of both the type and relative amount of the excipient used.

Besides surface texture, excipient particle size also plays an important role in the fine particle generation as shown by budesonide, where the highest fine particle fraction was obtained with small-sized (<32 μm) lactose as the carrier (39). Additionally, fine particle excipients such as fine lactose or polyethylene glycol were reported to improve the performance of carrier-based protein dry powder aerosols (40). However, there are some cases where carriers improved total powder emission but reduced the percent of active powders in the aerosol (41). To be useful carriers, the excipients must be physically stable. The important physicochemical characteristics for drug carrier selection are discussed in Ref. 42.

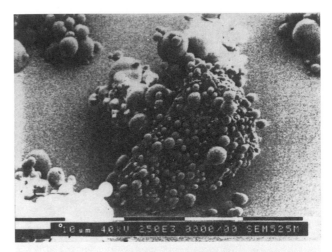

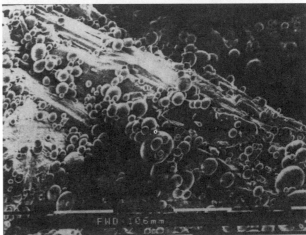

Fig. 1 An example of excipient as carrier for drug particles. Scanning electron micrographs showing adhesion of recombinant human deoxyribonuclease I (rhDNase) particles to lactose (*top*) and mannitol (*bottom*).

In addition to being used as carrier, excipients can enhance the aerosol performance by cospray-drying with the active ingredient. In this case, instead of being external to the drug particles, the excipient exists with the active ingredient in the same particle. For example, using sodium chloride as a crystalline excipient, the fine particle fraction of rhDNase in the aerosol was increased linearly with the amount of excipient present (38). The enhancement was correlated with the degree of crystallinity of the powder in Fig. 2.

As pointed out at the beginning, excipients are not the active ingredients and should be physiologically inert. However, a special use of excipients in dry powder aerosols has been for bronchial provocation testing in asthmatics (43, 44) and for the enhancement of mucociliary clearance in both normal and asthmatic subjects (45, 46). In both cases they acted as the active

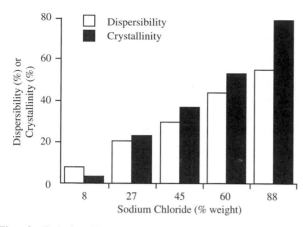

Fig. 2 Relationship between dispersibility (expressed as percent weight of particles less than 7 μm in the aerosol) and crystallinity (by X-ray powder diffraction) of rhDNase powders with different sodium chloride contents. (Adapted from Ref. 38.)

ingredients. The excipients are osmotic agents such as sodium chloride and mannitol. They change the osmolarity of the airway fluid, leading to the physiologic effects of enhanced clearance in the lungs or bronchoconstriction in hyperresponsive subjects.

EXCIPIENTS IN SPRAY-DRIED POWDERS

Spray-drying is a process where a drug solution is atomized to fine droplets followed by evaporation in a stream of warm air to form dry particles (47). The properties of the spray-dried products are controlled by both the process and formulation parameters (48). During the process, the active ingredients are subjected to mechanical shears from atomization and heat stress from the drying air at elevated temperature. Because of the tremendous surface area exposure of the atomized droplets, the drug will also be subjected to degradations such as oxidation and surface denaturation. Excipients can be used as stabilizers or protectants against degradation of the active ingredients. Autoxidation of the analgesic and anti-inflammatory agent aminopyrine was eliminated by excipients such as antioxidants, chelating agents, and clay (49, 50). Denaturation of the model protein (β-Galactosidase was prevented in the presence of trehalose as an excipient (51). Sucrose was found to minimize the degradation product methemoglobin when oxyhemoglobin was spray-dried (52). Recombinant human growth hormone (rhGH), degraded by aggregation resulting from surface denaturation during spray-drying, was successfully stabilized by the

surfactant polysorbate 20 (53). Lactose has been found to protect spray-dried rhDNase against aggregation during storage (54, 55). As a cospray-dried excipient, sodium chloride was reported to increase the dispersibility of the spray-dried rhDNase powder to form aerosols for inhalation (38).

Excipients such as colloidal silica have been reported to increase the flow of spray-dried aminopyrine-barbital powders (49). In contrast, formulations of spray-dried salicylic-acid-containing gelatin and polyvinyl alcohol as excipients were less free-flowing (56). Gum arabic and polyvinylpyrrolidone prevented the sublimation of salicylic acid during spray-drying. For vitamin E acetate, the cospray-dried excipients affected both the powder flowability and drug release properties. Hydroxypropyl cellulose improved the drug release properties; Aerosil™ (colloidal silica) enhanced the powder flow. A balance between these two physical parameters was achieved with approximately 6:1 weight ratio of cellulose to Aerosil (57).

Although it does not effectively protect ascorbic acid against oxidative degradation, colloidal silicon dioxide was found to increase the yield of spray-dried powder (58).

For polymorphic compounds, such as sulfa drugs, talc excipients induced polymorphic transformation of sulfamethoxazole during the process of microencapsulation by spray-drying (59).

Particle size and true density of spray-dried sodium salicylate were affected by binder excipients (56). Drug distribution in spray-dried tolbutamide particles was dependent on the disintegrant excipients used. The drug distributed throughout the particles with low-substituted hydroxypropyl cellulose as excipient but only deposited on the surface with pregelatinized corn starch (60).

Excipients like dibutyl phthalate were used as plasticizers for controlled-release microspheres of theophylline and sulfamethazine prepared by spray-drying (61). Likewise, citric acid was used as plasticizer for spray-dried sodium carboxymethyl cellulose and hydroxypropylmethyl cellulose microspheres containing theophylline (62). Excipients were found to affect the release rate of theophylline with citric acid and triethylene citrate giving the slowest and fastest rate, respectively, as compared with polyethylene glycol and glycerin excipients.

EXCIPIENTS IN CONTROLLED RELEASE SOLID DOSAGE FORMS

Polymeric excipients are commonly used for controlled-release formulations either as a coating around a drug core by microencapsulation or as a matrix in which the drug is embedded. Depending on the release profile requirement, polymeric excipients are traditionally classified as hydrophilic or hydrophobic. Some representative coating materials include water-soluble resins (e.g, gelatin, starch, polyvinylpyrrolidone, water-soluble celluloses), water-insoluble resins (e.g., polymethacrylate, silicones, water-insoluble celluloses), waxes and lipids (e.g., paraffin, beeswax, stearic acid), enteric resins (e.g., shellac, cellulose acetate phthalate) (63). (Further details on polymers for controlled release systems can be found under "Biopolymers for Controlled Drug Delivery" in the first edition of this encyclopedia series.) Here the focus is on some recent applications of excipients in biologicals.

Live rotavirus vaccine was developed for oral delivery to prevent infections by the virus in young children (64). However, incorporation of live rotavirus into poly (DL-lactide-co-glycolide) microspheres or alginate micro-capsules was reported to result in a significant loss of rotavirus infectivity. The loss was reduced by stabilization of the rotavirus vaccine with an excipient blend of cellulose, starch, sucrose, and gelatin at a mass ratio of 30:30:30:10 in granules or tablets (64).

Transforming growth factor (TGF)-betal, a cytoprotec-tant against the toxicity caused by cell cycle-specific drugs, was encapsulated in alginate beads as a potential oral delivery system to release TGF-betal in the gastrointestinal tract. However, the TGF-betal was interacting with alginate, which prevented the release of the protein. Polyacrylic acid, as a polyanion excipient, was used to shield the TGF-betal from interacting with the alginate (65).

Glucose at concentrations >10% was used to achieve adequate reconstitution of freeze-dried biodegradable poly-Σ-caprolactone nanoparticles with conservation of the encapsulated cyclosporin A (66). Glucose and trehalose were also found to be the most efficient cryoprotectors for the lyophilization process, whereas trehalose was used for spray-drying, in the production of solid lipid nanoparticles (67).

Tetanus toxoid (the vaccine for tetanus) encapsulated in polyester microspheres was produced for single-injection immunization (68, 69). The entrapment efficiency of the protein vaccine was significantly improved by coencapsu-lation with excipients such as trehalose and (γ-Hydro--Hydroxypropyl cyclodextrin. However, these excipients did not impart stabilizing effect on tetanus toxoid. In contrast, bovine serum albumin was found to be the most prominent stabilizer for protein in the body after administration by injection.

It is important to point out that the stabilizing effects of excipients were sometimes reported for the formulations in vitro rather than in the in vivo conditions. However, the degree of retention of the native protein structure in the dry state may not be a general indication of stability for the 'wetted' solid within polymer controlled-release devices in the body. In the case of tetanus toxoid, it was shown that the extent of structural alternations in the presence of 1:5 (gram excipient:gram protein) sodium chloride, sorbitol, or polyethylene glycol did not correlate with stability conferred toward moisture-induced aggregation (70).

Surfactant and polyethylene glycols (PEG) excipients have been used in microencapsulation of macromolecules for various effects. For example, Tween 20, at the critical micelle concentration and at a molar concentration of protein:surfactant of 1:0.018 or larger, was found to increase the encapsulation efficiency of β-Lactoglobuline in poly (DL-Lactide-co-glycolide) microspheres (71). The initial burst release was reduced with increasing Tween 20 concentration, and the effect was attributed to reduction of the number of pores and channels inside the microspheres. For gene therapy, the release of biologicals encapsulated in microspheres can be signifi-cantly improved by adding surfactant during micro-encapsulation, as recently exemplified by the enhancing effect of polyvinyl alcohol on the release of adenovirus from PLGA microspheres (72). PEG 400 has been used to improve the stability of the protein, nerve growth factor (NGF) during the microencapsulation by a double emulsion method. It stabilized the protein by reducing the contact with the organic solvent in the process. Furthermore, the presence of NaCl in the microencapsu-lation process has been shown to modify the microsphere structures, leading to a reduction of the initial release rate of NGF (73).

EXCIPIENTS AND FORMULATION INCOMPATIBILITY

During formulation design some excipients may be incompatible with the active ingredient or with other excipients. Excipient incompatibility problems are, in fact, widely published and date back to the mid-1950s. For example, as a tableting excipient, lactose could react via its aldehyde group with both primary (1) and secondary (74) amines by the Maillard-type condensation reaction. Sorbitol, another excipient sugar, is hygroscopic at relative humidity >65%, which should thus be avoided during manufacturing. Calcium salts are other widely used tableting excipients. However, calcium carbonate is incompatible with acids or acidic drugs because of the acid–base chemical reaction. Calcium salts are also incompatible with tetracyclines because of the formation of calcium–tetracycline complexes. Details of reactivities and incompatibilities of individual excipients are given in Ref. 1. Incompatibility attributable to excipients is commonly studied under accelerated testing conditions or using thermal analyses such as differential scanning calorimetry. However, the results of this rapid testing could be misleading and thus of very limited value (75).

Besides direct excipient–drug interactions, excipients can lead to instability of the active ingredient by an indirect role through moisture distribution. Residual water content is known to affect the stability of solid dosage forms and powders (76). Decomposition of cephalothin sodium and benzylpenicillin potassium decomposition in freeze-dried preparation was believed to be partly attributed to the effect of water binding to excipients (4). The degradation rate of cephalothin sodium increased with the water content of excipients corn starch and celluloses (77). The results were correlated with the water mobility in the presence of the excipients (4, 77). A study of the effect of various excipients on the solid-state crystal transformation of the antimalarial compound mefloquine hydrochloride revealed that microcrystalline cellulose promoted the transformation from form E into form D (78). However, methylcellulose, hydroxyethylcellulose, β-Cyclodextrin, crospovidone, and hydrous lactose had no effect. The effect was again explained by the difference in the water uptake behavior by the excipients. Aspirin was formulated with a sugar diluent containing approximately 8% moisture, which did not cause instability problems (79). This was ascribed to the moisture present in the formulation being unavailable to react with the aspirin. The availability of moisture associated with excipients in a formulation can thus be manipulated to control the hydration rate of the active ingredient as in the case of nitrofurantoin, with crystalline lactose giving the fastest and microcrystalline cellulose giving the slowest rate (80). The rate of hydrolysis of methylprednisolone sodium succinate was higher when cofreeze-dried with mannitol than with lactose (81). This correlated with the rate of crystallization of mannitol in the formulation and its subsequent effect on the water distribution in the solid. The stabilizing potency of excipients on recombinant human albumin against aggregation also correlated with the water-sorbing capacity of the excipients (27).

Instability attributable to excipient-mediated water distribution in solids and powders has been explained by excipient physical properties (21, 82–84). Crystalline materials will not uptake moisture until the deliquescent point is reached. In contrast, amorphous excipients will absorb water until their glass transition temperatures fall below the ambient temperature when the mobility of the molecules has increased so much that excipient crystallization will occur to expel the absorbed water from the crystal lattice. Before crystallization, these excipient materials will act as buffers or sorbents to hold the excess moisture which, depending on the water activity, may not be accessible to the active ingredient that is thus be protected from moisture-mediated decomposition. However, when excipient crystallization occurs, the expelled water will become available to react, leading to instability of the drug.

CONCLUSION

Although excipients are the nonactive ingredients, they are indispensable for the successful production of acceptable solid dosage forms. The important roles played by excipients in tablets and capsules, freeze-dried, and spray-dried powders, as well as powder aerosol formulations, were discussed. Some recent applications of excipients in controlled, release formulations for biologicals were also highlighted. Finally, incompatibility problems attributable to excipients were considered with an emphasis on the indirect role of excipients through moisture distribution.

REFERENCES

1. Wade, A., Weller, P.J., Eds.; *Handbook of Pharmaceutical Excipients*, 2nd Ed.; American Pharmaceutical Association: Washington DC, 1994.
2. Bandelin, F.J. Compressed Tablets by Wet Granulation. *Pharmaceutical Dosage Forms: Tablets*, 2nd Ed.; Lieberman, H.A., Lachman, L., Schwartz, J.B.; Eds.; Marcel Dekker, Inc.: New York, 1989; 1.
3. Pikal, M.J. Freeze-Drying of Proteins. Part I: Process Design. BioPharmacology **1990**, 18–27.
4. Oguchi, T.; Yamashita, J.; Yonemochi, E.; Yamamoto, K.; Nakai, Y. Effects of Saccharides on the Decomposition of Cephalothin Sodium and Benzylpenicillin Potassium in Freeze-Dried Preparations. Chem. Pharm. Bull. **1992**, *40*, 1061–1063.
5. Williams, N.A.; Guglielmo, J. Thermal Mechanical Analysis of Frozen Solutions of Mannitol and Some Related Stereoisomers: Evidence of Expansion During Warming and Correlation With Vial Breakage During Lyophilization. J. Parenteral Sci. Technol. **1993**, *47*, 119–123.
6. Pikal, M.J. Freeze –Drying of Proteins. Part II: Formulation Selection. BioPharmacology **1990 October,** 26–30.
7. Crommelin, D.J.A., Sindelar, R.D., Eds.; *Pharmaceutical Biotechnology* Harwood Academic Publishers: The Netherlands, 1997; 72–74.

8. Carpenter, J.F.; Pikal, M.J.; Chang, B.S.; Randoph, T.W. Rational Design of Stable Lyophilized Protein Formulations: Some Practical Advice. Pharm. Res. **1997**, *14*, 969–975.

9. Arakawa, T.; Prestrelski, S.J.; Kenney, W.C.; Carpenter, J.F. Factors Affecting Short-Term and Long-Term Stabilities of Proteins. Adv. Drug Delivery Rev. **1993**, *10*, 1–28.

10. Quan, C.; Wu, S.; Hsu, C.; Canova-Davis, E. Protein Sci. **1995**, *4* (suppl), 490T.

11. Vemuri, S.; Yu, C.-D.; Roosdorp, N. Effect of Cryoprotectants on Freezing, Lyophilization and Storage of Lyophilized Recombinant Alpha1–Antitrypsin Formulations. PDA J. Pharm. Sci. Technol. **1994**, *48*, 241–246.

12. Frank, F. Long-Term Stabilization of Biologicals. Biotechnology **1994**, *12*, 253–256.

13. Izutsu, K.; Yoshioka, S.; Terao, T. Decreased Protein–Stabilizing Effects of Cryoprotectants Due to Crystallization. Pharm. Res. **1993**, *10*, 1232–1237.

14. Pikal, M.J.; Dellerman, K.M.; Roy, M.L.; Riggin, R.M. The Effects of Formulation Variables on the Stability of Freeze-Dried Human Growth Hormone. Pharm. Res. **1993**, *8*, 427–436.

15. Carpenter, J.F.; Prestrelski, S.J.; Dong, A. Application of Infrared Spectroscopy to Development of Stable Lyophilized Protein Formulations. Eur. J. Pharmacol. Biopharmacol. **1998**, *45*, 231–238.

16. Chan, H.-K.; Ongpipattanakul, B.; Au-Yeung, J. Aggregation of Rh DN ase Occurred During the Compression of KBr Pellets Used for FTIR Spectroscopy. Pharm. Res. **1996**, *13*, 238–241.

17. Hageman, M.J. Water Sorption and Solid-State Stability of Proteins. *Stability of Protein Pharmaceuticals, Part A*; Ahern, T.J., Manning, M.C.; Eds.; Plenum Press: New York, 1992; 273–309.

18. Hsu, C.C.; Ward, C.A.; Pearlman, R.; Nguyen, H.M.; Yeung, D.A.; Curley, J.G. Determining the Optimum Residual Moisture in Lyophilized Protein Pharmaceuticals. Dev. Biol. Standard **1992**, *74*, 255–271.

19. Yoshioka, S.; Aso, Y.; Kojima, S. Determination of Molecular Mobility of Lyophilized Bovine Serum Albumin and (γ-Globulin by Solid-State ^{1}H NMR And Relation to Aggregation–Susceptibility). Pharm. Res. **1996**, *13*, 926–930.

20. Separovic, F.; Lam, Y.H.; Ke, X.; Chan, H.-K. A Solid-State NMR Study of Protein Hydration and Stability. Pharm Res. **1998**, *15*, 1816–1821.

21. Chan, H.-K.; Au-Yeung, J.K.-L.; Gonda, I. Water Distribution in Freeze-Dried Solids Containing Multiple Components. Pharm. Res. **1996**, *13* (suppl), S-216.

22. Katakam, M.; Banga, A.K. Aggregation of Insulin and Its Prevention by Carbohydrate Excipients. PDA J. Pharm. Sci. Technol. **1995**, *49*, 160–165.

23. Bush, L.; Webbs, C.; Bartlett, L.; Burnette, B. The Formulation of Recombinant Factor IX: Stability, Robustness, and Convenience. Sem. in Hematol. **1998**, *35* (suppl 2), 18–21.

24. Luckel, B.; Bodmer, D.; Helk, B. A Strategy for Optimizing the Lyophilization of Biotechnology Products. Pharm. Sci. **1997**, *3*, 3–8.

25. Chang, S.B.; Beauvais, R.M.; Dong, A.; Carpenter, J.F. Physical Factors Affecting the Storage Stability of Freeze-dried Interleukin-1 Receptor Antagonist: Glass Transition and Protein Conformation. Arch. Biochem. Biophys. **1996**, *331*, 249–258.

26. Jang, J.W.; Kitamura, S.; Guillory, J.K. The Effect of Excipients on Glass Transition Temperatures for FK 906 in the Frozen and Lyophilized States. PDA J. Pharm. Sci. Tech. **1995**, *49*, 166–174.

27. Costantino, H.R.; Langer, R.; Klibanov, A.M. Aggregation of a Lyophilized Pharmaceutical Protein, Recombinant Human Albumin: Effect of Moisture and Stabilization by Excipients. Biotechnology **1995**, *13*, 493–496.

28. Prestrelski, S.J.; Arakawa, T.; Carpenter, J.F. Separation of Freezing-and Drying-Induced Denaturation of Lyophilized Proteins Using Stress-Specific Stabilization. II. Structural Studies Using Infrared Spectroscopy. Arch. Biochem. Biophys. **1993**, *303*, 465–473.

29. Ford, A.W.; Dawson, P.J. The Effect of Carbohydrate Additives in the Freeze-Drying of Alkaline Phosphatase. J. Pharm. Pharmacol. **1993**, *45*, 86–93.

30. Bell, L.N.; Hageman, M.J.; Muraoka, L.M. Thermally Induced Denaturation of Lyophilized Bovine Somatotropin and Lysozyme As Impacted Moisture and Excipients. J. Pharm. Sci. **1995**, *84*, 707–712.

31. Heller, M.C.; Carpenter, J.F.; Randolph, T.W. Protein Formulation and Lyophilization Cycle Design: Prevention of Damage Due to Freeze-Concentration Induced Phase Separation. Biotechnol. Bioeng. **1999**, *63*, 166–174.

32. Kreilgaard, L.; Frokjaer, S.; Flink, J.M.; Randolph, T.W.; Carpenter, J.F. Effects of Additives on the Stability of Recombinant Human Factor XIII During Freeze-Drying and Storage in the Dried Solid. Arch. Biochem. Biophys. **1998**, *360*, 121–134.

33. Clark, A.R. Medical Aerosol Inhalers: Past, Present, and Future. Aerosol Sci. Technol. **1995**, *22*, 374–391.

34. Ganderton, D. The Generation of Respirable Clouds from Coarse Powder Aggregates. J. Biopharm. Sci. **1992**, *3*, 101–105.

35. Kassem, N.M.; Ganderton, D. The Influence of Carrier Surface on the Characteristics of Inspirable Powder Aerosols. J. Pharm. Pharmacol. **1990**, *42*, 11.

36. Mackin, L.A.; Rowley, G.; Fletcher, E.J. An Investigation of Carrier Particle Type, Electrostatic Charge and Relative Humidity on In-Vitro Drug Deposition from Dry Powder Inhaler Formulations. Pharm. Sci. **197**, *3*, 583–586.

37. Cipolla, D.C.; Clark, A.R.; Chan, H.-K.; Gonda, I.; Shire, S.J. Assessment of Aerosol Delivery Systems for Recombinant Human Deoxyribonuclease. STP Pharma. Sci. **1994**, *4*, 50–62.

38. Chan, H.-K.; Clark, A.R.; Gonda, I.; Mumenthaler, M.; Hsu, C. Spray Dried Powders and Powder Blends of Recombinant Human Deoxyribonuclease (rhDNase) for Aerosol Delivery. Pharm. Res. **1997**, *14*, 431–437.

39. Steckel, H.; Muller, B.W. In Vitro Evaluation of Dry Powder Inhalers II: Influence of Carrier Particle Size and Concentration on in Vitro Deposition. Int. J. Pharm. **1997**, *154*, 31–37.

40. Lucas, P.; Anderson, K.; Staniforth, J.N. Protein Deposition from Dry Powder Inhalers: Fine Particle Multiplets As Performance Modifiers. Pharm. Res. **1998**, *15*, 562–569.

41. French, D.L.; Edwards, D.A.; Niven, R.W. The Influence of Formulation on Emission, Deaggregation and Deposition of

Dry Powders for Inhalation. J. Aerosol Sci. **1996**, *27*, 769–783.

42. Byron, P.R.; Naini, V.; Phillips, E.M. Drug Carrier Selection Important Physicochemical Characteristics, *Respiratory Drug Delivery V*; Dalby, R.N., Byron, P.R., Farr, S.J., Eds.; Interpharm Press: Illinois, 1996; 103–113.

43. Anderson, S.D.; Brannan, J.; Spring, J.; Spalding, N.; Rodwell, L.; Chan, H.-K.; Gonda, I.; Walsh, A.; Clark, A.R. A New Method for Bronchial Provocation Testing in Asthmatic Subjects Using a Dry Powder of Mannitol. Am. J. Crit. Care Med. **1997**, *156*, 758–765.

44. Chew, N.Y.K.; Chan, H.-K. Dispersion of Mannitol Powders As Aerosols: Influence of Particle Size, Air Flow and Inhaler Device. Pharm. Res. **1999**, *16*, 1098–1103.

45. Daviskas, E.; Anderson, S.D.; Brannan, J.D.; Chan, H.-K.; Eberl, S.; Bautovich, G. Inhalation of Dry Powder Mannitol Increases Mucociliary Clearance. Eur. Respir. J. **1997**, *10*, 2449–2454.

46. Brannan, J.D.; Anderson, S.D.; Koskela, H.; Chew, N. Responsiveness to Mannitol in Asthmatic Subjects With Exercise– And Hyperventilation-Induced Asthma. Am. J. Respir. Crit. Care Med. **1998, in press**, *158*.

47. Masters, K. *Spray Drying Handbook*, 4th Ed.; Wiley & Sons: New York, 1985.

48. Wendel, S.; Celik, M. An Overview of Spray-Drying Applications. Pharm. Technol. **1997**, (Oct), 124–156.

49. Kawashima, Y.; Lin, S.Y.; Ueda, M.; Takenaka, H.; Ando, Y. Direct Preparation of Solid Particulates of A minopyrin–Barbital Complex (Pyrabital) from Droplets by a Spray-Drying Technique. J. Pharm. Sci. **1983**, *72*, 514–519.

50. Kawashima, Y.; Lin, S.Y.; Ueda, M.; Takenaka, H. Preparation of Solid Particulates of Amino–Pyrine-Barbital Complexes (Pyrabital) Without Autooxidation by a Spray Drying Technique. Drug Dev. Ind. Pharm. **1983**, *9*, 285–302.

51. Broadhead, J.; Rouan, EdmondS.K.; Hau, I.; Rhodes, C.T. The Effect of Process and Formulation Variables on the Properties of Spray Dried Galactosidase. J. Pharm. Pharmacol. **1994**, *46*, 458–467.

52. Labrude, P.; Rasolomanana, M.; Vigneron, C.; Thirion, C.; Chaillot, B. Protective Effect of Sucrose on Spray Drying of Oxyhemoglobin. J. Pharm. Sci. **1989**, *78*, 223–229.

53. Mumenthaler, M.; Hsu, C.C.; Pearlman, R. Feasibility Study on Spray-Drying Protein Pharmaceuticals: Recombinant Human Growth Hormone and Tissue-Type Plasminogen Activator. Pharm. Res. **1994**, *11*, 12–20.

54. Clark, A.R.; Dasovich, N.; Gonda, I.; Chan, H.-K. The Balance Between Biochemical and Physical Stability for Inhalation Protein Powders: RhDNase As An Example. *Respiratory Drug Delivery V*; Dalby, R.N., Byron, P.R., Farr, S.J., Eds.; Interpharm Press: Illinois, 1996; 167–174.

55. Chan, H.-K.; Gonda, I. Solid State Characterization of Spray-Dried Powders of Recombinant Human Deoxyribonuclease (rhDNase). J. Pharm. Sci. **1998**, *87*, 647–654.

56. Kawashima, Y.; Matsuda, K.; Takenaka, H. Physicochemical Properties of Spray-Dried Agglomerated Particles of Salicylic Acid and Sodium Salicylate. J. Pharm. Pharmacol. **1972**, *24*, 505–512.

57. Takeuchi, H.; Hsaaki, T.Niwa; Hino, T.; Kawashima, Y.; Uesugi, K.; Kayano, M.; Miyake, Y. Preparation of Powdered Redispersible Vitamin E Acetate Emulsion by Spray-Drying Technique. Chem. Pharm. Bull. **1991**, *39*, 1528–1531.

58. Moura, T.F.; Gaudy, D.; Jacob, M.; Terol, A.; Pauvert, B.; Chauvet, A. Vitamin C Spray Drying: Study of the Thermal Constraints. Drug Dev. Ind. Pharm. **1996**, *22*, 393–400.

59. Takenaka, H.; Kawashima, Y.; Lin, S.Y. Polymorphism of Spray-Dried Microencapsulated Sulfamethoxazole With Cellulose Acetate Phthalate and Colloidal Silica, Montmorillonite, or Talc. J. Pharm. Sci. **1981**, *70*, 1256–1260.

60. Takeuchi, H.; Handa, T.; Kawashima, Y. Enhancement of the Dissolution Rate of a Poorly Water-Soluble Drug (tolbutamide) by a Spray-Drying Solvent Deposition Method and Disintegrants. J. Pharm. Pharmacol. **1987**, *39*, 769–773.

61. Palmieri, G.F.; Wehrle, P.; Stamm, A. Evaluation of Spray-Drying As a Method to Prepare Microparticles for Controlled Drug Release. Drug. Dev. Ind. Pharm. **1994**, *20*, 2859–2879.

62. Wan, L.S.; Heng, P.W.; Chia, C.G. Citric Acid As a Plasticizer for Spray-Dried Microcapsules. J. Microencapsulation **1993**, *10*, 11–23.

63. Baker, J.A. Microencapsulation. *The Theory and Practice of Industrial Pharmacy*, 3rd Ed.; Lachman, L., Lieberman, H.A., Kanig, J.L., Eds.; Lea & Febiger: PA, 1986; 415–416.

64. Duncan, J.D.; Wang, P.X.; Harrington, C.M.; Schafer, D.P.; Matsuoka, Y.; Mestecky, J.F.; Compans, R.W.; Novak, M.J. Comparative Analysis of Oral Delivery Systems for Live Rotavirus Vaccines. J. Controlled Release **1996**, *41*, 237–247.

65. Mumper, R.J.; Hoffman, A.S.; Puolakkainen, P.A.; Bouchard, L.S.; Gombotz, W.R. Calcium-alginate Beads for the Oral Delivery of Transforming Growth Factor-Beta1 (TGF-Beta1): Stabilization of TGF-Beta1 by the Addition of Polyacrylic Acid Within Acid-Treated Beads. J. Controlled Release **1994**, *30*, 241–251.

66. Molpeceres, J.; Aberturas, M.R.; Chacon, M.; Berges, L.; Guzman, M. Stability of Cyclosporin-Loaded Poly-Sigma-Caprolactone Nanoparticles. J. Microencapsulation **1997**, *14*, 777–787.

67. Muller, R.H.; Dingler, A.; Weyhers, H.; Muhlen, A.Zur; Mehnert, W. Solid Lipid Nanoparticles—A Novel Carrier Systems for Cosmetics and Pharmaceutics. Pharmazeutische Industrie **1997**, *59*, 614–619.

68. Johansen, P.; Men, Y.; Audran, R.; Corradin, G.; Merkle, H.P.; Gander, B. Improved Stability and Release Kinetics of Microencapsulated Tetanus Toxoid by Coencapsulation of Additives. Pharm. Res. **1998**, *15*, 1103–1110.

69. Audran, R.; Men, Y.; Johansen, P.; Gander, B.; Corradin, G. Enhanced Immunogenicity of Microencapsulated Tetanus Toxoid With Stabilizing Agents. Pharm. Res. **1998**, *15*, 1111–1116.

70. Constantino, H.R.; Schwendeman, S.P.; Griebenow, K.; Klibanov, A.M.; Langer, R. The Secondary Structure and Aggregation of Lyophilized Tetanus Toxoid. J. Pharm. Sci. **1996**, *85*, 1290–1293.

71. Rojas, J.; Pinto-Alphandary, H.; Leo, E.; Pecquet, S.; Couvreur, P.; Fattal, E. Optimization of the Encapsulation

and Release of Beta-Lactoglobulin Entrapped Poly (DL-l actide-co-glycolide) Microspheres. Int. J. Pharm. **1999**, *183*, 67–71.

72. Matthews, C.B.; Jenkins, G.; Hilfinger, J.M.; Davidson, B.L. Poly- L-Lysine Improves Gene Transfer With Adenovirus Formulated in PLGA Microspheres. Gene Ther. **1999**, *6*, 1558–1564.

73. Pean, J.-M.; Boury, F.; Venier-Julienne, M.-C.; Menei, P.; Proust, J.-E.; Benoit, J.-P. Why Does PEG 400 Coencapsulation Improve NGF Stability and Release from PLGA Biodegradable Microspheres. Pharm. Res. **1999**, *16*, 1294–1299.

74. Wirth, D.D.; Baertshi, S.W.; Johnson, R.A.; Maple, S.R.; Miller, M.S.; Hallenbeck, D.K.; Gregg, S.M. Maillard Reaction of Lactose and Fluoxetine Hydrochloride a Secondary Amine. J. Pharm. Sci. **1998**, *87*, 31–39.

75. Monkhouse, D.C.; Maderich, A. Whither Compatibility Testing. Drug Dev. Ind. Pharm. **1989**, *15*, 2115–2130.

76. Zografi, G. Status of Water Associated With Solids. Drug Dev. Ind. Pharm. **1988**, *14*, 1905–1926.

77. Aso, Y.; Yoshioka, S.; Terao, T. Effect of the Binding of Water to Excipients As Measured by ²H-NMR Relaxation Time on Cephalothin Decomposition Rate. Chem. Pharm. Bull. **1994**, *42*, 398–401.

78. Kitamura, S.; Chang, L.-C.; Guillory, J.K. Polymorphism of Mefloquine Hydrochloride. Int. J. Pharm. **1994**, *101*, 127–144.

79. Snavely, M.J.; Price, J.C.; Jun, H.W. The Stability of Aspirin in a Moisture Containing Direct Compression Tablet Formulation. Drug Dev. Ind. Pharm. **1993**, *19*, 729–738.

80. Otsuka, M.; Matsuda, Y. The Effect of Humidity of Hydration Kinetics of Mixtures of Nitrofurantoin Anhydride and Diluents. J. Pharm. Bull. **1994**, *42*, 156–159.

81. Herman, B.D.; Sinclair, B.D.; Milton, N.; Nail, S.L. The Effect of Bulking Agent on the Solid-State Stability of Freeze-Dried Methylprednisolone Sodium Succinate. Pharm. Res. **1994**, *11*, 1467–1473.

82. Zografi, G.; Grandolfi, G.P.; Kontny, M.J.; Mendenhall, D.W. Prediction of Moisture Transfer in Mixtures of Solids: Transfer Via the Vapor Phase. Int. J. Pharm. **1988**, *42*, 77–88.

83. Saleki-Gerhardt, A.; Stowell, J.G.; Byrn, S.R.; Zografi, G. Hydration and Dehydration of Crystalline and Amorphous Forms of Raffinose. J. Pharm. Sci. **1995**, *84*, 318–323.

84. Chan, H.-K.; Au-Yeung, K.-L.; Gonda, I. Development of a Mathematical Model for the Water Distribution in Freeze-Dried Solids. Pharm. Res. **1999**, *16*, 660–655.

85. Wade, A., Weller, P.J.; Eds.; *Handbook of Pharmaceutical Excipients*, 2nd Ed.; American Pharmaceutical Association: Washington, DC, 1994.

86. Lieberman, H.A., Lachman, L., Schwartz, J.B., Eds.; *Pharmaceutical Dosage Forms: Tablets*, 2nd Ed.; Marcel Dekker, Inc.: New York, 1989.

EXCIPIENTS—SAFETY TESTING

Marshall Steinberg

International Pharmaceutical Excipients Council-Americas, Arlington, Virginia

Florence K. Kinoshita

Hercules Incorporated, Arlington, Virginia

INTRODUCTION

The safety issues concerning pharmaceutical excipients can be classified into three categories: quality, toxicology, and improper use (1). Various regulatory directives address the quality category. In addition, the International Pharmaceutical Excipient Council's (IPEC) guideline publications address this issue by following the Organization of International Standardization (ISO) 9000 structure. IPEC is an industry association with worldwide membership that includes over 200 pharmaceutical, chemical, and food processing firms that develop, manufacture, sell, and use pharmaceutical excipients. IPEC comprises three regional organizations located in the United States, Europe, and Japan each with the same objectives.

Quality

The aforementioned IPEC guidelines that address quality include:

- Good Manufacturing Guide for Bulk Pharmaceutical Excipients
- Good Manufacturing Practices (GMP) Audit Guideline for Distributors of Bulk Pharmaceutical Excipients
- IPEC-Americas Significant Change Guide for Bulk Pharmaceutical Excipients
- GMP Audit Guideline for Suppliers of Bulk Pharmaceutical Excipients
- New Excipient Safety Evaluation Guidance
- IPEC-Americas Guide for the Development of an Impurity Profile
- Format and Required Content of Certificates of Analyses

The IPEC-Americas Safety Guidelines (modified) are presented as an information chapter in United States Pharmacopoeia (USP) 24/NF 19 (2). The Good Manufacturing Guide or Practices for Bulk Pharmaceutical Excipients also has been published as an information chapter in USP 24/NF 19. The guideline also serves as a basis for the World Health Organization (WHO) guidance to its national members (3). The intention of IPEC is to ensure that these guidelines reflect the concerns and intentions of responsible parties in the United States, the European Union (EU), and Japan. In other words, the guidelines are harmonized so that excipients that meet the requirements of a harmonized monograph can be sold and used in these three areas of the world. The use of these and other national guidelines ensure the quality of excipients.

These guidelines, using an ISO 9000 format, not only provide a way to assess whether systems are in place, but provide a means for evaluating the effectiveness of the systems. They also provide guidance on how to conduct an audit of a manufacturing operation that produces excipients (4) and in turn, give guidelines on auditing their distribution and repackaging (5).

International Conference on Harmonization Residual Solvent Guidance

Excipient impurity profiles and how to evaluate this important aspect of excipient manufacture, particularly in light of the International Conference on Harmonization (ICH) guidance published in 1999 (6), also are addressed. Care must also be taken that residual solvent levels do not exceed those proscribed in the ICH Guidance for Residual Solvents published in 1999. Solvents are divided into three classes:

1. *Class 1 solvents: Solvents to be avoided.* These include known human carcinogens, strongly suspected human carcinogens, and environmental hazards.
2. *Class 2 solvents: Solvents to be limited.* These include nongenotoxic animal carcinogens or possible causative agents of other irreversible toxicity, such as neurotoxicity or teratogenicity and solvents suspected of other significant but reversible toxicities.

3. *Class 3 solvents: Solvents with low toxic potential.* These include solvents with low toxic potential to man; no health-based exposure limit is needed. Class 3 solvents have permitted daily exposures of 50 mg or more per day.

IPEC Significant Change Guidance

Two areas of concern to excipient makers and users have been those of significant change and certificates of analyses. Any change by the manufacturer of an excipient that alters an excipient's physical or chemical property from the norm or that is likely to alter the excipient's performance in the dosage form is considered significant (7). Regardless of whether there is a regulatory requirement to notify the local regulatory authority, the manufacturer has an obligation to notify its customers of significant change so that the customer can evaluate the change on the customer's products. The Significant Change Guidance establishes uniform considerations for evaluating significant changes involving the manufacture of bulk excipients. The types of changes that might be considered include:

Site
Scale
Equipment
Process
Packaging
Specifications

The requirement for evaluating the impact of change on the excipient begins at the processing step from which GMP compliance begins, as noted in the IPEC Good Manufacturing Guide or Practices Guide for Bulk Pharmaceutical Excipients, or later in the process.

The evaluation criteria in the guideline include:

1. Changes in the chemical properties of the excipient owing to the change
2. Changes in the physical properties of the excipient owing to the change
3. Changes in the impurity profile of the excipient owing to the change
4. Changes in the functionality of the excipient owing to the change
5. Changes in the moisture level of the excipient owing to the change
6. Changes in the bioburden of the excipient owing to the change

The guideline also provides for consideration of objective criteria when considering changes to the impurity profile of an excipient as a result of any change. IPEC-Americas has developed a guide for the preparation of an impurity profile for excipients. The profile addresses the following:

1. All specified organic impurities
2. Unidentified organic impurities at or above 0.1% whether specified or not, unless the impurity has an established pharmacological effect or is known to be unsafe at a lower level
3. Residual solvents
4. Inorganic impurities
5. Toxic impurities

The content of the impurity profile varies with the nature of the excipient, the raw materials used in its manufacture, and its chemical composition. Changes are considered significant whenever a new impurity is introduced at or above the 0.1% concentration or when an impurity previously present at or above 0.1% disappears.

IPEC Certificate of Analysis Guidance

The second issue involves the certificate of analysis that the manufacturer must provide to the formulator when shipping the excipient. Most often, a certificate of analysis does not contain information developed as a result of analysis of the specific batch of material being delivered. The analysis may have either been conducted on previous individual batches or on a mixture of aliquots of previous batches. No guidelines regarding exactly what should be found in the certificate and how it should be presented have been established. This is addressed in the guideline (8). At the time of this writing, the frequency of sampling has not been resolved with the U.S. Food and Drug Administration (FDA). Some believe that in the face of no significant changes it should not be necessary to sample each manufactured batch, but that there is a need only for sufficient sampling to ensure that statistical significance of sampling results can be met. What to do if the manufacturing process is continuous rather than a batch process would fall under the same criteria except that the sampling frequency would probably be based on time/volume rather than batches.

EXCIPIENT USAGE

There are roughly 8000 "nonactive" ingredients being used in food, cosmetics, and pharmaceuticals worldwide (1). In 1996, approximately 800 excipients were used in marketed pharmaceutical products in the United States (1). Although the FDA maintains a "list" of inactive ingredients, the EU and other European countries do not have official published lists, although steps are being taken to rectify this situation.

Few excipients are manufactured specifically for pharmaceutical use. Many are manufactured for other purposes (e.g., food, cosmetics, paint thickeners, construction, etc.). For their use in pharmaceuticals, additional quality, functionality, and safety requirements must be met.

Improper Use of Excipients

The improper use of excipients is addressed, to a certain extent, by the package inserts found in the formulated products. The challenge is to educate consumers and health providers to read and comply with the information contained in these inserts.

DEFINITION OF AN EXCIPIENT

For toxicological purposes, it may be inappropriate to define excipients as inert ingredients. It may be more appropriate to define an excipient (9) as "Any substance other than the active drug or pro-drug which has been appropriately evaluated for safety and is included in a drug delivery system to either:

1. Aid processing of the system during manufacture
2. Protect, support, or enhance stability, bioavailability
3. Assist in product identification
4. Enhance any other attribute of the overall safety and effectiveness of the drug product during storage and use."

As the fourth definition indicates, excipients include a multiplicity of activities from mold releasers to absorption enhancers, and more recently include substances that permit large molecule (e.g., proteins) to be absorbed from the gastrointestinal tract without degradation. Most actions by an excipient are mechanical rather than pharmacological.

APPROVAL MECHANISMS FOR EXCIPIENTS

Currently, regulatory agencies have not established safety-testing guidelines specifically for excipients (10–13). Under U.S. law, a new pharmaceutical excipient, unlike an active drug, has no regulatory status unless it can be qualified through one or more of the approval mechanisms available for components used in finished drug dosage forms. These approval mechanics include:

- Generally Recognized As Safe (GRAS) determination pursuant to 21 Code of Federal Regulations (CFR) 182, 184, and 186
- Approval of a food additive petition under 21 CFR 171
- As contained in a New Drug Application (NDA) approval for a specific drug product and for a particular function or use in that dosage form

Within the EU there is a directive that makes it clear that new chemical excipients will be treated in the same way as new actives (14).

TOXICITY TESTING

The very nature of excipients, for the most part, represents unique problems in testing for toxicity. The actions sought for many excipients are mechanical rather than physiological. Exceptions to this are flavors (12). A most desirable description of some excipients would include being pharmacologically inert and mechanically functional. An alternative would be one where the toxic dose was so high as to be meaningless while still retaining functionality requirements through a range of high and low doses. The acceptable risk for a traditional excipient, when compared to an active principle in a formulation, is generally several orders of magnitude different. Unless an excipient has some very unique properties, it is unlikely that a new excipient would be developed that did not have a large safety factor for toxicity and side effects under conditions of use.

As excipients become more complex and are required to perform functions not required in the past, it is conceivable that a distinction will have to be made between excipients and what might be termed "co-drugs." The use of monoclonal antibodies to deliver an active principle to a specific tissue site might be considered an example of this diversity.

In 1994, as part of the IPEC-Americas program to obtain stand-alone status for excipients, a safety committee was formed. The committee was composed of men and women from a variety of medical and chemistry disciplines who were directed to develop safety-testing guidelines for new excipients. These guidelines were published in 1996 (12). At that time, regulations in most developed countries did not address registration of an excipient as a separate entity. For example, the drug master file for an excipient in the United States is reviewed only as part of the NDA process. Inherent to the current process is the assumption that the use of an excipient in an approved drug dosage form ensures its acceptance in other dosage forms and its ultimate inclusion in the National Formulary (NF). The NF monographs provide standards/specifications for identity, purity, and analysis. Priority for inclusion is given to formulations with approved NDAs and those approved for use in foods. The FDA favors the use of commercially established excipients, such as food additives and substances that have been designated GRAS.

The guidelines developed by IPEC-Americas (12) provide for a tier approach to required testing. The tests to be conducted are based upon the route of application of the

formulated drug and the duration of use. A base set of data is required for all candidate excipients. The guidelines require a review of the chemical and physical properties of the excipient and a review of the scientific literature, exposure conditions (including dose, duration, frequency, route, and user population), and absence or presence of pharmacological activity.

Alternatives to the use of living animals are encouraged wherever these procedures have been validated. The information will provide sufficient information upon which to base a safety judgment and the data will be acceptable to a regulatory agency. The studies should also follow the appropriate legal and professional codes (15) in the conduct of all tests and should meet the Good

Table 1   Summary IPEC-America safety testing guidelines

	Routes of exposure for humans:					
Tests	Oral	Mucosal transdermal/ injectable	topical	Inhalation/ intranasal		Ocular
Baseline toxicity data						
Acute oral toxicity	R	R	R	R	R	R
Acute dermal tox.	R	R	R	R	R	R
Acute inhalation tox.	C	C	C	C	R	C
Eye irritation	R	R	R	R	R	R
Skin irritation	R	R	R	R	R	R
Skin sensitization	R	R	R	R	R	R
Acute parenteral tox.	—	—	—	R	—	—
Application site eval.	—	R	R	R	R	—
Pulmonary sensitization	—	—	—	—	R	—
Phototoxicity/allergy	—	—	R	—	—	—
Bacterial gene mutation	R	R	R	R	R	R
Chromosomal damage	R	R	R	R	R	R
ADME—intended route	R	R	R	R	R	R
28-day toxicity (2 species) intended route	R	R	R	R	R	R
Additional data: Short- or intermediate-term repeated use						
90-day toxicity (most appropriate species)	R	R	R	R	R	R
Embryo-fetal toxicity	R	R	R	R	R	R
Additional assays[a]	C	C	C	C	C	C
Genotoxicity	R	R	R	R	R	R
Immunosupression (3)	R	C	C	R	R	R
Additional data: Intermittent long-term or chronic use						
Chronic toxicity (rodent Nonrodent)	C	C	C	C	C	C
1-generation reproduction	R	R	R	R	R	R
Photocarcinogenicity	—	—	C	—	—	—
Carcinogenicity	C	C	C	C	C	C

Note: R, required; C, conditional
[a]Additional assays are dependent on the judgment of the data evaluator. They may include, but are not limited to screening for endocrine modulators or tests to determine if findings in animals are relevant to humans.
(From Ref. 12, p. 53.)

Laboratory Practices of the agency-(ies) to which the data will be submitted.

The base set of data is designed to provide fundamental information regarding acute toxicity by the oral route and/or intended dose route (Table 1). Skin and eye irritation testing should be conducted irrespective of the route of use of the candidate excipient. These data are intended to protect researchers during the research and production life of the material.

Absorption/distribution/metabolism/excretion/pharmacodynamics are considered fundamental data, as are mutagenicity tests (e.g., Ames test, in vivo chromosome aberration test, and mouse micronucleus test). Twenty-eight day repeated dosing studies in two species by appropriate route(s) also should be performed in a rodent and a nonrodent species, respectively.

One of the unique aspects of the IPEC approach is that not all tests are required. Some of the tests are conditional upon findings in other test procedures. Specific attention is paid to the route of exposure as well as to tests that might be required as potential exposure duration is increased. Emphasis is placed on the fact that the route of exposure for the test animals should be the same as the route of exposure anticipated in humans. Strict attention is paid to the type of exposure. For example, a protocol for study of a product intended for inhalation therapy that results in prolonged exposure of up to several hours per day will differ from that used to evaluate a material that would be used in a product resulting in exposure to several metered doses each day. Some tests may have to be conducted using a route of exposure different from the intended use route. This may be due to the nature of the test animal (e.g., reproductive tests in rabbits may require that the dosage route be other than inhalation, if inhalation is to be the route of use of the formulation containing the excipient).

The IPEC-Americas publication emphasizes that untrained people should not use its guidelines. In addition, the guidelines are not to be used as a checklist. They are to be used by professionals qualified to make the necessary judgments concerning what is referred to as "Conditional" tests. The conduct of these conditional tests is dependent on the results obtained from other required tests. It was considered that given the specificity of some of the cellular and subcellular techniques available and the variety of test animals being developed, that the traditional long-term imprecise test procedures may produce irrelevant information compared to that available from other test procedures. Also, some chemical families produce false positive or questionable results in certain species and the development of these types of data only serve to confound and require additional testing to clarify the questionable results.

It is conceivable that some excipients may not require the standard 2-year, two rodent species carcinogenicity studies. Such excipients include those that are not absorbed (or are rapidly metabolized and/or rapidly excreted), that do not exhibit toxicity in 90-day studies, and those that are negative for genotoxicity. This is the approach taken by the IPEC-Americas Safety Committee and one of the reasons that the 1996 peer-reviewed journal publication (12) indicates that the conduct of rodent carcinogenicity studies is conditional. The carcinogenicity studies that are conditional are the traditional 50 animals/sex/group rodent studies conducted for 18 or 24 months or variations thereof. The decision to make these tests conditional was also predicated on the fact that other models, that provided adequate information upon which to base a safety judgment regarding carcinogenic potential, were available.

GENETICALLY ENGINEERED ANIMAL MODELS

The use of genetically engineered animals has the potential to supplant some of the traditional long-term (2-year) rodent studies. Mouse models have been developed for use as mechanistic models in cancer research. Potential alternatives to the 2-year rodent oncogenicity bioassay include the p53 knockout mouse and the Tg.AC mouse (16).

The use of these mouse models is based on the observation that human neoplasms commonly demonstrate molecular alterations in tumor suppressor genes and/or oncogenes. In normal tissues, tumor suppressor genes (such as p53 and Rb) serve as negative regulators of cell proliferation. Inactivation or loss of tumor suppressor activity through gene mutation or deletion results in loss of this critical regulatory function and may lead to uncontrolled cell proliferation.

Loss of tumor suppressor gene is the most common genetic alteration found in human cancers. Deletion of one or both alleles of p53 (p53 knockout mice) increases the incidence of neoplasia and decreases latency of tumor development. When p53 knockout mice are exposed to genotoxic agents, they rapidly develop neoplasms in a range of tissues. Sensitive targets in p53 mice are often comparable to those in "normal" mice and hence, their utility as a model.

The Tg.AC mouse is used as a skin tumorigenesis model, and when exposed to phorbol ester tumor promoters and other nongenotoxic agents, is rapidly induced. When fully validated, a test battery, including the

Table 2 Summary of IPEC-Europe excipient testing guidelines

Tests	Oral	Mucosal	Transdermal	Dermal/topical	Parenteral	Inhalation/intranasal	Ocular
Step 0							
ADME	R	R	R	R	R	R	R
Step 1 (Basic set)							
Acute oral toxicity (intended route)	R	R	R	R	R	R	R
Eye irritation	—	R	R	R	R	R	R
Skin irritation	—	R	R	R	R	R	R
Skin sensitization	R	R	R	R	R	R	R
Acute parenteral toxicity	—	—	—	—	R	—	—
Application site evaluation	—	R	R	R	R	—	—
Pulmonary sensitization	—	—	—	—	—	C	—
Phototoxicity/photo-allergy	—	—	C	C	—	—	—
Ames test	R	R	R	R	R	R	R
Chromosome damage	R	R	R	R	R	R	R
Micronucleus	R	R	R	R	R	R	R
4 weeks toxicity	R	R	R	R	R	R	R
2(species)—intended route							
Step 2							
90-day toxicity (most appropriate species)	R	R	R	R	R	R	R
Teratology (rat and rabbit)	R	R	R	R	R	R	R
Genotoxicity assays	R	R	R	R	R	R	R
Step 3							
6—9 months chronic toxicity (Rodent, nonrodent)	C	C	C	C	C	C	C
Segment 1	R	R	R	R	R	R	R
Segment III	C	C	C	C	C	C	C
Photocarcinogenicity	—	—	C	C	—	—	—
Carcinogenicity	C	C	C	C	C	C	C

Note: R, required C, conditional.
(From the IPEC Europe Safety Committee. The Proposed Guidelines for the Safety Evaluation of New Excipients. European Pharmaceutical Review, Nov 1997.)

heterozygous p53 knockout mouse and the Tg.AC mouse, may provide a model which will identify both genotoxic and nongenotoxic carcinogens and reduce the in-life time to conduct studies for carcinogenicity to as little as 6 months.

SUMMARY

The tests suggested by IPEC-Americas are summarized in Table 1 (12). The "R" represents required tests and the "C" represents tests that are conditional based on intended use and the results of previous tests. The tests suggested by IPEC-Europe (18) are found in Table 2 and differ slightly from Table 1. The decision whether or not to perform "C" labeled tests requires the judgment of a trained professional. Both IPEC test models are also predicated on obtaining chemical, pharmacological, and physical data from other investigators involved in the development of candidate excipients. Information developed by chemists, pharmacologists, and other disciplines is invaluable in estimating the hazards associated with a new compound.

Testing in humans, using the IPEC-Americas model, either as part of a clinical trial or as a stand-alone procedure, should be conducted as soon as warranted by the animal data. Critical evaluation of the base- set data may support the use of a candidate excipient intended for use once or twice in a lifetime. If one conducts the studies listed in Table 1, section 2, critical evaluation of the data may support the use of the new excipient in a variety of products intended for limited repeated intake, for example an antibiotic. If the Absorption, Distribution, Metabolism, Excretion/Pharmacokinetics (ADME/PK) studies show that the excipient is not absorbed, review of the other data may permit inclusion in a product intended to be used for 30–90 consecutive days. For longer-term usage, the tests listed in Table 1, section 3 must be considered. One-generation reproduction studies must be conducted to assess any excipient-induced effects/disturbances in mating behavior, development/ maturation of gametes, fertility, and preimplantation/ implantation loss of embryos. Should the data continue to support some concern for either reproductive or developmental toxicity, a segment III study might be appropriate (3, 19, 20).

Specific details regarding test methodology are not provided in the guideline. Test procedures generally recognized by experts and the regulatory agencies should be used. Each test should be designed to address a specific issue and the data should be evaluated accordingly. Care should be taken when evaluating animal data to ensure that toxicological findings are not unique to the particular test species and therefore not relevant to the human experience.

Finally, it is important that a material being evaluated for safety is the same as that which will be used in pharmaceutical preparations. The manufacturer of the excipient must follow GMPs. A complete audit trail must be available from the time of manufacture until the product is made available to the consumer. IPEC-Americas has developed a third-party audit program that follows the guidelines enumerated above. The program is conducted by the International Pharmaceutical Excipients Audits, Inc. (IPEA) and is the only program of its type that focuses only on the quality of pharmaceutical excipients.The program is designed to prevent problems with excipients, such as the one that occurred in Haiti in 1996, where 80 children died because the glycerol in their cough medication was mostly glycol.

Ultimately, the safety of an excipient in a formulation requires the following:

1. That the excipient being used is the same excipient that was tested for safety.
2. The test procedures were adequate to evaluate safety and are acceptable to relevant regulatory authorities.
3. The excipient is as specified.
4. The formulated pharmaceutical is used as specified.
5. The concentration of the excipient in the formulation takes into account appropriate test data.

REFERENCES

1. De Jong, H.J. The Safety of Pharmaceutical Excipients. *Therapie* **1999**, *54* (11).
2. The United States *Pharmacopoeia 24/National Formulary 19; 2000.*
3. Principles for the Safety Assessment of Food Additives and Contaminants in Food. World Health Organization. Environ. Health Criter. **1987**, *70*.
4. *Good Manufacturing Practices Guide for Bulk Pharmaceutical Excipients*; The International Pharmaceutical Excipients Council: Arlington, VA, 2000.
5. *The International Pharmaceutical Excipients Council Guideline for Distribution of Bulk Pharmaceutical Excipients; 2000.*
6. Guideline for Residual Solvents, *International Conference on Harmonization; 1999.*
7. IPEC-Americas Significant Change Guide for Bulk Pharmaceutical Excipients, The International Pharmaceutical Excipients Council of the Americas, 2000.
8. Guidance on the Required Content and Format of Certificates of Analysis, The International Pharmaceutical Excipients Council of the Americas, 2000.

9. Blecher, L. Excipients: The Important Components. Pharm. Process **1993**.

10. Cooper, J. Inert Components of Pharmaceutical Preparations. Drug Dev. Ind. Pharm. **1979**, *5*, 293.

11. Smith, J.M.; Dodd, T.R.P. Adverse Drug Reactions. Acute Poisoning Review **1982**, *1*, 93.

12. Steinberg, M.; Borzelleca, J.F.; Enters, E.K.; Kinoshita, F.K.; Loper, A.; Mitchell, D.B.; Tamulinas, C.B.; Weiner, M.L. A New Approach to the Safety Assessment of Pharmaceutical Excipients. Regul. Toxicol. Pharmacol. **1996**, *24* (2), 149.

13. Steinberg, M. ICH Guidelines and Safety: An Update. Pharm. Tech. **1999**.

14. E.U. Directive 75/318 European Economic Community, 1995.

15. Guiding Principles in the Use of Animals in Toxicology Society of Toxicology, 1996.

16. *Life Sciences News Letter*; ITT Research Institute: Chicago IL, 2000.

17. Moreton, C.R. New Excipients: From Idea to Market. Eur. Pharma. Rev. **1997**, *2* (3).

18. The IPEC Europe Safety Committee. The Proposed Guidelines for the Safety of New Excipients. Eur. Pharm. Rev. **1997**, November.

19. Bass, R.; Ulbrich, B.; Hildebrandt, A.G.; Weissinger, J.; Doi, O.; Baeder, C.; Fumero, S.; Harada, Y.; Lehmann, H.; Manson, J.; Neubert, D.; Omori, Y.; Paimer, A.; Sullivan, F.; Takayama, S.; Tanimura, T. Draft Guideline on Detection of Toxicity of Reproduction for Medicinal Products. Adv. Drug React. Toxicol. Rev. **1991**, *9* (J), 127.

20. Toxicological Principles for the Safety Assessment of Direct Food Additives and Color Additives Used in Foods, Redbook II: Draft, *U.S. Food and Drug Administration (USFDA), Bureau of Foods; 1993*.

21. Weiner, M.L.; Kotloskie, L.A. *Excipient Toxicity and Safety*; Marcel Dekker, Inc.: New York, 1999.

EXCIPIENTS FOR PHARMACEUTICAL DOSAGE FORMS

Patrick J. Crowley
Luigi G. Martini
GlaxoSmithKline, Harlow, United Kingdom

INTRODUCTION

Medicinal dosage forms, regardless of composition or mode of use, must meet the following requirements that underpin efficacy, safety, and quality:

1. Contain an accurate dose
2. Be convenient to take or administer
3. Provide the drug in a form for absorption or other delivery to the target
4. Retain quality throughout the shelf life and usage period
5. Be manufactured by a process that does not compromise performance and that is reproducible and economical.

Few if any active pharmaceutical ingredients have properties that allow incorporation in units that meet all these criteria. Therefore, it is necessary to add other materials to make good any shortfalls. Consequently, virtually every medicinal product is a combination of the drug substance and excipients. These are indispensable components of medicinal products and, in most cases comprise the greatest proportion of the dosage unit. It goes without saying that knowledge of the composition, function, and behavior of excipients is a prerequisite to the successful design, development and manufacture of pharmaceutical dosage forms.

The requirements listed above can be considered the prime reasons for including excipients in dosage forms since they relate directly to product performance. Issues such as regulatory acceptability, environmental effects and impact on cost of the product are also important selection criteria.

A single chapter cannot do justice to the richness and complexity of the possibilities and constraints associated with using excipients to transform a drug to a dosage form. Each topic merits a chapter, possibly a complete volume in its own right. This chapter provides a general overview of the issues involved in selecting and evaluating excipients. More detailed accounts of individual applications, performance, and associated issues may be found in the references.

ACCURACY OF DOSE

Where the active ingredient is very potent (i.e., dose is low), it may be necessary to disperse the drug in a "diluent" or bulking agent. Otherwise, quantities being filled into capsules or dies for tableting may be so low that normal filling and other process variations translate to excessive variation in unit drug content. Likewise, low-dose medications for inhalation as dry powders may have the drug dispersed in or otherwise associated with an inert "carrier" or flow aid. For a diluent to function in this way it must form a homogenous blend with the drug. Otherwise accuracy of dose cannot be guaranteed (1).

Water may be considered a "diluent" in liquid presentations as it provides the required dose in a volume that can be accurately dispensed or administered. It is also invariably present in medications for topical or transdermal application. Water can be one of the most problematic companion materials in a dosage form because of its capability to promote hydrolysis, act as a vehicle for other molecular interactions, or simply be a medium for microbial growth. Such properties illustrate how a material that resolves one problem may pose others that in turn require the presence of additional excipients.

Liquid or semisolid preparations may require the presence of ancillary excipients to effect solvation or dispersion of the active ingredient. In particular, formulations containing drugs in the suspended state may require viscosity-enhancing agents or other additives to ensure that the drug remains homogenously dispersed. Otherwise, the accuracy of the dose may be compromised.

USER OR PATIENT CONVENIENCE

Drugs that are bitter or otherwise unpalatable, and administered as oral liquids may be unacceptable, particularly to younger patients. Compliance and therefore efficacy may be compromised unless the product can be made more palatable. Thus, sweeteners, flavors, or taste-masking agents may be present in liquid oral products, in chewable dosage forms, and in effervescent or dispersible tablets that are constituted as liquids prior to use (2).

Some drugs given by injection cause local pain due to high volume, tonicity, pH, etc. An additive that evinces a local anesthetic effect may relieve such discomfort. Benzyl alcohol is employed for this purpose.

RELEASE OF DRUG FROM THE DOSAGE FORM

Once a medication is ingested, applied to a target area, or otherwise administered, the drug must leave the dosage form for absorption or other delivery to the target. This may involve the following:

1. Dissolution in the gastrointestinal (GI) tract following oral dosage;
2. Partitioning to the skin in the case of topical or transdermal preparations;
3. Passage to pulmonary or nasal cavities (inhalation products).

Excipients can ensure that such delivery is expeditious and consistent. Their presence may be even more crucial with more esoteric forms that must be delivered to a tissue, organ, or even specific cells. Researchers are developing excipients that act as "homing devices" to guide drugs to designated targets. Such approaches will be discussed later in this chapter.

In its simplest form, designing "release" into a dosage form involves adding a disintegrant to the tablet or capsule formulation so that on ingestion the compact breaks up and drug is released for dissolution and absorption. In the case of hydrophobic drugs, dissolution may be aided by wetting agents. More complex release patterns involve using excipients to modify release from the dosage form to delay onset of action or otherwise modify the pharmacokinetics of the drug, thereby maximizing efficacy or minimizing side effects.

Excipients can influence delivery from topical and transdermal medications. The propensity of the drug to migrate from the formulation to the application surface is affected by factors such as lipophilicity of the vehicle, drug solubility in the formulation, and effects of additives on the barrier properties of the skin or mucosal surface.

ORAL ABSORPTION ENHANCEMENT

Oral absorption is indirectly aided by excipients that promote release of drug from the dosage form, or help dispersion and dissolution prior to passage to the systemic circulation. Excipients that promote absorption per se are less widely used. However, lipids have been used to enhance absorption of hydrophobic active ingredients. Dissolution or dispersion of drug in such materials provides a substrate for lipolysis, resulting in an emulsion of drug and lipid that provides enhanced surface area for dissolution and absorption (3).

Lipids such as oleic acid or its salts are reported to slow gastric emptying and also act as an "ileal brake." This allows longer time for dissolution and absorption in the small intestine (4, 5). Citric acid and other organic acids also have been shown to slow gastric emptying (6). However, the levels required for such effects may be impractical for most dosage forms.

The small intestine is drained by the hepatic portal vein, making the liver the first "port of call" for orally absorbed drugs. Therefore, high hepatic metabolism will compromise systemic availability. Formulation to enhance lymphatic absorption offers the potential for avoiding such first-pass metabolism. It could also target anticancer agents to lymphatic carcinomas (7). Table 1 lists various materials and associated therapeutic agents that have been formulated for lymphatic delivery.

Oleic acid has been used in a novel approach to boost the bioavailability of propranolol (Fig. 1). The effect was ascribed to preferential uptake by the lymphatic system and avoidance of the extensive first-pass metabolism that would follow passage through the hepatic portal system (8). Formulation with triglycerides also enhanced lymphatic absorption of the antimalarial drug halofantrine (9). However, the low lymph/blood flow ratio limits lymphatic absorption to drugs that are highly lipophilic (log P > 5) and that have significant solubility in long-chain triglycerides (>50 mg/mL).

Strategies to breach physical and enzymatic barriers in the intestinal epithelium that hinder passage to the systemic circulation have included enhancing paracellular flux by disrupting "tight junctions" (10, 11). Inhibition of the P-glycoprotein (PGP) that ejects unrecognized or unwanted materials also has been studied (12). Certain lipids are reported to be PGP inhibitors but there are no reports of successful application to commercial products or use in clinical trials.

Yet another approach to intestinal absorption enhancement concerns the inhibition of intestinal Cytochrome P450 3A4, an enzyme responsible for the prehepatic metabolism of many drugs. Grapefruit juice is reported to be a powerful inhibitor of this enzyme and is known to enhance the bioavailability of cyclosporin, triazolam, nifedipine, and other drugs. Studies have been carried out to identify the components in grapefruit juice that evince

Table 1 Drug carriers for lymphatic targeting

Lymphotropic carrier	Drug	Type of interaction
Dextran sulphate	Bleomycin	Ion-pair
Dextran	Mitomycin C	Covalent binding
β-Cyclodextrin oligomer	1-Hexylcarbamoyl-5-fluorouracil	Hydrophobic inclusion
L-Lactic acid oligomer microsphere	Aclarubicin, cisplatin	Incorporation
Gelatin microsphere	Mitomycin C	Incorporation
Intrinsic protein complex	Vitamin B$_{12}$	Complex
Styrene-maleic acid anhydrideco-polymer	Neocartinostation	Covalent binding
Lipsome	Ara-C	Encapsulation
S/O emulsion	5-Fluorouracil, Bleomycin	Encapsulation
Lipid mixed micelle	Inteferon, TNF	Hydrophobic binding
Chylomicron, LDL	Cyclosporine, vitamin A, coenzyme Q, DDT	Incorporation
	Ethynylesteradiol 3-cyclopententyl ether	
Carbon colloid	Mitomycin C, Aclarubicin	Hydrophobic adsorption

(From Ref. 7.)

this effect (13, 14). It could be argued that inclusion of such materials (thought to be flavinoids), as "excipients" in the dosage form would lead to not only more complete but also more consistent systemic levels by counteracting inconsistencies brought about by enzyme inhibitors in food and drink (such as grapefruit juice). Time will tell whether the ongoing interest in this area will lead to new "excipients" that modulate absorption in this way.

Excipients that are bioadhesive or that swell on hydration can promote absorption by increased contact with epithelial surfaces, by prolonging residence time in the stomach, or by delaying intestinal transit. Cellulose ethers, gums of natural origin, and synthetic acrylic acid polymers have been evaluated for such purposes. The range of materials available and their differing viscoelastic and rheological behaviors mean that it is possible, by

judicious admixture, to develop delivery units with balanced properties so that adhesion, density, hydration, drug release rate, etc. can be tailored to the drug in question and the physiological characteristics of the target delivery site (15).

Enhancers for Other Modes of Absorption

Many physical and enzymatic barriers can prevent successful delivery of active pharmaceutical ingredients by noninvasive, nonoral routes. It is not surprising, therefore, that there is great interest in excipients that can overcome such obstacles.

Transdermal delivery is a case in point. The skin, particularly the stratum corneum presents a formidable barrier to diffusion. Materials used to enhance its permeability have ranged from simple solvents such as ethanol or propylene glycol to aromatic chemicals such as terpenoids. Such penetration enhancers appear to work by disrupting the lipid domains in the stratum corneum that reduce permeability (16). A bespoke penetration enhancer, laurocapram (Azone), was developed in the late 1970s for use in transdermal delivery but its use in commercial products appears to be limited (17).

Entry via nasal or buccal mucosa allows the delivery of peptides or other labile drugs that are highly potent (low-dose drugs) and that do not have steep dose-response relationships. Absorption enhancement requires increased contact time and reduced clearance rate (in the case of nasal delivery), thereby optimizing conditions for mucosal diffusion. Excipients that enhance nasal absorption include

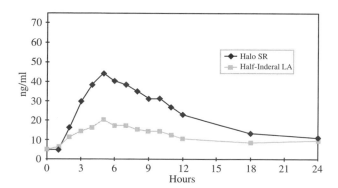

Fig. 1 Effect of oleic acid on propranolol bioavailability. (From Ref. 8.)

phospholipids to enhance mucosal permeability and agents that imbibe water and become mucoadhesive (e.g., glyceryl mono oleate). In addition, the gelling agents hydroxypropyl cellulose and polyacrylic acid promote absorption of insulin in dogs (18). These findings, however, have not been used to find a commercially viable product for intranasal delivery of insulin, presumably due to insulin's narrow therapeutic index. However, intranasal delivery systems for calcitonin, a macromolecule with a much safer dose-response relationship, have been commercialized.

EXCIPIENTS FOR DRUG TARGETING

The 1990s saw an explosion in knowledge and understanding of the roles that natural mediators play in physiological and pathological processes. At the same time, biotechnology has made it feasible to manufacture such mediators relatively cheaply and in large quantities, thereby affording possibilities for use as therapeutic agents. However, effective delivery remains a formidable challenge from the efficacy, safety, and patient-convenience perspective. Most natural mediators are highly potent, extremely labile, and may need to be delivered to a specific organ or cellular target. Conventional oral dosage is not usually feasible due to the hostile environment and enzymatic barriers along the GI tract. Parenteral administration is hardly desirable for chronic therapy. Therefore, many biotechnology products need to be combined with materials that afford protection against destruction, reduce elimination rate, or target a specific site so that activity is enhanced and toxicity minimized. The level of interest and activity in this area supports the view that more effective delivery systems are required if the promise of biotechnology is to be realized. Hence, it is likely that the search for absorption-enhancing excipients for such materials will continue unabated.

Carriers for biopharmaceutical therapeutic agents range from well-established excipients of natural origin to custom-made synthetic materials with putatively enhanced protective or targeting features. Natural or semisynthetic materials predominate however. Sources as diverse as primitive marine plants (chitosans and alginates), plant or animal phospholipids (egg and seed lecithin), and mammalian collagens (gelatin) are being mined for useful delivery or targeting aids, as well as for components of complex formulations such as microemulsions or liposomes. The wide use of biological materials may mean that Mother Nature produces more suitable biopolymers than the synthetic chemist. More plausibly, it may reflect the need for long and expensive safety evaluation of novel synthetic materials prior to use in man. This hinders timely evaluation other than in vitro or animal models.

More esoteric materials that confer target specificity include glycoproteins, recombinant proteins, or monoclonal antibodies (19). To date, clinical performance of such carrier systems has been disappointing. Further refinement of concepts and materials may be necessary before the performance matches the promise.

Attenuated adenoviruses have been used as vectors where delivery to cell nuclei is required (e.g., in gene medicine). It is a moot point whether these or other targeting or carrier materials are "excipients" part of a prodrug or something in-between. The boundaries between "active" and "inactive" materials are much less clear in such cases. The traditional approach of evaluating a novel entity in its own right in animal safety programs and then formulating with "inert" materials is inappropriate with sophisticated delivery systems because of the important effect of the adjuvant on disposition and kinetics of the active ingredient.

EXCIPIENTS AS STABILIZERS

Product quality can be compromised during manufacture, transport, storage or use. The causes of deterioration can be manifold and product-specific. They include microbial spoilage or chemical transformation of the active or physical changes that alter performance in vivo. Deterioration can compromise safety or make the medication less attractive, which means it may not be used. Excipients can contribute to or cause such changes unless carefully screened for possible interactions in preformulation studies.

Cases where excipients have the opposite effect and stabilize labile drugs are less common. Nevertheless, they have been shown to reduce degradation rates of drugs that are photolabile, oxidizible, or degradable consequent to inter- or intramolecular reactions (20). Stablization strategies include the following:

1. Formulation with an excipient whose light absorption spectrum overlaps that of the photolabile drug. This is the so-called spectral overlay approach;
2. Using an antioxidant in formulations that are susceptible to degradation by oxidation. This approach has been particularly successful in vitamin-containing products
3. Using an excipient that "hinders" association of groups in the same molecule, in adjacent molecules, or in the vehicle that can interact and cause degradation. There

are several reports of cyclodextrins effecting such "steric stabilizations." Polyethylene glycol also has been shown to stabilize an ointment formulation by preventing formation of inactive rearrangement products.

Less esoteric but equally important stabilizers include preservatives in liquid products to prevent microbial growth and buffers to provide an environment conducive to good stability where degradation is pH-related. Chelating agents also are used as stabilizers to prevent heavy metals from catalyzing degradation.

EXCIPIENTS AS PROCESS AIDS

The vast majority of medicinal products are manufactured by high-speed, largely automated processes for reasons that are related as much to safety and quality as to cost of goods. Excipients that aid in processing include the following:

1. The almost universal use of lubricants such as stearates in tablets and capsules to reduce friction between moving parts during compression or compaction;
2. Excipients that aid powder flow in tablet or capsule manufacture. Materials such as colloidal silica improve flow from hopper to die and aid packdown in the die or capsule shell. Accuracy and consistency of fill and associated dose is thereby improved
3. Compression aids to help form a good compact, whether on dry granulation (slugging) prior to tableting or on tablet compression. Most are derived from plant, animal, or mineral origin (microcrystalline cellulose, lactose, or magnesium carbonate)
4. Agents such as human or bovine serum albumin that are used in the manufacture of biotechnology-based products. These avoid adsorption of the protein to flexible tubing, filters, and other process equipment
5. Stabilizers to protect the drug from processing conditions that might otherwise be deleterious. It is common to use "cryoprotectants" such as sugars, polyhydric alcohols or dextrans in lyophilized parenteral biotechnology products to prevent inactivation during freezing. A similar approach has also been used to prevent liposomal aggregation and leakage (21).

"Flow aids" also can help performance in cases where the delivery device is an integral part of the medication. Products for pulmonary delivery are often formulated as dry powders that are inhaled via the oral cavity. The fine-particle nature of the medicinal agent, which may be vital for efficient delivery to the

bronchial target area, militates against good flow. Materials such as lactose or mannitol (of appropriate particle size) can enhance flow or act as a "carrier" from the dose unit (usually a capsule) through the inhalation delivery device to the oral cavity on inspiration. They are widely used for these purposes in inhalation formulations of anti-asthmatic agents such as salbutamol and budesonide (22, 23). The recombinant therapeutic proteins human deoxyribonuclease (used to treat cystic fibrosis) and human granulate colony stimulating factor (g-CSF) are also formulated with "carriers" to aid pulmonary delivery (24).

The adherence of very fine particles to larger ones can solve segregation problems when mixing powders containing particles of differing size or shape. If the fine particles can associate with their larger companions due to some surface effect, "ordered mixing" ensues and homogeneity is assured during subsequent processing (25).

Process aids do not usually contribute to the performance of the dosage form in terms of quality or in vivo performance. Indeed, lubricants, because of their hydrophobic nature, can hinder disintegration and dissolution of solid dosage forms unless the level and mode of incorporation is carefully characterized and controlled. Thus, in addition to drug-excipient interactions, the potential for interexcipient competition and incompatibility must be considered and studied.

DRUG–EXCIPIENT INTERACTIONS

Despite the earlier account of excipients acting as stabilizers, it is fair to state that there are far more cases on record of excipients adversely affecting quality. Degradation may be caused by interaction between functional groups in the excipient and those associated with the drug. Many small-molecule drugs contain primary, secondary, or tertiary amino groups and these have the propensity to interact with aldehydic groups in sugars or volatile aldehydes present as residues. Chemical interaction can result in degradation of the drug substance to inactive moieties with loss of efficacy where degradation is excessive. Even when degradation is modest, it is possible that the formed degradation products may compromise safety.

Physical interactions between drug and excipient also can compromise quality. Adsorption of drug by microcrystalline cellulose resulted in drug dissolution being less than complete (26). Interaction between chloramphenicol stearate and colloidal silica during grinding led to polymorphic transformation (27).

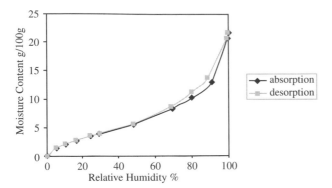

Fig. 2 Water vapor sorption isotherm for microcrystalline cellulose at 25°C. (From Ref. 30.)

Excipients may contribute to degradation even when not directly interacting with active moieties. Soluble materials may alter pH or ionic strength, thereby accelerating hydrolytic reactions in liquid presentations. Such effects may be accentuated during processing. For instance, sterilization by autoclaving, while of short duration, may cause significant degradation product formation because of the high temperature involved. Dextrose is widely used in parenteral nutrition solutions or as a tonicity modifier in other parenterals. Sterilization by autoclaving can cause isomerization to fructose and formation of 5-Hydroxymethyl furfulaldehyde in electrolyte-containing solutions (28). At the other extremes of processing, succinate buffer was shown to crystallize during the freezing stage of lyophilization, with associated reduction of pH and unfolding of gamma interferon (29). It is important to identify and characterize such "process stresses" during dosage-form development and tailor processing conditions accordingly.

Microcrystalline cellulose is a partially depolymerized cellulose that is part-crystalline/part noncrystalline and hygroscopic. Adsorbed water is not held in any "bound" state but will rapidly equilibrate with the environment during processing or storage (30) (Fig. 2). Thus, it is possible that in a dosage form, water can be sequestrated by a more hygroscopic active ingredient. If the drug is moisture sensitive, degradation may follow. Stabilization may be possible by drying prior to use, but loss of water may make it a less effective compression aid (31).

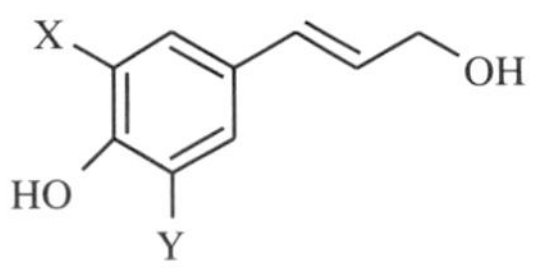

Microcrystalline cellulose may also contain low levels of nonsaccharide organic residues. These emanate from lignin, a cross-linked biopolymer made up primarily of the three allylic alcohols/phenols in the wood chip starting material (Fig. 3) (32).

It is also possible that degradation products of these phenols, or free radical combinations, may be present, with potential for chemical interaction with the drug.

This focus on residues associated with microcrystalline cellulose is not to denigrate it as an excipient. It is and will remain a most valuable formulation aid that can help compression, disintegration, and flow, as well as acting as a general diluent in solid-dose formulation (33). It can also be a useful additive in liquid products. Indeed, the knowledge available on microcrystalline cellulose interactions probably reflects the level of interest in such a useful material. Rather, the intent is to illustrate how excipients, or residues contained in them, can interact with active ingredients in a number of ways. The first commandment for the formulator is arguably to "know your drug," but it is also important to be aware of the composition, residues, and other behaviors of excipients.

STABILITY OF EXCIPIENTS

Excipients can lose quality over time. Oils, paraffins, and flavors oxidize; cellulose gums may lose viscosity. Polymeric materials used in film coating or to modify release from the dosage form can age due to changes in glass transition temperature. This can lead to changes in elasticity, permeability, and hydration rate and associated changes in release properties or appearance (34).

Preservatives such as benzoic acid or the para hydroxybenzoates are volatile and can be lost during product manufacture if the process involves heating. Loss during product storage is also feasible if containers are permeable to passage of organic vapors. Acetate buffer is volatile at low pH and can be lost during the drying stages of lyophilization. Such behaviors reinforce the need to know the behaviors of excipients as well as of the active ingredient so that appropriate processing, storage conditions, and "use by" periods are stipulated where necessary.

IMPURITIES IN EXCIPIENTS

Excipients, like drug substances contain process residues, degradation products or other structural deviants formed during manufacture. Historically, it was not unusual for

X & Y = H : *p*-coumaryl alcohol
X = OMe, Y = H : coniferyl alcohol
X & Y = OMe : sinapyl alcohol

Fig. 3 Potential residues in microcrystalline cellulose.

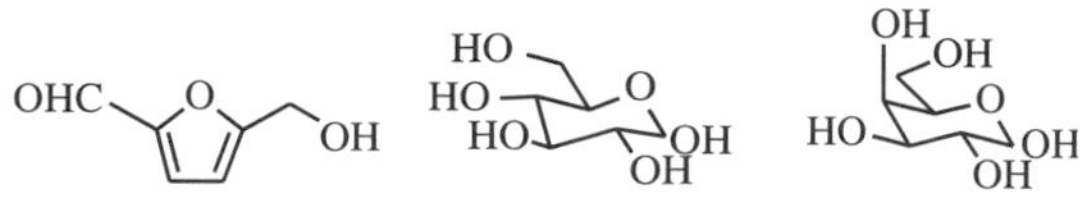

5-Hydroxymethylfurfural   glucose   galactose

Fig. 4   Potential residues in lactose.

Table 2   Potential residues in common excipients

Excipient	Residue
PVP, Polysorbates, benzyl alcohol	Peroxides
Magnesium stearate, fixed oils, paraffins	Antioxidants
Lactose	Aldehydes, reducing sugars
Benzyl alcohol	Benzaldehyde
Polyethylene glycol	Aldehydes, peroxides, organic acids
Microcrystalline cellulose	Lignin, hemicelluloses

adulterants to be added to "bulk up" the commodity. Thankfully, a combination of better analytical techniques, vendor certification programs, and quality audit systems should mean that adulteration is largely a thing of the past. However, constant vigilance is necessary. As recently as 1996, renal failure in children in Haiti was ascribed to use of glycerol contaminated with diethylene glycol in a liquid paracetamol product (35).

Residues in excipients can affect quality and performance by interacting with the drug or other key components. Reducing sugar impurities in mannitol were responsible for the oxidative degradation of a cyclic heptapeptide (36).

Lactose is one of the most widely used excipients in tablet manufacture. It is available in a number of different forms, differing in hydration and crystal states. Isolation and purification may involve treatment with sulphur dioxide (37). However, there are no reports of complications from residues of this powerful oxidizing agent.

Lactose is a disaccharide comprised of glucose and galactose units. These reducing sugars are reported to be present in spray dried lactose (38), as is the hexose degradent 5-hydroxymethyl furfural (39). This aldehyde has the potential for additional reactions with primary amino groups, Schiff Base formation and color development (Fig. 4) (40).

Drugs containing secondary amine groups also can be degraded. Maillard reaction products have been reported in capsules containing lactose and the antidepressant fluoxetine (41). This reaction is also reported extensively in publications concerned with the food industry. High temperatures and low moisture contents associated with food processing induces caramelization of sugars and oxidation of fatty acids to aldehydes, lactones, ketones, alcohols, and esters (42, 43). It would not be surprising if such degradation products were generated in the same materials used in pharmaceutical dosage forms. Unfortunately, most pharmacopoeial monographs do not list such organic contaminants. Also, some excipient vendors are reluctant to share information on residues and contaminants with customers. The pharmaceutical industry generally represents only a small proportion of business for such commodity providers. Hence, it is difficult to be persuasive on the need for individualized standards and controls. Therefore, the following list (Table 2) cannot be

considered as comprehensive because of this unsatisfactory state of affairs.

Excipient residues may also compromise safety or tolerance. Wool fat or lanolin derived from sheep wool may contain low levels of insecticides from sheep treated for parasites. These insecticide levels are probably too low to cause direct toxicity, but may cause allergic reactions when lanolin in cosmetics or topical medicaments is applied to the skin.

Paradoxically, excipient residues such as antioxidants may inadvertently act as stabilizers of the drug substance. Unheralded removal by the vendor or replacement by a different type of stabilizer could precipitate an unheralded product stability crisis leading to recall from the market. Such a possibility highlights the need for agreed change control systems between the pharmaceutical manufacturer and the excipient vendor.

SAFETY OF EXCIPIENTS

Although excipients have traditionally been considered "inert," it is now well accepted that some carry the potential for untoward effects. These can range from the inconvenient to the serious, be general or patient-specific, and may or may not be dose-related. The effect may be ascribable to the excipient itself or to a residue from the starting material or the process of manufacture.

Lactose is one of the most widely used tablet excipients. However, 5–10% of the population of the United Kingdom suffers from lactose malabsorption (44), nor is there reason to suppose that this percentage is lower in other countries. Lack of the lactase enzyme leads to fermentation by colonic bacteria, with formation of lactic acid and carbon dioxide causing stomach cramps, diarrhea, and vomiting (45). Whether such clinical symptoms are manifest following ingestion of the levels normally present in dosage forms is not known, but such phenomena may sometimes explain minor side effects regularly reported during the monitoring that accompanies volunteer Phase I studies.

Malabsorption of the cereal protein gluten is another potential source of untoward effects from excipients. This condition demands a gluten-free diet. Most starches utilized in medicinal products are now gluten-free but gluten-containing materials have been used as film formers in miscroencapsulated products (46). There is also a possibility that gluten could be present in excipients that utilize cereal derivatives as starting materials or bases (e.g., dry powder flavors that sometimes use maltodextrin bases).

Sucrose is a very effective sweetener, particularly for liquids dosed to children. Its propensity to cause dental caries and the complications it poses in the management of diabetes may have contributed to its progressive removal from medicinal products despite its continuing widespread use in foods and confectionery. Sorbitol is another excellent sweetening agent and has been used as a replacement for sucrose in oral liquid products. It has the propensity to cause diarrhea and flatulence, although the effect may only be manifest at high doses. However, there may be additive effects (e.g., if it is formulated with active ingredients that are also associated with GI intolerance, such as antibiotics).

Synthetic sweeteners have had checkered careers as excipients (47). Cyclamate was banned in the United States following reports of carcinogenicity and withdrawal of generally regarded as safe (GRAS) status in 1969. It remains banned despite additional studies to clarify safety and attempts at reinstatement. It remains acceptable in Europe.

Saccharin is equally controversial. It also is suspected as being a carcinogen due to cyclohexylamine formation, possibly by gut flora, on ingestion (48). It was banned as a food additive by the Food and Drug Administration (FDA) in 1977, but has remained available consequent to regular congressional moratoria on the proposed ban. It is not permitted in Canada except for diabetic beverages and foods.

The flavoring agent sodium glutamate is sometimes used to flavor protein supplements or liver extracts. Flushing, headache, and chest pain have been ascribed to its presence, albeit after food intake rather than medication. This is the background to the so-called Chinese restaurant syndrome (49).

Aspartame is a newer sweetener/flavor enhancer but it too may cause angiodema and urticaria. It is contra-indicated in patients suffering from phenylketone urea, as hydrolysis can lead to formation of phenylalanine.

Aspartame also can hydrolyze in solution to form a diketopiperazine derivative and can participate in Michael-type addition reactions with olefines susceptible to nucleophilic attack. The products of such interactions, if they occur, will be drug and formulation-specific, and it is likely that their safety characteristics will be unknown (45).

The use of benzyl alcohol as a local anesthetic was previously discussed. It is also used as a preservative in parenteral dosage forms. However, there is some evidence that benzyl alcohol is neurotoxic and its use is contra-indicated in the United Kingdom in children under 3 years of age (50).

The literature is replete with reports of various allergic-type reactions to preservatives (parabens, chlorocresol), antioxidants (propyl gallate, metabisulphite), surfactants and solvents. The list is too long to be discussed in this article but Ref. 48 contains a very useful compilation and discussion of immunotoxic events seen with various dosage form additives.

Many of these studies involved application of copious amounts to animal skin or to human volunteers in Phase I studies. Others concerned reports of reactions in people suffering from pre-existing allergic conditions. Reports of side effects must, therefore, be viewed from such perspectives and the possibilities for side effects weighed against the widespread use of the same materials in food, confectionery, cosmetic, and household products as well as in medicines. This is not to belittle the hypersensitivity and other reported reactions but unless these are put into context, there may be further constraints on excipient usage and unrealistic demands for "totally inert" formulation adjuvants.

Adverse reactions may be caused by the excipient per se but by a residue. HIV infection in humans and spongiform encephalopathies in cattle have raised the specter of viral transmission by materials as diverse as human and bovine serum albumin, lactose, gelatin, fatty acids, or their salts, as well as polyols such as glycerol. It is generally accepted that screening procedures for blood donors and the heat treatment usually employed for sterilizing human serum albumin (minimum 10 h at 60°C), originally introduced to guard against hepatitis infection, provides good lethality against the HIV virus. However, the prions associated with spongiform ence-phalopathies are so resistant to heat and other forms of sterilization that removal is more problematic. Conse-quently, the use of vegetable sources for fatty acid and organic alcohol-type excipients is becoming more common. Whether gelatin capsules will be replaced by starch or cellulose gum-based alternatives (for the same reason) remains to be seen.

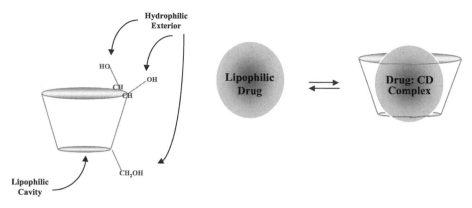

Fig. 5 Mechanism of solubilization by cyclodextrins. (Reproduced from CyDex Inc.)

NOVEL EXCIPIENTS

It might be expected that the increased knowledge of pathological processes and drug-receptor dynamics, along with the relentless pressure for manufacturing efficiencies and economies of scale that have been the hallmark of the 1990s, would also demand and generate new and better formulation aids. This has not happened. Indeed, some have implied that excipients available in 2000 A.D. are not very different from those that were available in 2000 B.C. (51). While clearly calculated to amuse, the assertion contains a grain of truth. Only a handful of novel excipients have emerged over the past 20 years.

The reasons for this are not difficult to understand. Like novel pharmacological agents, a novel excipient must go through numerous safety and metabolic evaluation processes before it can be used in humans. In essence, it would be necessary to apply for a Type 4 Drug Master File in the United States, or a Certificate of Suitability in European Union (EU) countries (50). Such safety and filing programs are expensive and time-consuming. Furthermore, it is difficult to prove "lack of activity" in any material. Excipients are not subject to prescription or pharmacovigilance monitoring, therefore, they need to be "squeaky clean" before "blanket approval" is forthcoming. While a novel excipient can be evaluated at the same time as a novel drug, few organizations wish to put their investment in a novel drug at risk by partnering it with an unproven excipient.Therefore, novel excipients are likely to remain scarce commodities. However, a number of materials considered as "novel" are evincing interest as formulation aids.

Cyclic Glucose Polymers

Cyclodextrins are not new molecular entities. They were first reported a century ago. However, it is only relatively

recently that their potential as formulation aids has been recognized. Their capability to stabilize labile drugs has already been mentioned. They can also be used to solubilize highly insoluble molecules as, with the insertion of the drug in the annulus, the complex largely acquires the solubility characteristics of the cyclodextrin (52) (Fig. 5). Inclusion complexes have also been used to successfully mask taste or odor, reduce sublimation of drugs with high volatility (53), and enhance thermal stability (54).

The so-called parent cyclodextrins viz the alpha, beta, and other forms (Fig. 6) have properties that may have prevented widespread use as formulation adjuvants. The moderate solubility and the perceived need to form molar complexes meant that their use would be limited to low-dose, highly potent compounds. Furthermore, β-Cyclodextrin in particular could not be used parenterally because of renal nephrotoxicity. This was ascribed to its low solubility possibly associated with the propensity to form a molecular complex with cholesterol in vivo and precipitate in the proximal renal tubule. Thus, the potentially most useful application viz dissolution of poorly soluble compounds for injection could not be countenanced. However, β-Cyclodextrin is currently a well-established excipient in oral dosage forms and has recently been allocated monographs (as Betadex) in the European Pharmacopoeia (EP) 2000 and in the U.S. National Formulary, NF 19.

It is also encouraging that derivatized cyclodextrins with greater solubility are now available. The hydroxypropyl and sulphobutyl ether derivatives of β-Cyclodextrin (Fig. 7) have much greater solubilities than the parent material. Indeed, sulphobutyl ether was deliberately developed for use with parenterals in the knowledge that many novel drug substances are poorly soluble. Both these forms have been subjected to comprehensive safety evaluation programs (parenteral in the case of the sulphobutyl ether), and Drug Master Files have been lodged with the FDA. Such

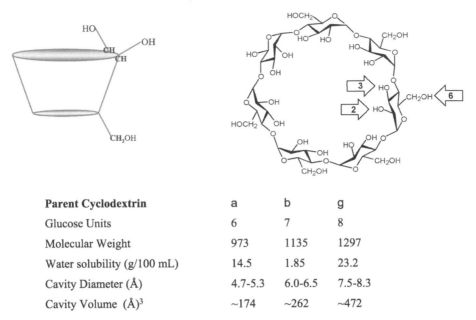

Parent Cyclodextrin	a	b	g
Glucose Units	6	7	8
Molecular Weight	973	1135	1297
Water solubility (g/100 mL)	14.5	1.85	23.2
Cavity Diameter (Å)	4.7-5.3	6.0-6.5	7.5-8.3
Cavity Volume (Å)^3	~174	~262	~472

Fig. 6 Properties and functional groups of some cyclodextrins. (Reproduced from CyDex Inc.)

initiative and commitment on the part of the manufacturers of these newer agents is particularly praiseworthy in light of the costly safety evaluation programs. It may well be that with the availability of such "more suitable" cyclodextrins, they will find a valuable niche in the armamentarium of the formulation scientist. The references cited below comprise two excellent reviews of the promise, properties, and limitations of cyclodextrins (55, 56).

Thus, cyclodextrins are a family of excipients, each with somewhat different properties that allow the possibility of matching individual cyclodextrins to specific drugs to compensate for a deficiency or to aid performance in some way.

Fluorocarbons

The replacement of chlorofluorocarbon (CFC) propellants with the nonozone-depleting hydrofluorocarbons (HFCs) merit mention for two reasons. First, it illustrates how environmental impact can be an important selection

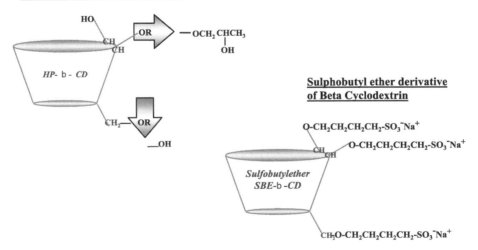

Fig. 7 Functional groups of novel cyclodextrins. (Reproduced from CyDex Inc.)

criterion at a time when "green" issues are high profile. Second, HFCs were developed and evaluated for safety and delivery capability by a consortium of pharmaceutical companies, with costs shared and evaluation programs defined by prior agreement between end-users and propellant manufacturers. Such collaboration could be employed usefully in the future to develop novel excipients for delivery or targeting. The benefits would undoubtedly accrue to all.

Polymeric Targeting or Delivery Aids

Many publications, particularly from academic institutes, contain information concerning synthetic or semisynthetic polymers, which are designed to enhance targeting or delivery properties. However, evaluation of the effect of such material on performance has been invariably confined to in vitro work or perhaps studies in rodents. Clearance for use in humans has not been obtained. Therefore, these substances cannot be considered as excipients that are readily available to the formulation technologist.

If few novel delivery materials become available in the future, the formulation scientist may have to rely on using mixtures of established excipients that, in combination, have properties that are "greater than the sum of the parts" in terms of viscoelasticity, diffusivity, tissue/organ specificity or other desirable targeting or delivery features. Such approaches seem likely to provide considerable scope for creative approaches, and for the formulation technologist, it should be an exciting and fulfilling road to travel.

EXCIPIENT SELECTION

The nature and properties of the active ingredient dictate the choice of an excipient, the dosage form to be elaborated, and the process by which it is manufactured. It is also important to know the patient group and clinical condition. The mode of use of the medication and the envisaged dose must also be considered. Candidate excipients should then be evaluated to demonstrate that they function in the manner intended (do what they are meant to do) and do not adversely interact with the drug, or with other excipients. Obviously, they should not have any pharmacological effect and should not otherwise compromise safety or tolerance.

It is also necessary to consider the regulatory status of excipients and any country-specific requirements or constraints. The U.S. and Japanese regulatory agencies

publish lists of excipients used in medicinal products (57, 58). The materials listed in these compendia can generally be considered suitable for administration by the route for which they are already being used. For materials with no history of previous use, evidence must be provided that they do not compromise patient safety nor induce any other undesirable effects.

SOURCING EXCIPIENTS

Excipients can be crucial determinants of product performance and quality. Thus, they should be sourced directly from a reputable vendor who has quality systems in place to ensure consistent manufacture and control. Procurement from brokers is to be discouraged. Auditing such providers for the presence of quality systems and controls should be the norm, particularly if they are new suppliers to the pharmaceutical industry. A validation program should be put in place to establish reliability of the supply source (59). This program should take the following into account:

1. The nature of the excipient and medicinal product in which it will be used
2. The conditions under which the materials are manufactured and controlled
3. The nature and status of the supplier, and his understanding of the Good Manufacturing Practice (GMP) requirements of the pharmaceutical industry
4. The Quality Assurance system of the manufacturer. Excipients, unlike active ingredients, are not currently subject to regulatory control in terms of GMP unless they are novel materials (in which case preapproval inspection for GMP compliance is necessary). However, the Guide to Good Manufacturing Practice for Bulk Pharmaceutical Excipients, elaborated by the International Pharmaceutical Excipients Councils (IPEC) of Europe and the U.S. while not having any regulatory status, provides much useful information on quality systems and is a good reference for performing audits of excipient facilities (60, 61).

A particular drug or dosage form may have features that rely on the presence of excipients for stabilization, delivery, or other performance parameters. Alternatively, the excipient may need to have additional features to render it suitable for the product in question (e.g., density, absence of a particular residue, etc.). In such cases it may be necessary to agree to extra quality tests and limits over and above those demanded by pharmacopoeias or applied by the vendor.

It is also prudent to be aware of the materials, reagents, and solvent used in the manufacture of the excipient and consider potential interactions between such residues and the active ingredient. It may also be advisable to agree to a Change Control notification procedure with the vendor, to avoid the introduction of new materials in the manufacture of the excipient without prior consideration of the possible impact on the medicinal product.

CONCLUSION

Traditional attitudes that viewed excipients as "inert" materials are long outmoded. It is now well accepted that they are not merely place fillers but can be true "partners" of the active ingredient in many medicinal products and have the potential to enhance or possibly adversely affect performance. As such, their choice, quality control, mode of inclusion, stability, and performance characteristics merit the same attention as the active ingredient. Thus, knowledge of excipients, their foibles, and requirements for handling, processing, and storage are powerful assets in the armamentarium of the pharmaceutical technologist.

REFERENCES

1. Orr, N. Quality Control and Pharmaceutics of Uniformity of Content of Medicines Containing Potent Drugs with Special Reference to Tablets. *Progress in the Quality Control of Medicines*; Deasy, P.B., Timoney, R.F., Eds.; Elsevier Press: Amsterdam, 1981; 193–256.
2. Roy, G.M. Taste Masking in Oral Pharmaceuticals. Pharm. Technol. (USA) **1994**, *18*, 84–90.
3. Hutchinson, K. Formulation of Softgels for Improved Oral Delivery of Hydrophobic Drugs. *Excipients and Delivery Systems for Pharmaceutical Formulations*; Royal Society of Chemistry: Cambridge, 1995; 133–147.
4. Bates, T.R.; Sequira, J.A. Bioavailability of Micronized Griseofulvin from Corn Oil: In Water Emulsion, Aqueous Suspension and Commercial Tablet Dosage Forms. J. Pharm. Sci. **1975**, *64*, 793–797.
5. Brown, N.J.; Read, N.W.; Richardson, R.D.; Bogentoft, C. Characteristics of Lipid Substances Activating the Ileal Brake in the Rat. Gut **1990**, *31*, 1126–1129.
6. Hunt, J.N.; Knox, M.T. The Slowing of Gastric Emptying by Four Strong Acids and Three Weak Acids. J. Physiol. **1972**, *222*, 187–208.
7. Muranishi, S. Drug Targeting towards Lymphatics. Adv. Drug Res. **1991**, *21*, 1–37.
8. Barnwell, S.G.; Gauci, L.; Harris, R.; Attwood, D.; Littlewood, G.; Guard, P.; Pickup, M.E.; Barrington, P. J. Controlled Release **1994**, *28* (1–3), 306–309.
9. Porter, C.H.; Charman, S.A.; Charman, W.N. Lymphatic Transport of Halofantrine in the Triple-Cannulated Anaesthetized Rat Model: Effect of Lipid Vehicle Dispersion. J. Pharm. Sci. **1996**, *85* (4), 351–361.
10. Muranishi, S. Absorption Enhancers. Crit. Rev. Drug Carrier. Syst. **1990**, *7* (1), 1–33.
11. Swenson, E.S.; Curatola, W.J. Means to Enhance Penetration 2. Intestinal Permeability Enhancement for Protein Peptides and Other Polar Drugs: Mechanisms and Potential Toxicity. Adv. Drug. Del. Rev. **1992**, *8* (1), 39–92.
12. Hidalgo, I.J. Cultured Epithelial Cell Models. *Models for Assessing Drug Absorption and Metabolism*; Plenum Press: New York and London, 1996; 35–48.
13. Hukkinen, S.K.; Varhe, A.; Oikkola, K.T.; Neuvonen, P.J. Plasma Concentrations of Triaxolam are Increased by Concomitant Ingestion of Grapefruit Juice. Clin. Pharmacol. Ther. **1995**, *58* (2), 127–131.
14. Edwards, D.J.; Bellevue, F.H.; Woster, P.M. Identification of 6′ 7′ Dihydroxybergamotin, a Cytochrome P450 Inhibitor in Grapefruit Juice. Drug Metab. Dispos. **1996**, *24* (12), 1287–1290.
15. Zaman, M.; McAllister, M.; Martini, L.G.; Lawrence, M.J. The Physicochemical and Biological Factors Influencing Bioadhesion. Pharm. Tech. Eur. **1999**, *11* (8-Biopharm. Suppl.), 52–60.
16. Hadgraft, J.; Walters, K.A. Skin Penetration Enhancement. J. Dermatol. Treat. **1994**, *5* (1), 43–47.
17. Wiechers, J. Excipients in Topical Drug Formulations. Man. Chem. **1998**, 17–21.
18. Rogerson, A.; Parr, G.D. Nasal Drug Delivery. *Routes of Drug Administration*; Florence, A.T., Salole, E.G., Eds.; Wright: London, 1990; 1–29.
19. Hnatyszyn, H.J.; Kossovsky, N.; Gelman, A.; Sponsler, E. Drug Delivery Systems for the Future. PDA J. Pharm. Sci. Technol. **1994**, *48* (5), 247–254.
20. Crowley, P.J. Excipients as Stabilizers. Pharm. Sci. Tech. Today **1999**, *2* (6), 237–243.
21. Carpenter, J.F.; Crowe, J.H. Modes of Stabilization of a Protein by Organic Solutes during Dessication. Cryobiol. **1988**, *25*, 459–470.
22. Ganderton, D. The Generation of Respirable Clouds from Coarse Powder Aggregates. J. Biopharm. Sci. **1992**, (3), 102–105.
23. Steckel, H.; Muller, B.W. In Vitro Evaluation of Carrier Particle Size and Concentration on In Vitro Deposition. Int. J. Pharm. **1997**, *154*, 31–37.
24. Chan, H.K.; Clark, A.R.; Gonda, I.; Mumenthaler, M.; Hsu, C. Spray Dried Powders and Powder Blends of Recombinant Human Deoxyribonuclease (rhDNase) for Aerosol Delivery. Pharm. Res. **1997**, *14* (4), 431–437.
25. Cook, P.; Hersey, J.A. Powder Mixing in the Tableting of Fenfluramine Hydrochloride: Evaluation of a Mixer. J. Pharm. Pharmacol. **1974**, *26*, 298–303.
26. Senderoff, R.I.; Mahjour, M.; Radebaugh, G.W. Characterization of Adsorption Behavior by Solid Dosage Form Excipients in Formulation Development. Int. J. Pharm. **1992**, *83*, 65–72.
27. Forni, F.; Coppi, G.; Iannuccelli, V.; Vandelli, M.A.; Cameroni, R. The Grinding of the Polymorphic Forms of Chloramphenicol Stearic Ester in the Presence of

Colloidal Silica. Acta. Pharmaceutica. Suecica. **1988**, *25* (3), 173–180.

28. Buxton, P.C.; Jahnke, R.; Keady, S. Degradation of Glucose in the Presence of Electrolytes during Heat Sterilization. Eur. J. Pharm. Biopharm. **1994**, *40* (3), 172–175.

29. Lam, X.M.; Constantino, H.R.; Overcashier, D.E.; Nguyen, T.H.; Hsu, C.C. Replacing Succinate with Glycollate Buffer Improves the Stability of Lyophilised Gamma Interferon. Int. J. Pharm. **1996**, *142*, 85–95.

30. Hollenbeck, G.R.; Peck, G.E.; Kildsig, D.O. Application of Immersional Calorimetry to Investigation of Solid–Liquid Interaction: Microcrystalline Cellulose-Water System. J. Pharm. Sci. **1978**, *67* (11), 1599–1606.

31. Khan, K.A.; Musikabhumma, P.; Warr, J.P. The Effect of Moisture Content of Microcrystalline Cellulose on the Compression Properties of Some Formulations. Drug Dev. Ind. Pharm. **1981**, *7*, 525–538.

32. Lewis, N.G.; Davin, L.B.; Sarkanen, S. *The Nature and Function of Lignins: Comprehensive Natural Products Chemistry*; Pinto, B.M., Ed.; Pergamon Press: Oxford, 1999; 3, Ch. 18.

33. Jivraj, M.; Martini, L.G.; Thomson, C.M. An Overview of the Different Excipients Useful for the Direct Compression of Tablets. Pharm. Sci. Technol. Today **2000**, *3* (2), 58–62.

34. Guo, J.H. Aging Processes in Pharmaceutical Polymers. Pharm. Sci. Tech. Today **1999**, *2* (12), 478–483.

35. Anonymous. Morbidity and Mortality Weekly Reports **1996**, *45* (30).

36. Dubost, D.C.; Kaufman, J.; Zimmerman, J.A.; Bogusky, M.J.; Coddington, A.B.; Pitzenberger, S.M. Characterization of a Solid State Reaction Product from a Lyophilized Formulation of a Cyclic Heptapeptide: A Novel Example of an Excipient-Induced Oxidation. Pharm. Res. **1996**, *12*, 1811–1814.

37. Stabilization of Crystalline Lactose, Netherlands Patent Application: NL 8301220 A 841101(DMV-Campina B.V., Netherlands). Patent Application, NL 83-1220 830407.

38. Brownley, C.A., Jr.; Lachman, L. Preliminary Report on the Comparative Stability of Certified Colorants with Lactose in Aqueous Solution. J. Pharm. Sci. **Jan. 1963**, *52*, 86–93.

39. Brownley, C.A., Jr.; Lachman, L. Browning of Spray-Processed Lactose. J. Pharm. Sci. **April, 1964**, *53*, 452–454.

40. Janicki, C.A.; Almond, H.R., Jr. Reaction of Haloperidol with 5-(Hydroxymethyl)-2-Furfuraldehyde: An Impurity in Anhydrous Lactose. J. Pharm. Sci. **1974**, *63*, 41–43.

41. Wirth, D.D.; Baertschi, S.W.; Johnson, R.A.; Maple, S.R.; Miller, M.S.; Hallenbeck, D.K.; Gregg, S.M. Maillard Reaction of Lactose and Fluoxetine Hydrochloride, A Secondary Amine. J. Pharm. Sci. **1998**, *87*, 31–39.

42. Aidrian, J. The Maillard Reaction. *Handbook of the Nutritive Value of Processed Food*, Rechcigl, M., Ed.; CRC Press: Boca Raton, FL, 1982; 1, 529–608.

43. Danehy, J.P. Mailliard Reactions: Non-Enzymic Browning in Food Systems with Specific Reference to the Development of Flavor. Adv. Food Res. **1986**, *30*, 77–138.

44. Neale, G. The Diagnosis, Incidence and Significance of Disaccharidase Deficiency in Adults. Proc. Royal Soc. Med. **1968**, *61*, 1099–1102.

45. Weiner, M., Bernstein, I.L., Eds. Adverse Effects: Bulk Materials. *Adverse Reactions to Drug Formulation Agents*; Marcel Dekker, Inc.: New York, 1989; 89–113, Ch. 6.

46. Weiner, M., Bernstein, I.L., Eds. Adverse Effects: Bulk Materials. *Adverse Reactions to Drug Formulation Agents*; Marcel Dekker, Inc.: New York, 1989; 121–128, Ch. 7.

47. Pinco, R.G. Hurdling International Barriers to Existing and New Excipients. World Pharm. Stand. Rev. **1991**, *2*, 14–19.

48. Smith, J.M.; Dodd, T.R.P. Adverse Reactions to Pharmaceutical Excipients. Adv. Drug React. Pois. Rev. **1982**, *1*, 93–142.

49. Taylor, S.L.; Dormedy, E.S. The Role of Flavoring Substances in Food Allergy and Intolerance. Adv. Food Nutrition Res. **1998**, *42*, 1–44.

50. Saiki, J.H.; Thompson, S.; Smith, F.; Atkinson, R. Paraplegia Following Intrathecal Chemotherapy. Cancer **1972**, *29* (2), 370–374.

51. Robertson, M.I. Regulatory Issues with Excipients. Int. J. Pharm. **1999**, *187*, 273–276.

52. Staniforth, J.N. Design and Use of Tableting Excipients. Drug Dev. Ind. Pharm. **1993**, *19* (17/18), 2273–2308.

53. Loftsson, T.; Brewster, M. Pharmaceutical Applications of Cyclodextrins. 1. Solubilisation and Stabilization. J. Pharm. Sci. **1996**, *85*, 1017–1025.

54. Duchene, D.; Vaution, C.; Glomot, F. Cyclodextrins: Their Value in Pharmaceutical Technology. Drug Dev. Ind. Pharm. **1986**, *12* (11/13), 2193–2215.

55. Cwiertnia, B.; Hladon, T.; Stobieki, M. Stability of Diclofenac Sodium in the Inclusion Complex with β-Cyclodextrin in the Solid State. J. Pharm. Pharmacol. **1999**, *51* (11), 1213–1218.

56. Stella, V.J.; Thompson, D.O. Cyclodextrins-Enabling Excipients: Their Present and Future Use in Pharmaceuticals. Crit. Rev. Ther. Drug Carrier Syst. **1997**, *14* (1), 1–104.

57. Stella, V.J.; Rajewski, R.A. Cyclodextrins: Their Future in Drug Formulation and Delivery. Pharm. Res. **1997**, *14* (5), 556–567.

58. *Inactive Ingredients Guide* Division of Drug Information Resources; United States Food & Drug Administration Center for Drug Evaluation Research (CDER): Rockville, MD, Jan 1996.

59. *Japanese Pharmaceutical Excipients Directory 1996* Japanese Pharmaceutical Excipients Council, Eds.; Yakuji Nipo, Ltd.: Tokyo, MHW, Japan, 1996.

60. *Rules and Guidance for Pharmaceutical Manufacturers and Distributors*; Medicines Control Agency (UK), HMSO: London, 1997, Section 5, Annex 8.

61. Mervcill, A. A Good Manufacturing Practices Guide for Bulk Pharmaceutical Excipients. Pharm. Technol. (USA) **1995**, *19*, 34–40.

62. Weiner, M., Bernstein, I.L., Eds. *Adverse Reactions to Drug Formulation Agents (A Handbook of Excipients)*; Marcel Dekker, Inc.: New York, 1989.

63. Kibbe, A.J., Ed. *Handbook of Pharmaceutical Excipients*, 3rd Ed.; Pharmaceutical Press: London, 2000.

64. *Inactive Ingredients Guide* Division of Drug Information Resources; United States Food & Drug Administration, Center for Drug Evaluation Research (CDER), Rockville, MD, Jan 1996.

65. *Japanese Pharmaceutical Excipients Directory 1996*, Japanese Pharmaceutical Excipients Council, Eds.; Yakuji Nipo Ltd.: Tokyo, 1996.

EXCIPIENTS—THEIR ROLE IN PARENTERAL DOSAGE FORMS

Sandeep Nema
Pharmacia Corporation, Skokie, Illinois

Ron J. Brendel
Mallinckrodt, Inc., St. Louis, Missouri

Richard J. Washkuhn
Lexington, Kentucky

INTRODUCTION

The term pharmaceutical excipient or additive denotes compounds that are added to the finished drug product for a variety of reasons. Most often excipients are major components of the drug product, with the active drug molecule present in a small percentage. Excipients also have been referred to as inactive or inert isngredients to distinguish them from the active pharmaceutical ingredients. However, in many instances excipients may not be as inert as some scientists believe. Several countries have restrictions on the type or the amount of excipient that can be included in the formulation of parenteral drug products due to safety issues. For example, in Japan, amino mercuric chloride, or thimerosal use is prohibited, even though these excipients are present in several products in the United States.

As defined in the *European Pharmacopoeia* (EP) 1997 and the *British Pharmacopoeia* (BP) 1999, "Parenteral preparations are sterile preparations intended for administration by injection, infusion, or implantation into the human or animal body" (1, 2). However, for the purposes of this article, only sterile preparations for administration by injection or infusion into the human body will be surveyed. Injectable products require a unique formulation strategy. The formulated product has to be sterile, pyrogen free, and in the case of solutions, free of particulate matter. No coloring agent may be added solely for the purpose of coloring the parenteral preparation. Preferably, the formulation should be isotonic, and depending on the route of administration, certain excipients may not be allowed. For a given drug, the risk of an adverse event may be higher or the effects may be difficult to reverse if it is administered as an injection versus a nonparenteral route, since the injected drug bypasses natural defense barriers. The requirement for sterility demands that the excipient be able to withstand terminal sterilization or aseptic processing. These factors limit the choice of excipients available to the formulator.

Generally, a knowledge of which excipients have been deemed safe by the Food and Drug Administration (FDA) or are already present in a marketed product provides increased assurance to the formulator that these excipients will probably be safe for their new drug product. However, there is no guarantee that the new drug product will be safe as excipients are combined with other additives and/or with a new drug molecule, creating unforeseen potentiation or synergistic toxic effects. Regulatory bodies may view favorably an excipient previously approved in an injectable dosage form and will frequently require less safety data. A new additive in a formulated product will always require additional studies adding to the cost and timeline of product development.

In Japan, if the drug product contains an excipient with no precedence of use in that country, then the quality and safety attributes of the excipient must be evaluated by the Subcommittee on Pharmaceutical Excipients of the Central Pharmaceutical Affairs Council concurrently with the evaluation of the drug product application (3). Precedence of use means that the excipient has been used in a drug product in Japan, and will be administered via the same route and in a dose level equal to or greater than the excipient in question in the new application.

This chapter is a comprehensive review of the excipients included in the injectable products marketed in the United States, Europe, and Japan. A review of the literature indicates that only a few articles that specifically deal with the selection of parenteral excipients have been published (4–9). However, excipients included in other sterile dosage forms not administered parenterally, such as solutions for irrigation, ophthalmic or otic drops, and ointments, will not be covered.

Several sources of information were used to summarize the information compiled in this chapter (4–7, 10–14). Formulation information on the commercially available injectable products was entered in a worksheet. Tables presented in this chapter are condensed from this worksheet. Each table is categorized based on the primary function of the excipient in the formulation. For example, citrates are classified as buffers and not as chelating agents, and ascorbates are categorized as antioxidants, although they can serve as buffers. This classification system minimizes redundancy and provides a reader-friendly format. The concentration of excipients is listed as percent weight by volume (w/v) or volume by volume (vol%). If the product was listed as lyophilized or powder, the percentages were derived based on the reconstitution volume commonly used. The tables list the range of concentration and examples of products containing the excipient, especially those that use an extremely low or high concentration.

TYPES OF EXCIPIENTS

Solvents and Cosolvents

Table 1 list solvents and cosolvents used in parenteral products. Water for injection is the most common solvent but may be combined or substituted with a cosolvent to improve the solubility or stability of drugs (15, 16). The dielectric constant and solubility parameters are among the most common polarity indices used for solvent blending (17, 18). Ethanol and propylene glycol are used either alone or in combination with other solvents in more than 50% of parenteral cosolvent systems. Surprisingly, propylene glycol is used more often than polyethylene glycols (PEGs) in spite of its higher myotoxicity and hemolyzing effects (19–22). The hemolytic potential of cosolvents is as follows (19):

$$\text{Dimethyl acetamide} < \text{PGE400} < \text{Ethanol}$$
$$< \text{Propylene glycol}$$
$$< \text{Dimethyloxide}$$

It is possible that the presence of residual peroxide from the bleaching of PEG or the generation of peroxides in PEG may result in the degradation of the drug in the cosolvent system. It is important to use unbleached and/or peroxide–free PEGs in the formulation.

Oils such as safflower and soybean are used in total parenteral nutrition products, where they serve as a fat source and as carriers for fat-soluble vitamins. The *U.S. Pharmacopeia* (USP) requirement for injectable oils is as follows:

A. Fixed oils (of vegetable origin)

- Saponification value (185–200)
- Iodine number (79–128). (*The Japanese Pharmacopoeia* (*JP*) recommends value between 79–137.)

Table 1 Solvents and cosolvents

Excipient	Frequency	Range	Example
Almond oil	1	ND	Poison Ivy Extract (Parke Davis)
Benzyl benzoate	3	20–44.7% w/v	Delestrogen® 40 mg/ml (Bristol Myers) 44.7% w/v
Castor oil	1	ND	Delestrogen® 20 mg/ml (Bristol Myers) 44.7% w/v
Cottonseed oil	2	73.6–87.4% w/v	Depo-Testadiol® (Upjohn) 87.4% w/v
N,N-Dimethylacetamide	2	6–33% w/v	Busulfex® (Orphan Medical) 33%
Ethanol	26	0.6–100%	Prograf (Fujisawa) 80 vol%, Alprostadil (Bedford Lab) 100%
Glycerin (glycerol)	12	1.6–70% w/v	Multitest CMI® (Pasteur Merieux) 70% w/v
Peanut oil	1	ND	Bal in Oil® (Becton Dickinson)
Polyethylene glycol			
PEG	5	0.15–50%	Secobarbital sodium (Wyeth-Ayerst) 50%
PEG 300	3	50–65%	VePesid® (Bristol Myers) 65% w/v
PEG 400	3	18–67 vol%	Busulfex® (Orphan Medical) 67%
PEG 600	1	5% w/v	Persantine® (Dupont-Merck)
PEG 3350	5	0.3–3%	Depo-Medrol® (Upjohn) 2.95% w/v
Poppyseed oil	1	ND	Ethiodol® (Savage)
Propylene glycol	29	0.2–80%	Ativan® (Wyeth-Ayerst) 80%
Safflower oil	2	5–10%	Liposyn II® (Abbott) 10%
Sesame oil	6	100%	Solganal Inj.® (Schering)
Soybean oil	4	5–20% w/v	Intralipid® (Clintec) 20%
Vegetable oil	2	ND	Virilon IM Inj.® (Star Pharmaceuticals)

ND, No data available.

- Test for unsaponifiable matter
- Test for free fatty acid
- Solid paraffin test at 10°C
- Acid value NMT 0.56 (*JP* only)

B. Synthetic mono-and diglycerides of fatty acids (which are liquid and remain so when cooled to 10°C)

- Iodine number (<140)
- Solid paraffin test at 10°C

The oils also are used to dissolve drugs with low aqueous solubility and provide a mechanism to slowly release drug over a long period of time. Deterioration of fixed oils, which leads to rancidity and production of free fatty acids, must be avoided in injectable products. Also the fixed oils or fatty acid esters must not contain mineral oil or paraffin which the body cannot metabolize.

Polymeric and Surface Active Compounds

Table 2 includes a broad category of excipients whose fun ction in formulation could be as follows:

1. To impart viscosity or act as suspending agents such as carboxy methyl cellulose, sodium carboxy methyl cellulose, acacia, Povidone, hydrolyzed gelatin, and sorbitol.

2. To act as solubilizing, wetting, or emulsifying agents such as Cremophor EL, sodium desoxcholate, Polysorbate 20 or 80, PEG 40 castor oil, PEG 60 castor oil, sodium dodecyl sulfate, lecithin, or egg yolk phospholipid.

3. To form gels such as when aluminum monostearate is added to fixed oil to form a viscous or gel-like suspension medium.

Polysorbate 80 is the most common and versatile solubilizing, wetting and emulsifying agent. Again, one must be concerned about the level of residual peroxides present in polysorbates and protecting them from air to prevent further oxidation (23). Polysorbate 80 is polyoxyethylene sorbitan ester of oleic acid (unsaturated fatty acid) while polyoxyethylene Polysorbate 20 is sorbitan ester of lauric acid (saturated fatty acid). Thus, stability differences could occur in the drug product formulated with Polysorbate 80 versus Polysorbate 20. One example is Neupogen® which when exposed to a high concentration of Polysorbate 20 exhibited substantially less oxidation than when exposed to a similar concentration of Polysorbate 80 (24).

Table 2   Solubilizing, wetting, suspending, emulsifying, or thickening agents

Excipient	Frequency	Range	Example
Acacia	2	7%	Tuberculin Old Test® (Lederle) 7%
Aluminum monostearate	1	2%	Solganal Inj.® (Schering) 2%
Carboxy methyl cellulose	4	0.50–0.55%	Bicillin® (Wyeth-Ayerst) 0.55%
Caboxy methyl cellulose, sodium	19	0.15–3.0%	Nutropin Depot® (Genentech) 3%
Cremophor EL[a]	3	50–65% w/v	Sandlmmune® (Sandoz) 65% w/v
Desoxycholate sodium	1	0.4% w/v	Fungizone® (Bristol Myers) 0.41% w/v
Egg yolk phospholipid	3	1.2%	Intralipid® (Clintec) 1.2%
Gelatin, Hydrolzyed	1	16% w/v	Cortone® (Merck) 16% w/v
Lecithin	8	0.4–1.2% w/v	Diprivan® (Zeneca) 1.2% w/v
Pluronic F-68	1	—	Fluosol® (Alpha Therapeutics)
Polyoxyethylated fatty acid	2	7–12% w/v	AquaMephyton® (Merck) 7% w/v Aquasol A parenteral® (Astra) 12%
Polysorbate 80 (Tween 80)	48	0.004–100%	Taxoterer® (Aventis) 100%
Polysorbate 20 (Tween 20)	9	0.01–0.4%	Calcijex® (Abbott) 0.4%
PEG 40 castor oil[b]	1	11.5 vol%	Monistat® (Janssen) 11.5 vol%
PEG 60 castor oil[c]	1	20% w/v	Prograf® (Fujisawa) 20% w/v
Povidone (Polyvinyl pyrrolidone)	7	0.5–0.6% w/v	Bicillin®(Wyeth-Ayerst) 0.6% w/v
Sodium dodecyl sulfate (Na lauryl sulfate)	1	0.018% w/v	Proleukin® (Cetus) 0.018% w/v
Sorbitol	3	25–50%	Aristrospan® (Fujisawa) 50 vol%

[a]Cremophor EL, Etocas 35, polyethoxylated castor oil, polyoxyethylene 35 castor oil.
[b]PEG 40 castor oil, polyoxyl 40 castor oil, castor oil POE-40, Croduret 40, polyoxyethylene 40 castor oil, Protachem CA-40.
[c]PEG 60 hydrogenated castor oil, Cremophor RH 60, hydrogenated castor oil POE-60, Protachem CAH-60.

Table 3 Chelating agents

Excipient	Frequency	Range	Example
Calcium disodium EDTA[a]	9	0.01–0.1%	Wydase® (Wyeth-Ayerst) 0.1% w/v
Disodium EDTA	38	0.01–0.11%	Calcijex® (Abbott) 0.11% w/v
Sodium EDTA	1	0.20%	Folvite® (Lederle) 0.20%
DTPA[b]	1	0.04%	Magnevist® (Berlex) 0.04%

[a]EDTA = Ethylenediaminetetraacetic acid.
[b]DTPA = Diethylenetriaminepentaacetic acid; pentetic acid.

Chelating Agents

Only a limited number of chelating agents are used in parenteral products (Table 3). They serve to complex heavy metals and therefore can improve the efficacy of antioxidants or preservatives. Citric acid, tartaric acid and some amino acids also can act as chelating agents. There have been some misunderstandings concerning the use of EDTA (as calcium salt) as an approved injectable product in Japan. Currently in Japan, some drug products that contain calcium disodium EDTA are on the market and this excipient is also listed as an official excipient (see Table 11). An advantage of calcium EDTA over tetrasodium salt is that calcium EDTA does not contribute sodium and does not chelate as much calcium from the blood.

A complexing agent should not be used in metalloprotein formulations, where the protein subunits are held by the metal (25). The EDTA, in rare instances, can increase the oxidation rate due to binding of the EDTA–metal complex to protein, resulting in site-specific generation of radicals (26).

Antioxidants

Antioxidants are used to prevent the oxidation of active substances and excipients in the finished product. There are three main types of antioxidants:

1. *True antioxidants*: They act by a chain-termination mechanism by reacting with free radicals, e.g., butylated hydroxytoluene.
2. *Reducing agents*: They have a lower redox potential than the drug and get preferentially oxidized, e.g.,

Table 4 Antioxidants and reducing agents

Excipient	Frequency	Range	Example
Acetone sodium bisulfite	4	0.2–0.4% w/v	Novocaine® (Sanofi-Winthrop) 0.4% w/v
Ascorbate (sodium/acid)	8	0.1–4.8% w/v	Vibramycin® (Pfizer) 4.8% w/v
Bisulfite sodium	31	0.02–0.66% w/v	Amikin® (Bristol Myers) 0.66% w/v
Butylated hydroxy anisole (BHA)	3	0.00028–0.03% w/v	Aquasol A® (Astra) 0.03% w/v
Butylated hydroxy toluene (BHT)	3	0.00116–0.03% w/v	Aquasol A® (Astra) 0.03% w/v
Cystein/Cysteinate HCl	3	0.07–1.3% w/v	Acthrel® (Ferring) 1.3% w/v
Dithionite sodium (Na hydrosulfite, Na sulfoxylate)	1	0.10%	Numorphan® (Endo Lab) 0.10%
Gentisic acid	1	0.02% w/v	OctreoScan® (Mallinckrodt) 0.02% w/v
Gentisic acid ethanolamine	1	2%	M.V.I. 12® (Astra) 2%
Glutamate monosodium	2	0.1% w/v	Varivax® (Merck) 0.1% w/v
Formaldehyde sulfoxylate sodium	9	0.02–0.5% w/v	Terramycin solution (Pfizer) 0.5% w/v
Metabisulfite potassium	1	0.10%	Vasoxyl® (Glaxo-Wellcome) 0.10%
Metabisulfite sodium	32	0.02–1% w/v	Intropin® (DuPont) 1% w/v
Monothioglycerol (Thioglycerol)	6	0.1–1%	Terramycin solution (Pfizer) 1%
Propyl gallate	2	0.02%	Navane® (Pfizer) 0.02%
Sulfite sodium	7	0.05–0.2% w/v	Enlon® (Ohmeda) 0.2% w/v
Tocopherol alpha	1	0.005% w/v	AmBisome® (Fujisawa) 0.005%
Thioglycolate sodium	1	0.66% w/v	Sus-Phrine® (Forest) 0.66% w/v

ascorbic acid. Thus, they can be consumed during the shelf-life of the product.

3. *Antioxidant synergists*: These enhance the effect of antioxidants, e.g., EDTA.

Table 4 summarizes the antioxidants, their frequency of use, concentration range, and examples of products containing them. Sulfite, bisulfite, and metabisulfite constitute the majority of antioxidants used in parenteral products despite several reports of incompatibility and toxicity (27, 28). Butylated hydroxy anisole, butylated hydroxy toluene, alpha tocopherol, and propyl gallate are primarily used in semi/nonaqueous vehicles because of their low aqueous solubility (29). Ascorbic acid/sodium ascorbate may serve as an antioxidant, buffer and chelating agent in the same formulation. Some amino acids such as cysteine also function as effective antioxidants.

The Committee for Proprietary Medicinal Products (CPMP) guideline calls for a full explanation and justification for including antioxidants in the formulation (30). It further states that antioxidants should only be included in a formulation if it has been proven that their use cannot be avoided. Thus, it is imperative to first try inert gas (nitrogen or argon) in the headspace to prevent oxidation. If the antioxidant has to be included, its concentration must be justified in terms of efficacy and safety. Antioxidants such as sulfites and metabisulfites are especially undesirable.

Some antioxidants possess antimicrobial properties, such as propyl gallate and butylated hydroxy anisole, which are somewhat effective against bacteria. Butylated hydroxy toluene has demonstrated some antiviral activity. Compatibility of antioxidants with the drug, packaging system and the body should be studied carefully. For example, tocopherols may be absorbed onto plastics;

ascorbic acid is incompatible with alkalis, heavy metals, and oxidizing materials such as phenylephrine, and sodium nitrite; and propyl gallate forms complexes with metal ions such as sodium, potassium and iron.

Preservatives

Benzyl alcohol is the most common antimicrobial preservative present in parenteral formulations (Table 5). This observation is consistent with other surveys (6, 31). Parabens are the second most common preservatives. Surprisingly, thimerosal is also common, especially in vaccines, even though some individuals are sensitive to mercurics. Several preservatives can volatilize easily (such as benzyl alcohol, and phenol) and, therefore, should not be used for lyophilized dosage form. Chlorocresol is purported to be a good preservative for parenterals, but our survey did not find any examples of commercial products containing chlorocresol. The British Pharmaceutical Codex and Martindale list chlorocresol as a preservative to be used in multidose aqueous injections at concentrations of 0.1% but no examples of injectable products have been provided (32, 33).

Antimicrobial preservatives are allowed in multidose injections to prevent growth of microorganisms that may accidentally enter the container during withdrawal of the dose. However, they are discouraged from being used in single-dose injections in the United States while the EP and BP allow aqueous preparations, that are manufactured using aseptic techniques, to contain suitable preservatives. It should be emphasized that preservatives should never be used as a substitute for inadequate good manufacturing practices (GMP). BP and EP prohibit antimicrobials from single-dose

Table 5 Antimicrobial preservatives

Excipient	Frequency	Range	Example
Benzalkonium chloride	1	0.02% w/v	Celestone Soluspan® (Schering) 0.02% w/v
Benzethonium chloride	4	0.01%	Benadryl® (Parke-Davis) 0.01% w/v
Benzyl alcohol	85	0.75–10%	Progesterone (United Res) 10%
Chlorbutanol	18	0.25–0.5%	Codine phosphate (Wyeth-Ayerst) 0.5%
m-Cresol	5	0.1–0.35%	Humalog® (Lilly) 0.35%
Myristyl gamma–picolinium chloride	2	0.0195–0.169% w/v	Depo-Provera® (Pharmacia-Upjohn) 0.169% w/v
Paraben methyl	52	0.05–0.18%	Inapsine® (Janssen) 0.18% w/v
Paraben propyl	44	0.01–0.1%	Xylocaine w/ Epinephrine (Astra) 0.1% w/v
Phenol	50	0.2–0.5%	Calcimar® (Rhone-Poulanc) 0.5% w/v
2-Phenoxyethanol	4	0.50%	Havrix® (SmithKline Beecham) 0.50% w/v
Phenyl mercuric nitrate	3	0.001%	Antivenin® (Wyeth-Ayerst) 0.001%
Thimerosal	48	0.003–0.012%	Atgam® (Pharmacia-Upjohn) 0.01%

Table 6 Maximum permissible amount of preservatives and antioxidants

Excipient	Maximum limit in USP
Mercurial compounds	0.01%
Cationic surfactants	0.01%
Chlorobutanol	0.50%
Cresol	0.50%
Phenol	0.50%
Sulfur dioxide or an equivalent amount of the sulfite, bisulfite, or metabisulfite of potassium or sodium	0.20%

injections where the dose volume is greater than 15 mL or if the drug product is to be injected via intracisternal, or any route which gives access to the cerebrospinal fluid (CSF). Toxicity is the primary reason for minimizing the use of antimicrobial preservatives. For example, many individuals are allergic to mercury preservatives while benzyl alcohol is contraindicated in children under the age of 2. USP has also placed some restrictions on the maximum concentration of preservatives allowed in the formulation to address toxicity and allergic reactions (Table 6). The World Health Organization (WHO) has set an estimated total acceptable daily intake for sorbate (as acid, calcium, potassium and sodium salts) as not more than 25 mg/kg body weight. The efficacy of the preservative should be assessed during product development using Antimicrobial Preservative Effectiveness Testing (PET) (34–36). Thus, an aqueous-preserved parenteral product can be used up to a maximum of 28 days after the container has been opened (37). Obviously, 28 days has to be justified by performing PET on the finished product in the final package. On the other hand, unpreserved products preferably should be used immediately following opening, reconstitution, or dilution.

Buffers

Buffers are added to a formulation to adjust the pH in order to optimize solubility and stability. For parenteral preparations, the pH of the product should be close to physiologic pH. The selection of buffer concentration (ionic strength) and buffer species is important. For example, 5–15 mM of citrate buffers are used in the formulation but increasing buffer concentration to >50 mM will result in excessive pain on subcutaneous injection and toxic effects due to the chelation of calcium in the blood.

Buffers have maximum buffer capacities near their pK_a. For products that may be subjected to excessive temperature fluctuations during processing (such as sterilization or lyophilization), it is important to select buffers with a small ΔpK_a/°C. Thus, Tris, whose ΔpK_a/°C is large (−0.028/°C), the pH of buffer made at 25°C will change from 7.1 to 5.0 at 100°C. This may dramatically alter the stability or solubility of the drug. Similarly, the best buffers for a lyophilized product may be those that show the least pH change upon cooling, that do not crystallize out, and that can remain in the amorphous state protecting the drug. For example, replacing succinate with glycolate buffer improves the stability of lyophilized interferon-γ (38). During the lyophilization of mannitol that contains succinate buffer at pH 5, monosodium succinate crystallizes, reducing the pH and resulting in the unfolding of interferon-γ. This pH shift is not seen with glycolate buffer.

Table 7 lists buffers and chemicals used to adjust the pH of formulations and the product pH range. Phosphate, citrate, and acetate are the most common buffers used in parenteral products. Mono- and diethanolamines are added to adjust pH and form corresponding salts. Hydrogen bromide, sulfuric acid, benzene sulfonic acid, and methane sulfonic acids are added to drugs which are salts of bromide (Scopolamine HBr, Hyoscine HBr), sulfate (Nebcin, Tobramycin sulfate), besylate (Tracrium Injection, Atracurium besylate) or mesylate (DHE 45 Injection, Dihydroergotamine mesylate). Glucono delta lactone is used to adjust the pH of Quinidine gluconate. Benzoate buffer, at a concentration of 5%, is used in Valium Injection. Citrates are a common buffer that can have a dual role as chelating agents. The amino acids lysine and glycine, function as buffers and stabilize proteins and peptide formulations. These amino acids are also used as lyo-additives and may prevent cold denaturation. Lactate and tartrate are occasionally used as buffer systems. Acetates are good buffers at low pH, but they are not generally used for lyophilization because of potential sublimation of acetates.

Bulking Agents, Protectants, and Tonicity Adjusters

Table 8 lists additives that are used to modify osmolality, and as bulking or lyo/cryoprotective agents. Dextrose and sodium chloride are used to adjust tonicity in the majority of formulations. Some amino acids such as glycine, alanine, histidine, imidazole, arginine, asparagine, and aspartic acid are used as bulking agents for lyophilization and also can serve as stabilizers, and/or as buffers.

Table 7 Buffers and pH-adjusting agents

Excipient	pH Range	Example
Acetate		
Sodium	3.7–4.3	Syntocinon® (Novartis)
Acetic acid	3.7–4.3	Syntocinon® (Novartis)
Glacial acetic acid	3.5–5.5	Brevibloc® (Ohmeda)
Ammonium	6.8–7.8	Bumex Injection® (Roche)
Ammonium sulfate	—	Innovar® (Astra)
Ammonium hydroxide	—	Triostat® (Jones Medical)
Arginine	7.0–7.4	Retavase® (Boehringer)
Aspartic acid	5.7–6.4	Pepcid® (Merck)
Benzene sulfonic acid	3.25–3.65	Nimbex® (Glaxo Wellcome)
Benzoate Sodium/acid	6.2–6.9	Valium® (Roche)
Bicarbonate	5.5–11.0	Cenolate® (Abbott)
Boric acid/sodium		Comvax® (Merck)
Carbonate, sodium	5.0–11.0	Hyperab® (Bayer)
Citrate		
Acid	3.0–5.5	DTIC-Dome® (Bayer)
Sodium	3.5–6.5	Amikin® (Bristol Myers)
Disodium	—	Cerezyme® (Genzyme)
Trisodium	—	Cerezyme® (Genzyme)
Diethanolamine	9.5–10.5	Bactim IV® (Roche)
Glucono delta lactone	5.5–7.0	Quinidine Gluconate(Lilly)
Glycine/glycine HCl	6.4–7.2	Hep-B Gammagee® (Merck)
Histidine/histidine HCl	6.5	Doxil® (Sequus)
Hydrochloric acid	6.0–7.6	Amicar® (Immunex)
Hydrobromic acid	3.5–6.5	Scopolamine (UDL)
Lactate sodium/Acid	2.7–5.7	Innovar® (Janssen)
Lysine (L)	—	Eminase® (Roberts)
Maleic acid	3.0–5.0	Librium® (Roche)
Meglumine	6.5–8.0	Magnevist® (Berlex)
Methanesulfonic acid	3.2–4.0	DHE-45® (Novartis)
Monoethanolamine	8.0–9.0	Terramycin (Pfizer)
Phosphate		
Acid	6.5–8.5	Saizen® (Serono Labs)
Monobasic potassium	6.7–7.3	Zantac® (Glaxo-Wellcome)
Monobasic sodium[a]	6.0–8.0	Pregnyl® (Organon)
Dibasic sodium[b]	6.7–7.8	Zantac® (Glaxo-Wellcome)
Tribasic sodium	—	Synthroid® (Knoll)
Sodium hydroxide	Broad range	Optiray® (Mallinckrodt)
Succinate sodium/Disodium	5.0–6.0	AmBisome® (Fujisawa)
Sulfuric acid	3.0–6.5	Nebcin® (Lilly)
Tartrate sodium/acid	2.7–6.2	Methergine® (Novartis)
Tromethamine	6.0–7.5	Optiray® (Mallinckrodt)

[a]Sodium biphosphate, sodium dihydrogen phosphate, or Na dihydrogen orthophosphate.
[b]Sodium phosphate, disodium hydrogen phosphate.

Monosaccharides (dextrose, glucose, maltose, lactose), disaccharides (sucrose, trehalose), polyhydric alcohols (inositol, mannitol, sorbitol), glycols (PEG 3350), Povidone (polyvinylpyrrolidone, PVP) and proteins (albumin, gelatin) are commonly used as lyo-additives.

Hydroxyethyl starch (hetastarch) and pentastarch, which are currently used as plasma expanders in commercial injectable products such as Hespan and Pentaspan, also are being evaluated as protectants during freeze-drying of proteins.

Table 8 Bulking agents, protectants, and tonicity adjusters

Excipient	Example
Alanine	Thrombate III® (Bayer)
Albumin	Bioclate® (Arco)
Albumin (human)	Botox® (Allergan)
Amino acids	Havrix® (Smith Kline Beecham)
Arginine (L)	Activase® (Genentech)
Asparagine	Tice BCG® (Organon)
Aspartic acid (L)	Pepcid® (Merck)
Calcium chloride	Phenergan® (Wyeth-Ayerst)
Cyclodextrin-alpha	Edex® (Schwartz)
Cyclodextrin-gamma	Cardiotec® (Squibb)
Dextran 40	Etopophos® (Bristol Myers)
Dextrose	Betaseron® (Berlex)
Gelatin (cross-linked)	Kabikinase® (Pharmacia-Upjohn)
Gelatin (hydrolyzed)	Acthar® (Rhone-Poulanc Rorer)
Lactic & glycolic acid copolymers	Lupron Depot® (TAP)
Glucose	Iveegam® (Immuno-US)
Glycerine	Tice BCG® (Organon)
Glycine	Atgam® (Pharmacia-Upjohn)
Histidine	Antihemophilic Factor, human (Am. Red Cross)
Imidazole	Helixate® (Armour)
Inositol	OctreoScan® (Mallinckrodt)
Lactose	Caverject® (Pharmacia-Upjohn)
Magnesium chloride	Terramycin Solution (Pfizer)
Magnesium sulfate	Tice BCG® (Organon)
Maltose	Gamimune N® (Bayer)
Mannitol	Elspar® (Merck)
Polyethylene glycol 3350	Bioclate® (Arco)
Polylactic acid	Lupron Depot® (TAP)
Polysorbate 80	Helixate® (Armour)
Potassium chloride	Varivax® (Merck)
Povidone	Alkeran® (Glaxo-Wellcome)
Sodium chloride	WinRho SD® (Univax)
Sodium cholesteryl sulfate	Amphotec® (Sequus)
Sodium succinate	Actimmune® (Genentech)
Sodium sulfate	Depo-Provera® (Pharmacia-Upjohn)
Sorbitol	Panhematin® (Abbott)
Sucrose	Prolastin® (Bayer)
Trehalose (alpha, alpha)	Herceptin® (Genentech)

PVP has been used in injectable products as a solubilizing agent, a protectant and as a bulking agent. Only pyrogen-free grade, with low molecular weight (K value less than 18) should be used in parenteral products to allow for rapid renal elimination. PVP not only solubilizes drugs such as rifampicin, but it also can reduce the local toxicity as seen in oxytetracycline injection.

Many proteins can be stabilized in the lyophilized state if the stabilizer and protein do not phase separate during freezing or the stabilizer does not crystallize out.

In the case of Neupogen® (GCSF), the original formulation was modified by replacing mannitol with sorbitol to prevent the loss of activity of liquid formulation in case of accidental freezing (24). Mannitol crystallizes if the solution freezes while sorbitol remains in an amorphous state protecting GCSF. Similarly, it is useful that the drug remains dispersed in the stabilizer upon freezing of the solution. Thus, Cefoxitin, a cephalosporin, is more stable when freeze-dried with sucrose than with trehalose, although the glass transition temperature and structural relaxation time is much greater for trehalose than sucrose (39). FTIR data indicated that the trehalose–cefoxitin system phase separated into two nearly pure components, resulting in no protection (stability). Similarly, dextran was not found to be as useful a cryoprotectant for protein as sucrose because dextran and protein underwent phase segregation as the solution started to freeze. The mechanism of cryoprotection in the solution has been explained by the preferential exclusion hypothesis (40).

Trehalose is a nonreducing disaccharide composed of two D-glucose monomers. It is found in several animals that can withstand dehydration and therefore was suggested as a stabilizer of drugs that undergo denaturation during spray or freeze-drying (41). Herceptin® (Trastuzumab) is a recombinant DNA-derived monoclonal antibody (MAb) that is used for treating metastatic breast cancer. The MAb has been stabilized in the lyophilized formulation using α,α-trehalose dihydrate. Trehalose has also been used as a cryoprotectant to prevent liposomal aggregation and leakage. In the dried state, carbohydrates such as trehalose, and inositol, exert their protective effect by acting as a water substitute (42).

Additives may have to be included in the formulation to adjust the specific gravity. This is important for drugs that upon administration may come in contact with CSF. CSF has a specific gravity of 1.0059 at 37°C. Solutions that have the same specific gravity as that of CSF are termed isobaric, while those solutions that have specific gravity greater than that of CSF are called hyperbaric. Upon administration of a hyperbaric solution in the spinal cord, the injected solution will settle and will affect spinal nerves at the end of the spinal cord. For example, Dibucaine hydrochloride solution (Nupercaine® 1:200) is isobaric, while Nupercaine 1:500 is hypobaric (specific gravity of 1.0036 at 37°C). Nupercaine heavy solution is made hyperbaric by addition of 5% dextrose solution, and this solution will block (anesthetize) the lower spinal nerves as it settles in the spinal cord.

Special Additives

Special additives serve special functions in pharmaceutical formulations (Table 9). The following is a summary of special additives along with their intended use:

1. Calcium gluconate injection (American Regent) is a saturated solution of 10% w/v. Calcium D-saccharate tetrahydrate 0.46% w/v is added to prevent crystallization during temperature fluctuations.
2. Cipro IV® (Ciprofloxacin, Bayer) contains lactic acid as a solubilizing agent for the antibiotic.
3. Premarin Injection® (Conjugated Estrogens, Wyeth-Ayerst Labs) is a lyophilized product that contains simethicone to prevent the formation of foam during reconstitution.
4. Dexamethasone acetate (Dalalone DP, Forest, Decadron-LA, Merck) and Dexamethasone sodium phosphate (Merck) are available as a suspension or a solution. These dexamethasone formulations contain creatine or creatinine as additives.
5. Adriamycin RDF® (Doxorubicin hydrochloride, Pharmacia-Upjohn) contains methyl paraben, 0.2 mg/mL to increase dissolution (43).
6. Ergotrate maleate (Ergonovine maleate, Lilly) contains 0.1% ethyl lactate as a solubilizing agent.
7. Estradurin Injection® (Polyestradiol phosphate, Wyeth-Ayerst Labs) uses Niacinamide (12.5 mg/ml) as a solubilizing agent. Hydeltrasol® also contains niacinamide. The concept of hydrotropic agents to increase water solubility has been tried on several compounds, including proteins (44, 45).
8. Aluminum, in the form of aluminum hydroxide, aluminum phosphate or aluminum potassium sulfate, is used as adjuvant in various vaccine formulations to elicit an increased immunogenic response.
9. Lupron Depot Injection® is lyophilized microspheres of gelatin and glycolic–lactic acid for intramuscular (IM) injection. Nutropin Depot consists of poly-lactate–glycolate microspheres.
10. Gamma cyclodextrin is used as a stabilizer in Cardiotec® at a concentration of 50 mg/mL.
11. Alprostadil (Edex®, Schwartz) is a lyophilized product of Prostaglandin E_1 in α-cyclodextrin inclusion complex. The complex has better stability and aqueous solubility than the drug itself.
12. Itraconazole (Sporanox®, Janssen) is solubilized as a molecular inclusion complex using hydroxypropyl-β-cyclodextrin.
13. Sodium caprylate (sodium octoate) has antifungal properties, but it is also used to improve the stability of albumin solution against the effects of heat. Albumin solution can be pasteurized by heating at 60°C for 10 h in the presence of sodium caprylate. Acetyl tryptophanate sodium is also added to albumin formulations.
14. Meglumine (N-methylglucamine) is used to form in situ salt. For example, diatrizoic acid, an X-ray contrast agent, is more stable when autoclaved as meglumine salt than as sodium salt (46). Meglumine is also added to Magnevist®, a magnetic resonance contrast agent.
15. Tri-n-butyl phosphate is present as an excipient in human immune globulin solution (Venoglobulin®). Its exact function in the formulation is not known, but it may serve as a scavenging agent.

Table 9 Special additives

Excipient	Example
Acetyl tryptophanate	Human Albumin (American Red Cross)
Aluminum hydroxide	Recombivax HB® (Merck)
Aluminum phosphate	Tetanus Toxoid Adsorbed (Wyeth-Ayerst)
Aluminum potassium sulfate	TD Adsorbed Adult (Pasteur Merieux)
ε-Aminocaproic acid	Eminase® (Roberts)
Calcium D-saccharate	Calcium Gluconate (American Regent)
Caprylate sodium	Human Albumin (American Red Cross)
8-Chlorotheophylline	Dimenhydrinate® (Steris)
Creatine	Dalalone DP® (Forest)
Creatinine	Decadron® (Merck)
Cholesterol	Doxil® (Sequus)
Cholesteryl sulfate sodium	Amphotec® (Sequus)
Alpha-cyclodextrin	Edex® (Schwartz)
Gamma-cyclodextrin	Cardiotec® (Squibb)
Hydroxypropyl beta cyclodextrin	Sporanox® (Janssen)
Distearyl Phosphatidylcholine	DaunoXome® (Nexstar)
Distearyl Phosphatidylglycerol	MiKasome® (NeXstar)
L-Alpha-Dimyristoylphosphatidylcholine	Abelcet® (The Liposome Co.)
L-Alpha-Dimyristoylphosphatidylglycerol	Abelcet® (The Liposome Co.)
Dioleoylphosphatidylcholine (DOPC)	DepoCyt® (Chiron)
Dipalmitoylphosphatidylglycerol (DPPG)	DepoCyt® (Chiron)
MPEG-distearoyl phosphoethanolamine	Doxil® (Sequus)
Diatrizoic acid	Conray® (Mallinckrodt)
Ethyl lactate	Ergotrate maleate (Lilly)
Ethylenediamine	Aminophylline (Abbott)
L-Glutamate sodium	Kabikinase® (Pharmacia-Upjohn)
Hydrogenated soy phosphatidylcholine	Doxil® (Sequus)
Iron ammonium citrate	Tice BCG® (Organon)
Lactic acid	Cipro IV® (Bayer)
D,L-Lactic and glycolic acid copolymer	Zoladex® (Zeneca)
Meglumine	Magnevist® (Berlex)
Niacinamide	Estradurin® (Wyeth-Ayerst)
Paraben methyl	Adriamycin RDF® (Pharmacia-Upjohn)
Protamine	Insulatard NPH® (Novo Nordisk)
Simethicone	Premarin Injection® (Wyeth-Ayerst)
Saccharin sodium	Compazine Injection® (Smith Kline Beecham)
Tri-n-butyl phosphate	Venoglobulin® (Alpha Therapeutic)
Triolein	DepoCyt® (Chiron)
von Willebrand factor	Bioclate® (Arco)
Zinc	Lente Insulin® (Novo Nordisk)
Zinc acetate	Nutropin Depot® (Genentech)
Zinc carbonate	Nutropin Depot® (Genentech)
Zinc oxide	Humalog® (Lilly)

16. von Willebrand factor is used to stabilize recombinant antihemophilic factor (Bioclate®).
17. Maltose serves as a tonicity adjuster and stabilizer in immune globulin formulation (Gamimune N®).
18. Epsilon amino caproic acid (6-amino hexanoic acid) is used as a stabilizer in anistreplase (Eminase Injection®).

19. Zinc and protamine have been added to insulin to form complexes and control the duration of action.

The FDA has published the "Inactive Ingredient Guide" which lists all excipients in alphabetical order (14). Each ingredient is followed by the route of administration, and

Table 10 List of excipients from the 1996 FDA Inactive Ingredient Guide

Benzyl chloride	Poloxamer 165
Butyl paraben	PEG 4000
Caldiamide sodium	Polyoxyethylene fatty acid esters
Calteridol calcium	Polyoxyethylene sorbitan monostearate
Cellulose (microcrystalline)	Polyoxyl 35 castor oil
Deoxycholic acid	Polysorbate 40
Dicyclohexyl carbodiimide	Polysorbate 85
Diethyl amine	Potassium hydroxide
Disofenin	Potassium phosphate, dibasic
Docusate sodium	Sodium bisulfate
Edamine	Sodium chlorate
Exametazime	Sodium hypochloride
Gluceptate sodium	Sodium iodide
Gluceptate calcium	Sodium pyrophosphate
Glucuronic acid	Sodium thiosulfate, anhydrous
Guanidine HCl	Sodium trimetaphosphate
Iofetamine HCl	Sorbitan monopalmitate
Lactobionic acid	Stannous chloride
Lidofenin	Stannous fluoride
Medrofenin	Stannous tartrate
Medronate disodium	Starch
Medronic acid	Succimer
Methyl boronic acid	Succinic acid
Methyl cellulose	Sulfurous acid
Methylene blue	Tetrakis (1-isocyano-2-methoxy-2-methyl-propionate) copper (I) Tc
N-(Carbamoyl-methoxy polyethylene glycol 2000)-1,2- distearoyl	Thiazoximic acid
N-2-Hydroxyethyl piperazine *N'*-2' ethane sulonic acid	Urea
Nioxime	Zic acetate
Nitric acid	Zinc chloride
Oxyquinoline	2-ethyl hexanoic acid
Pentate (DTPA) calcium trisodium	PEG vegetable oil

in some cases, the range of concentration used in the approved drug product. However, this list does not provide the name of commercial product(s) corresponding to each excipient. Table 10 summarizes all the excipients included in the "Inactive Ingredient Guide" that do not appear in the Physician's Desk Reference (PDR), GenRx, or Handbook of Injectable Drugs.

Similarly, in Japan the "Japanese Pharmaceutical Excipients Directory" is published by the Japanese Pharmaceutical Excipients Council, with the cooperation and guidance of the Ministry of Health and Welfare (47). This directory divides the excipients into:

1. *Official.* Those 590 excipients that have been recognized in the JP, Japanese Pharmaceutical Codex, and Japanese Pharmaceutical Excipients, and

for which testing methods and standards have been determined. Table 11 summarizes official excipients used in parenteral products.

2. *Nonofficial Excipients.* These 522 excipients are used in pharmaceutical products sold in Japan and will be included in the official book or in supplemental editions. The nonofficial excipients, used in parenteral products, are listed in Table 12.

REGULATORY PERSPECTIVE

The International Pharmaceutical Excipients Council (IPEC) has classified excipients into the following four classes, based on available safety testing information (48):

Table 11 Official Japanse pharmaceutical excipients

Name	Uses	Administration route
Acacia	Diluent, dispersing agent	im
Acetic acid	Buffer agent, solvent, stabilizer	iv, im, sc
L-Alanine	Stabilizer	iv, im,
Aluminum monostearate	Dispersing agent, stabilizer, vehicle	other inj.
Aluminum potassium sulfate	pH adjustment, stabilizer	im, sc
Aminoacetic acid	Buffering agent, solubilizer, stabilizer, suspending agent, vehicle	iv, im, sc, ic
Anhydrous citric acid	Buffer agent, pH adjustment, solubilizing agent, stabilizer	iv, im, other inj.
Anhydrous disodium hydrogen phosphate	Buffering agent, pH adjustment, solubilizer, stabilizer, suspending agent	iv, im, sc, other inj.
Anhydrous sodium dihydrogen phosphate	Buffering agent, pH adjustment, stabilizer	iv, im, other inj.
Arginine hydrochloride	Buffering agent, solubilizing agent, stabilizer	iv, im, sc
Ascorbic acid	Antioxidant, buffering agent, Stabilizer	iv, im, sc, ia
L-Aspartic acid	Solubilizer, stabilizer, vehicle	iv, im
Benzylkonium chloride	Buffering agent, preservative, stabilizer	
Benzethonium chloride	Dispersing agent, preservative, stabilizer	iv, im, other inj.
Benzoic acid	Buffering agent, preservative, stabilizer	iv, im
Benzyl alcohol	Preservative, solubilizer, solvent, stabilizer	iv, im, sc, ic, other inj.
Benzyl benzoate	Antiseptic, solubilizer, solvent	im
Calcium bromide	Isotonicity, stabilizer	iv
Calcium chloride	Isotonicity, suspending agent	iv
Calcium disodium edetate	Stabilizer	iv, ic, ia, is, other inj
Calcium gluconate	Buffering agent, stabilizer	iv, im, sc
Calcium oxide	Solubilizing agent	iv
Calcium D-saccharate	Stabilizer	iv
Camellia oil	Solvent	im, sc
Carmellose sodium	Emulsifying agent, solubilizing agent, stabilizer, suspending agent	im, ic, sc, other inj.
Castor oil	Solubilizer, solvent	im
Chlorobutanol	Buffering agent, preservative	iv, im, sc
Citric acid	Antioxidant, buffering agent, pH adjustment, preservative, solubilizing agent, stabilizer	iv, im, sc, ia,
Concentrated glycerin	Isotonicity, solubilizer, stabilizer	iv, im, sc
Creatinine	Buffering agent, stabilizer	iv, im, ic, sc, other inj.
Cresol	Preservative	iv, im, sc
L-Cystine	Stabilizer	iv
Dehydrated ethanol	Solubilizer, solubilizing agent, solvent	iv, im, sc
Dextran 40	Stabilizer, vehicle	iv, im
Dextran 70	Stabilizer	sc
Dibasic potassium sulfate	Buffering agent, pH adjustment	iv, im, sc
Dibasic sodium citrate	Buffering agent, vehicle	iv
Dibasic sodium phosphate	Buffering agent, pH adjustment, solubilizing agent, stabilizer, vehicle	iv, im, sc, ia, is, ic, other inj.
Dilute hydrochloric acid	Buffering agent, pH adjustment, solubilizer, stabilizer	iv, im, sc
N, N-Dimethylacetamide	Solvent	iv

(Continued)

Table 11 Official Japanese pharmaceutical excipients (*Continued*)

Name	Uses	Administration route
Glucose	Buffering agent, isotonicity, solubilizer, stabilizer, vehicle	iv, im, sc, ic
Glycerin	Dispersing agent, isotonicity, preservative, solubilizing agent, solvent, stabilizer, suspending agent, vehicle	iv, im, sc, other inj.
Heparin sodium	Stabilizer	iv
L-Histidine	Stabilizer	iv
Hydrochloric acid	pH adjustment, solubilizing agent, stabilizer	iv, im, sc, ia, is,ic, other inj.
N-Hydroxyethyl lactamide solution	Solubilizing agent	iv
Hydroxypropylcellulose	Emulsifying agent, solubilizer, stabilizer, suspending agent, vehicle	im
Isotonic sodium chloride solution	Isotonicity, solvent	iv, im, sc, ia, ic, other inj.
Lactic acid	Buffering agent, pH adjustment, solubilizer, stabilizer,	iv, im, sc
Lactose	Dispersing agent, suspending agent, vehicle	iv, im, sc, ia, ic, other inj.
Lidocaine	Solubilizing agent, solvent	iv, im
L-Lysine-L-Glutamate	Solubilizing agent, stabilizer	iv
Lysine hydrochloride	Stabilizer	iv
Macrogol 400 (PEG 400)	Solubilizing agent	iv
Macrogol 4000 (PEG 4000)	Isotonicity, solubilizer, solvent, stabilizer, suspending agent, vehicle, wetting agent	iv, im, sc
Magnesium chloride	Isotonicity, solubilizing agent, stabilizer	iv
Magnesium gluconate	Stabilizer	iv
Magnesium sulfate	Stabilizer	iv, im, sc
Maleic acid	Buffering agent, pH adjustment, stabilizer	im
Maleic anhydride	Solubilizer, stabilizer	iv
Maltose	Stabilizer	iv, im, sc, ic, other inj.
D-Mannitol	Isotonicity, solubilizing agent, stabilizer	iv, im, sc, ic, other inj.
Meglumine	pH adjustment, solubilizing agent	iv
Meprylcaine hydrochloride	Soothing agent	iv, im, sc
Methanesulfonic acid	pH adjustment	im, sc
L-Methionine	Stabilizer	dental inj.
Methyl parahydroxybenzoate	Preservative, stabilizer	iv, im, sc, ic, other inj.
Monobasic potassium phosphate	Buffer agent, isotonocity, pH adjustment, solubilizing agent, stabilizer	iv, im, sc, ic
Monoethanolamine	Buffer agent, pH adjustment, solubilizer, stabilizer	iv
MonopotassiumL-Glutamate monohydrate	Preservative, stabilizer	sc
Monosodium L-Glutamate monohydrate	Buffer agent	iv, im, sc
Nicotinamide	Isotonicity, solubilizing agent, stabilizer	iv, im, sc, other inj.
Peanut oil	Solubilizer, solvent, suspending agent, vehicle	im
Peptone, caesin	Stabilizer	sc
Phenol	Antiseptic, preservative	ic, im, sc, ic, othe inj.

(*Continued*)

Table 11 Official Japanse pharmaceutical excipients (*Continued*)

Name	Uses	Administration route
Disodium edetate	Antioxidant, antiseptic, preservative, stabilizer	iv, ia, other inj.
Phosphoric acid	Buffer agent, isotonicity, pH adjustment, solubilizing agent, stabilizer	iv, im, sc
Polyoxyethylene hydrogenated castor oil 60	Dispersing agent, emulsifying agent, solubilizing agent, stabilizer, surfactant, suspending agent, vehicle	iv, im, sc
Polyoxyethylene hydrogenated castor oil 51	Dispersing agent, emulsifying agent, solubilizing agent	iv, im, sc, is
Polyoxyethylene [160] Polyoxypropylene [30] glycol	Dispersing agent, emulsifying agent, solubilizer, stabilizer, suspending agent, vehicle, surfactant, wetting agent	iv
Polysorbate 80	Dispersing agent, emulsifying agent, solubilizer, surfactant, stabilizer, suspending agent, vehicle, wetting agent	iv, im, sc, ic, other inj.
Potassium sulfate	Stabilizer	local anesthetic inj.
Powdered acacia	Dispersing agent, suspending agent	im, sc
Propylene glycol	Dispersing agent, isotonicity, preservative, solubilizer, solvent, stabilizer, suspending agent, vehicle, wetting agent	iv, im, sc
Propyl parahydroxybenzoate	Antiseptic, preservative, stabilizer	iv, im, sc, ic, other inj
Protamine sulfate	Prolongating agent	sc
Purified gelatin	Base, stabilizer, suspending agent, vehicle	iv, im, sc
Purified soybean lecithin	Dispersing agent, emulsifying agent, solubilizer, stabilizer	iv
Purified yolk lecithin	Emulsifying agent	iv
Sesame oil	Base, solubilizing agent, solvent, stabilizer, vehicle	iv, im, sc, other inj.
Sodium acetate	Buffer agent, pH adjustment, solubilizing agent, stabilizer	iv, im, sc, other inj.
Sodium acetyl tryptophan	Stabilizer	iv, sc
Sodium benzoate	Antiseptic, buffer agent, preservative, solubilizer, stabilizer	im
Sodium bicarbonate	Buffer agent, isotonicity, pH adjustment, solubilizer, stabilizer	iv, im, sc, is, ic, other inj.
Sodium bisulfite	Antioxidant, isotonicity, stabilizer	iv, im, sc, other inj.
Sodium bromide	Isotonicity	iv, im, sc
Sodium caprylate	Stabilizer	iv, sc
Sodium carbonate	Buffer agent, pH adjustment, solubilizing agent, stabilizer	iv, im, sc
Sodium chloride	Base, buffering agent, isotonicity, solubilizer, stabilizer, suspending agent, vehicle	iv, im, sc, ia, is
Sodium chondroitin sulfate	Stabilizer	iv
Sodium citrate	Antiseptic, buffer agent, isotonicity, pH adjustment, solubilizer, stabilizer	iv, im, sc, ic, ia, is, other inj.
Sodium desoxycholate	Solubilizing agent	ic, iv, is
Sodium dihydrogen phosphate dihydrate	Buffer agent, isotonicity, pH adjustment, stabilizer	iv, im, sc, ia, is, other inj.
Sodium formaldehydesulfoxylate	Stabilizer, isotonicity, pH adjustment	iv, im
Sodium hydroxide	Solubilizer	iv, im, sc, ia, ic, other inj.

(*Continued*)

Table 11 Official Japanse pharmaceutical excipients (*Continued*)

Name	Uses	Administration route
Sodium salicylate	Antiseptic, preservative, solubilizing agent, stabilizer	iv, im, sc
Sodium thiomalate	Antioxidant, stabilizer	im
Sodium thiosulfate	Solubilizer, stabilizer	iv, im, sc
Sorbitan sesquioleate	Base, emulsifying agent, solubilizing agent, stabilizer, surfactant, vehicle	iv, im
D-Sorbitol	Dispersing agent, isotonicity, plasiticizer, preservative, solubilizing agent, stabilizer	iv, im, sc, other inj.
D-Sorbitol solution	Base, isotonicity, solubilizing agent, stabilizer, vehicle	im, sc, other inj
Soybean oil	Base, solubilizer, solvent, vehicle	iv
Stannous chloride	Reducing agent	iv
Sucrose	Base, stabilizer, vehicle	iv, sc
Tartaric acid	Buffering agent, pH adjustment, solubilizing agent, stabilizer, vehicle	iv, im
Thimerosal	Preservative	iv, im, sc
Thioglycolic acid	Solubilizing agent, stabilizer	iv, im, sc
Tribasic sodium phosphate	Buffering agent, pH adjustment	iv, im, sc
Trometamol (Tromethamine)	Buffering agent, solubilizing agent, stabilizer	iv, im, sc, ia, is, ic
Urea	Solubilizing agent, stabilizer, wetting agent	iv, im, sc
Water for injection	Solubilizer, solvent	iv, im, sc, ia, is, ic, other inj.
Xylitol	Isotonicity, stabilizer, vehicle	iv, im, other inj.
Zinc acetate	Stabilizer	sc
Zinc chloride	Stabilizer	im, sc
Zinc oxide	Dispersing agent, stabilizer, vehicle	sc

1. *New chemical excipients*: Require a full safety evaluation program. The estimated cost of safety studies for a new chemical excipient is approximately $35 million over 4–5 years. European Union (EU) directive 75/318/EEC states that new chemical excipients will be treated in the same way as new actives. In the United States a new excipient requires a Drug Master File (DMF) to be filed with the FDA. Similarly, in Europe a dossier needs to be established. Both the DMF and dossier contain relevant safety information. The IPEC Europe has issued a draft guideline (Compilation of Excipient Masterfiles Guidelines) which provides guidance to excipient producers on how to construct a dossier that will support a Marketing Authorization Application (MAA) while maintaining the confidentiality of the data.

2. *Existing chemical excipient—first use in man*: Implies that animal safety data exist since data may have been used in some other application. Additional safety information may have to be gathered to justify its use in humans.

3. *Existing chemical excipient*: Indicates that it has been used in humans but change in route of administration (say from oral to parenteral), new dosage form, higher dose, etc. may require additional safety information.

4. *New modifications or combinations of existing excipients:* A physical interaction NOT a chemical reaction. No safety evaluation is necessary in this case.

Simply because an excipient is listed as Generally Recognized As Safe (GRAS) does not mean that it can be used in parenteral dosage form. The GRAS list may include materials that have been proven safe for food (oral administration) but have not been deemed safe for use in an injectable product. This makes it difficult for the formulation development scientist to choose additives during the dosage form development.

Many pharmacopeial monographs for identical excipients differ considerably with regards to specifications, test criteria, and analytical methods. Thus, if a pharmaceutical manufacturer is going to supply a product

Table 12 Non-official Japanese pharmaceutical excipients

Excipients	Uses	Administration
Aluminum chloride	Potentiating agent	im, sc
Aluminum hydroxide	Adsorbent	sc, im
Aminoethyl sulfonic acid	Buffer, isotonicity, stabilizer, vehicle	iv, im
Ammonium acetate	pH adjusting agent	im
Anhydrous stannous chloride	Reducing agent	iv
L-Arginine	Buffer, stabilizer, solubilizer	iv, im, sc
Asepsis sodium bicarbonate	Stabilizer	iv
Butylhydroxyanisol	Antioxidant, stabilizer	iv
m-Cresol	Preservative	iv, im, sc, ic
L-Cysteine	Stabilizer	iv
Cysteine hydrochloride	Antioxidant, stabilizer	iv, im
Dichlorodifluoromethane	Propellant	iv
Diethanolamine	Buffer, solubilizer, stabilizer	iv
Diethylenetriaminepentaacetic acid	Stabilizer	iv
Ferric chloride	Stabilizer	iv
Highly purified yolk lecithin	Emulsifier	iv
Human serum albumin	Preservative, stabilizer	iv, im, sc
Hydrolyzed gelatin	Stabilizer	sc
Inositol	Stabilizer, vehicle	iv, im
Lidocaine hydrochloride	Soothing agent	im
D,L-Methionine	Stabilizer	im, sc
Monobasic sodium phosphate	Buffer, isotonicity, adjust pH	iv, im, sc
Oleic acid	Dispersing agent, solvent	iv
Phenol red	Coloring agent	sc
Polyoxyethylene castor oil	Base, emulsifying agent, solubilizing agent, stabilizer	iv
Polyoxyethylene hydrogenated castor oil	Base, emulsifying agent, solubilizer, stabilizer, suspending agent, vehicle	iv
Polyoxyethylene sorbitan monolaurate	Emulsifying agent, solubilizing agent, surfactant	iv, im, sc
Potassium pyrosulfite	Stabilizer	iv, sc, im
Potassium thiocyanate	Stabilizer	iv
Purified soybean oil	Solubilizer	iv
Sodium acetate, anhydrous	Buffer, pH adjuster, solubilizing agent, stabilizer	im
Sodium carbonate, anhydrous	Buffer, solubilizing agent	iv, im, ic
Sodium dihydrogen phosphate monohydrate	Buffering agent	ic
Sodium gluconate	Stabilizer, vehicle	iv, im
Sodium pyrophosphate, anhydrous	Dispersing agent, isotonicity, stabilizer	iv, im, is
Sodium sulfite	Antioxidant, stabilizer	iv
Sodium thioglycolate	Antioxidant, stabilizer	iv, im, sc
Sorbitan esters of fatty acids	Emulsifying agent, solubilizing agent, surfactant, stabilizer, suspending agent, vehicle	iv
Succinic acid	pH adjusting agent	iv
α-Thioglycerol	Antioxidant	iv, im, sc
Trienthanolamine	Buffer, pH adjuster, solubilizing agent, stabilizer	iv
Zinc chloride solution	Stabilizer	sc

throughout the world, the manufacturer will have to repeat testing on the same excipient several times in order to meet USP, JP, EP, BP, and other pharmacopoeias. EP, JP and USP are the main driving bodies within the International Conference on Harmonization (ICH) that are working on several of the commonly used excipients in order to achieve a single monograph for each excipient. For example, benzyl alcohol undergoes degradation by a free radical mechanism to form benzaldehyde and hydrogen peroxide. The degradation products are much more toxic than the parent molecule. The *USP*, *JP*, and *EP* require three different chromatographic systems to test for organic impurity (mainly benzaldehyde). The harmonized monograph of benzyl alcohol will eliminate unnecessary repetition, which does not contribute to the overall quality of the product (49). The following 11 pharmacopoeial tests can be substituted by a single gas chromatography (GC) method:

EP:
- Benzaldehyde, related substance (GC)
- Halogenated compounds and halides (colorimetric test)
- Assay (hydroxyl value)

JP:
- Limit test for benzaldehyde
- Limit test for chlorinated compounds
- Distillation rangeAssay (hydroxyl value)

NF/USP:
- Benzaldehyde (HPLC)
- Halogenated compounds and halides (colorimetric test)
- Organic volatile impurities (GC)
- Assay (hydroxyl value)

The harmonization process is just beginning and is a major step in the right direction.

Another area where regulatory bodies are focusing their attention is the manufacturing process used to produce excipients. The IPEC has undertaken major initiatives to improve the quality of additives and has published "Good Manufacturing Practices Guide for Bulk Pharmaceutical Excipients" (50). The excipients may be manufactured for the food, cosmetic, chemical, agriculturo, or pharmaceutical industries, and the requirements for each area are different. The purpose of this guide is twofold: 1) to develop a quality system framework that can be used for suppliers of excipients and which will be acceptable to the pharmaceutical industry, and 2) to harmonize the requirements in the United States, Europe, and Japan.

The United States, Europe, and Japan require that all excipients be declared on the label if the product is an injectable preparation. The European guide for the label and package leaflet also lists excipients, that have special issues. These are addressed in an Annex (51). Table 13 contains a summary of some of these ingredients, which are commonly used as parenteral excipients and the corresponding safety information that

should be included in the leaflet. Similarly, 21 CFR 201.22 requires prescription drugs containing sulfites to be labeled with a warning statement about possible hypersensitivity. An informational chapter in USP ⟨1091⟩ entitled "Labeling of Inactive Ingredients" provides guidelines for labeling of inactive ingredients present in dosage forms.

CRITERIA FOR THE SELECTION OF EXCIPIENT AND SUPPLIER

During the development of parenteral dosage forms, the formulator selects excipients that will provide a stable, efficacious, and functional product. The choice, and the characteristics of excipients should be appropriate for the intended purpose.

An explanation should be provided with regard to the function of all constituents in the formulation, with justification for their inclusion. In some cases, experimental data may be necessary to justify such inclusion, e.g., preservatives. The choice of the quality of the excipient should be guided by its role in the formulation and by the proposed manufacturing process. In some cases, it may be necessary to address and justify the quality of certain excipients in the formulation (52).

Normally, a pharmaceutical development report is written in the United States, which should be available at the time of Pre-Approval Inspection (PAI). The development report contains the choice of excipients, their purpose and levels in the drug product, compatibility with other excipients, drug or package system, and how they may influence the stability and efficacy of the finished product.

The following key points should be considered in selecting an excipient and its supplier for parenteral products:

1. Influence of excipient on the overall quality, stability, and effectiveness of drug product.
2. Compatibility of excipient with drug and the packaging system.
3. Compatibility of excipient with the manufacturing process. For example, preservatives may be adsorbed by rubber tubes or filters, acetate buffers will be lost during lyophilization process, etc.
4. The amount or percentage of excipients that can be added to the drug product. Table 6 summarizes the maximum amount of preservatives and antioxidants allowed by various pharmacopoeias.

Table 13 Excipients for label and corresponding information for leaflet

Name	Information on leaflet
Arachis oil	Whenever arachis oil appears, peanut oil should appear beside it (because some individuals are sensitive to peanuts)
Benzoic acid and benzoates	It may increase the risk of jaundice in newborn babies
Benzyl alcohol	Contraindicated in infants or young children; up to 3 years old
Boric acid its salts and esters	Contraindicated in infants or young children; up to 3 years old
Dimethyl sulfoxide	Can cause stomach upset, diarrhea, drowsiness, and headache
Lactose	Unsuitable for people with lactose insufficiency, galactos emia, or glucose/galactose malabsorption syndrome
Organic mercury compounds	Can cause kidney damage
Parahydroxybenzoate and their esters	Known to cause urticaria. Generally delayed type reactions, such as contact dermatitis
Phenylalanine	Harmful for people with phenylketonuria
Polyethoxylated castor oils	Warning for parenterals only—hypersensitivity, drop in blood pressure, inadequate circulation, dyspnea, hot flushes
Potassium	For products administered iv—can cause pain at the site of injection or phlebitis
Sodium	May be harmful to people on low sodium diet
Sorbitol	Unsuitable in hereditary fructose intolerance
Sucrose (saccharose)	Unsuitable in hereditary fructose intolerance, glucose/galactose malabsorption syndrome, or sucrase-isomaltase deficiency
Sulphites (metabisulphites)	Can cause allergic-type reactions including anaphylactic symptoms and bronchospasm in susceptable people, especially those with a history of asthma or allergy
Urea	For products given iv—may cause venous thrombosis or phlebitis

5. Route of administration. The *USP*, *EP*, and *BP* do not allow preservatives to be present in injections intended to come in contact with brain tissues or CSF. Thus intracisternal, epidural, and intradural injections should be preservative free. Also, it is preferred that a drug product to be administered via intravenous (iv) route be free of particulate matter. However, if the size of the particle is well controlled, like in fat emulsion or colloidal albumin or amphotericin B dispersion, it can be administered by iv infusion.

6. Dose volume. All LVPs and those SVPs where the single dose injection volume can be greater than 15 ml are required by the EP/BP to be preservative free (unless justified). The USP recommends that special care be observed in the choice and the use of added substances in preparations for injections that are administered in volumes exceeding 5 ml.

7. Whether the product is intended for single or multiple dose use. According to USP, single dose injections should be free of preservative. The FDA takes the position that even though a single dose injection may have to be aseptically processed, the manufacturer should not use a preservative to prevent microbial growth. European agencies have taken a more lenient attitude on this subject.

8. The length or duration of time that the drug product will be used once the multidose injection is opened.
9. How safe is the excipient?
10. Does the parenteral excipient contain very low levels of lead, aluminum, or other heavy metals?
11. Does a dossier or DMF exist for the excipient?
12. Has the excipient been used in humans? Has it been used via a parenteral route and in the amount and concentration that is being planned?
13. Has the drug product that contains this excipient been approved throughout the world?
14. What is the cost of the excipient and is it readily available?
15. Is the excipient vendor following the IPEC GMP guide? Is the vendor ISO 9000 certified?
16. Will the excipient supplier certify the material to meet USP, BP, EP, JP, and other pharmacopoeias?
17. Has the supplier been audited by the FDA or the company's audit group? How did it fare?

Presence of impurities in excipients can have a dramatic influence on the safety, efficacy or stability of the drug product. Monomers or metal catalysts used during a polymerization process are toxic and can also destabilize the drug product if present in trace amounts. Due to safety concerns, the limit of vinyl chloride (monomer) in polyvinyl pyrrolidone is nmt 10 ppm, and for hydrazine (a side product of polymerization reaction) nmt 1 ppm. Monomeric ethylene oxide is highly toxic and can be present in ethoxylated excipients such as PEGs, ethoxylated fatty acids, etc.

The FDA has issued a guidance suggesting that animal-derived materials such as egg yolk lecithin, and egg phospholipid) used in drug products, originating from Belgium, France, and the Netherlands between January and June 1999 should be investigated for the presence of dioxin and polychlorinated biphenyls. The contamination in the animal-derived product was probably due to contaminated animal feed.

Excipients manufactured by fermentation processes, such as dextrose, citric acid, mannitol, and trehalose, should be specially controlled for endotoxin levels. Mycotoxin (highly toxic metabolic products of certain fungi species) contamination of an excipient derived from natural material has not been specifically addressed by regulatory authorities. The German health authority issued a draft guideline in 1997 where a limit was specified for Aflotoxins M_1, B_1, and the sum of B_1, B_2, G_1, and G_2 in the starting material for pharmaceutical products.

Heavy metal contamination of excipients is a concern, especially for sugars, phosphate, and citrate. Several rules have been proposed or established. For example, the EP sets a limit of nmt 1 ppm of nickel in polyols. California Proposition 65 specifies a limit of nmt 0.5 μg of lead per day per product (53). Similarly, the FDA has proposed a guideline that would limit the aluminum content for all LVPs used in TPN therapy to 25 μg/L (54). Furthermore, it requires that the maximum level of aluminum in SVPs intended to be added to LVPs and pharmacy bulk packages, at expiration date, be stated on the immediate container label.

Physical and chemical stability of the excipient should be considered in assigning a reevaluation date. Since many drug products have a small amount of active and a comparatively high amount of excipients, degradation of even a small percentage of excipient can lead to levels of impurities sufficient to react or degrade a large percentage of active material. For example, benzyl alcohol decomposes via free radical mechanism in the presence of light and oxygen, to form benzaldehyde (x% of benzaldehyde is approximately equivalent to 1/3 x% of hydrogen peroxide). Hydrogen peroxide can rapidly oxidize sulfhydryl groups of amino acids such as cysteine present in peptides or proteins.

It is essential that adequate research and thought be given in the selection of a pharmaceutical excipient

supplier. It is not uncommon for the supplier to change its manufacturing process to make products more efficiently (i.e., less costly). Normally, excipients are low-value, high-volume products that are used by several industries. The pharmaceutical industry, in general, is not the major customer of excipients (in terms of volume of material purchased). For example, the pharmaceutical industry uses approximately 20% of gelatin produced. Of this 20%, most is for production of oral dosage forms. The parenteral portion is approximately 5% of this 20%. Therefore, it is extremely important that the drug manufacturer has a contract with the excipient supplier, that prohibits the supplier from making any change in the process/quality of the material without informing their customers well in advance. Also, the pharmaceutical manufacturer should investigate all the alternate sources that could be used in case of an emergency. A change in the supplier should not be made without consulting the pertinent regulatory bodies, since such an event may require prior regulatory approval.

The pharmaceutical manufacturer should have an active Vendor Certification Program. The manufacturer also should assure that the vendor is ISO 9000 certified. An audit of the excipient manufacturer is essential, since the pharmaceutical industry is ultimately responsible for the quality of the drug product that includes the excipient(s) as one of the components. The IPEC GMP guide may be used as an audit tool, since it is written in the format of ISO 9000 using identical nomenclature and paragraph numbering. The audit may ensure that the quality is being built into the excipient that may be difficult to measure later by quality control on receipt of the material. This is especially true for parenteral excipients where not only chemical, but also microbiological attributes are critical. Bioburden and endotoxin limits may be needed for each of the excipients and several guidelines are available to establish the specifications (55, 56).

Recent events in Haiti highlight the importance of assuring the quality of excipients to the same degree that one normally does for active ingredients. From November 1995 through June 1996, acute anuric renal failure was diagnosed in 86 children. This was associated with the use of diethylene glycol-contaminated glycerin used to manufacture acetaminophen syrup (57).

SAFETY ISSUES

Reference 58 is an excellent resource on the safety and adverse reaction to several excipients. Sensitization reactions have been reported for the parabens, thimerosal, and propyl gallate. Sorbitol is metabolized to fructose and can be dangerous when administered to fructose-intolerant patients. Table 13 also lists safety concerns.

Progress in drug delivery systems and new proteins/peptides being developed for parenteral administration has created a need to expand the list of excipients that can be safely used. An informational chapter included in the USP 24, presents a scientifically based approach for safety assessment of new pharmaceutical excipients (59). This chapter is based on the excipient safety evaluation guidelines prepared by The Safety Committee of the International Pharmaceutical Excipient Council, with appropriate redaction. Table 14 summarizes the approach in developing a new excipient.

Currently, there are some concerns regarding Transmissible Spongiform Encephalopathies (TSE) via animal-derived excipients such as gelatin. TSEs are caused by prions that are extremely resistant to heat and normal sterilization processes. TSEs have a very long incubation time with no cure and include diseases such as the following:

- Scrapies in sheep and goats
- Bovine spongiform encephalopathy (BSE), otherwise known as Mad Cow Disease, in cattle
- Kuru disease in humans
- Creutzfeld-Jacob disease (CJD) in humans, which has been attributed to repeated parenteral administration of growth hormone and gonadotropin derived from human pituitary glands.

Several guidelines have been issued that address the issue of animal-derived excipients and scientific principles to minimize the possible transmission of TSEs via medicinal products (60, 61). The current situation indicates that there are negligible concerns for lactose, glycerol, fatty acids, and their esters, but the situation is less clear for gelatin. In this scenario, if one has a choice, then it may be beneficial to select nonanimal-derived excipients. The use of bovine serum albumin (BSA) or human serum albumin (HSA) is of concern because they can be derived from virus-contaminated blood. The risk of TSEs from excipients can be greatly reduced by controlling the following parameters:

1. Source of animal should be from countries where BSE has not been reported.
2. Animals used should be young.
3. Category III or IV animal tissue should be used in manufacture (60).
4. A production process that is likely to destroy TSE agents should be utilized.

Table 14 Summary of safety evaluation of excipient

Tests	Injectable route[a]
Baseline toxicity data	
Acute oral toxicity	Required
Acute dermal toxicity	Required
Acute inhalation toxicity	Conditional
Eye irritation	Required
Skin irritation	Required
Skin sensitization	Required
Acute injectable toxicity	Required
Application site evaluation	Required
Phototoxicity/photoallergy	Required
Genotoxicity assays	Required
ADME/PK-intended route	Required
28-day toxicity (2 species) intended route	Required
Additional data: Short or intermediate term repeated use	
90-day toxicity (most appropriate species)	Required
Embryo-fetal toxicol	Required
Additional assays	Conditional
Genotoxicity assays	Required
Immunosuppression assays	Required
Additional data: Intermittent long-term or chronic use	
Chronic toxicity (rodent, nonrodent)	Conditional
Reproductive toxicity	Required
Photocarcinogenicity	Conditional
Carcinogenicity	Conditional

[a]Term injectable includes routes such as iv, sc, intrathecal, etc.

Amendment to the European Commission directive 75/318/EEC would require manufacturers to provide a "Certificate of Suitability" or the underlying "scientific information" in the form of a marketing variation to attest that their pharmaceuticals are free of TSEs.

FUTURE DIRECTION

Several new excipients are being evaluated in order to increase the solubility or improve the stability of parenteral drugs. Cyclodextrins have been tried for the above reasons. Currently, there are two FDA approved parenteral products that have utilized α and γ-cyclodextrins. β-cyclodextrin is unsuitable for parenteral administration because it causes necrosis of the proximal kidney tubules upon IV and subcutaneous administration (62). Hydroxypropyl β-cyclo-dextrin (HPβCD) and sulfobutylether β-cyclodextrin

(SBE-7-β-CD) have shown the most promise. Captisol™ is the trade name of SBE-7-β-CD and is anionic. Currently, two Captisol™ based small molecule IV and IM drug formulations are in Phase III clinical trials in the United States. One parenteral formulation that utilizes HPβCD (Cavitron®) is in Phase II/III clinical trials, and another (Sporanox) has been approved by the FDA. Manufacturers of HPβCD and SBE-7-β-CD have established a DMF with the FDA. A detailed review of cyclodextrins was recently published (63, 64). It should be noted, however, that cyclodextrin also can accelerate the degradation of drug product (65) and can sequester preservatives, rendering them ineffective (66).

Chitosan, β-1,4-linked glucosamine, is a naturally occurring, biodegradable, nontoxic polycationic biopolymer. It is being investigated for its potential as a cross-linked matrix of microspheres to deliver antineoplastic drugs. Because of its charge, it can trap several drugs and can bind strongly with cancer cells, thereby minimizing drug toxicity and enhancing therapeutic efficacy (67). Chitosan also has been shown to stabilize liposomes.

Biodegradable polymeric materials such as polylactic acid, polyglycolic acid, and other poly-alphahydroxy acids have been used as medical devices and as biodegradable sutures since the 1960s (68). Currently, the FDA has approved for marketing, only devices made from homopolymers or copolymers of glycolide, lactide, caprolactone, p-dioxanone, and trimethylene carbonate (69). Such biopolymers are finding increased application as a matrix to deliver parenteral drugs for prolonged delivery (70). At least four drug products—Lupron Depot®, Decapeptyl®, Nutropin Depot®, and Zoladex®—have been approved. These four drug products are microspheres in PLG, polylactic acid (PLA), or the PLGA matrix. Polyglycolic acid (PGA) is highly crystalline (approximately 50%) with a high melting point (220–225°C). PLA can be produced by the polymerization of L-lactic acid (LPLA), D-lactic acid (DPLA), or a blend of D- and L- lactic acid (DLPLA). LPLA is 37% crystalline while DLPLA, is amorphous. The degradation time of LPLA is much slower than that of DPLA requiring more than 2 years. By copolymerizing lactic and glycolic acid, polymeric matrices with a wide range of properties (tensile strength, crystallinity, and degradation rate) can be obtained. Decapeptyl® is approved in France and is a microsphere for IM administration. It contains drug in a matrix of PLGA and Carboxymethyl cellulose with mannitol and polysorbate 80.

Polyanhydrides degrade primarily by surface erosion and possess excellent in vivo compatibility. In 1996 the FDA approved a polyanhydride-based drug delivery system to the brain of chemotherapeutic agent BCNU, which is currently being manufactured by Guilford Pharmaceutical, Inc.

Several phospholipid-based excipients are finding increased application as solubilizing agents, emulsifying agents, or as components of liposomal formulation. The phospholipids occur naturally and are biocompatible and biodegradable. Examples include egg phosphatidylcholine, soybean phosphatidylcholine, hydrogenated soybean phosphatidylcholine (HSPC), DMPC, DSPC, DOPC, DSPE, DMPG, DPPG, and DSPG. Spartaject™ technology uses a mixture of phospholipids, to encapsulate poorly water-soluble drugs, to form micro-suspensions that can be injected intravenously. Busulfan® drug product uses this technology and is currently undergoing Phase I clinical trials. Many liposomal and liposomal-like formulations (DepoFoam®) are either approved (Depo-Cyt®) or are undergoing clinical trials to reduce drug toxicity, improve drug stability, prolong the duration of action, or to deliver drug to the central nervous system (71). Two amphotericin formulations have been approved in the United States, They are liposomal, or a lipid complex between the antifungal drug and positively charged lipid. Amphotec® is a 1:1 molar ratio complex of amphotericin B and cholesteryl sulfate while Abelcet® is a 1:1 molar complex of amphotericin B with phospholipids (seven parts of L-α-dimyristoylphosphatidylcholine and L-α-dimyristoylphosphatidyl glycerol).

Poloxamers or pluronics are block copolymers comprised of polyoxyethylene and polyoxypropylene segments. They exhibit reverse thermal gelation and are being tried as solubilizing, emulsifying, and stabilizing agents. Thus, a depot drug delivery system can be created using pluronics whereby the product is a viscous injection that gels upon IM injection (72). Pluronics can prevent protein aggregation or adsorption/absorption and can help in the reconstitution of lyophilized products. Pluronic F68 (Polaxamer-188), F38 (Poloxamer-108), and F127 (Poloxamer-407) are the most commonly used pluronics. For example, liquid formulation of human growth hormone and Factor VIII can be stabilized using pluronics. Fluosol® is a complex mixture of perfluorocarbons, with a high oxygen-carrying capacity emulsified with Pluronic F-68, and various lipids. It was recently approved by the FDA for adjuvant therapy to reduce myocardial ischemia during coronary angioplasty. A highly purified form of Poloxamer 188 (Flocor™), intended for IV administration, is undergoing Phase III clinical trials for various cardiovascular diseases. Purification of Poloxamer 188 has been shown to reduce nephrotoxicity.

1185

Poloxamers and other polymeric materials such as albumin may coat the micro- or nano particle, alter their surface characteristics and reduce their phagocytosis and opsonization by the reticuloendothelial system following IV injection. Such surface modifications often result in prolongation in the circulation time of intravenously injected colloidal dispersions (73). Poloxamers also have been used to stabilize suspension such as NanoCrystal™ (74).

The first successful development of an injectable perfluorocarbon-based commercial product was achieved by the Green Cross Corporation in Japan, when it made Fluosol-DA®, a dilute (20% w/v) emulsion based on perfluorodecalin and perflurotripropylamine emulsified with potassium oleate, Pluronic F-68, and egg yolk lecithin. These perfluorocarbons are inert and also can be used to formulate nonaqueous preparations of insoluble proteins and small molecules (75). Perfluorocarbons also have been approved by the FDA for use in one ultrasound contrast agent, Optison®, which is administered via the IV route. Optison® is a suspension of microspheres of HSA with octafluoropropane. Heat treatment and sonication of appropriately diluted human albumin, in the presence of octafluoropropane gas, is used to manufacture microspheres in the Optison® injection. The protein in the microsphere shell makes up approximately 5–7 (wt%) of the total protein in the liquid. The microspheres have a mean diameter range of 2.0–4.5 μm with 93% of the microsphere being less than 10 μm.

Sucrose acetate isobutyrate (SAIB) is a high viscosity liquid system that converts into free-flowing liquid when mixed with 10–15% ethanol (76). On subcutaneous or IM injection, the matrix rapidly converts to a water-insoluble semi-solid, that is capable of delivering proteins and small molecules for a prolonged period. SAIB is biocompatible, and biodegrades to natural metabolites. This is a fairly new matrix and three INDs have been filed for veterinary applications. It has not been used in humans.

Several other biodegradable, biocompatible, injectable polymers are being investigated for drug delivery systems. They include polyvinyl alcohol, block copolymer of PLA–PEG, polycyanoacrylate, polyanhydrides, cellulose, alginate, collagen, gelatin, albumin, starches, dextrans, hyaluronic acid and its derivatives, and hydroxyapatite (77).

REFERENCES

1. Parenteral Preparations. *European Pharmacopoeia*, 3rd Ed.; Council of Europe: Strasbourg, 1997; 1765.
2. Parenteral Preparations. *British Pharmacopoeia*; Stationary Office: London, 1999; II, 1575.
3. Uchiyama, M. Regulatory Status of Excipients in Japan. Drug Inf. J. **1999**, *33*, 27–32.
4. Nema, S.; Washkuhn, R.J.; Brendel, R.J. Excipients and their Use in Injectable Products. PDA J. Pharm. Sci. Technol. **1997**, *51* (4), 166–71.
5. Wang, Y.J.; Kowal, R.R. Review of Excipients and pHs for Parenteral Products Used in United States. J. Parenter. Sci. Technol. **1980**, *34* (6), 452.
6. Powell, M.F.; Nguyen, T.; Baloian, L. Compendium of Excipients for Parenteral Formulations. PDA J. Pharm. Sci. Technol. **1998**, *52* (5), 236–311.
7. Wang, Y.J.; Hanson, M.A. Parenteral Formulations of Proteins and Peptides: Stability and Stabilizers. J. Parenter. Sci. Technol. **1988**, *42* (supplement), S4–S26.
8. Boylan, J.C.; DeLuca, P.P. Formulation of Small Volume Parenterals. *Pharmaceutical Dosage Forms: Parenteral Medications*, 2nd Ed.; Avis, K.E., Lieberman, H.A., Lachman, L., Eds.; Marcel Dekker, Inc.; New York, 1992; 1, 173–48.
9. Strickley, R.G. Parenteral Formulations of Small Molecules Therapeutics Marketed in the United States (1999)--Part 1. PDA J. Pharm. Sci. Technol. **1999**, *53* (6), 324–349.
10. *Physician's Desk Reference*, Medical Economics Co.: Montvale, 1994, 1996, 1998 & 1999.
11. Trissel, L.A. *Handbook on Injectable Drugs*, 10th Ed.; American Society of Health-System Pharmacists, Inc.: Bethesda, 1998.
12. Kibbe, A.H. *Handbook of Pharmaceutical Excipients*, 3rd Ed.; The Pharmaceutical Press: London, 2000.
13. Mosby's, GenRx (Ed.) 8th Ed. Mosby-Year Book, Inc.: St. Louis MO, 1998.
14. Inactive Ingredient Guide, Division of Drug Information Resources, Food & Drug Administration, CDER, January 1996.
15. Sweetana, S.; Akers, M.J. Solubility Principles and Practices for Parenteral Drug Dosage Form Development. PDA J. Parenter. Sci. Technol. **1996**, *50* (5), 330–342.
16. Yalkowsky, S.H.; Roseman, T.J. Solubilization of Drugs by Cosolvents. *Techniques of Solubilization of Drugs*; Marcel Dekker, Inc.: New York, 1981; 91–134.
17. Rubino, J.T.; Yalkowsky, S.H. Cosolvency and Cosolvent Polarity. Pharm. Res. **1987**, *4* (3), 220–230.
18. Hancock, B.C.; York, P.; Rowe, R.C. The Use of Solubility Parameters in Pharmaceutical Dosage Form Design. Int. J. Pharm. **1997**, *148*, 1–21.
19. Reed, K.W.; Yalkowsky, S. Lysis of Human Red Blood Cells in the Presence of Various Cosolvents. J. Parenter. Sci. Technol. **1985**, *39* (2), 64.
20. Brazeau, G.A.; Fung, H. Use of an In-vivo Model for the Assessment of Muscle Damage from Intramuscular Injections: In-vitro–In-vivo Correlation and Predictability With Mixed Solvent Systems. Pharm. Res. **1989**, *6* (9), 766.
21. Brazeau, G.A.; Cooper, B.; Svetic, K.A.; Smith, C.L.; Gupta, P. Current Perspectives on Pain Upon Injection of Drugs. J. Pharm. Sci. **1998**, *87* (6), 667.
22. Yalkowsky, S.H.; Krzyzaniak, J.F.; Ward, G.H. Formulation-Related Problems Associated with Intravenous Drug Delivery. J. Pharm. Sci. **1998**, *87* (7), 787.
23. Johnson, D.M.; Gu, L.C. Autoxidation and Antioxidants. *Encyclopedia of Pharmaceutical Technology*; Swarbrick, J., Boylan, J.C., Eds.; Marcel Dekker, Inc.: NY, 1988; 1, 415–449.

24. Herman, A.C.; Boone, T.C.; Lu, H.S. Characterization, Formulation, and Stability of Neupogen® (Filgrastim), a Recombinant Human Granulocyte-Colony Stimulating Factor. *Formulation, Characterization, and Stability of Protein Drugs: Case Histories*; Pearlman, R., Wang, Y.J., Eds.; Plenum Press: NY, 1996; 9, 325.

25. Fatouros, A.; Osterberg, T.; Mikaelsson, M. Recombinant Factor VIII SQ: Influence of Oxygen, Metal Ions, pH and Ionic Strength on its Stability in Aqueous Solution. Int. J. Pharm. 1997, *155*, 121–131.

26. Stadtman, E.R. Metal Ion Catalyzed Oxidation of Proteins: Biochemical Mechanism and Biological Consequences. Free Radical Biol. Med. 1990, *9*, 315.

27. Munson, J.W.; Hussain, A.; Bilous, R. Precautionary Note for Use of Bisulfite in Pharmaceutical Formulations. J. Pharm. Sci. 1977, *66* (12), 1775–1776.

28. Enever, R.P.; Po, A.L.W.; Shotton, E. Factors Influencing Decomposition Rate of Amitriptyline Hydrochloride in Aqueous Solution. J. Pharm. Sci. 1977, *66* (8), 1087–1089.

29. Akers, M.J. Antioxidants in Pharmaceutical Products. J. Parenter. Sci. Technol. 1982, *36* (5), 222–228.

30. *Note for Guidance on Inclusion of Antioxidants and Antimicrobial Preservatives in Medicinal Products* CPMP: January 1998.

31. Dabbah, R. The Use of Preservatives in Compendial Articles. Pharmacopeial Forum 1996, *22* (4), 2696.

32. *Martindale: The Extra Pharmacopoeia*, 31st Ed.; Royal Pharmaceutical Society: London, 1996; 1128.

33. *British Pharmaceutical Codex*; Royal Pharmaceutical Society: London, 1973; 100.

34. USP ⟨51⟩ Antimicrobial Effectiveness Testing. *United States Pharmacopeia*; 24; US Pharmacopeial Convention, Inc.: Rockville, 2000, 1809.

35. Efficacy of Antimicrobial Preservation. *European Pharmacopoeia*, 3rd Ed.; Council of Europe: Strasbourg, 1997; 286.

36. Dabbah, R. Harmonization of Microbiological Methods–A Status Report. Pharmacopeial Forum 1997, *23* (6), 5334–5344.

37. *Note for Guidance on Maximum Shelf-life for Sterile Products for Human Use After First Opening or Following Reconstitution* ; CPMP: July 1998.

38. Lam, X.M.; Costantino, H.R.; Overcashier, D.E.; Nguyen, T.H.; Hsu, C.C. Replacing Succinate with Glycolate Buffer Improves the Stability of Lyophilized Interferon-γ. Int. J. Pharm. 1996, *142*, 85–95.

39. Pikal M.The Correlation of Structural Relaxation Time With Pharmaceutical Stability Freeze-Drying of Pharmaceuticals and Biologicals Conference Brownsville VT Sept. 23–26 1998.

40. Arakawa, T.; Kita, Y.; Carpenter, J.F. Protein–Solvent Interactions in Pharmaceutical Formulations. Pharm. Res. 1991, *8* (3), 285–291.

41. Miller, D.P.; Anderson, R.E.; de Pablo, J.J. Stabilization of Lactate Dehydrogenase Following Freeze-Thawing and Vacuum-Drying in the Presence of Trehalose and Borate. Pharm. Res. 1998, *15* (8), 1215–1221.

42. Carpenter, J.F.; Crowe, J.H. Modes of Stabilization of a Protein by Organic Solutes During Desiccation. Cryobiology 1998, *25*, 459–470.

43. Baumann, T.J.; Smythe, M.A.; Kaufmann, K.; Miloboszewski, Z.; O'Malley, J.; Fudge, R.P. Dissolution Times of Adriamycin and Adriamycin RDF. Am. J. Hosp. Pharm. 1988, *45*, 1667.

44. Jain, N.K.; Jain, S.; Singhai, A.K. Enhanced Solubilization and Formulation of an Aqueous Injection of Piroxicam. Pharmazie 1997, *52* (12), 942–946.

45. Meyer, J.D.; Manning, M.C. Hydrophobic Ion Pairing: Altering the Solubility Properties of Biomolecules. Pharm. Res. 1998, *15* (2), 188–192.

46. Wang, Y.J.; Dahl, T.C.; Leesman, G.D.; Monkhouse, D.C. Optimization of Autoclave Cycles and Selection of Formulation for Parenteral Product, Part II: Effect of Counter-Ion on pH and Stability of Diatrizoic Acid At Autoclave Temperatures. J. Parenter. Sci. Technol. 1984, *38* (2), 72.

47. Japan Pharmaceutical Excipient Council, Eds. *Japanese Pharmaceutical Excipients Directory 1996*; Yakuji Nippo, Ltd.: Tokyo, 1996.

48. Excipients in Pharmaceutical Dosage Forms: The Challenge of the 21st Century Conference Proceedings Nice France May 14–15 1998.

49. Benzyl Alcohol. Pharmacopeial Forum Sept.–Oct. 1995, *21* (5), 1240.

50. USP ⟨1078⟩ Good Manufacturing Practices for Bulk Pharmaceutical Excipients. *United States Pharmacopeia*, 24 Ed.; US Pharmacopeial Convention, Inc.: Rockville, 2000; 2040.

51. Excipients in the Label and Package Leaflet of Medicinal Products for Human Use. *The Rules Governing Medicinal Products in the European Union*; Guidelines: Medicinal Products for Human Use, European Commission: September 1997; 3B.

52. *Note for Guidance on Development Pharmaceutics* Committee for Proprietary Medicinal Products (CPMP): July 1998.

53. Paul, W.L. Excipient Intake and Heavy Metals Limits. Pharmacopeial Forum 1995, *21* (6), 1629.

54. Aluminum in Large and Small Volume Parenterals Used in Total Parenteral Nutrition. Federal Register January 5 1998, *63* (2), 176–185.

55. *Guideline on Validation of the Limulus Amebocyte Lysate Test as an End-Product Test for Human and Animal Parenteral Drugs, Biological Products, and Medical Devices*; Food & Drug Administration: December 1987.

56. Opalchenova, G.A. Comparison of the Microbial Limit Tests in the British, European, and United States Pharmacopeias and Recommendation for Harmonization. Pharmacopeial Forum 1994, *20* (4), 7872–7877.

57. US Department of Health and Human Services. Morbidity and Mortality Weekly Report. August 2 1996, *45* (30), 649–650.

58. Weiner, M.; Bernstein, I.L. *Adverse Reactions to Drug Formulation Agents: A Handbook of Excipients*; Marcel Dekker, Inc.: New York NY, 1989.

59. USP ⟨1074⟩ Excipient Biological Safety Evaluation Guidelines. *United States Pharmacopeia*, 24 Ed.; US Pharmacopeial Convention Inc.: Rockville, 2000; 2037.

60. Note for Guidance on Minimizing the Risk of Transmitting Animal Spongiform Encephalopathy Agents Via Medicinal Products. *CPMP*; April 21, 1999.

61. The Sourcing and Processing of Gelatin to Reduce the Potential Risk Posed by Bovine Spongiform Encephalo-

pathy (BSE) in FDA-Regulated Products for Human Use, Guidance for Industry, US Dept. of Health and Human Services, FDA, Sept. 1997.

62. Frank, D.W.; Gray, J.E.; Weaver, R.N. Cyclodextrin Nephrosis in the Rats. Am. J. Pathol. **1976**, *83*, 367.

63. Stella, V.J.; Rajewski, R.A. Cyclodextrins: Their Future in Drug Formulation and Delivery. Pharm. Res. **1997**, *14* (5), 556–567.

64. Thompson, D.O. Cyclodextrins-Enabling Excipients: Their Present and Future Use in Pharmaceuticals: Critical Reviews in Therapeutic Drug Carrier Systems. **1997**, *14* (1), 1–104.

65. Loftsson, T.; Johannesson, H.R., Die Pharmazie **1994**, *49*, 292–293.

66. Lehner, S.J.; Muller, B.W.; Seydel, J.K. Effect of Hydroxylpropyl-Beta-Cyclodextrin on the Antimicrobial Action of Preservatives. J. Pharm. Pharmacol. **1994**, *46*, 186–191.

67. Felt, O.; Buri, P.; Gurny, R. Chitosan: A Unique Polysaccharide for Drug Delivery. Drug Develop. Ind. Pharm. **1998**, *24* (11), 979–993.

68. Jain, R.; Shah, N.H.; Malick, A.W.; Rhodes, C.T. Controlled Drug Delivery by Biodegradable Poly(Ester) Devices: Different Preparative Approaches. Drug Develop. Ind. Pharm. **1998**, *24* (8), 703–727.

69. Middleton, J.C.; Tipton, A.J. Synthetic Biodegradable Polymers as Medical Devices. Med. Plastics Biomaterial **1998**, *5* (2).

70. Pettit, D.K.; Lawter, J.R.; Huang, W.J.; Pankey, S.C.; Nightlinger, N.S.; Lynch, D.H.; Schuh, J.A.C.L.; Morrissey, P.J.; Gombotz, W.R. Characterization of Poly(glycolideco-D,L-lactide)/Poly(D,L-lactide) Microspheres for Controlled Release of GM-CSF. Pharm. Res. **1997**, *14* (10), 1422–1430.

71. Katre, N.V.; Asherman, J.; Schaefer, H. Multivesicular Liposome (DepoFoam™) Technology for the Sustained Delivery of Insulin-Like Growth Factor-I. J. Pharm. Sci. **1998**, *87* (11), 1341–1346.

72. Wang, P.; Johnston, T.P. Sustained-Release Interleukin-2 Following Intramuscular Injection in Rats. Int. J. Pharm. **1995**, *113* (1), 73–81.

73. Moghimi, S.M. Mechanisms Regulating Body Distribution of Nanospheres Conditioned with Pluronic and Tetronic Block Co-Polymers. Adv. Drug Deliv. Rev. **1995**, *16*, 183–193.

74. Zheng, J.Y.; Bosch, H.W. Sterile Filtration of NanoCrystal™ Drug Formulations. Drug Develop. Ind. Pharm. **1997**, *23* (11), 1087–1093.

75. Knepp, V.M.; Muchnik, A.; Oldmark, S.; Kalashnikova, L. Stability of Nonaqueous Suspension Formulations of Plasma Derived Factor IX and Recombinant Human Alpha Interferon at Elevated Temperatures. Pharm. Res. **1998**, *15* (7), 1090–1095.

76. Sullivan, S.A.; Gilley, R.M.; Gibson, J.W.; Tipton, A.J. Delivery of Taxol and Other Antineoplastic Agents from a Novel System Based on Sucrose Acetate Isobutyrate. Pharm. Res. **1997**, *12* (11), 291.

77. Gombotz, W.R.; Pettit, D.K. Biodegradable Polymers for Proteins and Peptide Drug Delivery. Bioconjugate Chem. **1995**, *6*, 332–351.

EXPERT SYSTEMS IN PHARMACEUTICAL PRODUCT DEVELOPMENT

Raymond C. Rowe
Ronald J. Roberts
AstraZeneca, Macclesfield, Cheshire, United Kingdom

INTRODUCTION

The process of formulation, whether it be for oral products (e.g., tablets and capsules), parenterals [e.g., intravenous (iv) injections], or any one of the myriad of pharmaceutical products, is generically the same. The process begins with some form of product specification and ends with the generation of one or more formulations that meet the requirements. Although the formulation consists of a list of ingredients and their proportions together with some processing variables where appropriate, the specification can vary considerably from one application to another. In some cases it may be very specific, expressed in terms of a performance level when subjected to a specific test, or quite general. It may also contain potentially conflicting performance criteria that the formulator may need to redefine in the light of experience. Figure 1 shows a typical formulation process broken down into its constituent tasks and subtasks (1).

In designing a formulation, the formulator must take into account the properties of the active ingredient as well as possible chemical interactions between it and the other ingredients added to improve processibility and product properties since these may result in chemical instability. There may even be interactions between added ingredients, leading to physical instability. Commercial factors as well as the policy of the industry toward ingredient usage are important influences, as are production factors in the intended markets. The formulator may also routinely access databases on previous formulations as well as make use of mathematical models. During the formulation process, specific tests may need to be run to evaluate the properties of the proposed formulation and an analysis of zunexpected results may lead to an adjustment of the ingredients and/or their levels.

TECHNOLOGY

There is a wide divergence of views as to what defines an expert system. Examples include the following:

1. "An expert system is a knowledge-based system that emulates expert thought to solve significant problems in a particular domain of expertise" (2).
2. "An expert system is a computer program that draws on the knowledge of human experts captured in a knowledge base to solve problems that normally require human expertise" (3).

In its simplest form, an expert system has three major components: 1) an interface, a monitor, and keyboard that allow two-way communication between the user and the system; 2) a knowledge base where all the knowledge pertaining to the domain is stored; and 3) an inference engine where the knowledge is extracted and manipulated to solve the problem at hand. Inferencing strategies may be either forward chaining, which involves the system reasoning from data and information gained by consultation from the user to form a hypothesis, or backward chaining, which involves the system starting with a hypothesis and then attempting to find data and information to prove or disprove the hypothesis. Both strategies are included in most expert systems.

Knowledge in any domain takes the form of facts and heuristics; the former being valid, true, and justifiable by rigorous argument, the latter (often referred to as rules of thumb) being the expert's best judgment in any particular circumstance and hence justifiable only by example. Associated with these are the terms data and information, the former referring to facts and figures, the latter being data transferred by processing such that the data are meaningful to the person receiving the information. Knowledge can, therefore, be regarded as information combined with heuristics and rules. It is the objective of the knowledge engineer to acquire or elicit this knowledge and structure it in a computer-readable format.

Knowledge acquisition is probably one of the most difficult stages in the development of an expert system. It is both time-consuming and tedious as well as being expensive and often difficult to manage. However, it is a necessary element in the building of an expert system and, if done well, will undoubtedly lead to potentially useful systems. The basic model of knowledge acquisition is one of a team process whereby the knowledge engineer

Encyclopedia of Pharmaceutical Technology

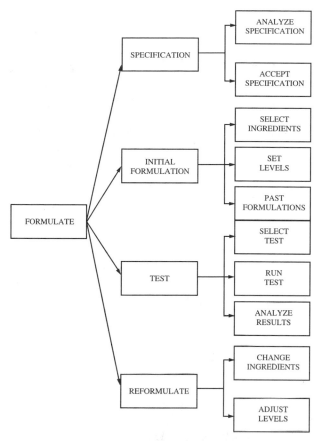

Fig. 1 Tasks and subtasks in the formulation process. (From Ref. 1.)

mediates between the expert(s), the users, and the knowledge bases. The knowledge engineer must acquire or elicit knowledge from not only the expert(s) but also from all the other potential sources, including written documents (research reports, reference manuals, and operating procedures policy statements) as well as consultants, users, and managers. In the case of experts, knowledge is usually acquired through face-to-face interviews. While this process is tedious and can place great demands on both the expert and knowledge engineer, it requires little equipment (e.g., tape recorder or notebook), is highly flexible, and often yields a considerable amount of useful information. At all times, there must be empathy between the participants and in many cases it is helpful to have two knowledgeable engineers present at the interview.

A technique that is often used in the acquisition process is the rapid prototyping approach. In this approach, the knowledge engineer builds a small prototype system as early as possible. This is then shown to both the expert and user, who can suggest modifications and additions. Here the system grows incrementally as more information and

knowledge are gained. This methodology has been used successfully in the development of systems for the formulation of pharmaceuticals.

Once acquired, there are many ways of representing the knowledge in the knowledge base, including production rules, frames, semantic networks, decision tables, and trees and objects (2). Probably the most common methodology is the production rule, which expresses the relationship between several pieces of information by way of conditional statements that specify sections under certain sets of conditions, for example:

IF	(condition 1)
AND	(condition 2)
OR	(condition 3)
THEN	(action)
UNLESS	(exception)
BECAUSE	(reason)

Each rule implements an autonomous piece of knowledge and is easy to understand. Unfortunately, complex knowledge can require large numbers of rules, causing the system to become difficult to manage. The decision as to which method of knowledge representation should be adopted is dependent primarily on the complexity of the domain.

Expert systems can be developed using either conventional computer languages, special purpose languages, or with the assistance of development shells or tool-kits. Conventional languages such as PASCAL and C have the advantages of wide applicability and full flexibility to create the control and inferencing strategies required. They also are well supported and easy to customize. However, considerable amounts of time and effort are needed to create the basic facilities.

Specialized languages, such as LISP (a recursive language and the primary one for artificial intelligence research), PROLOG (a language based on first-order predicate logic), and SMALLTALK (an object-orientated language), have been used extensively in the development of expert systems. They have the advantages of applicability and flexibility of the conventional languages but are faster to implement.

Expert system shells and tool kits are sets of computer programs written in either conventional or specialized languages that can form an expert system when loaded with the relevant knowledge. They compromise on applicability and flexibility but allow more rapid development. Many offer basic facilities, including the means to prepare and store knowledge as a set of rules and to make deductions by chaining the rules together in an inferential process.

Shells differ in their secondary characteristics, such as user interfaces, operating speeds, the method of knowledge representation, and the associated algorithmic and arithmetic computational facilities. It is not surprising, therefore, that formulation is a highly specialized task that requires specific knowledge and often years of experience. This kind of expertise is not easily documented and hence, senior formulators often spend considerable amounts of time training new personnel. In addition, retirement or personnel moves can lead to a loss of irreplaceable commercial knowledge. Computer technology in the form of expert systems provides an affordable means of capturing this knowledge and expertise in a documented form available to all.

One such shell of specific importance in product formulation is Product Formulation Expert System (PFES), now termed Formulogic, developed by Logica UK Ltd. Formulogic a reusable software kernel and associated methodology to support the generic formulation process. It arose from research work during the mid-1980s and is now used for a variety of formulation support tools across a range of industry sectors, most notably pharmaceuticals (4, 5).

Formulogic is designed specifically for building formulation systems. Its formulation capability is generic, i.e., it is not specific to any particular domain. Individual formulation applications are developed using the shell by defining characteristics of the domain and the corresponding approach to formulation. The end result is a decision support tool for formulators that provides assistance in all aspects of the formulation development process. Formulogic provides the expert system developer with the knowledge representation structures that are common to most product formulation tasks so that a new application can be developed rapidly and efficiently. The architecture of Formulogic comprises three levels—the Physical Level, the Task Level, and the Control Level.

The Physical Level contains all the "nuts and bolts" of the formulation domain in a number of information sources, including a database. The Physical Level is accessed from the Task Level via a query interface. The physical net contains the domain knowledge in a number of objects. An object consists of a set of attributes, each of which may have zero or more values. The objects are arranged in a classification hierarchy. Subobjects, which descend from another object, inherit their attributes and values.

The Task Level is where the formulation problem-solving activity takes place. The formulation process is driven via the generation of a hierarchy of tasks. A task represents some well-defined activity. The hierarchy has an indefinite number of task levels. Domain knowledge about the formulation application is distributed throughout the hierarchy, with more abstract knowledge represented towards the top of the hierarchy and more specific knowledge toward the bottom.

The task decomposition allows the problem-solving process to be largely decoupled between tasks and also facilitates reasoning about subtasks. An important principle is that tasks plan about and directly manipulate only their immediate subtasks. Recursive application of this principle is the key to integrated behavior of a formulation system as a whole. The task tree is built on dynamically, depending upon the specification at hand as the problem-solving process proceeds. This is different to the object hierarchy where the structure is fixed for a particular domain.

Agendas, a particularly important class of objects used for communication between tasks, also are part of the Task Level. Agendas are important because the user exercises control over the formulation process principally through their manipulation. For parallel reasoning and backtracking by the user it is necessary to maintain more than one world. A world contains a formulation object and specification object together with agendas (in other words, a complete description of the state of the formulation process at any one time). Tasks run on a world or set of worlds; it is meaningless for tasks to run without reference to worlds.

Tasks perform their function by the execution of processes. Each task contains several types of processes. The precondition process assesses whether or not the task can play a sensible role in the current context. The action process performs the primary work of the task, which can include scheduling subtasks to be run next. The monitor process executes between each of the subtasks, typically to assess their result. Finally, the postcondition process assesses the success of the task as a whole immediately prior to completion.

Each process consists of a set of production rules; a rule is said to fire if its condition is true and its exception is false. When a rule fires, its action is executed. The reason is for information only and is not interpreted by Formulogic.

Rules are assigned a priority that reflects the order in which they should be considered. When executing a rule set, rules are tried in order until no more rules can fire. To find a suitable rule, Formulogic orders the rules first on priority and then on specificity. The first rule having a true condition and false exception is fired, and its action executed. The process of finding the next rule that can fire then starts all over again. To avoid looping, rules are only allowed to fire once with the same set of variable bindings.

The Control Level is concerned with the mechanics of running the Task Level. It contains no domain knowledge and requires no design amendment when a new formulation system is built. Although the Task Level decides which tasks need running and the order in which they should run, the Control Level deals with the mechanics of actually running them and of passing control to them.

The typical functionality of a completed application is as follows:

1. The user enters the product specification, which forms the starting point of the formulation. In a tablet formulation, for example, this would consist of the drug details (unless already known to the system) and the dose.
2. Formulogic steps through a series of tasks to select ingredients and determine their quantities based on the product specification. It achieves this by following the rules and other knowledge that have been built into the system during development. An initial formulation is produced.
3. If the system performs reformulation in addition to producing initial formulations, then the user can enter the test results that have been performed on the product. Formulogic will then determine what kinds of problems with the formulation are indicated by the test results. The user can agree with the system's analysis of the problems or modify them as he or she sees fit. It uses the problem summary to make recommendations about what ingredients need to be added or what quantities need to be altered, and again the user can override the recommendations if he or she wishes. Once the user is happy with the recommendations, Formulogic will produce a modified formulation that meets the new requirements.

At any point during a session, the user can ask for an explanation of the results, browse the system's knowledge, or revert to an earlier stage of the process to modify the specification and obtain another formulation. The user can also save formulations (along with their associated product specifications) and generate printed reports.

APPLICATIONS

The first recorded reference to the use of expert systems in pharmaceutical product formulation was by Bradshaw on the April 27, 1989, in the London Financial Times (6), closely followed by an article in the autumn of the same year by Walko (7). Both refer to the work then being undertaken by personnel at ICI/Zeneca Pharmaceuticals (now AstraZeneca), United Kingdom (UK) and Logica UK Ltd. to develop expert systems for formulating pharmaceuticals using Formulogic. Since that time,

several companies and academic institutions have reported on their experiences in this area (Table 1). This article will review these applications.

The Boots System

Although not strictly developed for pharmaceutical formulation, this system has been included since it is the only one known for formulating topicals. It was developed to assist formulators in the formulation of sun care products—a highly skilled occupation requiring 3–4 years of experience to attain a reasonable level of experience.

Implemented with the use of Formulogic, the system, called SOLTAN, uses knowledge captured by interviewing senior formulators. Ingredients, processes, and relationships of the formulation are represented in a way that reflects their groupings and associations in the real world. In addition, existing information sources, such as databases, are presented in a frame-based semantic network that can be manipulated by the problem-solving knowledge of the domain. Tasks are structured in a hierarchy that is built up dynamically depending on the specification at hand as the problem-solving process proceeds. Knowledge about the formulation is distributed throughout the task hierarchy, with strategic knowledge represented toward the top of the hierarchy and tactical knowledge towards the bottom.

The system was originally developed to formulate sun oils (solutions of ultraviolet absorbers in emollients) but has been rapidly extended, with the incorporation of basic emulsion technology, to cover oil-in-water lotions. Subsequently, the system has been further expanded to incorporate water-in-oil, oil-in-water, and water-in-silicone

Table 1 Published applications of product formulation expert systems in pharmaceuticals

Company/institution	Domain	Development tool
Boots Company	Topicals	Formulogic
Cadila Laboratories (India)	Tablets	PROLOG
University of Heidelberg	Aerosols	C/SMALLTALK
	Tablets	
	Capsules	
	Injections	
University of London/ Capsugel	Capsules	C
Sanofi Research	Capsules	Formulogic
Zeneca Pharmaceuticals	Tablets	Formulogic
	Parenterals	
	Film coatings	

creams and lotions. It can now be used to formulate all types of skin care products, not just sun care products (8). The system won second prize in the UK DTI Manufacturing Intelligence Awards in 1991. It is the only system for which the developers have given details of costings and quantitative benefits.

The Cadila System

Cadila Laboratories Ltd. of Ahmedabad, India have developed an expert system for the formulation of tablets for active ingredients based on their physical, chemical, and biological properties (9). The system first identifies the desirable properties in the excipients for optimum compatibility with the active ingredient and then selects those that have the required properties based on the assumption that all tablet formulations comprise at least one binder, one disintegrant, and one lubricant. Other excipients such as diluents (fillers) or glidants are then added as required.

Knowledge is acquired through "active collaboration" with domain experts over a period of 6–7 months. It is structured in two knowledge bases in a spreadsheet format. In the knowledge base concerning the interactions between active ingredients and excipients, the columns represent the properties of the excipients with descriptors of "strong," "moderate," and "weak." The rows represent the properties of the active ingredients, e.g., functional groups (primary amines, secondary amines, highly acidic etc.), solubility (very soluble, freely soluble, soluble, sparingly soluble, slightly soluble, very slightly soluble, insoluble), density (low, moderate, high), etc. Each cell in the spreadsheet then represents the knowledge of the interaction between the various properties. Production rules derived from this knowledge are in the following forms:

IF	(functional group of active ingredient is "primary/secondary amine")
THEN	(add "strong" binder)
AND	(add "strong" disintegrant)
AND	(avoid lactose)

or

IF	(functional group of active ingredient is "highly acidic")
THEN	(add "moderate" binder)
AND	(add "moderate" disintegrant)
AND	(avoid starch)

or

IF	(active ingredient is soluble)
THEN	(add "weak" binder)
AND	(add "weak" disintegrant)

A similar approach is used for the knowledge base concerning the excipients, where the columns now represent details (e.g., name, minimum, maximum, and normal concentrations) of the excipients and the rows their properties (e.g., type and the descriptors—strong, moderate, and weak). Each cell in the spreadsheet then represents the name and the amount to be added to the formulation.

The system, written in PROLOG, is menu-driven and interactive with the user. The user is first prompted to input all the known properties of the new active ingredient. If the properties have descriptors, the user can select the appropriate ones. All information can be edited to correct errors. The expert system then consults the knowledge bases, suggesting compatible excipients and a formulation. If the latter is unacceptable, the system provides alternative formulations with explanations. All formulations can be stored along with explanations, if necessary. The user is able to update the knowledge base via an interface with a spreadsheet. An example of a formulation generated for the analgesic drug paracetamol, or acetaminophen, (dose 500 mg) is shown in Table 2. It is interesting to note that the diluent/filler is unnamed; it can be assumed that it will not be lactose since the relevant production rule indicates that there would be an interaction with the secondary amine in paracetamol. Furthermore, an examination of formulations on the market indicates that

Table 2   An example of a tablet formulation for the analgesic drug paracetamol as generated by the Cadila system

Input		
Dose	500 mg	
Functional group	Secondary amines	
Solubility	Sparingly soluble	
Density	Moderate	
Hygroscopicity	Moderate	
Dissolution	Slow	
Desired tablet weight	570 mg	
Output		
Active agent	Paracetamol	500.0 mg
Binder	Pregelatinized starch	43.7 mg
Disintegrant	Sodium starch glycolate	5.0 mg
Lubricant	Stearic acid	2.5 mg
Diluent/filler	Unnamed	20.0 mg
	Tablet weight	571.2 mg

(From Ref. 9.)

none contain lactose and that some contain mixtures of maize starch, sodium starch glycolate, stearic acid, magnesium stearate, and microcrystalline cellulose, adding further credibility to the Cadila system.

When first implemented, the prototype system had 150 rules, but this has expanded rapidly to approximately 300 rules in order to increase reliability. This is expected to increase further over time. The system is regarded as being highly successful, providing competitive advantage to the company (9).

The Galenical Development System

The Galenical Developmental System (GSH) was developed by personnel in the Department of Pharmaceutical and Biopharmaceutics and the Department of Medical Informatics at the University of Heidelberg, Germany. It is designed to provide assistance in the development of a range of formulations, starting from the chemical and physical properties of an active ingredient. The project was initiated in 1990 under the direction of Stricker (10), and in the interim has been extensively revised and enhanced (11, 12). Originally implemented using object-oriented C on a workstation, the system was recently upgraded using SMALLTALK V running under the Windows operating system on a personal computer.

Various forms of knowledge representation are used depending on the type of knowledge. Knowledge about objects (e.g., functional groups in the active ingredient, excipients, processes, etc.), their properties, and relationships are represented in frames using an object-oriented approach. Causal relationships are represented as rules, functional connections as formulas, and procedural knowledge as algorithms. The system currently has knowledge bases for aerosols, IV injection solutions, capsules (hard-shell powder), and tablets (direct compression). Each knowledge base incorporates information on all aspects of that dosage formulation (e.g., properties of the excipients to be added, compatibility, processing operations, packaging, and containers and storage conditions), with each aspect given a reliability factor (Sicherheitsfaktor) to indicate its accuracy/reliability. In the original version of the system values for each factor varied between 0 and 9 (10); however, values between 0 and 1 are used currently. The values are propagated using the arithmetic minimum rule and are not used for any decisions. They only serve as indicators of the accuracy/reliability of the knowledge.

The approach used in the system is the decomposition of the overall process into individual distinct development steps, with each step focusing on one problem associated

with a subset of its specifications or constraints for the formulation. A problem is considered solved if its predicted outcome satisfies its associated constraints. The problems are worked through in succession, with care being taken that any solution should not violate any constraints from previous steps. For simplicity, the developers imposed a predefined ordering onto the development steps, providing a backtracking mechanism to go back to a previous step or abort. This ordering minimizes dependency between development steps, which might result in an action causing a constraint previously satisfied to be violated. It also reduces the complexity of the problem to be solved.

The procedural model for one development step (e.g., for the choice of an excipient) is shown in Fig. 2. In any development step the first decision is whether or not to proceed with any action since the problem may have already been solved in previous steps. This is done by comparing the predicted or relevant properties of the current formulation with the initial specification. If the answer is negative, then further action is required; if positive, the problem has been solved. Once this has been decided, actions need to be defined and ranked. Knowledge for this is by means of hierarchically structural rule sets to form a decision tree where each leaf node consists of a subgroup of actions and each branch a rule. The rules in a rule set are ordered as the simplest and most straightforward way of handling conflict. Ranking numbers are used as the basis for the selection strategy. The concept is to search for the best alternative in terms of the highest score, these being the sum of the values of the constants to be resolved within the development step (e.g., solubility, compressibility, etc.) and their weights indicating their respective importance (11, 12). It should be noted that this method of ranking is different from that used originally by Stricker et al. (10), where the lowest score was regarded as the best alternative.

Once the action is selected, the decision is checked in terms of whether or not the measure has adverse effects on the active ingredient in terms of physical or chemical incompatibility. This does not necessarily mean a rejection of the action since knowledge of compatibility is generally of a qualitative nature with little quantification to denote severity. Hence, the overall decision is left to the user.

The amounts of excipients to be used are calculated by formulae with rule-based mechanisms for selecting the appropriate formula. A rule-based mechanism is also used to determine the appropriate function for predicting the property of the intermediate formulation. This is necessary for checking whether or not the original specifications have been satisfied and the action is successful. If

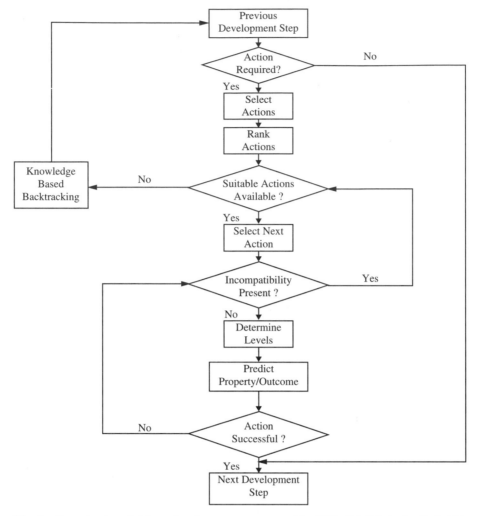

Fig. 2 Procedural model for a development step as used in GSH. (Modified after Ref. 12.)

negative, the chosen action is rejected and the next action in the ranking is tried. It is possible that none of the ranked actions is successful. If this is the case, then knowledge-based backtracking is used to determine which of the previous development steps to return to. Usually, background pharmaceutical knowledge is applied to determine why the current development step was unsuccessful, and a new development step that can solve the root cause of the problem is chosen.

In any expert system, explanations of the decisions made are important, both for instruction of the user and for maintenance of the system. Explanations in GSH take several forms. There are explanations for the development steps and their ordering provided by the designer of the knowledge base. Detailed explanations of the rules activated, formulae used, or individual scores of actions can be generated if required, and canned text and literature references are provided for general knowledge.

A simplified task structure for generating an iv injection solution is shown in Fig. 3. The input to the system includes all the known properties of the active ingredient to be formulated (e.g., solubility, stability, impurities, pK_a, presence/absence of functional groups, etc.) with user-defined labels that relate the specific drug property to the required product property. Use of the system results in the production of four packages—the product formulation, the production method, the recommended packaging and storage conditions, and predicted product properties. All the outputs are provided with reliability factors. An example for an IV injection solution of the cardiac drug digoxin is shown in Table 3, and an example for a hard gelatin capsule of the antifungal drug griseofulvin is shown in Table 4. Comparison of a 0.1 mg. commercial formulation of digoxin with that shown in Table 3 indicates that the same cosolvent is used (1,2-propandiol, presumably to enhance solubility) and ethanol. However,

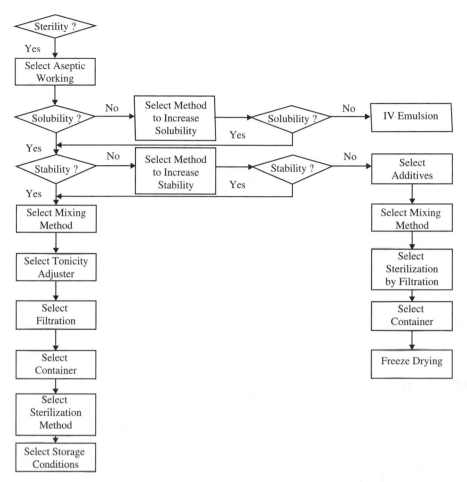

Fig. 3 Structure of the expert system described by Stricker et al. (10) for the formulation of intravenous injection solutions.

the commercial formulation is more sophisticated since it also contains a buffer (disodium hydrogen phosphate/citric acid).

At present, knowledge bases for aerosols, IV injection solutions, hard gelatin capsules, and direct compression tablets have been completed. Other knowledge bases for coated forms, granules, freeze-dried formulations, and pellets are in different stages of development. Trials have demonstrated that the system proposes formulations that are acceptable to formulators, and in December 1996, the system was first introduced for field trials in a pharmaceutical company.

The University of London/Capsugel System

This system is designed to aid the formulation of hard gelatin capsules (13–15). It was developed as part of a Ph.D. program by Lai, Podczeck, and Newton at the School of Pharmacy, University of London, and was supported by Daumesnil of Capsugel, Switzerland, together with personnel from the University of Kyoto, Japan and the University of Maryland, United States. The system (Fig. 4) is unique in that its knowledge base is broad and contains the following:

1. A database of literature references associated with the formulation of hard gelatin capsules, which is permanently updated through monitoring of current literature.
2. Information on excipients used and their properties. This database currently contains information on 72 excipients and is frequently updated. Data can be retrieved via a menu.
3. An analysis of marketed formulations from Germany, Italy, Belgium, France, and the United States. This is used to identify trends in formulation and identify guidelines on the use of excipients. Currently, the database contains information on 750 formulations of 250 active ingredients. It is frequently updated and data can be retrieved via a menu.

Table 3 An example of an intravenous injection solution formulation for the
cardiac drug digoxin as generated by GSH

Formulation		
Active	Digoxin	0.1 mg
Solvent 1	1,2-Propandiol	0.5 mL
	Water for injection to	1.0 mL

Packaging
Brown glass ampules

Product properties

Properties	Specification	Actual	R.F.[a]
Active (mg)	0.095	0.098	1.0
Volume (mL)	1.0	1.0	1.0
pH	3–9	7.0	1.0
Freezing point depression (°C)	0.5–20	13.2	0.8
Shelf life at 25°C (years)		5.0	1.0
Decomposition at 25°C (mol)		1.8	0.7

[a]R.F., reliability factor.
(From Ref. 10.)

4. Experience and nonproprietary knowledge obtained over a period of 18 months from a group of industrial experts from Europe, the United States, and Japan.
5. Results from statistically designed experiments that identify factors that influence the filling and in vitro release performance of model active ingredients.

The system uses production rules with a decision tree implemented in C, coupled with a user interface through which the user can access both the databases and develop new formulations. To assist in collecting all necessary input data, a questionnaire has been designed. Called the expert system input package, it requires information on the physical properties of the active ingredient (e.g., dose, particle shape, particle size, solubility, wettability, adhesion to metal surfaces, melting point, and bulk density), compatibility of the active ingredient with excipients (e.g., fillers/diluents, disintegrants, lubricants, glidants, and surfactants), and properties of excipients used by the user and manufacturing conditions (e.g., capsule sizes, fill weights, densification techniques, granulation techniques) used by the user.

From this data the system uses a variety of methods to evaluate and predict properties of mixtures of the active ingredient and the excipients. For instance, it uses Carr's compressibility index (16) to predict the flow properties that are used to give an indication of the ability to produce a uniform blend, and the Kawakita equation (17) to predict a maximum in the volume reduction of the powder

Table 4 An example of a hard gelatin capsule formulation for the antifungal drug griseofulvin as generated by GSH

Formulation		
Active	Griseofulvin	150.0 mg
Diluent	Microcrystalline cellulose (PH102)	199.2 mg
Lubricant	Magnesium stearate	3.5 mg

Production process
High shear mixer for deagglomeration, premix, and main mix.
Add lubricant, planetary mixer at 12 rpm for 3 min.
Capsule-filling machine type 1.

Packaging
Foil blisters (PVC and aluminum foil)

(From Ref. 12.)

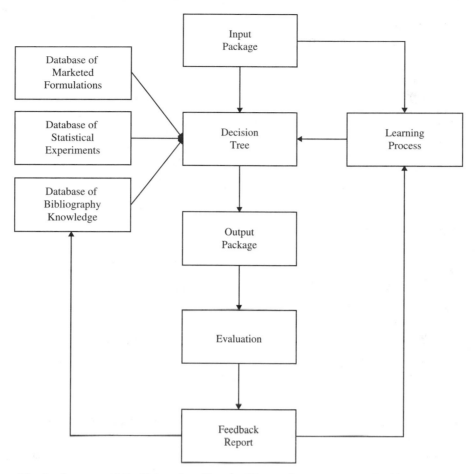

Fig. 4 Structure of the University of London/Capsugel system as described by Lai et al.

achievable by the application of low pressure. The packing properties are obviously important to give the volume that a given weight of powder occupies in order to indicate the size of capsule shell that can be used. When wet granulation is offered as the preferred method of densification, the system only offers advice on the choice of a granulating liquid and binder; no choice on the granulation procedure is offered.

The system provides an output package that includes a formulation (Table 5) with any necessary powder processing and filling conditions, the required capsule size, a statistical design to quantitatively optimize the formulation, specification of excipients used, recommended tests to validate the formulation, and a complete documentation of the decision process.

An interesting addition to the system is a semiautomatic learning tool. This monitors user habits and collects data about the use of excipients. Statistical analysis is performed on these data, allowing agreed alterations to be made to the database. The user is also asked to reply to a

questionnaire regarding the recommended formulation and its performance. The data are analyzed by the expert system founder group, and provide the background for further alterations and developments.

Field trials have proved that the system does provide reasonable formulations (18).

The Sanofi System

Personnel at the Sanofi Research Division of Philadelphia recently developed an expert system for the formulation of hard gelatin capsules based on specific preformulation data of the active ingredient (19). Using Formulogic, the system generates one first-pass clinical capsule formulation with as many subsequent formulations as desired to accommodate an experimental design. The latter are produced as a result of the user overruling decisions made by the system.

Knowledge acquisition is obtained by meetings between formulators, with a knowledge engineer present as a

Table 5 An example of a hard gelatin capsule formulation for a model drug as generated by the university of londoncapsugel system

Tablet properties (*inputs*)

Dose (mg)	50.0
Solubility	Insoluble
Particle size (μm)	5.0
Minimum bulk density (g ml^{-1})	0.4
Tapped bulk density (g ml^{-1})	0.7
Carr's compressibility (%)	42.857

Formulation

		wt%	mg/capsule
Active	Drug	39.7	50.0
Filler	Starch:lactose (1:2)	56.8	71.6
Disintegrant	Croscarmellose sodium	2.0	2.5
Lubricant	Magnesium stearate	1.0	1.3
Surfactant	Sodium lauryl sulfate	0.5	0.6
Capsule weight			126.0
Capsule size			No. 4

(From Refs. 13 and 14.)

consultant. Meetings are limited to 2 h, with minutes being taken and reviewed by all attendees. Meetings are specific to one topic defined in advance. A rapid prototyping approach is used to generate the expert system.

Knowledge in the system is structured using the strategies implemented in Formulogic, i.e., objects and production rules. The latter are as follows:

Tasks are scheduled dynamically. An outline of the task structure used is given in Fig. 5.

IF	(electrostatic properties of a drug are problematic)
THEN	(add glidant)
UNLESS	(glidant has already been added)

The user is first prompted to enter specified preformulation data on the active ingredient (e.g., acid stability, molecular weight, wettability, density, particle size, hygoscopicity, melting point, solubility, etc.) and known excipient incompatibilities together with the required dose. At the initial formulation task, the capsule size is selected together with the process and milling requirements. The excipient classes are selected, with some excipients being excluded, others prioritized, and their amounts determined. At the display reports task, three reports are provided, one providing the preformulation data as given, the second giving the recommended formulation, including the amounts of the excipients and processing/milling requirements, and the third providing the explanation of the decisions and reasoning used by the system. On the

first-pass through the system, the selection of the possible processing, milling, and excipient options are automatic. On subsequent passes, the selections are optional, allowing the user to generate a number of formulations.

An example of a formulation generated by this system, for the nonsteroidal anti-inflammatory drug naproxen, is given in Table 6. This example, as well as others, was considered acceptable by experienced formulators for manufacture and initial stability evaluation.

Unfortunately, the authors (19) do not provide any further details on the state of the system except to imply that formulation evaluation and preformulation tasks could be accommodated with the possible development for other formulation types such as tablets, liquids, and creams.

The Zeneca Systems

Work on expert systems within ICI/Zeneca Pharmaceuticals (now AstraZeneca) began in April 1988, with the initiation of a joint project between the Pharmaceutical and Corporate Management Services departments to investigate the use of knowledge-based techniques for the formulation of tablets. Since that time, work has proceeded with the successful development of expert systems for formulating tablets, parenterals, and tablet film coatings. All have been implemented using Formulogic from Logica UK Ltd., although elements of the system developed for

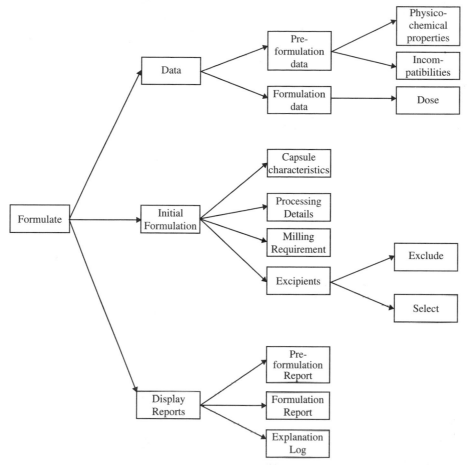

Fig. 5 Task structure for the formulation of hard gelatin capsules as used by Bateman et al. (19).

tablet film coatings were originally prototyped using a rule induction tool to produce decision trees.

Delivery of the first usable system for tablet formulation was in January 1989 (20, 21). All the knowledge was acquired from two primary experts in the field of tableting—one with extensive heuristic knowledge and the other with extensive research knowledge—and structured into Formulogic using specialist consultancy support. Consultancy time for the initial system was in the order of 30 man days, 20% of which was involved in three 2-day visits to the laboratories, incorporating three 90-min interviews with the experienced formulator plus members of the research group, the demonstration of prototype systems, and the validation of the previously acquired knowledge with the expert and other members of the department. Sixty percent of the time was involved in system development and 20% in writing the final report.

After commissioning and extensive demonstration to management and formulators throughout the company during 1989, the system was enhanced by the addition of a

link to a database in January 1990, and the installation of a formulation optimization routine in September 1990. A major revision was initiated in February 1991, following a significant change in formulation practice. Total consultancy time for these enhancements was of the order of 30 man-days. In August 1991, the system was completed and handed over to the formulators both in the United Kingdom and the United States.

The completed system is shown in Fig. 6 (20). It is divided into three stages: 1) the entry of the data, product specification, and strategy; 2) the identification of the initial formulation; and 3) the formulation optimization as a result of testing the initial formulation. The sequence is as follows:

1. The user enters all the relevant physical, chemical, and mechanical properties (e.g., solubility, wettability, compatibility with excipients, and deformation behavior) of the new active ingredient to be formulated into the database. The data may be

Table 6 An example of a hard gelatin capsule formulation for the antiinflammatory drug naproxen as generated by the system described by Bateman et al.

Selected drug properties (inputs)		
Molecular weight		230.26
Melting point (°C)		155
Solubility in water (mg ml^{-1})		0.01
Wettability		Poor
Water stability		Poor
Photostability		Poor
Susceptible to hydrolysis		No
Primary/secondary amines		No
Hygroscopicity		Class 1
Poured density (g cm^{-3})		0.366
Electrostatic problems		No
Unmilled particle size (μm)		36
Formulation		
Active	Naproxen	100 mg
Diluent	Lactose (hydrous)	224 mg
Disintegrant	Microcrystalline cellulose (PH105)	60 mg
Surfactant	Sodium lauryl sulfate	4 mg
Lubricant	Talc	12 mg
Production information		
Milling	Jet milling of drug	
Capsule	Size 0 colored opaque	
Process	Direct blend	

Explanation log
A colored opaque capsule used because drug is unstable to light.
Drug requires milling as it has a medium particle size and is insoluble.
A surfactant is required because drug has poor wettability.

(From Ref. 19.)

numerical or symbolic (e.g., for solubility in water the data can be entered as mg ml^{-1} or as the descriptors "soluble," "partially soluble," "insoluble," etc. The data are obtained from a series of proprietary preformulation tests carried out on the active ingredient as received (i.e., 5 g of the drug milled to a specified particle size). These tests include excipient compatibility studies whereby the drug is mixed with the excipient and stored under specified conditions of temperature and humidity for one week, the proportion of drug remaining being analyzed by HPLC and expressed as a percentage. The deformation properties essential for the evaluation of compactibility are assessed using yield pressure and strain rate sensitivity measured via a compression simulator (22).

2. The user enters the proposed dose of the active ingredient and a target tablet weight is calculated using both a formula determined from an extensive study of

previously successful formulations and certain rules governing minimum weights for ease of handling and maximum weights for ease of swallowing.

3. The user selects a strategy dependent on the number of fillers (one or two).

4. The system selects the filler(s), disintegrant, binder, surfactant, glidant, and lubricant, and their recommended concentrations based on a combination of algorithms, formulae, and mixture rules governing their compatibility and functionality. Tasks in this process are dynamically scheduled depending on the problem to be solved. If the system is unable to decide between two excipients, both of which satisfy all the embedded rules, then the user is asked to select a preference.

5. The recommended initial formulation is displayed, including final tablet weight, recommended tablet diameter calculated compression properties, and all relevant data (Table 7). This is normally printed for inclusion in a laboratory notebook, file, etc. If required,

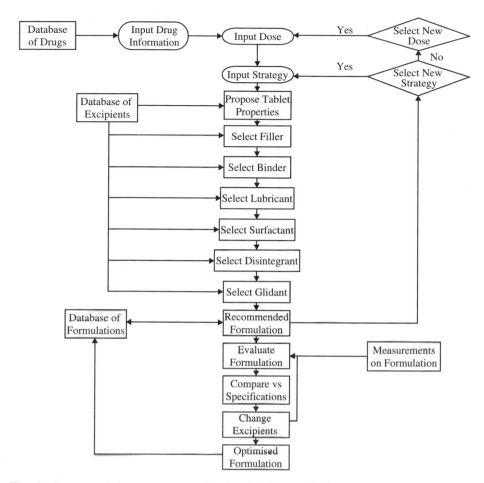

Fig. 6 Structure of the expert system developed by Rowe (20) for the formulation of tablets.

the data may be stored in a database for future reference, necessary if the formulation optimization route is used.

6. The user enters results from testing tablets prepared using the initial formulation. These may include disintegration time, tablet strength, tablet weight variation, and presence of any defects (e.g., capping, lamination, etc.). The results are compared with specifications, and any problems identified are confirmed with the user. Recommendations for modifications to the formulation are then listed. This routine is fully interactive with the user, who is asked to confirm or contradict/change the advice given.

7. After agreement is reached, the system modifies the formulation accordingly and displays it as described earlier. This routine may be used as many times as required; each time, the system iterates on the previously modified formulation.

Two "help" routines are embedded in the system, one to provide on-line help in the use of the system, the other to provide an insight into the rationale behind adoption of the specific rules/formulae/algorithms used. The user is able to browse the knowledge base at will but is not able to edit it without privileged access. Explanations for any recommendations made by the system can be easily accessed, if required. Hypertext links are used throughout. Two screen images from the system are shown in Fig. 7 to illustrate the operation of the system.

The system is well used and is now an integral part of the development strategy for tablet formulation. To date, it has successfully generated formulations for more than 40 active drugs. In many cases, the initial formulations have been acknowledged as being on a par with those developed by expert formulators. Consequently, the formulation optimization routine is now considered redundant and is used very rarely.

Following the successful implementation of the tablet formulation expert system, a request was made for the development of a similar system for parenteral formulations. This project was initiated in April 1992, and

Table 7 Examples of tablet formulations for a model drug as generated by the system described by Rowe

Drug properties (inputs)

Solubility (mg ml^{-1})	0.1
Contact angle	82°
Yield pressure (MPa)	50
Strain rate sensitivity (%)	50
+ Excipient compatibilities	

Formulation

		Quantity (mg)	Quantity (mg)
Active	Drug A	50.0	150.0
Filler	Lactose monohydrate	166.9	–
Filler	Dicalcium phosphate dihydrate	–	165.7
Disintegrant	Croscarmellose sodium	4.8	7.0
Binder	Polyvinylpyrrolidone	4.8	–
Binder	Hydroxypropylmethyl cellulose	–	7.0
Surfactant	Sodium lauryl sulfate	0.7	1.1
Lubricant	Magnesium stearate	2.4	3.5
Tablet weight		230.0	335.0

Predicted properties	Formulation	
	50 mg	150 mg
Tablet diameter (mm)	8.0	10.0
Yield pressure (MPa)	139	238
Strain rate sensitivity (%)	20.8	5.1

(From Ref. 20.)

completed in August 1992 (23). The structure of the system is shown in Fig. 8. It is designed for formulating a parenteral for either clinical or toxicological studies in a variety of species (dog, man, mouse, primate, rabbit, or rat) by a variety of routes of administration (iv, intramuscular, subcutaneous, interperitoneal), supplied in either a single or multidose container. Knowledge was acquired from two domain experts using a series of interviews. The sequence is as follows:

1. The user enters all known data on the solubility (aqueous and nonaqueous), stability in specified solutions, compatibility, pK_a, and molecular properties of the active ingredient (molecular weight, log P, etc.). As with the system for tablet formulation, the data may be numerical or symbolic. All relevant properties of additives used in parenteral formulation (e.g., buffers, antioxidants, chelating agents, antimicrobials, and tonicity adjusters) are present in the knowledge base.
2. The selection first attempts to optimize the solubility/ stability of the active drug at a range of pH using a variety of formulae and algorithms together with specific rules before selecting a buffer to achieve that

pH. If problems still exist with solubility and stability, then formulation variants (e.g., oil-based or emulsion formulations—not implemented in the present system) are recommended.
3. The system then selects additives, depending on the specification required (e.g., an antimicrobial will only be added if a multidose container is specified or a tonicity adjuster will only be added if the solution is hypotonic). The selection strategy is generally on the basis of ranking with some specific rules.
4. The recommended formulation is displayed with all concentrations of the chosen ingredients expressed as percentage weight by volume (w/v) together with the calculated tonicity, proposed storage conditions, and predicted shelf life (Table 8). Specific observations on the sensitivity of the formulation to metals, hydrolysis, light, and oxygen also are included. This is normally printed for inclusion in a laboratory notebook, file, etc. If required, the formulation may be stored in a database for future reference.

As with the system developed for tablet formulations, this system contains extensive "Help" routines. No

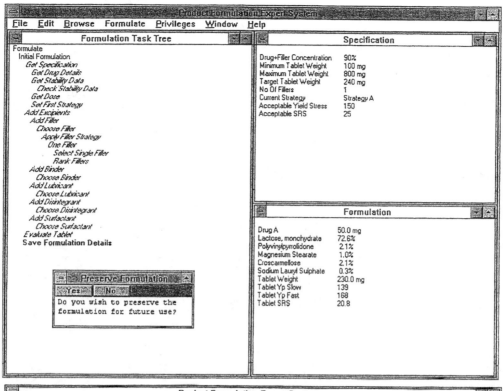

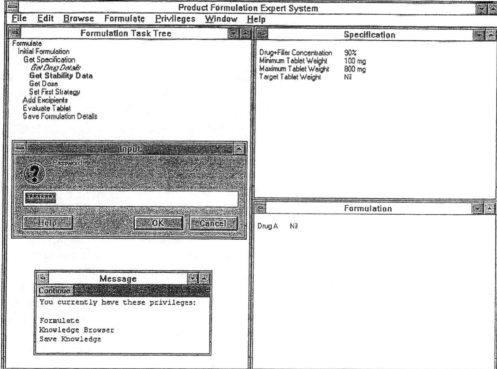

Fig. 7 Screen images for the tablet formulation expert system as described by Rowe (20). (a) Shows user interface with windows for the formulation task tree, specification, formulation, and current task. Tasks are displayed in various formats—current task in highlighted or bold text, completed in italics, and future in standard text. (b) Shows the security of the system. The input of a password displays the user privileges.

Table 8 An example of a formulation of an intravenous injection for clinical trials in man as generated by the system described by Rowe et al.

Drug properties (inputs)		
Drug type		Acid
pK_a		4.5, 3.5
Molecular weight		458.5
Solubility (mg ml^{-1})	pH 3.0	0.5
	pH 4.0	1.5
	pH 5.0	7.0
	pH 7.0	40.0
Sensitivity	Light, metal, oxygen	
Formulation		Quantity (% w/v)
Active	Drug (10 mg/ml)	1.00
Buffer	Disodium hydrogen phosphate anhydrous	0.87
Buffer	Hydrochloric acid	q.s.
Chelating agent	Disodium edetate	0.02
	Water for injection to	100.00
Predicted solution properties		
pH	7.4	
Tonicity	Hypertonic (1.6)	
Storage temperature (°C)	25	
Atmosphere for filling	Nitrogen	
Shelf life (years)	>5	

(From Ref. 23.)

formulation optimization routines are included, although a routine to develop a placebo formulation to match the active formulation is included. The system is used to recommend parenteral formulations for a wide range of investigational drugs.

Work on expert systems in the specific domain of tablet film coating was initiated in April 1990, using a rule induction tool in order to develop a system for the identification and solution of defects in film-coated tablets. Although not strictly a formulation expert system, the developed system did contain knowledge whereby a given formulation known to cause defects could be modified to provide a solution. The completed system described by Rowe and Upjohn (24, 25) is a perfect illustration of fault diagnosis with a rule-based decision tree including both forward and backward chaining. Total development time was approximately 1 man-month using both documented knowledge (26) and expert assistance.

The system (Fig. 9) is divided into three parts: identification, solution, and information/references. In the first part, a question and answer routine is used to ascertain the correct identification of the defect. The decision tree used for this process is shown in Fig. 10.

At this point, the user is asked to confirm the decision by comparing the defect with a picture or photographs stored in the database. In the second part, the user is asked to enter all relevant process conditions and formulation details regarding the best way of solving the defect. This may be a change in the process conditions, as in the case of defects occurring with an already registered formulation, or a change in the formulation, as in the case of defects occurring at the formulation development stage. In the third part, the user is able to access data and knowledge regarding each defect. These are in the form of notes, photographs, and literature references connected by hypertext links.

In 1994, due to the successful implementation of both this system and that used to formulate tablets, it was decided to initiate work on a new system that would recommend film-coating formulations for the generated tablet formulations, combined with a reformulation routine based on the film defect diagnosis system (27). The structure of the new system is shown in Fig. 11. The knowledge for the system was acquired by interviewing two domain experts, one with extensive heuristic knowledge and the other with extensive research knowledge. The sequence is as follows:unital)

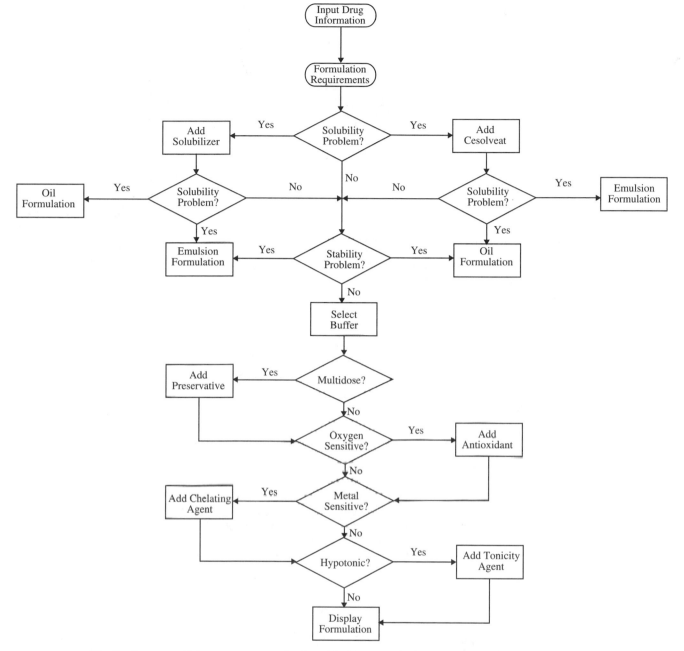

Fig. 8 Structure of the expert system developed by Rowe et al. (23) for the formulation of parenterals.

1. The user enters details of the tablet formulation (e.g.,dose of active ingredient and all excipients) together with all tablet properties (e.g., diameter, thickness, strength, friability, color, shape, and the presence/ absence of intagliations).
2. The user enters specifications for the film coating formulation (i.e., immediate release/controlled release, enterosoluble, white or colored).
3. The system first checks that there are no inconsistencies between the input details and the required specification (e.g., tablets with high friabilities are extremely difficult to film coat). If positive, a warning is displayed.
4. The system calculates the surface area of the tablet and selects the required polymer at the recommended level to form a film of reasonable thickness.

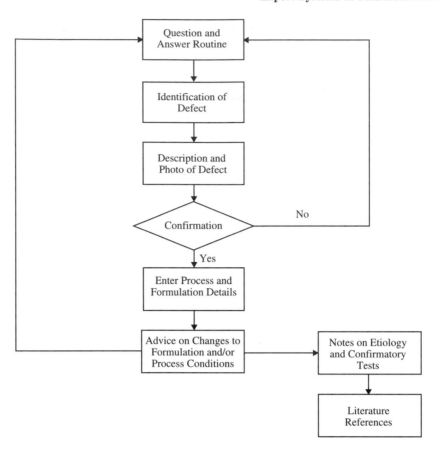

Fig. 9 Structure of the expert system for the identification and solution of film coating defects as described by Rowe and Upjohn (24, 25).

Table 9 An example of a formulation of a white film coating for a tablet of a model drug as generated by the system described by Rowe et al.

Tablet properties (inputs)		
Tablet core formulation	Drug A 50 mg	
Punch shape	Normal concave	
Weight (mg)	230	
Diameter (mm)	8.0	
Thickness (mm)	3.5	
Surface area (cm^2)	1.49	
Formulation	mg/tab	mg/cm^2
Polymer Hydroxypropyl methylcellulose (6 cps)	6.14	4.12
Plasticizer Polyethylene glycol (PEG 400)	1.23	0.82
Pigment Titanium dioxide (Anatase)	5.63	3.78
Predicted film properties		
Thickness (μm)	45	
Opacity (%)	94.9	
Crack velocity (ms^{-1})	5.71	

(From Ref. 27.)

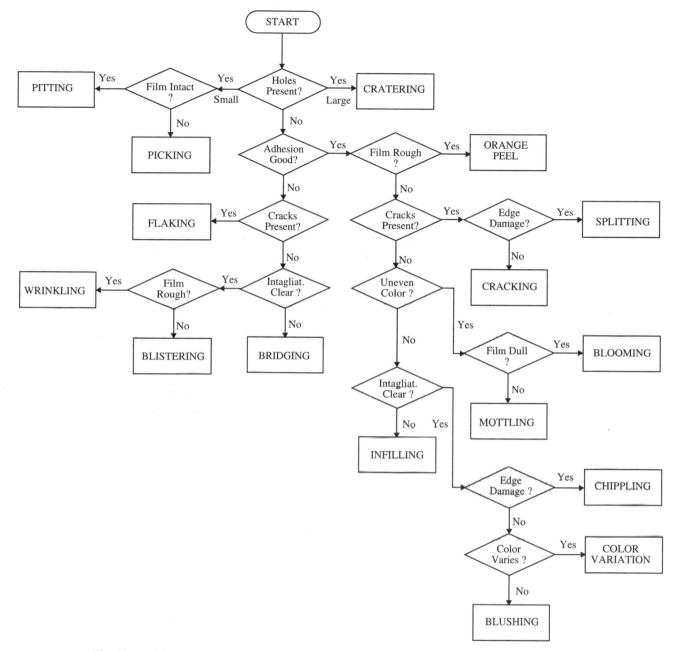

Fig. 10 A decision tree for the identification of film defects on film-coated tablets. (From Ref. 25).

5. The system selects a plasticizer and checks that there are no stability/compatibility problems. If positive, the user is asked to select an alternative plasticizer.

6. The system defines the target opacity of the film coating and decides if an opaque coating is required. The opacity is assessed by means of the contrast ratio defined as the ratio of the reflectance of the film when viewed with a black background to that viewed with a white background (the higher the value the more opaque the film) (28, 29). If positive and the

specification has been set as white, the system uses specifically developed algorithms (30, 31) to calculate if the target specification can be achieved within certain predefined formulation limits of the volume concentration of titanium dioxide and film thickness. If negative, thc user is provided with a series of options to continue with the predefined limits, change the limits, or select a colored film coating.

7. The system selects the pigments to achieve the target specification and determines the amount of water

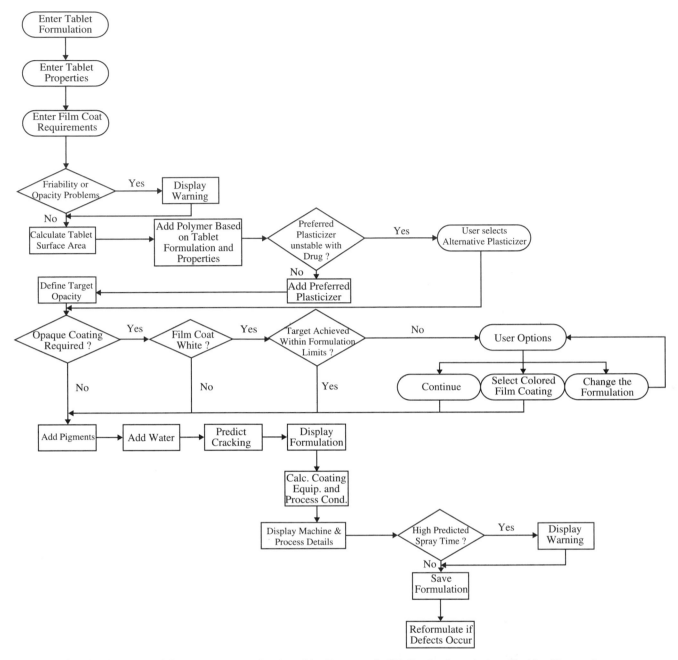

Fig. 11 Structure of the expert system developed by Rowe et al. (27) for the formulation of tablet film coatings.

(the system has been developed for aqueous film coating only).

8. The system accesses a simulation program written in C to predict the cracking propensity of the film formulation (32–34).

9. The recommended formulation is displayed (Table 9) and includes predicted film thickness, opacity, and cracking propensity. Standard machine settings and process details also are displayed with warnings

if the total spray time is judged to be excessive. This is normally printed for inclusion in a laboratory notebook or file. If required and in particular if reformulation is likely to be necessary, the data may be stored in a database for future reference.

10. If a reformulation is necessary due to the presence of defects after coating, then the system uses a modified form of the defect diagnosis system to recommend changes in the formulation and/or process conditions.

This system has proved successful in initial trials, especially in the formulation of opaque films for drugs that are either unstable to light or colored, producing mottled tablets. The calculations concerning the achievement of the target opacity within predefined limits have enabled formulators to make informed decisions regarding the use of white or colored film coatings. The system is now an integral part of the development strategy for film-coated tablets and now has a common database with the tablet formulation system.

BENEFITS

Expert systems have many benefits. These include the following:

1. *Knowledge protection and availability.* The existence of a coherent, durable knowledge base not affected by staff turnover (20). The developers of the University of London/Capsugel system have reported the benefit of being able to use knowledge from experts from many industrial companies in Europe, the United States, and Japan (14, 15). The developers of both the Cadila and the Sanofi systems have reported the benefit of the prompt availability of information and the rapid access to physical chemical data of both drugs and excipients, reducing the time spent searching the literature (9, 19).
2. *Consistency.* All systems generate robust formulations with increased certainty and consistency. This is seen as a distinct benefit where regulatory issues are important.
3. *Training aid.* All systems have been used to provide training for both novice and experienced formulators. The developers of the SOLTAN system have stated that experienced formulators use their expert systems to expose themselves to new raw material combinations with which they are not familiar. Bateman et al. (19) suggested the documentation used in the development of the Sanofi system be adapted to train novice formulators.
4. *Speed of development.* Reduction in the duration of the formulation process has been reported by many (8, 9, 20). Wood (8) reported that formulators who use SOLTAN can produce a formulation in 20 min that might otherwise have taken 2 days. Ramani et al. (9) reported a 35% reduction in the total time needed to develop a new tablet formulation.
5. *Cost savings.* Cost savings can be achieved not only by reducing the development time but also by the more effective use of materials, especially if material cost and controls are included in the system. Ramani et al. (9) reported that use of their system has been a benefit in planning the purchase and stocking of excipients.

The developers of SOLTAN reported that formulations generated by their system are cost effective not only for savings in raw material costs but also because fewer numbers of ingredients are used as compared to traditional formulations. Several users have also reported a decrease in the size of raw material inventories since their expert systems only use those materials specified in the database.

6. *Freeing experts.* The implementation of expert systems in product formulation has inevitably allowed expert formulators to devote more time to innovation (8, 20). The developers of the SOLTAN system reported that the time saved using their expert system typically releases about 30 days of formulating time per year per formulator. Of course, experienced formulators originally involved in training also will have more time to devote to innovation.
7. *Improved communication.* Rowe (20) reported that expert systems in his company have provided a common platform from which to discuss and manage changes in working practice and to identify those critical areas requiring research and/orrationalization. The developers of SOLTAN reported that use of their system has made them scrutinize the way in which they formulated products, highlighting shortfalls from the ideal. They also report that they have discovered previously unknown relationships between ingredients and properties in their products. The benefit of an expert system in promoting discussion also was reported by Bateman et al. (19).

Of all the systems in product formulation, only one has provided costings and undertaken a cost benefit analysis. The developers of SOLTAN estimated the overall cost of their system to be £10,400 for hardware and software, £6000 for consultancy, and £9000 for expert's time, making a total of £25,400. Annual cost savings in the region of £200,000 were reported, delivering a payback of approximately 3 months.

It is interesting to note that where expert systems have been implemented in product formulation, early skepticism among potential users has generally changed to a mood of enthusiastic participation. It is unlikely that expert systems will ever replace expert formulators, but as a decision support tool they are invaluable, delivering many measurable and intangible benefits.

CONCLUSION

Expert systems have been developed by a number of pharmaceutical companies and academic institutes in order to cover the most common formulation types. Only those that have been mentioned in the open literature have been discussed, although it is generally known that SmithKline Beecham, Glaxo Wellcome, Eli Lilly, and Pfizer also have developed systems. It is possible that many more systems exist, but reticence with regard to publication abounds, and it is difficult to estimate exactly the number developed.

ACKNOWLEDGMENTS

This article has been abstracted from *Intelligent Software for Product Formulation* by R.C. Rowe and R.J. Roberts (1998), with permission from Taylor and Francis Ltd., London.

REFERENCES

1. Bold, K. Expertensysteme Unterstutzen Bei der Produkt-formulierung. Chem. Ztg. **1989**, *113* , 343–346.
2. Sell, P.S. *Expert Systems—A Practical Introduction*; Camelot Press: Basingstoke, 1985.
3. Partridge, D.; Hussein, Ch.M. *Knowledge-Based Information Systems*; McGraw Hill: New York, 1994.
4. Turner, J. Manufacturing Intelligence. **1991**, *8* , 12–14.
5. Bentley, P. Product Formulation Expert System. *Intelligent Software for Product Formulation*; Rowe, R.C., Roberts, R.J., Eds.; Taylor and Francis: London, 1998; 27–41.
6. Bradshaw, D. The Computer Learns from the Experts. Financial Times London **April 27th 1989**, *26*.
7. Walko, J.Z. Turning Dalton's Theory into Practice. Innovation **1989**, *18*, 24.
8. Wood, M. Expert Systems Save Formulation Time. Lab-Equipment Digest **Dec. 1991**, *17–19*.
9. Ramani, K.V.; Patel, M.R.; Patel, S.K. An Expert System for Drug Preformulation in a Pharmaceutical Company. Interfaces **1992**, *22* (2), 101–108.
10. Stricker, H.; Haux, R.; Wetter, T.; Mann, G.; Oberhammer, L.; Flister, J.; Fuchs, S.; Schmelmer, V. Das Galenische Entwicklungs-System Heidelberg. Pharm. Ind. **1991**, *53*, 571–578.
11. Stricker, H.; Fuchs, S.; Haux, R.; Rossler, R.; Rupprecht, B.; Schmelmer, V.; Wiegel, S. Das Galenische Entwicklungs-System Heidelberg-Systematische Rezepturentwicklung. Pharm. Ind. **1994**, *56*, 641–647.
12. Frank, J.; Rupprecht, B.; Schmelmer, V. Knowledge-based Assistance for the Development of Drugs. IEEE Expert **1997**, *12* (1), 40–48.
13. Lai, S.; Podczeck, F.; Newton, J.M.; Daumesnil, R. An Expert System for the Development of Powder Filled Hard Gelatin Capsule Formulations. Pharm. Res. **1995**, *12* (9), S150.
14. Lai, S.; Podczeck, F.; Newton, J.M.; Daumesnil, R. An Expert System to Aid the Development of Capsule Formulations. Tech. Eur. **1996**, *8* (9), 60–68.
15. Newton, J.M.; Podczeck, F.; Lai, S.; Daumesnil, R. The Design of an Expert System to Aid the Development of Capsule Formulations. *Formulation Design of Oral Dosage Forms*; Hashida, M. Ed.; Yakugyo-Jiho: 1998, 236–244.
16. Carr, R. Evaluating Flow Properties of Solids. Chem. Engineer **1965**, *18*, 163–168.
17. Ludde, K.H.; Kawakita, D. Die Pulverkompression. Pharmazie **1996**, *21*, 393–403.
18. Kashihara, T.; Yoshioka, M. Assessment in Japanese Focus Group. *Formulation Design of Oral Dosage Forms*; Hashida, M., Ed.; Yakugyo-Jiho: 1998; 244–253.
19. Bateman, S.D.; Verlin, J.; Russo, M.; Guillot, M.; Laughlin, S.M. The Development and Validation of a Capsule Formulation Knowledge-Based System. Pharm. Technol. **1996**, *20* (3), 174–184.
20. Rowe, R.C. An Expert System for the Formulation of Pharmaceutical Tablets. Manufacturing Intelligence **1993**, *14*, 13–15.
21. Rowe, R.C. Expert Systems in Solid Dosage Development. Pharm. Ind. **1993**, *55* , 1040–1045.
22. Rowe, R.C.; Roberts, R.J. The Mechanical Properties of Powders. *Advances in Pharmaceutical Sciences*; Ganderton, D., Jones, T., McGinity, J., Eds.; Academic Press: New York, 1995; 7, 1–62.
23. Rowe, R.C.; Wakerly, M.G.; Roberts, R.J.; Grundy, R.U.; Upjohn, N.G. Expert System for Parenteral Development. J. Pharm. Sci. Technol. **1995**, *49*, 257–261.
24. Rowe, R.C.; Upjohn, N.G. An Expert System for Identifying and Solving Defects on Film-Coated Tablets. Manufacturing Intelligence **1992**, *12*, 12–13.
25. Rowe, R.C.; Upjohn, N.G. An Expert System for The Identification and Solution of Film Coating Defects. Pharm. Tech. Int. **1993**, *5* (3), 34–38.
26. Rowe, R.C. Defects in Film Coated Tablets—Aetiology and Solution. *Advances in Pharmaceutical Sciences*; Ganderton, D., Jones, T., Eds.; Academic Press: New York, 1992; 6, 65–100.
27. Rowe, R.C.; Hall, J.; Roberts, R.J. Film Coating Formulation Using an Expert System. Pharm. Tech. Eur. **1998**, *10* (10), 72–82.
28. Rowe, R.C. The Opacity of Tablet Film Coatings. J. Pharm. Pharmac. **1984**, *36*, 569–572.
29. Rowe, R.C. Quantitative Opacity Measurements on Tablet Film Coatings Containing Titanium Dioxide. Int. J. Pharm. **1984**, *22*, 17–23.
30. Rowe, R.C. Knowledge Representation in the Prediction of the Opacity of Tablet Film Coatings Containing Titanium Dioxide. Eur. J. Pharm. Biopharm. **1995**, *41*, 215–218.
31. Rowe, R.C. Predicting Film Thickness on Film Coated Tablets. Int. J. Pharm. **1996**, *133*, 253–256.
32. Rowe, R.C.; Roberts, R.J. Simulation of Crack Propagation in Tablet Film Coatings Containing Pigments. Int. J. Pharm. **1992**, *78*, 49–57.
33. Rowe, R.C.; Roberts, R.J. The Effect of Some Formulation Variables on Crack Propagation in Pigmented Tablet Film Coatings Using Computer Simulation. Int. J. Pharm. **1992**, *86*, 49–58.
34. Rowe, R.C.; Rowe, M.D.; Roberts, R.J. Formulating Film Coatings with the Aid of Computer Simulations. Pharm. Technol. **1994**, *18* (10), 132–139.

EXPIRATION DATING

Leslie C. Hawley
Mark D. VanArendonk

Pharmacia Corporation, Kalamazoo, Michigan

INTRODUCTION

Expiration dating of pharmaceuticals corresponds to the determination of a retest period for drug substances and an expiration dating period or shelf-life for drug products. The shelf-life, or expiration dating period, of a drug product is defined as the time interval that a drug product is expected to remain within an approved shelf-life specification, provided that it is stored according to label storage conditions and that it is in the original container closure system. The Expiry/Expiration Date is the actual date placed on the container/labels of a drug product designating the time during which a batch of the drug product is expected to remain within the approved shelf-life specification if stored under defined conditions and after which it must not be used. To arrive at an expiration date, it must be determined first for how long and under what conditions a pharmaceutical formulation can meet all of its quality specifications. In general, this issue is answered through stability testing that monitors chemical and physical product attributes as a function of time, temperature, and other environmental factors. It is not the intent of this article to discuss the mechanics of starting a testing program or to provide an exhaustive discussion of all the testing requirements necessary to establish an expiration dating period. Rather, this discussion focuses on changes in worldwide regulatory requirements pertaining to expiration dating since the last edition of this publication (1), the statistical treatment of stability data to determine a shelf-life for a given drug product, the impact of postapproval changes on the expiration date of a drug product, and finally, a discussion of unresolved issues in expiration dating.

REGULATORY CONSIDERATIONS

Before 1990 there was no official harmonization of stability testing requirements for countries throughout the world. In the United States, the major reference documents outlining regulations or guidelines pertaining to expiration dating at that time were the Code of Federal Regulations (CFR) (2), the *United States Pharmacopeia* (USP) (3), and the 1987 FDA Guideline for Submitting Documentation for the Stability of Human Drug and Biologics (4). In Europe there was the European Community Guide to Good Manufacturing Practices for Medicinal Products (5), which contained minimal information pertaining to expiration dating. More extensive European guidelines at that time were found in the Note for Guidance, Stability Tests on Active Substances and Finished Products (6). In Japan, the primary reference for the determination of expiration intervals for the approval of a drug product was given in a guideline entitled, at that time, Draft Policy to Handle Stability Data Required in Applying for Approval to Manufacture (Import) Drugs (7) and Draft Guidelines on Methods to Perform Stability Test (8). Very little information pertaining to expiration dating was available for Zone III/IV countries. There were many similarities among the requirements for each of the regions of the world, but there were also many differences. Because the stability testing requirements for many countries and also the regulations pertaining to expiration dating periods were different, a systematic approach to establishing stability protocols adequate for worldwide registration and harmonization of expiration dates in the different regions of the world was virtually impossible.

Since 1990, significant gains in the harmonization of technical requirements for registration of pharmaceuticals for human use were achieved with the inception of the International Conference on Harmonization (ICH). The ICH convened for the first time in 1990, and the first draft of the ICH Tripartite Guideline on Stability Testing of New Drug Substances and Products was issued on March 23, 1992. In that Guidline, the stability testing requirements for the United States, European Union, and Japan are defined. Approved ICH guidances include (9):

Q1A   Stability Testing of New Drug Substances and Products
Q1B   Photostability Testing of New Drug Substances and Products

Q1C   Stability Testing for New Dosage Forms

Q5C   Stability Testing of Biotechnological Biological
       Products

Additional DRAFT ICH guidances currently in the early review stages are:

Q1D   Reduced Designs for Stability Testing of
       Medicinal Products
Q1E   Statistical Analysis and Data Evaluation

In addition, both European and U.S. regulators have published regional guidances that complement or supplement the ICH guidances regarding the stability requirements for establishing the expiration dating of pharmaceutical products. Harmonization of stability testing requirements for Climate Zone III/IV countries has also begun (10). Below, the stability testing requirements and regulations pertaining to expiration dating are broken down by major geographical regions.

United States

The current U.S. requirements pertaining to expiration dating and the stability testing necessary to establish expiration dates of pharmaceutical products are covered in the USP (11), The Code of Federal Regulations, the ICH guidances mentioned previously, and the Draft FDA Guidance for the Industry (12). The three relevant sections of the CFR cover: 1) where expiration dates must appear on a product (§201.17); 2) what products are required or exempted from having an expiration date (§211.137); and 3) requirements for stability tests and the testing program (§211.166). Because the pertinent sections of the CFR for human pharmaceuticals are brief, they are presented later in this article. The USP covers the same general information as the CFR. The FDA Draft Guidance for the Industry titled, Stability Testing of Drug Substances and Drug Products (12) has replaced the original guidance entitled, Guideline for Submitting Documentation for the Stability of Human Drugs and Biologics, published in February 1987. The guidance is intended to be a comprehensive document that provides information on all aspects of stability data generation and use. It references and incorporates substantial text from ICH Q1A, Q1C, Q1B, and Q5C. The guidance provides recommendations regarding the design, conduct, and use of stability studies necessary to establish expiration dates and to support various regulatory applications.

§201.17 DRUGS: LOCATION OF EXPIRATION DATE

When an expiration date of a drug is required, e.g., expiration dating of drug products required by §211.137 (see the next section) of this article, it shall appear on the immediate container and also the outer package, if any, unless it is easily legible through such outer package. However, when single-dose containers are packed in individual cartons, the expiration date may properly appear on the individual carton instead of on the immediate product container (43 FR 45076, Sept. 29, 1978).

§211.137 EXPIRATION DATING

1. To assure that a drug product meets applicable standards of identity, strength, quality, and purity at the time of use, it shall bear an expiration date determined by appropriate stability testing described in §211.166.
2. Expiration dates shall be related to any storage conditions stated on the labeling, as determined by stability studies described in §211.166.
3. If the drug product is to be reconstituted at the time of dispensing, its labeling shall bear expiration information for both the reconstituted and unreconstituted drug products.
4. Expiration dates shall appear on labeling in accordance with the requirements of §201.17 of this article.
5. Homeopathic drug products shall be exempt from the requirements of this section.
6. Allergenic extracts that are labeled "No U.S. Standard of Potency" are exempt from the requirements of this section.
7. New drug products for investigational use are exempt from the requirements of this section, provided they meet appropriate standards or specifications as demonstrated by stability studies during their use in clinical investigations. When new drug products for investigational use are to be reconstituted at the time of dispensing, their labeling shall bear expiration information for the reconstituted drug product.
8. Pending consideration of a proposed exemption, published in the Federal Register, September 29, 1978, the requirements in this section shall not be enforced for human over the counter (OTC) drug products if their labeling does not bear dosage limitations and if they are stable for at least 3 years as supported by appropriate stability data (43 FR 45077,

Sept. 29, 1978, as amended at 46 FR 56412, Nov. 17, 1981; 60 FR 4091, Jan. 20, 1995).

§211.166 STABILITY TESTING

1. There shall be a written testing program designed to assess the stability characteristics of drug products. The results of such stability testing shall be used in determining appropriate storage conditions and expiration dates. The written program shall be followed and shall include:

   - Sample size and test intervals based on statistical criteria for each attribute examined to assure valid estimates of stability
   - Storage conditions for samples retained for testing
   - Reliable, meaningful, and specific test methods
   - Testing of the drug product in the same container-closure system as that in which the drug product is marketed
   - Testing of drug products for reconstitution at the time of dispensing (as directed in the labeling), as well as after they are reconstituted.

2. An adequate number of batches of each drug product shall be tested to determine an appropriate expiration date and a record of such data shall be maintained. Accelerated studies, combined with basic stability information on the components, drug products, and container-closure system, may be used to support tentative expiration dates, provided full shelf-life studies are not available and are being conducted. Where data from accelerated studies are used to project a tentative expiration date that is beyond a date supported by actual shelf-life studies, there must be stability studies conducted, including drug product testing at appropriate intervals, until the tentative expiration date is verified or the appropriate expiration date determined.

3. For homeopathic drug-products, the requirements of this section are as follows:

   - There shall be a written assessment of stability, based at least on testing or examination of the drug product for compatibility of the ingredients and based on marketing experience with the drug product to indicate that there is no degradation of the product for the normal or expected period of use.
   - Evaluation of stability shall be based on the same container-closure system in which the drug-product is being marketed.

4. Allergenic extracts that are labeled "No U.S. Standard of Potency" are exempt from the requirements of this section (43 FR 45077, Sept. 29, 1978, as amended at 46 FR 56412, Nov. 17, 1981).

EUROPEAN UNION

In addition to the ICH, the Committee for Proprietary Medicinal Products, under the European Agency for the Evaluation of Medicinal Products (EMEA) (13), issued, in 1997 and 1998, a number of stability-related guidances to be used for establishing stability testing protocols for drug products to be filed in European countries. The documents complement and supplement the ICH guidelines and are listed below:

1. Reduced Stability Testing Plan-Bracketing and Matrixing: Annex to Note for Guidance on Stability Testing of New Drug Substances and Products (14)—CPMP/QWP/157/96
2. Note for Guidance on Maximum Shelf-Life for Sterile Products for Human Use After First Opening or Following Reconstitution (16)—CPMP/QWP/159/96
3. Note for Guidance on Declaration of Storage Conditions for Medicinal Products in the Products Particulars (17)—CPMP/QWP/609/96
4. Note for Guidance on Stability Testing of Existing Active Substances and Related Finished Products (18)—CMPM/QWP/556/96
5. Note for Guidance on Stability Testing for Type II Variation to a Marketing Authorization (19)—CPMP/QWP/576/96
6. Note for Guidance for In-Use Stability Testing of Human Medicinal Products—Annex to Note for Guidance on Stability Testing of Existing Active Substances and Related Finished Products and Note for Guidance on Stability Testing of Existing Active Substances and Related Finished Products—CPMP/QWP/2934/99

Japan

In addition to ICH guidelines, the specific Japanese stability testing requirements for establishing expiration dating are described in the regional guidelines. In particular, the Japanese Ministry of Health and Welfare (MHW) has issued a guidance entitled, *Handling of Data on Stability Testing Attached to Applications for Approval to Manufacture or Import Drugs* (22). For the most part, the MHW guidance complements the ICH guidelines. The MHW guidance provides more detailed requirements for "stress" testing than that found in the ICH and the guidances for stability testing used in United States or European Union (see above). In fact, specific stress testing conditions and testing duration and frequency are provided. In contrast, European Union and the U.S. regional guidances do not recommend specific testing conditions and schedules and specify that stress testing is usually accomplished during routine formulation and analytical methods development. This discrepancy between the regional requirements in Japan versus those in European Union and the United States is a notable opportunity for harmonization.

Climate Zone III/IV Countries

Currently countries in climate Zones III and IV are not member countries of the ICH, although it has been recommended by Grimm (14) that the ICH Tripartite Guideline be extended to include Zone III/IV countries. Needless to say, great strides in the harmonization of stability testing requirements and expiration dating for climatie Zone III and IV countries has begun. The definitive source on stability testing requirements can be found in a set of guidelines published by the World Health Organization, entitled, Guidelines for Stability Testing of Pharmaceutical Products Containing Well-Established Drug Substances in Conventional Dosage Forms (15). This document outlines the conditions and testing required for Zone III and IV countries. Also contained in that document are a list of recommended storage conditions to be prominently indicated on the label of pharmaceutical products distributed in climatie Zone III and IV countries. Another set of guidelines relevant to stability testing in climatie Zone III and IV is a document issued by MERCOSUL ("Mercado Comun del Sur" or "Common Market of the South"), entitled Pharmaceutical Products Stability (10). The MERCO-SUL document was specifically intended for use as a guidance for designing stability testing programs by countries that are members of MERCUSOL, Argentina, Paraguay, Uruguay, and Brazil. The stability testing requirements described in the MERCOSUL guidelines essentially match the conditions and testing requirements in the WHO document. The stability testing requirements for Zone III and IV, for which the WHO guidelines are considered the definitive requirements, are just now being implemented throughout the industry to support marketing of pharmaceutical products in climatie Zone III and IV countries.

STATISTICAL DETERMINATION OF SHELF-LIFE FROM LONG-TERM STORAGE DATA

The current approach to analyzing stability data to predict shelf-life involves statistical analysis of long-term storage data. The accelerated data are generally used as supportive data. In particular, it is recommended in ICH Q1A, CPMP QWP/556/96, and the FDA Draft Guidance that a shelf-life of a drug product be determined by the point at which the 95% one-sided confidence limit for the mean degradation curve intersects the acceptable lower specification limit. Typically, statistical analysis to determine shelf-life is applied to at least 12 months of long-term storage data on three production scale batches of drug product. Data from individual batches are first treated by least-squares fitting. The true line representing degradation behavior is not known a priori, but it is estimated by least-squares analysis. The confidence interval about the least-squares line from fitting the stability data is also obtained. As noted above, it is the intercept between the line representing the confidence limit and the upper or lower registration limit that yields the expiration period. If the application of appropriate statistical tests to the slopes and zero time intercepts of the regression lines for the individual batches indicate that the batch-to-batch variability is small (e.g., p values for level of significance of rejection of more than 0.25), and therefore, the data pool, it is advantageous to then combine all the data into one overall estimate for shelf-life. If it is inappropriate to combine data from several batches, the overall expiration dating period is determined by the minimum time a batch may be expected to remain within acceptable and justified limits (9, 12). Detailed information about the statistical evaluation of long-term stability data using regression analysis, tests for batch similarity, and data pooling is described in Carstensen (16), Wessels (17), Lin (18), Bancroft (19), and the FDA guidance (12).

Software packages that handle the statistical evaluation of stability data per the ICH or FDA guidelines are sold commercially. Also, the FDA has developed and makes available its own drug formulation stability test program, STAB, which can be downloaded from the FDA website (20). This statistical approach to calculating the expiry dating period from long-term data applies to new drug substances and their products (9, 12) as wellas products containing established unstable substances (15).

Often the expiration dating period determined by the statistical analysis described above results in extrapolation of the regression lines to times for which there are no stability data available. For extrapolation beyond the observed range to be valid, the assumed degradation relationship must continue to apply through the estimated expiration dating period. As stated in the FDA *Draft Guidance on Stability Testing* (13), an expiration dating period assigned in this manner should always be justified and supported by accelerated test data and is considered tentative until confirmed through full long-term stability data from at least three production batches reported through annual reports. For known stable products, a more flexible approach is taken. According to the WHO guideline (15), one may directly assign a 24-month shelf-life to a product provided that the active ingredient is stable i.e., stability studies have been performed per tabulated accelerated test conditions for Zones II and IV with no significant changes; supporting data indicate that similar formulations have been assigned a shelf-life of 24 months or more; and the manufacturer continues to perform real-time studies until the proposed shelf-life has elapsed. For products (simple dosage forms) covered under ANDAs, the FDA also permits a direct assignment of a shelf-life as long as 24 months at labeled storage conditions if the accelerated stability data at 0, 1, 2, and 3 months and available long-term stability data are satisfactory (12). CPMP guideline QWP/556/96, however, does not follow this approach, and suggests a statistical analysis of real-time data for the determination of shelf-life, even for existing drug substances and products (13).

How the actual expiration date is calculated from the expiration dating period determined from the statistical analysis described above is also of importance. The FDA draft guidance and CPMP/QWP/486/95 both state that the computation of expiration period of the drug product should begin no later than the time of release of the batch (12, 13). The date of release generally should not exceed 30 days from the production date regardless of packaging date (12). If the release date of the lot fails the 30-day test, a different standard applies in fixing the expiration period. In such cases, the expiration date is calculated from within 30 days of the manufacture of the lot, rather than from the release date (12, 13, 21). If the expiration date includes only a month and year, the product should meet specifications through the last-day-of-that-month guidance (21). The data generated in support of the assigned expiration dating period should be from long-term studies under the storage conditions recommended in the labeling (12).

Arrhenius analysis, described below, of multitemperature data cannot be used alone to set a definitive shelf-life at a different temperature than that for which long-term data are available. This is primarily because discrepancies in degradation mechanisms at different temperatures makes the Arrhenius law invalid for prediction of a definitive shelf-life from accelerated data. Although Arrhenius analysis is not used as a primary method for proposing a tentative expiration dating period based on accelerated data, application of this analysis to accelerated data can be used as supportive data in conjunction with extrapolation of long-term data. As described below, Arrhenius analysis can be used to anticipate the impact of storage condition or climate zone on the expiration dating interval.

IMPACT OF STORAGE CONDITION OR CLIMATIC ZONE ON EXPIRATION DATING INTERVAL

Arrhenius analysis of a given degradation process yields a relationship between temperature and rate constant. The results of such an analysis can be useful in predicting the impact of changes in storage conditions or climatie zone on expiration dating interval of a given drug-product. In particular, Arrhenuis analysis can be used to predict the relationship between the expiration dating period and the label storage conditions. In practice a given formulation and container/–closure system may have different expiration periods assigned to them, depending on where, i.e., in which "climate zone," they are being marketed. The Arrhenius relationship between temperature and rate constant is derived below.

For zero-order processes, by which many chemical reactions can be modeled, the rate of disappearance of the reactant A is constant and independent of its concentration, as shown in Eq. 1:

$$-dA/dt = k \tag{1}$$

Solving Eq. 1 yields Eq 2:

$$A = A_o - kt \tag{2}$$

where,

A = the amount of A remaining at time t,
A_o = the initial amount of A, and
k = rate constant.

For reactions following zero-order kinetics, a plot of A versus t yields a straight line whose slope is equal to $-k$.

For first-order processes, the rate of disappearance of the reactant A is proportional to the concentration of A at any time t, as shown Eq. 3.

$$-dA/dt = kA \qquad (3)$$

The solution of the Eq. 3 yields Eq. 4:

$$\ln A/A_o = -kt \qquad (4)$$

or

$$lnA = -kt + lnA_o$$

For stability data that follows first-order kinetics, a plot of lnA versus t will yield a straight line whose slope is k. The rate constant k, in almost all cases, is a function of the temperature T. For most pharmaceutical products, as T is increased, the rate constant and, therefore, the rate of degradation increases. This is the basis for the well known Arrhenius relationship that states that for a given chemical reaction, the empirical relationship between k and T may be described as in Eq. 5:

$$k = b_o e^{-E/RT} \qquad (5)$$

or

$$\ln k = \ln b_o - E/RT$$

where,

$T =$ Kelvin temperature,
$E =$ activation energy,
$R =$ ideal gas constant, and
$b_o =$ constant depending on the molecule of interest.

If a particular kinetic process follows Arrhenius' Law, then a plot of lnk versus $1/T$ will yield a straight line with a slope of E/R.

A good example of the application of Arrhenius analysis is a pharmaceutical product whose shelf-life is limited by degradation of the active ingredient A. Using stability-indicating assays, the loss of A with time at 25°C has been shown to follow zero-order kinetics between 100 and 90% of the labeled amount. In addition, data from accelerated studies at 40, 50, and 60°C show the same zero-order behavior. If the rate constants from the 25, 40, 50, and 60°C experiments follow Arrhenius' Eq. 5, then from the straight line plot of lnk vs. $1/T$ for component A in this matrix, the rate constant at any temperature in the data range may be obtained by interpolation. Thus, knowing k for any temperature and the time to be spent at that temperature, the stability performance may be calculated by Eq. 2. In other words, Arrhenius analysis can be used to predict

an expiration date at any temperature owing to storage or climatie zone under which the Arrhenius behavior is valid. Although useful for obtaining an understanding of the impact of temperature changes on expiration dating, Arrhenius analysis breaks down when the degradation mechanisms occurring at one temperature are different from the degradation mechanisms occurring at other temperatures.

Grimm has used the Arrhenius relationship to determine "predictive factors" that can be used to predict the shelf-life at long-term storage in various climate zones from accelerated data (14). For example, the degradation rate at 40°C can be determined by multiplying the time it takes the drug to degrade by 5% at 25 or 30°C by "predictive factors" for those temperatures. Using an activation energy of 83 kJmole^{-1} Grimm derives predictive factors of 5 and 3.3 for 25 and 30°C, respectively. Obviously, the use of "predictive factors" is only an approximation and breaks down when Arrhenius behavior at different temperatures is not followed.

Impact of Post-Approval Changes on Expiration Dating Period

Often, after a pharmaceutical drug product and its associated dating period and storage condition have been approved, there is a desire to change some aspect of the product (e.g., production process, formulation, packaging, etc.). When a postapproval change occurs, the expiration dating period approved for the original product must be justified for the product after the postapproval change. To justify an expiration date after a postapproval change has been made, various amounts of new or different stability testing are required. Since the last edition of this article, there has been significant activity in the development of new regulations and refinement of existing regulations corresponding to stability testing required for postapproval changes.

The *ICH Topic Q1C; Stability Testing: Requirements for New Dosage Forms* is an annex to the parent ICH guidance (issued 5/1997) Q1A and addresses the recommendations for the data that should be submitted regarding stability of new dosage forms by the owner of the original application after the original submission for new active substances and medicinal products. In the United States, the FDA has issued *Scale-Up and Post-Approval Changes* (SUPAC) guidelines that dictate the stability testing requirements for various postapproval changes for U.S. filings. The available SUPAC guidances are listed below (23):

1. SUPAC-IR: Immediate-Release Solid Oral Dosage Forms: Scale-Up and Post-Approval Changes: Chemistry, Manufacturing and Controls, In Vitro Dissolution Testing, and In Vivo Bioequivalence Documentation (Manufacturing Equipment Addendum Issued 1/1999).
2. SUPAC-MR: Modified Release Solid Oral Dosage Forms Scale-Up and Postapproval Changes: Chemistry, Manufacturing and Controls: In Vitro Dissolution Testing and In Vivo Bioequivalence Documentation (Issued 10/6/97, Manufacturing Equipment Addendum Issued 1/1999).
3. SUPAC-SS: Nonsterile Semisolid Dosage Forms; Scale-Up and Post-Approval Changes: Chemistry, Manufacturing and Controls; In Vitro Release Testing and In Vivo Bioequievalence Documentation (Issued 5/1997; Posted 6/16/1997, Addendum Issued 12/1998).

In Europe, two regulations have been introduced to address "variations" to medicinal products, Regulation (EEC) No. 541/95 and 542/95. For the implementation of the procedures set out by these regulations, a number of guidances have been prepared and an application form for a variation to a marketing authorization has been issued.

In the United States, the approach for determination of stability testing required for a given change follows a tiered approach, with more additional stability data obviously being required for more significant postapproval changes (SUPAC reference). Table 1, reproduced from the FDA Guidance on Stability Testing, describes the five stability data package types required to support a postapproval change.

For each type of postapproval change, the above table is used to help determine what type of Stability Data Package should be filed. A discussion of the type of Stability Data Package necessary for different changes is found in the FDA Draft Guidance for Stability Testing (12) and dosage form-specific information is available in the SUPAC guidances listed above. For certain changes no prior approval is needed, and a Changes-Being-Effected supplement can be filed. This is not the case in Europe, where all postapproval changes require an amendment to be approved before marketing medicinal product manufactured with post-approval change.

EXTENSIONS OR REDUCTIONS IN EXPIRATION DATING

Often after extensive stability data have been collected, there is a desire to change the expiration dating of a product. In particular, the available stability data support either an extension or a reduction in the expiration date approved in the original filing. Changes in expiration dating is covered in the FDA guidance.

For example, the methods for obtaining an extension is outlined in the FDA guidance (12):

Table 1 Stability data package types to support a postapproval change

Stability data package	Stability data at time of submission	Stability commitment
Type 0	None	None beyond the regular annual batches
Type 1	None	First (1) production batch and annual batches thereafter on long-term stability studies
Type 2	Three months of comparative accelerated data and available long-term data on 1 batch[a] of drug product with the proposed change	First (1) production batch[b] and annual batches thereafter on long-term stability studies[c]
Type 3	Three months of comparative accelerated data and available long-term data on 1 batch[a] of drug product with the proposed change	First (3) production batch[b] and annual batches thereafter on long-term stability studies[c]
Type 4	Three months of comparative accelerated data and available long-term data on 3 batches[a] of drug product with the proposed change	First 3 production batch[b] and annual batches thereafter on long-term stability studies[c]

[a]Pilot scale batches acceptable.
[b]If not submitted in the supplement.
[c]Using the approved stability protocol and reporting data in annual reports.

1. Can be described in an annual report if criteria set forth in the approved protocol are met. In this case, the extension of the expiration dating period must be based on full long-term stability data obtained from at least three production batches (21 CFR 314.70).
2. A prior approval supplement is necessary to extend a tentative expiration date based on three pilot-scale batches. The expiration dating remains tentative until confirmed with full long-term data from at least three production batches.

The methods for shortening an expiration date is through a Changes-Being Effected supplement (21 CFR 314.70 or 21 CFR 601.12).

UNRESOLVED ISSUES FOR THE NEW MILLENNIUM

Two major issues still require attention: first, complete harmonization of stability testing requirements throughout the world remains to be achieved. In particular, benefits could be obtained by harmonizing the "stress" testing requirements for different ICH member countries, complete harmonization of stability testing requirements for all Zone III/IV countries, and more extensive harmonization of stability testing conditions between Zone III/IV countries, where 30C/70%RH is the long-term storage condition for stability studies, and ICH member countries, where 30C/60%RH is the intermediate storage condition. The second unresolved issue is worldwide harmonization of label storage statements. Because the ultimate objective of a stability study is to predict a product's shelf-life at a particular label storage condition, it makes sense that label storage statements be harmonized much the way stability testing requirements have been harmonized. Unfortunately, this is not the case. Q1A suggests that labeling be based on each country's requirements. These requirements are different for most countries. For example, label statements in the United States satisfy the USP, whereas in Europe, no labeling is required. In Japan, labeling is necessary only if the product's stability is less than 3 years. In the WHO guidance, labeling is also defined by the requirements of the country. As can be seen, harmonization of label storage statements still needs to be accomplished. More thorough harmonization of stability testing requirements throughout the world and worldwide harmonization of label storage statements is highly desirable to streamline stability testing programs designed to support a global marketplace.

CONCLUSIONS

Worldwide harmonization of stability testing requirements has made significant progress, but it is still not complete (e.g., labeling requirements are country-specific). In the last decade, the ICH guidances and complementary regional guidelines have significantly enhanced the level of harmonization of stability testing requirements for Europe, Japan, and the United States. The WHO guideline for stability testing of pharmaceutical products containing well established drug substances in conventional dosage forms and the MERCOSUR guidance have begun to accomplish harmonization of stability testing requirements in Zone III/IV. There is still a considerable amount of harmonization to be achieved in Zone III/IV countries. As Zone III/IV countries continue to harmonize, it will be interesting to see whether a new intermediate condition is adopted by the ICH that replaces 30C/60%RH, which would allow worldwide harmonization of testing requirements to support determination of expiration dating periods for each of the four climate zones of the world.

REFERENCES

1. VanArendonk, M.; Dukes, G.R. Expiration Dating. *Encyclopedia of Pharmaceutical Technology*; Swarbrick, J., Boylan, J.C., Eds.; Marcel Dekker, Inc.: New York, 1995; 5, 379–394.
2. Federal Register 601. January 15, 1971.
3. U.S. Pharmacopeia XXII. *National Formulary XVII*; U.S. Pharm. Convention, Inc.: Rockville, MD, 1990; 10.
4. Guideline for Submitting Documentation for the Stability of Human Drugs and Biologics, U.S. Department of Health and Human Services, Food and Drug Administration, Center for Drugs and Biologics, Washington, DC, 1987.
5. Guide to Good Manufacturing Practices for Medicinal Products. The Rules Governing Medicinal Products in the European Community, Vol. IV. Luxembourg: Office for Official Publications of the European Communities: Luxembourg, 1989.
6. Stability Tests on Active Substances and Finished Products, Notes for Guidance Concerning the Application of Section F of Part I of the Annex to Directive 75/318/EEC. III/66/87-EN, Rev. 4, Brussels, 1988, 7.
7. Notification No. 698, Pharmaceutical Affairs Bureau, Japanese Ministry of Health and Welfare, Tokyo, 1980.
8. Draft Policy to Handle Stability Data Required in Applying for Approval to Manufacture (Import) Drugs and Draft Guidelines on Methods to Perform Stability Test, Ministry of Health and Welfare: The First Evaluation and

Registration Division, Pharmaceutical Affairs Bureau, 1990.

9. http://www.ifpma.org/ich5q.html#stability (accessed April 2000).

10. MERCSUL/GMC/P.RES No. 53/96.

11. U.S. Pharmacopeia XXIV. *National Formulary XIX*; U.S. Pharm. Convention, Inc.: Rockville, MD, 2000.

12. http://www.fda.gov/cder/guidance/1707dft.pdf (accessed April 2000).

13. http://www.eudra.org/emea.html (accessed April 2000).

14. Grimm, W. Extensions of the International Conference on Harmonization Tripartite Guideline for Stability Testing of New Drug Substances and Products to Countries of Climatic Zones III and IV. Drug Dev. Ind. Pharm. **1998**, *24*, 313–325.

15. WHO Technical Report Series 863, World Health Organization Geneva, Switzerland, 1996

16. Carstensen, J.T.; Nelson, E.W. J. Pharm. Sci. **1976**, *65*, 311.

17. Wessels, P., et al. Statistical Evaluation of Stability Data for Pharmaceutical Products for Specification Setting. Drug Dev. Ind. Pharm. **1997**, *23*, 427–439.

18. Lin, K.K.; Lin, T-Y.D.; Kelley, R.E. Stability of Drugs: Room Temperature Tests. *Statistics in the Pharmaceutical Industry*; Buncher, C.R., Tsay, J.-Y., Eds.; Marcel Dekker, Inc.: New York, 1994; 419–444.

19. Bancroft, T.A. Analysis and Inference for Incompletely Specified Models Involving the Use of Preliminary Test(s) of Significance. Biometrics **1964**, *20* (3), 427–442.

20. http://www.fda.gov (accessed April 2000).

21. Washington Drug Letter, No. 36. 1999, *31*.

22. Handling of Data on Stability Testing Attached to Applications for Approval to Manufacture of Import Drugs, Notification No. 413; Pharmaceutical Affairs Bureau, Japanese Ministry of Health and Welfare, Tokyo, 1992.

23. http://www.fda.gov/guidance/1721fnl.pdf (accessed April 2000).

EXTRUSION AND EXTRUDERS

J.M. Newton

University of London, London, United Kingdom

INTRODUCTION

Extrusion is the process of forming a raw material into a product of uniform shape and density by forcing it through an orifice or die under controlled conditions. An extruder consists of two distinct parts: a delivery system which transports the material and sometimes imparts a degree of distributive mixing, and a die system which forms the material into the required shape. Extrusion may be broadly classified into molten systems under temperature control or semisolid viscous systems. In molten extrusion, heat is applied to the material in order to control its viscosity to enable it to flow through the die. Semisolid systems are multiphase concentrated dispersions containing a high proportion of solids mixed with a liquid phase. Extrusion is achieved by formulation to control the viscosity of the semisolid mass.

Extrusion is a continuous process that affords a consistent product at high throughput rates. The process has diverse applications in a range of industries utilizing extrusion equipment specifically designed or adapted to form a particular product. A description of the different types of extruders is given here, along with details that illustrate the versatility of extrusion processing.

THEORY AND CHARACTERIZATION OF EXTRUSION

The various types of extruders have the common feature of forcing the extrudate from a wide cross section through the restriction of the die. The force required and the characteristics of the extrudate produced are dependent on the rheological properties of the extrudate, the design of the die, and the rate at which the material is forced through the die. The theoretical approach to understanding the systems, therefore, is generally associated with dividing the process of flow into three sections: 1) entry into the die, 2) flow through the die, and 3) exit from the die.

Extrusion is dependent on the material, and the technique varies with the material studied. With regard to pharmaceuticals, most systems consist of particles dispersed in a fluid and, although consideration will be given to plastics, the main emphasis is on paste extrusions. These differ in the fact that a fluid is present between solid particles. The relative position of solid and liquid can change during the various stages of the extrusion process, and hence produce effects different from those associated with single-phase systems.

If the die is considered as a simple capillary flow, the relationship between the rate of shear (γ) and die wall shear stress (τ_w) can be described by Eq. 1:

$$\tau_w = \gamma P \cdot R/2L \tag{1}$$

where P is the pressure drop across the length of capillary L and radius R. Corrections for entrance effects modify this equation by considering an increase in the length of the capillary to give Eq. 2:

$$\tau_w = \gamma P/2(L/R + n_b) \tag{2}$$

where n_b is the Bagley entrance correction (1). Determination of n_b can be made by measuring the pressure necessary to force extrudate through dies of different length-to-radius (L/R) ratio. Extrapolation of the graphs to zero pressure values gives the value of n_b as the intercept on the L/R axis (1).

Han and Charles (2) found experimentally that the exit pressure is actually above atmospheric pressure and proposed modification of Eq. 2 to Eq. 3 corrected for exit pressure losses:

$$\tau_w = (\gamma P - P_e)/2(L/R + n_b) \tag{3}$$

where P_e is the exit pressure. This value is difficult to determine and, because it is considerably lower than the pressure loss upstream and through the die, it is usually neglected. The upstream pressure loss can be considerable and can be determined as the intercept on the pressure axis at zero L/R ratio (the Bagley equation), giving Eqs. 4 and 5:

$$\tau_w = (P_T - P_0)R/2L \tag{4}$$

$$P_T = P_0 + 2\tau_w(L/R + n_b) \tag{5}$$

The upstream pressure loss includes pressure losses due to kinetic energy, head effects, elastic losses, and turbulence. Harrison (3) found for a series of pharmaceutical systems that the value of P_0 increases with increasing rate of passage through the die.

Encyclopedia of Pharmaceutical Technology

Rheological Curves

In addition to determination of the upstream pressure loss P_0 and the end correction n_b, Eq. 5 can be seen to provide a value for the shear stress τ_w in such systems. The slope of the graph P_T versus. L/R has a gradient of $2\tau_w$; that is, the die-wall shear stress. The rate of shear at the die wall—$(dv/dr)_w$—can be derived from the Hagen–Poiseuille's law, as in Eq. 6:

$$(dv/dr)_w = 4Q/R^3 \tag{6}$$

where Q is the volumetric flow rate and R the radius of the die. This assumes that the flow is Newtonian. If this is not the case, Jastrzebski (4) suggested that a correction should be made for the rate of shear, as in Eq. 7:

$$-(dv/dr)_w = \left(\frac{3n' + 1}{n'}\right)\frac{Q}{\pi R^3} \tag{7}$$

where n' is the degree of non-Newtonian flow; it is determined from the gradient of the graph of log-shear stress as a function of the log apparent shear rate. Wilkinson (5) has also indicated that these equations assume that: 1) the flow is laminar, 2) there is no slip at the die wall, and 3) the rate of shear depends only on the shear stress at the point of measurement and is independent of time.

Determination of shear rate versus shear stress curves by application of the ram extruder allow characterization of the rheological properties of the extruded material according to the basic type of curve, as expressed by Eqs. 8–11.

Newtonian:

$$\sigma_{w = \gamma'}\eta \tag{8}$$

where η is the apparent viscosity and γ' is the rate of shear.

Bingham body:

$$\tau_w = \sigma_y + \gamma'U \tag{9}$$

where σ_y is the stress necessary to be exceeded before Newtonian flow commences, yield value, and U is the plastic viscosity.

Power-law model:

$$\tau_w = K\gamma^{n'} \tag{10}$$

where K is the power-law viscosity constant and n' is the degree of non-Newtonian flow. For values of n' less than 1, the material becomes less viscous with increasing shear rate (shear thinning), and for values of n' greater then 1, the viscosity increases with increasing shear rate (shear thickening).

Herschel–Buckley model:

$$\tau_w = \tau_y + K\gamma^n \tag{11}$$

which allows for a system that has a yield value and a shear rate dependent on viscosity.

The application of these types of flow curves requires homogeneous materials that do not change in consistency with extrusion. Harrison et al. (6) found this not to be the case, and suggested that this was due to the presence of plug flow within the extrudate bulk and slip flow at the die wall.

The inability of the standard rheological models to quantitatively describe the process of flow into, through, and out of the die requires an alternative treatment. From a study of ceramic catalyst pastes, Benbow and Ovensten (7) and Benbow (8) assumed that there was broad plug flow at the center of the extrudate, with shearing occurring within a thin liquid layer at the die wall. Assuming that this layer behaves as a Newtonian liquid of thickness x and viscosity η, and that the initial shear stress to induce flow is τ_0, the total die-wall shear stress τ_w at a given extrudate velocity V is given by Eq. 12:

$$\tau_w = \tau_0 + (\eta/x)V \tag{12}$$

The values of η and x cannot be determined directly and, therefore, Benbow et al. (9) introduced the term β, the die land viscosity factor, to replace η/x, as in Eq. 13:

$$\tau_w = \tau_0 = \beta V \tag{13}$$

Incorporation of this expression into Eq. 4 yields:

$$P_\tau = P_0 + 2(L/R)(\tau_0 + \beta V) \tag{14}$$

The value of τ_0 can be determined by plotting the extrusion pressure against the extrudate velocity V for extrusion through dies of constant value of L. The extrapolated value of extrusion pressure at $V = 0$ gives the value P_{0v0} at zero velocity, as shown by Eq. 15:

$$P_{\tau v0} = P_{0v0} + 2(L/R)\tau_0 \tag{15}$$

Thus, a graph of $P_{\tau v0}$ versus L/R provides the value of τ_0 as equal to half the slope. The value of β can be calculated by rearranging Eq. 14 to Eq. 16:

$$\beta = \left(P_{\tau_w} - P_{0w}\right) - \left(P_{\tau v0} - P_{0v0}\right)2(L/R)V \tag{16}$$

where P_{τ_w} is the total extrusion pressure at extrudate velocity V, and P_{0_w} is the upstream pressure loss at extrudate velocity V.

Further characterization of the system was suggested by Benbow (8) and Benbow and Bridgwater (10) in terms of a yield value σ_y associated with the convergence of flow from the wide cross section of the feed to the narrow cross section of the die. This takes the form of Eq. 17:

$$P_0 = \sigma_y \ln(A_0/A) \tag{17}$$

where A_0 is the initial cross-sectional area and A that of the die. If the original and final cross sections are circular, Eq. 18 holds:

$$P_0 = 2\sigma_y \ln(D_0/D) \tag{18}$$

where D_0 and D are the barrel and die diameters, respectively. For materials that deform plastically and are time independent, the value of σ_y can be calculated from the intercept of the pressure axis divided by twice the natural log reduction ratio (D_0/D) for plots of P against L/R.

By combining this concept with those expressed above, Benbow et al. (9) and Benbow and Bridgwater (10) further modified the Bagley equation to Eq. 19:

$$P_T = 2(\sigma_{y0} + \alpha V) \ln(D_0/D) + 2(L/R)(\tau_0 + \beta V) \tag{19}$$

If the die land velocity factor β varies with the extrusion rate or the liquid layer at the die wall is non-Newtonian, Eq. 19 must be further modified to Eq. 20:

$$P_\tau = 2\sigma_y \ln(D_0/D) + 2(L/R)(\tau_0 + \beta^* V^{l-n}) \tag{20}$$

where β^* is a modified power-law constant and n the degree of non-Newtonian flow. If the flow velocity into the die is also dependent on the velocity of flow, Benbow et al. (9) and Benbow and Bridgwater (10) propose replacement of the yield value δ_y, by two empirical parameters, the initial die entry yield stress σ_{y0} and the die-entry yield-stress velocity factor α. Substituting in Eq. 18 gives Eq. 21:

$$P_0 = 2(\sigma_{y0} + \alpha V) \ln (D_0/D) \tag{21}$$

The fully corrected Bagley equation now becomes Eq. 22:

$$P_T = 2(\sigma_{y0} + \alpha V) \ln(D_0/D) + 2(L/R)(\tau_0 + \beta V) \tag{22}$$

The value of σ_{y0} can be obtained as the intercept from the derived zero-velocity graph of P_{0v0} as a function of L/R. The value of α, for a given system, is obtained from Eq. 23:

$$\alpha = \left(P_{0_w} - P_{v0}\right)/(2 \ln(D_0/D)V) \tag{23}$$

where P_{0_w} and P_{0v0} are obtained as described previously.

If the systems are treated as polymer melts instead of as paste (i.e., homogenous systems with no fluid migration during extrusion), further characterization of the wet masses can be achieved (11). The flow of melts through a capillary rheometer can be considered to show flow streamlines converging and then accelerating, which according to Cogswell (12), is extensional flow. He separated the flow field into shear and tensile deformation and then described their calculation from the following equations:

$$TS = \frac{3}{8}(n + 1)P_0 \tag{24}$$

where TS is the tensile stress (i.e., stretching), n is the power law index, and P_0 is the die-entrance press drop,

$$ESR = \frac{4\pi\gamma}{3(n + 1)} = \frac{\gamma}{2} \tan \theta \tag{25}$$

where ESR is the tensile stretch rate, τ is the shear stress at the die wall, γ is the shear strain rate, and θ is the half angle of natural convergence.

$$EV \frac{TS}{ESR} \tag{26}$$

where EV is the apparent extensional (elongational) viscosity.

Such an approach depends on the flow fitting the power law model (i.e., Eq. 10), and that flow is not dominated by wall slip.

In addition to elongation flow, material can also exhibit elastic behavior. Two parameters that have been proposed (13, 14) to quantify this property are (1) recoverable shear RS and (2) compliance C. These can be derived from:

$$RS = \frac{P}{4\pi} \tag{27}$$

and

$$C = \frac{P}{4\tau^2} \tag{28}$$

Chohan (14) has used these to study the flow of branched polyethylene melt, and while what is exactly implied by these terms at high stretch rates is not clear, they are undoubtedly related to the elastic behavior of the material. The higher the values of each, the greater will be the elastic nature of the material.

MEASUREMENT OF RHEOLOGICAL PROPERTIES

The application of the theoretical treatment depends on the ability to measure the extrusion force and rate. Most commercial extruders do not allow for these types of measurement. Normal rheological equipment, such as cup-and-bob or cone-and-plate, do not have a suitable geometry or instrumentation to handle materials of the consistency normally used. A ram extruder is a suitable experimental design.

The ram extruder, designed by Benbow and Ovenston (7), operates on a prefilled system and is used for experimental and small-scale extrusion (Fig. 1). It consists of a stainless steel barrel (2.54 cm internal diameter, approximately 20 cm in length), which acts as the material reservoir. The base is constructed to enable interchangeable dies, with central capillaries of varying dimensions to be bolted on. A rubber ring is inserted between the barrel and die to ensure a watertight connection. The piston, or ram, is a stainless steel rod that fits loosely into the barrel. A fluon ring positioned at its lower end provides a low-friction seal to prevent material escaping above the point where the piston moves down the barrel. The extrusion is a noncontinuous operation; first the material (50–100 g) is packed into the barrel and partially consolidated to a plug by inserting the piston. It is possible to add temperature control to the barrel to extrude materials that are thermosensitive. The barrel-and-die assembly is mounted on a rigid metal C-piece,

and a load is applied to the piston sufficient to extrude the material through the die. The ram extruder can be used in conjunction with an instrumented press. The piston is attached to the cross-head that may be driven down at various constant rates, and its displacement monitored by an attached displacement transducer. Output from this and the load cell is fed into an x–y chart recorder or computer. This arrangement enables the force acting on the material during extrusion to be recorded as a function of the displacement of the piston, and a force–displacement profile is produced.

A typical extrusion mixture produces three distinct regions, as shown in Fig. 2. In the compression stage, the piston descends into the barrel and consolidates the material into a plug prior to flow. This results in a large change in displacement accompanied by a small change in load. Eventually, the material is compressed to its minimum volume and maximum density. At this point, the pressure builds up while the material density is maintained. This is shown in the profile by a large increase in load accompanied by a minimal change in displacement. At the end of the compression stage, the pressure applied to the mass increases until it is high enough for the material to yield and commence flow. This is followed by a period of steady-state flow in which the force required to maintain the extrusion remains constant as the displacement increases. Forced flow occurs when steady-state flow can no longer be maintained. It leads to a gradual rise in extrusion force with displacement. This occurs often toward the end of the extrusion and is caused by the close proximity of the ram tip to the die face.

The force–displacement profile is altered by varying one of the extrusion parameters, such as the die diameter, L/R, or extrusion rate. For a given mixture, the relationship between the steady-state extrusion force, the die L/R at constant die diameter, and the extrusion rate can be represented graphically, as shown in Fig. 3. This is known as the Bagley plot (1). Used in this way, the extruder operates on a principle similar to that of a capillary rheometer, and expressions derived from capillary rheometry (described previously) may be used to characterize the properties of the wet powder mass. After conversion of the steady-state force values to pressure values, the slope of the relationship between the pressure and L/R is numerically equivalent to twice the value of the mean die-wall shear stress (according to Eq. 4). Plotting these values against the corresponding apparent die-wall shear rates (derived from Eq. 6) results in a flow curve that is unique for a particular wet-mass formulation (Fig. 4). The materials exhibit non-Newtonian flow and shear-thinning properties.

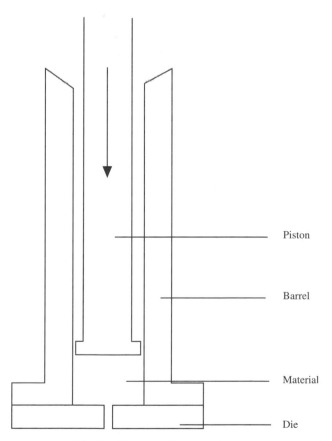

Fig. 1 Diagram of a ram extruder.

Piston

Barrel

Material

Die

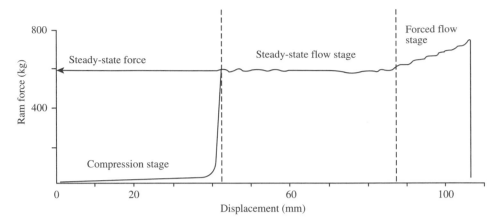

Fig. 2 Force–displacement profile for microcrystalline cellulose–lactose–water mixture.

PRACTICAL CHARACTERIZATION OF EXTRUSION SYSTEMS

The expression of the extrusion properties of pharmaceutical systems by numerical values could aid formulation. To be able to apply the theoretical approaches described previously, it is important to ensure that the restrictions of the systems are considered. One major problem with paste systems is that when subjected to pressure, there is phase separation resulting in variations in the composition of the mass as it is being extruded. This can be detected by collecting the extrudate and measuring its water content (15, 16). Alternatively, magnetic resonance imaging has been used to quantify the water distribution within the barrel (17) and within the extrudate (18).

The extent to which die-wall slip is involved can be assessed by using dies of different lengths and diameters. An important characteristic that can be observed in the extrudate is its quality in terms of surface structure. Harrison et al. (19) have shown how this can vary from a smooth, regular surface via a rough, "shark-skinned" extrudate. There is obvious need to prevent this

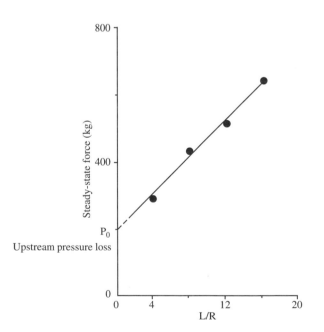

Fig. 3 Steady-state extrusion force as a function of the length-to-radius ratio of the die for microcrystalline cellulose–lactose–water (5:5:6) at constant die diameter (1.5 mm) and extrusion rate (20 cm/min).

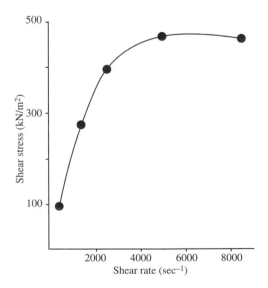

Fig. 4 Typical shear stress-shear rate flow curve for an extrusion mixture containing 50% microcrystalline cellulose extruded through a 1.5-mm diameter die.

phenomenon if extrudate of the correct quality is to be produced. The occurrence of the surface defects is associated with both the composition of the material and the operating conditions (e.g., die length and diameter and the rate of extrusion) (Fig. 5). Raines et al. (20) were able to relate the quality of the surface of the extrudate to the value of the yield stress at zero velocity δ_{y0}, in that those systems with a high value were smooth and regular while those with low values were shark-skinned.

Of the systems studied, most pastes show non-Newtonian behavior. This has important consequences for extruder design and operating conditions as material that are shear-rate dependent require careful handling. To date, most reported rheological investigations indicate that paste systems are shear thinning (i.e., their viscosity decreases with an increase in shear rate) (Fig. 4). Their extent of property can be quantified by obtaining the value of n', the slope of the log shear-rate/log shear-stress graph. There is also some evidence that paste systems show plug flow (i.e., the central core of the extrudate moves at a constant velocity), while there is a thin layer of moisture at the die wall where shear takes place (21).

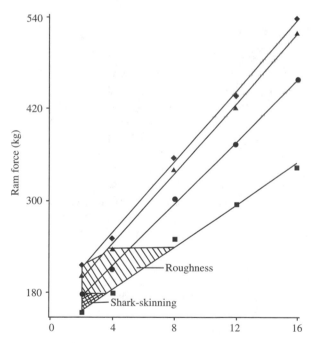

Fig. 5 A graph of ram force as a function of length-to-radius ratio, depicting conditions under which surface defects occur when extruding microcrystalline cellulose–lactose–water (5:5:6). Die diameter = 1.5 mm; ram speed cm/min: ■, 5; ●, 10; ▲, 20; ◆, 40.

FORMULATION

Extrusion mixtures are formulated to produce a cohesive plastic mass that remains homogeneous during extrusion. The mass must possess inherent fluidity, permitting flow during the process and self-lubricating properties as it passes through the die. The resultant extrudate must remain nonadhesive to itself and retain a degree of rigidity so that the shape imposed by the die is retained. Precise formulation requirements depend upon subsequent processing. Extrudate that is simply to be cut to short lengths to form cylindrical granules that are dried in a fluid-bed drier can be less rigid than extrudate intended for complex processing such as spheronization, where the extrudate undergoes a series of subtle shape changes.

The requirements for spheronization of the cylindrical extrudate are as follows:

1. The extrudate must possess sufficient mechanical strength when wet, yet it must be brittle enough to be broken down to short lengths in the spheronizer, but not to be so friable that it disintegrates completely. To achieve a narrow size distribution of spheres, the extrudate is ideally reduced to cylindrical rods of uniform length equal to approximately one and a half times their diameter (22).
2. The extrudate must be sufficiently plastic to enable the cylindrical rods to be rolled into spheres by the action of the friction plate in the spheronizer.
3. The extrudate must be nonadhesive to itself in order that each spherical granule remains discrete throughout the process.

A typical extrusion mixture might contain the following ingredients:

Drug	50–90%
Extrusion aid	
Microcrystalline cellulose, bentonite	5–90%
Binder	
Polyvinylpyrrolidone (PVP)	
Sodium carboxymethylcellulose (SCMC)	
Hydroxypropyl methylcellulose (HPMC)	
Fluid	
Water or solvent	

Extrusion offers the advantage of incorporating a relatively high proportion of active ingredient, up to 90%, in the final product. However, the physicochemical properties of the drug determine to a large extent the maximum quantity that can be included in a particular formulation. An extrusion aid is essential; microcrystalline cellulose is commonly used (23). The function of microcrystalline cellulose is two-fold: it controls the movement of water through the wet powder mass during extrusion, and modifies the rheological properties of the other ingredients in the mixture, conferring a degree of plasticity which allows it to be readily extruded. This interaction with the liquid phase is both a physical and chemical phenomenon. The microscopic structure of microcrystalline cellulose is a random aggregation of filamentous microcrystals that create a high internal porosity and a large surface area, approximately 130–270 m^2/g (24). This provides highly absorbent and moisture-retaining characteristics that are often unaffected by the extrusion process. This could be the essential quality that makes microcrystalline cellulose a unique material for extrusion. Bentonite and kaolin also have been used. Inclusion of 5–10% can significantly improve the extrusion properties of mixtures containing high proportions of drug. Recent work (25) has shown that it is possible to reduce the quantity of microcrystalline cellulose by adding glyceryl monostearate.

Additional ingredients may or may not be necessary. A binder increases plasticity and reduces extrudate friability, particularly when the content of microcrystalline cellulose is low. Natural or synthetic polymers, such as gelatin, PVP, or SCMC, may be incorporated into the mixture as a solid during dry mixing or in solution in the liquid phase. Commercial preparations of microcrystalline cellulose that are already combined with polymers are available. Examples include Avicel RC and Avicel CL grades of microcrystalline cellulose combined with SCMC (FMC Corporation). Variations in the type of microcrystalline cellulose significantly change the rheological properties of the mixture, and therefore, the extrusion characteristics (20). The differences between shear stress–shear rate flow curves of mixtures of microcrystalline cellulose–lactose–water (5:5:6) containing different particle sizes of microcrystalline cellulose and different quantities of SCMC are distinct but different. Inclusion of a polymer in the wet mass produces marked rheological differences. This has implications in the choice of formulations, since the extrudates formed from these various microcrystalline cellulose mixtures behave differently during subsequent processing, such as cutting, spheronization, and drying.

The mixture of dry ingredients is blended with water or a solvent such as ethanol (26) to form a dense cohesive mass suitable for extrusion. The liquid content of the wet powder mass and its distribution are highly critical and should be controlled so that they produce an extrudate that posses the ideal characteristics. In general, these wet mixes have a much higher moisture content, typically 20–30 wt%, than is required for conventional (tablet)

granulations, the aim being to produce as dense a material as possible for passing through the extruder. Fluffy and incompletely wetted masses feed poorly and cause problems by creating excessive pressure and friction within the equipment. On spheronizing, they tend to produce large quantities of fines, and the "dry" extrudate is insufficiently plastic, forming dumbbell-shaped or ovoid pellets which never round off into spheres. On the other hand, if the mixture is too wet, it produces an extrudate that adheres to the spheronizer plate and to itself. This product tends to aggregate uncontrollably or at best produce spheres of wide-size distribution as the material is transferred from pellet to pellet via the plate motion.

The possible processability of different drugs by this approach has not yet been fully established. It is not possible to relate the pK_a, and freezing point depression, or to relate the ability to produce uniform pellets from a spheronization grade of microcrystalline cellulose (27). However, a relationship between the water solubility and the water level required by a formulation for equal parts of a series of model drugs and microcrystalline cellulose has been established (28).

INDUSTRIAL APPLICATIONS

Plastics

Extrusion technology is extensively applied in the plastics and rubber industries where it is one of the most important fabrication processes. Examples of products made from extruded polymers include pipes, hoses, insulated wires and cables, plastic and rubber sheeting, and polystyrene tiles. The most common extruder employed is the single-screw type (Fig. 6) with either cold or hot feed, which requires the polymer to be heated prior to processing. The extruder consists of a rotating screw inside a stationary cylindrical barrel. The barrel is often manufactured in sections that are bolted or clamped together. Usually, the inner surface of the barrel is grooved to reduce slippage and increase pumping capability. An end-plate die, connected to the end of the barrel, determines the configuration of the extruded product.

The extruder is conventionally divided into three sections: feed zone, transition zone, and metering zone. Resin granules are fed from a hopper directly into the feed section, which has deeper flights or flights of greater pitch. This geometry enables the feed material to fall easily into the screw for conveying along the barrel. The pellets are transported as a solid plug to the transition zone where they are mixed, compressed, melted, and

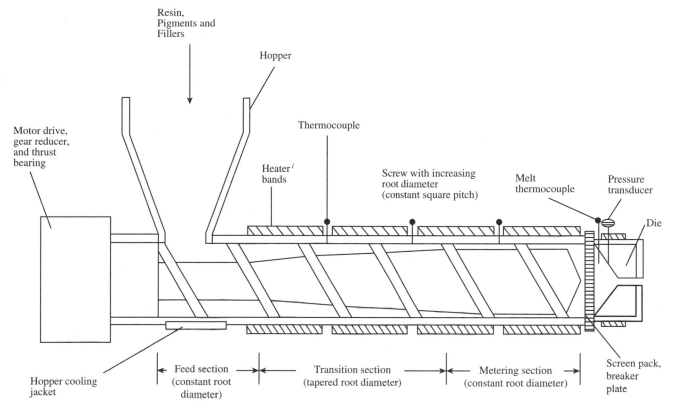

Fig. 6 Component parts of a single-screw extruder.

plasticized. Compression is developed by decreasing the thread pitch but maintaining a constant flight depth or by decreasing flight depth while maintaining a constant thread pitch (29). Both methods result in increased pressure as the material moves along the barrel. Most of the heat required to melt the material is supplied by the heat generated by friction as the resin granules are sheared between the rotating screw and the wall of the barrel. Additional heat may be supplied by electric heaters mounted on the barrel. The melt moves by circulation in a helical path by means of transverse flow, drag flow, pressure flow, and leakage: the latter two mechanisms reverse the flow of material along the barrel. The material reaches the metering zone in the form of a homogeneous plastic melt suitable for extrusion. For an extrudate of uniform thickness, flow must be consistent and without stagnant zones right up to the die entrance. The function of the metering zone is to reduce pulsating flow and ensure a uniform delivery rate through the die cavity. Some applications require a strainer plate fitted between the extruder and die plate to remove solid impurities or lumps of incompletely melted resin.

Polymers with a wide range of viscoelastic and melt viscosities cannot be processed with a single screw. Most

commercial extruders are, therefore, modular in design, providing a choice of screws or interchangeable sections that alter the configuration of the feed, transition, and metering zones. This makes it possible to modify the process to meet particular requirements, for example, from a standard to a high shear or high output extrusion. Modified screw designs allow the extruder to perform a mixing role in addition to extrusion, so that the material can be colored and blended. The various screw and die designs available and practical considerations of thermoplastic extrusion are reviewed by Whelan and Dunning (30). Extrusion processing requires close monitoring of the various parameters that affect polymer extrusion: viscosity, variation of viscosity with shear rate and temperature, elasticity, extensional flow, and slippage of the material over hot metal surfaces. Equations used to describe flow are included in the section on the "Theory and Characterization of Extrusion" presented earlier. Recent advances in the design and operation of extruders allow in-process monitoring and control of parameters, such as the temperature in the extruder, head, and die; pressures in extruder and die; wall thickness and other dimensions; "haul-off" speed and extrusion speed; and power consumption.

The process described above is known as profile or line extrusion in which the shape of the extrudate is determined by the die. The extruded profile proceeds horizontally to the cutoff equipment, which controls its length. It is then cooled to a solid state, usually by spraying with or immersion in water, and passed through a haul-off unit. Finally, it is cut to the required length or coiled. The downstream auxiliaries (e.g., such as haul-off equipment for handling the extrudate stream, collection machinery for winding or coiling continuous lengths of tubing or profiles, cropping and cooling equipment, and systems for monitoring the diameter and wall thicknesses of pipes on-line) are as important as the extruder itself (30, 31). Tubes and pipes and other solid cross-sections are mainly produced by profile extrusion. Profiles may be further processed, for example, as in film extrusion, blow molding, or injection molding (32).

Film extrusion

The polymer melt is extruded through a long slit die onto highly polished cooled rolls that form and wind the finished sheet. This is known as cast film. Plastic packaging film is also formed by blow extrusion, where tubular film is produced by extruding the melt, usually vertically, through an annular-shaped slit die. The extruded tube is inflated by air to form a large cylinder. The bubble is cooled externally by an airstream directed onto its surface and is collapsed on passing between a pair of rollers before being wound up. Film made by the casting process generally has better optical properties than blown film, but is less strong mechanically. Cast films usually require edge trimming at additional cost.

Blow molding

The plastic is heated to a melted or viscous state and a section of molten polymer tubing (parison) is extruded usually downward from the die head into an open mold. The mold is closed around the parison, sealing it at one end. Compressed air is blown into the open end of the tube, expanding the viscous plastic to the walls of the cavity, thus forming the desired shape of the container. The material cools in the cavity and solidifies. The mold is opened and the molding is removed. This technique is used for the manufacture of bottles, toys, and large containers.

Injection molding

The molten plastic is extruded into a cavity mold at high pressure. The material cools in the cavity and solidifies. The mold is then opened and the article is removed. Very intricate configurations can be obtained by this technique

(e.g., to provide intricate and strong components for the electronic, telecommunications, and clock-making industries).

Plastics that are commonly processed by extrusion include acrylics (polymethacrylates, polyacrylates) and copolymers of acrylonitrile; cellulosics (cellulose acetate, propionate, and acetate butyrate); polyethylene (low and high density); polypropylene; polystyrene; vinyl plastics; polycarbonates; and nylons. The material properties and extrusion properties have been reviewed by Whelan and Dunning (30). Additives that may be included to modify or enhance properties (33) include lubricants and antislip agents to assist processing during extrusion; plasticizers to achieve softness and flexibility; stabilizers and antioxidants to retard or prevent degradation; and dyes and pigments.

Food

In principle, any food that can be formed into a paste can be processed by an extruder. Food extrusion has been utilized since the 1930s for pasta production. Modern equipment and processing techniques allow the manu-facture of complex products in a variety of shapes and sizes. Raw materials such as cereals, oil seed, and protein, along with carbohydrates and water mixtures, can be converted into products such as meat substitutes, pet foods, and snack meals. A widely used and versatile technique combines cooking and extrusion in a so-called extrusion cooker (34). It has the potential to manufacture a range of novelty or specialty products, such as breakfast cereals (expanded and shaped cereals), shaped and filled snacks, protein-fortified and precooked pasta products, and precooked meat pieces for convenience foods. The process is highly economical, and provides mixing, high temperature–short duration cooking, texturizing, and shaping of the food in one step. The equipment closely resembles the screw extruders used in the processing of thermoplastics. The screw is designed to create varying zones along the barrel, allowing the food substance to be processed in stages. The solid and liquid starting materials are fed from a hopper to the feed zone of the extruder and conveyed to the transition zone. Here the materials may be compressed, mixed, sheared, and heated to form a viscous plastic dough. In the metering zone, the plastic mass is subjected to further heating and shearing before being pumped into the die to form the shaped product. The pressure drop on leaving the die causes superheated water to flash off the molten material. If the dough contains starch, gelatinization will result in an expanded porous product with a crunchy texture (35). Finally, the product may be cut, shaped by passing through rollers, dried, and packed.

The viscosity of the dough may vary more than an order of magnitude during the extrusion cooking process as a result of changes in shear rate, temperature, moisture content, and induced physicochemical changes such as protein denaturation, polysaccharide gel formation, and reorientation of molecules (36). For this reason, success in food extrusion requires accurate monitoring and control of feed rate, screw speed, temperature, and moisture to produce and control desired product characteristics. Knowledge of the viscous rheology of the food mixture in the metering section immediately prior to extrusion is of particular importance. However, this is not easily predicted since, unlike the case of homogeneous or simple mixtures of polymers where the major change is melting, food doughs are of such complexity that the exact chemical composition and structure cannot readily be determined. Efforts have been made to develop semiempirical models derived from plastics extrusion to describe the apparent viscosity of cooking doughs, which may be useful in evaluating food formulations (37, 38). Remsen and Clarke (36) used an Instron capillary viscometer and amylograph to describe the relationship between the viscosity of a typical soy flour dough and the applied shear rate, temperature, and time–temperature history. Fletcher et al. (39) investigated the viscous dough rheology of maize mixtures as a function of the extrusion variables (pressure, shear, and temperature). They used an instrumented single-screw extruder fitted with slit dies, and related the results to the product properties. The advantage with this method is that the food material receives a deformation history corresponding to the extrusion cooking process, which is otherwise difficult to replicate in a laboratory rheometer.

Animal Feed Production

In the animal feed industry, extrusion is applied as a means of producing pelletized feeds, commonly in the form of short cylindrical rods of 4–8 mm in diameter. Pellets are a convenient means of precisely controlling the animal's diet. They offer several advantages (40). The quantity of feed the animal receives is better controlled by pellets than a loose-mix feed, and a complex diet of controlled composition is easily produced. The pellet feed can contain as many as 30 single ingredients mixed in the correct proportions. The animal is obliged to chew pellet feed with improved palatability and therefore, digestion. During extrusion, the feed mixture is compressed, resulting in a densified product that requires less storage space.

Pellets are prepared from a mixture of raw materials of varying chemical composition (starch, oil, fiber, and moisture) and physical characteristics (particle size, bulk density, and moisture-retention properties). The composition of a typical poultry feed is often complex (41). The raw material properties determine the quality of pellet formation. Equipment performance and pellet quality (friability, size uniformity) can be improved by a small amount of extrusion or pelleting aid (binders, lubricants) (42). Additives commonly used in the feed industry include molasses with binding properties when activated by steam; fatty acid lubricants to reduce product–metal friction when extruding or pressing through long dies; lignosulfates (organic materials derived from lignin in trees that improve pellet quality and throughput rates); and mineral binders, such as ball clay and bentonite, or cellulose binders, such as sodium carboxymethylcellulose. It should be noted that in small quantities cellulose binders can improve the pelleting process and reduce pellet friability.

The pelleting process (40) consists of blending and conditioning the feed mixture immediately prior to pressing, pressing itself, cutting of the pellets, and cooling. The complexity of the feed mixture, composed of a number of ingredients of different particle sizes and densities in varying proportions, requires thorough blending to ensure homogeneity. The product is conditioned by adding moisture, typically up to 15%, and heating to a controlled temperature in order to gelatinize the starch or convert it to simple sugars. This reaction causes the starch to act as a binder and converts the meal into a physical state suitable for pressing. The most efficient means of conditioning and heating is by steam. Optimal conditioning parameters, moisture content of the material, temperature, and duration of heating depend on the composition of the mixture (42). For example, high starch–low fiber meals require temperatures of 80–85°C, whereas feeds that contain heat-sensitive ingredients, such as milk and sugar, have a temperature limit of 55°C (39).

Extrusion Pressing

According to Sebestyen (40), pellet mills may be classified into disk-die presses or ring-die pellet mills. In the former, the die consists of a circular plate resting in the horizontal plane into which holes are drilled in a regular pattern. A set of rollers move around the upper surface of the disk, sweeping the meal in their path through the holes and compressing it to form pellets or cubes. Rotating adjustable knives located beneath the disk cut the extrudate to an appropriate length. In another design, the plate revolves while the rollers and knives remain fixed.

Ring-type pellet mills have a radially arranged die resting in the horizontal plane with rollers rotating and revolving along the inner surface. The rolls are offset from the die face, leaving a slight clearance that allows buildup of a thin product layer, optimizing throughput efficiency. The peripheral velocity of the rollers depends upon the die diameter; that is, higher speeds are required for smaller-diameter holes and lower speeds for larger-diameter holes.

Cooling

On leaving the extruder, the warm pellets are pliable and prone to abrasion and deformation. Therefore, a final processing stage is required to harden the pellets (40). Cooling equipment placed directly beneath the mill employs ambient or chilled air to reduce the temperature and remove excess moisture from the final product.

PHARMACEUTICAL INDUSTRY

Extrusion processes are applied within the pharmaceutical industry to produce a variety of dosage forms such as suppositories, implants, and granulations.

The large-scale manufacture of suppositories and pessaries uses either the fusion method where the drug is dispersed in a molten base and the mixture poured into molds to solidify, or the cold compression method (43, 44). In the latter process, the medicament and cold-grated base, usually theobroma oil or witepsol base, are intimately mixed and placed in a cylinder. The mass is extruded by means of a piston through small holes that connect with the mold. The cavities are filled by pressure with the mass which is prevented from escaping by movable end plates. The plates are removed and the suppositories ejected by further extrusion. The extrusion equipment is chilled to prevent melting of the

components due to the heat generated by the friction of compression.

The most important application of extrusion in the pharmaceutical industry is in the preparation of granules or pellets of uniform size, shape, and density that contain one or more drugs. The process involves a preliminary stage in which dry powders, drug, and excipients are mixed by conventional blenders, followed by addition of a liquid phase and further mixing to ensure homogeneous distribution (Fig. 7). The wet powder mass is extruded through cylindrical dies or perforated screens with circular holes, typically 0.5–2.0 mm in diameter, to form cylindrical extrudates. These may be further processed, for example, by cutting and drying to yield granules, or by spheronization (24) to yield spherical granules followed by drying. The spheroids are usually coated with a polymer to control the rate of drug release and filled into hard gelatin capsules to yield a multiple-unit dosage form.

Extruders Used for Pharmaceuticals

Commercial extruders may be classified according to the die design and the feed mechanism that transports the material to the die region.

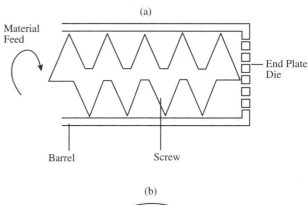

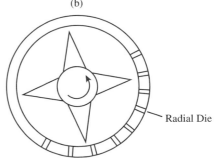

Fig. 8 Screw extruder with (a) end-plate die and (b) radial-screen die.

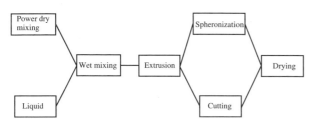

Fig. 7 Schematic of extrusion processing in the pharmaceutical industry.

E

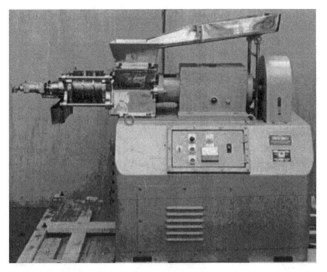

Fig. 9 Twin-screw extruder with radial-screen die. (Manufactured by Fuji Pauldal Company, Japan.)

Screen extruders

Screen extruders utilize a screw-feed mechanism consisting of single or twin helical screws rotating in a barrel to convey the damp mass from a feed hopper to the die zone. The die consists of a thin steel plate perforated with numerous holes, which is positioned radially or axially to the screw feed (Fig. 8). The advantages of this arrangement are high continuous throughput rates, from 5 kg/h of wet mass for a laboratory-scale single-screw extruder, up to 800 kg/h for a larger twin-screw design. The screens are easily cleaned and interchanged; they have holes of varying diameter beginning at 0.5 mm and are available commercially. The disadvantage of this type of equipment, however, is that the screw mechanism can exert a high pressure on the material, generating excessive friction and heat as the wet mass passes between the screw and barrel. This is particularly the case with axially orientated dies. These extruders tend to have a high dead volume that contains stagnant material between the feed screws and the screen. Consideration should be given to this if the wet powder mass contains ingredients that are unstable when wetted with water. The low L/R of the die holes can also result in low compaction in the extrudate and distortion of the surface finish, known as shark-skinning. This problem can sometimes be overcome by varying the throughput rate, which will be discussed later.

The twin-screw design and radial-die screen assembly of an extruder manufactured by the Fuji Paudal Company of Japan is shown in Fig. 9. Water can be circulated

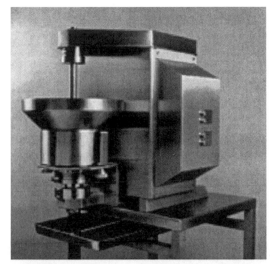
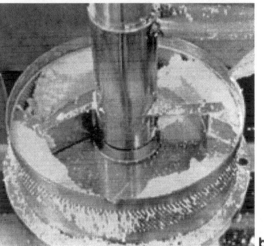
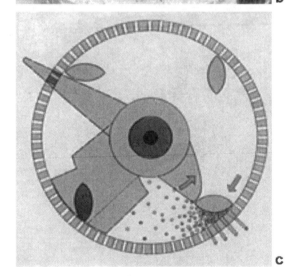

Fig. 10 The NICA system radial-screen extruder. (a) Assembled unit. (b) Dismantled to show extrusion mechanism. (c) Cross section indicating working principle.

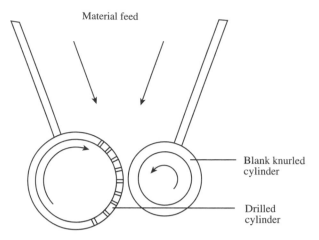

Material feed

Blank knurled cylinder

Drilled cylinder

Fig. 11 The rotary-cylinder-type extruder.

through the hollow extrusion rotors to maintain a constant temperature in the extrusion zone. This is a useful facility when processing heat-sensitive materials and for controlling temperature, extrudate moisture levels, and viscosity. Interchangeable screens are available with die holes ranging from 0.5 to 1.5 mm in diameter, allowing the production of a wide range of extrudates. Explosion-proof motors, with fixed or variable speed drive, are fitted for safe processing of wet masses granulated with inflammable solvents. All components in contact with process materials are constructed of high-grade stainless steel. An additional feature is the option of fitting an axial die plate in cases where a denser extrudate is required.

A screen extruder that operates with a novel mechanism is the Nica System Extruder (Fig. 10), manufactured in Sweden. It consists of a radial screen encircling an extrusion rotor and a rotating disk fitted with angled impeller blades or baffles. Above this is a counterrotating central feed blade. Speeds of both the extrusion rotor and the feed blade are variable. Material, such as gravity fed from a hopper, is swept into the blades and pressed through the holes in the screen, According to the manufacturer, there are several advantages to this equipment. First, pressure is exerted on only a small quantity of mass and only at the point of extrusion; that is, just between the baffles and the screen. Second, temperature increase is minimal, and a moisture gradient between the wet mass and extrudate is avoided. Because of this, cooling facilities are not necessary. The dead volume, located in front of each baffle, is limited and may be as low as 15 g per baffle. A small extruder with output up to 4 kg/min is available for development and small-scale production.

For larger production, an extruder with output of up to 12 kg/min is available.

Rotary-cylinder extruder

The working principle of this machine is based on two counterrotating cylinders (Fig. 11). The granulating cylinder is perforated and acts as the die. The diameter and the L/R of the holes can be varied. The holes are spaced further apart and are drilled rather than of punched sheet construction as in the screen-type extruders. The other cylinder is solid and acts as a pressure cylinder. Material is gravity fed from a hopper to the die region between the cylinders and adheres to the knurled surface of the solid cylinder, building up a thin layer that is pressed through the die cylinder. Although the extrusion is a continuous process, actual material flow though each hole is intermittent due to the rotation of the die. Pressure is built up in the perforations, which compacts the wet mass and forces the extrudate to the interior of the cylinder. This pressure is dependent upon the diameter and the length of the perforations. Hence, with die holes of high L/R, this system can achieve good densification of the wet powder mass. This is important in giving the most granules mechanical strength and stability for further processing. Another advantage is the lack of a dead zone, which is limited to the thin layer of material adhering to the pressure cylinder. Since the cylinders only apply pressure to a small quantity of material in the feed zone, there is little tendency for creating moisture gradients. However, cleaning of the granulating cylinder can be troublesome. The material remaining in the die holes can be difficult to dislodge, particularly when the L/R is high. Furthermore, the granulating cylinders are expensive because of the high costs of drilling stainless steel.

A cylinder extruder manufactured by Alexanderwerk (Germany) is shown in Fig. 12. With this equipment, the feed stock material can be metered to the working area. On the smallest machines this is accomplished by a rotary-table feed hopper. On larger machines, the feed rate is controlled by screw feeders sited through the feed hopper. The throughput rate depends on the diameter and L/R of the die holes, as well as on the feed rate. Laboratory-scale extruders with a throughput range of 30 to 50 kg/h use granulation cylinders 70 mm in diameter. Production-scale equipment with a larger granulating cylinder (186 mm diameter) can achieve an output of 100–105 kg/h. Interchangeable cylinders with die holes of 1.0–5.0 mm are available. A multiple-unit assembly consisting of three parallel

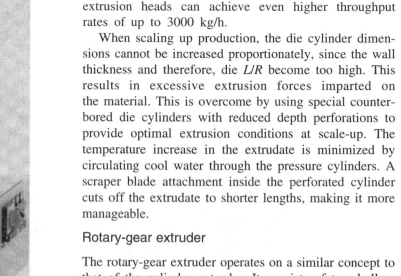

extrusion heads can achieve even higher throughput rates of up to 3000 kg/h.

When scaling up production, the die cylinder dimensions cannot be increased proportionately, since the wall thickness and therefore, die L/R become too high. This results in excessive extrusion forces imparted on the material. This is overcome by using special counterbored die cylinders with reduced depth perforations to provide optimal extrusion conditions at scale-up. The temperature increase in the extrudate is minimized by circulating cool water through the pressure cylinders. A scraper blade attachment inside the perforated cylinder cuts off the extrudate to shorter lengths, making it more manageable.

Rotary-gear extruder

The rotary-gear extruder operates on a similar concept to that of the cylinder extruder. It consists of two hollow counterrotating gear cylinders with counterbored dies, described by the manufacturer (Bepex, Berwind Corporation) as nozzles, that are drilled into the cylinders between the teeth (Fig. 13). The material, gravity fed from a hopper, is drawn in by the toothed cylinders and pushed through the nozzles into the center of the cylinders, where scrapers cut off the extrudate. The product is compacted as it passes through the nozzles, and thereby forms a dense extrudate. The density depends on the nozzle L/D (the ratio of nozzle length to nozzle diameter). Higher throughput rates can be attained with this type of extruder, since output is achieved through both rotating-gear wheels. The equipment and the gear-toothed cylinders are shown in Fig. 13b.

Interchangeable gear cylinders are available with variable nozzle L/D ratios by counterboring from the inside of the rollers to reduce the die length or by using replaceable nozzle inserts to increase the die length. The diameter of the holes can be varied from 1.0 to 10.0 mm to produce a range of pellet sizes. The throughput rate can be controlled by varying the cylinders' rotation speed and the corresponding feed rate. Throughput capacity ranges from 20 kg/h for the small-scale laboratory extruders to approximately 1000 kg/h for production equipment. For large equipment or materials with poor flow characteristics, agitators can be installed in the hopper to prevent bridging; special hoppers with conical feed screws fitted with additional wipers are used for highly viscous products. The machine can be furnished with cooling equipment, circulating water through the compaction gears for processing materials that need temperature control. An alternative pharmaceutical gear extruder, similar in design to the above, has recently been marketed by G.B. Caleva Ltd., United Kingdom.

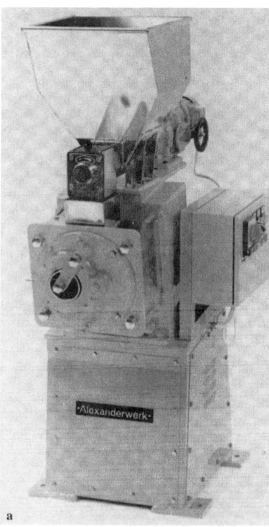

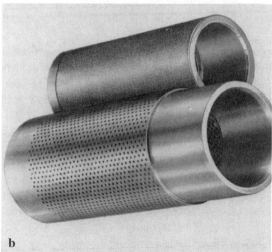

Fig. 12 The cylinder extruder, manufactured by Alexanderwerk, Germany. (a) Laboratory-scale extruder. (b) Die cylinder and pressure cylinder.

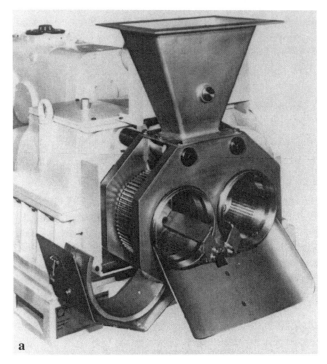

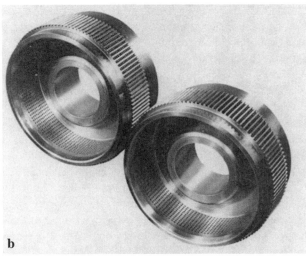

Fig. 13 (a) Rotary-gear extruder. (b) Gear-toothed cylinders.

Ram extruder

Industrial ram extruders are commonly used in the plastics and rubber industries for the preparation of warm strip feed for large cold-fed screw extruders and for forming strips or slugs for feeding injection molding and compression molding machines. They are used in the extrusion of specialized substances that require critical in-process control or that are not readily amenable to processing by screw extruders. Examples include the extrusion of waxlike substances such as coloring crayons,

dental waxes, and rocket propellant, and in the extrusion of moist powders and claylike materials, such as blackboard chalks. Ram extrusion allows control of parameters, such as temperature, size, and weight of extrudate. An example of a high performance ram extruder, as manufactured by Borwell International Ltd., United Kingdom, is shown in Fig. 14. It consists of a chrome-plated barrel positioned in a thermostatically controlled storage tunnel. A range of dies can be fitted to the extruder head. Material is loaded into the barrel by manual or mechanical means and vacuum is applied to eliminate air from the system. The material is extruded by means of an hydraulically powered ram, with the hydraulic (oil) fluid being passed through a special valve system to sense changes in the plasticity of the material and compensate ram pressure to achieve an even extrusion through the hole. A multispeed cutter mounted on a fly wheel severs the extrudate at the die face. The volume of the extrudate is a function of the cut speed and the set ram speed, and can be controlled to a high degree of accuracy within ±1%. A continuous operation is possible with the help of a twin barrel and ram arrangement in which material is fed to each barrel in turn by a screw system. Various sizes of extruder are available, from 4.5-L barrel capacity up to 80 L, offering production rates up to a maximum of 800 kg/h.

Choice of extruder

The selection of the extruder design is based on the principal requirements of the extrudate and the nature of further processing. For the production of uniform granules to be dried in a fluid-bed drier, a low-compaction system, such as that provided by the various types of screen extruders may be suitable. Cylinder or gear-type extruders may be more appropriate when aiming for a densified extrudate, such as that required for spheronization. Ram-extrusion systems, which allow precision control of extrudate density, size, and shape, are ideal for the extrusion and forming of pharmaceutical polymers of the type used for subdermal implants.

Consideration should be given to the availability of small-scale equipment, which is vital for development work prior to scale-up on pilot- or production-scale machines. Equipment choice is not necessarily based on maximum throughput rate, since the subsequent processing stages (e.g., cutting, spheronization, and drying) are batch processes and are therefore, a rate-limiting factor in production. Since extrusion is a continuous process, it allows adequate production rates for most purposes with any of the above mentioned extruder types.

The equipment must comply with the code of Good Manufacturing Practice (GMP) standards within the

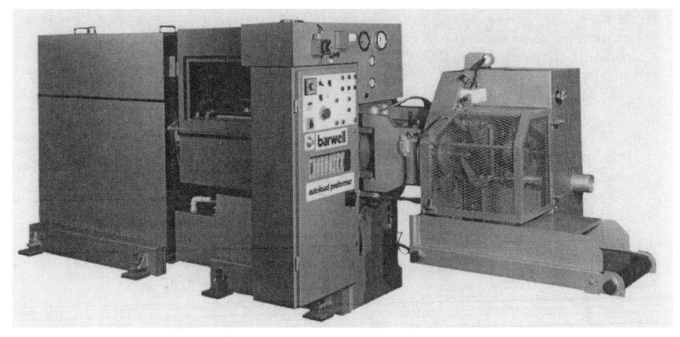

Fig. 14 The Barwell ram extruder.

pharmaceutical industry. Machines should be constructed of durable material with smooth surfaces to discourage adhesion of extraneous material and facilitate cleaning. Materials used for equipment construction must not affect the product. They should be corrosion resistant and able to withstand cleaning disinfectants. All surfaces and parts in contact with the product must therefore be of high-grade stainless steel and designed to exclude contamination of process material or product by lubricant during manufacture. Controls should be accessible by means of recessed contact buttons.

NOMENCLATURE

A_0	initial cross-sectional area
A	die cross-sectional area
C	compliance
D	die diameter
D_0	barrel diameter
$(dv/dr)_w$	rate of shear at the die wall
ESR	tensile stretch rate
EV	apparent elongational viscosity
K	power law viscosity constant
L	length of capillary (die)
n	degree of non-Newtonian flow (power law index)
n_b	Bagely entrance correction
P	pressure drop along die
P_e	die exit pressure
P_0	upstream pressure loss
P_{0_w}	pressure drop at zero velocity
P_T	total pressure drop
P_{t_v}	pressure drop at velocity v
Q	volumetric flow rate of extradate
R	radius of capillary (die)
RS	recoverable shear
T	tensile stress
U	plastic viscosity
V	extrudate velocity
x	thickness of Newton liquid layer
α	die entry yield stress velocity factor
β	die and velocity factor
γ	rate of shear
η	apparent viscosity
σ_y	yield value
σ_{y_0}	yield value at zero velocity
θ	half angle of convergence
τ	shear stress
τ_0	die wall shear stress at zero velocity
τ_w	die wall shear stress
τ_y	shear stress to be exceeded before flow commences

REFERENCES

1. Bagley, E.B. J. Appl. Phys. **1957**, *28*, 624–627.
2. Han, C.D.; Charles, M. Trans. Soc. Rheol. **1971**, *15*, 371–384.
3. Harrison, P.J. *Extrusion of Wet Powder Masses*; University of London: 1982.
4. Jastrzebski, Z.D. I & E C Fundamentals, **1967**, *6*(3), 445–454.
5. Wilkinson, W. *Non-Newtonian Fluids*; Pergamon Press: London, 1960.
6. Harrison, P.J.; Newton, J.M.; Rowe, R.C. J. Pharm. Pharmacol. **1984**, *36*, 796–798.
7. Benbow, J.J.; Ovenston, A. Trans. Br. Cer. Soc. **1968**, *67*, 543–567.
8. Benbow, J.J. Chem. Eng. Sci. **1971**, *26*, 1467–1473.
9. Benbow, J.J.; Oxley, E.W.; Bridgwater, J. Chem. Eng. Sci. **1987**, *42*, 2151–2162.
10. Benbow, J.J.; Bridgwater, J. Chem. Eng. Sci. **1987**, *42*, 915–919.
11. Cohan, R.K.; Newton, J.M. Int. J. Pharm. **1996**, *131*, 201–207.
12. Cogswell, F. Polym. Eng. Sci. **1972**, *12*, 64–72.
13. Bealy, J.M.; Wisbren, K. *Rheology of Molten Plastics Processing*; Van Norstrand: New York, 1990.
14. Chohan, R.K. J. Appl. Polym. Sci. **1994**, *54*, 487–494.
15. Beart, L.; Remon, J.P.; Knight, P.; Newton, J.M. Int. J. Pharm. **1992**, *86*, 187–192.
16. Tomer, G.; Newton, J.M. Int. J. Pharm. **1999**, *182*, 71–77.
17. Tomer, G.; Newton, J.M.; Kinechesh, P. Pharm. Res. **1999**, *16*, 666–671.
18. Tomer, G.; Mantle, M.D.; Gledden, L.F.; Newton, J.M. Int. J. Pharm. **1999**, *189*, 19–28.
19. Harrison, P.J.; Newton, J.M.; Rowe, R.C. J. Pharm. Pharmacol. **1985**, *37*, 81–83.
20. Raines, C.L.; Newton, J.M.; Rowe, R.C. Extrusion of Microcrystalline Cellulose. *Rheology of Food, Pharmaceutical and Biological Materials with General Rheology*; Carter, R.E., Ed.; Elsevier Applied Science: London, 1990; 268–287.
21. Harrison, P.J.; Newton, J.M.; Rowe, R.C. J. Pharm. Pharmacol. **1984**, *36*, 796–798.
22. Fielden, K.E. *Extrusion and Spheronization of Microcrystalline Cellulose/Lactose Mixtures*; University of London: 1987.
23. Newton, J.M. Extrusion/Spheronization. *Powder Technology and Pharmaceutical Processing*; Ghulia, D., Delevil, M., Paercelt, Y., Eds.; Elsevier Biomedical: Amsterdam, 1994; 391–401.
24. Battiste, O.A. *Microcrystalline Polymer Science*; McGraw-Hill: London, 1975.
25. Basit, A.; Newton, J.M.; Lacey, L.F. Pharm. Dev. Tech. **1999**, *4*, 499–505.
26. Tufvesson, C.; Lindberg, N.O.; Olbjer, L. Drug Develop. Ind. Pharm. **1987**, *13* (9–11), 1891–1913.
27. Jover, I.; Podczeck, F.; Newton, J.M. J. Pharm. Sci. **1990**, *85*, 700–705.
28. Lustig-Gustafsson, C.; Johal, H.K.; Podczeck, F.; Newton, J.M. Eur. J. Pharm. **1999**, *8*, 147–152.
29. Johnson, P.S. *Developments in Extrusion Science and Technology*; Polysay Ltd.: South Samia, Ontario, Canada, 1982.
30. *The Dynisco Extrusion Processors Handbook*; Whelan, T., Dunning, D., Eds.; London School of Polymer Technology, Polytechnic of North London: London, 1988.
31. Smoluk, U.R. Modern Plastics Mt. **1988**, *18* (12), 49–56.
32. Schott, H. Polymer Science. *Physical Pharmacy—Physical Chemical Principles in the Pharmaceutical Sciences*; Martin, A., Swarbrick, J., Cammarata, A., Eds.; Ch. 22; Lea & Febiger: Philadelphia, 1983.
33. Giles, R.L.; Pecina, R.W. Plastic Packaging Materials. *Remmingtons Pharmaceutical Sciences*; Gennaro, A.R., Ed.; Ch. 81; Mack Publishing Co.: Easton, PA, 1985.
34. Senouci, A.; Smith, A.; Richmond, P. Chem. Eng. **1985**, *417*, 30–33.
35. Owusu-Ansah, J.; Van de Voort, F.R.; Stanley, D.W. Can. Inst. Food Sci. Technol. I. **1984**, *17* (2), 65–70.
36. Remsen, C.H.; Clark, J.P. J. Food Process Eng. **1978**, *2*, 39–64.
37. Harmann, D.V.; Harper, J.M. Food Sci. **1974**, *39*, 1009–1104.
38. Harper, J.M. Crit. Rev. Food Sci. Nutr. **1979**, *11* (2), 155–215.
39. Fletcher, S.I.; McMaster, T.J.; Richmond, P.; Smith, A.C. Chem. Eng. Cornmun. **1985**, *32*, 239–262.
40. Sebestyen, E. Flour and Animal Feed Milling **1974**, *156* Oct, 24–25, Nov. 1974, 22–25; Dec. 1974, 16–18.
41. Young, L.R.; Pfost, H.B.; Feyerherm, A.M. Trans. Am. Soc. Agr. Eng. **1963**, *50*, 144–151.
42. Payne, J.D. Milling Feed Fert. **1978**, *161*, 34–41.
43. Anschel, J.; Lieberman, H.A. Suppositories. *The Theory and Practice of Industrial Pharmacy*; Lachman, L., Lieberman, H.A., Kanig, J.L., Eds.; Ch. 8; Lea & Febiger: Philadelphia, 1976.
44. Hadgraft, J.W. Rectal Administration. In *Bentley's Textbook of Pharmaceutics*; Rawlins, E.A., Ed.; Ch. 25; Bailliere Tindall: London, 1977.

FILTERS AND FILTRATION

Maik W. Jornitz

Sartorius Group, Germany

INTRODUCTION

The separative process of filtration is widely used within the biopharmaceutical industry to remove contaminants from liquids, air, and gases, such as particulate matter but especially microorganisms. Microorganism removal is either required to achieve a sterile filtrate or, if the pharmaceutical product is thermally sterilized, to reduce the bioburden and, therefore, avoid elevated levels of endotoxins—the debris of gram-negative organisms (1).

There are many filter configurations within the industry, such as sheet or modular depth filter types for prefiltration purposes, flat filter membranes mainly for microbial detection and,specifications, and, most commonly, filter cartridges containing either depth filter fleeces or membrane filters. Such membrane filters are available in a large variety of membrane polymers for different applications. These materials are discussed later in the chapter.

Sterilizing grade membrane filters are defined by the FDA Guideline on Sterile Drug Products Produced by Aseptic Processing (2) by being able to retain 10^7 Brevundimonas diminuta (formerly Pseudomonas diminuta) organisms per square centimeter of filtration area at a differential pressure of 2 bar (3). Such retention efficiency has to be validated, using the actual drug product and the process parameters, due to the possibility of an effect to the filters compatibility and stability and/or the microorganisms size and survival rate (4, 5). Performing these so-called product bacteria challenge tests became a regulatory demand (6) and, therefore, belong to a standard filter validation. Before these challenge tests can be performed, several parameters, for example, bactericidal effects of the product, have to be evaluated. The recently published PDA Technical Report 26 (7) describes the individual parameters—the possible effects and mechanisms to be used to perform challenge tests. Additionally, the report discusses filtration modes, sterilization, and integrity testing.

FILTER TYPES

One can differentiate filters in different distinctive types, commonly in membrane and depth filters. Depth filters retain contaminants within the depth of the filter matrix. Contaminants have to move through the tortuous path of the fiber matrix and eventually will collide with a fiber and separate from the medium. Due to the depth retention, such filters have a very high dirt-load capacity and are able to separate a high load of contaminants of different sizes. Depth filters are utilized for coarse particle removal, polishing filtration, and, especially, to protect final membrane filters reverse osmosis or deionizing units. Depth filters can greatly enhance the membrane filter's total throughput capability. Therefore, before utilizing a filtration process in a new application, filterability trials are commonly performed to evaluate the optimal prefilter–final filter combination to achieve the lowest cost per liter ratio and highest yield. Initial filterability tests are done with 47-mm composites (flat filter discs of the filter cartridge device to be used). Having found the optimal combination of prefilter retention to final filters pore size, pleated small-scale devices are used to achieve appropriate filter sizing parameters. Filterability trials are performed with automatic test rigs, which utilize a balance as a load cell to measure the filtrate collected. Commonly, the balance is connected to a computer system, which uses a specific software showing the flow rate, total throughput, and differential pressure graphs and offer a report including such.

As depth filters retain contaminants within the fiber matrix, membrane filters are surface retentive filters and, therefore, have the distinct disadvantage to clog faster. The filter industry, therefore, pleats such membranes to install a higher effective filtration area into a filter device. Still, such effort has its limitation, due to a maximum allowable pleat density. Having reached the limit, the only option is the use of prefilters or membranes of different pore sizes to gain a fractionate retention and, therefore, a prolonged lifetime of the filter. Some membrane filter configurations have such membrane or depth filter prefilters built into the filter cartridge. This is convenient for the filter user in respect to lowered hardware costs. Additional prefilter housings are not necessary. In comparison to depth filters, membrane filters have a narrow pore size distribution, which results in a by far sharper retention rate. Pore size ratings are facilitated to differentiate membrane filters

Copyright © 2002 by Marcel Dekker, Inc. All rights reserved.

and the performance of such. Commonly, a sterilizing grade filter is labeled 0.2 μm when it retains 10^7 B.diminuta/cm^2. Another advantage and necessity of membrane filters is the fact that these are integrity testable. Therefore, flaws or defects can be detected, which is critical, due to the function of membrane filters, mainly in separating microorganisms from pharmaceutical solutions.

Membrane filters are made in a wide variety of pore sizes (Fig. 1). The effective pore size for membranes vary, and membranes can be used in reverse osmosis (RO), nanofiltration (NF), ultrafiltration (UF), and microfiltration (MF). RO membranes are widely used in water treatment to remove ionic contaminations from the water. These membranes have an extreme small pore size and, therefore, require excellent pretreatment steps to reduce any fouling or scaling of the membrane, which would reduce the service lifetime. RO membranes are used by extensive pressures on the upstream side of the filter membrane to force the liquids through the pores.

The retention ratings of UF filters are also not measured in pore size but rather in MWCO (molecular weight cut-off), i.e., the molecular weight of the substance to be retained. UF filter systems are most often used in cross-flow (tangential flow) systems. The feed stream is directed over the actual membrane to diminish blockage of the membrane. Depending on the pressure conditions, the fluid (permeate) penetrates through the membrane, whereby the remaining fluid is recirculated (retentate). UF filter systems find applications in concentration, diafiltration, and removal steps within pharmaceutical downstream processing. MF can be used as dead-end filtration (the feed is directed to the membrane, resulting into a filtrate, separated from the contaminant) or tangential flow mode. The tangential flow characteristic for MF is commonly used for cell or cell debris removal in downstream processing. MF membranes typically differ from UF membranes in

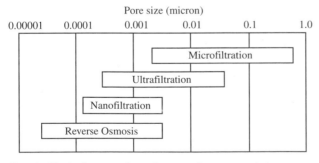

Fig. 1 Typical pore sizes for membranes used in reverse osmosis, nanofiltration, ultrafiltration, and microfiltration.

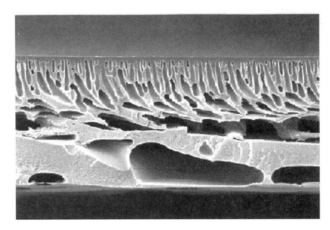

Fig. 2 Skin layer structure of a UF membrane. (Courtesy of Sartorius AG.)

the morphology of the membrane's cross-sectional cut. The symmetry of sterilizing-grade microfilters usually ranges from being uniform to being slightly asymmetric. Ultrafilters, on the other hand, are highly asymmetric, with the rejecting layer consisting of a tight skin (0.5–10 to μm thick) supported by a thick spongy structure of a much larger pore size (Fig. 2).

MF is used in a large variety of filtration applications, from fine cut prefiltration to sterilizing grade filtration in aseptic processing. Often sterilizing grade filters are the terminal step before filling or final processing of the drug product. MF is available for air and gas applications and liquid clarification or sterilization. For the different applications, specific membrane configurations and materials have been developed.

FILTER MATERIALS

There are a variety of different depth filter and membrane filter materials used within the pharmaceutical processes. Depth filter are fibrous materials: for example, Polypropylene, Borosilicate, or Glassfibre fleeces (Fig. 3). Borosilicate and Glassfibre materials are highly adsorptive and commonly used to remove colloidal substances, like iron oxide from water or colloidal haze from sugar solutions.

Prefilters can also contain membranes instead of fibrous depth filter material. Such membrane material are commonly mixesters of cellulose or pure cellulose acetate. The cellulose mixester filter material contains a high degree of cellulose nitrate, which again is highly adsorptive. Such prefilters have a very sharp retention rating and, therefore, are used in applications in which the

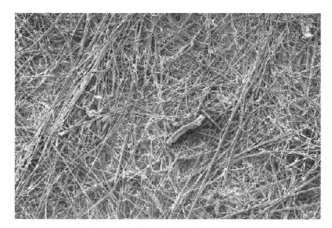

Fig. 3 SEM of the random fiber matrix of a depth filter. (Courtesy of Sartorius AG.)

contaminant has a narrow size distribution and/or a sterilizing grade filter has to be protected, due to the fact that such a filter cannot be changed during the filtration process. Membrane prefilters, when blocked, can be

exchanged during the filtration process, due to the final filter downstream.

Most commercial UF and NF membranes and many MF membranes are made by the phase-inversion process, where a polymer is dissolved in an appropriate solvent along with appropriate pore-forming chemical agents. The polymer solution is cast into a film, either on a backing or freestanding, and then the film is immersed in a nonsolvent solution that causes precipitation of the polymer. Such membranes are Polyamides, such as Nylon, Polyethersulfon (PESU), or Polyvinyldienefluoride (PVDF). Cellulosic membranes, such as cellulose nitrate, acetate, or regenerated cellulose, are casted as a cellulose–water–solvent mixture onto a belt and transported through heated tunnels. The resulting evaporation process produces the porous structure of the membrane seen in Fig. 4.

Other techniques for membrane formation include stretching the polymeric film, commonly Polytetrafluoroethylene (PTFE), while it is still in a flexible state and then annealing the membrane to "lock in" and strengthen the

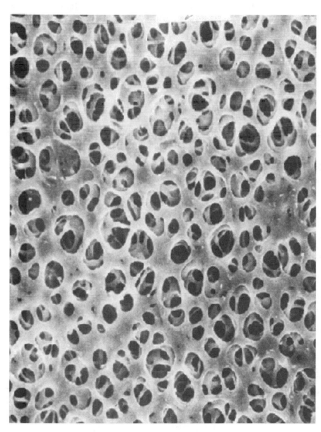

Fig. 4 Porous structure of Celluloseacetate. (Courtesy of Sartorius AG.)

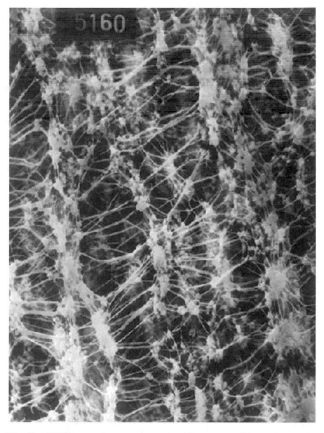

Fig. 5 PTFE membrane structure. (Courtesy of Sartorius AG.)

pores in the stretched membrane. The stretching process results into a distinctive membrane structure of PTFE nodes, which are interconnected by fibrils, (Fig. 5).

PTFE membranes are highly hydrophobic and, therefore, are used as air filters. Air filters have to be highly hydrophobic to avoid water blockage due to moisture or condensate, especially after steam sterilization of these filters. Water blockage could be detrimental, if the filter is, for example, used in a tank venting application to overcome condensation vacuum of a nonvacuum resistant tank. If the filter would not allow a free flow of air into the tank, it may implode. Therefore, vent filters for this application have to be chosen and sized with care. PTFE membranes are also highly mechanical and thermal resistant, which is required, because such filters are used over several months, withstanding multiple steam-sterilization cycles. Especially in large-scale fermentation, these filters are used over several months, avoiding unwanted infections of the fermenter's or bioreactor's cell line.

Finally, track-etched MF membranes are made from polymers, such as polycarbonate and polyester, wherein electrons are bombarded onto the polymeric surface. This bombardment results in "sensitized tracks," where chemical bonds in the polymeric backbone are broken. Subsequently, the irradiated film is placed in an etching bath (such as a basic solution), in which the damaged polymer in the tracks is preferentially etched from the film, thereby forming cylindrical pores. The residence time in the irradiator determines pore density, and residence time in the etching bath determines pore size. Membranes made by this process generally have cylindrical pores with very narrow pore-size distribution, albeit with low overall porosity. Furthermore, there always is the risk of a double hit, i.e., the etched pore becomes wider and could result in particulate penetration. Such filter membranes are often used in the electronic industry to filter high-purity water.

Table 1 lists the different membrane polymers available and the advantages and disadvantages, which depend on the properties of the polymer. The table shows that there is no such thing as a membrane polymer for every application. Therefore, filter membranes and the filter performance have to be tested before choosing the appropriate filter element.

FILTER CONSTRUCTION

Filters are available in several constructions, effective filtration areas, and configurations. Depending on the

individual process, the filter construction and setup will be chosen to fit its purpose best. Most commonly used for RO filters are tubular devices, so-called spiral wound modules due to the spiral configuration of the membrane within the support construction of such device. UF systems can be found as a spiral wound module, a hollow fiber, or a cassette device. The choice of the individual construction depends on the requirements and purposes towards the UF device. Similar to the different membrane materials, UF device construction has to be evaluated in the specific applications to reach an optimal functioning of the unit. Microfilters and depth filters can be lenticular modules or sheets but are mainly cylindrical filter elements of various sizes and filtration areas, from very small scale of 300 cm^2 to large scale devices of 36 m^2. A 10-inch high cylindrical filter element can be seen in Fig. 6.

These filter elements are installed into stainless steel filter housings by pushing the double O-ring cartridge adapter into the housing base plate recess. The filter housing is then assembled and connected, and the filter is flushed with water and steam-sterilized, either by in-line steaming or autoclaved. If filter housings are not available or not preferred, disposable filters can be used. The filter element is welded into a plastic housing, usually Polypropylene, and after every filtration process, discarded. The advantage of such a disposable filter device is the reduced cleaning validation effort, and the user does not come in contact with the filtered product. Such disposable filters can be autoclaved, but not in-line steam-sterilized, due to the pressure–temperature ratio of the housing polymer. Most often, such disposable filters are used for scale-up filtration tests, due to the ease of use and the availability of a band of effective filtration areas.

FILTER VALIDATION

Pharmaceutical processes are validated processes to assure a reproducible product within set specifications. Equally important is the validation of the filters used within the process, especially the sterilizing grade filters, which, often enough, are used before filling or the final processing of the drug product. In its Guideline on General Principles of Process Validation, 1985 (8), and Guideline on Sterile Drug Products Produced by Aseptic Processing, 1987 (2), the FDA makes plain that the validation of sterile processes is required by the manufacturers of sterile products.

Sterilizing grade filters are determined by the bacteria challenge test. This test is performed under strict

Table 1 Advantages and disadvantages of various membrane polymers

Membrane material	Advantages	Disadvantages
Cellulose acetate	Very low nonspecific adsorption (nonfouling) High flow rates and total throughputs	Limited pH compatibility Not dry autoclavable
Cellulose nitrate (nitrocellulose)	Good flow rate and total throughputs	High nonspecific adsorption Limited pH compatibility Not dry autoclavable
Regenerated cellulose	Very low nonspecific adsorption (nonfouling) Very high flow rates and total throughputs	Limited pH compatibility Not dry autoclavable
Modified regenerated cellulose	Very low nonspecific adsorption (nonfouling) Moderate flow rates and total throughputs, especially with difficult to filter solutions Broad pH compatibility	Ultrafilters not dry autoclavable
Nylon 66	Good solvent compatibility Good mechanical strength Broad pH compatibility Dry autoclavable	High nonspecific protein adsorption Low hot-water resistance Moderate flow rate and total throughput
Polycarbonate	Good chemical compatibility	Moderate flow rates Low total throughputs Difficult to produce
Polyethersulfone	High flow rates and total throughputs Broad pH compatibility	Moderate-to-low nonspecific adsorption, depending on surface modifications. Limited solvent compatibility

(Continued)

Table 1 Advantages and disadvantages of various membrane polymers (*Continued*)

Membrane material	Advantages	Disadvantages
Polypropylene	Excellent chemical resistance High mechanical resistance	Hydrophobic material High nonspecific adsorption due to hydrophobic interactions
Polysulfone	High flow rates and total throughputs Broad pH compatibility	Moderate-to-high nonspecific adsorption Limited solvent compatibility
Polytetrafluoro-ethylene	Excellent chemical resistance High mechanical resistance	Hydrophobic material High nonspecific adsorption due to hydrophobic interactions High-cost filter material
Polyvinylidene-difluoride	Low nonspecific adsorption Dry autoclavable Good solvent compatibility	Moderate flow rate and total throughput Hydrophobic base, made hydrophilic by chemical surface treatment; may lose hydrophilic modification due to chemical attack High-cost filter material

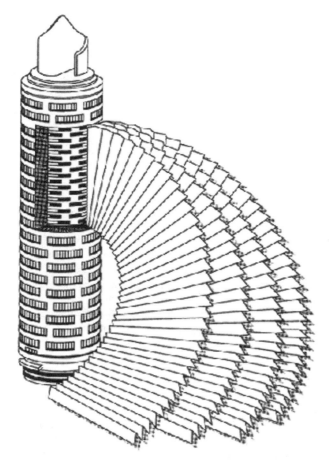

Fig. 6 10-inch standard filter element with pleated membrane and protection fleeces. (Courtesy of Sartorius AG.)

parameters and a defined solution (ASTM F 838-83) (3). In any case, the FDA nowadays also requires evidence that the sterilizing grade filter will create a sterile filtration, no matter the process, fluid or bioburden, found (6, 9). This means that bacteria challenge tests have to be performed with the actual drug product, bioburden, if different or known to be smaller than B. diminuta and the process parameters. The reason for the requirement of a product bacteria challenge test is threefold. First, the influence of the product and process parameters to the microorganism has to be tested. There may be cases of either shrinkage of organisms due to a higher osmolarity of the product or prolonged processing times. Second, the filter's compatibility with the product and the parameters has to be tested. The filter should not show any sign of degradation due to the product filtered. Additionally, rest assurance is required that the filter used will withstand the process parameters; e.g., pressure pulses, if happening, should not influence the filter's performance. Third, there are two

separation mechanisms involved in liquid filtration: sieve retention and retention by adsorptive sequestration (1, 8, 10–12). In sieve retention, the smallest particle or organism size is retained by the biggest pore within the membrane structure. The contaminant will be retained, no matter the process parameters. This is the ideal. Retention by adsorptive sequestration depends on the filtration conditions. Contaminants smaller than the actual pore size penetrate such and may be captured by adsorptive attachment to the pore wall. This effect is enhanced using highly adsorptive filter materials, for example, Glassfibre as a prefilter or Polyamide as a membrane. Nevertheless, certain liquid properties can minimize the adsorptive effect, which could mean penetration of organisms. Whether the fluid has such properties and will lower the effect of adsorptive sequestration and may eventually cause penetration has to be evaluated in specific product bacteria challenge tests. Table 2 shows the advantages and disadvantage of both separation mechanisms.

Before performing a product bacteria challenge test, it has to be assured that the liquid product does not have any detrimental, bactericidal or bacteriostatic, effects on the challenge organisms. This is done utilizing viability tests. The organism is inoculated into the product to be filtered at a certain bioburden level. At specified times, the log value of this bioburden is tested. If the bioburden is reduced due to the fluid properties, a different bacteria challenge test mode becomes applicable (7). If the reduction is a slow process, the challenge test will be performed with a higher bioburden, bearing in mind that the challenge level has to reach 10^7 per square centimeter at the end of the processing time. If the mortality rate is too high, the toxic substance is either removed or product properties are changed. This challenge fluid is called a placebo. Another methodology would circulate the fluid product through the filter at the specific process parameters as long as the actual processing time would be. Afterwards, the filter is flushed extensively with water and the challenge test, as described in ASTM F838-38, performed. Nevertheless, such a challenge test procedure would be more or less a filter compatibility test.

Besides the product bacteria challenge test, tests of extractable substances or particulate releases have to be performed (7, 8, 13). Extractable measurements and the resulting data are available from filter manufacturers for the individual filters. Nevertheless, depending on the process conditions and the solvents used, explicit extractable tests have to be performed. These tests are commonly done only with the solvent used with the drug product but not with the drug ingredients themselves, because the drug product usually covers any extractables during measurement. Such

Table 2 Advantanges and disadvantages of separation mechanisms

Retention mechanism	Advantages	Disadvantages
Sieve retention	Reliable at worst case product properties Reliable separation even at high flows and pressure conditions Blockage, i.e., exhaustion, can be determined No unspecific adsorption, minimal loss of desired product, and little adsorptive fouling	Retentive only at the specific pore size rating
Adsorptive sequestration	It is possible to retain particles smaller than the filter's indicated pore size Separation of colloidal substances is possible In some case, pyrogens can be removed	Highly influenced by product specific properties Separated particles can be shed by varying process conditions Saturation of the active sites cannot be determined, no warning Unspecific adsorption will result in product losses and fouling Lower reliability in terms of absolute separation

tests are conducted by the validation services of the filter manufacturers using sophisticated separation and detection methodologies, as GC-MS, FTIR, and RP-HPLC. These methodologies are required, due to the fact that the individual components possibly released from the filter have to be identified and quantified. Elaborate studies, performed by filter manufacturers, showed that there is neither a release of high quantities of extractables (the range is ppb to max ppm per 10-inch element) nor have toxic substances been found (13).

Particulates are critical in sterile filtration, specifically of injectables. The USP 24 (*United States Pharmacopoeia*) and BP (*British Pharmacopoeia*) quote specific limits of particulate level contaminations for defined particle sizes. These limits have to be kept and, therefore, the particulate release of sterilizing grade filters has to meet these requirements. Filters are routinely tested by evaluating the filtrate with laser particle counters. Such tests are also performed with the actual product under process conditions to proove that the product, but especially process conditions, do not result in an increased level of particulates within the filtrate.

Additionally, with certain products, loss of yield or product ingredients due to adsorption shall be determined (14, 15). For example, preservatives, like benzalkoniumchloride or chlorhexadine, can be adsorbed by specific filter membranes. Such membranes need to be saturated by the preservative to avoid preservative loss within the actual product. This preservative loss, e.g., in contact lens solutions, can be detrimental, due to long-term use of such solutions. Similarly, problematic would be the adsorption of required proteins within a biological solution. To optimize the yield of such proteins within an application, adsorption trials have to be performed to find the optimal membrane material and filter construction.

Cases that use the actual product as a wetting agent to perform integrity tests require the evaluation of product integrity test limits (7, 17). The product can have an influence on the measured integrity test values due to surface tension, or solubility. A lower surface tension, for example, would shift the bubble point value to a lower pressure and could result in a false negative test. The solubility of gas into the product could be reduced, which could result in false positive diffusive flow tests. Therefore, a correlation of the product as a wetting agent to the, water wet values has to be done, according to standards set by the manufacturer of the filter. This correlation is carried out by using a minimum of three filters of three filter lots. Depending on the product and its variability, one or three product lots are used to perform the correlation. The accuracy of such a correlation is enhanced by automatic integrity test machines. These test machines measure with highest accuracy and sensitivity and do not rely on human judgement, as with a manual test (7). Multipoint diffusion testing offers the ability to test the filter's performance and, especially, to plot the entire diffusive flow graph through the bubble point. The individual graphs for a water-wet integrity test can now be compared to the product wet test and a possible shift evaluated. Furthermore, the multipoint diffusion test enables the establishment of an improved statistical base to determine the product wet versus water-wet limits (16, 17).

FILTER INTEGRITY TESTING

Sterilizing grade filters require testing to assure the filters are integral and fulfill their purpose. Such filter tests are called integrity tests and are performed before and after the filtration process. Sterilizing grade filtration would not be admitted to a process if the filter would not be integrity tested in the course of the process. This fact is also established in several guidelines, recommending the use of integrity testing, pre- and post-filtration. This is not only valid for liquid but also for air filters.

Examples of such guidelines are:

1. FDA *Guideline on Sterile Drug Products Produced by Aseptic Processing* (1987): Normally, integrity testing of the filter is performed after the filter unit is assembled and prior to use. More importantly however, such testing should be conducted after the filter is used in order to detect any filter leaks or perforations that may have occurred during filtration.

2. *The Guide to Inspections of High Purity Water Systems, Guide to Inspections of Lyophilization of Parenterals*, and also the CGMP document 212.721 Filters state the following:

   a. The integrity of all air filters shall be verified upon installation and maintained throughout use. A written testing program adequate to monitor integrity of filters shall be established and followed. Results shall be recorded and maintained as specified in 212.83.
   b. Solution filters shall be sterilized and installed aseptically. The integrity of solution filters shall be verified by an appropriate test, both prior to any large-volume parenteral solution filtering operation and at the conclusion of such operation before the filters are discarded. If the filter assembly fails the test at the conclusion of the filtering operation, all materials filtered through it during that filtering operation should be rejected. Rejected materials may be refiltered using filters

whose integrity has been verified provided that the additional time required for refiltration does not result in a total process time that exceeds the limitations specified in 212.111. Results of each test shall be recorded and maintained as required in 212.188(a)

3. ISO 13408-1 *First Edition, 1998-08-1, Aseptic Processing of Health Care Products*, Part 1: General requirements: Section 17.11.1 Investigation, m. pre- and post-filter integrity test data, and/or filter housing assembly:

   20.3.1. A validated physical integrity test of a process filter shall be conducted after use without disturbing the filter housing assembly. Filter manufacturer's testing instructions or recommendations may be used as a basis for a validated method. Physical integrity testing of a process filter should be conducted before use where process conditions permit. "Diffusive Flow," "Pressure Hold," and "Bubble Point" are acceptable physical integrity tests.
   20.3.2. The ability of the filter or housing to maintain integrity in response to sterilization and gas or liquid flow (including pressure surges and flow variations) shall be determined.

4. USP 23, 1995, P. 1979. *Guide to Good Pharmaceutical Manufacturing Practice* (Orange Guide, U.K., 1983):

   PDA (Parenteral Drug Association), Technical Report No. 26, *Sterilizing Filtration of Liquids* (March 1998):

Integrity tests, such as the diffusive flow, pressure hold, bubble point, or water intrusion tests, are nondestructive tests, which are correlated to the destructive bacteria challenge test with $10^7/cm^2$ B. diminuta (1, 8). Derived from these challenge tests, specific integrity test limits are established, which are described and documented within the filter manufacturers' literature. The limits are water-based; i.e., the integrity test correlations are performed using water as a wetting medium. If a different wetting fluid, such as a filter or membrane configuration, is used, the integrity test limits may vary. Integrity test measurements depend on the surface area of the filter, the polymer of the membrane, the wetting fluid, the pore size of the membrane, and the gas used to perform the test. Wetting fluids may have different surface tensions, which can depress or elevate the bubble point pressure. The use of different test gases may elevate the diffusive gas flow. Therefore, appropriate filter validation has to be established to determine the appropriate integrity test limits for the individual process.

Bubble Point Test

Microporous membranes will fill their pores with wetting fluids by imbibing that fluid in accordance with the laws of capillary rise. The retained fluid can be forced from the filter pores by air pressure applied from the upstream side. The pressure is increased gradually in increments. At a certain pressure level, liquid will be forced first from the set of largest pores, in keeping with the inverse relationship of the applied air pressure P and the diameter of the pore, d, described in the bubble point equation:

$$P = \frac{4\gamma \cos \theta}{d} \qquad (1)$$

where γ is the surface tension of the fluid, θ is the wetting angle, P is the upstream pressure at which the largest pore will be freed of liquid, and d is the diameter of the largest pore.

When the wetting fluid is expelled from the largest pore, a bulk gas flow will be detected on the downstream side of the filter system (Fig. 7). The bubble point measurement determines the pore size of the filter membrane, i.e., the larger the pore the lower the bubble point pressure. Therefore, filter manufacturers specify the

bubble point limits as the minimum allowable bubble point. During an integrity test, the bubble point test has to exceed the set minimum bubble point.

Diffusion Test

A completely wetted filter membrane provides a liquid layer across which, when a differential pressure is applied, the diffusive airflow occurs in accordance with Fick's law of diffusion (Fig. 8). This pressure is called test pressure and commonly specified at 80% of the bubble point pressure. In an experimental elucidation of the factors involved in the process, Reti (18) simplified the integrated form of Fick's law to read as follows:

$$N = \frac{DH(p_1 - p_2)}{L} \cdot \rho$$

where N is the permeation rate (moles of gas per unit time), D is the diffusivity of the gas in the liquid, H is the solubility coefficient of the gas, L is the thickness of liquid in the membrane (equal to the membrane thickness if the membrane pores are completely filled with liquid), P ($p_1 - p_2$) is the differential pressure, and ρ is the void volume of the membrane, its membrane porosity, commonly around 80%.

The size of pores only enter indirectly into the equation; in their combination, they comprise L, the thickness of the

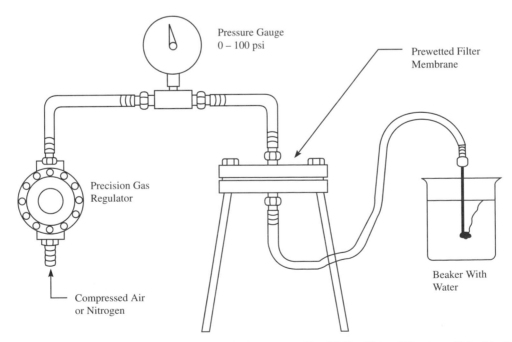

Fig. 7 Manual bubble point test set-up. (Reprinted from Technical Report No. 26, Sterilizing Filtration of Liquids © 1998 by PDA.)

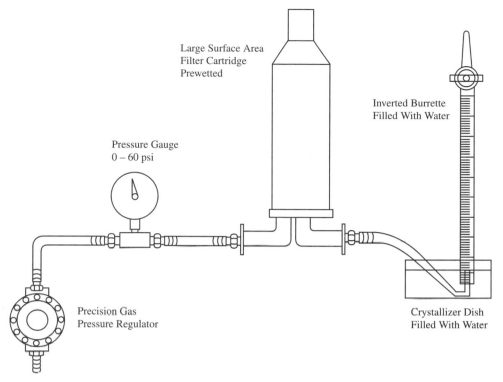

Fig. 8 Manual diffusive flow test set-up. (Reprinted from Technical Report No. 26, Sterilizing Filtration of Liquids © 1998 by PDA.)

liquid layer, the membrane being some 80% porous. The critical measurement of a flaw is the thickness of the liquid layer. Therefore, a flaw or an oversized pore would be measured by the thinning of the liquid layer due to the elevated test pressure on the upstream side. The pore or defect may not be large enough that the bubble point comes into effect, but the test pressure thins the liquid layer enough to result into an elevated gas flow. Therefore, filter manufacturers specify the diffusive flow integrity test limits as maximum allowable diffusion value. The larger the flaw or a combination of flaw, the higher the diffusive flow.

Pressure Hold Test

The pressure hold test is a variant of the diffusive airflow test (19). The test set-up is arranged as in the diffusion test except that when the stipulated applied pressure is reached, the pressure source is valved off (Fig. 9). The decay of pressure within the holder is then observed as a function of time, using a precision pressure gauge or pressure transducer.

The decrease in pressure can come from two sources: 1) the diffusive loss across the wetted filter. Because the upstream side pressure in the holder is constant, it decreases progressively as all the while diffusion takes place through the wetted membrane; and 2) the source of pressure decay could be a leak of the filter system set-up.

An important influence on the measurement of the pressure hold test is the upstream air volume within the filter system. This volume has to be determined first to specify the maximum allowable pressure drop value. The larger the upstream volume, the lower will the pressure drop be. The smaller the upstream volume, the larger the pressure drop. This also means an increase in the sensitivity of the test, and also an increase of temperature influences, if changes occur. Filter manufacturers specify maximum allowable pressure drop values.

Water Intrusion Test

The water intrusion test is used for hydrophobic vent and air membrane filters only (20–23). The upstream side of the hydrophobic filter cartridge housing is flooded with water. The water will not flow through the hydrophobic membrane. Air or nitrogen gas pressure is then applied to the upstream side of the filter housing above the water level to a defined test pressure. This is done by way of an automatic integrity tester. A period of pressure stabilization takes place over time frame, by the filter manufacturer's recommendation, during which the

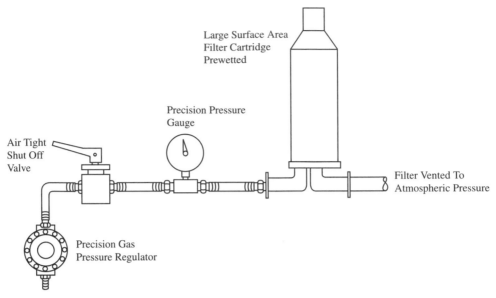

Fig. 9   Manual pressure-hold test set-up. (Reprinted from Technical Report No. 26, Sterilizing Filtration of Liquids © 1998 by PDA.)

cartridge pleats adjust their positions under imposed pressures. After the pressure drop thus occasioned stabilizes, the test time starts, and any further pressure drop in the upstream pressurized gas volume, as measured by the automatic tester, signifies a beginning of water intrusion into the largest (hydrophobic) pores, water being incompressible. The automated integrity tester is sensitive enough to detect the pressure drop. This measured pressure drop is converted into a measured intrusion value, which is compared to a set intrusion limit, which has been correlated to the bacteria challenge test. As with the diffusive flow test, filter manufacturers specify a maximum allowable water intrusion value. Above this value, a hydrophobic membrane filter is classified as nonintegral.

REFERENCES

1. *Filtration in the Biopharmaceutical Industry*; Meltzer, T.H., Jornitz, M.W., Eds.; Marcel Dekker, Inc.: New York, 1998.
2. FDA, Center for Drugs and Biologics and Office of Regulatory Affairs. *Guideline on Sterile Drug Products Produced by Aseptic Processing*; 1987.
3. *Standard Test Method for Determining Bacterial Retention of Membrane Filters Utilized for Liquid Filtration, Standard F838-83*; Revised 1988 American Society for Testing and Materials (ASTM), 1983.
4. Meltzer, T.H.; Jornitz, M.W.; Mittelman, M.W. Surrogate Solution Attributes and Use Conditions: Effects on Bacterial Cell Size and Surface Charges Relevant to Filter Validation Studies. PDA J. Sci. Technol. **Jan/Feb 1998**, *52* (1).
5. Levy, R.V. The Effect of PH, Viscosity, and Additives on the Bacterial Retention of Membrane Filters Challenged With Pseudomonas Diminuta. In *Fluid Filtration: Liquid*; American Society for Testing and Materials (ASTM): Washington DC, 1987; II.
6. *Validation of Microbial Retention of Sterilizing Filters*; PDA Special Scientific Forum: Bethesda, MD, July 1995; 12–13.
7. Technical Report No. 26, Sterilizing Filtration of Liquids. PDA J. Pharm. Sci. Technol. **1998**, *52* (S1).
8. FDA, Center for Drugs and Biologicals and Office of Regulatory Affairs. *Guideline on General Principles of Process Validation*; Washington, DC, September 1985.
9. Jornitz, M.W.; Meltzer, T.H. *Sterile Filtration—A Practical Approach*; Marcel Dekker, Inc.: New York, 2001.
10. Tanny, G.B.; Strong, D.K.; Presswood, W.G.; Meltzer, T.H. Adsorptive Retention of Pseudomonas Diminuta by Membrane Filters. J. Parent. Drug Assoc. **1979**, *33*, 40–51.
11. Emory, S.F.; Koga, Y.; Azuma, N.; Matsumoto, K. The Effects of Surfactant Types and Latex-Particle Feed Concentration on Membrane Retention. Ultrapure Water **1993**, *10* (2), 41–44.
12. Osumi, M.; Yamada, N.; Toya, M. Bacterial Retention Mechanisms of Membrane Filters. PDA J. Pharm. Sci. Technol. **1996**, *50* (1), 30–34.
13. Reif, O.W.; Sölkner, P.; Rupp, J. Analysis and Evaluation of Filter Cartridge Extractables for Validation in Pharmaceutical Downstream Processing. PDA J. Pharm. Sci. Technol. **1996**, *50*, 399–410.
14. Hawker, J.; Hawker, L.M. Protein Losses During Sterilization by Filtration. Lab. Practises **1975**, *24*, 805–814.

15. Brose, D.J.; Henricksen, G. A Quantitative Analysis of Preservative Adsorption on Microfiltration Membranes. Pharm. Tech Europe **1994**, 42–49.

16. Waibel, P.J.; Jornitz, M.W.; Meltzer, T.H. Diffusive Airflow Integrity Testing. PDA J. Pharm. Sci. Tech. **1996**, *50* (5), 311–316.

17. Jornitz, M.W.; Brose, D.J.; Meltzer, T.H. Experimental Evaluations of Diffusive Airflow Integrity Testing. PDA J. Parenter. Sci. Technol. **1998**, .

18. Reti, A.R. An Assessment of Test Criteria in Evaluating the Performance and Integrity of Sterilizing Filters Bull. J. Parenter. Drug Assoc. **1977**, *31* (4), 187–194.

19. Madsen, R.E., Jr.; Meltzer, T.H. An Interpretation of the Pharmaceutical Industry Survey of Current Sterile Filtration Practices. PDA J. Pharm. Sci. Technol. **1998**, *52* (6), 337–339.

20. Jornitz, M.W.; Waibel, P.J.; Meltzer, T.H. The Filter Integrity Correlations. Ultrapure Water **1994 Oct.**, *59–63*.

21. Meltzer, T.H.; Jornitz, M.W.; Waibel, P.J. The Hydrophobic Air Filter and the Water Intrusion Test. Pharm. Tech. **1994**, *18* (9), 76–87.

22. Tarry, S.W.; Henricksen, G.; Prashad, M.; Troeger, H. Integrity Testing of EPTFE Membrane Filter Vents. Ultrapure Water **1993**, *10* (8), 23–30.

23. Tingley, S.; Emory, S.; Walker, S.; Yamada, S. Water-Flow Integrity Testing: A Viable and Valida-table Alternative to Alcohol Testing. Pharm. Tech. **1995**, *19* (10), 138–146.

FLAME PHOTOMETRY

Thomas M. Nowak

Abbott Laboratories, Abbott Park, Illinois

INTRODUCTION

The use of flame photometry as a quantitative tool can be traced to work by Kirchhoff and Bunsen in the early 1860s (1). Its modern history begins, however, in the 1940s, when instruments became available that successfully addressed the problems of reproducible sample introduction and detection. Flame photometry soon developed into a reliable analytical technique for the determination of several cations of pharmaceutical interest, notably sodium, potassium, and lithium. The technique is useful in the analysis of bulk drugs, dosage forms, and clinical samples such as blood and urine.

This article focuses primarily on "traditional" low-temperature flame photometry. High-temperature flame photometry has evolved into separate techniques, typically identified by their temperature sources (e.g., inductively coupled plasma-atomic emission spectrometry, ICP-AES 2). Some references to other related analytical tools, including high-temperature flame photometry, are made here to establish perspective.

PRINCIPLE OF OPERATION

Flame photometry, as with other spectrophotometric techniques, takes advantage of the unique spectral properties of each element when it is energized about its ground state to an excited state. When the energized electrons return to their ground state, they emit light at discrete wavelengths. The emitted light is optically filtered and photometrically detected. Quantification is based on a calibration curve of emission of intensity versus analyte concentration.

The analyte is introduced as a homogeneous solution into the flame as an aerosol. The flame provides sufficient energy to yield free gaseous atoms in the ground state. The amount of energy provided by the flame additionally allows a small faction of available atoms to be energized above the ground state. Typically, the flame is produced using a mixture of air and propane (or air and butane), which provides a temperature of approximatley 1900°C (3). In high-temperature flame photometry, the percentage of atoms is increased. In both high- and low-temperature flame photometry, the atoms of interest are energized as a result of the temperature of the flame, furnace, or plasma. This is in contrast to atomic absorption spectrophotometry, which uses light of a discrete wavelength to energize the analyte atoms. The temperature of the flame in atomic absorption is primarily used to yield a sufficient name of free atoms in their ground state.

The general viability of low-temperature flame photometry depends on two factors. First, the alkali and alkaline earth metals of analytical interest (sodium, potassium, lithium, cesium, rubidium, magnesium, calcium, strontium, and barium) reach their excited states at relatively lower temperatures than do most other elements. Second, the emission wavelengths offer enough resolution such that optical filtering can be accomplished at a relatively low cost.

INSTRUMENTATION AVAILABLE

The first commercially available flame photometer was introduced in the 1940s by the Perkin–Elmer Corporation. In 1948, Beckmann Instruments, Inc., introduced a flame attachment that could be used with their popular model D. U. spectrophotometer (1). By the late 1950s, instruments had been developed that used lithium as an internal standard to maximize precision. Autodilution features and microprocessor-controlled operations became widely used options in the 1970s. The most recent significant development was the introduction of cesium as the internal standard, by Instrumentation Laboratory, Inc. (Figs. 1–3). This development makes concurrent lithium determinations more practical.

With the use of fuels that produced hotter flames, earlier flame photometers became useful for analyzing elements beyond the alkali and alkaline earth metals. The development of atomic absorption spectrophotometers in the late 1960s provided the analytical chemist with a better tool for many of these applications. Later developments in high-temperature flame photometry narrowed the analytical applications

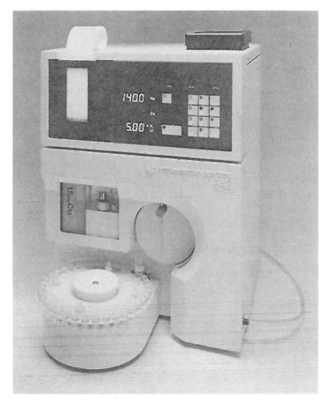

Fig. 1 Flame photometer using cesium as the internal standard. (Courtesy of Instrumentation Laboratory, Inc.)

of low-temperature flame photometry even further. The utility of the flame photometer to the clinical chemist, however, was not diminished until the development of ion-selective electrode (ISE) analyzers, which began in the mid-1970s. Although the niche for traditional flame photometers has narrowed, owing to the emergence of other technologies, flame photometry is the method of choice in a variety of applications.

APPLICATIONS

The analysis of clinical samples represents a typical application of flame photometry. Concentrations of sodium, potassium, and lithium in blood and urine are well within instrument working ranges. The specificity of the technique is a distinct advantage. Automated models of flame photometers, available during the past 25 years, are typically designed to serve the needs of the clinical chemist. Instrument calibration protocols are built into instruments to facilitate the timely analysis of sodium, potassium, and lithium in clinical samples.

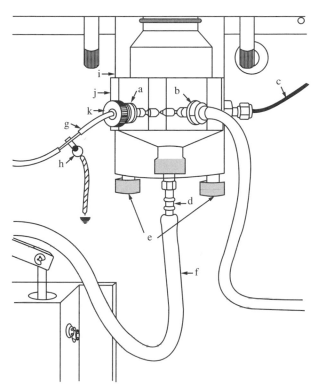

Fig. 2 Atomizer of IL 943 Flame Photometer; a) sample orifice assembly; b) air orifice; c) gas tube assembly; d) atomizer bowl drain; e) atomizer thumb screws; f) U-tube; g) sample injection nozzle tubing; h) ground fitting; i) top atomizer assembly; j) bottom atomizer assembly; k) adjustment for aspiration rate setting. (Courtesy of Instrumentation Laboratory, Inc.)

Other applications in the scope of pharmaceutical analysis include the analysis of sodium and potassium in injectable formulations and of trace amounts in bulk drugs, in dissolution experiments, and in content uniformity testing (4).

There are at least 14 USP, NF, or BP bulk drug monographs that use flame photometry either to control sodium potassium as an impurity or to assay for the primary ion (Table 1) (5, 6). An external standard method procedure is referenced in both the USP and the EP. The USP chapter, "Flame Photometry for Reagents," first appeared in USP XVII (1965) (7).

There are at least 25 USP or BP formulation monographs that use flame photometry to assay ions of interest (Table 2) (8). This technique is applicable to a variety of situations because of the relatively low cost per sample (in analyst time, instrument capital expense, and testing supplies); reasonable precision (typical relative standard deviation values are 0.6% for sodium, 1% for potassium, and 2% for lithium); low sample volume

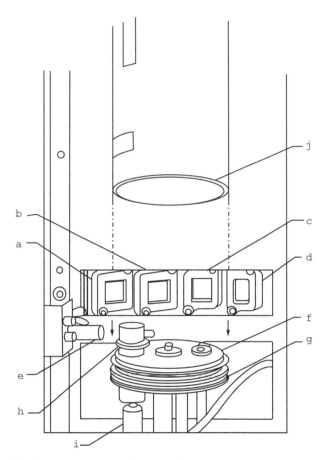

Fig. 3 Flame housing of IL 943 flame photometer; a) sodium filter, 589 nm; b) potassium filter, 776 nm; c) lithium filter, 670 nm; d) cesium filter, 852 nm; e) ignition detector; f) burner assembly; g) rubber gasket; h) spark electrode; i) ignition coil wire; j) chimney. (Courtesy of Instrumentation Laboratory, Inc.)

Table 1 USP, NF, or EP bulk drug monographs

Monograph	Assay
Cellulose sodium phosphate, USP	11% sodium
Chlorophyllin copper complex sodium, USP	6% sodium
Lithium carbonate, EP	0.03% sodium
Lithium carbonate, USP	0.1% sodium
Lithium citrate, USP	Lithium
Lithium hydroxide, USP	Lithium
Magaldrate, USP	0.11% sodium
Polacrilin potassium, NF	Potassium
Potassium acetate, EP	0.5% sodium
Potassium acetate, USP	0.03% sodium
Potassium chloride, EP	0.1% sodium
Potassium citrate, EP	0.3% sodium
Potassium nitrate, EP	0.1% sodium
Sodium chloride, EP	0.05% potassium

requirements (as low as 10 μl in some cases); and ease of operation.

COMMON SOURCES OF ANALYTICAL ERROR

In most applications, interferences are rare. Each new matrix requires some investigation, however, because problems can occur, especially when one element is to be determined in the presence of a large excess of another element. In a typical analysis, a liquid sample is diluted in a 1:100 or 1:200 ratio with diluent containing a lithium or cesium salt. Adequate dilution of a sample represents one of the most effective means of overcoming interference problems. Generally, samples are diluted to contain less than 10% by weight of total solids (not including the dilution with internal

standard). If dilution does not eliminate interference, atomic absorption should be used. It offers advantages for the determination of magnesium, calcium, and zinc in many matrices (9, 10). In some instances, however, sample pretreatment can make it possible to obtain good results with flame photometry (11).

With the development of ion-selection electrode technology (ISE), a means became available to directly measure (no dilution) sodium and potassium in the presence of clinical samples containing a significant amount of protein or lipids. Because of nonaqueous components in the sample matrix, the volume occupied by sodium and potassium ions is less than the total volume of the sample. When using a technique that requires dilution (flame photometry) or utilizes dilution (indirect-ISE), a lower concentration is observed than that obtained with direct-ISE. In as much as the bias can be clinically significant (up to 7% in some instances) it is important that the method used be taken into account (12, 13).

THE FUTURE

Low-temperature flame photometry is a mature technology and not likely to see many significant new applications. Advances in high-temperature flame photometry and atomic absorption techniques appear, well-suited to most of the new challenges in elemental analysis. Indeed, most of the pioneer commercial suppliers of flame photometry instrumentation have abandoned the market. Clinical laboratories are using ion-selective electrode analyzers more and more for

Table 2   USP, NF, or EP bulk drug monographs

Monograph	Use
Anticoagulant citrate phosphate dextrose adenine solution, USP	Sodium
Citric acid, magnesium oxide, and sodium carbonate irrigation, USP	Sodium assay
Half-strength lactated Ringer's and dextrose injection, USP	Sodium and potassium assay
Lactated Ringer's injection, USP	Lithium assay
Lithium carbonate capsules, USP	Lithium assay
Lithium carbonate tablets, USP	Lithium assay
Lithium carbonate extended-release tablets, USP	Lithium assay
Lithium citrate syrup, USP	Lithium assay
Modified lactated Ringer's and dextrose injection, USP	Sodium and potassium assay
Multiple electrolytes and dextrose injection type 4, USP	Sodium assay
Oral rehydration salts, BP	Sodium and potassium assay
Potassium and sodium bicarbonates and citric acid effervescent tablets, USP	Sodium and potassium assay
Potassium chloride and glucose intravenous infusion, BP	Potassium assay
Potassium chloride and sodium chloride intravenous infusion, BP	Sodium and potassium assay
Potassium chloride in sodium chloride injection, USP	Sodium and potassium assay
Potassium chloride in dextrose and sodium chloride injection, USP	Sodium and potassium assay
Potassium chloride, sodium chloride, and glucose intravenous infusion, BP	Sodium and potassium assay
Potassium citrate and citric acid oral solution, USP	Potassium assay
Protein hydrolysate injection, USP	Sodium and potassium assay
Ringer's injection, USP	Sodium and potassium assay
Ringer's irrigation, USP	Sodium and potassium assay
Sodium acetate injection, USP	Sodium assay
Sodium citrate and citric acid oral solution, USP	Sodium assay
Tricitrates oral solution, USP	Sodium and potassium assay
Tromethamine for injection, USP	Sodium and potassium assay

sodium, potassium, and lithium determinations. A core of existing applications, however, will support the viability of low-temperature flame photometry into the foreseeable future.

REFERENCES

1. Gardiner, K.W. Flame Photometry. *Physical Methods in Chemical Analysis*; Berl, W.G., Ed.; Academic Press: New York, 1972; III.
2. DiPietro, E.S.; Bashor, M.M.; Stroud, P.E.; Smarr, B.J.; Burgess, B.J.; Turner, W.E.; Neese, J.W. Sci. Total Environ. **1988**, *74*, 249–262.
3. Dean, J.A. *Flame Photometry*; McGraw-Hill: New York, 1960.
4. Soltero, R.A. Clin. Chem. **1985**, *31* (6), 1094.
5. *United States Pharmacopeia, The National Formulary*, 24th Rev.; 19th Ed., National Publishing: Philadelphia, 1999.
6. *European Pharmacopoeia 2000*; 3rd Ed., European Department for the Quality of Medicines: Strasbourg France, 1999.
7. *The United States Pharmacopeia XVII*; Mack Printing Co: Easton, PA, 1965.
8. *British Pharmacopoeia, 1998*; Her Majesty's Stationery Office: London, 1999; Version 2.1.
9. Williams, W.D. Flame Photometry and Atomic Absorption Spectrophotometry. *Practical Pharmaceutical Chemistry*, 3rd Ed.; Beckett, A.H., Stenlake, J.B., Hayworth, A., Eds.; Athlone Press: University of London, 1976; 2, 297–310.
10. Oberdier, J.O. Atomic Absorption Spectrophotometry. *Encyclopedia of Pharmaceutical Technology*; 1st Ed.; Swarbrick, J., Boylan, J.C., Eds.; Marcel Dekker, Inc.: New York, 2000; 1.
11. Nielsen, I. J. Clin. Chem. Clin. Biochem. **1986**, *24* (5), 353–354.
12. Burnett, D.; Ayers, G.J.; Rumjen, S.C.; Woods, T.F. Ann. Clin. Biochem. **1988**, *25* (1), 102–109.
13. Worth, H.G.J. Ann. Clin. Biochem. **1985**, *22* (4), 343–350.

FLAVORS AND FLAVOR MODIFIERS

John M. Lipari
Thomas L. Reiland
Abbott Laboratories, Abbott Park, Illinois

INTRODUCTION

The use of flavors and flavor modifiers to improve the taste and aroma of foods and pharmaceuticals is an art that dates back several centuries. In large measure, the practice is still the same today and, except for the advent of new semisynthetic flavoring agents with improved stability, the field has remained relatively unchanged. In the analytical arena, the story is different. Sophisticated instrumentation methods have been developed to characterize, purify, and manufacture flavoring agents that are similar, in many respects, to those occurring in nature. The technology continues to evolve at an accelerated pace, resulting in several stable, potent, and unique flavors, which are now available to target both foods and pharmaceuticals. This article discusses flavors and flavoring agents typically used in industry and highlights formulation variables that could affect the performance of flavors in finished products. Where necessary, pertinent literature for further reading is cited.

DEFINITION OF FLAVOR

Flavor is the complex effect of three components: taste, odor, and feeling factors. It is usually associated with the pleasure of savoring food or beverages and has, subsequently, suffered from considerable imprecision in definition. Flavor is a sensation with multidimensional components involving subjective and objective perceptions. The sensory perceptions are both qualitative as well as quantitative and, therefore, can be measured. *Webster's New Collegiate Dictionary* defines flavor as the "... quality of something that affects the sense of taste, ... the blend of taste and smell sensations evoked by a substance in the mouth." This definition is correct, but incomplete, and should be redefined to include feeling factors.

Taste

Taste consists of four primary sensations: sweet, sour, bitter, and salty. Correspondingly, there are four different kinds of taste buds. These sensations are elicited by the tongue and interpreted by the brain. Certain areas of the tongue respond more readily to specific tastes (1) than others. Sweet sensations are most easily detected at the tip of the tongue, whereas bitter ones are most readily detected at the back of the tongue. Sour sensations occur at the sides of the tongue, but salty sensations are usually detected at both the tip and at the sides of the tongue. During ingestion, taste buds react to soluble substances. The resulting sensations are transmitted to the brain by the ninth cranial (glossopharyngeal) nerve. The tenth and twelfth cranial nerves participate in this sensory reaction, but their role is limited (2).

Odor

The odor component of flavor is due to conscious or subconscious reactions to volatile substances, without which most foods would be lacking in taste appeal. By closing the nostrils while eating a mouthful of some flavored substance and immediately following this with another mouthful with the nostrils open, it may be shown that food could be rendered tasteless, as is often experienced by people suffering from the effects of a head cold.

There are many varieties of odorants, but a universally accepted structure–activity relationship of these has not been established. Yet, there is evidence that odor may involve specific receptor interactions (3), suggesting that structural properties of odorants may be important in eliciting specific odor sensations.

Feeling Factors

"Mouth feel" factors are critical in flavor perception. Examples include astringency, pepper bite, menthol cooling, and texture (e.g., softness or hardness as in candy). Sensations, such as crunch after biting into a crisp stick of celery or an apple, contribute to the overall flavor of foods. These mouth feel factors are also important in improving the organoleptic qualities of pharmaceuticals.

Encyclopedia of Pharmaceutical Technology
Copyright © 2002 by Marcel Dekker, Inc. All rights reserved.

FLAVORING AGENTS

Flavoring agents may be classified as natural, artificial, or natural and artificial (N&A) by combining the all-natural and synthetic flavors (4). Pharmaceutical flavors are available as liquids (e.g., essential oils, fluid extracts, tinctures, and distillates), solids (e.g., spray-dried, crystalline vanillin, freeze-dried cinnamon powders, and dried lemon fluid extract), and pastes (e.g., soft extracts, resins, and so-called concretes, which are brittle on the outside and soft on the inside). Liquid flavors are by far the most widely used because they diffuse readily into the substrate. They are available both as oily (e.g., essential oils) or nonoily liquids. Their texture is generally dependent on the solvent within which they are prepared. Fluid extracts may contain a single ingredient or a variety of compounded ingredients. Tinctures are obtained by maceration or percolation of specific herbs and spices in alcohol.

Essential oils boil at elevated temperatures, but many cannot be directly distilled without decomposition. Vacuum, steam, and fractional or molecular distillation are often used for their manufacture. Fractional distillation removes traces of water, resinous materials, colors, terpenes, and sesquiterpenes from the distillate. This process improves solubility and enhances flavor intensity. Sesquiterpeneless oils are more soluble than terpeneless oils because of the removal of head and tail fractions (e.g., waxy residues). Most common sesquiterpeneless oils used in the pharmaceutical industry include oil of orange and oil of lemon.

Oils and juices are obtained from plant sources by expression. Citrus essential oils are almost exclusively obtained by this method. Thoroughly washed unripe citrus fruits are cold pressed manually, or mechanically, to rupture oil cells in the rind. The oil is collected by draining and centrifuging. Manual operation is labor intensive and has been replaced by machines.

Natural Flavoring Agents

Natural ingredients have been used since antiquity to flavor foods and to make early "medicines" palatable. Honey was and remains a sweetener and flavoring agent. Wine was used as a crude infusorial in medicinal herbs. Modern use of natural flavors in pharmaceuticals is limited, because they are often unstable and their quality is unpredictable from season to season. The most commonly used natural flavors are terpeneless citrus oils, which are stable if well protected from light and air. A variety of other natural flavors are used in the food and pharmaceutical industries; some of the more common flavors are described below.

Anise (*Pimpinella anisum,* Umbelliferae)

Anise is a herbaceous annual cultivated extensively in Europe. The essential oil is obtained by steam distillation of dried fruits (seeds). The distillate is a clear-to-pale yellowish oil. It solidifies at low temperatures and has a characteristic sweet licorice-like odor and flavor. Its main constituents include anethol (approximately 90%), methylchavicol, *p*-methoxyphenylacetone, and acetic aldehyde. Anise oil is used frequently at concentrations of up to approximately 3000 ppm in liquid preparations.

Cardamon (*Elettaria cardamomum,* Zingiberaceae)

Cardamon is cultivated in India and Sri Lanka. The essential oil is obtained by steam distillation of comminuted seeds to yield a greenish-yellow liquid with a warm, spicy, aromatic odor and flavor. The main constituents of the oil are limonene, cineol, D-α-terpineol, and terpinyl acetate. Cardamon is generally used at concentrations of approximately 5–50 ppm.

Wild Cherry (*Prunus serotina,* Rosaceae)

Wild cherry is a large tree, native to southern Canada. It is widespread in the United States and Europe. The bark, small branches, and twigs are used to prepare the fluid extract and tincture. The main constituent of wild cherry extract is the glucoside prunasin, which on enzymatic hydrolysis yields prussic acid, glucose, and benzaldehyde. Also present are coumarin, phytosterols, benzoic acid, and fatty acids (e.g., oleic, linoleic, and palmitic acids). It has a characteristic sweet, tart, cherry-like flavor. Wild cherry bark extract is commonly used at concentrations of approximately 50–800 ppm in foods and pharmaceuticals.

Lemon (*Citrus limonum,* Rutaceae)

Lemon is an evergreen shrub or tree native to the Far East; it was introduced to the Mediterranean regions at the time of the Crusades. The leaves, fruits, and rind are used either whole or pressed in foods and in liquid or solid pharmaceutical products. The essential oil of lemon is obtained by cold expression. Approximately 40 constituents have been identified, with 90% being limonene. Fluid extracts and tinctures are obtained from the dried peel.

Lemon petitgrain is obtained by steam distillation of the leaves. For flavoring, it must be terpeneless. The main constituents are D-α-pinene, camphene, D-limonene, dipentene, L-linalol, nerol, and citral. Lemon petitgrain oil is used in a wide variety of applications. Typical concentrations range from 1 to 35 ppm. The essential oil and extract of lemon are generally used at higher concentrations that may range up to 1000 and 10,000 ppm, respectively. All lemon oil derivatives have the characteristic lemon odor and a slightly bitter flavor.

Orange, Bitter (*Citrus aurantium,* Rutaceae)

Bitter orange is a tall tropical tree that can grow up to approximately 10 m (33 ft.) high. The tree is native to the Far East and is cultivated extensively throughout the Mediterranean, Guinea, the West Indies, West Africa, and Brazil. The leaves and twigs produce essential petitgrain oil following steam distillation. *Neroli bigarade* essential oil is produced from the blossoms by steam distillation. The peel is expressed and steam distilled to produce essential oil of orange. The main constituent of orange oil is D-limonene, with various acids, aldehydes, and diesters. Essential oil of orange is widely used in foods and pharmaceuticals at concentrations of up to 500 ppm.

Orange, Sweet (*Citrus sinensis, var. aurantium dulcis,* Rutaceae)

Sweet orange is an evergreen tree that grows to approximately 6 m (20 ft.) high. It is generally of oriental origin and is cultivated extensively in the Mediterranean, Florida, and California. A petitgrain oil is obtained from the leaves and twigs, but its production is low because of limited use, primarily in the perfumery industry.

Essential oil of sweet orange is obtained by expression. Its physical–chemical properties (e.g., specific gravity, optical rotation, and refractive index) vary according to origin. The oil contains more than 90% limonene, in addition to relatively high quantities of decylic, octylic, nonylic, and dodecylic aldehydes, and citral esters. It has a characteristic odor and a mildly bitter, astringent flavor; it is generally used at concentrations of up to 500 ppm.

Peppermint (*Mentha piperita,* Labiatae)

Peppermint is a herbaceous plant that grows to approximately 81 cm (32 in.) high. The essential oil is obtained by steam distillation of the flowering plant tops. It is cultivated in Europe, North and South America, and

Japan. The main constituents of the essential oil are α- and β-pinene, limonene, cineol, ethyl amylcarbinol, menthone, menthol, isomenthol, menthyl acetate, and piperitone. It has a strong mint odor with a sweet balsam taste masked by a strong cooling effect. It is widely used in foods, as well as in liquid pharmaceuticals, to 8000 ppm.

Artificial Flavoring Agents

Unlike natural flavoring agents, synthetic flavors are usually stable. The development of synthetic flavors paralleled the development of instrumental analysis, in which active ingredients in natural flavors are identified and reconstructed synthetically with reasonable accuracy. Exact duplication of a natural flavor is, however, difficult because often minor components are the most important contributors to the overall flavor profile. These minor components are not easily identified. For example, the major components of vanilla are vanillin and ethyl vanillin. However, the flavor nuances of the vanilla bean have never been successfully matched in artificial (synthetic) vanilla.

Natural and Artificial (N&A) Agents

In N&A flavor systems, natural flavors are combined with synthetic ingredients to enhance flavor balance and fullness. These flavors are generally classified according to type and taste sensation. Table 1 contains a list of N&A flavor components that elicit various sensory properties, all of which are commonly used in food and drug compounding. It is not an exhaustive list because manufacturers regard their flavor formularies as proprietary. Many N&A flavors may be chemically and structurally similar, but vary significantly in taste and aroma. Similar flavors from various vendors might vary significantly in composition. Of interest is the fact that a relatively small change in chain length can have a profound impact on flavor type. Minor changes, such as the conversion of allyl benzoate to cyclohexyl esters (e.g., a caproate or valerate), transform a basic cherry flavor to peach or pineapple.

In situ conversion of essential N&A flavor components from one molecular form to another, as a result of ion pairing, is common in food and drug products. Therefore, the inadvertent conversion of flavors between types during drug formulation studies (e.g., effect of pH, salts, and temperature) can present a serious challenge in flavor-quality assessment. The fact that one and the same N&A flavor component can deliver several flavor and odor impressions implies that a blend of several flavor compounds would be preferable. Such blends show improved stability. In addition, flavor impressions from

Table 1   Primary taste and flavor characteristics of typical flavor ingredients

Ingredient	Sweet	Bittersweet	Bitter	Flavor characteristic
		Primary taste		
Allyl benzoate		X		Cherry
Allyl caproate		X		Pineapple
Allyl cyclohexylbutyrate		X		Pineapple
Allyl cyclohexylcaproate		X		Peach/apricot
Allyl cyclohexylvalerate		X		Apple
Allyl phenoxyacetate		X		Honey/pineapple
Anethol	X			Anise
Anisyl alcohol	X			Peach
Anisyl formate	X			Strawberry
Benzyl isobutyrate	X			Strawberry
Benzyl salicylate	X			Raspberry
Cinnamaldehyde		X		Cinnamon/melon
Cinnamyl anthranilate		X		Grape
Citral		X		Lemon
Citronellyl formate		X		Plum
Cyclohexyl caproate		X		Peach/cognac
Decyl formate	X			Grape
Diacetyl	X			Butter
Diphenyl ether	X			Black currant
Ethyl valerate		X		Banana/apple
Eugenol			X	Clove buds
Geraneol			X	Rose-like
α-Ionone	X			Raspberry
Isoamyl salicylate		X		Strawberry
Isobutyl anthranllate		X		Grape/strawberry
Isopropyl valerate		X		Apple
Linalyl anthranilate	X			Orange
Methyl ionone	X			Raspberry/currant
Methyl propionate	X			Black currant
Methyl undecyl ketone		X		Coconut
Musk ambrette	X			Peach
Nerol			X	Rose-like
Neryl acetate	X			Raspberry
Neryl butyrate	X			Cocoa
Propenyl guaethol	X			Vanilla
Propyl isobutyrate	X			Pineapple
Rhodinol			X	Rose
Santalyl acetate		X		Apricot
Terpenyl butyrate		X		Plum
Tetrahydrofurfuryl proprionate		X		Chocolate/apricot
Vanillylidene acetone		X		Vanilla
Yara yara	X			Strawberry

N&A flavor blends are usually not dominated by a single component. For these reasons, single natural and artificial flavor ingredients are seldom, if ever, used alone in a finished product.

Tables 2 and 3 list the components thus far qualitatively identified (4) in two common fruits, the raspberry and the strawberry. These tables illustrate the complexity in compounding synthetic systems to mimic natural types. For this reason, there has been a steady rise in the use of N&A flavors, in addition to their superior performance, when compared to natural flavors. Also, the quality and uniformity of the N&A flavor is greater than that of natural

Table 2   Natural components of raspberry aroma

Acids	Carbonyls	Esters	Alcohols
Acetic	Acetaldehyde	Butyl acetate	1-Butanol
Butyric	Acetone	Ethyl acetate	*trans*-2-Buten-l-ol
Caproic	Acetyl methyl carbinol	Ethyl butyrate	Ethanol
Caprylic	Acrolein	Ethyl crotonate	Geraniol
Formic	Diacetal	Ethyl propionate	1-Hexanol
2-Hexenoic	β, β-Dimethylacrolein	2-Hexenyl acetate	*cis*-3-Henen-l-ol
3-Hexenoic	Hexanal	2-Hexenyl butyrate	Methanol
Isobutyric	2-Hexenal	Hexyl acetate	3-Methyl-3-buten-l-ol
Isovaleric	*cis*-3-Hexenal	Hexyl butyrate	1-Pentanolol
Propionic	4-(*p*-Hydroxyphenyl)-2-butanone	Isoamyl acetate	1-Penten-3-ol
Valeric	α-Ionone	Isopropyl butyrate	
	β-Ionone	Methyl butyrate	
	2-Pentanone	Methyl caproate	
	2-Pentanal	Methyl caprylate	
	Propanal	Propyl acetate	

(From Ref. 4.)

flavors, and lower concentrations of N&A flavors are often used to achieve the same effect as obtained with natural flavors. Table 4 shows a typical formulation of a commercial N&A strawberry flavor. It contains a small proportion of natural flavors; the bulk of the ingredients are synthetic.

Another advantage of N&A flavors is the broad spectrum of flavoring agents from which the formulator can develop an entirely new flavor system that is unique, not available naturally. A flavor extensively used in foods and pharmaceutical products is tutti-frutti—bubble gum (Table 5).

In summary, there are a variety of flavor types: natural, synthetic, and semisynthetic. Appropriate use concentrations depend on many factors, including product characteristics, such as composition, physical state, shelf life, pH, processing temperature, storage conditions, and reactivity of components. Flavor concentrations also depend on the market sector for which the product is targeted. The age of the user and the mode of use are two examples of user-dependent variables that have significant bearing on the type, concentration, and nature of the flavor selected for product development.

FLAVOR SELECTION IN PHARMACEUTICAL PREPARATIONS

A number of criteria are used to select flavors during formulation. Different flavor concentrations produce highly subjective sensations. Specific requirements for balance and fullness are dependent, in part, on the drug substance and the physical form of the product. For this reason, when selecting a flavor system, the compounding pharmacist must take into account several variables upon which a desired response would depend. Some of these are product texture (e.g., viscosity of formulation, solid or liquid), water content, base vehicle or substrate, and taste of the subject drug. Notable specific examples to consider are:

- Immediate flavor identity from the formulation as it is ingested;
- Compatible mouth feel factors and rapid development of a fully blended flavor in the mouth during ingestion of the product;
- Absence of "off" notes in the mouth and a mild transient aftertaste during ingestion of the product.

The selection of a flavor system, thus, requires an extensive evaluation of a number of organoleptic qualities. Vehicle components within which the drug is presented have a significant bearing on the performance of the flavor system. Of these, the sweetener is perhaps the most relevant.

Sweeteners

The most commonly used sweeteners are sucrose, glucose, fructose, sorbitol, and glycerin. Using sucrose (sugar) as a standard, with 100 units of sweetness, Table 6 lists the

F

Table 3 Natural components of strawberry aroma

Acids	Esters	Alcohols
Acetic	Butyl acetate	Benzyl alcohol
Benzoic	Ethyl acetate	1-Borneol
Butyric	Ethyl acetoacetate	Butanol
Caproic	Ethyl benzoate	2-Butanol
Cinnamic	Ethyl butyrate	Ethanol
Formic	Ethyl capronate	2-Heptanol
Isobutyric	Ethyl cinnamate	Hexanol
Isovaleric	Ethyl crotonate	trans-2-Hexanol
α-Methylbutyric	Ethyl formate	p-Hydroxyphenyl-2-ethanol
Propionic	Ethyl isobutyrate	Isoamyl alcohol
Salicylic	Ethyl isovalerate	Isobutanol
Succinic	Ethyl α-methylbutyrate	Isofenchyl alcohol
n-Valeric	Ethyl propionate	Methanol
Isovaleric	Ethyl salicylate	1-Pentanol
	Ethyl valerate	Penten-l,3-ol
	trans-2-Hexenyl	Phenyl-2-ethanol
	trans-2-Hexynl acetate	n-Propanol
	Hexyl acetate	DL-α-Terpineol
	Hexyl butyrate	cis-Terpineol hydrate
	Isoamyl acetate	
	Isopropyl butyrate	
	Methyl acetate	
	Methyl butyrate	
	Methyl capronate	
	Methyl isobutyrate	
	Methyl-α-methylbutyrate	
	Propyl acetate	

Carbonyl compounds		**Others**
Acetaldehyde		Acetals
Acetophenone		Acetoin
Acetone		γ-Decalactone
Acrolein		1,1-Diethoxyethane
n-Butanal		1,1-Dimethoxyethane
Crotonal		Dimethoxymethane
Diacetyl		Dimethyl sulfide
2-Heptanone		Hydrogen sulfide
cis-3-Hexal		1-Ethoxy-l-propoxyethane
Methyl-3-butanone		Maltal
2-Pentanone		1-Methoxy-l-ethoxyethane
2-Pentanal		Methyl sulfide

(From Ref. 4.)

relative intensities of other sweeteners. Sweetness intensity changes with concentration. It has been estimated (5) that the sweetness of glucose relative to cane sugar is 53 at a concentration of 8% but increases to 88 at a concentration of 35%. Sweetener intensity increases with concentration but reaches a maximum where feeling factors become more prominent. Sugar (sucrose), at a concentration of 30%, is intensely sweet. Yet, its sweet intensity at concentrations 50% or higher is not perceptibly different, although distinct mouthfeel characteristics (e.g., syrupy, salivation) become pronounced. This is due to osmotic effects on mucous membranes within the oral cavity.

Glycerin, glucose, sorbitol, and sucrose have limited use in solid dosage forms (e.g., tablets) because the materials are hygroscopic. Mannitol is used more often in

Table 4 A typical formula composition of natural and artificial strawberry flavor

Ingredient	Parts by weight
Amyl acetate	34.0
Amyl butyrate	15.0
Anethole	1.5
Butyric acid	15.0
Cinnamyl valerate	9.5
Diacetyl	10.0
Ethyl amyl ketone	15.0
Ethyl cinnamate	52.0
Ethyl methylphenylglycidate	260.0
Ethyl valerate	60.0
Lemon essential oil	1.0
Maltol	70.0
Methyl heptene carbonate	0.5
Neroli essential oil	0.5
γ-Undecalactone	58.5
α-Ionone	6.5
Amyl valerate	15.0
Jasmine absolute	85.0
Cinnamyl isobutyrate	7.0
Cognac essential oil	1.5
Ethyl acetate	50.0
Ethyl butyrate	30.0
Ethyl heptylate	2.5
Ethyl propionate	15.0
Hydroxyphenyl-2-butanone	0.5
Methyl anthranilate	6.5
Methyl cinnamate	35.5
Methyl salicylate	6.5
Orris resinoid	1.5
Vanillin	70.0
Solvent {ethylene glycol ethyl ester}	1060.0
Total	2000.0

(From Ref. 4.)

Table 5 Formula and composition of natural and artificial tutti-frutti flavor

Ingredient	Parts by weight
Amyl acetate	300.0
Amyl butyrate	48.0
Ethyl butyrate	36.0
α-Ionone	120.0
Jasmine absolute (10 % in alcohol)	0.1
Lemon essential oil	1.0
Orris resinoid	80.0
Imitation rose (10 % in alcohol)	28.0
Rum ether	100.0
γ-Undecalactone	18.0
Vanillin	11.0
Alcohol (solvent)	257.0
Total	1000.0

(From Ref. 4.)

The artificial sweeteners, cyclamate and aspartame, are about 30 $\times$ as sweet as sugar, but like saccharin, their sweet-bitter profiles are concentration dependent. Aspartame does not have a significant bitter aftertaste when compared to saccharin and has gained in popularity. Cyclamates were banned in the 1970s because of carcinogenic concerns, which have, subsequently, been shown to be overstated.

Monoammonium glycyrrhizinate has a lingering sweet aftertaste, which can be exploited for taste-masking products with a mildly bitter aftertaste. It is also effective in enhancing chocolate flavor. Glycerin is commonly used for its solvent effect on many compounds, as well as its humectant effect. Sugar syrups promote significant "cap-locking"—the crystallization of the sugar on the cap and bottle thread, but the addition of glycerin (10–20%) minimizes this effect. Glycerin is seldom used as a single sweetener in pharmaceuticals because it has a characteristic mouth-warming and burning effect.

Flavor Enhancers and Potentiators

Flavor enhancers are used universally in the food and pharmaceutical industries. Sugar, carboxylic acids (e.g., citric, malic, and tartaric), common salt (NaCl), amino acids, some amino acid derivatives (e.g., monosodium glutamate—MSG), and spices (e.g., peppers) are most often employed. Although extremely effective with proteins and vegetables, MSG has limited use in pharmaceuticals because it is not a sweetener. Citric acid

tablet manufacture. Besides being less hygroscopic, it has a negative heat of solution. For this reason, chewable tablets containing mannitol have a pleasant cooling sweet taste, which complements flavor quality. The artificial sweetener saccharin is widely used in foods and pharmaceuticals. It is approximately 350 $\times$ as sweet as sugar. It is sweet at very low concentrations (equivalent to about 5–10% sugar) but bitter at higher concentrations. Approximately 20% of the population are "saccharin sensitive;" that is, they perceive saccharin to be bitter even at low concentrations. Upon repeated tasting, saccharin becomes less sweet and increasingly bitter. By the third or fourth tasting, solutions of relatively low concentrations are often no longer sweet to the saccharin-sensitive person.

Table 6 Intensity values for frequently used sweeteners

Sweetener	Intensity
Sorbitol	60
Mannitol	50
Hydrogenated starch hydrolysate	30–40
Maltitol solution	70–80
Maltitol	90
Xylitol	100
Erythritol	60–70
Glycerin	55–75
Sucrose	100
Fructose	117
Maltose	30

(From SPI Polyols, Inc., Polyols Comparison Chart, Revised 6/99.)

is most frequently used to enhance taste performance of both liquid and solid pharmaceutical products, as well as a variety of foods. Other acidic agents, such as malic and tartaric acids, are also used for flavor enhancement. In oral liquids, these acids contribute unique and complex organoleptic effects, increasing overall flavor quality. Common salt provides similar effects at its taste threshold level in liquid pharmaceuticals. Vanilla, for example, has a delicate bland flavor, which is effectively enhanced by salt.

Taste-Masking Agents

The flavoring industry has many proprietary products purported to have excellent taste-masking properties (4), which have been used with some success. Yet, there are a number of natural and artificial flavors that can be generally described to possess similar taste-masking effects (Table 7).

Table 7 Agents for masking and complementing the basic tastes

Basic taste	Masking agent
Sweet	Vanilla, bubble gum, grape, other fruits
Acid	Lemon, lime, orange, cherry, grapefruit
Metallic	Berries, mints, grape, marshmallow, gurana
Bitter	Licorice, coffee, chocolate, mint, grapefruit, cherry, peach, raspberry, orange, lemon, lime

Of the many tastes that must be masked in pharmaceuticals, bitterness is most often encountered; to mask it completely is difficult. A tropical fruit has been used for centuries in central Africa to mask the bitter taste of native beers. This so-called "miracle berry" contains a glycoprotein that transiently and selectively binds to bitter taste buds. Due to stability challenges, attempts to isolate the compound for commercial exploitation have been unsuccessful. Yet, many fruit syrups are relatively stable in pharmaceuticals if formulated with antimicrobial preservative agents. Syrups of cinnamon, orange, citric acid, cherry, cocoa, wild cherry, raspberry, or glycyrrhiza elixir can be used to effectively mask salty and bitter tastes in a number of drug products (6). The extent to which taste-masking may be achieved is not usually predictable due to complex interactions of other flavor elements in these products. The degree to which bitterness may be masked by these agents ranks in a descending order: cocoa syrup is most effective, followed by raspberry syrup, cherry, cinnamon, compound sarsaparilla, citric acid, licorice, aromatic elixir, orange, and wild cherry.

Sour and metallic tastes in pharmaceuticals also can be reasonably masked. Sour substances containing hydrochloric acid are most effectively neutralized with raspberry and other fruit syrups. Metallic tastes in oral liquid products (e.g., iron) are usually masked by extracts of gurana, a tropical fruit. Gurana flavor is used at concentrations ranging from 0.001 to about 0.5% and may be useful in solid products as well (e.g., chewable tablets and granules).

FLAVOR MODIFICATION TECHNOLOGIES

Solubility-Limiting Methods

Many drugs are reasonably soluble in water and ionize extensively at physiologic pH. Drugs with an offensive taste usually demonstrate negative organoleptic properties after dissolving in saliva during ingestion. Chemical modification, such as derivatization or lipophilic counterion selection, where possible, may be an effective method for reducing aqueous solubility and taste. This is exemplified by erythromycin, a partially soluble, bittertasting macrolide anti-infective. The solubility of erythromycin monohydrate is approximately 2 mg/mL in water at a pH of approximately 7. When converted to erythromycin ethylsuccinate, the aqueous solubility of the drug is less than 50 μg/mL. This form is practically tasteless as a ready-made liquid or a chewable tablet. The rate of dissolution in body fluids (e.g., saliva) may be further reduced by controlling formulation pH, solids content, and temperature. This technique can be applied to a number of drugs whose taste profiles are dependent on aqueous solubility.

Vesicles and Liposomes

Host–guest systems (7) (e.g., phospholipids and certain surfactants) form spherical or ellipsoidal, closed, bilayer structures called vesicles. These structures often comprise several compartments within which a drug could be trapped, either as a solution or a dispersion. Under various conditions, these vesicles form closed systems, which are ideal vehicles for taste masking or for modulated release of drug in vivo. It is a challenge to formulate drugs with these flavor-masking methods without altering the regulatory status of the product (e.g., chemical designation of the active substance, in vitro dissolution kinetics, physical or chemical stability, and bioavailability). Various manufacturers (e.g., American Lecithin Company, Oxford, Connecticut) offer a complete line of phospholipids (purified and solubilized in various carrier systems) for use in the food and pharmaceutical industries.

Microencapsulation and Coated Systems

Recently, a great deal of attention has been focused on the usefulness of coated fine particles in achieving pharmaceutical objectives. By coating drug particles with an appropriate polymer system, desirable properties can be imparted to the dosage form, eliminating undesirable properties, such as taste. Coating drug particles significantly modulates drug release while improving taste, stability, and other handling characteristics (e.g., flow and compression). Commercial particle coaters make it possible to coat fine drug particles, achieving slow release and taste masking in oral formulations. Examples for which particle coating has been used to introduce unique line extensions to the marketplace include Theo-Dur® and Depakote Sprinkle®. In the case of Theo-Dur®, theophylline is sprayed onto sugar beads followed by a polymer to control drug release. By encapsulating a drug substance, this process prevents interaction of the drug with taste receptors, thus eliminating bitterness. Other frequently used microencapsulation methods include spray drying, spray congealing, coacervation and phase separation, interfacial polymerization, and extrusion.

Complexation and Chemical Modification

The use of ion exchange resins to form drug adsorbates for sustained release (8, 9) was closely associated with Strasenburgh Laboratories, an affiliate of Pennwalt Corporation, which was granted several patents in this area (10, 11). Their first significant application involved amphetamine adsorbed onto a sulfonic acid cation exchange resin (Biphetamine®) for use in appetite suppression (12). Over the years, several products have been introduced commercially since the initial work with amphetamine (13–16); examples include Ionamin® (phentermine: Medeva Pharmaceuticals, Inc.), Tussionex® (hydrocodone polistirex and chlorpheniramine polistirex: Medeva Pharmaceuticals, Inc.), and a variety of cough-cold products, including phenylpropanolamine, chlorpheniramine, and dextromethorphan (17). This technology is applicable to taste masking as well.

The mechanism of drug release from the sustained–release complex (e.g., an ion exchange resinate consisting of a drug with a bitter taste) is ideal for liquids, when formulated either as granules for reconstitution or ready-made suspensions. By retaining a low counter-ion concentration in the product, almost all of the drug may be retained in the matrix, so that upon ingestion, ions of the body trigger the release mechanism through a dynamic equilibration process. Slow equilibrating complexes that provide low diffusivity of drug to the taste buds (e.g., low aqueous solubility of the drug) can eliminate bitterness and other offensive organoleptic drug properties. Other complexation phenomena employed in formulation work for flavor enhancement are: inclusion complexes (e.g., cyclodextrins and their derivatives), matrices, and physical complexes with waxy substances (e.g., polyethylene glycols).

More recently, pharmaceutical manufacturers have introduced various technologies for coating drug particles with semipermeable polymeric membranes designed to provide controlled release in vivo. Coatings of neat drugs and their adsorbates (18–21) combined controlled–release characteristics with the benefit of taste masking, caused by the effective reduction of dissolved drug concentrations in the mouth. Taste evaluation of a variety of these preparations showed a significant reduction in bitterness (19–21), suggesting that coatings and adsorbates have potential in the flavor enhancement of drugs with offensive tastes.

CONCLUSIONS

The use of flavors and flavor modifiers in pharmaceutical formulations is of considerable importance in promoting drug products. Flavors are also key factors in promoting patient compliance, because products with offensive taste are likely to be objectionable. Taste sensations are, however, wholly subjective, and of the many objective methods thus far used, none can adequately and completely characterize taste and aroma sensations without some bias.

It is also certain that a fair proportion of the population is indifferent to taste and lacks the acuity necessary for distinguishing small differences in taste and aroma between samples (22, 23). Furthermore, clear flavor performance differences can be obtained during pharmaceutical product development, by techniques designed to promote taste acceptance. The use of flavors, flavor modifiers, and other methods for flavor enhancement, such as physical and chemical manipulations of drugs, may be potential methods for the development of products with superior market preference characteristics.

ACKNOWLEDGMENTS

The authors are grateful to Akwete L. Adjei and Richard Doyle for their contributions to the 1st Edition of this article and to Tracy B. Lynch for her assistance in the final preparation of this manuscript.

REFERENCES

1. Beidler, L.M. *Olfaction and Taste*; Zotterman, Y., Ed.; Pergamon Press, Inc.: New York, 1963.
2. Pfaffmen, C.J.J. Neurophysiol. **1955**, *18*, 429–444.
3. Amerine, M.A.; Pangborn, R.M.; Roessler, E.B. *Principles of Sensory Analysis of Food*; Academic Press: New York, 1965; 193–206.
4. Furia, E., Bellanca, N., Eds. *Fenaroli's Handbook of Flavor Ingredients*; CRC Press: Cleveland OH, 1971.
5. Renner, H.D. Confect. Prod. **1939**, *5*, 255–256.
6. In *Remington's Pharmaceutical Sciences*; Gennaro, A.R., Ed.; Ch. 69 Mack: Easton, PA, 1980.
7. Fendler, J.H. Membrane Mimetic Chemistry. Chem. Eng. News **1984 Jan 2**, 25–38.
8. Martin, G.J. *Ion Exchange and Adsorption Agents in Medicine*; Little, Brown, & Co.: Boston, MA, 1955.
9. Calmon, C.; Kressman, T.R.E. *Ion Exchangers in Organic and Biochemistry*; Interscience: New York, 1957.
10. Keating, J.W. US Patent 2,990,332, 1961; US Patent 3,143,465, 1964.
11. Hays, E.E. US Patent, 3,035,979, 1962.
12. Deeb, G.; Becker, B. Absorption of Sustained-Release Oral Amphetamine Preparations in the Rat. Toxicol. Appl. Pharmacol. **1960**, *2*, 410.
13. Swift, J.G. A Study of Sustained Ionic Release Antihistamines. Arch. Int. Pharmacodyn. **1960**, *124*, 341.
14. Wulff, O.J. Prolonged Antitussive Action of a Resin-Bound Noscapine Preparation. Pharm. Sci. **1965**, *54*, 1058.
15. Brudney, N. Ion-exchange Resin Complexes in Oral Therapy. Can. Pharm. J. **1959**, *59*, 245.
16. Schlichting, D.A. Ion Exchange Resin Salts for Oral Therapy I. J. Pharm. Sci. **1962**, *51*, 134.
17. Raghunathan, Y.; Amsel, L.; Hinsvark, O.; Bryant, W. Sustained-release Drug Delivery System I: Coated Ion-Exchange Resin System for Phenylpropanolamine and Other Drugs. J. Pharm. Sci. **1981**, *70*, 379.
18. Borodkin, S. US Patent 3,947,572, 1976.
19. Borodkin, S.; Sundberg, D. US Patent 3,594,470, 1971.
20. Borodkin, S.; Sundberg, D.P. J. Pharm. Sci. **1971**, *60*, 1523.
21. Borodkin, S.; Yunker, M.H. Interaction of Amine Drugs with a Polycarboxylic Acid Ion-Exchange Resin. J. Pharm. Sci. **1970**, *59*, 481.
22. Cameron, C.W. *The Taste Sense and the Relative Sweetness of Sugars and Other Sweet Substances*, Scientific Report Series No. 9, Sugar Research Foundation, Inc.: New York, 1947.
23. *Flavor Quality: Objective Measurement*; Symposium, Division of Agricultural and Food Chemistry; American Chemical Society: Washington, D.C., 1976.

FURTHER READING

Flavor: Its Chemical, Behavioral, and Commercial Aspects. In *Proceedings of the Arthur D. Little, Inc., Flavor Symposium, 1977*; Apt, C.M., Ed.; Westview Special Studies in Science and Technology: Boston, MA, 1977.
Basic Principles of Sensory Evaluation; ASTM Special Technical Publication, No. 433; American Society for Testing and Materials: Philadelphia, PA, 1973.
Correlation of Subjective-Objective Methods in the Study of Odors and Taste; ASTM Special Technical Publication, No. 440; American Society for Testing and Materials, Philadelphia, PA, 1968.
Food Acceptance Testing Methodology; Advisory Board on Quartermaster Research and Development; National Academy of Sciences-National Research Council: Chicago, IL, 1954.
Fenaroli's Handbook of Flavor Ingredients; Furia, E., Bellanca, N., Eds.; CRC Press: Cleveland, OH, 1971.
Gorman, W. *Flavor, Taste and the Psychology of Smell*; Charles C. Thomas: Springfield, IL, 1964.
Moncrieff, R.W. *The Chemical Senses*; Leonard Hill: London, 1967.
Modifying Bitterness; Roy, Glenn, Ed.; Technomic Publishing Company, Inc.: Lancaster, PA, 1997.
Flavor Quality: Objective Measurement. Scanlan, ACS Symposium Series, Scanlan, R.A., Ed.; American Chemical Society: Washington, D.C., 1977; 51.

FLOW PROPERTIES OF SOLIDS

Stephen A. Howard

Purdue Pharma L.P., Ardsley, New York

INTRODUCTION

The preparation of essentially all dosage forms involves the handling of solid materials. Among all finished products, solid dosage forms are the most predominant in terms of volume and value. The importance of solid-handling properties, especially flow properties, cannot not be overemphasized. The flow properties of solids have great impact on the tableting and encapsulation processes since these dosage form manufacturing processes require the flow of powder materials from a storage container to filling stations, such as tablet dies or capsule fillers. Weight uniformity of course is dependent on the uniform and rapid flow of powders. The flow properties of solids also have great influence on the mixing and demixing of powders that take place before tableting or encapsulation. As is pointed out by Von Behren (1) in process steps affected by the flowability of formulations include mix uniformity and flow and of course the weight and pressure settings used. It should also be pointed out that the speed of production is also greatly affected by the formulation's flow characteristics. For the final product, Von Behren (1) lists, weight, content uniformity, hardness and disintegration/dissolution as being affected by formulation flow.

Different flow properties are required at different stages of processing and should be carefully taken into consideration during formulation and process validation. Kinetics of mixing is influenced by the physical state of the active constituent (2). Particle size of excipients has a significant effect on the content uniformity of ethinyl estradiol powder mixes and tablets. As the particle sizes of excipients increase, the degree of mixing decreases. The more free-flowing the excipient, the more abrasive the particle, facilitating the breakdown of drug agglomerates (3). On the other hand, segregation studies carried out in a two-dimensional segregation cell suggest that materials with good flow show demixing tendencies, whereas powder blends with poor flow are less apt to separate (4). Fast flow is not always helpful in weight uniformity of the finished product. Hauer et al. (5) showed that none cohesive free flowing powders gave poorer capsule fill uniformity since they were less cohesive and flowed out of the dosators. Knowing your process and determining the characteristics needed to optimize that process is critical.

Characterization of powders is essential to quality control of raw materials, active or excipient, in order to maintain product uniformity. Flow-property studies of powder materials facilitate the scientific design of formulations and processing equipment, such as the design of mass-flow hoppers. This article reviews the flow properties of powder materials. The factors affecting the flow properties of solids are briefly discussed first, followed by measurement of flow properties.

FACTORS INFLUENCING THE FLOW OF SOLIDS

Nature of Powders and Granulations

Powders are generally considered as two-phase assemblies of discrete particles with interactions between gas and solid internal surfaces. A material is classified as a powder if it is composed of dry, discrete particles with a maximum dimension of less than 1000 μm according to British Standard 2955 (6). Powders differ from other physical states of matter since they are nonhomogenous in nature but consist of discrete solid particles of different sizes and shapes interdispersed with a gaseous phase. Powders are similar to solids in that they can exhibit both elastic recovery and brittle fracture. Unlike solids, however, powders can expand or contract when stressed. Preconditioning can change the nature of the material. The condition and duration preconditioning forces are applied to a powder can determine if and how a powder will flow. Under stress, powders can flow like a liquid. However, unlike liquids, they do not flow if the stresses are too small. When powder materials do flow, the stresses are not dependent on the rate of flow as they are with a liquid. In order to characterize the properties of an assembly of particles or a bulk mass, the collective properties of constituent particles within their gaseous environment must be determined. The solid-handling properties of a bulk mass are influenced by any factor that can have an effect on the particle–particle interactions of constituent particles. Factors associated with the nature of the particles

Encyclopedia of Pharmaceutical Technology

and their surfaces such as size, shape, surface morphology, packing conditions, and interparticle forces must therefore be considered. To make the situation more complex, the interparticle forces can be of a number of types: mechanical forces, surface tension, electrostatic forces, van der Waals forces, solid-bridge forces, or plastic welding forces; none of these can be readily quantified. The properties and phenomena associated with an assembly of particles are (7):

- Particle size distribution and specific surface area;
- Particle shape distribution;
- Cohesion, strength, and adhesion;
- Packing properties (bulk density, porosity);
- Rate and compressibility of packing;
- Flowability and failure properties;
- Segregation; and
- Angle of internal friction. A combination of these properties determines the behavior of bulk material.

Particle Size and Size Distribution

All matter interacts. As the dimensions of particles increase and the particles change in nature, the forces acting on them change. Fine powder particles less than 100 μm in diameter are acted upon primarily by surface forces. Particles above 1000 μm in diameter are governed by gravitational forces. Therefore, the balance of interaction forces determines powder behavior. With relatively small particles, the flow through an orifice may be restricted because the cohesive forces between the particles are of the same magnitude as gravitational forces. Since the latter forces are a function of the diameter raised to the third power, they become more significant as the particle size increases and flow is facilitated. Too large a particle however with respect to the orifice through which it has to flow can cause arching that can block flow from hopper or into a die or capsule dosator. The properties of solids that determine the magnitude of particle–particle interactions have been reviewed (8, 9).

In general larger particle flow faster than smaller particles. In the TSI Aero-Flow brochure (10) two sieved fractions of lactose, one larger than 38 μm and one less than 38 μm, were compared to the unfractionated lactose. As expected the fine fraction showed the poorest flow while the larger fraction showed the best flow characteristics in the Aero-Flow rotating drum tester while the unfractionated sample was between the two extremes. With wider particle distributions and gravimetric test methods such as flow from a hopper, density differences can be a determining factor until the cohesive nature of the fine particles decrease flow. Particle size and size

distribution has been systematically investigated for their effects on flow using a flat-bottom flowmeter (11). Increase in the content of fines increases the flow rate to a maximum value, followed by a decrease in flow rate if the content of fines is further increased. For a given concentration of fines, the flow rate increases to a maximum as the diameter of the fines decreases to approximately 90 μm; further reduction in fine diameter reduces the flow rates. Equations of the Brown–Richards type relationship are adequate for modeling the static flow in such systems. Equation (1) relates the flow rate Q to powder density ρt and circular aperture diameter D_A:

$$D_A K[4Q/60\pi \cdot \rho t \cdot \sqrt{g}]^{1/n} \tag{1}$$

where K and n are material-dependent constants and g is the gravitational force.

In a similar study of the factors influencing the flow of lactose granules, a strong negative correlation was found between the flow rate of granules and proportion of particles less than 150 μm (100 mesh) in size (12).

A decrease in particular size of salicylic acid resulted in a decrease in the angle of internal flow Ψ, which was derived empirically as a measure of cohesiveness (13). The value of Ψ was found to be dependent on the relative proportion and particle size of salicylic acid and lactose when blends of these powders were studied. Geoffroy and Carstensen (14) have used shear cell measurements of sodium chloride, granular dicalcium phosphate (DiTab) and hydroxyapatite (TriTab) to examine the affect particle size has on the constants in the shear cell. They modified the Warren–Springs equation (Eq. 5 found in the Shear Cell section of this article) which relates cohesion and tensile strength of cohesive powders. They showed that cohesion stress (C) is related to tangential force (T) by the equation $C = \alpha T^\beta$ where α and β are constants dependent on the materials used. They also demonstrated relationship of α to particle diameter. They incorporated this into the Warren–Springs equation so that particle size could be better accounted for in analyzing shear cell data.

Shape Factors and Surface Morphology

Particle sizes combined with shape factors have been the subject of many of the recent studies regarding flow of solids. Sphericity, circularity, surface-shape coefficient, volume-shape coefficient, and surface-volume-shape coefficient are some of the most commonly used shape factors. It is generally accepted that the flowability of powders decreases as the shapes of particles become more irregular. Efforts to relate various shape factors to powder bulk behavior have become more successful recently, primarily because of the fact that shape characterization techniques and methods for physically sorting particles of different shapes are improving. This is primarily thanks to the use of fractal geometry.

Fractal geometry was developed by B.B. Mandelbrot and was most fully described in a 1983 text (15). Fractal geometry essentially describes the space filling ability of a rugged line or surface by adding a fractional number to the to the topological dimension of a system as illustrated in Fig. 1. Brian Kaye and co-workers have extended Mandelbrot's concepts to describe the structure of rugged shaped powder grains and later to the distribution function of a powder (16–19). The use of fractal geometry and chaos theory has been used to develop a test method, using a rotating drum (10, 18, 19) and this test method will be described later in the article.

Hickey and Concessio (20) studied a series of powders of pharmaceutical interest using a vibrating spatula. In all of the powders studied, mass flow rates increased as the particle size increased. Sodium chloride, which did not exhibit fractal behavior (very low fractal number), showed no irregular flow patterns. Lactose, cromolyn sodium and charcoal that did exhibit fractal behavior at low stride lengths, demonstrated irregular flow patterns. Kaye in unpublished data described the avalanching behavior of five lactose powders. Though similar in particle size, the various lactose samples showed different morphology and different avalanche behavior. Brittain (21) tested anhydrous and fast flow lactose, using Carr index and showed that the Fast-Flo lactose yielded higher flow capacity. He attributed this to the morphology of the two materials and the rounded edges in the Fast-Flo material. Cartillier and Tawashi (22) also related the flow properties and packing characteristics of seven different lactose powders as measured by the angle of repose and flow through an orifice to particle morphology, especially micro morphology as determined through a scanning electron

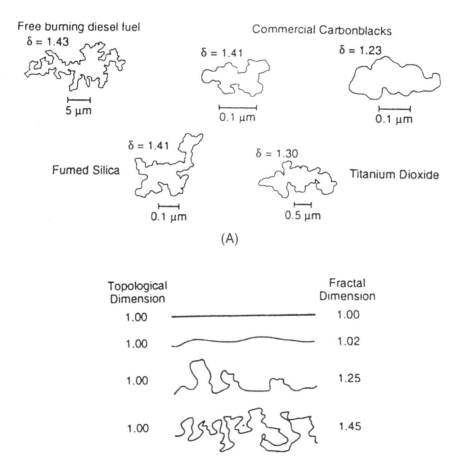

Fig. 1 (A) Profiles of fumed pigment fine particles where the fractal dimension, δ, describes the ruggedness of the profile. (B) Four lines with identical topological dimensions with varying degrees of ruggedness as seen from their corresponding fractal dimensions. (From Ref. 18.)

microscope, and expressed in various parameters including fractal dimensions.

The angle of repose of granules prepared by five different methods was found to be primarily a function of surface roughness. The Hausner ratio (discussed later) has been related to the morphological properties of sands (23).

The shapes of components being mixed have a great impact on the mixing rate and the physical stability of the resultant mixture. Lactose and calcium carbonate of different particle shapes were mixed in a Y-cone mixer. The time required to achieve an acceptable standard deviation of mixing o_A increased with the irregularity of the particles of both components, and the mixtures containing irregularly shaped particles segregated less on subsequent vibration (24).

Some work has shown a direct correlation between shape factor and the flow properties of powders. The flowability of fine powders, as measured by a shear-cell as well as by Carr's method, was found to increase with increasing sphericity, where the sphericity is indicated by a shape index Ψ approaching one, as measured by an image analyzer (25). Huber and co-workers (26) derived an equuation in which flow rate was correlated to the volume specific surface as measured by laser diffractometry. Reasonable predictions were made for individual powders as well as binary and ternary mixtures.

Moisture and Static Charge

The affect of humidity can vary drastically from powder to powder. Absorbed moisture in solids can exist either in the unbound state or as part of crystal structure. It exerts its effect directly by changing the surface properties of the particle. It can also affect flow properties indirectly and permanently through the formation of granules, which are held, together by solid bridges generated by hydration and dehydration of a binder. The process of wet granulation can be viewed as an intentional use of moisture (or other organic liquid) in controlling powder flow properties. Moisture significantly influences powder flowability as measured by the tensile strength of powders by forming liquid bridges. The increase in tensile strength has been translated into increase in torque or power consumption in a mixer and has been utilized for the monitoring of wet-granulation processes. At higher moisture content and higher packing densities, liquid bridges may progress from pendular to funicular bonds. The effect of moisture varies, depending on the degree of packing or the porosity of the powder bed. For a porous and cohesive material, flowability is not affected by moisture since the moisture can penetrate to the inside of particles without the formation of liquid bridges. A single lot of microcrystalline cellulose NF was placed in various humidity conditions and the moisture content determined through loss of drying (27). Flow parameters were determined through the compressibility index determined by tap density and also through the use of a shear cell. It was shown that increased moisture decreased flow and that once the moisture content of the microcrystalline cellulose exceeded 5% its flow was predicted to be poor. Differences in flow rates of microcrystalline cellulose through an orifice were attributed partially to differences in moisture contents that affected cohesiveness (28). Cohesiveness of two grades of microcrystalline cellulose (Avicel PH101 and Emcocel) measured with a sandwich rheometer, peaks at approximately 20–25 wt% moisture content. Avicel was found to be more cohesive than Emococel at a moisture content less and 30 wt%, whereas at higher moisture content the cohesive behavior was comparable (29).

Very low moisture can hinder flow since you are more likely to develop electrostatic charging. Particles acquire static charge most commonly through grinding, attrition, and collision, a phenomenon generally known as triboelectrification. Surface charge can also be generated by the sudden separation of their closely contacted, dissimilar surfaces, as in the case of sieving, mixing, or the movement of dry particles through a hopper or over a belt. Excipient powders are generally charged negatively in contact with metal or glass surfaces, whereas many are charged positively in contact with plastic surfaces (30). Most pharmaceutical excipients have low resistivity and therefore lose electrostatic charge through earth leakage relatively quickly. Electrostatic charge interactions can be controlled with beneficial results in terms of improved physical stability of normally unstable, segregating systems. Physical stability can be improved with or without permanent electrification (31).

Powder Cohesion and Storage Compaction

The storage condition a powder is placed under will have a great affect on the flow characteristics it exhibits. As stated in recent article by Marinelli (32) "as a solid remains at rest in a bin or hopper, it can become more cohesive and difficult flowing." Hopper and bin load levels, vibratory forces, time in storage, temperature of storage as well as the intrinsic cohesiveness of the material will alter its flow characteristics. Shear cells have been designed to measure the cohesion of materials under load and after preconditioning. The nature of these tests and how they work is described in more detail later on in this chapter.

Effects of Temperature

The cohesion of powder as measured in a Jenike or annular shear cell decreases as the temperature is decreased (33). This is attributed to the reduction in plasticity and in the inability of asperities on the surface of neighboring particles to form welded bonds as the temperature of the sample is lowered (34). Similarly, flow rates of powdered sugars and fatty acids through a circular orifice decrease with increasing temperature (35). An increase in tensile strength of powders is also observed for lactose and griseofulvin with increasing temperature and explained on the same basis (36). Pilpel (37) noted that an important property of a powder determining whether or not it was sensitive to temperature changes when studying flow behavior was its homologous temperature. The homologous temperature for any given material is the investigational temperature as a fraction of the melting point of the material in absolute degrees (Kelvin). Stearic acid that has a melting point of 343 K when tested at 25°C (298 K) would have a homologous temperature of 298/343 K equal to 0.87. In his investigations Pilpel found that powders started to have less flowability at homologous temperatures above 0.9. As you would suspect materials with lower melting points will have more flow problems than would higher melting point solids. Pilpel also noted that when powders that would not flow out of a funnel at room temperature were cooled to −25°C they flowed easily.

MODELS OF HOPPER FLOW

The design of hoppers and bins has been studied extensively in the last 35 years especially in the mining, food and chemical industry. Due to the large volumes of powders handled in these industries the design of storage and handling materials are a major investment. During the late 1950s and early 1960s Jenike employed a soil mechanics approach to powder handling, developing a logical, theoretical basis for bulk solids flow (38). In general, two flow patterns can be used to describe material flow through a hopper, although systems exist in between. When materials flow by gravity, the entire content of the hopper moves together and the material discharges on a first-in first-out basis. This is the case of mass flow. When the movement is restricted to a central region, leaving a relatively stationary zone in the periphery, the situation is known as funnel flow or core flow. Alternatively, flow blockage occurs by doming or bridging where a stable arch is formed across the outlet of a hopper (Fig. 2a). With highly cohesive powders or poorly designed hoppers when the gate is opened only the material above the opening

flows out and then no further flow occurs. This is an extreme funnel flow condition known as rat holing or piping (Fig. 2b). Mechanical and structural arches are stable obstructions formed when particles come together to form a weight bearing arch, much in the same way a stone bridge is formed. This type of arch can be avoided by making sure the opening is of sufficient width to allow the particles to pass through. For cones the rule of thumb is that the opening should be six to eight times the largest particle size (39), 10 times has been mentioned by Jenike (38). The more troublesome arch is a cohesive arch. This type of arch is formed through compaction and cohesion of the material in the hopper. Bates (40) defines cohesive arching as "the formation of a stable flow obstruction over an outlet or within a flow channel due to the bulk strength of the material exceeding the unconfined failure strength at which the span of the arch would collapse because of the stresses acting on the mass." The design of a mass-flow hopper is based on the postulate that gravity flow of a solid in a channel takes place, provided that the yield strength that the solid develops as a result of consolidation is insufficient to support an obstruction to flow. The calculations for hopper dimension are based on an assumption of the stress pattern that may exist in the hopper in the static condition that is expressed as a flow factor (ff), which is the ratio of the maximum principal stress at two difference points, as shown by

$$ff = \frac{\text{Maximum principal stress encountered within the hopper}}{\text{Maximum principal stress at free surface}} \quad (2)$$

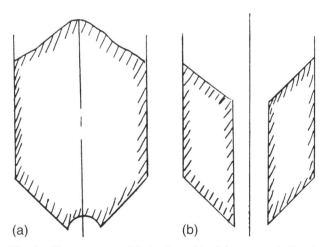

Fig. 2 Flow patterns: (a) doming; (b) piping or rat holing in obstructed flow.

The hopper design, therefore, requires the maximum principal stress at the outlet to be greater than the unconfined yield stress of the powder material. The two stresses may be compared graphically by plotting the flow function of the material (FF) and the flow factor of the hopper (ff) on the same fc vs. σ_m plot. The point at which the hopper stress and the material strength are equal is known as the *"critical unconfined yield stress;"* it must be determined when calculating the size of the hopper outlet. The hopper flow factor is obtained from figures described by Jenike (38) and come from shear cell measurements described later on in this chapter.

If the hopper-flow factor lies above the powder-flow function, cohesive arching is not possible with the material in that hopper. If the hopper factor lies below the powder-flow function, arching of material in the hopper is possible even for large-outlet sizes.

Various shear cells have been developed to aid in obtaining the needed information to determine the functions necessary to design mass flow hoppers, bins and silos. In addition to powder shear, wall friction testing (41, 42) and compressibility (43) as well as other testing all enter into hopper design. This chapter can only briefly touch on the theories and test methods that go into hopper design. Various recent texts (44–46) give a much more in depth treatment of the subject. Various web sites such as www. powderandbulk.com have been the source of updates in this area.

Prescott and Hossfeld (47) have written an article relating hopper design directly to pharmaceuticals, most specifically to the tabletting process. Mechanisms of segregation in the hopper are discussed and case histories of how hopper designs and inserts, which aid flow, can help solve these problems. Since the hoppers for tablet presses as well as capsule filling equipment are specifically designed for this equipment and since in the pharmaceutical industry a variety of materials must be handled by the same equipment, the use of inserts might be a relatively inexpensive fix for flow problems. Bates (48) discusses the use of inserts in hoppers and Troxel (49) also discusses the use of mechanical flow aids such as vibrators, air cannons as well as chemical flow aid, which are discussed in the next section.

FLOW ENHANCERS (GLIDANTS)

To improve the flowability of powders and granulations, a small amount of a flow agent, or glidant, is often added, usually in powder form. Commonly used glidants are colloidal silicone dioxide, talc, and starch. Several postulates have been proposed for the mechanism of glidant action (50–52).

- Dispersion of static charge from the surface of host particles;
- Distribution of glidant in the host particles;
- Preferential adsorption of gases and vapors otherwise adsorbed onto the host particle;
- Physical separation of particles and subsequent reduction in van der Waals interaction; and
- Adsorption of glidant particles to granulation surfaces in such a way that friction between particles and surface rugosity are minimized.

The effects of a glidant on the flowability of a powder depend on many factors, such as physical and chemical affinity for the powder, the average particle size and shape in relation to those of the powder, concentration of the glidant and degree of mixing, as well as the moisture content. To be effective, in general, the glidant particles should be very much smaller than those of the host powder in order to coat them completely, smoothing out irregularities in their shape, and reducing the frictional and adhesive forces that operate between them. In almost all systems, there is an optimum concentration above which the glidant ceases to be effective. If too much is added, powder flowability may decrease, and it is therefore necessary to control the addition carefully for the best results. Glidants probably have mainly a mechanical action. They adhere to the surfaces of host powders, smoothing out irregularities and reducing their tendency to interlock mechanically during movement and flow. If the particles of the glidants are assumed to be spherical in shape with a radius r and are uniformly closely packed to those of the host, which are also assumed to be spherical with the radius R, optimum flow should occur when the mixture contains approximately $(2\pi r(R + r)^2 100/R^3 \sqrt{3}\%\text{w/w})$ of a glidant (53). A 100-μm powder requires about 3% of a 1-μm glidant, which is in reasonable agreement with experimental observations. The type of glidant, the mixing factors, and the nature of the formulation all will have affects on the reliability of this equation.

Colloidal Silcion dioxide is an agent that has been commonly used as a glidant. Flow rate, density, as well as other related measurements, were conducted on four different excipients. The addition of 1% colloidal silicon dioxide increased the flow of the poorer flowing excipients but had lesser affects on the exipients that were of larger size and were better flowing (54). Increasing amounts of chlorpromazine hydrochloride markedly decreased the flow characteristics of all the various blends. The particle size of the excipient blend seemed to grow larger with the addition of the chlorpromazine hydrochloride since it is believed that the drug stuck to the surface of the excipients. The addition of 1% collodial silicon dioxide negated the negative affects of the drug. The addition of the collodial silicon dioxide decreased the particle size increases caused by the addition of drug. It is believed therefore that a possible mechanism of the silicon dioxide was to prevent the drug from coating the excipient particles and reducing flow. Scanning electron microscopy corroborated this conclusion. In another work (55) the amount of silicon dioxide was varied from 0–2%. It was shown that 0.5% addition of the glidant caused a marked reduction to the weight deviation of tablets produced on a single punch tablet press. The standard deviation of tablet weight did not further reduce when greater than 0.5% of colloidal silicon dioxide was added to the formulation showing a limit to its effectiveness. In a recent article (56), 2% colloidal silicon dioxide was shown to be affective in improving the flow of micronized ibuprofen powder in powder layering.

Magnesium stearate, which is better know as a lubricant, has also been shown to have glidant properties. Shear cell studies with eight different materials with varying size and shape showed that the optimum amount of magnesium stearate that affected flow was related directly to particle size (57). In another study mixing time and type of mixer had a marked affect on the flow of lactose containing 1% magnesium stearate (58). These experiments demonstrate that magnesium stearate becomes increasingly affective as a glidant as it coats the material. The surface area needed to be covered and the shear and duration of the mixing are primary variables in determining the optimal glidant concentration of magnesium stearate.

MEASUREMENTS OF FLOW PROPERTIES

Flow Through an Orifice

During the manufacture of tablets, granulations must first flow through a stationary orifice, the outlet of a hopper, followed by flowing into moving orifices, that is, tablet dies. The first type of flow, static flow, has been investigated extensively. Equations developed for modeling static flow, W_s, through an orifice of diameter P, are often based on the Brown–Richards equation and are written as

$$W_S = f(d)P^{b(d)} \qquad (3)$$

Generally f and n denote "function of" and $n(d)$ is generally 2.5. Moreover n has also been shown to be a function of the particle diameter d. Conditions for static flow where the Brown–Richards equation is applicable are the following (59):

- The flow rate decreases as the particle size is increased;
- The orifice size is at least six times greater than the particle size;
- The granulation height is at least two times greater than the orifice diameter; and
- The ratio of the orifice diameter to granulation hopper diameter is less than 0.5.

The dimensions of a flowmeter should therefore be carefully considered prior to its construction. For example, a flat-bottom flowmeter with a diameter of 6.0 cm, and circular orifices with diameters of 1.428, 0.925, and 0.635 cm and a column height exceeding 18 cm were employed as reported by Danish and Parrott (11). For a flowmeter consisting of a hopper with interchangeable attachments, a top-loading balance with output capabilities, and a digital analog converter, a strip-chart recorder was employed in the evaluation of formulations (60). Criteria for acceptance of prototype formulations were developed, including uniform flow of > 200 g/min through a 30° cone, and low through a 12.7-mm straight-bore attachment of 7 > 2000 g/min.

Some formulations can flow too well and upper limits are required based on the capacity of the tablet press under consideration.

A flowmeter is generally capable of measuring the flow rate of powders that flow well. For cohesive materials the minimum orifice diameter necessary to induce free flow was reported to be a better index of flowability (61).

Several studies were conducted to investigate the relationship between the orifice flow rate and the failure properties of powder materials. It was indicated that a simple linear relationship between flow rate and tensile strength would exist only when the powder system is sufficiently cohesive to produce measurable tensile strength of a consolidated powder but sufficiently free-flowing to produce a gravity flow under an unknown and changing consolidation state (62). For less easily flowing powders the hopper may be vibrated to facilitate flow in order to measure flow rates.

A flow device was developed with movable orifices that attempted, through the geometry of the system, to eliminate wall friction as a factor (63). Most consistent results were obtained when a stainless steel cylinder was used as the main hopper. The orifice was a movable end piece with different size holes. In order to select the best excipients for the direct compression of microtablets a funnel flow device, using interchangeable orifices was used. The lengths of the orifices were also varied to keep the angle of inclination constant (64). It was shown that flow rates could be estimated even for narrow orifices. The Carr index and Hausner ratios, which will be discussed in the next section, of the excipients was also determined and used in the excipient evaluation. In a more recent paper (65) a funnel method was used to evaluate a number of sustained release theophylline microtablet formulations. Colloidal silicon dioxide was added to the nonflowing granulations and then measurements were taken. The angle of repose was also measured for all of these formulations. A number of papers in the last 10 years, in addition to the ones already discussed, use flow rate measurements to evaluate pharmaceutical formulations and excipients (66–73) and almost all combine the hopper flow measurements with other measurements, such as angle or repose and Carr Index. In summary, flowmeters are a practical way of screening powders with good flow and distinguishing good flowing materials from poorer flowing materials. Since all materials don't flow well enough for evaluation, flowmeter measurements are often used in combination with other measurements for formulation flow evaluation.

Empirical Measurements of Powder or Granular Properties

A number of tests such as contact angle, bulk density, and tap density are relatively simple tests that, though not direct measurements of flow, have been found often to be predictive of the flow characteristics of materials. This is because these measurements are highly dependent on particle size and shape and the cohesive nature of the material, all of which are chief variables in the flowability of solids. These tests are commonly used in combination and are still routinely being conducted and related to flow in every-day pharmaceutical development.

Angle of Repose and Other Handling Angles

If a powder is allowed to flow onto a flat surface, a pile or heap of powder is formed. A material that is not cohesive and flows well, spreads out, forming a low heap. More cohesive materials form higher heaps, which are less spread out. The angle of repose is defined as the angle of the free surface of a pile of powder to the horizontal plane. Pharmaceutical powders give two main types of angle of repose: the poured angle, which is the angle measured on a pile poured freely onto a flat surface; and the drained angle, which is the angle measured on the conical surface of powder in a flat-bottomed container, if the powder is discharged through an orifice in the base. The poured angle of repose can be determined by any

device that allows a standard method of pouring the powder onto the flat surface and measuring the angle of the resulting heap. A protractor is commonly used or the base of the heap is controlled and the height of the heap is measured (Fig. 3) (74).

The drained repose angle is obtained with flow devices as described previously. The measurement is affected by the degree of consolidation of the material in the hopper. The drained angle is usually larger than the poured angle for the same powder. Just as the flow rate is affected by the size of the orifice and the particle size of the powder, so is the drained angle. Pilpel (75), recognizing the effect wall friction could have on the drained angle, reported on a device in which the powder is initially placed in a large container with a built-in platform. The powder is allowed to flow out at the bottom, leaving an undisturbed conical heap on the platform, thus eliminating wall friction from the measurement. Carstensen et al. (76) demonstrated that the frictional force between the support base and the granulation plays a significant part in the repose angle of a heap of granules on a plane surface. This means that even the Pilpel device as well as poured-angle measurements would be affected by frictional factors. Jones and Pilpel (77) tested a number of devices and showed that the measurements obtained were highly dependent on the device. In a review article (78), Pilpel states that since the angular properties of powders are so dependent on the details of measurements, they are useful only in a qualitative manner. For this reason, the shear cell has replaced the repose angle measurement as a quantitative method to detect the cohesive characteristics of powder.

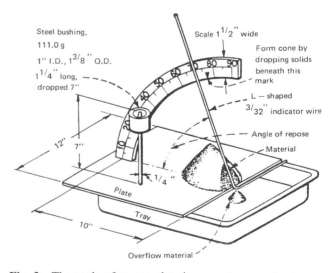

Fig. 3 The angle-of-repose plate incorporates a protractor, an indicator wire, and a jarring device for angle-of-fall tests. (From Chem. Engi. **1965**, *18*, 164.)

In addition to measurements of poured and drained repose angles, several other handling angles have been utilized. By placing the powder on a smooth surface (slide) and finding the minimum slope that causes the powder to slide, the angle of the slide is obtained. It is highly dependent on the material over which it slides (79), and can be useful in designing hoppers or conveyers. Another angle that has been utilized is the angle of spatula, which is measured by lifting powder with a flat spatula and measuring the angle the heap of powder forms with the spatula surface. Carr (74) standardized this method and utilized it with several other parameters to characterize powders. Characterization numbers are discussed later. The angle of spatula serves as a very simple but rough method of characterizing a powder with respect to flow. A vibrating spatula has also been used in recent years and this will also be discussed in a later section (20, 80).

Dahlinder et al. (61) developed a new device to measure the drained angle of repose. It consists of a split cylinder, which contains a flat circular platform. To measure the angle of repose, the cylinder is filled with powder. The cylinder is split, allowing the powder to fall into a heap on the platform. This device is similar to Pilpel's (75) but eliminates wall friction during the flow by utilizing the split cylinder to initiate flow. Dahlinder tested sodium chloride, microcyrstalline cellulose, and aspirin powder as well as lactose, lactose-cornstarch, and aluminum hydroxide-magnesium carbonate granules. The resulting angle-of-repose measurements were reproducible (relative standard deviation about 2%). The authors concluded that this method could be used to characterize even fairly cohesive materials. Nyqvist and Nicklasson (81) utilizing Dahlinder's repose-angle device tested direct-compression lactose containing small concentrations of various actives and found a linear relationship of the angle of repose to the coefficient of tablet-weight variation. Nyqvist (82) found that when testing penicillin granulations the Dahlinder repose-angle results did not give any specific ranking order for the pure drug substance or the granulation. In contrast, annular shear cell data were able to predict the flow behavior for tablet production. Most recently Parrott (83) utilized a poured angle measurement to compare Soludex, a corn-based maltodextrin, to nine commercial excipients. He also used flow through a fixed orifice, and found that the flowmeter represented the flow of the materials better than the repose angle. However, several ingredients did not flow at all through the orifice, and the angle of repose represented the only comparative value for the 10 excipients investigated.

Heistand (8) and Carstensen (84) related the repose angle to the intrinsic cohesion and frictional coefficient of powders. As mentioned previously, the dependence on the technique used makes this method much less reliable for this purpose than a shear cell. In addition, the repose angle does not quantitatively treat the compressive forces of the flow process in the same way as the shear cell. As Pilpel mentioned (79), angular tests are applicable to relatively free-flowing powders containing particles larger than 100 μm. Such powders cannot be investigated in the scientifically more satisfactory shear cell and tensile strength test apparatus because of their low cohesion and tensile strength. Furthermore, the particles become crushed on consolidation. Today angular measurements continue to be used with mixed results, as shown by the previous examples. The test, usually in combination with other tests, provides a simple and sometimes useful method for monitoring the characteristics of powders and granules for quality control purposes.

Packing Properties and Bulk Densities

The bulk density of a powder is obtained by dividing its mass by the bulk volume it occupies. The volume includes the spaces between particles as well as the envelope volumes of the particles themselves. The true density of a material (i.e., the density of the actual solid material) can be obtained with a gas pycnometer. The bulk density of a powder is not a definite number like true density or specific gravity but an indirect measurement of a number of factors, including particle size and size distribution, particle shape, true density, and especially the method of measurement. Although there is no direct linear relationship between the flowability of a powder and its bulk density, the latter is extremely important in determining the capacity of mixers and hoppers and providing an easily obtained valuable characterization of powders.

Aerated bulk density

This is the bulk density of a powder after it has been allowed to aerate, that is, in most cases flow. A number of commercial devices are used to obtain this value. These devices allow the powder to flow from a fixed height, usually through a set of screens, into a container of fixed volume. An excess of powder is used and cleared from the top of the container, the tared container is then weighed. The bulk density is the weight of the powder divided by the volume of the container. The device can be as complex as a series of vibrating screens or as simple as pouring powder through a screen into a tared graduated cylinder. The cylinder is placed on a tapping device to measure the tap or, as Carr (74) defines it, the packed bulk density. Some tap the cylinder three times in order to level the powder and get a more uniform result. The leveling of the powder can also be critical in other devises. The author utilized a device known as a Scott volumeter in which powder is passed through a series of glass baffles before falling into a tared cubical container. The excess powder is removed, so that the powder is flush with the container top. Considerable operator variability between tests has been noted, and it was found that the pressure in removing the excess powder varied between operators; this was the chief source of variability. A standard wiper method was developed and solved the problem.

Tapped or compressed bulk density

Tap density is the bulk density of a powder which has been compacted by tapping or vibration following a specified procedure. A large number of machines are available to measure tap density; some use a fixed volume of powder and some a fixed weight of powder. The sample is dropped (tapped) a set distance at a set frequency for a fixed number of times. Vibrators of known frequency have also been used for compaction. A simple device, developed by Neumann in 1953 (85) is shown in Fig. 4. It uses a cut cam, which allows the powder to drop exactly 1 cm each revolution. In tap devices the machine can be set to stop after a certain number of taps and the volume is measured. The sample is usually tapped or vibrated until an equilibrium volume is obtained and at that point the final tap density is determined. The rate of tap density can also be measured by recording the density after a given number of taps or vibrating for a given amount of time, and repeating the process until no change in volume occurs.

Density and flow

Carr (74) reported that the more a material is compacted in a compaction or tap bulk density test, the poorer its flow properties. He defines compressibility C by

$$\%C = 100(P - A)/P \qquad (4)$$

where P is the final tap or compacted bulk density and A the aerated bulk density. A more commonly used term is the Hausner ratio, which is simply P/A, the final tap density divided by the aerated bulk density. This ratio was introduced by Hausner in 1967 (86) to characterize metal powders, but is commonly used today for pharmaceutical powders. The higher the Hausner ratio, the poorer the flow. Neumann (52) reported that the higher the rate of packing (fewer taps to reach equilibrium), the better the flowability. He also experimented with weights to compact the powder. He plotted the log of the relative volume obtained with a given weight vs. the log of the weight used; linear plots are produced. Chowhan and Chow (87)

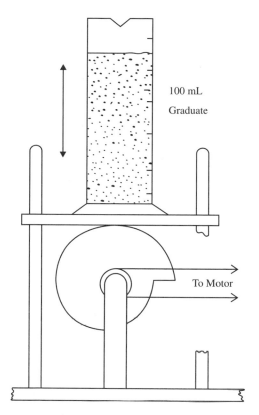

Fig. 4 Tapping device. (From Ref. 85.)

used a modified version of Neumann's device in which they placed loosely packed powders and powder mixtures in cylindrical containers and applied a series of loads to the surface of the powder beds. They tested a drug with various excipients and plotted the log of the relative volume vs. the log of the relative weight utilized. They also obtained linear plots and called the intercept on the relative volume axis the powder-consolidating ratio. This value yielded a linear correlation with weight variation for capsules filled on a Zanasi capsule-filling machine.

Varthalis and Pilpel (88) derived a relationship between tensile strength and packing rate with lactose and paracetamol and, alternatively, lactose and oxytetracycline. From this relationship they developed a measure of powder flow and packing in terms of the "angle of internal flow," an empirically derived parameter, for the rate of change of bulk density with tamping. Newton and Bader (13) utilized this parameter and related it to the fill weight of capsules containing aspirin and lactose. Attempts to relate it to in vitro release of the aspirin were not successful. In the first of a series of articles regarding lactose coated with nonionic surfactant, Sakr and Pilpel (89) utilized tap density to explain the surface effects of the coating. Yamashiro et al. (90) used very short tap intervals (stopped and measured after one or two taps) to test an equation stating that the number of taps divided by the relative volume of the powder after these taps is linearly related to the number of taps. When this relationship holds, the flow rate of a material can be related to the proportionality constants.

In conclusion, tap-density methods are a quick and inexpensive way to characterize materials. A strictly empirical relationship exists between the degree of compaction and powder flow. If viewed in this light, tap density can be a useful measurement technique.

CLASSIFICATION SYSTEMS

In 1965 Carr (74) proposed a characterization system that has been used extensively to classify pharmaceutical powders and granulations. The method consists of a point system that weighs four factors equally, giving each a maximum of 25 points with a maximum of 100 for a perfectly flowing material. The first measurement is the angle of repose. A diagram of the apparatus used by Carr and a discussion of angle of repose appear earlier (Fig. 3). According to Carr, the contact angle is a simple and easy method of indirectly measuring the following properties affecting flow: shape, size, porosity, cohesion, fluidity, surface area, and bulk density. The second factor, also discussed previously, is compressibility as obtained from tap density. Carr defined compressibility by Eq. 4 and claimed that the percent compressibility indirectly provides an excellent representation of uniformity in size and shape, deformability, surface area, cohesion, and moisture content.

The third factor in Carr's characterization scheme is the angle of spatula. As mentioned previously, Carr designed a special method for measuring this angle. According to him, the angle of spatula is an indirect measure of cohesion, surface area, size, shape, uniformity, fluidity, porosity, and deformability.

The last factor is either the cohesion or the coefficient of uniformity. Cohesion is used with powders (very fine particles) or with materials on which an effective cohesion force can be measured. The uniformity coefficient is used with granular and powdered granular materials on which an effective surface cohesion cannot be measured.

The procedure for finding the apparent surface cohesion involves determining the retention of material on a nest of 250-, 150-, and 74-μm (60-, 100-, and 200-mesh) screens over a bottom pan. A weight of 2 g of test powder is recommended to be placed on the 250-μm (60-mesh) screen, followed by vibrating the nest of screens for

20–120 s. The amount of material left on each screen is weighed and rated in points or percentage. Accordingly: each 0.1 g on the 250-μm (60-mesh) screen corresponds to five points or 5%; each 0.1 g on the 150-μm (100-mesh) screen corresponds to three points; and each 0.1 g on the 74-μm (200-mesh) screen corresponds to one point. If the entire amount of material passes through the 74-μm (200-mesh) screen, the cohesion is zero. Electrostatic attraction of some particles and the tendency of smaller particles to adhere to larger particles can skew the result. The particle must be 74-μm (200-mesh) material in order for the test to be attempted.

The uniformity coefficient is arrived at by dividing the width of the sieve opening that passes 10% of the sample. It is determined from a screen analysis of the material. The more uniform a mass of particles is in both size and shape, the more flowable it is likely to be.

The point score for the evaluation of flowability of dry solids is given in Table 1. In order to measure the flowability of a powder utilizing this method, each test is made and the points can be found in the table. The total number of points would place the sample into one of the seven categories in the left column of the table. Because of its simplicity and the fact that commercial devices are available to conduct these tests (this test is ASTM test designation D 6393-99), this system is widely used in the pharmaceutical industry both in preformulations, formulation research, and in quality control.

Other classification systems are used less frequently. Carr (74) also devised a system to classify materials as to their floodability. He defines the floodability of a material as its tendency to flow like a liquid because of the natural fluidization of a mass of particles by air. In order to so classify a material, the flowability is determined utilizing the method just described. This value is equivalent to a measurement Carr calls the angle of fall, angle of difference, and dispersibility. Though referred to in any of the papers mentioned here, this system is much less utilized then the flowability measurements. Geldart (91) reported on a characterization system of powders according to their ability to aerate and later Molerus (92) modified this system. In a more recent symposium this method of powder classification was examined (93–95).

As mentioned in previous sections of this article, the Carr index as well as other empirical tests such as the Hausner ratio continue be used, often in combination with other tests to characterize and predict the flow of pharmaceutical excipients and formulations. In addition to papers already discussed in this article a number of papers have appeared in the more recent pharmaceutical literature in which these methods have been used to classify the flow characteristics of pharmaceutical

Table 1 Point scores for evaluation of flowability of dry solids

Flowability and performance	Angle of repose		Compressibility		Angle of spatula		Uniformity coef.[a]		Cohesion[b]	
	Deg.	Points	%	Points	Deg.	Points	Units	Points	%	Points
Excellent, 90–100 pts.	25	25	5	25	25	25	1	25		
Aid not needed	26–29	24	6–9	23	26–30	24	2–4	23		
Does not arch	30	22.5	10	22.5	31	22.5	5	22.5		
Good, 80–89 pts.	31	22	11	22	32	22	6	22		
Aid not needed	32–34	21	12–14	21	33–37	21	7	21		
Does not arch	35	20	15	20	38	20	8	20		
Fair, 70–79 pts.	36	19.5	16	19.5	39	19.5	9	19		
Aid not needed, but vibration may be necessary	37–39	18	17–19	18	40–44	18	10–11	18		
	40	17.5	20	17.5	45	17.5	12	17.5		
Passable, 60–69 pts.	41	17	21	17	46	17	13	17		
Borderline, material may hang up	42–44	16	22–24	16	47–59	16	15–16	16		
	45	15	25	15	60	15	17	15	<6	15
Poor, 40–59 pts.	46	14.5	26	14.5	61	14.5	18	14.5	6–9	14.5
Agitation and vibration required	47–54	12	27–30	12	62–74	12	19–21	12	10–29	12
	55	10	31	10	75	10	22	10	30	10
Very poor, 20–39 pts.	56	9.5	32	9.5	76	9.5	23	9.5	31	9.5
More positive agitation needed	57–64	7	33–36	7	77–89	7	24–26	7	32–54	7
	65	5	37	5	90	5	27	5	55	5
Very, very poor, up to 19 pts.	66	4.5	38	4.5	91	4.5	28	4.5	56	4.5
Special agitation and hopper design required	67–89	2	39–45	2	92–99	2	29–35	2	51–79	2
	90	0	>45	0	>99	0	>36	0	>79	0

[a] Used with granular and powdered granular materials.
[b] Used with powders or where an effective cohesion can be measured.
(From Chem. Eng. **1965**, *18*.)

powders (93–101). Sugar based excipients (96), granulated lactitol (101), microcrystalline cellulose codried with β-cyclodextrins (100) and various phyllosilicate powders such as bentonites (97) were characterized through Carr index measurements. With the phyllosilicate powders the authors noted that hopper flow values were of little use due to very high standard deviations and the angle of repose measurements and Carr index and Huasner Ratio were considered more relevant to their characterization. In the microwave drying of high shear granulations, the Carr index decreased with increasing microwave power due possibly to an increase in dust formation (98). Hausner ratio and slowing of the rate of taping was used to show that moisture increased the interparticular friction of Avicel PH 302 99). Angle of repose along with flow through multi size orifices were used to characterize the flow of several dextrins (93). Another example of the use of Carr's indexing method is given in a paper by Vennat

et al. (102) where the flowability and floodability index of a group of direct-compression excipients and procyanidins are reported. The material was tested in the commercial Hosokawa powder characteristic tester. Only angle of repose and taped and bulk densities were used to classify the rheology of Avicel PH-200 and Cellactose (94, 95).

In summary, Carr's flow characterization method is frequently used for characterizing powders. No one method alone gives a total picture of flow and hence a combination of methods is often used. If known forces are being utilized during the flow process, a shear cell would be the method of choice when a scientifically based characterization is needed. If granulations are being tested with good flow characteristics, a flowmeter might be the method of choice. A combination of empirical tests, for example, Carr's flowability test, would be very useful as a simple screening device or as a quality control test for multiple lots. The selection of the method should be based on the amount of information needed and the material to be tested, and may be more importantly, the equipment available.

SHEAR CELLS

The flow through an orifice is an excellent method to compare materials with good flow. Pharmacy, however, most often deals with cohesive powders that do not readily flow. The flow of these materials is increased by employing force feeders, resulting in a dynamic process. Angle-of-repose measurements that do not utilize force and that are often a measurement of stagnant powder have therefore limited application. Shear testers, that measure the frictional characteristics of a powder bed under load, yield valuable information with regard to powder flow in high-speed tablet- and capsule-filling equipment.

Data Treatment

A number of different types of shear cells are discussed in this section. Each of these cells is designed to condition the powder under a known force, and measure the force needed to shear the powder bed under a load force equal to or less than the original conditioning force. For each conditioning force, the force needed to shear the bed for a series of loads is plotted against the load force in a similar manner in which a frictional coefficient is determined for a nonpowdered material. Such a plot is known as a yield locus (Fig. 5), and it is often obtained for a number of different conditioning forces. Thus, if the forces acting on a material in a given process can be approximated, intrinsic information regarding the frictional and cohesive nature of the material can be obtained that should have great relevance to real processes.

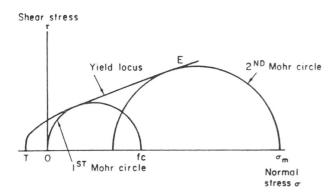

Fig. 5 Mohr circle construction to obtain the major normal stress, σ_m, and the unconfined field stress, fc. (From Ref. 78.)

The most common method of treating shear data is the Mohr circle analysis, also shown in Fig. 5. The x-axis represents the stress normal to the shearing power (load stress), and the y-axis represents the shear stress. The curve represents the yield locus for a cohesive solid. The intersections of the Mohr circles are drawn in such a way that they are tangent to the yield locus. These circles represent the total forces on the powder bed at the point of shear for any direction. The point at which the Mohr-circle-drawn tangent to the upper end of the yield locus (2nd Mohr circle) intersects the x-axis at the highest point is known as the principal normal stress σ_m. This value represents the maximum normal stress under which the powder was consolidated before it yielded and changed volume. Drawing a Mohr circle that is tangent to the yield locus and passes through the origin gives a value known as the unconfined yield locus fc (the point where the Mohr circle intersects with x-axis). This value represents the maximum principal stress acting on a free surface necessary to cause failure. Jenike (38) related this value to the strength of an arch in a hopper. For a cohesive solid, the intersection of the yield locus with the y-axis (shear stress) is considered the cohesion of the powder for that yield locus. The point at which the yield locus intersects the negative x-axis is considered the tensile strength of the material compressed under the normal load used to generate the locus. Most often a series of conditioning forces is used, giving a series or "family" of yield loci (Fig. 6a). A plot of the unconfined yield locus fc vs. the principal consolidating force for a series of yield loci has been used by Jenike (38) as a flow (or failure) function. Each of these values has been used to classify material as to their flowability.

Eq. 5 describes the yield locus. As early as 1965, Eq. 5 was established empirically from a study of the shapes of yield loci for more than 30 powders (103):

$$\ln[\tau/C] = (1/\eta)\ln[(\sigma + T)/T] \qquad (5)$$

where τ is the shear stress, σ the normal stress, T the tensile strength, C the cohesion, and n the shear index. It is often referred to as the Warren–Springs equation and has been confirmed by numerous authors (104–106). Earlier in this article it was mentioned that Geoffroy and Carstensen (14) modified this equation taking particle size of the material into affect. Hiestand (106) states that the Warren–Springs equation is suitable for describing the yield locus for failure in shear. However, contrary to common usage, the term T is not the tensile strength but the internal cohesion, the magnitude of which may be much less than the tensile strength. As stated by Hiestand, this is contrary to the common usage of the equation. He based his conclusion primarily on experimental data with sitosterols. In contrast,

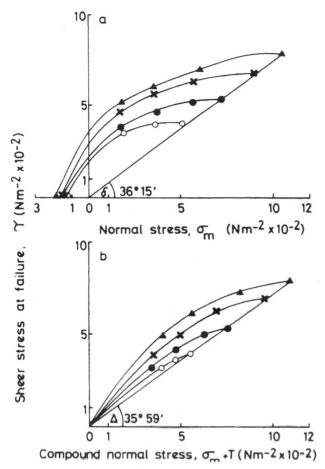

Fig. 6 Families of yield loci for lactose powder coated with 0.5 × 10⁻⁵ mol g⁻¹ of light paraffin at 20°C. P_f ▲, 0.346; ×, 0.282; •, 0.279; ○, 0.261; (a) normal stress; (b) compound stress. (From Ref. 107.)

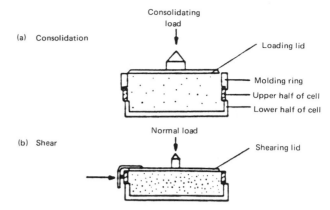

Fig. 7 The Jenike shear cell. (From York, P. Int. J. Pharm. **1980**, *6*, 101.)

Irono and Pilpel (107) modified the treatment of the shear data (Fig. 6b). In this figure they added tensile strength values obtained independently in the tensile-strength measuring to the normal load in the shear cell loci plots.

The actual method used to treat the data varies with respect to the nature of the shear cell utilized. Direct measurements of the various functions such as tensile strength and unconfined yield strength have been taken. The following section describes the methods being utilized and their advantages and disadvantages and how they have been applied to the flow of pharmaceutical powders. A detailed description of data evaluation is not included. Several excellent reviews of shear and tensile measurement are available and can be found in the references. Johanson, who teamed with Jenike in conducting much important work in the field, has published an interesting historical perspective of the field (108).

Jenike Shear Cell

This instrument was developed first for soil testing and adapted by Jenike to measure cohesive powders and relate the data to hopper flow and hence hopper design. This is essentially the standard cell (Fig. 7) and the basis of much of the data solids-handling work. It is split horizontally; the lower half is fixed and the upper half is moveable at a constant low rate. The cells are first filled with sample and then consolidated by placing a load on the loading lid (Fig. 7a) and rotating the lid backward and forward through a slight angle. The loading lid and molding ring are removed and the powder scrapped level with the top of the upper half of the cell. The shearing lid is placed in position and the cell is sheared by moving the upper half over the lower fixed portion. The load is equal to or lower than the consolidated load. The process is repeated with the same consolidating load but with lower shearing loads until the yield locus is obtained. If a family series of yield loci are to be developed, a series of consolidating forces are used. A flow-factor plot should be based on at least three consolidation pressures. Needless to say, this process is extremely time-consuming and tedious. Another disadvantage is that correct consolidation of the sample is difficult to achieve. For this reason the results may be very operator-dependent. Correct consolidation is generally established by preliminary experiments, which examine the shape of the stress—strain curve obtained during shearing. Despite these difficulties, the Jenike shear cell has been used extensively and is commercially available. A number of papers have appeared in the pharmaceutical literature describing utilization of this device (103–116). Doelker (109) in comparing various microcrystalline cellulose types states that techniques such as the Hausner ratio and Carr index are poorly reproducible and can be compared only if determined by

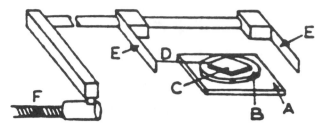

Fig. 8 The plate-type shear cell. Key: (A) lower plate; (B) template; (C) upper plate; (D) tow line; (E) cantilever strain gauge; (F) screw jack. (From York, P. Int. J. Pharm. **1980**, *6*, 100.)

the same authors. He states "A more trustworthy method for evaluating the flow characteristics of cohesive powders is to use shear cells." He goes on to review various flow measurements of microcrystalline cellulose as well as other commonly used direct compression excipients.

Plate-Type Shear Cell

Nash et al. (117) and later Hiestand et al. (118,119) developed a very simple test device that can be easily constructed (Fig. 8) and was used to evaluate pharmaceutical powders. The powder is placed between two plates, usually with the surface in contact with the powder consisting of sandpaper or other rough surface to ensure that the powder shears in the bed rather than at the surface of the plate. A consolidating weight is placed on the upper plate. Final consolidation is achieved by shearing, using very short movements in such a way that a reading from the strain gauge is obtained. This is repeated until the shear force, read on a chart recorder, reaches a plateau value. A lower weight is then placed on the upper plate and a lower point in the yield locus is obtained through a single shear movement. The entire process must be repeated for each point in the yield locus.

As with the Jenike cell, this process is time-consuming. Amidon and Houghton (111), however, used a single yield locus with this cell for comparative purposes. Hiestand et al. (120), in comparing this apparatus to the Jenike cell, claimed that this simple shear cell can be used to provide characterization of the unconfined yield strengths of powders. The results from the two devices are not identical. However, as much as the Hiestand device requires less powder and the consolidation step is more automated and consistent, it provides an inexpensive alternative to the Jenike-type cell to characterize pharmaceutical powders. Amidon and Houghton used the cell to examine the effect of moisture

on the powder flow properties of microcrystalline cellulose (27).

Ring or Annular Shear Cell

The ring or annular shear cell, was developed by Carr and Walker (121) as early as 1968. In recent years this tester has undergone a number of modifications. Peschl (122, 123) has developed an annular shear cell in which the sample and shear cell consists of a full circle. This contrasts to the earlier cells that have a band of sample on the outer portion of the circle. This was done to eliminate wall friction. It is also rotated very slowly, since at low speed, velocity variability becomes more negligible in the shear measurement. In this way a full ring can be utilized and speed differences in the outside and inside of the ring become negligible. Schulze (124–126) made the latest modifications to the ring cell tester (Schulze tester RST – 01.01). In the Schulze ring shear tester the sample is placed in an outer circular channel. An angular lid, which is attached to a crossbeam, lies on top of the sample. Small bars are attached to the bottom side of the lid and the bottom of the cell to prevent the powder from sliding against the lid or the bottom. The shear cell is rotated while the lid is prevented from rotating by cross beams attached to fixed beam. The movement of the cell with respect to the fixed lid causes the powder bed to shear and load cells attached to tie rods measure the force needed to initiate this. To exert weight on the sample, weights are hung from a crossbeam. This can be done during the shearing and conditioning of the powder sample. The cell can also be removed and time consolidation can be conducted by placing weights on the sample out side of the test device, in a similar mannner to that with the Jenike cell. An automatic version of this tester (126) has been developed in which the computer can automatically add loading to the sample and condition it. The instrument can be operated in a manual, semiautomatic or totally computer run mode. Both the earlier annular shear cells, the Peschl or Schulze's RST –01.01 cell have several important advantages over the Jenike-type cell. They offer a constant area of shear. Handling is easier and consolidation and shear are quicker, since after the bed is consolidated, a full locus can be generated without reconsolidating after each load. The consolidation process becomes more automated and uniform, eliminating much of the operator variability in the measurement process. Peschl reported a relationship between tablet weight variation and internal friction as measured by his device (122, 123). The Peschl shear tester has been utilized for shear testing and quality control of pharmaceuticals by at least one U.S. pharmaceutical company as well as in Europe. Nyqvist (82, 127) and

Nyqvist and Nicklasson (81) utilized an annual shear cell with direct-compression lactose and various actives as well as high-dose penicillin products and found that the device was an excellent predictor of flow on a tablet press as related to tablet weight variation. From the shear-cell data it was actually possible to predict the frequency of tablet machine adjustment on a rotary tablet press in the production of penicillin products (82). In 1985 Baichwal and Augsburger (128) employed an annual shear cell to quantify the amount of friction between pharmaceutical powders with various lubricants and a smooth metal surface. More recently Podczeck and Miah (57) used a commercial version of a Carr annular shear cell to measure the flow factors for unlubricated and lubricated powders. Schulze (125, 126) demonstrated the ability to differentiate the flow function of lactose with and without the presence of 1% active drug. This same laboratory has also produced a ring shear tester to measure wall friction of bulk solids (129). Schulze (130) provides an excellent review of all the previously mentioned shear devices as well as contact angle, and paddle type testers, to be discussed later in this chapter. He also lists several devices not included in this discussion.

Bi- and Triaxial Shear Cells and Other Related Tests

There are several shear tests as well other related tests, which have been used in bulk solids handling and in the design of hoppers and silos but have not been used extensively to study pharmaceuticals. The monoaxial shear tester, Johanson Hang-up Indicizer and compressibility test are examples of test devices that have been used in the bulk handling industries and are described in Schulze's chapter (130). Enstad and Feise (131) further discuss the uniaxial shear tester which tests powder compacted in one direction. The major discussion in their chapter (131) is a discussion of biaxial shear testers. Though not mentioned in the pharmaceutical literature, this test has received a good deal of attention in the recent powder technology literature with the development of a number of new test devices in the 1990s. There are essentially three types of biaxial testers, those being rigid boundary, flexible boundary, and mixed boundary testers. The rigid boundary tester is the one used most for the measurement of mechanical behavior of particulate solids. The sample is brick shaped and the set-up insures that the sample will always retain a rectangular cross-section. In the flexible tester the walls are flexible and made of rubber. Pressure can be exerted via air pressure by inflating chambers within the flexible walls. The mixed boundary

system has only been used at very high pressure with primarily sand. Shearing at constant volume, testing time of loading and varying the direction of loading, and measuring the affects on the stress and strain relationships in the bed are the chief function of this test method. Most of the work with this tester has been with limestone and sand and the results have been used in the design of hoppers. The triaxial shear tester, which was introduced into soil mechanics in the 1920s, has not been used to characterize pharmaceutical powders to any great extent but has been discussed in the powder-handling literature. Luong (132) provides a review of this test method. Kolymbas and Wu (133) gives an extensive discussion of the experimental techniques and the potential errors occurring with the device and how to adjust for them. In a triaxial tester the sample is subjected to pressure in three directions, a pressure chamber usually keeps two of which constant. The cells discussed previously were biaxial with pressure by the normal load and in the direction of shear. In the triaxial shear cell, the sample is placed in a cylindrical rubber membrane and enclosed by rigid end cups. The sample is consolidated by maintaining the same pressure in all three directions, which does not induce shear but volumetric strain. Pressure is usually exerted at the end cups with some sort of a piston that moves in one direction while the pressure chamber maintains the pressure in the other directions. The pressure changes and the volume changes are monitored in all directions. A Mohr-circle treatment of the data is usually made. Certain factors, which are used to evaluate materials, are more directly obtained with this device than with biaxial test devices. The triaxial shear device is still primarily a research tool, and many variations have been constructed. It is less appropriate for flow measurement of pharmaceuticals since it is designed for relatively high pressures.

Johanson (134) developed a very simple device they called the Johanson Indicizer system, or the Johanson Hang-up Indicizer, which they claim can predict material bridging in a hopper. This device was reviewed by Bell et al. (135). In private conversations Johanson stated that they have employed this device with a number of pharmaceuticals. It simply compacts very small amounts of powder into a potential bridge and measures the force to break the bridge and allow the powder to flow. It is not designed to give any detailed information on the powder but only provides a test for powder bridging. This device is commercially available.

Tensile strength can be obtained from shear measurements via the Warren–Springs equation or through extension of the yield locus. The direct measurement of the tensile strength of powders with the help of commercial split-cell devices is common. The powder is consolidated to a known density, usually through weights. One half of the cell is stationary and the other half is movable on a low-friction surface. The force needed to separate the powder bed at a given density is recorded. In general, a straight-line log–log relationship exists between the tensile strength and the packing fraction (density of sample divided by the true density). Hiestand et al. (106) stated that no method, using loosely packed powder beds, as just described, is highly successful. For this reason, he measured the tensile strength of compacts. Despite his opinion, the measurement of the tensile strength of powder beds continues to be utilized by pharmaceutical scientists. Chowhan and Yang (136) found a linear relationship between tensile strength and the coefficient of variation of the fill weight of capsules. In a separate paper (62) they reported that the flow rate of powder mixtures containing simple glidants, such as corn starch and microcrystalline cellulose, at different concentrations is linearly related to tensile strength. Ho et al. (110) on the other hand, found no relationship between tensile strength and tablet weight variation for a number of direct-compression excipients

In general tensile strength is not used alone to predict flow. Danjo et al. (25) utilized tensile strength measurement, shear cell measurement, and Carr's flow factor to investigate the effect of particle shape on powder flow.

In summary, various shear and tensile strength measuring devices have been developed, and many are commercially available. Though they are more complex and often more difficult to use than the other methods, they yield data on a more scientific basis, which allows a mechanistic approach to flow problems.

AVALANCHE BEHAVIOR AND POWDER RHEOMETERS

Earlier in this article, in the section on the Affect of Particle Shape, the principle of fractal geometry was introduced. As discussed previously Hickey and Concessio (20) utilized fractal analysis to characterize flow of pharmaceutical powders, using a vibrating spatula. Crowder and Hickey developed a vibratory spatula device that was able to obtain flow data much more rapidly (137). Using this device and fractal geometry, they were able to quantify the differences in the flow properties of sprayed and nonspray dried lactose (80). Kaye et al. also used the vibratory flow of solids to measure avalanches down a shoot (18, 19). Eventually Kaye et al. would use a rotating drum method (138) to study solid flow through avalanching behavior. This device is commercially

available (10) as the Aero-Flow™ automated powder flowability analyzer and is being used in the pharmaceutical industry today.

The theoretical basis for this device can be found in fractal dimensions and deterministic chaos theory. Kaye (139) uses a term know as "fractal dimensions in space" in which he treats fractal data not as a physical structure but as a pattern of events that can be used to describe chaotic systems. He describes deterministic chaos, in the same text, as an interaction of events, which are described by deterministic physics. The interaction of the events become so complex that the system may as well be chaotic. For this reason he has combined fractal analysis with chaos theory to develop an understanding of dynamic particle flow. Hickey and Concessio (140) used this same

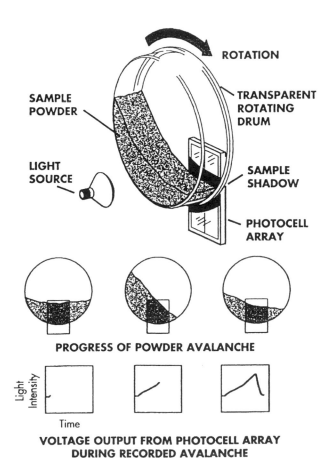

Fig. 9 Descriptive drawing of a rotating drum avalanche test device. This device is commercially available as the TSI Aero-Flow automated powder flowability analyzer. The top pictures the device. The progress of powder avalanche shows the position of the powder in the drum as the drum is rotated and the lower voltage output shows the output of the device during each drum rotation. (From Ref. 10.)

approach in characterizing lactose, using a rotating drum device. In their device they utilized a video camera to measure the dynamic angle of repose with time. The commercial device developed by Kaye works, using light transmission and a series of photocells to measure the light transmission. The device can be seen in Fig. 9.

As can be seen in Fig. 9 the powder is placed in the drum and the drum is allowed to rotate. The powder lifts up and when the dynamic angle of repose is exceeded, the powder sample will avalanche downward. The movement of the powder blocks the photocells from obtaining light and a voltage output, which can be related to the avalanching of the powder is recorded (Fig. 9). A set of data for lactose can be seen in Fig. 10(141).

The flowability of materials according to the literature is related to the mean time for avalanching to occur. The shorter the time the more free flowing. The scatter is related to cohesiveness (10) or an irregularity factor (143). Lower scatter values would indicate a less cohesive material and would predict more regular flow while greater scatter would be indicative of a more cohesive material and the increased likely hood of irregular flow patterns. The example in Fig. 10 shows a lactose sample that was sieved into two fractions: one above 38 μm and one below 38 μm. The middle data is from unfractionated lactose. As can be seen from Fig. 10 that as expected the finer material

had a larger mean and larger scatter showing it to be a poorer flowing material. The larger fraction showed the shortest mean time to avalanche and the smallest scatter showing that it would be the better flowing material. As expected the unfractionated lactose yielded data in between the two fractions. The flow properties of various lots of lactose monohydrate and paracetamol were studied using the Aero-Flo device and lot to lot variations were noted (142). Trobridge et al. (143) tested five grades of lactose with a variable commercial automated drum tester and found that the mean time to avalanche correlated well with flow performance on a tablet press when the drum speed was 180 s/rotation (spr). When the speed of rotation was set at 200 spr slippage was observed with one of the lactose grades and a different rank order was obtained. It was concluded that the fixed speed unit data identified the two optimal formulations but did not distinguish between marginal flow and no flow, but the variable speed unit did. Crowder and Hickey (144) reviewed the physics of powder flow as related to pharmaceutical solids. Included in the article is a section, which explains many of the terminology of complex systems. They include a discussion of avalanching measurement and the use of chaos theory in measuring flow including rotating drum devices. Included in the discussion is powder and granular mixing as well as milling, neither of which is covered in

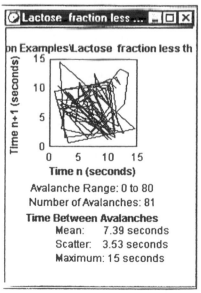

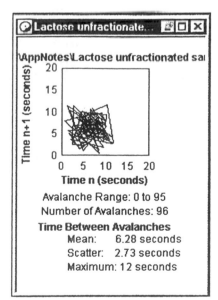

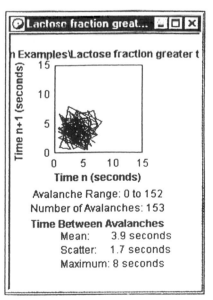

<38 microns   **Powder Blend**   **>38 microns**

Fig. 10 Rotating drum avalanche data from a TSI Aero-Flow automated powder flowability analyzer. The first frame shows the data output for lactose, which passed through a 38-μm screen (less than 38-μm). The output data for the original lactose sample (not screened) is shown in the middle frame. The last frame shows the flow data for the lactose sample remaining on the 38-μm screen (greater than 38-μm). (From Ref. 10.)

this article, but is also effected by or affect the flow characteristics of solids.

Paddle or blade rheometers are commonly used in to measure the shear of liquids. Brabender (145) developed such a system for solids in which a plate compacts the solid and the torque to initiate turning is measured. Podczek (146, 147) has tested seven different suppliers' microcrystalline cellulose with a new commercial blade type rheometer. In their experiments they were able to measure very small differences between these lots, which they related to actual capsule filling and tablet experiences. The measuring device is commercially available and is now marketed as the FT3 Powder Rheometer (148). (Podczeck articles list the instrument as Wet and Dry Powder Rheometer Fingerprint, ManUmit Products Ltd., Bourne End, U.K.) In this instrument the powder is placed in a circular vessel with a closed bottom. The blade enters the powder and moves downward or upward in a helical motion while the force on the blade shaft is recorded. The helical path along which the blade moves is dependent on the axial and rotational speeds and the direction the blade rotates. The angle of approach the blade makes with the powder can be varied, and the direction and angle of the measurement will allow the measurement of compaction, shear and slicing of the powder bed (terms and conditions defined in Podczek's papers). The torque data is treated so as to give theoretically the largest torque exerted by the whole powder column on the rotor blade for a defined test condition. In this way powder shear can be measured under a variety of shear conditions, including various downward compaction modes and upward expansion modes. Podczek (146, 147) found that a downward compaction mode was most sensitive to small differences in the behavior of the various microcrystalline cellulose samples. These differences were not apparent using the Carr compressibility index. Other conditions such as slicing the bed was much less discriminatory. Freeman (149) reported on testing this device with talcum, zinc oxide, and an un-named pharmaceutical. By testing a material and finding the proper test conditions, this device could provide a simple and highly sensitive control test since it is relatively operator independent and yields quantitative values.

CONCLUSION

The final question that should be answered regarding these test methods is which one or ones should you use. Velasco et al. (150) compared data from static angle of repose, dynamic angle of repose, Carr compressibility index, flow meter, and ring shear test for Ludipress® and Maltrin® M 150 and found a good correlation between all the methods. Tan and Newton (151) compared Carr compressibility, Hausner ratio, angle of repose, and the Jenike flow factor and demonstrated good correlation between all the test methods for five pharmaceutical excipients. They found no correlation between the angle of internal flow and the angle of effective friction. As mentioned previously, differences were seen from slow avalanche results, and faster avalanche results, and other physical measurements (143). As discussed above, rheometer measurements at different conditions (146, 147) and physical measurements for the same powders didn't always correlate.

Two very recent papers compare a number of flow measurement techniques and use statistics for comparison and to devise a new flow index. Lee et. al. (152) compared results from avalanche testing, Carr's compressibility index and critical orifice diameter for six pharmaceutical excipients. Statistical analysis established that there are relationships and similarities between the ranking of powder flow properties between these three methods. They also used a dual approach, which combines visual observation of the type of motion of the powder bed in rotation with the numerical descriptors such as mean time to avalanche and scatter. They found this dual approach was found to be more accurate in the assessment of powder flow than using the numerical descriptors alone. Taylor et al. (153) tested 41 pharmaceutical blends including pure excipients and active blends, using a vibrating spatula, avalanching, critical orifice, angle of repose, and compressibility index. An empirical composite index was established and powder flow was ranked in accordance with formulator experience. Principal components analyses of the angle of repose, percent compressibility, and critical orifice of the powders were also performed. Using principal components analysis, the results of these three tests were statistically weighted to provide a weighted composite index that the authors showed to be the best predictor of flow for these pharmaceuticals. The vibrating spatula and avalanche data were not consistent with formulator experience and cited vendor references for flow. The authors stated that the results of these two test methods might have more relevance if they had used further data treatment such as fractal analysis.

The process of solid flow is extremely complex and dependent on many material and process variables. The answer to the question of which is the best method to use is therefore dependent on your process and what you are trying to predict or measure and select the method or combination of methods that best meets your needs.

REFERENCES

1. Von Behren, Dale, A. Physical Characterization of Excipients in Practice. Pharm. Technol. **1996**; 87–89, June.
2. Cartilier, L.H.; Moës, A. Effect of Flowing Adjuvants on the Homogeneity and the Kinetics of Mixing of Low Dosage Cohesive Powder Mixtures. Drug Dev. Ind. Pharm. **1986**, *12* (8, 9), 1203–1218.
3. Sallam, E.A.; Orr, N.A. Studies Relating to the Content Uniformity of Ethinylestradiol Tablets 10 μg: Effect of Particle Size of Excipients. Third Expo./Congr. Int. Technol. Pharm. **1983**, *2*, 28–37.
4. Samyn, J.C.; Murphy, K.S. Experiments in Powder Blending and Unbending. J. Pharm. Sci. **1974**, *63*, 370–375.
5. Hauer, V.B.; Remmele, T.; Züger und Sucker, H. Gezieltes Entwickeln und Optimieren von Kapselformulierungen mit Einer Instrumentierten Dosierröhrchen-Kapselabfüllmaschine. Pharm. Inc. 55 Nr. 5 **1993**, .
6. British Standard 2955, British Standards Institute, London, 1958.
7. Standly-Wood, N. WS-16, Powder and Bulk Solids Conference and Exhibitions, Chicago, 1989.
8. Hiestand, E.N. Powders: Particle–Particle Interactions. J. Pharm. Sci. **1966**, *35*, 1325–1344.
9. Carstensen, J.T.; Ertell, C.; Geoffrey, J.-M. Physico-Chemical Properties of Particulate Matter. Drug Dev. Ind. Pharm. **1993**, *19* (1, 2), 195–219.
10. *TSI Aero-Flow*™ *Automated Powder Flowability Analyzer*, TSI Inc.
11. Danish, F.Q.; Parrott, E.L. Flow Rates of Solid Particulate Pharmaceutical. J. Pharm. Sci. **1971**, *60*, 548–554.
12. Gold, G.; Duvall, R.N.; Palermo, B.T.; Slater, J.G. Powder Flow Studies III. J. Pharm. Sci. **1968**, *57*, 667–671.
13. Newton, J.M.; Bader, F. The Angle of Internal Flow as Indicator of Filling and Drug Release Properties of Capsule Formulations, J. Pharm. Pharmacol. **1987**, *39*, 164–168.
14. Geoffroy, J.-M.; Carstensen, J.T. Modified Warren-Springs Equation, Powder Technol. **1993**, *76*, 135–140.
15. Mandelbrot, B.B. *The Fractal Geometry of Nature*; Freeman, W. Ed.; San Francisco, 1983.
16. Kaye, B.H. *Characterization of Powders and Aerosols*; Wiley-VCH: Weinheim, 1999.
17. Kaye, B.H. *Chaos and Complexity: Discovering the Surprising Patterns of Science and Technology*; VCH: Weinheim, 1993.
18. Kaye, B.H. Characterizing the Flowability of Powder Using the Concepts of Fractal Geometry and Chaos Theory. Part. Part. Syst. Charact. **1997**, *14*, 53–66.
19. Kaye, B.H. A New Approach to Powder Rheology. Pharm. Technol. **March**, 1994;116–126, .
20. Hickey, A.J.; Concessio, N.M. Flow Properties of Selected Pharmaceutical Powders from a Vibrating Spatula. Part. Part. Syst. Charact. **1994**, *11*, 457–462.
21. Brittain, H.G. Raw Materials. Drug Dev. and Ind. Pharm. **1989**, *15* (13), 2083–2103.
22. Cartilier, L.H.; Tawashi, R. Effect of Particle Morphology on the Flow and Packing Properties of Lactose. S.T.P. Pharma Sci. **1993**, *3* (3), 213–220.
23. Pitkin, C.; Carstensen, J.T. Effect of Particle Shape on Some Bulk Solid's Properties. Drug Dev. Ind. Pharm. **1990**, *16* (1), 1–12.
24. Wong, L.W.; Pilpel, N.J. Effect of Particle Shape on the Mixing of Powders. J. Pharm. Pharmacol. **1990**, *42*, 1–6.
25. Danjo, K.; Kinoshita, K.; Kitagawa, K.; Lid, I.K.; Sunada, H.; Otsuka, A. Chem. Pharm. Bull. **1989**, *37* (11), 3070–3073.
26. Huber, G.M.W.; Becker, R.; Müller, R.H. Zusammenhang zwischen Fließeigenschaften und Oberfläche Pulverförmiger Rezepturen. Pharm. Ind. **1994**, *56* (4), 389–392.
27. Amidon, G.E.; Houghton, M.E. The Effect of Moisture on the Mechanical and Powder Flow Properties of Microcrystalline Cellulose. Pharm. Res. **1995**, *12* (6), 923–929.
28. Doelker, E.; Mordier, D.; Iten, H.; Humbert-Droz, P. Comparative Tableting Properties of Sixteen Microcrystalline Celluloses. Drug Dev. Ind. Pharm. **1987**, *13* (9–11), 1847–1875.
29. Heng, P.W.S.; Staniforth, J.N. The Effect of Moisture on the Cohesive Properties of Microcrystalline Celluloses. J. Pharm. Pharmacol. **1987**, *40*, 360–362.
30. Staniforth, J.N.; Rees, J.E. Electrostatic Charge Interactions in Ordered Powder Mixes. J. Pharm. Pharmacol. **1982**, *34*, 69–76.
31. Staniforth, J.N. British Pharmaceutical Conference Science Award Lecture 1986 Order out of Chaos. J. Pharm. Pharmacol. **1987**, *39*, 329–334.
32. Marinelli, J. Factors that Impact a Bulk Solid's Flowability, (Internet). 2000; 1–2.
33. York, P.; Pilpel, N. Effect of Temperature on the Frictional, Cohesive, and Electrical Conducting Properties of Powders. Mater. Sci. Eng. **1972**, *9* (5), 281–291.
34. Pilpel, N.; Britten, J.R. Effects of Temperature on the Flow and Tensile Strengths of Powders. Powder Technol. **1979**, *22* (1), 33–44.
35. Onyekweli, A.O.; Pilpel, N. Cooling as a Possible Method for Increasing the Flowability of Certain Pharmaceutical and other Powders. J. Pharm. Pharmacol. **1980**, *32*, 120–125.
36. Jayasinge, S.S.; Pilpel, N.; Harwood, C.F. Effect of Temperature and Compression on the Cohesive Properties of Particulate Solids. Mater. Sci. Eng. **1970**, *5* (5), 287–294.
37. Pilpel, N. Cool Powders Run Fast. New Scientist *1981*;313–315.
38. Jenike, A.W. Storage and Flow of Solids. Bull. *123* **1964**, Utah Engineering Experimental Station, University of Utah, Salt Lake City.
39. Marinelli, J. Mass Flow Design Considerations? (Arching—Part 1), (Internet). 2000; 1–2.
40. Bates, L. Flow in Bulk Storage Bins, (Internet). 2000;1–4.
41. Marinelli, J. Wall Friction Effects, (Internet). 2000; 1–3.
42. Marinelli, J. How Wall Friction Effects Hopper Angles, (Internet). 2000; 1–3.
43. Marinelli, J. Compressibility —What is it? (Internet). 2000; 1–3.
44. Brown, C.J., Nielson, J., Eds.; *Silos Fundamentals of Theory, Behaviour and Design,* E & FN Spon: London and New York, 1998.
45. Marinelli, J.; Carson, J.W. Bulk Powders. *Encyclopedia of Chemical Technology*, 4th Ed.; 1996; 19, 1114–1141.

46. Mulcahy, D.E., Ed. *Materials Handling Handbook*, 1998.
47. Prescott, J.K.; Hossfeld, R.J. Maintaining Product Uniformity and Uninterrupted Flow to Direct-Compression Tableting Presses. Pharm. Technol. **1994**, *18* (6), 98–114.
48. Bates, L. The Use of Inserts in Hoppers, (Internet). Powder and Bulk Dot Com2000, 1–3.
49. Troxel, T.G. Flow Aids—What to Use and when to Use them. Powder/Bulk Solids Adv. Dry Process2000, 12–16.
50. Jones, T.M. Symposium on Powders, Society of Cosmetic Chemists of Great Britain, Dublin, Ireland, 1969
51. Peleg, M.; Mannheim, C.H. Effect of Conditioners on the Flow Properties of Powdered Sucrose. Powder Technol. **1972**, *7*, 45–50.
52. Neumann, B.S. *Advances in Pharmaceutical Sciences*. Bean, H.S., Beckett, A.H., Charles, J.E., Eds.; Academic Press: London, 1965, 2, 181–207.
53. Jones, T.M.; Pilpel, N. Some Physical Properties of Lactose and Magnesia. J. Pharm. Pharmacol. **1965**, *17*, 440.
54. Borerro, J.M.; Muñoz Ruiz, A.J.; Jiménez-Castellanos, M.R. Relationship between the Flow Characteristics and the Intrinsic Factors of Chlorpromazine Hydrochloride and its Mixtures with Diluents as Direct Compression Formulations. Boll. Chim. Farmaceutico. Anno. **1994**, *133* (5), 294–300.
55. Chang, R.-K.; Leonzio, M.; Hussain, M.A. Effect of Colloidal Silicone Dioxide on Flowing and Tableting Properties of an Experimental, Crosslinked Polyalkylammonium Polymer. Pharm. Dev. Technol. **1999**, *4* (2), 285–289.
56. Nastruzzi, C.; Cortesi, R.; Esposito, E.; Genovesi, A.; Spadoni, A.; Vecchio, C.; Menegatti, E. Influence of Formulation and Process Parameters on Pellet Production by Powder Layering Technique. AAPS Pharm. Sci. Tech. **2000**, *1* (2), 1–22.
57. Podczeck, F.; Miah, Y. The Influence of Particle Size and Shape on the Angle of Internal Friction and the Flow Factor of Unlubricated and Lubricated Powders. Elsevier Int. J. Pharm. **1996**, *144*, 187–194.
58. Van Ooteghem, M.; De Winter, B.; Ludwig, A. Influence of the Mixing Conditions on the Flow Properties of Powders to be Filled into Hard Gelatin Capsules. Acta Pharm. Jugosl. **1998**, *38*, 287–295.
59. Laughlin, S.; Carstensen, J.T. Relationship between Flow Rates of Granular Powders through Stationary and Moving Orifices. J. Pharm. Sci. **1981**, *70*, 711–713.
60. Joyce, M.A.; Liebert, R.T.; Carter, R.W. Eastern Regional Meeting, American Association of Pharmaceutical Scientists, Atlantic City, NJ, 1988.
61. Dahlinder, L.E.; Johansson, M.; Sjogren, J. Comparison of Methods for Evaluation of Flow Properties of Powders and Granulates. Drug Dev. Ind. Pharm. **1982**, *8* (3), 455–461.
62. Chowhan, Z.T.; Yang, I.C. Powder Flow Studies IV. Tensile Strength and Orifice Flow Rate Relationships of Binary Mixtures. Int. J. Pharm. **1983**, *14*, 231–242.
63. Muñoz-Ruiz, A.J.; Jiménez-Castellanos, M.R. Integrated System of Data Acquisition for the Measurement of Flow Characteristics. Pharm. Technol. Int. 1993; 21–26.
64. Flemming, J.; Mielck, J.B. Requirements for the Production of Microtablets: Suitability of Direct-Compression Excipients Estimated from Powder Characteristics and Flow Rates. Drug Dev. Ind. Pharm. **1995**, *21* (19), 2239–2251.
65. Rey, H.; Wagner, K.G.; Wehrlé; Schmidt, P.C. Development of Matrix-Based Theophylline Sustained-Release Microtablets. Drug Dev. Ind. Pharm. **2000**, *26* (1), 21–26.
66. Moneghini, M.; Carcano, A.; Perissutti, B.; Rubessa, F. Formulation Design Studies of Atenolol Tablets. Pharm. Dev. Technol. **2000**, *5* (2), 297–301.
67. Faham, A.; Prinderre, P.; Farah, N.; Eichler, K.D.; Kalantzis, G.; Joachim, J. Hot-Melt Coating Technology. I. Influence of Compritol 888 Ato and Granule Size on Theophylline Release. **2000**, *26* (2), 167–176.
68. Fernández-Arévalo, M.; Vela, M.T.; Rabasco, A.M. Rheological Study of Lactose Coated and Acrylic Resins. Drug Dev. Ind. Pharm. **1990**, *16* (2), 295–313.
69. Timmins, P.; Delargy, A.M.; Minchom, C.M.; Howard, J.R. Influence of Some Process Variables on Product Properties for a Hydrophilic Matrix Controlled Release Tablet. Eur. J. Pharm. Biopharm. **1992**, *38* (3), 113–118.
70. Mollan, M.J., Jr.; Çelik, Characterization of Directly Compressible Maltodextrins Manufactured by Three Different Processes. Drug Dev. Ind. Pharm. **1993**, *19* (17, 18), 2335–2358.
71. Onunkwo, G.C.; Udeala, O.K. Studies of *Rauwolfia vomitoria* Root III. Flow Properties of R. vomitoria Granulations. S.T.P. Pharma Sci. **1995**, *5* (4), 296–301.
72. Goracinova, K.; Klisarova, L.; Simov, A.; Fredro-Kumbaradzi, E.; Petruševska-Tozi, L. Characterization of Fluid Bed Prepared Granulates with Verapamil Hydrochloride as Active Substance. Acta. Pharm. **1996**, *46*, 147–153.
73. Gohel, M.C.; Patel, L.D.; Modi, C.J.; Jogani, P.D. Functionality Testing of a Coprocessed Diluent Containing Lactose and Microcrystalline Cellulose. Pharm. Technol.1999; 44–46, Yearbook.
74. Carr, R.L., Jr. Classifying Flow Properties of Solids. Chem. Eng. **1965**, *7*, 163–167.
75. Pilpel, N. Flow Properties of Non-Cohesive Powders. Chem. Process Eng. **1965**, *46*, 167.
76. Carstensen, J.T.; Lai, T.Y.F.; Toure, P.; Sheridan, J. Repose Angles as a Function of the Supporting Surface. Int. J. Pharm. **1980**, *5*, 157–160.
77. Jones, T.M.; Pilpel, N. Some Angular Properties of Magnesia and their Relevance to Material Handling. J. Pharm. Pharmacol. **1966**, *18* (Suppl.), 182–189.
78. Pilpel, N. Cohesive Pharmaceutical Powders. *Advances in Pharmaceutical Sciences*; Bean, H.S., Beckett, A.H., Charles, J.E. Eds.; Academic Press: London, 1971, 3, 179–219.
79. Augenstein, D.A.; Hogg, R. An Experimental Study of the Flow of Dry Powders over Inclined Surfaces. Powder Technol. **1978**, *19*, 205–215.
80. Crowder, T.M.; Hickey, A.J. An Instrument for Rapid Powder Flow Measurement and Temporal Fractal Analysis. Part. Part. Syst. Charact. **1999**, *16*, 32–34.
81. Nqvist, H.; Nicklasson, M. Flow Properties of Compressible Lactose Containing Small Quantities of Drug Substances. Drug Dev. Ind. Pharm. **1985**, *11* (4), 745–759.
82. Nqvist, H. Measurement of Flow Properties in Large Scale Tablet Production. Int. J. Pharm. Tech. Prod. Mfr. **1984**, *5* (3), 21–24.

83. Parrott, E.L. Comparative Evaluation of a New Direct Compression Excipient, Soludex 15. Drug Dev. Ind. Pharm. **1989**, *15* (4), 561–583.

84. Carstensen, J.T. *Solid Pharmaceutics: Mechanical Properties and Rate Phenomena*; Academic Press: New York, 1980.

85. Neuman, B.S. Ch. 10. *Flow Properties in Disperse Systems*; Herman, J.J., Ed.; North-Holland Publishing Co. Amsterdam, 1953.

86. Hausner, H.H. Friction Conditions in a Mass of Metal Powder. Int. J. Powder Metall. **1967**, *3* (4), 7–13.

87. Chowhan, Z.T.; Chow, Y.P. Evaluation of Pharmaceutical Availability from the Calculation of Drug Levels and Release Profiles. Int. J. Pharm. **1980**, *4*, 317–326.

88. Varthalis, S.; Pilpel, N. Anomalies in Some Properties of Powder Mixtures. J. Pharm. Pharmacol. **1976**, *28*, 415–419.

89. Sakr, F.M.; Pilpel, N. The Tensile Strength and Consolidation of Lacose Coated with Non-Ionic Surfacetants II-Tablets. Int. J. Pharm. **1982**, *10*, 43–56.

90. Yamashiro, M.; Yuasa, Y.; Kawakita, K. An Experimental Study on the Relationship between Compressibility, Fluidity and Cohesion of Powder Solids at Small Tapping Numbers. Powder Technol. **1983**, *34* (2), 225–231.

91. Geldart, D. Types of Gas Fluidization. Powder Technol. **1973**, *7* (5), 285.

92. Molerus, O. Interpretation of Geldart's Type A, B, C and D Powders by Taking into Account Interparticle Cohesion Forces. Powder Technol. **1982**, *33* (1), 81–87.

93. Munoz, R.; Velasco, A.; Antequera, M.V.; Monedero Perales, M.; del Carmen, J.-C.; Ballesteros, M.R. Powder Flow and Compression Characteristics of Dextrins for Direct Compression. Congr. Int. Technol. Pharm. **1992**, *4*, 131–139.

94. Flores, L.E.; Arellano, R.L.; Esquivel, J.J.D. Lubricant Susceptibility of Cellactose and Avicel PH-200: A Quantitative Relationship. Drug Dev. Ind. Pharm. **2000**, *26* (3), 297–305.

95. Flores, L.E.; Arellano, R.L.; Esquivel, J.J.D. Study of Load Capacity of Avicel PH-200 and Cellactose, Two Direct Compression Excipients, Using Experimental Design. Drug Dev. Ind. Pharm. **2000**, *26* (4), 465–469.

96. Mulderrig, K.B. Placebo Evaluation of Selected Sugar-Based Excipients. Pharm. Technol. **2000**, *24* (5), 34–42.

97. Viseras, C.; López-Galindo, A. Characteristics of Pharmaceutical Grade Phyllosilicate Powders. Pharm. Dev. Technol. **2000**, *5* (1), 47–52.

98. Kiekens, F.; Córdoba-Díaz; Remon, J.P. Influence of Chopper and Mixer Speeds and Microwave Power Level during the High-Shear Granulation Process on the Final Granule Characteristics. Drug Dev. Ind. Pharm. **1999**, *25* (12), 1289–1293.

99. Nicholas, V.; Chambin, O.; Andrès; Rochat-Gonthier, M.-H.; Pourcelot, Y. Preformulation: Effect of Moisture Content on Microcrystalline Cellulose (Avicel PH-302) and its Consequences on Packaging Performances. Drug Dev. Ind. Pharm. **1999**, *25* (10), 1137–1142.

100. Tsai, T.; Wu, J.-S.; Ho, H.-O.; Sheu, M.-T. Modification of Physical Characteristics of Microcrystalline Cellulose by Codrying with β-Cyclodextrins. J. Pharm. Sci. **1998**, *87* (1), 117–122.

101. Armstrong, N.A. Direct-Compression Characteristics of Granulated Lactitol. Pharm. Technol. 1998; 84–92.

102. Vennat, B.; Gross, D.; Pourrat, A.; Pourrat, H. A Dosage Form for Procyanidins High-dose Tablets by Direct Compression. S.T.P. Pharma. **1988**, *4* (5), 378–383.

103. Ashton, M.D.; Cheng, D.C.H.; Farley, R.; Valentin, F.H.H. Some Investigations into the Strength and Flow Properties of Powders. Rheol. Acta **1965**, *4* (3), 206–217.

104. Eaves, T.; Joness, T.M. Rheol. Acta, **1971**, *10*, 127–134.

105. Kocova, S.; Pilpel, N.A. Failure Properties of Lactose and Calcium Carbonate Powders. Powder Technol. **1972**, *5* (6), 329–343.

106. Heistand, E.N.; Poet, C.B. Tensile Strength and Compressed Powders and an Example of Incompalibility as End-point and Shear Yield Locus. J. Pharm. Sci. **1974**, *63* (4), 605–612.

107. Irono, C.I.; Pilpel, N. Effects of Paraffin Coatings on the Shearing Properties of Lactose. J. Pharm. Pharmacol. **1982**, *34*, 480–485.

108. Johanson, J.R. Theory of Bulk Solids Flow a Historical Perspective. Int. J. Bulk Solids Storage in Silos **1987**, *3* (1), 1–15.

109. Doelker, E. Comparative Compaction Properties of Various Microcrystalline Cellulose Types and Generic Products. Drug Dev. Ind. Pharm. **1993**, *19* (17, 18), 2399–2471.

110. Ho, R.; Bagster, D.F.; Crooks, M.J. Flow Studies on Directly Compressible Tablet Vehicles. Drug Dev. Ind. Pharm. **1977**, *3* (5), 475–487.

111. Amidon, G.E.; Houghton, M.E. Powder Flow Testing in Preformulation and Formulation Development. Pharm. Manu.July 1985; 21–31.

112. Kata, M. Shear Cell Investigation of Powder Mixtures Containing Micronized Drugs. Acta Pharm. Technol. **1979**, *25* (3), 203–216.

113. Laloge, M.; Chulia, D.; Guillemoteau, J.Y.; Verain, A. S.T.P. Pharma. **1988**, *4*, 319–324.

114. Cohard, C.; Gonthier, Y.; Chulia, D.; Verain, A. Comparative Rheological Study of Different Materials with the Jenike Shear Cell. J. Pharm. Belg. **1984**, *39* (4), 209–216.

115. Chulia, D.; Verian, A. Une Nouvelle Cellule a Cisaillement Adaptee Aux Problemes Pharmaceutiques, (A New Shear-cell Adapted to Pharmaceutical Problems). Ann. Pharm. Franc. **1983**, *41*, 15–24.

116. Sanz Urgoti, E.; Vasquez Lopez, F. Reologia De Materiales Pulverulentos – I. Aproximacion a su Estudio. Cienc. Ind. Farm. **1986**, *5*, 350–353.

117. Nash, J.J.; Leiter, G.G.; Johnson, A.P. Ind. Eng. Chem. Prod. Res. Dev. **1965**, *4*, 140.

118. Hiestand, E.N.; Wilcox, C.J. Some Measurements of Friction in Simple Powder Beds. Pharm. Sci. **1968**, *57*, 1427.

119. Hiestand, E.N.; Wilcox, C.J. Shear Cell Measurements of Powders: Proposed Procedures for Elucidating the Mechanistic Behavior of Powder Beds in Shear. J. Pharm. Sci. **1969**, *58*, 1403.

120. Hiestand, E.N.; Valvani, S.C.; Peot, C.B.; Strzelinski, E.P.; Glasscock, J.F. Shear Cell Measurements of Powders: Determination of Yield Loci. J. Pharm. Sci. **1973**, *62* (9), 1513–1517.

121. Carr, J.F.; Walker, D.M. Annular Shear Cell for Granular Materials. Powder Technol. **1968**, *1*, 369–373.
122. Peschl, I.A.S.Z. Quality Control of Powders for Industrial Application. Powder Handling Process **1989**, *1* (4), 357–363.
123. Peschl, I.A.S.Z. Quality Control of Powders for Industrial Application, Proceeding of the 14th Annual Meeting Powder and Bulk Solids Rosemont, IL: May 1989, 517–536
124. Schulze, D. Development - Application of a Novel Ring. Aufbereitungs-Technik **2000**, *35* (10), 524–535.
125. Schulze, D. Flowability and Time Consolidation Measurements Using a Ring Shear Tester. Powder Handling Process **1996**, *8* (3), 221–226.
126. Schulze, D. *First European Symposium Process Technology in Pharmaceutical and Nutritional Sciences*; 1998, 276–285.
127. Nqvist, H. Int. J. Pharm. Prod. Mfr. **1984**, *5* (1), 13–17.
128. Baichwal, A.R.; Augsburger, L.L. Development and Validation of a Modified Annular Shear Cell to Study Frictional Properties of Lubricants. Int. J. Pharm. **1985**, *26*, 191–196.
129. Behres, M.; Klasen, C.-J.; Schulze, D. Development of a Shear Cell for Measuring the Wall Friction of Bulk Solids with a Ring Shear Tester. Powder Handling Process **1998**, *10* (4), 405–409.
130. Schulze, D. Ch. 2.2. *Measurements of the Flowability of Bulk Solids, Silos, Fundamentals of Theory, Behaviour and Design*; Brown, C.J., Nielson, J., Eds.; E. & FN Spon: London and New York, 1998; 18–52.
131. Enstad, G.G.; Feise, H. Ch. 2.3. *Flow Property Testing of Particulate Solids by Uniaxial and Biaxial Testers*; Brown, C.J., Nielson, J., Eds.; E. & FN Spon: London and New York, 1998; 53–64.
132. Luong, M.P. Ch. 2.4. *Reflections on Triaxial Testing, Rheology and Flowability, Silos, Fundamentals of Theory, Behaviour and Design*; Brown, C.J., Nielson, J., Eds.; E. & FN Spon: London and New York, 1998; 65–75.
133. Kolymbas, D.; Wu, W. Recent Results of Triaxial Tests with Granular Materials. Powder Technol. **1990**, *60* (2), 99–119.
134. Johanson, J.R. The Johanson Indicizer™ System vs. the Jenike Shear Tester. Bulk Solids Handling **1992**, *2*, 237–240.
135. Bell, T.A.; Ennis, B.J.; Grygo, R.J.; Scholten, W.J.F.; Schenkel, M.M. Practical Evaluation of the Johanson Hang-up Indicizer. Bulk Solids Handling **1994**, *14* (1), 117–125.
136. Chowhan, Z.T.; Yang, I.C. Powder Flow Studies III: Tensile Strength, Consolidation Ratio, Flow Rate and Capsule Filling–Weight Variation Relationships. J. Pharm. Sci. **1981**, *70* (8), 927–930.
137. Crowder, T.M.; Hickey, A.J. A Semiconductor Strain Gauge Based Instrument for Rapid Powder Flow Rate Measurement. Respiratory Drug Delivery **1998**, *6* 297–298.
138. Kaye, B.H.; Gratton-Liimatainen, J.; Faddis, N. Studying the Avalanching Behaviour of a Powder in a Rotating Disc. Part. Part. Syst. Charact. **1995**, *12*, 232–236.
139. Kaye, B. Moving and Storing Powders. Book in Preparation.
140. Hickey, A.J.; Concession, N.M. Chaos in Rotating Lactose Powder Beds. Part. Sci. Tech. **1996**, *14*, 15–25.
141. Kaye, B.H. Sampling and Characterisation Research: Developing Two Tools for Powder Testing. Powder and Bulk Eng. **1996**.
142. Trowbridge, L.; Grimsey, I.; York, P. Assessing Powder Flow from Avalanching Behaviour. *Pharmaceutical Technology*; School of Pharmacy, University of Bradford: BRADFORD BD7 1DP, API Ref. Lib. #80.
143. Trowbridge, L.; Williams, A.C.; York, P.; Worthington, V.L.; Dennis, A.B. A Comparison of Methods for Determining Powder Flow: Correlation with Tableting Performance. Pharm. Res. **1997**, *14* (11 (supplement)), 415.
144. Crowder, T.M.; Hickey, A.J. The Physics of Powder Flow Applied to Pharmaceutical Solids. Pharm. Techno. **2000**, *24* (2), 50–58.
145. Brabender, O.H.G. Duisburg: Flowability Test, Specification Sheet No. 2124, 1982.
146. Podczeck, F. Rheological Studies of the Physical Properties of Powders Used in Capsule Filling—Part I. Pharm. Technol. Europe **1999**, *11* (9), 16–24.
147. Podczeck, F. Rheological Studies of the Physical Properties of Powders Used in Capsule Filling—Part II. Pharm. Technol. Europe **1999**, *11* (10), 34–42.
148. TheNew FT3 Powder Rheometer—Freeman Technology.
149. Freeman, R.The Flowability of Powders, International Conference on Powder and Bulk Solids Handling, 2000.
150. Velasco, A.; Muñoz-Ruiz, A.J.; Perales, M.C.; Muñoz, N.; Jiménez-Castellanos, M.R. Evaluation of an Adequate Method of Estimating Flowability According to Powder Characteristics. Int. J. Pharm. **1994**, *103*, 155–161.
151. Tan, S.B.; Newton, J.M. Powder Flowability as an Indication of Capsule Filling Performance. Int. J. of Pharm. **1990**, *61*, 145–155.
152. Lee, Y.S.L.; Poynter, R.; Podczeck, F.; Newton, J.M. Development of a Dual Approach to Assess Powder Flow from Avalanching Behavior. AAPS Pharm. Sci. Tech. **2000**, *1* (3), 1–14, Article 21 (http://www.pharmscitech.com).
153. Taylor, M.K.; Ginsburg, J.; Hickey, A.J.; Gheyas, F. Composite Method to Quantity Powder Flow as a Screening Method in Early Tablet or Capsule Formulation Development. AAPS Pharm. Sci. Tech. **2000**, *1* (3), 1–21, Article 18 (http://www.pharmscitech.com).

FOOD AND DRUG ADMINISTRATION: ROLE IN DRUG REGULATION

Roger L. Williams
U.S. Pharmacopeia, Rockville, Maryland, U.S.A.

OVERVIEW

With a FY2000 budget of $395 billion and employees numbering over 61,000, the Department of Health and Human Services (DHHS) is one of the largest departments in the administrative branch of the United States Government. It is responsible for the activities of 11 operating divisions,[a] including the Food and Drug Administration (FDA) (1). Although FDA's budget and staff are comparatively small (FY2000 $1.1 billion and 9000 employees), FDA has broad authority and impact. FDA regulates approximately $1 trillion worth of products that are sold in the United States, accounting for about 25% of products purchased by consumers annually and affecting some 95,000 businesses whose manufactured goods fall under FDA regulation. FDA activities work to assure that: 1) foods are safe and wholesome; human and veterinary drugs, human biological products, and medical devices are safe and effective; cosmetics are safe; and radiation-emitting consumer products are safe; 2) regulated products are honestly, accurately, and informatively represented; and 3) regulated products are in compliance with FDA regulations and guidelines, noncompliance is identified and corrected, and any unsafe or unlawful products are removed from the marketplace.

FDA is directed by the Commissioner of Food and Drugs whose appointment by the DHHS Secretary is subject to confirmation by the United States Senate. The Office of the Commissioner includes eight subsidiary offices. These are Chief Counsel; Equal Opportunity; Administrative Law Judge; Senior Associate Commissioner; International and Constituent Relations; Policy, Planning, and Legislation; Management and Systems; and Science Coordination and Communication. In addition, the Office of the Commissioner directs the activities of five Centers that are responsible for many of the primary regulatory activities of the Agency. These are the Center for Biologics Evaluation and Research (CBER); the Center for Devices and Radiologic Health; the Center for Drug Evaluation and Research (CDER); the Center for Food Safety and Applied Nutrition; and the National Center for Toxicological Research. The first three of these Centers direct activities that result in the availability of many therapeutic products—drugs, biologics, and devices—to treat and prevent human disease. The Commissioner of Food and Drugs also directs the activities of the Office of Regulatory Affairs, which is responsible for FDA's enforcement activities and oversees the activities of more than 1100 field inspectors.

FDA activities are complex, challenging, science-based, and continually changing to meet societal needs and expectations. This article provides a brief overview of these activities, with the understanding that careful study and analysis may be needed to fully understand and adhere to the science, technical and legal conditions that underlie FDA's actions. Many articles and books have been published delineating FDA's statutory and regulatory mandates, to which the reader is referred (2a, 2b, 2c). FDA's web page at http://www.fda.gov also provides additional useful information.

LEGISLATION

The Food, Drug, and Cosmetic Act

FDA operates in accordance with provisions of the Federal Food, Drug, & Cosmetic Act (FFDCA) (3) the Public Health Service Act (4), and other laws (5). Although the principle regulatory agency for food and drugs, FDA works cooperatively with other federal agencies, such as the Environmental Protection Agency and the Department of Agriculture, and with state governments. Regulation of food and drugs by FDA dates back almost 100 years to passage of the Federal Food and Drugs Act in 1906. This law was enacted because of widespread concern about patent medicines and food quality in the US. It created

---

[a]The remaining are the National Institutes of Health, the Centers for Disease Control and Prevention, the Agency for Toxic Substances and Disease Registry, the Indian Health Service, the Health Resources and Services Administration, the Substance Abuse and Mental Health Services Administration, the Agency for Healthcare Research and Quality, the Health Care Financing Administration, the Administration for Children and Families, and the Administration on Aging.

important concepts that continue to the present, namely, that foods and drugs marketed in the United States should not be misbranded, i.e., should not make unsubstantiated claims or otherwise present misleading information, and should not be adulterated. The next major drug regulatory legislation after 1906 was the FFDCA itself, which was enacted in 1938 in response to the Elixir of Sulfanilamide tragedy. Using the excipient diethylene glycol to solubilize the sulfa drug, sulfanilamide, the Elixir was a potent nephrotoxin that killed over 100 children and adults. It was marketed without provision of any kind of information to FDA. In response, the 1938 law created a safety standard that requires performance of adequate tests using reasonable methods to demonstrate that a product is safe. An important feature of the 1938 legislation was and remains a requirement for premarket provision of safety information to FDA, with authority given to the Agency to confirm that the information did in fact support a determination of a safety. The 1938 approach was based on notification instead of premarket approval. If an applicant did not hear from the FDA within 60 days of filing an application it could market the product. The 1938 legislation also established the general approach, still current, that FDA for the most part responds to data developed by sponsors and applicants. FDA usually does not by itself develop data for a regulatory submission, although it frequently engages in sampling and testing of unapproved and approved products. The 1938 legislation introduced other approaches that continue to this date. For example, the concept that certain therapeutic products should bear adequate directions for use and that, in certain instances, some products may be administered only by prescription (Rx Legend) was introduced in the 1938 legislation. This distinction between Rx and over-the-counter (OTC) drugs was further elaborated in the 1951 Durham–Humphrey amendments to the FFDCA.

Many major amendments have been made to the FFDCA since 1938. The most important of these were the 1962 Harrison–Kefauver amendments that arose as a result of the thalidomide tragedy. These amendments created many provisions that form the basis for modern drug regulation by the Agency. The legislation established a premarket process that allows the FDA to judge the safety and efficacy of drugs before they can be legally marketed. It also created a requirement for submission of an Investigational New Drug (IND) application to allow distribution and study of an unapproved new drug. To document efficacy of a new drug, the legislation created an 'efficacy standard' requiring substantial evidence of effectiveness based on adequate and well-controlled efficacy studies submitted by an applicant. The 1962 legislation also stated that drugs be produced in

accordance with current Good Manufacturing Practices and expanded substantially the information required in product labeling.

Beyond the 1938 establishing legislation and the 1962 amendments, many other significant legislative changes to the FFDCA have occurred. These include the 1972 Drug Listing Act (established a notification process for commercially marketed products); the 1976 Medical Device Act (created Class I, II, and III types of devices based on risk, with premarket clearance required for Class III); the Drug Price Competition and Patent Term Restoration Act of 1984 (finalized approaches that allow marketing of therapeutically equivalent generic drugs coupled with patent term extension and exclusivity provisions to reward innovation); the Orphan Drug Act of 1983 (creates incentives to develop drugs for rare diseases); the Drug Export Act of 1996 (allows export of unapproved products with certain stipulations); the Prescription Drug Marketing Act of 1987 (protects again diversion of prescription drug products from well-controlled distribution channels); the Generic Drug Enforcement Act of 1993 (debars individuals convicted for illegal activities related to the approval of Abbreviated New Drug Applications); the Prescription Drug User Fee Act (requires payment for review of new drug and analogous applications and certain supplements, plus annual establishment and product fees); and the Dietary Supplement and Health Education Act of 1994 (creates a food category for dietary supplements and establishes a premarket notification process for dietary supplements entering the market after 1994). The most recent legislative amendments to the FFDCA, which also affects the Public Health Service Act, is the 1997 Food and Drug Administration Modernization Act (FDAMA) (6, 7). Many of the elements of drug regulation, as exemplified in the provisions of the FFDCA, have arisen as a result a finding of or concern for societal risk. In contrast, FDAMA was designed to address a somewhat different perception of risk, namely, that FDA reform was needed to accelerate the availability of new medicines. This perception arose from the belief that an excessively restrictive Agency could create risk by reducing the availability of new therapeutic products. FDAMA focused on improving all aspects of FDA's regulatory activities, including drugs (Title I), devices (Title II), foods (Title III), coupled with more general changes and requirements (Title IV). FDAMA codified many FDA initiatives previously expressed in regulations or guidance, including: 1) harmonization of measures to regulate the manufacture of drugs and biologics; 2) elimination of the need for insulin batch certification; 3) withdrawal of the distinction between antibiotics and drugs; 4) strategies to streamline approval of drug and antibiotic manufacturing changes; 5) reduction in the need for environmental assessments; and 6) FDA's rules on accelerated approval of specified investigational drugs. FDAMA also codified FDA's practice of allowing one clinical investigation as the basis for product approval in certain circumstances, while generally preserving the 1962 standard for more than one adequate and well-controlled studies to prove efficacy. FDAMA also changed FDA's policies in many important areas, including allowance of a firm to disseminate peer-reviewed journal articles about an off-label indication of its product with certain stipulations, and allowance of drug companies to provide economic information about their products to formulary committees, managed care organizations, and similar large-scale buyers of health-care products. FDAMA created a special exemption for pharmacy compounding with certain stipulations to prevent pharmaceutical manufacturing under the guise of compounding.

The Public Health Service Act

An additional important set of Federal laws, even older that the FFDCA, relates to the regulation of biologic products. Following the deaths of 12 children from poor quality diphtheria antitoxin, Federal laws were created in 1902 to require the licensing of biologic products. FDA now regulates these under the provisions of the Public Health Service Act, which defines a biologic product as "a virus, therapeutic serum, toxin, antitoxin, vaccine, blood, blood component or derivative, allergenic product, or analogous product, or arsphenamine or derivative or arsphenamine, applicable to the prevention, treatment or cure of a disease or condition of human beings." Biologic products are generally derived from living organisms. Because biologic products are also defined as "drugs" and/or "devices," they are subject to the adulteration, misbranding, and registration provisions of the FFDCA. The importance of the 1902 legislation expanded with availability of therapeutic products produced through recombinant biotechnology approaches. These products fall under the Public Health Service Act as "analogous products" and may be subject to the jurisdiction of CBER. Inter-center agreements at FDA allow review and approval of drugs and biologics produced through recombinant technology in other centers as well.

REGULATIONS

FDA implements the statutory provisions of the FFDCA and PHS Act and associated laws through regulations. Regulations are rules that generally have the force of law.

They provide more explicit information about how a business or manufacturer should conduct their operations and submit information to FDA to be in compliance with the law. For example, the stipulation for adequate and well controlled investigations stated in the 1962 amendments to the FFDCA was elaborated in a regulation that provide more explicit statements on what constitutes an adequate and well-controlled study. Other important regulations issued by FDA over the last several decades include the 1981 regulation Protection of Human Subjects; Informed Consent; Standards for Institutional Review Boards (clarifies or creates requirements for informed consent and institutional review boards to protect human subjects participating in FDA regulated research) and several regulations designed to accelerate the availability of investigational and approved drugs to treat life-threatening illnesses such as HIV and cancer (1987 Treatment Use of Investigational New Drugs, 1988 Procedures for Subpart E Drugs, 1992 Accelerated Approval, 1992 Parallel-Track Mechanism). A public process exists that allows interested parties to view and comment on preliminary (Announced Notice of Proposed Rule-Making) and draft (Proposed Rule-Making) FDA regulations before they are finalized (Final Rule). Provisions of the Federal Administrative Procedures Act govern the overall process, including the Agency's response to public comments. FDA regulations are published and updated annually in the Code of Federal Regulations (CFR).

GUIDANCES FOR INDUSTRY

FDA uses guidance documents as a means of communicating to regulated industry and the public at large about ways to meet its governing laws and implementing regulations. While guidance documents have been used over the years under many names, FDA began producing them regularly in the mid-1980s as one of three phases of a comprehensive effort to improve the IND/NDA process. Guidances assist sponsors and applicants in understanding how applications should be formatted and what they should contain, how regulated industry should comply with regulatory directives, how inspections should be conducted, and how to comply with many other regulatory activities. The use of guidances has increased as a result of international harmonizing activities, such as the International Conference on Harmonization of Technical Requirements for Registration of Pharmaceuticals for Human Use (ICH), the Veterinary International Conference on Harmonization for veterinary products, and the Global Harmonization Task Force for devices. To facilitate development, issuance, and use of guidance documents, the Agency published a 1997 Good Guidance Practices document (62 FR 8967) that articulated the purpose, definition, legal effects, procedures for development, standard elements, implementation, dissemination, and appeals for Agency guidances. As part of this effort, the FDA committed to publish semiannually possible guidance topics or documents for development or revision during the next year, and to seek public comment on additional ideas for new or revisions of existing guidance documents (63 FR 59317). Many guidances have been produced by FDA over the last several years to assist sponsors and applicants. Although FDA guidances do not have the force of law, they indicate the Agency's best judgment about the amount and type of information needed to satisfy the Agency's legal and regulatory requirements. Regulated industries and businesses do not need to follow guidance recommendations if they wish to employ alternative methods that are acceptable to FDA. In accordance with a requirement of the 1997 FDAMA legislation, FDA is converting its Good Guidance Practices document into a regulation (8).

GUIDANCES FOR REVIEWERS

While most FDA guidances are directed to regulated industries, some are directed to Agency review staff in the form of Good Review Practices documents. These guidances instruct FDA review staff on how to conduct a high quality, consistent, timely review of an application or supplement. Good Review Practices documents may be viewed as one element in a series of quality control elements for regulatory review processes that also include secondary and tertiary supervisory oversight of a primary review, review templates, training, internal standard operating procedures, and many other initiatives as well. Good Review Practices documents complement Agency guidances and are also developed in accordance with the Agency's Good Guidance Practices document. Although Good Review Practices documents and internal standard operating procedures are directed at agency staff, they are of substantial interest to regulated industry and serve as a means of promoting transparency about Agency functions to pharmaceutical sponsors and the public at large.

DRUG REGULATION AT FDA

The FFDCA defines drugs as "articles intended for use in the diagnosis, cure, mitigation, treatment, or prevention of disease in man or other animals" and "articles (other than

food) intended to affect the structure or any function of the body of humans or other animals." The therapeutic use defines whether an article is a drug. Thus, FDA may consider a food, cosmetic, and dietary supplement to be a drug if they are associated with a therapeutic claim. The FFDCA also defines a drug as an article recognized in the official United States Pharmacopeia, official Homeopathic Pharmacopeia of the United States or official National Formulary, or any supplement to these documents. The concept of new drugs arose with the 1938 legislation. FDA allows "grandfathered" drugs marketed in the United States prior to 1938 to remain in the market providing they are generally recognized as safe (GRAS) and effective (GRAE). After the 1938 and 1962 legislation, all new drugs require Agency review and approval before they can be marketed. Recognizing that "new drugs" may be considered by several FDA Centers, information about most new drugs, including both prescription pioneer, generic equivalents, and OTC drugs, is submitted in new drug applications (NDAs) or abbreviated new drug applications (ANDAs), and supplements and annual reports for these applications to CDER. Most of the following discussion thus relates to the regulation of new drugs as executed by this Center. Many elements considered in this discussion are also applicable to biologic products submitted to CBER. Note: Two licenses are necessary to manufacture and distribute some biological products—one for the product (Product Licensing Application/PLA) itself and one for the establishment where it is manufactured (Establishment Licensing Application/ELA). Others only require one application, termed a Biologics Licensing Application, which covers both the product and its manufacture.

DRUG DEVELOPMENT AND APPROVAL

Discovery, development, regulatory assessment with possible approval, and post-marketing manufacture, distribution, and marketing of a new drug is a complex series of activities that is highly resource intensive. Modern drug discovery and development occurs primarily in laboratories of the pharmaceutical industry and in academic and government research centers as well. The loss rate is large, with thousands of drugs screened in early laboratory and animal studies before a few are considered suitable for studies in humans. Information about early discovery and nonclinical animal studies is submitted to the Agency in an Investigational New Drug (IND) application. This part of the regulatory process relies on notification, so that a sponsor may proceed with clinical studies in humans if the Agency does not respond with

30 days of submission. Regulations giving provisions of the IND process are provided at 21 CFR 312 and in further agency guidances (e.g., the FDA guidance *Content and Format of INDs for Phase 1 Studies of Drugs, Including Well-Characterized Therapeutic Biotechnology-Derived Products* (9)). CDER receives approximately 1500 INDs each year, most of which represent individual investigator INDs. Approximately 400 of these are commercial ones submitted by pioneer manufacturers. A key provision of the IND process—and for many clinical studies of approved drugs as well—is the protection of human research subjects, which should occur according to the stipulations of the 1981 informed consent and institutional review board regulations.

After filing an IND, a sponsor conducts nonclinical and clinical studies to assess the safety, efficacy, and quality of an investigational new drug. Information from these studies is collected into an NDA and submitted to FDA for review. These studies involve characterization of the new drug for its important safety, efficacy, and quality attributes. The IND process may take many years and include scores of nonclinical and clinical studies. The studies move through discrete phases. The first phase (Phase 1) group of studies focus on safety coupled with pharmacokinetic and pharmacodynamic studies in small numbers of usually healthy subjects. The studies continue with patient studies to explore efficacy (Phase 2, sometimes termed proof of concept studies) and conclude with additional studies in larger numbers of patients to assess safety further and confirm efficacy (Phase 3). Many additional studies may be performed in association with these primary studies to assess the influence of concomitant medications (drug–drug interaction studies), bioavailability and bioequivalence, subpopulation effects, and other findings that may be useful to practitioners, patients, and consumers in understanding how to use the new drug optimally. While many drugs follow the sequences defined in Phases 1–3, this is not always the case. Depending on an investigational drug's intended indications, its safety profile, its therapeutic need and many other factors, many modications to the general sequence may occur.

Most NDAs and ANDAs are approved at FDA by CDER. In a single year, the Center approves approximately 100 NDAs, with approximately 30% of these representing previously unapproved new molecular entities (NMEs). The remainder represent line extensions, e.g., new dosage forms, new routes of administration. In addition, CDER approves many thousands of supplements to NDAs each year, most of which represent manufacturing changes but many of which represent supplements providing information about new uses (efficacy supplements) or additional safety information. CDER also has responsibility for considering annual reports that are required for each approved NDA and ANDA. With a review staff of approximately 1700, CDER is organized into several main units. One of the most important of these is the Office of Review Management that oversees the activities of five Offices of Drug Evaluation (I–V). These Offices in turn are responsible for the activities of 15 review divisions that are organized primary according to therapeutic groups and drug classes. For example, the Division of Cardio-Renal Drug Products reviews applications that are for new drugs used to treat cardiovascular and renal diseases. The Office of Review Management also comprises an Office of Biostatistics and an Office of Post-Marketing Drug Risk Assessment. The former office reviews statistical analyses in applications and supplements, while the latter office focuses on post-marketing adverse drug reports. A further primary unit in CDER is the Office of Pharmaceutical Science. This Office has responsibility for the Offices of New Drug Chemistry, Clinical Pharmacology and Biopharmaceutics, Office of Testing and Research, and Office of Generic Drugs. Addition administrative and regulatory activities in CDER, including those involving compliance, are handled at the level of the Center. CDER works closely with many Centers at FDA, including CBER and CDRH, and perhaps most notably with the Office of Regulatory Affairs, which is responsible for assuring that firms manufacture products in accordance with current Good Manufacturing Practices (cGMPs). Additional inspections to assure compliance with Good Laboratory Practices (GLPs) and Good Clinical Practices (GCPs) are conducted by CDER.

INDs and NDAs

From a science and technical standpoint, a good conceptual understanding has emerged in the last several decades about the IND processes that result, finally, in a safe, effective, and good quality new drug product. According to this understanding, a drug substance (active ingredient/active moiety and nonactive components, e.g., impurities, residual solvents) is combined with excipients to create a pharmaceutical product with defined identity, strength, quality, purity, and potency. An associated aspect of quality relates to product performance. Performance is assessed by product quality bioavailability and relative bioavailability (bioequivalence) studies. These studies measure the rate and extent of release of the active ingredient from a drug product and its subsequent availability to one or more sites of action. At these sites of action, the active ingredient and/or its metabolites produce the safety and efficacy outcomes reflected in product labeling. Safety, efficacy, and quality topics in drug development and regulation can be expressed via a set of questions (primary question, test to address the question, and confidence needed in analysis of test outcome) that allow a basis for mutual understanding. From a regulatory perspective, the first set of questions can usually be stated simply (does the new drug have good quality? is it safe? is it effective?). These are the questions that drive nonclinical and clinical characterization studies conducted during the IND period and that lead to a set of data that is submitted in an NDA. Following regulatory assessment and approval if indicated, these characterization studies result in product labeling that provide instructions for use by the practitioner for prescription drug products and by the patient and/or consumer for OTC products. With Agency approval, an applicant may manufacture, distribute, advertise, and sell the approved new drug product throughout the United States market.

An NDA submission includes the following six technical sections: 1) Clinical; 2) Human pharmacokinetics and bioavailability; 3) Chemistry, manufacturing and controls; 4) Microbiology; 5) Nonclinical pharmacology and toxicology; and 6) Statistics. Further information about some of these sections is considered briefly in the following sections. More detailed information is provided in FDA regulatory documents and in internet and print publications. Examples include *the CDER Handbook* (10) and a recently updated document entitled *From Test Tube to Patient: Improving Health through Human Drugs* (11).

Clinical Information

FDAs focus on efficacy began in 1962, was further elaborated in regulations, was modified by FDAMA, and has been considered in detail in an Agency guidance entitled *Providing Clinical Evidence of Effectiveness for Human Drug and Biological Products* (12). Data from clinical studies containing efficacy data are a primary component of any NDA. These data are judged by FDA review staff to establish effectiveness of a new drug for one or more indications. A core set of guidances, many developed in ICH, also provide basic recommendations on the conduct of clinical studies needed to establish efficacy. In addition, FDA has published many guidances that provide recommendations on clinical trial design approaches, therapeutic endpoints, and other factors to consider in planning clinical safety and efficacy studies for specific disease categories or drug classes. Depending on the drug class, therapeutic indication, and therapeutic need, FDA has substantial latitude in defining the types and amount of information needed to establish safety and efficacy. While full documentation of clinical benefit information, such as reduction in morbidity and mortality,

may be needed to support approval of many new drugs, FDA may rely on lesser information for investigational drugs where a critical therapeutic need exists. For example, FDA may rely on surrogate markets instead of clinical benefit markets to allow approval, with the understanding that additional clinical benefit information may be requested after marketing.

Unlike many other regulatory agencies, FDA encourages frequent meetings with sponsors during the IND period so that good communication occurs about the information that will be needed in an NDA. In the final analysis, this information must convince Agency review staff that adequate and well-controlled studies provide substantial evidence of effectiveness and that study results also show that a product is safe under the conditions of use in the proposed labeling. Overall, the benefits arising from use of the new drug product must outweigh its risks. Risk/benefit judgments are frequently challenging for the applicant, the FDA, and the public at large. For drugs used to treat benign, self-limited conditions, little risk may be tolerated. Larger degrees of risk may be acceptable for drugs used to treat serious and life-threatening illnesses. Both during and after approval, information about safety of a new drug is required through many Agency laws and regulations. During the IND period, many of these requirements are designed not only to provide information about adverse drug reactions but also to protect human subjects participating in clinical trials. After approval, the agency requires product manufacturers and certain health care facilities to report adverse drug events. FDA developed a MedWatch program with a common reporting form and contact points to facilitate reporting of serious adverse events by health care professionals and consumers. MedWatch covers not only new drug products regulated by CDER but also biologics and medical devices. Information from safety reporting may enter product labeling and otherwise impact on the availability of a new drug product to practitioners and consumers. Although rare, withdrawal of an approved new drug product from the market may occur if a pharmaceutical manufacturer and the FDA agree that its benefits no longer outweighs its risks.

Pharmacokinetic and Bioavailability Studies

Pharmacokinetic and bioavailability studies and other clinical pharmacology studies have taken on increasing importance in the set of nonclinical and clinical studies that are performed during the IND period. This has occurred in part as a result of increasing capability to measure an active ingredient/moiety and its metabolites in accessible biologic fluids over time (pharmacokinetic studies). It has also occurred with increasing capability to study the time course of drug effects (pharmacodynamics) relative to exposure, which can expressed in terms of either dose or systemic concentration. In addition, most investigational new drugs enter the clinic with a better mechanistic understanding of how positive and negative effects occur in relation to the pathophysiology of disease. A focus of these studies relates to an understanding of an optimal dosage regimen in the population and in an individual. Clinical pharmacology information supports adjustment in dosage regimens based on intrinsic (e.g., genetic polymorphisms, age, gender, height, body mass and composition, and organ dysfunction) and extrinsic factors (e.g., diet, smoking, alcohol intake, concomitant medications). Adjustments in a dosage regimen according to these factors have become of increasing importance. For example, several drugs have been withdrawn from the market in recent years because of dangerous adverse drug reactions (mibefradil, terfenadine, hismanal, cisapride). Dose optimization pharmacokinetic and pharmacodynamic studies, including subpopulation and drug–drug interaction studies, are now performed frequently, in addition to the more routine absorption, distribution, metabolism, excretion (ADME) pharmacokinetic studies that have been performed for many years. A good understanding of exposure–response relationships may also support risk/benefit judgments of safety/efficacy data.

Bioavailability and Bioequivalence

Product quality bioavailability and bioequivalence studies are also an important part of the information needed to support an FDA approval (13). For most orally administered drugs, BA and BE measures are frequently expressed in terms of systemic exposure measures such as area under the plasma concentration-time curve (AUC) and maximum concentration (C_{max}). These measures of systemic exposure link with safety and efficacy outcomes that may be expressed in terms of biomarkers, surrogate endpoints, or clinical benefit endpoints. Studies that can meet the intent of these regulations for orally administered and certain other drug products have been elaborated in greater detail in an FDA guidance entitled *Bioavailability and Bioequivalence Studies for Orally Administered Drug Products—General Considerations* (14). Bioavailability and bioequivalence studies document that the performance of a drug product is reliable and consistent. This is important not only as part of the new drug approval process but also in the presence of postapproval changes in the components and composition of an approved drug product and/or its method of manufacture. Depending on the magnitude of these changes, redocumentation of bioequivalence may be needed after approval. Relative BA

studies are useful in comparing the systemic exposure profiles of different dosage forms. In this context, BA information, sometimes together with pharmacokinetic and pharmacodynamic and other data, can be used to link the performance of two different dosage forms and assure comparable clinical outcomes.

Chemistry, Manufacturing and Controls, and Microbiology

During the IND period, sponsors characterize the drug substance and drug product sufficiently so that important quality attributes are established and controlled. This effort focuses on: 1) the drug substance, to assure identity and strength of the active ingredient(s) and to control impurities arising from production and/or degradation; 2) the drug product, to assure the identity and strength of the active ingredient(s) and to monitor degradants that may arise during manufacture and storage; 3) the container–closure system, to protect the drug product during storage; 4) stability testing to assure maintenance of quality attributes during shelf-life; and 5) container labeling. For sterile pharmaceutical products, special approaches are needed. Full understanding of the manufacturing processes for a finished drug product also requires an understanding and application of in-process controls and of the quality of manufacturing materials even when they are not present in the final drug product. Using characterization data, a sponsor develops a set of specifications to assure the identity, strength, quality, purity, and potency of the product and to allow batch release into the marketplace. A specification is defined as a list of tests, references to analytical procedures to evaluate those tests, and the appropriate acceptance criteria. Specifications allow a determination that a particular drug substance or drug product can be considered acceptable for its intended use. Specifications are needed for the drug substance, the drug product, and the container and closure. They may also be needed for intermediates, raw materials, reagents, and other components, including container and closure systems and in-process materials. Specifications are one part of a total control strategy for the drug substance and drug product designed to ensure product quality and consistency. Adherence to current Good Manufacturing Practices is an important part of this overall strategy. Based on characterization and specification setting processes, pioneer manufacturers compile information about the quality of starting materials and their manufacture into a finished dosage form. FDA chemists review this information to assure that critical quality attributes are controlled. In addition, the chemistry review also focuses on in-process controls and validation of analytical procedures and, for sterile drug products, process validation to assure sterility. Compendial drug substance and excipient monographs as well as general tests and procedures in the *United States Pharmacopeia and National Formulary (USP-NF)* are frequently cited in an NDA and considered during the chemistry review.

Nonclinical Pharmacology and Toxicology Studies

The purpose of nonclinical animal safety studies is to support estimation of initial starting doses in humans and to characterize toxic effects with regard to target organs, exposure, dose dependence, and reversability. This information is provided in a series of studies that focus on single and repeated dose toxicity, reproduction toxicity, genotoxicity studies, local tolerance studies and, for drugs with especial concern and/or that are intended for long-term use, on carcinogenicity. Other nonclinical studies in animals may focus on safety effects on vital organ systems and pharmacokinetic (ADME) studies. The timing of nonclinical studies is important to assure optimal and safe performance of clinical studies. A series of guidelines have become available through ICH that provide guidance on the types of nonclinical studies and their timing needed to support clinical studies of an investigational agent and product labeling for an approved new drug. These cover studies on the following general topics: carcinogenicity, genotoxicity, pharmacokinetics, toxicity, reproductive toxicity, study of biotechnology products, safety pharmacology, and timing of nonclinical and clinical studies. Because this information is required to allow advance of investigational studies in the clinic, it will be submitted in reports and updates during the IND process. It may be summarized and analyzed as well in the NDA.

Biostatistics

Nonclinical and clinical development of an investigational agent requires a series of exploratory and confirmatory studies that rely on adequate statistical analyses. Careful attention is needed with regard to the many aspects of trial design to assure unbiased, robust conclusions regarding safety and efficacy. Important elements of a statistical analysis are discussed in an FDA guidance entitled *Guidance on Statistical Principles for Clinical Trials* (15).

NDA Review

Review of the information in an NDA is conducted according to time frames that are stipulated by law. These time-frames vary depending on whether the drug merits a priority or standard review. Priority drugs represent a substantial advance over available therapy. FDA commits to reviewing these types of drugs within six months. Standard drugs are defined as having therapeutic qualities similar to an already marketed drug. FDA commits to reviewing these in 10–12 months. The outcome of the FDA's deliberations are expressed in action letters. If submitted information establishes the effectiveness and safety of the new drug, the FDA will issue an approval action letter that permits the applicant to market the approved new drug in the United States. If the information does not establish effectiveness and safety, FDA may issue a nonapprovable action letter with a request for further information. If satisfactory, this information may subsequently support FDA's issuance of an approval letter. Over the years, approximately 60–80% of NDAs are approved, with the number rising in recent years presumably as applicants develop a better understanding of the information needed in an application to establish safety, efficacy, and quality. As part of an approval, FDA may request that an applicant provide additional information as part of an approval commitment (Phase 4 studies).

To assist the Agency in its deliberations, FDA established a system of advisory committees in 1964. These committees review data and provide recommendations to the Agency about whether or not an approval should proceed, or whether some other Agency action is or is not appropriate. The Agency's advisory committees, which function generally under the 1972 Federal Advisory Committee Act, have been modified over the years. Some of these modifications occurred as result of a 1992 Agency requested review by the Institute of Medicine, which coincided with an internal Agency evaluation, and some were put in place in the 1997 FDAMA legislation. The Agency's current advisory committee system involves many committees that meet to discuss a new drug's safety and efficacy, a new indication for an already approved drug, or a special science topic or adverse event profile. FDA's advisory committees provide only recommendations, which the Agency usually follows but at times may not. Membership in an advisory committee is chosen to reflect a needed constituency for a given topic, and includes both consumer and industry representatives. Care is taken to avoid conflicts of interest, with exclusion of a member if needed or, if an individual's view is important, with waiver to allow participation according to specified criteria. Advisory committee charters must be renewed biennially by DHHS and the General Services Administration.

After an NDA is approved, a pharmaceutical manufacturer may promote and advertise the approved new drug in accordance with provisions of the FFDCA and its implementing regulations. An approved application may be supplemented with new safety, efficacy, or manufacturing information.

ABBREVIATED NEW DRUG APPLICATIONS

The 1984 Drug Price Competition and Patent Term Restoration amendments to the FFDCA created an abbreviated mechanism for the approval of generic copies of drug products approved for safety and efficacy via the NDA process. Provisions of the amendments and its implementing regulations require that a generic applicant demonstrate that its product is the same as that of the corresponding innovator drug (the reference listed drug) in terms of active ingredient(s), strength, dosage form, and route of administration. These stipulations are termed pharmaceutical equivalence. In addition, the applicant must demonstrate that the labeling of its proposed generic version is comparable to that of the innovator product and that the generic product is bioequivalent to the reference listed drug. With this approach, the requirement for extensive nonclinical and clinical testing for a generic product is frequently obviated. Information developed by a generic applicant is submitted for Agency review in an ANDA if acceptable, the application is approved and the generic copy is deemed interchangeable with the corresponding reference product under specified conditions of use. As part of the 1984 legislation, an extensive series of requirements regarding patent certification and exclusivity was developed. These approaches were part of a general intent of the 1984 legislation to balance incentives for innovation with the societal need for low-cost duplicates of pioneer products.

OVER-THE-COUNTER DRUG PRODUCTS

Based on distinctions created in the 1938 FFDCA and the 1951 Durham–Humphrey Act, new drugs are categorized as either prescription and nonprescription or OTC. OTC drug products are deemed sufficiently safe for self-use. While FDA applies the same standards of safety and efficacy to prescription and nonprescription new drugs, it regulates them in two ways. One is by a monograph system and the other is through switching a prescription drug approved under an NDA to nonprescription status (Rx to OTC Switch). The OTC monograph system arose out of a need to document efficacy for the many thousands of new drugs that had been approved for safety only between 1938 and 1962. This was accomplished through the Drug

Efficacy Safety Implementation (DESI) program. As part of the effort, FDA initiated an OTC Drug Review in 1972 that resulted in the development of over 100 monograph categories (e.g., antacids, laxatives) for over 500 active ingredients that were marketed between 1938 and 1962 in approximately 700,000 different dosage forms. A manufacturer may market an OTC product in one of these categories without submitting information to FDA providing the manufacture and marketing of the product conform to stipulations in the monograph and to *USP-NF* substance and product monographs if available. In addition, experience with a prescription drug after its approval may result in an understanding that its can be used safely and effectively without professional supervision. FDA has allowed this type of Rx to OTC switch, either for approved prescription new drugs or for new indications, on 66 occasions in the last five years.

THE *UNITED STATES PHARMACOPEIA*

Practitioners established the *United States Pharmacopeia* in 1820 to promote the availability of unadulterated and appropriately named and prepared therapeutic products. With the addition of an information component beginning in 1980, USP's role expanded from establishing standards for healthcare articles to providing useful information to assist practitioners, consumers, and patients in optimal use of therapeutic products. Section 201 (j) of the Federal Food, Drug and Cosmetic Act defines the *United States Pharmacopeia (USP)* and the *National Formulary (NF)* as official compendia. These texts provide quality standards for therapeutic products and excipients approved under the provisions of the Food, Drug & Cosmetic Act, and other therapeutic products as well. The availability of a *USP-NF* monograph requires that any drug marketed under the monograph name must comply with the specifications, irrespective of whether the article bears the *USP-NF* designation. Through the adulteration and misbranding provisions of the Food, Drug & Cosmetic Act, FDA can take enforcement action against firms whose drug products do not comply with a *USP* or *NF* standard. The letters "USP" or "NF" are not trademarked and can be utilized by companies for non-drug products if they wish as a representation of the quality of their products subject only, for the most part, to regulatory constraints. Manufacturers of drug are not required to comply with USP standards but if they choose not to do so they are required to label their product as "not USP" and indicate how their product differs on the container label. For the most part, manufacturers choose to adhere to USP standards rather than conform to this requirement.

ADDITIONAL INFORMATION

In regulating drugs, FDA is continually changing and growing as a result of societal needs, rapidly changing science and technology, and health care delivery challenges. It also must consider international activities and harmonization and carve-outs where regulatory focus is diminished or clarified. Key to all of FDA's activities is the availability of resources to allow performance of its statutory functions. Some of these issues are discussed briefly in the following paragraphs.

Resources

Until 1992, resources for FDA came from appropriated tax dollars allocated at the beginning of each year through budget processes of the Administration and Congress. In 1992, Congress enacted the Prescription Drug User Fee act (PDUFA) that authorized FDA to collect fees from the prescription drug industry to augment FDA's appropriated resources. The additional resources were to be used to expedite the review of NDAs and Biologics Licensing Applications (BLAs) so that prescription drug products could reach the marketplace more quickly. The first PDUFA program, termed PDUFA I, was enacted for a period of five years, ending in 1997. In that year, as part of FDAMA (Title 1/Subtitle A—Fees Relating to Drugs), PDUFA was reauthorized, as PDUFA II, for five more years. PDUFA I included performance goals for FDA that were coupled with FDA managerial reforms. Via fees charged for application review, more than 900 employees have been added to the Agency's new drug and biologics review programs. In 1999, approximately $125 million in user fees were collected from the pharmaceutical industry. With these resources, CDER and CBER have generally met or exceeded the performance objectives of PDUFA I and II. PDUFA II has increased both the resources available to the FDA as well the performance objectives, e.g., by 2002, when PDUFA II ends, 90 percent of standard original NDAs and BLAs filed during FY 2002 will be reviewed and acted on within 10 months of receipt.

PDUFA provides resources only for the review of NDAs, leaving many of areas and processes of the Center still supported by appropriated dollars. Failure to increase Agency appropriations in the last several years have left many non-PDUFA components at FDA with substantially lower funding at the end of the 1990s than at the beginning. While PDUFA resources are useful, consumer groups and other have expressed concern over both undue emphasis on review timeliness and industry influence, given that a substantial fraction of the budget for new drug reviews is now provided by industry. Recent market withdrawals have heightened this concern (16, 17), although FDA has provided data to indicate that market withdrawals diminished in frequency since PDUFA was introduced (18).

International Harmonization

FDA engages in many international activities that result in information exchange, working closely with the World Health Organization and in different types of bilateral, trilateral, and multilateral arrangements. One of the most substantial examples of this effort is ICH (19). A primary objective of ICH is to avoid duplicative animal and human testing and to come to a common understanding of technical requirements to support the registration processes in the three ICH nations/regions, which include the European Union, Japan, and the United States. ICH began in 1989 as a collaborative effort between representatives from the Food and Drug Administration working with representatives from the European Commission (at the time the Commission of the European Communities) and the Japanese Ministry of Health and Welfare, and also with representatives from the three corresponding pharmaceutical manufacturers associations, the Japanese Pharmaceutical Manufacturers Association, the US Pharmaceutical Research and Manufacturers of America, and the European Federation of Pharmaceutical Industries Associations. Observers to ICH include representatives from the World Health Organization (WHO), the European Free Trade Association, and Canada's Therapeutic Products Program. ICH has established a Steering Committee, which meets twice yearly, moving sequentially through each ICH area, to provide oversight to the ICH Expert Working Groups that focus on specific topics for harmonization. Secretariat support to ICH is provided by the International Federation of Pharmaceutical Manufacturers Association provides two representatives to the Steering Committee. The ICH Expert Working Groups focus on Efficacy (clinical safety and efficacy topics), Safety (nonclinical safety), Quality, and Regulatory Communications. ICH has established a process for guidance development that begins with identification of a topic area for harmonization, for which a concept paper is developed, collection of background information, and formation of an Expert Working Group to draft the guidance (Step 1). This initial process yields a draft guidance that moves through a multistep process that, if successful, yields a final guidance that becomes part of the regulatory machinery in the European Union, the United States, and Japan (Steps 2–5).

With this approach, ICH differs from guidances developed by the World Health Organization, which do not necessarily become binding on a regulatory agency. In the 10 years since its inception, ICH has resulted in the preparation of over 40 finalized guidelines and position papers that are designed to guide drug development and registration activities in the European Union, Japan, and the United States. A more recent focus of ICH has been the development of a Common Technical Document that will provide a core set of information to support an NDA or BLA in the US, and the corresponding application documents in Europe and Japan. ICH has confronted several issues and challenges during the initial 10 years of its existence. For example, ICH is highly resource intensive and has at times excluded interested parties and stakeholders. The issue of exclusion has been dealt with at least in part via the efforts of WHO, which has disseminated ICH draft and finalized guidelines to WHO Member States. In addition, at biennial meetings of WHO's International Conference of Drug Regulatory Authorities, presentations on the status of ICH topics has become an increasingly important part of the program.

Regulatory Control

A key question for any society is the scope of responsibility that it gives to its regulatory agencies. This scope is defined through legislative and administrative actions, through judicial decisions, and through regulatory action or inaction. In the last decade, legislative decisions have limited and/or clarified the scope of FDAs responsibilities in two important areas. Examples include the regulation of dietary supplements and pharmacy compounding. Before 1994, FDA regulated dietary supplements according to the provisions of the 1958 Food Additive Amendments to the FFDCA, which required pre-market safety review for all new ingredients, including dietary supplements. In the 1994 Dietary Supplement Health and Education Act (DSHEA), Congress added provisions to the FFDCA that eliminated requirements for pre-market documentation of safety for dietary supplements and dietary ingredients of dietary supplements (20). In accordance with the 1958 legislation, these requirements continue to apply to other new food ingredients or for new uses of old food ingredients. DSHEA and the 1990 Nutritional Labeling and Education Act (NLEA) also extended the definition of a dietary supplement from vitamins, minerals and, proteins to herbs or similar nutritional substances and substances such as ginseng, garlic, fish oils, psyllium, enzymes, glandulars, and mixtures of these. Many provisions of DSHEA are now being implemented via FDA regulations.

A particularly challenging one relates to regulations that distinguish between dietary supplement claims and drug claims. The FFDAC defines a drug as an article intended for use in the diagnosis, cure, mitigation, treatment, or prevention of disease in man or animals. A product may be subject to regulation as a drug if it makes a claim that is other than food, and it is intended to affect the structure or any function of the body of man or other animals. Manufacturers of a dietary supplement may claim an affect on the structure and function of the body as long as they do not make drug claims. FDA has been challenged to provide a clear distinction between drug and dietary supplement claims in product labeling. This challenge reflects the boundary between food and drug claims and relates to the limitations and/or clarification in the scope of FDA's responsibilities expressed in NLEA and DSHEA. This distinction is currently provided in an FDA regulation entitled Regulations on Statements Made for Dietary Supplements Concerning the Effect of the Product on the Structure or Function of the Body (21).

Section 127 of FDAMA added section 503A of the FFDCA to clarify the status of pharmacy compounding of a drug by a pharmacist or physician on a customized basis for an individual patient. Section 503A defines pharmacy compounding to allow exemptions from the Good Manufacturing Practices, full disclosure requirements, and new drug provisions of the FFDAC. To qualify for these exemptions, a compounded drug product must satisfy several requirements delineated in Section 127. The general objective of section 127 is to allow a pharmacist and or physician to engage in the legitimate practice of compounding and to clarify the distinction between compounding and pharmaceutical manufacturing that comes under the oversight of FDA.

SUMMARY

Drugs to prevent and/or treat disease are a critical component of the U.S. health care system. The U.S. total health care bill is well over $1 trillion, with medical products accounting for approximately 8% of this total expenditure. Both the total health care cost and the fraction of the cost represented by medical products is expected to rise substantially in the coming years. Availability of most medical products is regulated closely by FDA and is one activity in a complex set of activities by which a new drug reaches a patient. Generally, these activities may be viewed in terms of discrete yet overlapping efforts that include drug discovery, nonclinical and clinical development programs, regulatory assessment, and utilization.

Revolutionary changes are occurring in each of these four areas. Drug discovery is driven by an increasingly detailed understanding of human physiology and pathophysiology arising from the molecular biology revolution and many associated diagnostic and therapeutic advances. Molecular modeling and combinatorial chemistry combined with high through-put screens for positive and negative drug effects and biopharmaceutical properties have expanded the number of lead candidates for nonclinical and clinical development. An improved understanding of the mechanistic basis for drug absorption and disposition and drug action provides better information about drug safety and efficacy. The regulatory review process at FDA has become more timely, in part as a result of availability of resources from users' fees charged to pharmaceutical sponsors submitting NDAs for prescription drugs and certain supplements to these applications.

The utilization of drugs to maintain health and treat disease has undergone profound change in the medical community as a result of many factors, including the need to contain costs yet assure that patients have access to the latest medical treatments. Overarching these changes in discovery, development, assessment, and utilization have been revolutions in information technology, materials science, management, and many other areas. All activities associated with getting a medical product to a patient are further affected, sometimes profoundly, by national and international societal and political factors. The intensity with which FDA functions relates to countervailing forces that work to promote the availability of the latest medical products versus forces that work to focus on the safety of these products. Globalization of the pharmaceutical industry has resulted in a need to harmonize on regulatory requirements and recommendations for the development of a new drug product. From a public policy perspective, FDAMA represents societal encouragement, expressed through Congressional legislation, for FDA to act more rapidly in making regulatory decisions. Availability of users' fees has provided FDA with resources to achieve this objective. Changes arising from FDAMA and users' fees appear to represent a major transformation in societal thinking about drug regulation, which in the past has focused on an expectation the FDA should function as a gatekeeper to keep unsafe medical products and foods from the market. FDAMA and users' fees work to shift that focus to facilitation of the availability of medical and other products regulated by FDA. These changes arose in the decade of the 1990's as a result of many factors, including a long history of charges that FDA created a drug lag, availability of an increasing number of important new medical products, a rise in activism from patients with serious and life-threatening diseases such as AIDS and

cancer, and many other factors as well. As with all societal directives, opinions and forces may cause a a reversal in Agency approaches. Concerns are raised now about drug safety and certain market withdrawals of unsafe drugs and drug combinations. The charge, generally refuted by FDA (18), is that a more rapid regulatory process leads to the availability of unsafe medical products.

REFERENCES

1. FDA Mission Statement, http://www/fda/gov.
2a. Cooper, R.M., Ed.; *Food and Drug Law*, 5th Ed. Food and Drug Law Institute: Washington, DC, 1991.
2b. Beers, D.O. *Generic and Innovator Drugs—a Guide to FDA Approval Requirements*; Aspen Law Business: New York, 1998.
2c. Temple, R. Development of Drug Law, Regulations, and Guidance in the United States. *Principles of Pharmacology, Basic Concepts and Clinical Applications*; Munson, P.L., Ed.; Ch. 113 Chapman & Hall: New York, 1996, Revised Reprint.
3. 21 U.S.C. Sections, 321–397.
4. 42 U.S.C Sections 241 (Research and Investigations), 242 (a) (Controlled Substances), 2421 (International Cooperation), 262–263 (Biological Products), 264 (Interstate and Foreign Infectious Disease Control Functions that Relate to the Law Enforcement Functions of FDA) (1994), See also 21 C.F.R. 5.10 (a), 1998.
5. Horton, L. Mutual Recognition Agreements and Harmonization. Seton Hall Law Rev. **1998**, *29*, 692–735; Orphan Drug Act of 1983, Pub. L. No. 97-414, 96 Stat. 2049, 1983; Drug Price Competition and Patent Term Restoration Act of 1994, Pub. L. No. 98-417, 98 Stat. 1585, 1984; Food Drug Modernization Act of 1997, Pub. L. No. 105-115, 111 Stat. 2296, 1997.
6. Pub. L. No. 105-115, 111 Stat., 2296–1997.
7. FDAMA and Related Document, http://www.fda.gov/opacom/7modact.html.
8. Federal Register **2000**, *65* (30).
9. http://www.fda.gov/cder/guidance.
10. http://www.fda.gov/cder/handbook/index.htm.
11. http://www.fda.gov/cder/about/whatwedo/testtube.pdf.
12. http://www.fda.gov/cder/guidance–clinical/medical).
13. 21 Code of Federal Regulations 320.
14. http://www.fda.gov/cder/guidance/biopharmaceutics.
15. http://www.fda.gov/cder/guidance/91698.
16. Withdrawals of FDA-Approved Drugs Raise Questions. Mayo Clin. Health Letter **1998**, *16* (4).
17. Kleinke, J.D.; Gottlieb, S. Is FDA Approving Drugs Too Fast. BMJ **1998**, *70*, 405–406.
18. Friedman, M.A.; Woodcock, J.; Lumpkin, M.M.; Shuren, J.E.; Hass, A.E.; Thompson, L.J. The Safety of Newly Approved Medicines—Do Recent Market Removals Mean There is a Problem? JAMA **1999**, *281*, 1728–1734.
19. ICH information, http://www.ifpma.org/ich1.html.
20. A Summary of The Dietary Health Supplement and Education Act is Available. http://vm.cfsan.fda.gov/dms/dietsupp.html.
21. 21 CFR 101, Federal Register, **2000**, *65* (4), 1000–1050.

FREEZE DRYING

Michael J. Pikal
University of Connecticut, Storrs, Connecticut

INTRODUCTION

Freeze drying, also termed "lyophilization," is a drying process employed to convert solutions of labile materials into solids of sufficient stability for distribution and storage. A typical production scale freeze dryer consists of a drying "chamber" containing temperature-controlled shelves, which is connected to a "condenser" chamber via a large valve. The condenser chamber houses a series of plates or coils capable of being maintained at very low temperature (i.e., less than $-50°C$). One or more vacuum pumps in series are connected to the condenser chamber to achieve pressures in the range of 0.03–0.3 Torr in the entire system during operation. A commercial freeze dryer may have 10–20 shelves with a total load of the order of 50,000 vials. The objective in a freeze-drying process is to convert most of the water into ice in the *freezing stage*, remove the ice by direct sublimation in the *primary drying stage*, and finally remove most of the unfrozen water in the *secondary drying stage* by desorption. The water removed from the product is reconverted into ice by the condenser.

In a typical freeze-drying process, an aqueous solution containing the drug and various formulation aids, or "excipients," is filled into glass vials, and the vials are loaded onto the temperature-controlled shelves. The shelf temperature is reduced, typically in several stages, to a temperature in the vicinity of $-40°C$, thereby converting nearly all the water into ice. Some excipients, such as buffer salts and mannitol, may partially crystallize during freezing, but most "drugs," particularly proteins, remain amorphous. The drug and excipients are typically converted into an amorphous glass also containing large amounts of unfrozen water (15–30%) dissolved in the solid (i.e., glassy) amorphous phase. Thus, most of the desiccation actually occurs during the freezing stage of the freeze-drying process. After all water and solutes have been converted into solids, the entire system is evacuated by the vacuum pumps to the desired control pressure, the shelf temperature is increased to supply energy for sublimation, and primary drying begins. Due to the large heat flow required during primary drying, the product temperature runs much lower than the shelf temperature.

The removal of ice crystals by sublimation creates an open network of "pores," which allows pathways for escape of water vapor from the product. The ice–vapor boundary (i.e., the boundary between frozen and "dried" regions) generally moves from the top of the product toward the bottom of the vial as primary drying proceeds. Primary drying is normally the longest part of the freeze-drying process. Primary drying times of the order of days are not uncommon, and in rare cases, weeks may be required for a combination of poor formulation and suboptimal process design. Although some secondary drying does occur during primary drying (i.e., desorption of water from the amorphous phase occurs to a limited extent once the ice is removed from that region), the start of secondary drying is normally defined, in an operational sense, as the end of primary drying (i.e., when all ice is removed). Of course, because not all vials behave identically, some vials enter secondary drying whereas other vials are in the last stages of primary drying. When the judgment is made that all vials are devoid of ice, the shelf temperature is typically increased to provide the higher product temperature required for efficient removal of the unfrozen water. The final stages of secondary drying are normally carried out at shelf temperatures in the range of 25–50°C for several hours. Here, because the demand for heat is low, the shelf temperature and the product temperature are nearly identical.

As freeze-drying plants are very expensive and process times are often long, a freeze-dried dosage form is relatively expensive to produce. Indeed, because of both cost and ease of use, a ready-to-use solution is the preferred option for a parenteral dosage form, particularly if the solution can withstand terminal heat sterilization. When an aqueous solution does not have sufficient stability, the product must be produced in solid form. At least for small molecules, stability normally increases in the following order: solution < glassy solid < crystalline solid (1–3); this is likely a result of restricted motion in solids with the high degree of order in the crystalline solid limiting reactivity even further. As many pharmaceuticals cannot be produced on a commercial scale by crystallization, a glassy solid may be the only solid-state option.

Encyclopedia of Pharmaceutical Technology

Freeze drying (4–7) and spray drying (8–10) are drying methodologies in common use in the pharmaceutical industry, and are suitable for the production of glassy solids. Freeze drying is a low-temperature process. In general, a formulation can be dried to 1% water or less, without any of the product exceeding 30°C. Thus, conventional wisdom states that freeze-drying is less likely to cause thermal degradation than a high-temperature process such as spray drying. Historically, freeze-drying is the method of choice for products intended for parenteral administration. Sterility and relative freedom from particulates are critical quality attributes for parenterals. Largely because the solution is sterile filtered immediately before filling into the final container, and further processing is relatively free of exposure to humans, a freeze-drying process maintains sterility and particle-free characteristics of the product much more easily than do processes that must deal with dry powder handling issues, such as dry powder filling of a spray-dried or bulk-crystallized powder. Indeed, with modern robotics automatic loading systems (11), humans can be removed from the sterile processing area entirely, at least in principle. Furthermore, as the vials are sealed in the freeze dryer, moisture control and control of headspace gas can easily be controlled, an important advantage for products whose storage stability is adversely affected by residual moisture and/or oxygen. As the critical heat and mass transfer characteristics for freeze-drying are nearly the same at the laboratory scale as in full production, resolution of scale-up problems tends to be easier for a freeze-drying process than for spray drying, at least in our experience. Also, development of a freeze-dried product requires less material for formulation and process development, a particularly important factor early in a project.

While freeze-drying has a long history in the pharmaceutical industry as a technique for stabilization of labile drugs, including proteins, many proteins suffer irreversible change, or degradation, during the freeze-drying process (12–16). Even when the labile drug survives the freeze-drying process without degradation, the resulting product is rarely found perfectly stable during long-term storage, particularly when analytical techniques with a sensitivity to detect low levels of degradation ($\approx 0.1\%$) are employed. Both small molecules (1–3, 17) and proteins (18–21) show degradation during storage of the freeze-dried glass. In some cases, instability is serious enough to require refrigerated storage (18, 19, 22).

Stability problems are most often addressed by a combination of formulation optimization and attention to process control. Lyoprotectants are added for stability during the freeze-drying process as well as to provide storage stability, and the level and type of buffer is optimized. Optimization of the freezing process may be critical; control of product temperature during drying is critical for products that tend to suffer cake collapse during primary drying, and control of residual moisture is nearly always critical for storage stability. Formulation and process are interrelated: A bad formulation can be nearly impossible to freeze dry, and even with a well designed formulation, a poorly designed process may require more than a week to produce material of suboptimal quality. Although blind empiricism may, in time, yield an acceptable formulation and process, an appreciation for the materials science of amorphous systems and some understanding of heat and mass transfer relevant to freeze-drying are needed for efficient development of freeze-dried products. Obviously, one also requires at least a phenomenological understanding of the major degradation pathways specific to the drug under consideration.

The objective of this article is to present the scientific and engineering fundamentals most useful in the development of formulations and processes for the manufacture of freeze-dried pharmaceuticals. Generalizations are illustrated with specific examples from the literature, but no attempt is made to survey all published works. Most of the section on the freeze-drying process applies equally well to small molecules and proteins, whereas most of the section on formulation and stability is specific to proteins.

THE FREEZE-DRYING PROCESS

Freezing

Freeze concentration

The objective of freezing is to remove most of the water from the system by formation of ice and to convert all solutes into solids, either crystalline solids or a glass. Once the sample is a solid, primary drying may begin. As a sample is cooled, the system remains liquid well below the equilibrium freezing point, but with sufficient supercooling, nucleation of ice proceeds rapidly and growth of ice crystals begins. As liquid water converts to ice, all solutes are concentrated in the regions between ice crystals, ultimately concentrating until they crystallize or until the system increases in viscosity sufficiently to transform into a solid amorphous system, or glass. The example shown in Fig. 1 is representative of a solute that does not crystallize during freeze-drying. The system supercools about 10°C to a temperature of −15°C before ice nucleation becomes rapid enough to generate crystals

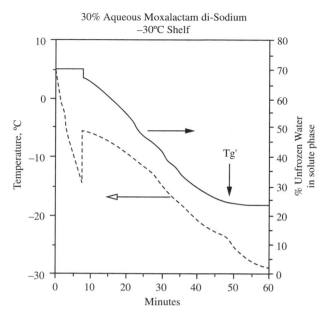

Fig. 1 Freeze concentration in an amorphous system. The product temperature is shown as a broken line whereas the percentage of unfrozen water is shown as a solid line. (From Ref. 6.)

of ice. The evolution of heat caused by the sudden crystallization of ice increases the sample temperature to roughly the equilibrium freezing point (−5°C). The sudden ice crystallization also results in a small but sharp decrease in the percentage of water in the solute phase (given on the right vertical axis). After the initial ice nucleation and crystallization at 10 min, the product cools with continuous conversion of water to ice, thereby decreasing the amount of water in the solute phase and increasing the concentration of solute in the remaining solution. When the product temperature reaches about −24°C, denoted as T_g', the concentration of water in the solute phase has been reduced to about 24%, and further reduction in water concentration is curtailed on the time scale of freezing, even though the sample temperature decreases further to about −30°C at the end of the freezing process at 60 min. Here, the solute phase has been concentrated from about 30% solute to about 76% solute, and most of the water has been separated from the solute phase as ice. Had the initial concentration been much lower, say 1%, the final concentration would still be 76%, although the freezing profile would differ quantitatively from that shown in Fig. 1. Clearly, most of the desiccation in a freeze-drying process occurs during the freezing process. While desiccation is indeed the objective, it must be recognized that concentration of all solutes during freezing will dramatically increase the probability of

bimolecular collisions, which could produce unexpected instability in the partly frozen system. If a system, initially at 1% solute, is susceptible to a second-order degradation reaction with an activation energy of 25 kcal/mol, a reduction in temperature from 5°C to −24°C would reduce the rate constant by a factor of 200, but an increase in concentration from 1% to 76% would increase the concentration factor in the rate equation by a factor of 5800, yielding a factor of 29 net increase in reaction rate. Although this example is an oversimplification, it is significant to note that increases in second-order degradation rates have been observed in model systems during freeze concentration (23).

T_g' is the temperature at which a sharp increase in baseline occurs during a differential scanning calorimeter (DSC) scan of a frozen solution, suggesting a sharp increase in heat capacity, and has been referred to as the glass transition temperature of the maximally concentrated freeze concentrate (24). A sharp decrease in electrical resistance of the frozen system is noted at the same temperature (25). Structural collapse of a cake structure in the dried region, indicating viscous flow, occurs during primary drying at the collapse temperature, denoted by $T_{c'}$, which is only slightly higher than T_g' (25). It is clear that T_g' corresponds to the temperature at which mobility in the system is manifested on an experimental timescale. Effectively, the system behaves as a solid below T_g'.

Various electrolytes, such as buffer salts and NaCl, if present in the formulation, will also concentrate during the freezing process. Such exposure to high concentrations of electrolytes (i.e., about 6 molal NaCl during freezing a 0.15 M NaCl solution) might contribute to the destabilization of the native conformation, thereby leading to degradation during freezing.

Crystallization of excipients and consequences

In the case of protein drugs, the drug does not crystallize, but other solute components may (or may not) crystallize, depending on their nature and concentration, other formulation components, and the details of the freezing process. High initial concentrations and slow freezing tend to favor crystallization. Depending on the intended role of the excipient, crystallization may be desirable or undesirable, and it may be important just when in the process crystallization does occur. For example, if mannitol is intended only as a bulking agent, and is not expected to play a role in stabilization of the drug, crystallization is desirable as crystalline mannitol can easily be freeze dried at high temperatures to give an elegant product, meaning a short freeze-drying cycle and freedom from product defects such as collapse. Here, the drug form is that of an amorphous coating on the crystalline mannitol, with stability properties normally close to that of a system freeze dried without the mannitol. If mannitol remains amorphous during freezing and crystallizes as the product temperature is increased in early primary drying, extensive vial breakage can occur (26). Conversely, if mannitol is intended to serve as a stabilizer during drying and/or storage, crystallization is undesirable. Complete crystallization yields a system equivalent to a physical mixture of glassy drug particles and crystalline mannitol, with no opportunity for a stabilizing interaction except at the phase boundary between the particles, no dilution of drug molecules, and no separation of "reactants" in the protein phase from the protein molecules. In short, any plausible stabilization mechanism requires that at least some of the mannitol remain molecularly dispersed in the amorphous drug phase. Of course, just as crystalline mannitol has some solubility in any liquid, mannitol will have a nonzero thermodynamic solubility in the drug phase. Thus, even if mannitol crystallization proceeds to thermodynamic equilibrium, a small amount of mannitol will remain in the drug phase. However, most of the stabilization potential of the mannitol will be lost upon crystallization. As mannitol does tend to crystallize nearly completely when present as the major formulation component, mannitol is generally a poor choice as a stabilizer for freeze drying.

Although buffers are included in a formulation to maintain constant pH, selective crystallization of the less soluble buffer component during freezing can result in massive pH shifts in the freeze concentrate. Figure 2 shows the pH changes observed during equilibrium freezing of several pure buffer systems (27). Freezing

was carried out while seeding with ice and crystalline buffer salts, so the data represent near-equilibrium behavior. Over the temperature range studied, the citrate buffer system showed no significant pH shift. The sodium phosphate buffer system shows a dramatic decrease in pH of about 4 pH units due to crystallization of the basic buffer component, $Na_2HPO_4 \cdot 2H_2O$. Conversely, the potassium phosphate system shows only a modest increase in pH of about 0.8 pH unit. Under nonequilibrium conditions (i.e., no seeding) and with lower buffer concentrations, the degree of crystallization is less, and the resulting pH shifts are moderated (28). Table 1 shows data accumulated (29, 30) during freezing of phosphate buffer solutions in large volumes at cooling rates intended to mimic freezing in vials. For the concentrated buffer solutions (100 mM), the frozen pH values are close to the equilibrium values given in Fig. 2. However, lowering the buffer concentration by an order of magnitude considerably reduces the pH shift observed during freezing. It should also be noted that the small pH shift for potassium phosphate buffer noted in Fig. 2 is a result of the starting pH being 7.5. As shown in Table 1, if the initial pH is 5.5, the 100 mM potassium phosphate buffer increases by 3.1 pH units during freezing. In short, the frozen system pH is near 8.7, regardless of whether the initial pH is 7.0 or 5.5. Clearly, if drug stability is sensitive to pH shifts, buffer crystallization must be avoided. In our experience, the best solution is to formulate such that the weight ratio of buffer to other solutes is very low (18, 22). However, the precise meaning of "very low" varies with the nature and amount of the other solutes as well as with the nature of the buffer.

Instability during freezing and T_g'

Most small molecules are stable during the freezing process, even though storage stability may be marginal. Proteins show a wide range of formulation-sensitive instability. Some proteins survive freezing with little or no

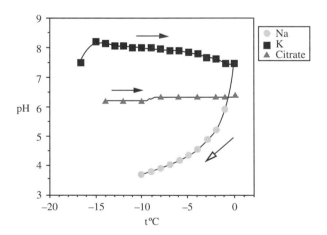

Fig. 2 Shifts in pH during freezing arising from buffer salt crystallization. Near-equilibrium conditions were achieved by seeding with ice and salt. circles: sodium phosphate; squares: potassium phosphate; triangles: citrate. (Data from Ref. 27.)

Table 1 Shifts in pH during nonequilibrium freezing with phosphate buffer systems

Concentration (mM)	Initial pH	Frozen pH	Δ pH
Sodium phosphate buffer			
100	7.5	4.1	−3.4
8	7.5	5.1	−2.4
Potassium phosphate buffer			
100	7.0	8.7	+1.7
100	5.5	8.6	+3.1
10	5.5	6.6	+1.1

(From Refs. 29 and 30.)

measurable loss in activity, whereas others are irreversibly deactivated by the freezing process (12–21, 31–33). An environment quite different from a dilute aqueous solution is created during freezing. All solute species are dramatically concentrated, ionic strength increases, the pH may shift, and above all, hydrophobic interactions that stabilize the native conformation in water are reduced or eliminated as bulk water is removed from the protein phase. In addition, just as proteins undergo thermal denaturation at elevated temperature, proteins also undergo spontaneous unfolding at very low temperature, called "*cold denaturation*" (34, 35). Estimated cold denaturation temperatures are often below the T_g' of a protein formulation and therefore of questionable relevance to freeze-drying. However, these estimates are based upon thermodynamic parameters measured in dilute aqueous solutions. The impact of perturbations caused by freeze concentration is largely unknown.

Because of these many freezing stresses that may decrease the free energy of denaturation, thermodynamic destabilization of the native conformation during freezing is not surprising. Indeed, it appears surprising that all proteins do not spontaneously unfold and degrade during freezing. However, for a destabilized protein to unfold and engage in subsequent irreversible reactions, the rate of unfolding must be fast relative to the timescale of freezing. Even in dilute aqueous solution at room temperature, protein unfolding may involve time constants of the order of hours (36, 37). In the freeze concentrate approaching T_g', at temperatures $\approx 30°C$ lower than room temperature and viscosities about 10 orders of magnitude greater than in a dilute aqueous solution, one would expect greatly reduced unfolding rates, perhaps sufficiently reduced to prevent degradation during freezing. Kinetic studies of unfolding near T_g' would resolve this question. Unfortunately, such data are not available. However, it has been argued on theoretical grounds that rate processes, in general, should be slowed greatly as the system temperature approaches a glass transition temperature (33). Experimental studies of three different reactions in frozen maltodextrin systems lend support to this view, although not all reactions show the same strong temperature dependence near a glass transition (38). As a general rule, it would seem prudent to minimize the time a protein spends in a freeze concentrate above T_g' (i.e., minimize freezing time), and primary drying should be carried out near or below T_g'. However, these precautions do not always guarantee stability.

Optimum freezing rate

Frequently, the freezing process is characterized by specification of freezing rate, where in most cases it is really the temperature change of the heat sink that is specified, or at best, the cooling rate of the solution is given. However, there are at least two freezing parameters that are needed to define the freezing process—the degree of supercooling and the rate of ice crystallization. The degree of supercooling is the difference between the equilibrium freezing point and the temperature at which ice crystals first form in the sample. The degree of supercooling determines the number of nuclei and, therefore, determines the number of ice crystals formed in the sample. A high degree of supercooling produces a large number of ice crystals, and as the total amount of water that freezes is fixed, the ice crystals produced after completion of freezing are small in size. Size of ice crystals impacts on process design and may also affect product quality, as will be discussed later. The rate of ice crystal growth determines the residence time of the product in a freeze-concentrated fluid state. A rapid growth rate minimizes the residence time, normally allowing less degradation during the freezing process. In practical freeze-drying applications, heat transfer limits the rate of ice growth. Therefore, in vials and pans where heat removal is through the container bottom, rapid ice growth is facilitated by a small fill volume to container area ratio (i.e., small fill depth) and good contact between the container bottom and the freeze dryer shelf. In general, rapid ice growth is also promoted by a low shelf temperature. However, if a warm vial with a large fill depth is placed directly on a very cold shelf, a very high degree of supercooling may be produced near the vial bottom before convective mixing cools the upper portion of the solution. Ice then forms near the vial bottom whereas the remainder of the solution remains completely liquid. Freezing then continues slowly from bottom to top as a freezing front. Such a freezing pattern normally produces a dried cake with two distinct structures: a region of very fine pores near the bottom, with most of the cake having very large pores due to the very large ice crystals that formed during advance of the freezing front. The product may be perceived as "lacking in elegance." At the least, a process designed to produce a fast freeze gives instead a slow freeze.

A high degree of supercooling produces small ice crystals and small pore size in the dried layer, which results in a high resistance to water vapor transport during primary drying (39). Consequently, long primary drying times result. Small ice crystals also mean a high specific surface area in the dried product, which decreases secondary drying time (40). These trends suggest that a moderate degree of supercooling is optimal. While the size of ice crystals would not normally be expected to impact on product quality, it is clear that if a protein were to denature at the aqueous ice interface, small ice crystals would mean a large interfacial area and more denaturation, perhaps leading to increased aggregation during freezing. There is now clear evidence that, at least in some cases, proteins may indeed denature at the aqueous–ice interface (41, 42).

In general, the optimum freezing process produces moderate and uniform supercooling and fast ice growth. Uniformity within a given vial avoids heterogeneous cake structure, and uniformity between vials minimizes variation in drying rates and sample temperatures. The combination of moderate supercooling and fast ice growth is difficult to achieve as, in usual practice, the cooling rate of the heat sink (i.e., the shelf) is the only controllable factor in freezing. A general procedure that normally gives satisfactory results may be summarized as follows. First, the product load is cooled to a temperature below the equilibrium freezing point but above the temperature where experience has demonstrated that ice nucleation does not occur (i.e., typically $\approx -5°C$), and the load is equilibrated at this temperature for a short time (i.e., 15–30 min). Next, the shelf temperature is decreased quickly toward the final temperature (i.e., to $-40°C$ at $\approx 1°C/min$). At least with a small fill depth (≈ 1 cm), ice nucleation usually occurs uniformly with moderate supercooling, yet ice growth proceeds relatively rapidly. When product temperature is monitored with temperature sensors in selected vials, the time at which all measured product temperatures are below a given temperature (i.e., time when the product is several degrees above the final shelf temperature) is recorded. Since vials containing temperature sensors often freeze sooner than the batch as a whole (43), the product load is allowed to soak for a fixed time (about an hour) to allow all vials to "catch up" and reach the desired temperature at which all product is in the solid state.

Primary Drying

Mass transfer resistance, product temperature, and drying rate

The effect of product temperature and mass transfer resistance on sublimation rate may be mathematically illustrated (39, 44) by expressing the sublimation rate per vial, dm/dt, in terms of the driving force for transport of water vapor from the ice–vapor interface to the chamber, $P_0 - P_c$,

$$\frac{dm}{dt} = \frac{P_0 - P_c}{R_p + R_s} \tag{1}$$

where P_0 is the equilibrium vapor pressure of ice at the temperature of the frozen product, P_c is the pressure in

the drying chamber, R_p is the resistance of the dried product layer, and R_s is the stopper resistance. As P_0 increases exponentially with temperature, it is obvious that the driving force for sublimation, and, therefore, also the sublimation rate, increases dramatically as the product temperature increases (about a factor of two per 5°C increase in temperature). The decrease in primary drying time with increasing product temperature is illustrated by Fig. 3. These data represent calculations based upon integration of Eq. 1 for a hypothetical (but typical) product at both a small (0.5 cm) and large (2.0 cm) fill depths. The value of chamber pressure used varies due to an attempt to maintain the condition $P_0 \gg P_c$, but yet employ chamber pressures near the optimum range for uniform heat transfer (≈ 0.1–0.2 Torr) when possible (44). At the lowest product temperatures, the chamber pressures selected are well below the optimum for uniform heat transfer, but much higher pressures would give very long drying times. At each temperature, drying time is roughly proportional to the square of the fill depth, and target temperatures below $-40°C$ become impractical for 2-cm fill depths.

It should be noted that Eq. 1 assumes that the gas in the vial is essentially 100% water vapor. Both theoretical and experimental evidence indicate that, during most primary drying conditions of practical interest, the gas in the vial and the gas in the drying chamber is nearly all water vapor, even when the chamber pressure is being controlled by an inert gas leak (44). The molar flow rate of inert gas (i.e., N_2) leaked into the drying chamber is generally much smaller than the molar flow rate of water

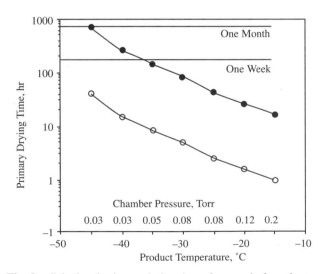

Fig. 3 Calculated primary drying times for a typical product as a function of product temperature. Open circles = 0.5-cm fill depth; filled circles = 2.0-cm fill depth.

vapor during primary drying, so the composition of gas in the drying chamber remains mostly water vapor. The inert gas "overwhelms" the vacuum pumps and, therefore, increases the total pressure in pumping system, which then causes a "back-up" of water vapor into the drying chamber.

Clearly, fast freeze-drying demands both high target product temperature and a small fill depth, which unfortunately is not always possible. To maintain product elegance, and in some cases to minimize degradation, primary drying must be carried out at product temperatures below the collapse temperature. As noted earlier, the collapse temperature and T_g' are closely related, with the collapse temperature normally being several degrees higher than T_g'. In practice, recognizing that not all vials freeze dry at exactly the same temperature, the target product temperature is chosen several degrees below the collapse temperature to provide a safety margin. A collapse temperature is a property of all components in the amorphous phase, and consequently the collapse temperature is highly formulation dependent (45, 46).

Although the product temperature is generally the most important factor in determining the rate of primary drying, product resistance is also an important parameter. The dried product resistance, R_p depends on the cross-sectional area of the product, A_p, by the relation $R_p = \hat{R}_p/A_p$, where $\hat{R}_p$ is the area normalized product resistance, which is independent of the sample area but depends on both the nature of the product and the thickness of the dried product. Thus, R_p depends on the container used in that A_p is fixed by the internal diameter of the vial. The units used for $\hat{R}_p$ (39, 44) are cm^2 Torr hr g^{-1}. With this choice of units, the numerical value of $\hat{R}_p$ represents the approximate time (in hours) to freeze dry a 1 cm thick sample at a temperature of $-20°C$, if the resistance would remain constant over the duration of primary drying. As one might expect, the resistance increases as the dry-layer increases in thickness, and therefore, resistance increases as primary drying proceeds. However, the relationship between resistance and thickness is not usually a direct proportion, although the resistance is often roughly linear in dry-layer thickness (39, 44).

Variation of product resistance with concentration is illustrated by the data in Fig. 4, where values of the mean product resistance, $\langle\hat{R}_p\rangle$, are given for various product types at different total solute concentrations. The mean product resistance is the mean resistance over a dry layer thickness interval of $0-1$ cm. The scatter reflects formulation-specific effects whereas the general trend with increasing concentration illustrates the tendency of higher concentrations to produce higher resistance and therefore, longer drying times. A typical value for the

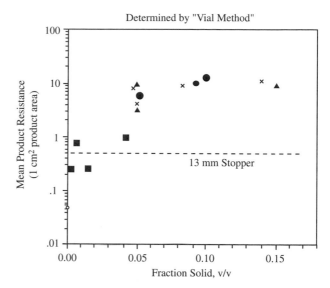

Fig. 4 Mean dry product resistance values for various products. Squares = proteins; filled circles = peptides; triangles = carbohydrates; open circle = pure ice; crosses (x) = miscellaneous types. (M.J. Pikal, Eli Lilly & Co., unpublished results.)

resistance of a small 13-mm finish stopper is shown as a straight line. Note that except for very dilute solutions, $R_p \gg R_s$.

Process control: Product temperature measurement

In most commercial freeze-drying processes, chamber pressure, shelf temperature, and time are the only controllable process parameters. Product temperature is not directly controlled. It is the balance between heat and mass transfer that determines the product temperature (47). Obviously, shelf temperature is important in determining the heat transfer and product temperature. However, because much of the heat is transferred through the gas phase (i.e., collisions of gas molecules with the hot shelf surface and the cold vial bottom), heat transfer as well as mass transfer (Eq. 1) is determined, in part, by the chamber pressure. Therefore, product temperature is determined by shelf temperature, chamber pressure, the heat-transfer characteristics of the vials, and the mass-transfer characteristics of the product and semistoppered vials.

Conventionally, product temperature is monitored in a small number of vials by placing temperature sensors at the bottom center of the vials. It is assumed that at least the average of the measured temperatures is representative of the rest of the vials. The trend in product temperature with time is often used to determine the end of primary drying. That is, when the measured product temperature shows a sharp increase near the anticipated end of primary drying, and begins to approach the shelf temperature, it is assumed that all ice in that vial has been removed. Generally, for that vial, this assumption is correct. When all vials containing temperature sensors are judged dry by this criterion, one might be tempted to assume that all vials in the batch are dry. This assumption is not generally correct. Vials containing temperature sensors are not representative of the batch as a whole. There exists a temperature and drying rate bias between the monitored vials and the rest of the batch. Monitored vials usually freeze sooner with less supercooling than does the batch as a whole (43). This effect is particularly significant in production where due to the particle-free environment, the introduction of a temperature sensor introduces a significantly higher level of heterogeneous nucleation sites, thereby causing nucleation of ice at a lower temperature than in vials without temperature sensors. Observations made during a production run on moxalactam are illustrated in Fig. 5 (43). Monitored vials supercool to around $-15°C$ and then begin freezing. The vials not monitored do not begin freezing until much later, at which time the product temperature must be close to the shelf temperature of $-25°C$. Thus, nonmonitored vials undergo a much greater degree of supercooling, have smaller ice crystals, smaller pores, more resistance to mass transfer, freeze dry at higher temperature, and require more time to dry than the rest of the vials. The temperature bias during primary drying is usually small, $\approx 1°C$, but the drying time bias is 10% of the primary drying time, which can be quite significant for long primary drying times (43). To compensate for this bias in drying time, a soak period of 10–15% of the primary drying time is imposed following the time when all monitored vials are judged dry. Only after this soak period is the shelf temperature increased for

secondary drying. Premature increase of the shelf temperature carries a high risk of collapse. Thus, although monitoring the temperature of the product in vials does provide some information on the progress of primary drying, the information provided is far from perfect!

Location of the monitored vials in the vial array on the shelf is also an important factor in recording representative data. Vials on the edge of an array (i.e., facing the dryer door or walls) normally are not representative of the vials in the interior of an array, which are surrounded by other vials (44). Due to differences in radiative heat transfer, such vials normally dry faster at a higher temperature. With a shelf temperature around 5°C, temperature bias is about 1°C, with drying time bias about 10% (44), and the effect increases in magnitude as the difference between shelf temperature and ambient temperature increases and chamber pressure decreases. However, to minimize the risk of loss of sterility in surrounding vials, the temperature sensors are frequently placed in vials on the edge of the vial array facing the door. Again, the monitored vials are not representative of the batch as a whole. Clearly, minimizing the risk of product contamination with microorganisms is extremely important. From a sterility assurance viewpoint, the ultimate low-risk process is achieved with fully automatic loading systems, which, in principle, can eliminate the need for human presence in the sterile block except in emergency situations. However, it is difficult—perhaps impossible—to place temperature sensors in product vials when using an automatic loading system. Given the problems noted above with the routine use of product temperature sensors, it would seem reasonable to employ product temperature sensors only in development and validation, where vials near the center of an array could be monitored. With a robust process and suitable validation data, it may be assumed that production batches would run with the same product temperature history as the development and validation batches. Thus, product temperature would not be monitored during routine manufacturing. The simplest process design involves using a fixed shelf temperature:chamber pressure:time program.

Designing an *efficient* and *robust* process based upon a fixed shelf temperature:chamber pressure:time program is not a difficult assignment when the primary drying time is short. For example, if the primary drying time of an average batch is 6 h, designing for worst case of perhaps twice the primary drying time of an average batch would extend the average process time by only 6 h; however, if the primary drying time of an average batch is 4 days, designing for worst case will result in a significant reduction of production capacity. By using methodology

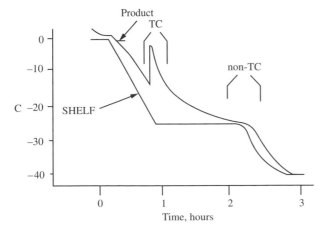

Fig. 5 Experimental observation of freezing bias: A production run of moxalactam di-sodium. (From Ref. 42.)

F

for remote sensing of the end point of primary drying (43), which will be discussed later, this process inefficiency can be virtually eliminated. Moreover, it is both possible and practical to monitor product temperature without placing temperature sensors in the product vials (48). This methodology, called manometric temperature measurement, is based on an analysis of the rate of pressure increase in the chamber when the valve separating the drying chamber from the condenser chamber is periodically quickly closed (and the pressure control system is deactivated) for a brief period of time (≈15 s). When the drying chamber is thus isolated from the condenser chamber, the chamber pressure increases due to four effects (Fig. 6): 1) sublimation at the ice–vapor interface at constant product temperature and transfer of water vapor through the dried cake; 2) dissipation of the temperature gradient in the frozen layer, thereby increasing the temperature at the ice-vapor interface; 3) heat flow from the shelf to the product, thereby increasing the temperature at the ice–vapor interface; and 4) natural air leaks from the surroundings into the chamber. The pressure rise data is fitted to a theoretical function to obtain the average product temperature at the ice–vapor interface. Effects 3 and 4 above both produce a linear increase in pressure with time whereas the other two effects are nonlinear. Effect 1 is dominant (Fig. 6), but a consideration of the other effects is necessary to obtain accurate product temperatures (48). Manometric temperature measurement gives

the temperature at the ice–vapor interface, which is the temperature relevant to collapse, and most important, gives a representative temperature of the product vials without risk of sterility compromise. The freeze dryer, however, must be computer-controlled so that product temperature data can be obtained in real time via mathematical analysis of the pressure rise data. Manometric temperature measurement can also be used to sense the endpoint of primary drying as well as providing accurate dried layer resistance data (48).

Process control and chamber pressure

Pressure control may be accomplished by one of three methods: controlled nitrogen leak, conductance control, or condenser temperature control. Pressure control by "controlled nitrogen leak" is accomplished by opening/closing a needle valve connected to a nitrogen source at atmospheric pressure in response to the deviation of the measured chamber pressure from the set point. Very fine pressure control, within ±5 mTorr, can easily be achieved. Typically, sterile nitrogen is leaked into the drying chamber, but equally fine pressure control is achieved by leaking nitrogen into the vacuum line near the vacuum pumps. Although, to my knowledge, no relevant data exists, current dogma suggests that leaking into the drying chamber is preferred because the risk of sterility compromise is less. Conductance control is based upon modulating the resistance of the chamber to condenser pathway by partially closing/opening the valve separating the drying chamber from the condenser chamber (49). One disadvantage of this technique is the inability to control pressure during secondary drying. Once evolution of water vapor slows to very low rates (during secondary drying), the chamber pressure will reduce to whatever ultimate vacuum the system will produce that day. Although control of chamber pressure to regulate heat input is only necessary in primary drying, one could argue that a process that does not control pressure throughout the process is not fully reproducible. In general, this argument is without scientific foundation, but there are special circumstances where product contamination by adsorption of volatile stopper impurities (or other foreign vapors in the freeze dryer) may occur, and such contamination is more serious at very low chamber pressures (50). Here, one would want to control chamber pressure in secondary drying at a somewhat elevated level (≈200 mTorr). Chamber pressure can also be controlled by control of condenser temperature, provided the freeze dryer design provides for fine control of condenser temperature (49). Control of condenser temperature controls the vapor pressure of ice on the condenser, thereby controlling the partial pressure of water in the drying chamber. Due to

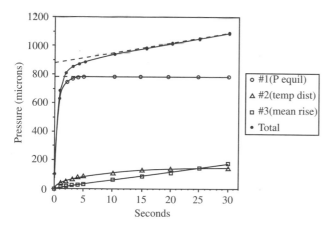

Fig. 6 Calculated contributions to the pressure rise in a manometric temperature measurement experiment. Calculations were made for a typical product with an initial ice temperature of −20°C, corresponding to an initial vapor pressure of 775 mTorr. Open circles = effect 1, sublimation; open triangles = effect 2, dissipation of temperature gradient; open squares = effect 3, heat flow from shelf to product; filled circles = sum of all effects. (Adapted from Ref. 48.)

natural air leaks and the finite pressure difference between condenser and chamber required for mass transfer, the controlled chamber pressure will be somewhat higher than the vapor pressure of ice on the condenser, perhaps 20–50 mTorr higher. Thus, to control chamber pressure at 200 mTorr, the condenser temperature would be controlled at a temperature around −35°C. With this mode of pressure control, the vapor in the drying chamber remains essentially 100% water vapor throughout the process, including secondary drying. Conversely, with pressure control by a nitrogen leak, the vapor changes from essentially 100% water vapor in primary drying to mostly nitrogen during secondary drying (Fig. 7). Thus, a process run with a nitrogen leak to provide pressure control is not necessarily the same as the corresponding process run with pressure control via control of condenser temperature. In general, the difference is not expected to be of practical significance. With a final product temperature of 25°C or greater in secondary drying, a chamber pressure of 200 mTorr pure water vapor produces a relative humidity of less than 0.8%, which is not high enough to impede secondary drying of most materials. However, chamber pressure control via condenser temperature control will not produce the change in gas composition noted in Fig. 7,

as the system passes from primary drying to secondary drying, which does limit the process control options for determining the end point of primary drying.

Process control: Effect of condenser performance

Depending upon dryer design and operating conditions, the condenser temperature may vary over a wide range. As long as the condenser temperature remains sufficiently low to allow control of the chamber pressure at the desired set point, the temperature of the condenser has no impact on the freeze-drying process (i.e., no change in any of the variables in Eq. 1). For example, if the chamber pressure is being controlled (via a nitrogen leak) at the target pressure of 0.10 Torr with a condenser temperature of −50°C, reduction of the condenser temperature to −70°C will have no effect on the process. Here, the reduced partial pressure of water at the condenser will be compensated by an increased partial pressure of nitrogen arising from an (automatic) increase in nitrogen leak rate. Although a detailed analysis of condenser performance is complex (49) and beyond the scope of this chapter, it should be noted that under conditions of very high sublimation rate, the condenser system may be overloaded, resulting in loss of pressure control (i.e., the chamber pressure increases beyond control). Unless the shelf temperature is sharply decreased, a "run-away" condition may develop with loss of product temperature control and ultimately, loss of the batch due to product collapse or ice melt. An overloaded condenser may reflect uneven ice build-up at the condenser plates caused by suboptimal design or operation, but may also arise from operation beyond the design capability of the refrigeration system (49). That is, the refrigeration system may not be able to remove heat from rapidly condensing water vapor (i.e., from very high sublimation rate) and yet maintain the condenser plate temperature low.

Process control: Determination of the end point of primary drying

Typically the shelf temperature setting used in primary drying is much lower than the shelf temperature required for efficient removal of residual water during secondary drying. Because an increase in shelf temperature before all vials have completed primary drying carries a high risk of product collapse, some indicator of the end of primary drying is needed for optimum process control. Of course, one can increase the temperature for secondary drying at a fixed time, but as discussed earlier, such a process is not an optimum one (i.e., the process is normally longer than necessary). Product temperature response is the most common indicator of the end of primary drying. Here, the time is noted when all product temperature sensors

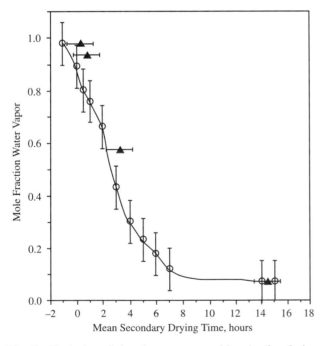

Fig. 7 Typical variation in gas composition in the drying chamber during secondary drying. Open circles: experimental values determined in a laboratory freeze dryer; filled triangles: theoretical values calculated from mass transfer theory and freeze dryer characteristics. (M.J. Pikal, Eli Lilly & Co., unpublished results.)

approach the shelf temperature being used in primary drying. Next, a delay time or soak period is introduced to compensate for the fact that the vials containing temperature sensors are not typical of the batch as a whole. After this delay time, the shelf temperature is increased from the primary drying setting to the setting used for secondary drying. As determination of the appropriate delay time is difficult, the delay times used are often quite arbitrary. The principle problem is that freezing bias normally differs considerably between development and manufacturing. Thus, the optimum delay time for manufacturing cannot be determined in most development laboratories. It is obvious that use of product temperature sensors to determine the end point of primary drying is not entirely satisfactory. As suggested earlier, manometric temperature measurement may be used to determine the end point of primary drying. A far simpler method is to base the determination of the end point upon a real time measurement of the vapor composition in the freeze dryer chamber. As primary drying ends, and the process passes into secondary drying, the composition of the vapor in the drying chamber shifts from nearly pure water vapor to nearly pure nitrogen (Fig. 7), assuming chamber pressure is being controlled via a nitrogen gas leak. A sensitive and inexpensive measurement of vapor composition is provided by an electronic moisture sensor with output in dew point or partial pressure of water (43, 51). An electronic moisture sensor has the sensitivity to determine presence of residual ice in less than 1% of the vials (43), and under some conditions can also be employed to determine the end point of secondary drying—i.e., when the residual moisture has been reduced to below the target levels (51).

Secondary Drying: Desorption of Water from the Freeze Concentrate

Product temperature control and glass transitions

The concept that one must maintain the product temperature below the collapse temperature during primary drying is now well accepted. Exceeding the collapse temperature will cause loss of product elegance, which will vary from moderate deformation and shrinkage to a complete melt and deposition along the walls and bottom of the vial. Structural collapse also may occur during secondary drying or during storage of the dried product, particularly if the dried product contains high levels of residual moisture, and the storage temperature is high. If the product temperature exceeds its glass transition temperature, cake shrinkage and deformation will occur. Such an event is a less common problem during secondary

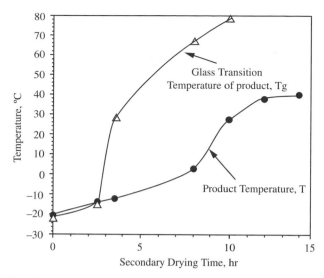

Fig. 8 Variation of glass transition temperature and product temperature for moxalactam di-sodium during secondary drying. (Calculated from data in Refs. 25 and 40.)

drying than is collapse during primary drying, largely because most secondary drying processes are extremely conservative during the early stage where a glass transition is most likely. As the water content of the amorphous phase decreases during drying, the glass transition temperature increases very sharply. Some representative data are shown in Fig. 8. If the shelf temperature remains at the setting used in primary drying for the first few hours of secondary drying, as is common practice, the glass transition temperature will nearly always rise much faster than will the product temperature. However, if one were to optimize secondary drying, and therefore, eliminate most of the dead time in early secondary drying, the potential for a glass transition would increase dramatically. Here, a knowledge of the glass transition temperature as a function of water content would be required for process optimization.

Optimum residual moisture

The optimum residual moisture for a given product must be established by empirical studies. Certainly, to eliminate the possibility of a structural collapse during storage, the water content needs to be low enough so that the glass-transition temperature is well above the highest temperature relevant to product distribution and storage. Moreover, in our experience with both small molecules and proteins, in-process degradation is generally relatively insensitive to the final moisture content, and storage stability normally improves as residual moisture decreases, although the relationship between stability and residual water is not

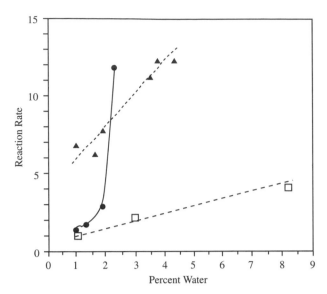

Fig. 9 The effect of residual water on the stability of freeze-dried proteins. Circles = human growth hormone deamidation and oxidation at 25°C, %/month (From Ref. 19); squares = aggregation of human serum albumin at 50°C, %/day (Ref. 52); triangles = hemoglobin oxidation at 23°C in a sucrose formulation, %/year (Ref. 53).

necessarily linear. Data for human growth hormone (hGH) formulated with glycine and mannitol (19), human serum albumin (52), and hemoglobin formulated with sucrose (53) illustrate the range of behavior normally encountered (Fig. 9). The rate of chemical degradation of hGH at 25°C (methionine oxidation and asparagine deamidation) increases in highly nonlinear fashion by nearly an order of magnitude as the moisture content varies from 1% to 2.5% (19); the rate of aggregation of human serum albumin increases linearly with increasing moisture content (52); and the rate of hemoglobin oxidation at room temperature doubles as the residual water content increases from 1% to 4% (53). Although the optimum moisture content for storage stability may be zero, the gain in stability between about 1% water and zero water content is often not sufficient to justify the additional processing complications in achieving and maintaining extremely low water contents. An exception is storage stability of a monoclonal antibody–vinca alkaloid conjugate formulation where stability is sensitive to very low levels of residual moisture (22).

The decrease in storage stability accompanied by an increase in residual moisture is often interpreted in terms of molecular mobility in the solid. That is, higher water content facilitates the mobility needed to support reactivity of the protein. One interpretation states that above monolayer levels of water, the protein has increased

conformational flexibility, and the additional water has the ability to mobilize water and other potential reactants in the amorphous protein phase (54). Both effects are expected to increase the rate of protein degradation. Alternatively, water plasticizes the amorphous phase, thereby lowering the glass transition temperature, T_g. Indeed, if sufficient water is present to lower T_g below the storage temperature, the amorphous phase would be in a fluid state, with greater mobility and greater reactivity than when stored below T_g in a glassy solid state. A system stored above its T_g would also suffer cake collapse and loss of pharmaceutical elegance. Although the monolayer and the glass transition interpretations are similar in that they both attribute the increased reactivity to water induced mobility in the amorphous phase, they differ in that a system above the monolayer level of water is not necessarily above the glass-transition temperature. Furthermore, as the level of water equivalent to monolayer coverage is essentially independent of temperature, the monolayer concept predicts that the trend in stability with water content is independent of temperature. For example, if monolayer coverage is equivalent to 10% water, protein reactivity would increase sharply above 10% water at all temperatures. Conversely, the glass transition interpretation states that the key stability variable is the difference between the glass transition temperature and the storage temperature, $T - T_g$. Here, reactivity increases sharply when $T > T_g$, so the sudden onset of reactivity depends on both T and the water content through the effect of water content on T_g.

Although most empirical and theoretical evidence suggest that storage stability improves monotonically as the water content decreases, we must also acknowledge the common assumption that there is a critical nonzero level of water that a protein requires for conformational stability in the freeze-dried solid, and therefore, some intermediate level of residual water would be optimum for stability. Although direct experimental evidence for this assumption is meager, some systems do have inferior stability when highly desiccated. Influenza virus is clearly less stable when the residual moisture deviates from the optimum 1.7% (55), but the direct relevance of this observation to protein formulations is uncertain. Aggregation of excipient-free tissue plasminogen activator at high temperature is faster at low water content (56), and aggregation of excipient-free hGH during storage at 25°C is faster in samples that, at some time in their history, have been highly desiccated (19).

Factors impacting drying rate

Water removal during secondary drying involves diffusion of water in the glassy solid, evaporation at the solid–vapor

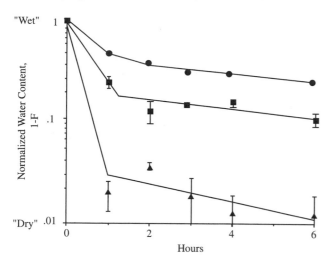

Fig. 10 Examples of the kinetics of secondary drying. Triangles = mannitol (crystalline); squares = poly (vinylpyrrolidone); circles = moxalactam di-sodium (amorphous). All solids were prepared by freeze-drying a 5% aqueous solution from a 1-cm fill depth, followed by hydration to a uniform moisture level of ≈7%. The quantity, F, is the fractional attainment of equilibrium, which corresponds to near zero water content. The secondary drying conditions were: product temperature = 18°C; chamber pressure = 200 mTorr. (From Ref. 40.)

boundary, and flow through the pore structure of the dried cake. During the early portion of secondary drying, water content is high, and the drying rate is high in spite of the relatively low temperature of the solid (40). An illustration of secondary drying kinetics under isothermal conditions is given in Fig. 10 (40) for samples initially about 7% water. Mannitol is crystalline whereas povidone and moxalactam are 100% amorphous. Even at the start of the experiment, the glass transition temperatures of povidone and moxalactam are well above the sample temperature of 18°C. Thus, water is being removed from either an essentially crystalline solid (mannitol) or glassy amorphous solids (povidone and moxalactam). The symbol F represents the fractional attainment of equilibrium, which in these experiments is near zero water content. Thus, $1-F$ represents a normalized water content with a value of unity representing no progress in drying. Although the quantitative aspects of drying behavior are obviously specific to the product, in each case, the water content is reduced sharply during the first 1–2 h, followed by a period of much lower drying rate. If the drying rate were directly proportional to the residual water content, drying kinetics would be first order, and the curves in Fig. 10 would be straight lines. A simple diffusion model based upon constant diffusion constant and constant area

for diffusion would also predict linear semilog drying curves (40). Obviously, the curves are not straight lines. The residual water content appears to approach a plateau level, which is specific to the product. For the mannitol data, the plateau level of residual water is very low (≈0.1–0.2%) and probably represents occluded water in the crystalline mannitol. For the amorphous samples, povidone and moxalactam, the plateau levels are quite high, ≈1% for povidone and ≈3% for moxalactam (i.e., a significant fraction of the water appears to be bound). However, calculations based upon equilibrium water desorption isotherms and the measured partial pressures of water in the drying chamber demonstrate that the residual water present at the end of 6 h is far above the equilibrium water content (40). Thus, the residual water is *not* bound in a thermodynamic sense, but rather is kinetically trapped, a result, at least in part, of decreasing effective surface area for desorption of water as the smaller more rapidly drying solid particles are dried (40). For a given product, the plateau level of water decreases as the drying temperature is increased, decreases as the specific surface area of the solid increases, but is relatively insensitive to the thickness of the dried cake (40).

Traditional freeze-drying practice has often used very low chamber pressures during secondary drying, presumably in the belief that the rate of secondary drying would be accelerated by the use of the low pressures. However, it is found (40) that the rate of secondary drying is insensitive to chamber pressure, at least with pressures in the range of 0–0.2 Torr (40). This empirical observation is consistent with the conclusion that the rate-limiting mass transfer process for drying an amorphous solid is either diffusion in the solid or evaporation at the solid–vapor boundary, probably the latter (40). As the use of very low pressures in secondary drying may facilitate contamination of the product by adsorption of impurity gases from the stopper or other sources (50), it is clear that relatively high chamber pressures (≈ 0.1–0.2 Torr) should generally be used for secondary drying. Of course, extremely high chamber pressures (≈1 Torr) should perhaps be avoided. With very high chamber pressures, flow of water vapor through the pore structure would become rate limiting, and the very high pressure would then decrease the rate of drying.

Changes in moisture content during storage

Often one employs a heroic secondary drying process to reduce the residual water content to very low levels only to find that the moisture content increases during storage. Although moisture transfer from ambient through the stopper is possible, the increase in moisture content is most

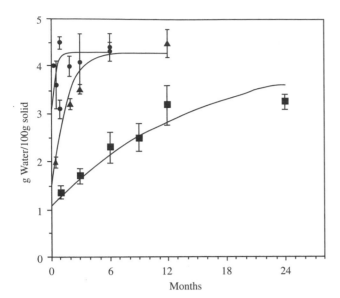

Fig. 11 Kinetics of water transfer from stoppers to 25 mg freeze dried lactose. The stoppers were 13 mm finish West 1816 gray butyl stoppers that were steam sterilized and vacuum dried for 1 hour. Circles = 40°C; triangles = 25°C; squares = 5°C. (From Ref. 57.)

often related to moisture release by the stopper (57). This phenomenon is illustrated in Fig. 11, where the time dependence of moisture content in 25 mg of freeze-dried lactose is given. Here, the stoppers were gray butyl stoppers that had been previously steam sterilized, followed by 1 h of vacuum drying to remove excess water. The symbols represent experimental data for 40°C, 25°C, and 5°C storage, and the smooth curves represent the best fit to a theoretical model (57). It should be noted that at least at 40°C and 25°C storage, the moisture content increases sharply from 1%, but then reaches a plateau value of about 4.3%, suggesting that equilibrium has been reached. That is, at the plateau value of 4.3% water, the activity of the water in the stopper is equal to the activity of water in the lactose and mass transfer ceases. In other studies, we have noted samples deliberately prepared to be initially of high water content have lost water during storage. In short, there is moisture equilibration between moisture in the stopper and moisture in the product that may either increase the moisture content of a dry product or decrease the moisture content of a wet product. The plateau or equilibrium level of water appears to be independent of temperature. The equilibrium values for 40°C storage and 25°C storage are identical, and the moisture content values for 5°C storage appear to be approaching the same equilibrium value of 4.3%. The rate of approach to equilibrium, however, is strongly temperature dependent. The equilibrium level of water is

strongly dependent upon the stopper treatment history. Stoppers vacuum dried for 8 h after steam sterilization allowed only a small increase in moisture content during storage. The equilibrium water content is lower for a higher mass of solid, and is slightly higher for a more hygroscopic product (57).

The moisture exchange between stopper and product may have important stability consequences. Absorption of moisture from the stopper may result in a product which has, after time, a moisture content high enough so that the glass transition temperature is below the storage temperature. Structural collapse will result, and stability of the product may well be compromised. Moreover, because the glass transition temperature often changes dramatically in a narrow range of water content, the onset of instability could be quite sudden. Moisture exchange may be moderated by extensive high temperature vacuum drying of the stoppers after steam sterilization. A better solution is to employ alternate rubber formulations that are less prone to release water to the product. Such stopper formulations are now available from several vendors.

FORMULATION AND STABILITY

Function of Excipients

Most freeze-dried products contain several components in addition to the drug or active component. These additional components, called excipients, are intended to serve a specific function, normally related to stability or process, and may constitute the major fraction of the freeze-dried solid.

With some products, the quantity of drug per vial is extremely small. Here, bulking agents such as mannitol or glycine are used to provide product elegance (i.e., satisfactory appearance) as well as to provide sufficient cake mechanical strength to avoid product blow-out. When a very dilute solution is freeze dried, the flow of water vapor during primary drying may generate sufficient force on the fragile cake to break the cake structure and carry some of the product out of the vial with the water vapor stream. Product blow-out normally occurs only when the solution to be freeze dried is very low in total solids (1% or less). Thus, with low dose drugs, a bulking agent may be a critical formulation component.

Collapse temperature modifiers are excipients that will increase the collapse temperature to allow more efficient freeze-drying without collapse. Such materials may also function as bulking agents and/or stabilizers. Dextran ($T_c = -10°C$), hydroxyethyl starch ($T_c = -10°C$), ficoll ($T_c = -20°C$), gelatin ($T_c = -8°C$) are examples.

Although none of these materials are commonly used in parenteral formulations, dextran and hydroxyethyl starch are used in large quantities as IV therapeutic agents, and therefore, would presumably be acceptable as excipients. Usually, the collapse temperature of a mixture is intermediate between the collapse temperatures of the individual components (58), but collapse temperatures of candidate formulations cannot be predicted with high accuracy.

Macroscopic collapse may often be avoided by use of a crystalline matrix component. Here a readily crystallizable component is added at a relatively high level (i.e., more than 50% of total solids and ideally much more) such that a crystalline matrix is formed. Freeze drying such a formulation amounts to freeze-drying with microscopic or partial collapse (i.e., complete collapse of the amorphous phase), but cake structure is maintained by the crystalline component. Thus, both elegance and good reconstitution time will be maintained, and the samples will normally dry to low residual water with ease. However, if collapse of the amorphous phase containing the protein leads to degradation, this method for circumventing collapse is not viable. Glycine and mannitol are commonly used as crystalline matrix components. This excipient function is, in reality, a special case of the use of a bulking agent.

Particularly with proteins, excipients are often added to prevent degradation, as for example, lyoprotectants, antioxidants, nonionic surfactants, metal ion chelators, and other proteins such as BSA in diagnostic products. In many cases, the stabilizer may also serve as a bulking agent. Glycine, mannitol, sucrose, and lactose are perhaps the most commonly used stabilizers. However, as lactose is a reducing sugar and commonly reacts with proteins, its use must be questioned. Both mannitol and glycine tend to crystallize, and are, therefore, generally poor choices as stabilizers when used alone. Sugars, in particular sucrose, are often effective lyoprotectants, as well as enhancers of storage stability.

Buffers are often added to control pH, but caution must be exercised when buffers are used in a formulation to be freeze dried. As discussed earlier, crystallization of either buffer component (acid or base) during freezing may cause a significant pH shift during freezing, thereby causing greater pH variation than would have been obtained in an unbuffered system.

Products intended for human use are occasionally formulated with NaCl or glycerol to make the reconstituted product isotonic. This practice is normally not a requirement for IV drugs, but can be quite important in minimizing pain on injection of subcutaneous and IM doses. In general, and in particular with proteins, isotonic adjustment is best accomplished by including the tonicity modifier in the diluent rather than in the freeze-dried product. Sodium chloride and glycerol can lower the collapse temperature significantly, and sodium chloride may cause aggregation of the protein during freeze drying.

With multidose products, there is a need for use of a preservative to prevent microbial growth during the period of product use. Mixtures of ethyl- and methyl-parabens are a common choice as are phenol and m-Cresol. As preservatives are used at extremely low levels (i.e., $\leq$0.1% w/w in solution), they normally would not alter the collapse characteristics of the formulation. However, since the preservative is not needed during the freeze-drying process, to keep the formulation for freeze-drying as simple as possible, preservatives are best introduced via the diluent intended for reconstitution.

Surfactants may be added at low levels (i.e., $\approx$0.05% w/w in solution) for several purposes. Surfactants may aid reconstitution if the drug does wet well, and surfactants are often added to low dose products to minimize losses due to surface adsorption. Surfactants may also be effective as stabilizers in low dose protein systems.

Relationships Between Formulation and Process

Particularly for freeze-dried products, formulation and process are interrelated. Properties of the formulation, in particular the collapse temperature, will have a significant impact on the ease of processing. An efficient process is one that runs a high product temperature. However, the temperature cannot be too high or product quality will be compromised. As the glass transition temperature depends on chemical composition of the amorphous phase, T_g' and collapse temperature are strongly formulation dependent. Collapse temperatures for common excipient systems vary from less than $-50°C$ to around $-10°C$ (Table 2).

The collapse temperature depends upon the composition of the amorphous phase, and crystallization of one or more components may significantly alter the collapse temperature. In this way, process variations that induce crystallization may alter the physical state of the formulation. For example, human growth hormone (hGH) formulated with glycine and mannitol in a hGH:glycine:mannitol weight ratio of 1:1:5 may form a completely amorphous system if frozen very quickly. Here, the collapse temperature is $-24°C$. However, a slower freeze allows crystallization of most of the mannitol, resulting in a collapse temperature greater than $-5°C$ (18). Another example is provided by the glycine:sucrose system (64–68) where glycine is present in excess of the sucrose. If frozen quickly, glycine remains

Table 2 Collapse temperature [T_c (°C)] and Glass Transition [T_g' (°C)] data for selected excipients[a]

Material	T_g' (°C)	Reference	T_c (°C)	Reference
Polymers				
BSA	−11	46		
Dextran	−10	46, 59	−10	60, 61
Ficoll	−19	59	−20	45
Gelatin	−9	59	−8	45
PVP (40k)	−20	59	−23	45
Saccharides and polyols				
Dextrose	−44	59		
Hydroxypropyl β-cyclodextrin			−18	60
Lactose	−28	46,59	−31	60, 61
Mannitol	−35, −28	46,59		
Raffinose	−27	62	−26	45
Sorbitol	−46	59	−45	45
Sucrose	−32, −35	46, 63	−34, −32	60, 61
Trehalose	−27, −29	46, 59	−34	60
Amino acids				
β-Alanine	−65	46		
Glycine	(−62)	64		
Histidine	−33	46		
Salts and buffer components				
Acetate, potassium	−76	46		
Acetate, sodium	−64	46		
CaCl$_2$	−95	46		
Citric acid	−54	46		
Citrate, potassium	−62	46		
Citrate, sodium	−41	46		
HEPES	−63	46		
NaHCO$_3$	−52	46		
Phosphate, KH$_2$PO$_4$	−55	46		
Phosphate, K$_2$HPO$_4$	−65	46		
Phosphate, NaH$_2$PO$_4$	−45	46		
Tris base	−51	46		
Tris HCl	−65	46		
Tris acetate	−54	46		
ZnCl$_2$	−88	46		

[a]Collapse temperature data were obtained with freeze-drying microscopy and T_g' data were obtained by DSC at roughly 10°C/min heating rates and represent mid-points of the glass transition region. Molecular weight is given for polymers when the data are sensitive to molecular weight. When significant differences exist between laboratories, both values are given. Values in parenthesis were estimated by extrapolation from noncrystallizing mixtures to the pure compound.

amorphous, and the glycine:sucrose freeze concentrate has a very low collapse temperature (i.e., roughly −45°C, depending upon the exact composition). However, if glycine is allowed to crystallize, the glass-transition temperature is essentially that of a sucrose freeze concentrate (i.e., about −34°C). Further, as the structure is maintained by the crystalline glycine, exceeding T_g' does not result in macroscopic collapse, and the system may be freeze dried without apparent collapse even at temperatures exceeding −15°C. Thus, crystallization can transform a formulation from one that is nearly

impossible to freeze dry in a commercial operation to one where freeze-drying is relatively easy. Clearly, if both glycine and sucrose are included in the formulation, the level of glycine must be either very low or very high relative to sucrose. If the level of glycine in the sucrose phase is very low, glycine will not crystallize but the impact on T_g' will be minimal. If the level of glycine is high, glycine can be induced to crystallize nearly completely (66, 68), thereby minimizing the level of glycine in the amorphous phase and maximizing the T_g' of the formulation.

The glass-transition temperature of a multicomponent amorphous system may be estimated from glass transition temperatures of the individual amorphous components (69). The simplest expression, commonly referred to as the Fox equation, is

$$\frac{1}{T_g} = \frac{w_i}{T_{gi}} + \frac{w_2}{T_{g2}} \qquad (2)$$

where w_i, is the weight fraction of component i and T_{gi} is the glass transition temperature of pure component i. Generalization of Eq. 2 to systems of more than two components is obvious. The effect of a second solute component on a formulation may be roughly calculated from Eq. 1 if T_{gi} in Eq. 2 is identified with T_g' of aqueous component i, and w_i are weight fractions of solute relative to the total mass of solute. Although Eq. 2 does not strictly apply to a freeze concentrate containing two (or more) solute components and water, such calculations from T_g' data are sufficiently accurate to be of practical use. For example, the effect of glycine on T_g' of aqueous sucrose systems (65) is fully consistent with Eq. 2.

Bulking Agents

General considerations

Bulking agents are intended to be inert and simply function as fillers to increase the density of the product cake. Product elegance is improved and product blow-out is prevented, but the bulking agent is not intended to provide enhanced chemical or physical stability of the drug substance. Amorphous excipients can function as bulking agents, but most amorphous excipients have relatively low collapse temperatures and therefore require low drying temperatures and long processing times. For example, although lactose has been used as a bulking agent, the relatively low collapse temperature ($-31°C$) requires long processing times. In addition, lactose is a reducing sugar and will chemically react with amine functionality, and therefore, cannot be used with many drugs. Although not in common use as a freeze-drying excipient, hydroxyethylstarch is an example of an inert amorphous additive with a high collapse temperature and therefore, could function as a bulking agent without requiring long processing times. However, hydroxyethyl-starch tends to undergo some cake shrinkage and cracking during drying and therefore, provides a less elegant product than do the common crystalline bulking agents, glycine and mannitol. Since sorbitol is simply an isomer of mannitol, one might expect sorbitol could serve as a bulking agent. However, sorbitol does not easily crystallize during freeze-drying, and amorphous sorbitol has a

collapse temperature around $-45°C$ (Table 2), thereby preventing its use at high levels in formulations for freeze-drying. Human serum albumin (HSA) or in diagnostic products, bovine serum albumin (BSA), have seen use as bulking agents and/or stabilizers. However, given current concerns regarding excipients isolated from human sources, use of HSA in new pharmaceutical products should be questioned. Mannitol is by far the most commonly used bulking agent. A mannitol-based formulation is elegant, reconstitutes quickly, and except for the potential of vial breakage (26, 70, 71), is generally easy to freeze dry without risk of product defects. Vial breakage is minimized by small fill depths, lower mannitol concentration, slow freezing, and avoiding freezing temperatures less than about $-25°C$ until crystallization is complete. Glycine functions well as a bulking agent. Glycine crystallizes easily to form an elegant product that reconstitutes quickly and does not induce vial breakage. However, a glycine cake is more fragile than a mannitol cake, and is generally perceived as being somewhat less elegant than a mannitol cake.

Polymorphism in crystalline bulking agents

In general, the polymorphism issue of greatest significance in freeze-drying is whether or not a given component is crystalline or amorphous. Which crystalline polymorph forms is usually of secondary importance. However, it should be noted that both mannitol and glycine do exhibit crystalline polymorphism in freeze-dried systems (72–75). The only crystal polymorphism issue of known significance is the formation of a hydrate of mannitol (73, 75). Under some conditions, not fully understood, mannitol forms a hydrate that does not easily desolvate to an anhydrate during secondary drying. Secondary drying at temperatures in excess of $50°C$ appear to be necessary to desolvate the hydrate. Thus, samples of freeze-dried mannitol may have high residual water content if secondary drying temperatures were moderate. If this residual water were to remain bound in the hydrate crystal lattice, the high residual water content would simply be a curiosity. However, during storage, particularly at elevated temperature, the hydrate slowly desolvates, thereby releasing water to the amorphous drug phase. Such a scenario may compromise storage stability, particularly during accelerated stability tests.

Conditions for crystallization of bulking agents

A number of factors are critical for crystallization of the bulking agent. First, the nature of the bulking agent is of obvious importance. Unless the bulking agent will readily crystallize from an aqueous system at ambient temperatures, crystallization during freezing is unlikely. Although both mannitol and glycine do readily crystallize during freezing, there are many other solutes that readily crystallize and are at least potentially acceptable as excipients for parenteral drugs. Mannitol and glycine are simply the most commonly used bulking agents. Crystallization is favored by higher concentrations of crystallizable solute, and perhaps most important, the bulking agent must be the major solute component to obtain reliable crystallization. The presence of high levels of other solutes, particularly those that remain amorphous, will generally impede or prevent crystallization of the bulking agent. As a general formulation rule, one should employ the crystallizable bulking agent at a concentration (weight percent) that is at least a factor of three greater than the sum of the concentrations of all other solute components. In addition, because resistance of the dry layer to flux of water vapor increases as the concentration of total solids increases, thereby prolonging primary drying, one should avoid total solids concentrations much above 100 mg/ml when possible. A rigid adherence to both of these rules would suggest that one would not employ a bulking agent if the drug concentration were much in excess of 25 mg/ml. Indeed, because a bulking agent is normally not needed to avoid product blow-out at drug concentrations above 25 mg/ml, one should question the use of bulking agents in such applications.

Surfactants

Generally, surfactants are employed to reduce surface adsorption losses of low-dose drugs, to improve wetting and reconstitution behavior, and to stabilize proteins during freezing. In nearly all applications, it is a nonionic surfactant that is used, and by far the most commonly used surfactant is polysorbate 80. However, it should be noted that the popularity of polysorbate 80 is due more to its extensive history of use and presumed greater acceptance by regulatory agencies than to its demonstrated superior performance in a given application. In practice, the surfactant level is very low, typically 0.01–0.1% w/v.

Proteins and surface active drugs often adsorb on filters, solution-processing equipment, and container surfaces, thereby producing loss of drug. Such losses are normally only of practical significance if the drug concentration is very low (i.e., when the total amount of drug loss is a significant percentage of the drug in solution). Addition of a low concentration of surfactant will frequently reduce the level of drug adsorption simply because the surfactant is preferentially adsorbed at the surfaces. With proteins, surface-adsorption effects may be considerably more

complex and damaging. Many proteins adsorb at interfaces, particularly the air–water interface, suffer a conformational change, desorb from the interface, and either refold or combine with other conformationally altered molecules, thereby leading to irreversible aggregation.

Human growth hormone aggregates extensively during shaking an aqueous solution, but this aggregation can be nearly eliminated by adding Polysorbate 20 to the formulation (76). It should be noted that although other surfactants (including polysorbate 80) were studied, Polysorbate 20 was the most effective stabilizer. In this study, all surfactant levels studied were above the surfactant critical micelle concentration (CMC), but the rate of aggregation decreases linearly as a function of increasing polysorbate 20:hGH mole ratio until it exceeds 2.0. This linearity provides a clue to the stabilization mechanism. As surfactant adsorption to the air–water interface would be expected to depend on the surfactant monomer concentration, and the monomer concentration is constant above the CMC, a stabilization mechanism involving adsorption of surfactant to the air–water interface would be expected to produce a roughly constant stabilization effect at all surfactant concentrations above the CMC. The data are not consistent with this prediction. However, it is known that polysorbate 20 binds to hGH with a stoichiometry of about 2.5 to 4 (77). Thus, it seems plausible that stabilization during shaking involves binding of surfactant to the surface of the protein (77).

Aggregation of hemoglobin during freeze–thaw is essentially eliminated by addition of polysorbate 80 at concentrations from 0.0125% to 0.1% (78). Without polysorbate 80, particle formation after five freeze–thaw cycles increased by more than an order of magnitude when freezing to $-20°C$ and by about a factor of five when freezing to $-80°C$. However, use of polysorbate 80 reduced particulate generation at both freezing temperatures to a level where particulate levels after freeze–thaw were not significantly different than before freezing. Attempts to demonstrate binding of the surfactant to hemoglobin were unsuccessful, suggesting that the stabilization mechanism does not involve binding to the protein. Rather, it was proposed that stabilization involves surfactant adsorption at the interface, thereby preventing the protein from adsorbing at interfaces.

Although one cannot always expect protein aggregation to be eliminated as effectively by addition of surfactant as demonstrated in the above examples, it is certainly prudent to test the effect of surfactants in situations where protein aggregation is a problem during freeze–thaw or during solution handling.

Stabilizers

Types of stabilizers

A stabilizer is simply a formulation component without physiological effect that is added to the formulation to maintain the physical or chemical stability of the drug substance. As discussed in the previous section, the function of a surfactant may be to stabilize, and as control of pH is often critical to stability, one might consider buffers to be stabilizers. However, in this section we will address stabilizers other than surfactants or buffers. Further, as most of the stabilization literature deals with proteins, our discussion will focus on proteins, although in principle many stabilization principles apply to small molecules as well.

Minimizing oxidation

Although oxidation is a very common degradation pathway in pharmaceutical systems, one might expect that oxidation problems in freeze-dried products would be easily solved by elimination of oxygen from the system during processing; that is, because the product is dried in a vacuum environment and the vials either sealed in vacuum or in an atmosphere of an inert gas (i.e., nitrogen), no oxygen will be present to support an oxidation reaction. Indeed, storage stability of human growth hormone is greatly improved in vials back-filled with nitrogen compared to vials back-filled with oxygen (19). However, significant oxidation was also observed in samples back-filled with nitrogen. In practice, complete elimination of oxygen from the solution being processed is unlikely, and some oxygen may well be trapped in the amorphous solute phase after freezing and not be completely removed during drying. Further, due to a variety of causes including diffusion from the atmosphere over time, oxygen content in the vial headspace may easily reach levels of about 1%. Even 1% oxygen in the vial headspace is sufficient, from a stoichiometric viewpoint, to produce substantial decomposition, particularly with high-molecular-weight drugs. For example, with a 5-mg dose of human growth hormone ($M = 22.5$ kD) in a 5-cc vial, 1% oxygen in the headspace represents a factor of ten excess of the oxygen required for complete oxidation of the protein.

As ground-state molecular oxygen is not particularly reactive, presence of oxygen is not the only requirement for a rapid oxidation reaction. Activation of molecular oxygen to more reactive species requires light (i.e., photoactivation to singlet oxygen, $^1O_2$), or presence of a reducing agent and trace levels of transition metal ions (i.e., iron and/or copper), which can then convert molecular oxygen into more reactive oxidizing agents

such as superoxide radical ($O_2\cdot^-$), hydroxyl radical ($\cdot OH$), or hydrogen peroxide (H_2O_2) (79). Transition metal ions are often present in excipients, and processing in stainless steel equipment can lead to significant iron contamination. As the role of the transition metal ion is catalytic, only trace levels are required. The reducing agent is consumed in the conversion of molecular oxygen into reactive oxygen species, so higher levels of reducing agent are required for significant degradation of a drug. However, higher levels could still represent contamination from impurities in the drug and/or excipients. In the example of 5 mg hGH, a low-molecular-weight reducing agent ($M \approx 100$) present at a level of 0.1% w/w of the amount of hGH could lead to oxidation of more than 10% of the protein. The reducing agent could also originate from a misguided attempt to suppress oxidation by addition of an antioxidant such as ascorbate. Ascorbate may function as an antioxidant in some circumstances but will also function as an effective prooxidant and reduce molecular oxygen to reactive oxygen species in the presence of transition metal ions such as iron or copper (79, 80). Finally, peroxides are common contaminants in polyethylene glycols and nonionic surfactants and can serve as the oxidant. Thus, at attempt to stabilize protein conformation by addition of these materials may well chemically destabilize if oxidation is a possible degradation pathway.

A number of amino acid residues are subject to oxidation. Metal-catalyzed oxidation of methionine to methionine sulfoxide and other products is perhaps the most common pathway. Oxidation of cysteine to form either nonnative intra- or intermolecular disulfide bonds is also common, and histidine residues are also easily oxidized in metal-catalyzed pathways, with tryptophan and tyrosine being degraded by light-catalyzed oxidations (79). Mechanisms are complex, and even with a given reaction such as methionine oxidation, the active oxygen species and reaction product(s) varies with the experimental conditions (79, 80); thus, stabilization is difficult. Certainly, oxygen content in the solution being processed should be minimized, and the product should be sealed in the freeze dryer with either vacuum or nitrogen in the headspace. Due to the negative impact of even small amounts of transition metal ions, prooxidants, and peroxides, the bulk drug substance and excipients need to have rigid specifications. Formulation pH and the type of buffer salt may also be important (80). The optimum conditions vary with the application, and some empirical screening experiments are necessary to optimize a given formulation.

Specific chemical components may also be added in an attempt to retard oxidation. The classical solution, addition of an antioxidant, must be approached with caution as the antioxidant may function as a prooxidant in a metal-catalyzed conversion of molecular oxygen into reactive oxygen species. Likewise, addition of a metal-complexing agent such as EDTA does not always retard oxidation. In fact, oxidation may be accelerated by complexing the transition metal (80). With most metal-catalyzed oxidations, the oxidation mechanism is a site-specific one, where the reduced form of the metal binds to a residue such as histidine on the protein and converts oxygen to reactive oxygen species at that site, which in turn oxidizes another residue nearby (81). In cases where complexation with EDTA facilitates oxidation, it is assumed that the EDTA–metal complex binds more strongly to the protein and is therefore more effective in generation of reactive oxygen species near a reactive residue (81). However, addition of EDTA does retard oxidation in some cases (82), and it would seem prudent to screen several complexing agents for impact on oxidation. Scavengers for reactive oxygen species, hydroxyl radical, $\cdot OH$, and singlet oxygen, $^1O_2$, may also retard oxidation (79, 83), but the results are highly specific to the system. For example, for iron-catalyzed oxidation of a methionine-containing peptide, thiourea was found effective for both ascorbate and dithiothreitol prooxidant systems but mannitol was effective only for the dithiothreitol prooxidant system (83).

Stabilization during freezing

In the context of proteins, stability has two distinct meanings. The term pharmaceutical stability refers to the ability of a protein to be processed, distributed, and used without irreversible change in primary structure, conformation, or state of aggregation. We refer to pharmaceutical instability as degradation. However, the phrase protein stability is also commonly used to describe the position of the equilibrium between native and unfolded conformations. If a protein formulation requires a high level of chemical denaturant, or a high temperature, to shift the equilibrium between native and unfolded in favor of the unfolded state, the protein is said to be stable. This meaning of stability I call "thermodynamic stability." Thermodynamic instability involves physical changes, somewhat analogous to a thermodynamic change of state. Pharmaceutical instability may be purely a result of a physical change (i.e., noncovalent aggregation), but may also involve changes in primary structure or, in other words, chemical degradation. Certainly, chemical transformations such as oxidation and deamidation are degradations as is aggregation to form insoluble precipitates.

Pharmaceutical stability and thermodynamic stability are not necessarily directly related. For example, a protein

may exhibit thermodynamic instability during freeze-drying and unfold, but if no irreversible reactions occur during storage or during reconstitution, the reconstituted protein may refold completely within seconds and, therefore, display perfect pharmaceutical stability. A protein that remains in the native state and is thermodynamically stable may still degrade via chemical reactions such as deamidation and oxidation over storage times of years, particularly if the reactive moiety is located on the protein surface. Conversely, thermodynamic instability may well be a prelude to degradation. Certainly, an unfolded protein could expose normally buried and protected methionine and asparagine residues to the solution environment and render these residues more reactive. Also, degradation via irreversible aggregation is believed to often proceed through unfolded or partially unfolded conformations as intermediates (84).

Many proteins survive the freeze-drying process with little or no degradation, whereas other proteins exhibit significant degradation and loss of activity during processing. Degradation during the freeze-drying process may arise during freezing and/or during drying, and it is useful to establish when in the process degradation occurs. As a measure of the degradation during freezing, freeze–thaw stability studies are carried out, and to estimate (roughly) the degradation during drying, stability during freeze-drying is compared to stability during freeze–thaw. The basic assumption is that degradation during thawing is comparable to degradation during reconstitution; therefore, the difference in activity between a freeze-dried–reconstituted sample and a freeze-thawed sample is a measure of the loss in activity during drying. This assumption is likely a reasonable approximation for a fast thawing process. One observation of particular significance is that some excipients stabilize during both freezing and drying (called lyoprotectants), whereas others stabilize only during freezing (called cryoprotectants) (41, 85, 86).

If degradation occurs only during freezing and practical variations in the freezing process do not eliminate the problem, it is obvious that a cryoprotectant system is required. However, as a number of distinct stresses may develop during freezing, the proper choice of cryoprotectant is not always obvious. Provided some information regarding the degradation pathway is available, the stabilization strategy could be quite specific. For example, if oxidation is suspected to be a major pathway, the recommendations regarding minimization of oxidation should be followed. If aggregation is a major problem, the use of nonionic surfactants should be considered, or if it is known that a change in pH caused by buffer crystallization is a problem, steps to minimize pH change during freezing need to be taken. Use of an alternative buffer system or simply use of very low levels of the buffer might well eliminate the pH change and solve the stability problem. Alternatively, addition of an excipient (i.e., sucrose or trehalose) that will interfere with buffer crystallization will also prevent excessive pH shift during freezing (41, 85, 86).

In addition to the specific stabilization strategies noted, one may also employ a general stabilization strategy that is based upon addition of components that normally increase the thermodynamic stability of the protein. That is, addition of a component that will increase the free energy of denaturation will moderate the effect of various freezing stresses that cause a decrease in the free energy of denaturation, with the net result that even during freezing, the native conformation will remain the dominant conformation and degradation will be reduced. The assumption is that increasing thermodynamic stability will also increase pharmaceutical stability. A number of solute types (i.e., amino acids, saccharides, polyols, polyethylene glycols, and some other classes) have been found effective both in increasing thermodynamic stability and in increasing pharmaceutical stability during freezing (85, 86). These solutes are referred to as excluded solutes because such solutes are present in lower concentration near the surface of a protein. The thermodynamic consequence of such exclusion is that the protein is preferentially hydrated, and the chemical potential of the protein is increased. It may be argued that the increase in the chemical potential will be much greater for the unfolded state than for the native state, thereby increasing the free energy of denaturation and stabilizing the native conformation (85, 86). Although the increase in protein chemical potential due to solute exclusion does not always correlate quantitatively with the effectiveness of that solute as a cryoprotectant, it would be prudent to test several pharmaceutically acceptable excluded solutes (i.e., glycine, mannitol, disaccharides, polyethylene glycols) as potential cryoprotectants in cases where freezing instability might involve conformational destabilization. Obviously, polyethylene glycols would not be a good choice if oxidation were an issue. For cryoprotection, it is the concentration of the cryoprotectant in solution that is the key concentration variable, regardless of the concentration of protein in the formulation. With nonpolymer excluded solutes, relatively high concentrations (i.e., 0.2–0.5 M) are normally required for effective cryoprotection (85).

Stabilization during drying

In addition to the stresses that develop during freezing, drying imposes an additional stress associated with

essentially complete removal of water. Indeed, the water substitute hypothesis (41, 85–87) is based upon the proposition that a significant thermodynamic destabilization occurs when the hydrogen bonding between protein and water is lost during the last stages of drying. The use of a water substitute as a lyoprotectant allows a hydrogen-bonding interaction between protein and the water substitute, which thermodynamically stabilizes the native conformation and preserves activity. A water substitute is a moiety that is capable of hydrogen bonding to the protein surface much as water and stabilizes via a thermodynamic mechanism; that is, stabilization is achieved by maintaining the free energy of unfolding very high such that essentially all of the protein is maintained in the native conformation. However, it must be recognized that most observations can also be rationalized in terms of a purely kinetic stabilization mechanism. In general, drying is conducted at temperatures sufficiently low that the protein exists in a glassy solid state where molecular mobility is greatly restricted. It may be argued (41) that a good stabilizer is a component that effectively couples protein dynamics to the dynamics of the glass such that even if the protein is destabilized thermodynamically, motion in the protein is too slow to allow significant unfolding during the drying operation. Thus, the protein conformation is stabilized regardless of the free energy of unfolding.

Nonreducing di- and tri-saccharides such as sucrose, trehalose, or raffinose are normally good drying stabilizers (41, 85, 86). They qualify as good water substitutes and also form glasses which, via hydrogen bonding, can couple protein dynamics to matrix dynamics. Under conditions of acid pH, particularly below pH 5, trehalose is a much more effective stabilizer than are sucrose or raffinose. Sucrose and raffinose hydrolyze to their reducing sugar components much more rapidly in the solid state than does trehalose, thereby leading to degradations initiated by reducing sugars (88). The key concentration variable in drying stabilization is the weight ratio (or mole ratio) of saccharide to protein, with the weight ratio of stabilizer to protein normally being between 1:1 and 10:1. The principle here is to insure that the protein is in a matrix of the stabilizer. Thus, with dilute protein systems, good stabilization can often be obtained at rather low concentrations of stabilizer. Here, it may be desirable to employ both a bulking agent such as glycine or mannitol, as well as a stabilizer. This strategy can yield both an elegant cake structure as well as optimal stability without the high solute concentrations than can slow primary drying.

Stabilization during storage

Although the destabilization stresses during storage remain much the same as the drying stresses, the time scale of storage is obviously much longer than the timescale of freeze-drying. In addition, the freeze-dried product is normally being stored well below its glass transition temperature, meaning molecular mobility is greatly restricted (41, 85, 86). Because of these differences, the dominant degradation pathway during storage may differ from the degradation pathway during freeze-drying. For example, deamidation of asparagine residues is a very common degradation pathway during storage but rarely is a problem during processing. This observation does not imply that deamidation is faster in the dry glassy solid than in solution, but rather is simply the result of the much longer time scale of storage. Indeed, because of the need to insure stability over the shelf life of about 2 years, storage stability normally presents a more serious problem than does stability during processing. Degradation during storage may arise from chemical degradation, such as oxidation and asparagine deamidation, and/or aggregation to noncovalent or covalent aggregates (41, 85, 86). Aggregation often means formation of a population of very large insoluble aggregates that precipitate from solution. It must be admitted, however, that the observation that the level of aggregation increases during storage does not necessarily mean that the bimolecular process of aggregation occurs in the solid state. It is also possible that only conformational changes occur during storage. Aggregation of a fraction of the conformationally modified protein could then occur instantaneously during reconstitution. The remaining fraction would then refold to the native conformation. As aggregation is normally measured in solution, it is not possible to determine just when the aggregation step actually does occur. When the amount of aggregation measured depends on the reconstitution procedure and/or the composition of the diluent (i.e., presence of surfactant) used to reconstitute (32), one would conclude that, at least in part, aggregation of (partially) unfolded protein occurs during reconstitution.

Stabilization strategies focus on three general factors: (1) specific chemical requirements, (2) physical state of the solid, and (3) structure of the protein. Depending on the degradation pathway(s) and mechanisms, any one or all of these factors could be critical. Certainly, if oxidation is a major degradation pathway, stabilization requires attention to the chemical composition of the system, including both the effects of impurities and addition of stabilizers as discussed earlier. Although pH has no real meaning in the solid state, the degree of ionization in the solid does reflect the pH of the solution from which the solid was prepared, and pH of the solution can be a major variable. Because differences in polarity of the environment between a dry solid and an aqueous solution may mean that the optimum pH for solid stability is somewhat different than the optimal pH for a solution, some solid-state screening experiments are necessary to define the precise optimum pH for stability of the freeze-dried solid.

The physical state of the system is of obvious importance. We freeze dry to increase storage stability relative to the solution state, assuming that the restricted molecular mobility of the solid state will lead to stabilization. In general, an amorphous solid (i.e., glass) is several orders of magnitude more stable than the corresponding aqueous solution, and at least with small molecules, crystalline drugs are much more stable than glasses (89). However, proteins cannot be crystallized during freeze-drying, so the only solid-state option is a glass. Forming a glass does not insure adequate stability. Pure dried proteins are glasses and often do not have sufficient stability for long-term storage at the temperatures of interest, and excipients are added to the formulation to stabilize. Because a physical mixture of protein and excipient will not provide additional stabilization, it is necessary that the proposed stabilizer system remain at least partially amorphous and in the same phase as the protein (41, 85, 86). Further, to avoid chemical reactions between the excipient and protein, the excipient system must be inert. The most common violation of inertness is the use of reducing sugars such as lactose in an attempt to stabilize the protein. For example, while lactose will stabilize hGH against aggregation, an adduct of lactose and hGH quickly forms during storage of the freeze-dried solid (18).

Drying also removes water, a reactant in a hydrolysis reaction, and stability is normally best at very low water content (41, 85, 86). However, the effect of residual

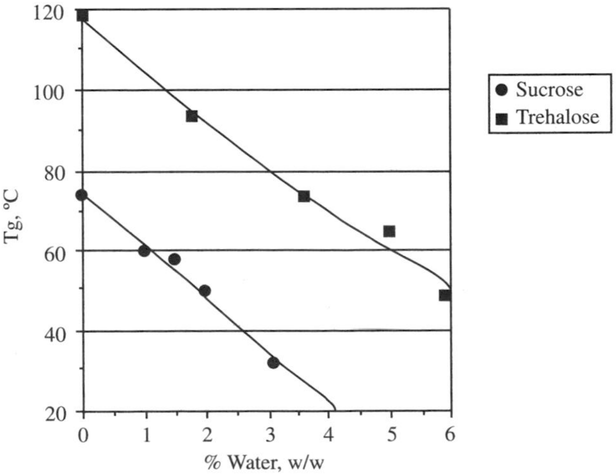

Fig. 12 The effect of residual water on the glass transition temperatures of sucrose and trehalose. (From Ref. 90.)

moisture on stability is far more complex than its possible role as a reactant. Residual water has a major effect on the physical state of the system in that increasing levels of residual moisture decreases the glass transition temperature of the amorphous system, thereby making the system less solid-like at a given temperature, and eventually causing the glass to transform into a fluid at the storage temperature. Figure 12 illustrates the effect of residual moisture on the glass transition temperature of two common stabilizers, sucrose and trehalose (90). For both examples, small amounts of residual water greatly depress the glass transition temperature, but since dry sucrose has a much lower glass transition temperature than does dry trehalose, the water content that gives a glass transition temperature at room temperature, W_g (25 °C), is much lower for sucrose. Thus, in applications where maintaining very low water

content is difficult, trehalose is a better choice for a stabilizer than is sucrose.

Generally, chemical and physical stability decrease sharply as the system enters the fluid state (41, 86, 91, 92). Chemical degradation of hGH in a trehalose formulation illustrates this behavior (92). The trehalose formulation shows a well-defined glass transition temperature with DSC, with the expected decrease in T_g as the water content is increased. The rate constant for chemical degradation is essentially independent of water content while the system remains glassy, but at least for the 50°C data, degradation increases sharply as increasing water content depresses the system glass transition temperature significantly below the storage temperature (Fig. 13). Rates of aggregation show essentially the same behavior (92). However, as stability is not sensitive to water content in the glassy state, stability is not correlated with $T-T_g$ below the glass transition temperature. The study of

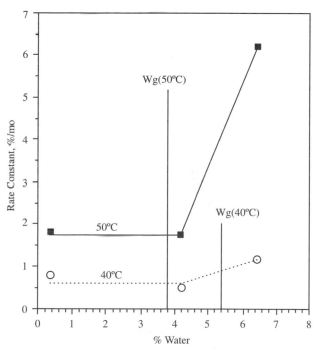

Fig. 13 Chemical degradation in freeze dried hGH formulated with trehalose as a function of water content at 40°C and 50°C. The pseudo first-order rate constant for degradation (%/month) is given for the combination of asparagine deamidation and methionine oxidation. The formulation is hGH:trehalose in a 1:6 weight ratio with sodium phosphate buffer (pH 7.4) at 15% of the hGH content. The highest moisture content samples were collapsed after storage at both 40°C (moderate collapse) and 50°C (severe collapse). The water content that reduces the glass transition temperature of the formulation to the storage temperature is denoted "Wg." Open circles = 40°C storage; filled squares = 50°C storage. (From Ref. 86.)

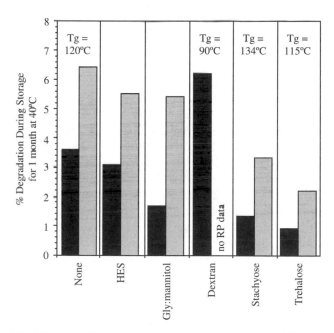

Fig. 14 The effect of excipients on the storage stability of freeze-dried human growth hormone (hGH). Samples were stored for 1 month at 40°C. Solid bars: aggregation (primarily dimer), shaded bar = chemical degradation via methionine oxidation and asparagine deamidation. The glass transition temperatures of the initial freeze-dried formulations are given above the bars when a glass transition temperature could be measured by DSC. The glycine:mannitol formulation is a weight ratio of hGH:glycine:mannitol of 1:1:5, the dextran formulation is 1:6 hGH:dextran 40, none means no stabilizer, and the others are 1:1 hGH:stabilizer. All formulations contain sodium phosphate buffer (pH 7.4) at 15% of the hGH content. Initial moisture contents are all ≈1%. (From Ref. 86.)

formulation effects on hGH stability suggests the same conclusion. Chemical and aggregation stability of hGH in several formulations is compared in Fig. 14 (92). The glycine:mannitol formulation is a 1:1:5 weight ratio of hGH:glycine:mannitol, where only the mannitol is crystalline. The other formulations are 100% amorphous. Hydroxyethyl starch (HES), stachyose, and trehalose are formulated in a 1:1 weight ratio of excipient:hGH, whereas the dextran formulation is 6:1 dextran:hGH. While the concept that an excipient system must remain at least partially amorphous to improve protein stability is not in question, it is clear that remaining amorphous is not a sufficient condition for stability. Apparent aggregation in the dextran formulation is greater than in the pure protein. Hydroxyethyl starch shows a slight improvement in stability over the pure protein, but is not nearly as effective as the glycine:mannitol formulation, and increasing the level of HES to 3:1 HES:hGH does not improve stability (92). Conversely, both stachyose and trehalose provide better stability than the glycine:mannitol system does, with trehalose superior to stachyose. All systems are glasses at the storage temperature of 40°C, and for those formulations where glass transition temperatures are available, it is clear that storage is well below the T_g, and there is no simple relationship between T_g and stability. Although one might speculate that a glass is more solid, and therefore more stable, the larger the difference between T_g and the storage temperature, the data are not consistent with this speculation. Comparing the stachyose and trehalose formulations, which are both 1:1 formulations with hGH, the T_g of the stachyose formulation is nearly 20°C higher than that of the trehalose formulation, but trehalose offers slightly better stability than does stachyose. These observations and other similar results (92) suggest that while it is necessary for the formulation to have a T_g well above the highest anticipated storage temperature for both elegance and stability reasons, stability well below T_g is not directly related to the precise difference between storage temperature and T_g.

The lack of a clear correlation between stability and T_g for systems well below T_g is not entirely unexpected. Molecular mobility slows greatly below T_g, but does not approach zero until some temperature much lower than T_g (41, 86). Thus, dynamics in the glass depend not only on the value of T_g but are also extremely sensitive to other characteristics of the glass as well as the thermal history of the glass (41, 93). Even if the major component of the glassy matrix (i.e., the sucrose) were to have essentially zero mobility (i.e., negligible translational and rotational motion), mobility of small molecules (i.e., diffusion of water) could still be significant, and mobility of potentially reactive groups on the protein (i.e., asparagine side chain)

could be sufficient to reorient into the transition state and react (41). Thus, it is not only necessary that the matrix itself be solid-like, but effective coupling between matrix mobility and the mobility critical for degradation is needed for solid-like stability behavior (41). Although the molecular characteristics required for effective coupling are not fully understood, it does seem that hydrogen bonding between protein and stabilizer provides one coupling mechanism (41, 86). Thus, disaccharides and trisaccharides are effective stabilizers.

With proteins, structure is also a critical stability variable. It is now common knowledge that proteins often suffer significant conformational changes on freeze-drying that may be moderated by addition of stabilizers to the formulation (41, 85, 86). In principle, different conformations may have different stability characteristics with the native conformation normally believed to represent the most stable conformation (41, 85, 86). Indeed data for rIL-2 show a strong correlation between storage stability and structure as measured by Fourier transform infrared spectroscopy (FTIR) (21), with a more native conformation associated with greater storage stability. Likewise, formulations of freeze-dried hGH having more native-like conformations are more stable to both aggregation and chemical degradation during storage (92). Thus, degradation of a protein in any given formulation is a function of the distribution and reactivites of the protein substates created during the freeze-drying process, with greater stability being associated with the more native-like substates. From this viewpoint, a good stabilizer is one that maximizes the population of native-like substates. Empirical evidence suggests that disaccharides perform this function quite well, regardless of what mechanism might be postulated to explain the observation (41, 85, 86).

In summary, guidelines for stabilization during storage involve the following principles: 1) optimize pH and address specific chemical effects such as oxidation; 2) disperse the protein in an inert glassy matrix with strong coupling between protein dynamics and matrix dynamics to form an amorphous phase such that at all residual water contents and storage temperatures of interest the protein phase will be well below its glass-transition temperature (note that this requires both protein and stabilizer exist in the same glassy phase); 3) employ a formulation (and process) such that the dried protein will retain the native conformation.

Retention of native conformation, coupling of protein mobility with matrix mobility, and formation of a single phase with the stabilizer all require an excipient that interacts, probably via hydrogen bonding, with the surface of the protein. Little or no interaction would likely lead to

Table 3 Glass transition temperatures, (T_g), of selected excipients measured by differential scanning calorimetry[a]

Compound	T_g (°C)	Reference
Citric acid	11	94
Glycine	($\approx$30)[b]	66
Lactose	114	95
Maltose	100	95
Mannitol	13	74, 96
Raffinose	114	95
Sorbitol	−1.6	96
Sucrose	75	95
Trehalose	118	95
Maltodextrin 860	169	95
PVP K90	176	95

[a]Consult the references for details of the techniques.
[b]Value in parentheses is extrapolated from mixtures using the Fox equation and is highly approximate.

phase separation, poor coupling of protein mobility with matrix mobility, and no opportunity for the excipient to stabilize the native conformation by either water substitution or immobilization of the protein. Disaccharides (i.e., sucrose and trehalose) and trisaccharides (i.e., raffinose) seem to satisfy these criteria and are generally good stabilizers. Polymers are generally much less effective. A product glass-transition temperature well above all anticipated storage conditions is an important product quality attribute. Glass transition temperatures of selected amorphous excipients are given in Table 3. Both trehalose and raffinose have much higher glass transition temperatures than does sucrose, and in this sense, would be better choices for stabilizers. However, as long as the residual water content is maintained low and the product is not plasticized by other low-molecular-weight formulation components, a sucrose formulation will be well below its glass-transition temperature at all practical storage temperatures. Due to a very low T_g, sorbitol should not be used as a major formulation component. Incomplete crystallization of glycine or mannitol may also lead to low product glass-transition temperatures. Lactose and maltose have high glass transition temperatures but are reducing sugars and, therefore, are poor stabilizer candidates. As noted earlier, applications at low pH pose problems for both sucrose and raffinose due to rapid hydrolysis to the reducing sugar components. Trehalose is a better choice for low pH applications.

As with drying stabilization, stabilization of a protein for storage with saccharides generally requires a weight ratio of stabilizer to protein between 1:1 and 10:1, with better stabilization at the higher excipient levels. At least for hGH, the rate constants for degradation (chemical

degradation and aggregation) decrease linearly on a plot of the logarithm of rate constant as a function of stabilizer:hGH weight ratio (92). With high dose products where the protein concentration in the fill solution is high, use of high ratios of stabilizer to protein may not feasible due to the extremely high concentration of stabilizer that would be required.

REFERENCES

1. Pikal, M.J.; Lukes, A.L.; Lang, J.E. Thermal Decomposition of Amorphous Beta-Lactam Antibacterials. J. Pharm. Sci. **1977**, *66*, 1312–1316.
2. Pikal, M.J.; Lukes, A.L.; Lang, J.E.; Gaines, K. Quantitative Crystallinity Determinations of Beta-Lactam Antibiotics by Solution Calorimetry: Correlations With Stability. J. Pharm. Sci. **1978**, *67*, 767–773.
3. Pikal, M.J.; Dellerman, K.M. Stability Testing of Pharmaceuticals by High-Sensitivity Isothermal Calorimetry at 25°C: Cephalosporins in the Solid and Aqueous Solution States. Int. J. Pharm. **1989**, *50*, 233–252.
4. Pikal, M.J. Freeze Drying of Proteins, Part I: Process Design. Biopharm. **1990**, *3* (8), 18–27.
5. Pikal, M.J. Freeze Drying of Proteins: Part II. Formulation Selection. Biopharm. **1990**, *3* (9), 26–30.
6. Pikal, M.J. Freeze Drying of Proteins: Process, Formulation, and Stability. In *Formulation and Delivery of Proteins and Peptides*; Cleland, J.L., Langer, R., Eds.; ACS: Washington DC, 1994; 120–133.
7. MacKenzie, A.P. Factors Affecting the Mechanism of Transformation of Ice into Water Vapor in the Freeze Drying Process. Ann. N. Y. Acad. Sci. **1965**, *125*, 522–547.
8. Broadhead, J.; Rouan, S.K.E.; Rhodes, C.T. The Spray Drying of Pharmaceuticals. Drug Dev. Ind. Pharm. **1992**, *18*, 1169–1206.
9. Mumenthaler, M.; Hsu, C.C.; Pearlman, R. Feasibility Study on Spray-Drying Protein Pharmaceuticals: Recombinant Human Growth Hormone and Tissue-Type Plasminogen Activator. Pharm. Res. **1994**, *11*, 12–20.
10. Masters, K. Applications of Spray-Drying in the Food Industry, in the Pharmaceutical-Biochemical Industry. In *Spray-Drying Handbook*; Longman Scientific and Technical: Esex UK, 1991; 491–676.
11. Parenteral Lyophilization Facilities: An Innovative Approach to Loading and Unloading Operations Proceedings of the International Congress, on Advanced Technologies for Manufacturing of Asceptic and Terminally Sterilized Pharmaceuticals and Biopharmaceuticals Basel Switzerland Feb. 17–19, 1992; 4–30.
12. Carpenter, J.; Crowe, J.; Arakawa, T. Comparison of Solute-Induced Protein Stabilization in Aqueous Solution and in the Frozen and Dried States. J. Dairy Sci. **1990**, *73*, 3627–3636.
13. Tanaka, R.; Takeda, T.; Miyajima, K. Cryoprotective Effect of Saccharides on Denaturation of Catalase by Freeze Drying. Chem. Pharm. Bull. **1991**, 1091–1094.
14. Hellman, K.; Miller, D.; Cammack, K. The Effect of Freeze Drying on the Quaternary Structure of L-Asparaginase

from Erwinia Carotovora. Biochim. Biophys. Acta. **1983**, *749*, 133–142.

15. Ressing, M.E.; Jiskoot, W.; Talsma, H.; van Ingen, C.W.; Beuvery, E.C.; Crommelin, D.J.A. The Influence of Sucrose, Dextran, and Hydroxyproply-β-Cyclodextrin as Lyoprotectants for a Freeze Dried Mouse IgG$_{2a}$ Monoclonal Antibody (MN12). Pharm. Res. **1992**, *9*, 266–270.

16. Izutsu, K.; Yoshioka, S. Stabilization of Protein Pharmaceuticals in Freeze Dried Formulations. Drug Stabil. **1995**, *1*, 11–21.

17. Bell, L.N.; Hageman, M.J. Differentiating Between the Effects of Water Activity and Glass Transition Dependent Mobility on a Solid State Chemical Reaction: Aspartame Degradation. J. Agric. Food Chem. **1994**, *42*, 2398–2401.

18. Pikal, M.J.; Dellerman, K.M.; Roy, M.L.; Riggin, R.M. The Effects of Formulation Variables on the Stability of Freeze Dried Human Growth Hormone. Pharm. Res. **1991**, *8*, 427–436.

19. Pikal, M.J.; Dellerman, K.M.; Roy, M.L. Formulation and Stability of Freeze Dried Proteins: Effects of Moisture and Oxygen on the Stability of Freeze Dried Formulations of Human Growth Hormone. Develop. Biol. Standard **1991**, *74*, 323–340.

20. Townsend, M.W.; DeLuca, P.P. Use of Lyoprotectants in the Freeze Drying of a Model Protein. Ribonuclease A. J. Parenter. Sci., Technol. **1988**, *42*, 190–199.

21. Prestrelski, S.J.; Pikal, K.A.; Arakawa, T. Optimization of Lyophilization Conditions for Recombinant Interleukin-2 by Dried-State Conformational Analysis Using Fourier-Transform Infrared Spectroscopy. Pharm. Res. **1995**, *12*, 1250–1259.

22. Roy, M.L.; Pikal, M.J.; Rickard, E.C.; Maloney, A.M. The Effects of Formulation and Moisture on the Stability of a Freeze Dried Monoclonal Antibody-Vinca Conjugate: A Test of the WLF Glass Transition Theory. Develop. Biol. Standard **1991**, *74*, 323–340.

23. Kiovsky, T.E.; Pincock, R.E. Kinetics of Reactions in Frozen Solutions. J. Am. Chem. Soc. **1966**, *88*, 7704–7710.

24. Franks, F. Freeze Drying: From Empiricism to Predictability. Cryo-Letters **1990**, *11*, 93–110.

25. Pikal, M.J.; Shah, S. The Collapse Temperature in Freeze Drying: Dependence on Measurement Methodology and Rate of Water Removal from the Glassy Phase. Int. J. Pharm. **1990**, *62*, 165–186.

26. Williams, N.A.; Dean, T. Vial Breakage by Frozen Mannitol Solutions: Correlation With Thermal Characteristics and Effect of Sterioisomerism, Additives, and Vial Configuration. J. Parenter. Sci. Technol. **1991**, *45*, 94–100.

27. Larsen, S.S. Studies on Stability of Drugs in Frozen Systems. Arch. Pharm. Chem. Sci. Ed. **1973**, *1*, 41–53.

28. Murase, N.; Franks, F. Salt Precipitation During the Freeze-Concentration of Phosphate Buffer Solutions. Biophys. Chem. **1989**, *34*, 293–300.

29. Gomez, G.; Rodriguez-Hornedo, N.; Pikal, M.J. Effect of Freezing on the pH Of Sodium Phosphate Buffer Solutions. Pharm. Res. **1994**, *11*, S-265, PPD 7364.

30. Szkudlarek, B.A.; Rodriguez-Hornedo, N.; Pikal, M.J. Analysis of pH Changes of Potassium Phosphate Buffer Salt Solutions During Freezing. Pharm. Res. **1994**, *11*, S-228, PPD 7215.

31. Arakawa, T.; Prestrelski, S.; Kinney, W.; Carpenter, J.F. Factors Affecting Short-Term and Long-Term Stabilities of Proteins. Adv. Drug Delivery Rev. **1993**, *10*, 1–28.

32. Carpenter, J.F.; Prestrelski, S.; Arakawa, T. Separation of Freezing- and Drying-Induced Denaturation of Lyophilized Proteins by Stress-Specific Stabilization: I. Enzyme Activity and Calorimetric Studies. Arch. Biochem. Biophys. **1993**, *303*, 456–464.

33. Franks, F.F. Product Stability During Drying. *BioPharm Conference, Proceedings 1993*; Advanstar Communications: Eugene Oregon, 1993; 78–87.

34. Franks, F. *Biophysics and Biochemistry at Low Temperature*; Cambridge University Press: London, 1985.

35. Privalov, P. Cold Denaturation of Proteins. Biochem. and Mol. Biol. **1990**, *25*, 281–305.

36. Tsong, T.Y.; Baldwin, R.L. Effects of Solvent Viscosity and Different Guanidine Salts on the Kinetics of Ribonuclease a Chain Folding. Biopolymers **1978**, *17*, 1669–1678.

37. Kiefhaber, T.; Quaas, R.; Hahn, U.; Schmid, F.X. Folding of Ribonuclease T$_1$. 1. Existence of Multiple Unfolded States Created by Proline Isomerization. Biochemistry **1990**, *29*, 3053–3061.

38. Lim, M.; Reid, D. Studies of Reaction Kinetics in Relation to The $T_g{}'$ Of Polymers in Frozen Model Systems. *Water Relationships in Food*; Levine, H., Slade, L., Eds.; Plenum Press: New York, 1991; 103–122.

39. Pikal, M.J.; Shah, S.; Senior, D.; Lang, J.E. Physical Chemistry of Freeze Drying: Measurement of Sublimation Rates for Frozen Aqueous Solutions by a Micro Balance Technique. J. Pharm. Sci. **1983**, *72*, 635–650.

40. Pikal, M.J.; Shah, S.; Roy, M.L.; Putman, R. The Secondary Drying Stage of Freeze Drying: Drying Kinetics as a Function of Temperature and Chamber Pressure. Int. J. Pharm. **1990**, *60*, 203–217.

41. Pikal, M.J. Mechanisms of Protein Stabilization During Freeze Drying and Storage: The Relative Importance of Thermodynamic Stabilization and Glassy State Relaxation Dynamics. In *Freeze Drying/Lyophilization of Pharmaceutical and Biological Products*; Rey, L., May, J., Eds.; Marcel Dekker, Inc.: 1999.

42. Chang, B.S.; Kendrick, B.S.; Carpenter, J.F. Surface-Induced Denaturation of Proteins During Freezing and its Inhibition by Surfactants. J. Pharm. Sci. **1996**, *85*, 1325–1330.

43. Roy, M.L.; Pikal, M.J. Process Control in Freeze Drying: Determination of the End Point of Sublimation Drying by an Electronic Moisture Sensor. J. Parenter. Sci. Technol. **1989**, 60–66.

44. Pikal, M.J.; Roy, M.L.; Shah, S. Mass and Heat Transfer in Vial Freeze Drying of Pharmaceuticals: Role of the Vial. J. Pharm. Sci. **1984**, *73*, 1224–1237.

45. MacKenzie, A.P. Basic Principles of Freeze Drying for Pharmaceuticals. Bull. Par. Drug Assoc. **1966**, *20*, 101–129.

46. Chang, B.S.; Randall, C.S. Use of Subambient Thermal Analysis to Optimize Protein Lyophilization. Cryobiology **1992**, *29*, 632–656.

47. Pikal, M.J. Use of Laboratory Data in Freeze Drying Process Design: Heat and Mass Transfer Coefficients and the Computer Simulation of Freeze Drying. J. Parenteral Sci., Technol. **1985**, *39*, 115–138.

48. Milton, N.; Nail, S.L.; Roy, M.L.; Pikal, M.J. Evaluation of Manometric Temperature Measurement as a Method of Monitoring Product Temperature During Lyophilization. PDA J. Pharm. Sci. Technol. **1997**, *51*, 7–16.

49. Kobayashi, M. Development of New Refrigeration System and Optimum Geometry of the Vapor Condenser for Pharmaceutical Freeze Dryers Proceedings of the 4th International Drying Symposium, Kyoto, Japan, July 9–12, 1984; Toei, R.R., Mujumdar, A., Eds.; *2*, 464–471.

50. Pikal, M.J.; Lang, J.E. Rubber Closures as a Source of Haze in Freeze Dried Parenterals: Test Methodology for Closure Evaluation. J. Parenter Drug Assoc. **1978**, *32*, 162.

51. Bardat, A.; Biguet, J.; Chatenet, J.; Courteille, F. Moisture Measurement: A New Method for Monitoring Freeze Drying Cycles. J. Parenter Sci. Technol. **1993**, *47*, 293–299.

52. Moreira, T.; Cabrera, L.; Gutierrez, A.; Cadiz, A.; Castellano, M. Role of Temperature and Moisture on Monomer Content of Freeze Dried Human Albumin. Acta Pharm. Nord. **1992**, *4*, 59–60.

53. Pristoupil, T.; Kramlova, M.; Fortova, H.; Ulrych, S. Haemoglobin Lyophilized With Sucrose: The Effect of Residual Moisture on Storage. Haematologia **1985**, *18*, 45–52.

54. Hageman, M.J. The Role of Moisture in Protein Stability. Drug Dev. Ind. Pharm. **1988**, *14*, 2047–2070.

55. Greiff, D. Protein Structure and Freeze Drying: The Effects of Residual Moisture and Gases. Cryobiology **1971**, *8*, 145–152.

56. Hsu, C.; Ward, C.; Pearlman, R.; Nguyen, H.; Yeung, D.; Curley, J. Determining the Optimum Residual Moisture in Lyophilized Protein Pharmaceuticals. Develop. Biol. Standard **1991**, *74*, 255–271.

57. Pikal, M.J.; Shah, S. Moisture Transfer from Stopper to Product and Resulting Stability Implications. Develop. Biol. Standard **1991**, *74*, 165–179.

58. MacKenzie, A.P. Collapse During Freeze Drying Qualitative and Quantitative Aspects. *Freeze Drying and Advanced Food Technology*; Goldblith, S.A., Rey, L., Rothmayr, W.W., Eds.; Academic Press: London, 1975; 277–307.

59. Her, L.M.; Nail, S.L. Measurement of Glass Transition Temperatures of Freeze-Concentrated Solutes by Differential Scanning Calorimetry. Pharm. Res. **1994**, *11*, 54–59.

60. Pikal, M.J.; Shah, S.; Unpublished Data Eli Lilly & Co.

61. MacKenzie, A.P.; as Cited in Ref. 4.

62. Slade, L.; Levine, H. Beyond Water Activity: Recent Advances Based on an Alternative Approach to the Assessment of Food Quality and Safety. Criti. Rev. Food Sci. Nutr. **1991**, *30*, 115–360.

63. Pikal, M.J.; Chang, L.Q.; Unpublished Data University of Connecticut.

64. Shalaev, E.Y.; Kanev, A.N. Study of the Solid-Liquid State Diagram of the Water–Glycine–Sucrose System. Cryobiology **1994**, *31*, 374–382.

65. Shalaev, E.; Malakhov, D.V.; Kanev, A.N.; Tuzikov, F.V.; Varaskin, N.D.; Vavilin, V.I. Study of the Phase Diagram Water Fraction of the System Water–Glycine–Sucrose by DTA and X-ray Diffraction Methods. Thermochim. Acta **1992**, *196*, 213–220.

66. Lueckel, B.; Bodmer, D.; Helk, B.; Leuenberger, H. Formulations of Sugars with Amino Acids or Mannitol-Influence of Concentration Ratio on the Properties of the Freeze-Concentrate and the Lyophilizate. Pharm. Develop. and Technol. **1998**, *3*, 325–336.

67. Suzuki, T.; Franks, F. Solid–Liquid Phase Transitions and Amorphous States in Ternary Sucrose–Glycine–Water Systems. J. Chem. Soc., Faraday Trans. **1993**, *89*, 3283–3288.

68. Kassraian, K.; Spitznagel, T.; Juneau, J.; Yim, K. Characterization of the Sucrose/Glycine/Water System by Differential Scanning Calorimetry and Freeze Drying Microscopy. Pharm. Develop. and Technol. **1998**, *3*, 233–239.

69. Hancock, B.C.; Zografi, G. The Relationship Between the Glass Transition Temperature and the Water Content of Amorphous Pharmaceutical Solids. Pharm. Res. **1994**, *11*, 471–477.

70. Williams, N.A.; Lee, Y.; Polli, G.P.; Jennings, T.A. The Effects of Cooling Rate on Solid Phase Transitions and Associated Vial Breakage Occurring in Frozen Mannitol Solutions. J. Parentes. Sci. and Tech. **1986**, *40*, 135.

71. Williams, N.A.; Guglielmo, J. Thermal Mechanical Analysis of Frozen Solutions of Mannitol and Some Related Steroisomers: Evidence of Expansion During Warming and Correlation with Vial Breakage During Lyophilization. J. Parenter Sci., and Technol. **1993**, *47*, 119–123.

72. Akers, M.J.; Milton, N.; Byrn, S.R.; Nail, S.L. Glycine Crystallization During Freezing: The Effects of Salt Form, pH, and Ionic Strength. Pharm. Res. **1995**, *12*, 1457–1461.

73. Yu, L.; Milton, N.; Groleau, E.; Mishra, D.; Vansickle, R. Existence of a Mannitol Hydrate During Freeze Drying and Practical Implications. J. Pharm. Sci. **1999**, *88*, 196–199.

74. Kim, A.I.; Akers, M.J.; Nail, S.L. The Physical State of Mannitol After Freeze Drying: Effects of Mannitol Concentration, Freezing Rate, and a Noncrystallizing Cosolute. J. Pharm. Sci. **1998**, *87*, 931–935.

75. Cavatur, R.K.; Suryanarayanan, R. Characterization of Phase Transitions During Freeze Drying by In Situ X-ray Powder Diffractometry. Pharm. Develop. and Technol. **1998**, *3*, 579–586.

76. Bam, N.B.; Cleland, J.L.; Yang, J.; Manning, M.C.; Carpenter, J.F.; Kelley, R.F.; Randolph, T.W. Tween Protects Recombinant Human Growth Hormone Against Agitation-Induced Damage Via Hydrophobic Interactions. J. Pharm. Sci. **1998**, *87*, 1554–1559.

77. Bam, N.B.; Randolph, T.W.; Cleland, J.L. Stability of Protein Formulations: Investigation of Surfactant Effects by a Novel EPR Spectroscopic Technique. Pharm. Res. **1995**, *12*, 2–11.

78. Kerwin, B.A.; Heller, M.C.; Levin, S.H.; Randolph, T.W. Effects of Tween 80 and Sucrose on Acute Short-Term Stability and Long-Term Storage at −20°C Of a Recombinant Hemoglobin. J. Pharm. Sci. **1998**, *87*, 1062–1068.

79. Li, S.; Schoneich, C.; Borchard, R. Chemical Instablity of Protein Pharmaceuticals: Mechanisms of Oxidation and Strategies for Stabilization. Biotech. Bioeng. **1995**, *48*, 490–500.

80. Li, S.; Schoneich, C.; Wilson, G.; Borchardt, R. Chemical Pathways of Peptide Degradation. V. Ascorbic Acid

Promotes Rather than Inhibits the Oxidation of Methionine to Methionine Sulfoxide in Small Model Peptides. Pharm. Res. **1993**, *10*, 1572–1579.

81. Stadman, E.R. Metal Ion-Catalyzed Oxidation of Proteins: Biochemical Mechanism and Biological Consequences. Free Radical Biol. Med. **1990**, *9*, 315–325.

82. Hall, P.; Roberts, R. Methionine Oxidation and Inactivation of α_1-Proteinase Inhibitor by Cu^{2+} And Glucose. Biochim. Biophys. Acta **1992**, *1121*, 325–330.

83. Li, S.; Schoneich, C.; Borchardt, R. Chemical Pathways of Peptide Degradation. VIII. Oxidation of Methionine in Small Model Peptides by Prooxidant/Transition Metal Ion Systems: Influence of Selective Scavengers for Reactive Oxygen Intermediates. Pharm. Res. **1995**, *12*, 348–355.

84. Brems, D.N. Solubility of Different Folding Conformers of Bovine Growth Hormone. Biochemistry **1988**, *27*, 4541–4546.

85. Carpenter, J.R.; Pikal, M.J.; Chang, B.S.; Randolph, T.W. Rational Design of Stable Lyophilized Protein Formulations: Some Practical Advice. Pharm. Res. **1997**, *14*, 969–975.

86. Pikal, M.J. Freeze Drying of Proteins. In *Peptide and Protein Delivery*; Lee, V.H.L., Ed.; *in press* Marcel Dekker, Inc.: New York.

87. Arakawa, T.; Kita, Y.; Carpenter, J.F. Protein –Solvent Interactions in Pharmaceutical Formulations. Pharm. Res. **1991**, *8*, 285–291.

88. Pikal, M.; Busse, J.; Kovach, P.; Unpublished Results Eli Lilly & Co.

89. Pikal, M.J. Impact of Polymorphism on the Quality of Lyophilized Products. In *Polymorphism in Pharmaceutical Solids*; Brittain, H.G., Ed.; Marcel Dekker, Inc.: New York, 1999.

90. Saleki-Gerhardt, A.; University of Wisconsin-Madison: 1993.

91. Duddu, S.; Zhang, G.; Dal Monte, P. The Relationship Between Protein Aggregation and Molecular Mobility Below the Glass Transition Temperature of Lyophilized Formulations Containing a Monoclonal Antibody. Pharm. Res. **1997**, *14*, 596–600.

92. Pikal, M.J.; Roy, M.L.; Rigsbee, D.R.; Unpublished Data Eli Lilly & Co.

93. Shamblin, S.L.; Tang, X.; Chang, L.; Hancock, B.C.; Pikal, M.J. Characterization of the Time Scales of Molecular Motion in Pharmaceutically Important Glasses. J. Phys. Chem. B. **1999**, *103*, 4113–4121.

94. Lu, Q.; Zografi, G. Properties of Citric Acid At the Glass Transition. J. Pharm. Sci. **1997**, *86*, 1374–1378.

95. Taylor, L.; Zografi, G. Sugar –Polymer Hydrogen Bond Interactions in Lyophilized Amorphous Mixtures. J. Pharm. Sci. **1998**, *87*, 1615–1620.

96. Yu, L.; Mishra, D.; Rigsbee, D. Determination of the Glass Properties of D-Mannitol Using Sorbitol as an Impurity. J. Pharm. Sci. **1998**, *87*, 774–777.

GELS AND JELLIES

Clyde M. Ofner III
University of the Sciences in Philadelphia, Philadelphia, Pennsylvania

Cathy M. Klech-Gelotte
McNeil Consumer Healthcare, Fort Washington, Pennsylvania

G

INTRODUCTION

The word "gel" is derived from "gelatin," and both "gel" and "jelly" can be traced back to the Latin *gelu* for "frost" and *gelare*, meaning "freeze" or "congeal" (1). This origin indicates the essential idea of a liquid setting to a solid-like material that does not flow, but is elastic and retains some liquid characteristics. The distinction between gel and jelly remains somewhat arbitrary, with some differences based on the field of application. The food industry uses the term "gelatin jelly" whereas the pharmaceutical industry uses the term "gelatin gel."

Use of the term "gel" as a classification originated during the late 1800s as chemists attempted to classify semisolid substances according to their phenomenological characteristics rather than their molecular compositions (2). At that time, analytical methods needed to determine chemical structures were lacking. The USP (3) defines gels (sometimes called jellies) as semisolid systems consisting of either suspensions made up of small inorganic particles, or large organic molecules interpenetrated by a liquid. Where the gel mass consists of a network of small discrete particles, the gel is classified as a two-phase system. Single-phase gels consist of organic macromolecules uniformly distributed throughout a liquid in such a manner that no apparent boundaries exist between the dispersed macromolecules and the liquid.

Single-phase gels and jellies can be described as three-dimensional networks formed by adding macromolecules such as proteins, polysaccharides, and synthetic macromolecules to appropriate liquids. In pharmaceutical applications, water and hydroalcoholic solutions are most common. Many polymer gels exhibit reversibility between the gel state and sol, which is the fluid phase containing the dispersed or dissolved macromolecule. However, formation of some polymer gels is irreversible because their chains are covalently bonded. The three-dimensional networks formed in two-phase gels and jellies are formed by several inorganic colloidal clays. Formation of these inorganic gels is reversible.

Gels are generally considered to be more rigid than jellies because gels contain more covalent crosslinks, a

higher density of physical bonds, or simply less liquid. Gel-forming polymers produce materials that span a range of rigidities, beginning with a sol and increasing in rigidity to a mucilage, jelly, gel, and hydrogel. Table 1 lists monographs for the 23 gel drug products, three jelly drug products, and three nondrug gels listed in the USP.

This review focuses mainly on water-based gels and jellies. Gel structure, the basis for understanding the physical properties associated with gels, is examined first, followed by the rheology of gels. Specific natural, semisynthetic, and synthetic gel-forming polymers and inorganic clays are then discussed along with their pharmaceutical applications.

GEL MICROSTRUCTURE

Substances that form aqueous gels are usually hydrophilic polymers capable of extensive solvation. At certain temperatures and polymer concentrations, and, in some cases, with the addition of ions, a three-dimensional network is formed. Although polymer gels vary considerably in chemical structure, they all behave as elastic solids at low applied stresses, even though they primarily consist of liquid. The differences in chemical composition, however, result in several types of gel microstructure. Pharmaceutical gels may be loosely categorized on the basis of the their network microstructure according to the following scheme suggested by Flory (2):

1. Covalently bonded polymer networks with completely disordered structures
2. Physically bonded polymer networks, predominantly disordered but containing ordered loci
3. Well-ordered lamellar structures, including gel mesophases formed by inorganic clays

Covalently Bonded Structures

Covalently crosslinked gel networks are irreversible systems. They are typically prepared from synthetic

Table 1 Gel and jelly monographs in the USP 24

Monograph title	Drug product or nondrug product
Aluminum Hydroxide Gel	Drug product
Aluminum Phosphate Gel	Drug product
Aminobenzoic Acid Gel	Drug product
Benzocaine, Butamben and Tetracaine Hydrochloride Gel	Drug product
Benzocaine Gel	Drug product
Benzoyl Peroxide Gel	Drug product
Betamethasone Benzoate Gel	Drug product
Silica Gel	Nondrug product
Clindamycin Phosphate Gel	Drug product
Desoximetasone Gel	Drug product
Desamethasone Gel	Drug product
Dimethyl Sulfoxide Gel	Nondrug product
Diclonine Hydrochloride Gel	Drug product
Erythromycin and Benzoyl Peroxide Topical Gel	Drug product
Erythromycin Topical Gel	Drug product
Flucinonide Gel	Drug product
Hydrocortisone Gel	Drug product
Hydroxypropyl Cellulose Ocular System	Drug product
Lidocaine Hydrochloride Jelly	Drug product
Metronidazole Gel	Drug product
Naftifine Hydrochloride Gel	Drug product
Phenylephrine Hydrochloride Nasal Jelly	Drug product
Porous Silica Gel	Nondrug product
Pramoxine Hydrochloride Jelly	Drug product
Salacylic Acid Gel	Drug product
Fluoride and Phosphoric Acid Gel	Drug product
Stannous Fluoride Gel	Drug product
Tolnaftate Gel	Drug product
Tretinoin Gel	Drug product

hydrophilic polymers in one of two ways, details of which may be found in a comprehensive treatise (4–6). Because the resulting gel matrices are often highly rigid, these gels have been classified as hydrogels.

In the first method of preparation, infinite gel networks arise from the nonlinear copolymerization of two or more monomer species, with one being at least trifunctional. Both the direction and position by which each polymer chain grows during the reaction are random, resulting in the final microstructure of these gels being completely disordered. The gel point for copolymerization between equimolar concentrations of two monomer species can be predicted using the modified Carothers equation (7):

$$\bar{X}_n = \frac{2}{(2 - \rho f_{av})}$$

where $\bar{X}_n$ is the number-average degree of polymerization, ρ is the fractional conversion, and f_{av} is the average functionality of the monomers involved. The gel point is

reached when $X_n \rightarrow \infty$, indicating that the critical conversion for gelation (ρc) is equal to $2/f_{av}$ (7). In practice, however, gel points tend to be overestimated by the equation.

The other method for preparing chemically crosslinked gel structures involves covalent crosslinking of individual linear or branched polymer chains, using a low concentration of crosslinking agent (5). The crosslinking ratio X, which is simply the mole ratio of crosslinking agent to polymer repeat units, can be used to characterize the resulting three-dimensional network.

Other parameters to characterize crosslinking are the equilibrium swelling ratio, the molecular weight between crosslinks, the so-called mesh size between crosslinks, and the crosslinking density (8). The equilibrium swelling ratio Q_m is the ratio of the volume of the swollen polymer to the volume of the dry polymer. It decreases as the extent of crosslinking increases. The molecular weight between crosslinks M_c, developed from the Flory equations for

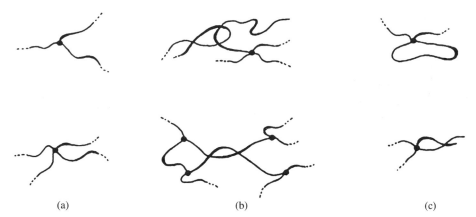

Fig. 1 Chemical and physical crosslinks associated with covalently bonded polymer gels. (a) Bi- and trifunctional chemical crosslinks; (b) simple and trapped physical entanglements; (c) ineffective chemically bonded loop and dangling ends.

equilibrium swelling (9), is also indirectly proportional to crosslinking extent. The mesh size ζ is an estimate of the distance between crosslinks based on the root-mean-square end-to-end distance of the random coil polymer between crosslinks. Estimates of the crosslinking density usually involve more rigorous treatments that require theoretical expressions (6). These models recognize the discrepancy between the amount of crosslinking agent added to the reaction and the number of effective chemical crosslinks actually produced, in addition to the presence of physical crosslinks formed by chain entanglements. If the crosslinking site is known, the covalent crosslinking density may be determined without theoretical models by chemical analysis of these sites (10). Examples of chemical and physical crosslinks, which may exist in a gel network of covalently linked linear chains, are illustrated in Fig. 1.

Physically Bonded Structures

Physically bonded gel networks are reversible systems; factors such as temperature and ion additives can induce a transition between the sol and gel phases. These gels are formed primarily by natural organic polymers (proteins and polysaccharides) and semisynthetic cellulose derivatives. Gels of some synthetic, hydrophilic polymers are also included in this class.

Polymer chains exist most often in the sol as random coils, which undergo conformational transitions to yield a gel (11). Such transitions may involve large ordered sections of one or more chains, which fold into a single, double, or triple helix. The three-dimensional network is then formed by cooperative association of several sections into higher ordered regions called junction zones (12). Many junction zones are dispersed throughout the

amorphous domains of the network, thus giving mechanical strength to the gel.

The microstructures of physically bonded gels are much more complex than those of the disordered, chemically crosslinked gels. The spatial arrangements assumed by polymer chains in forming junction zones may differ, as well as the secondary intermolecular forces that hold these zones together. The physical properties of gels, including rigidity, melting temperature, and yield point, are related to the type of junction zone formed. Several types have been identified or hypothesized; they are briefly reviewed here.

The particular organization of polymer chains in a junction zone depends on the chemical structure of the repeating unit. For example, sulfated polysaccharides (e.g., agar and κ-carrageenan) that contain an assortment of sulfated galactose residues form double helices, two or more of which aggregate into multihelical junction zones (12). However, the presence of a few contaminant residue units greatly reduces gelling ability. The residues produce kinks that effectively block helix formation in large sections of chains, indicating that steric fit is critical to gel formation (12). The microstructure of these gels is schematically represented in Fig. 2.

Gels composed of semisynthetic cellulose derivatives, including sodium carboxymethylcellulose, contain microcrystalline junction zones. Residual crystallinity in the form of chain bundles can survive the derivatization processing of cellulose (13). The bundles are connected through common chains to yield a gel, and the ultimate gel strength depends on the efficiency by which the bundles were previously dispersed throughout the sol (13). Furthermore, microcrystalline domains, forming between segments of stereoregular synthetic polymers such as polyvinyl alcohol (14), enhance the gel's rigidity.

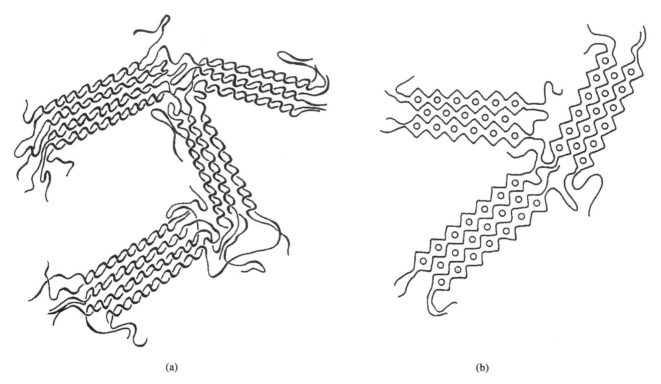

(a)   (b)

Fig. 2 Microstructures associated with physically bonded polymer gels. (a) Multihelical junction zones of agar gels; (b) egg-box model junction zones of calcium alginate gels.

Micelle-like junction zones are formed by methylcellulose and polyethyloxylene polypropyloxylene block copolymers (poloxamers). Although the polymers differ in chemical structure, both have hydrophobic regions in their chains: the di- and trimethyl-D-glucose residues of methylcellulose and the polypropyloxylene block of poloxamer. Another feature common to the two polymers is that their gels exhibit inverted thermal reversibility, that is, they gel with heating and melt with cooling. Both the inverted temperature behavior and the presence of hydrophobic regions in the polymers provide evidence for the formation of micelle-like junction zones (12, 15). Water molecules structured around the hydrophobic regions of polymer chains in a sol become disordered with increases in temperature. Newly exposed hydrophobic regions attract one another to form bonds, whereas hydrophilic areas rearrange to maximize their contact with the aqueous medium. The resulting micelle-like structures continue to grow in size and number at higher temperatures, leading eventually to gel formation.

Other junction zones require the presence of multivalent ions to form ion bridges between polymer chains. An egg box model was proposed by Grant et al. (16) for the formation of calcium alginate gels, in which calcium cations are cooperatively bound between ionized carboxyl groups located on the polyglucuronate sequences of alginic acid. The cations are coordinated in the interstices of ordered segments of the polysaccharide chains (Fig. 2b). Other mechanisms for the involvement of ions in gelation may be similar but less precisely understood. For instance, guar gum forms cohesive gels only in the presence of borate ions (17).

Finally, some physically bonded gel networks are held together by simple entanglement couplings between individual polymer chains rather than by large aggregate junction zones. Above a critical concentration, long chains of hydrophilic polymers, such as hyaluronic acid and carbomer, are apparently forced through the domains of other chains because of their large molecular volumes (18). An increasingly intertwined network occurs with higher polymer concentrations to produce a gel. Although these gels are highly disordered compared with other physically bonded gels that have ordered junction zones, they are considered here because they form reversible gel microstructures. Yet, some researchers believe (12) that ordered regions must be present to impart rigidity in entangled gels, but such regions may be relatively dispersed and unstable, making them difficult to identify. Others propose (19) that higher order exists from interchain bridging by complexation with solvent molecules.

Molecular associations between polymer segments occur through the cooperation of several intermolecular forces such as hydrogen bonding, van der Waals forces, and electrostatic attractive and repulsive forces. The disruption of junction zones is associated with a high activation energy, further indicating that many intermolecular forces cooperate to retain the structure of each junction (12).

Well-Ordered Gel Structures

Under suitable conditions, certain silica, alumina, and clay aqueus dispersions form rigid gels or lyogels. When clays belonging to the smectite class, such as bentonite, aluminum magnesium silicate, hectorite, and laponite, come into contact with water, they undergo interlayer swelling spontaneously, followed by osmotic swelling to produce a gel (20). The plate-like clay particles associate into an ordered, extended network for which two models have been described (21). The "house of cards" model is based on attraction between weak positively charged particle edges and negatively charged particle faces; edge-to-edge associations of particles into flat ribbons have also been proposed.

Highly ordered lamellar gel microstructures are formed by certain surfactants and mixtures of a surfactant and long-chain fatty alcohols in water. Using small angle X-ray scattering (SAXS), an ordered lamellar stack lattice model was proposed for the gel formed by 10% w/w cetostearyl alcohol containing 0.5% cetrimide surfactant (22). In contrast, the microstructure of a Brij 96 gel depends on the surfactants concentration. A hexagonal liquid-crystalline gel structure was detected by SAXS at concentrations of 40 to 60 wt% in water, whereas an extended lamellar structure was detected at higher concentrations (70 to 85 wt%) (23).

PHYSICAL PROPERTIES OF GELS AND JELLIES

The physical properties of gels and jellies can be classified into two groups: transitional properties (including gel point, retrogradation, and syneresis) and rheological properties (including rigidity, yield point, and rupture strength). The experimental techniques used to characterize these physical properties can be similarly classified (24). Spectrophotometric and thermal techniques are used to identify gel microstructures (physical junction zones) and their related transitional properties. For example, nuclear magnetic resonance (NMR) spectroscopy

measures the structural and dynamic characteristics of the polymer just prior to aggregation and gel formation, and circular dichroism (CD) spectroscopy measures the conformational changes of the polymer during network formation (e.g., helix–coil transitions). Mechanical techniques are used to determine rheological properties of gels. These techniques employ either small-deformation measurements that yield viscoelastic parameters or large-deformation measurements that generate complete stress-strain profiles, which include failure parameters.

Transitional Properties

Sol–gel transition (gel point)

Sol–gel transition may be dependent on polymer concentration or temperature. Spectrophotometric methods, as mentioned previously, are used to probe sol–gel transitions that depend on the critical gelling concentration. Thermal methods, including differential scanning calorimetry, are used to measure sol–gel transitions, or melting temperatures, of thermoreversible gels. A relationship for estimating the heat of gelation was derived by Eldrige and Ferry (25) in which the dependence of the sol–gel transition temperature on polymer concentration was considered.

The critical gelling concentration is the concentration below which no macroscopic gel is formed under the prevailing experimental conditions (24); rather, a sol is formed by the polymer and solvent. This concentration depends on polymer–polymer and polymer–solvent interactions, the hydrophilic–lipophilic character of the polymer, and the molecular weight and flexibility of the chain (26). Furthermore, polymers that require ions to form gels have critical gelling concentrations that depend on the concentration of these additives and many other variables. Table 2 lists ranges of minimal concentrations for substances to gel in water.

There are two thermal gel points associated with thermoreversible gels. Shifts in temperature may cause gel formation at the setting point or gel liquification at the melting point. In addition, temperature hysteresis may occur in some gels in which the gel-setting point is lower than the melting point. The hysteresis behavior indicates that junction zones constitute a family of associations rather than a set of identical crosslinkages (12). Agarose gels show temperature hysteresis; the gel sets at about 40°C and melts at about 90°C.

Physical aging

Most gels have structures that have not attained equilibrium; different preparative methods and conditions

Table 2 Gelling concentrations for substances used in pharmaceutical products

Substance	Gel-forming concentrations (wt %)	Required additives
Proteins		
Collagen	0.2–0.4[a]	
Gelatin	2–15	
Polysaccharides		
Agar	0.1–1	
Alginates	0.5–1	Ca^{2+}
	5–10	Na^+
K-Carrageenan	1–2	K^+
Gellum gum (low acetyl)	0.5–1	Ca^{2+}
Glycyrrhiza	2	
Guar gum	2.5–10	
	0.25	Borate ion
Hyaluronic acid	2	
Pectins (low methyoxy)	0.8–2	Ca^{2+}
Starch	6	
Tragacanth gum	2–5	
Semisynthetic polymers (cellulose derivatives)		
Carboxymethylcellulose	4–6	Na^+
	10–25	Na^+
Hydroxypropylcellulose	8–10	
Hydroxypropylmethylcellulose	2–10	
Methylcellulose	2–4	
Synthetic polymers		
Carbomer	0.5–2	
Poloxamer	15–50	
Poyacrylamide	4	
Polyvinyl alcohol	10–20	
Inorganic substances		
Aluminum hydroxide	3–5	
Bentonite	5	
Laponite	2	Electrolytes
Surfactants		
Cetostearyl alcohol	10	Cetrimide
Brij 96[b]	40–60	

[a] Adjusted to pH > 4 and warmed to 37°C.
[b] Brij 30–99 surfactants are polyoxyethylene-alkyl ethers.

influence the gel state. The gel physically ages as it moves toward equilibrium, making the history of a gel sample an important consideration when measuring physical properties. Aging reflects changes in gel microstructure, where noncovalent crosslinks are breaking and reforming. Furthermore, instabilities caused by the nonequilibrium state arise in some polymer gels; two examples are retrogradation and syneresis.

Retrogradation is the spontaneous reversion of a polymer solution to a gel on standing. Polyvinyl alcohol dissolved in water undergoes retrogradation, whereby the stereoregular chains form microcrystalline aggregates as the solution ages (14). Polyvinyl alcohol gels also retrograde, forming crystalline domains. Amylase, which is the linear polysaccharide fraction of starch, undergoes retrogradation, reducing the physical stability of starch solutions and gels over time.

Syneresis is the process whereby liquid is liberated spontaneously from the gel matrix. This instability arises from the nonequilibrium state of the gel established as it sets or because of a change in external conditions. At equilibrium, elastic contraction forces of polymer chains are usually balanced by solvent swelling forces, resulting from an osmotic pressure differential (27). With changes in temperature, for example, the osmotic pressure shifts, causing an elastic contraction of polymer chains. The contractive response squeezes excess liquid out of the matrix. Agar and carrageenan are examples of gels that exhibit syneresis.

Rheological Properties

Like the transitional physical properties, the rheological properties of gels are not easily characterized because they depend strongly on the attributes of the polymer, history of the gel sample, and experimental conditions. Most often, the apparent viscosity or gel strength increases with an increase in the effective crosslink density of the gel or in the concentration and average molecular weight of the polymer. However, a rise in temperature may increase or decrease the apparent viscosity, depending on the molecular interactions between the polymer and solvent. In addition, the direction of change in apparent viscosity may not be readily predictable when additives such as ions, nonelectrolytes, solvents or nonsolvents, and other compatible polymers are mixed with a gel.

Viscoelasticity

Under an applied stress, which is the force per unit area, ideal liquids flow and perfectly elastic solids deform. The rate of shear, $d\gamma/dt$, is the measure of liquid deformation (flow): viscosity η is a liquid's resistance to flow, strain γ is the measure of solid deformation, and the shear modulus G is the resistance to strain for stresses applied tangentially to the solid's surface. Clearly, gels are semisolids that have both solid and liquid character under stress—they are viscoelastic substances.

Depending on their rheological properties, physically bonded gels can be divided into three groups: entanglement networks, strong gels, and weak gels (24). Entanglement networks behave as dilute solutions when diluted below their critical gelling concentrations, whereas strong gels have stress–strain profiles that include rupture points. Examples of polymers that form entanglement networks are guar gum and hyaluronic acid; strong gels are formed by agar, calcium alginate, gelatin, and pectin.

Weak gels are also entanglement networks, but they undergo specific molecular interactions that increase their strength (24). Therefore, the rheological properties of weak gels are intermediate between those of entanglement networks and strong gels. Xanthan gum and carbomer are examples of polymers that form weak gels. Hyaluronic acid generally forms an entanglement network, but under specific conditions (pH 2.5 and 0.15 M salt), it forms a weak gel (28).

Types of flow

The flow associated with entanglement networks and weak gels can be readily measured with continuous-shear instruments, such as the Ferranti–Shirley cone and-plate viscometer. These instruments characterize the gel behavior over a range of shear rates; a complete rheogram is usually generated for a particular gel in order to identify its flow behavior. If the shear stress versus shear rate curve is concave toward the shear-rate axis, the gel exhibits pseudoplastic flow. The internal gel microstructure breaks down with increases in shear rate, which lowers the apparent viscosity (it "shear-thins" the gel). However, if a gel does not flow at low stresses, but only above a finite stress, it exhibits plastic flow. The yield point, which is a measure of gel strength, is the stress at which flow begins. In general, entanglement networks and weak gels exhibit pseudoplastic and plastic flow, respectively.

Entanglement networks and weak gels may exhibit thixotropy, or time-dependent flow, in addition to exhibiting either pseudoplastic or plastic flow. Thixotropy, which is noted in a rheogram as a hysteresis loop, occurs because the gel requires a finite time to rebuild its original structure that breaks down during continuous shear measurements. The degree of thixotropy depends on gel type, sample history, and experimental conditions.

Dynamic oscillatory techniques use small-deformation measurements to determine the viscoelastic properties of gels within the linear region. Unlike continuous shear instruments, oscillatory instruments (e.g., the Weissenberg rheogoniometer) have the advantage of not altering the gel microstructure because small deformations are made with a sinusoidally oscillating stress or strain. For an ideal elastic solid, the stress and strain are in phase, whereas for an ideal liquid, the stress and strain have a phase difference of 90°. Viscoelastic materials, including gels, have phase angles between 0 and 90°. The parameters obtained through oscillatory testing are the storage modulus G' which reflects solid-like properties, and the loss modulus G'', which reflects liquid-like properties. These moduli depend on the frequency of oscillation.

Details of both continuous shear and dynamic oscillatory testing of pharmaceutical semisolids, including gels, have been addressed in reviews (29, 30), where the fundamental viscoelastic principles are further developed along with a discussion of data analyses and interpretations.

Rigidity

The modulus of rigidity, or shear modulus (G), is defined as the ratio of shear stress to strain. It is a measure of a gel's ability to resist deformation. The minimum rigidity for a strong gel to resist deformation under its own weight is equal to about $g\rho l$ which is the product of the acceleration due to gravity (g), density (ρ), and a linear dimension (l) of the sample. Therefore, the minimum rigidity is about 100 Pa (10^3 dyn/cm) for a gel sample 1 cm long.

An empirical measure of gel rigidity is the measurement of gelatin gel strength, also known as Bloom strength. The procedure is described in the USP (31). It is the determination in a Bloom gelometer of the gram weight needed to depress a standardized plunger 4 mm into the surface of a 6.67% (w/w) gel after maturing the gel at 10°C for 17 h. The Bloom gelometer, however, has largely been replaced by the Stevens LFRA/Voland Texture Analyzer and the TA.XT2 Texture Analyzer (Micro Systems).

Rupture strength

Rupture strength is equal to the stress at which a strong gel ruptures or fails rather than undergoing further strain. The rupture strength is determined by large-deformation measurements on instruments such as the Instron tester, where a tensile stress is applied to the sample. However, strong gel samples can only be tested in tension if they can support their own weight (24), and most physically crosslinked gels are relatively weak, making this type of test difficult.

GEL-FORMING SUBSTANCES AND THEIR PHARMACEUTICAL USES

Gel-forming hydrophilic polymers are typically used to prepare lipid-free semisolid dosage forms, including dental, dermatological, nasal, ophthalmic, rectal, and vaginal gels and jellies. Gel vehicles containing therapeutic agents are especially useful for application to mucous membranes and ulcerated or burned tissues because their high water content reduces irritancy. Furthermore, these hydrophilic gels are easily removed by gentle rinsing or natural flushing with body fluids, reducing the propensity for mechanical abrasion. The superior optical clarity of synthetic polymer gels, such as those composed of poloxamer and carbomer, has led to the current interest in developing therapeutic ophthalmic gels.

Unconventional routes of drug administration by using gels and jellies are also being explored. Thus, two nasal jellies were developed and marketed. The intranasal vitamin B-12 gel, Nascobal (Schwarz Pharma), is used as a dietary supplement. The gel base is composed of a hydrophilic cellulose derivative, the exact nature of which is not disclosed. However, the gel is apparently odorless and nonirritating, and adheres well to the mucous

membrane. Neo-Synephrine Viscous (Sanofi Winthrop) is a water-soluble nasal jelly formulated with methylcellulose; it contains the decongestant phenylephrine hydrochloride.

In addition to serving as drug-containing vehicles, some gels have other important functions. For example, a soft, flexible gel applied to burned skin can prevent excessive water loss by forming a physical barrier. Ocular gel inserts are designed to lubricate the eye continuously and promote healing. Still other gels are intended for lubricating surgical and medical instruments in order to minimize local irritation.

Many gel-forming substances are available for preparing pharmaceutical gels and jellies. Although these substances share some common physical characteristics, the intended use may require gelling attributes of a certain substance or blend of substances. Table 3 lists the favorable properties of pharmaceutical gels for particular applications.

Proteins

Collagen

Collagen is the major connective tissue protein in animals. The collagen molecule is considered to be a block copolymer, formed with blocks of glycine (33%) and proline and hydroxyproline (23%), between blocks of the remaining amino acids (44%). Tropocollagen is the asymmetrical subunit of collagen, which is made up of three peptide chains wound in a triple helix. The nonhelical portions of collagen, so-called telopeptides, are susceptible to enzyme digestion. Native collagen is insoluble in water, but 2% to 3% may be solubilized in dilute acidic solutions. Collagen may also be solubilized by treatment with proteolytic enzymes, which digest the telopeptide portions (e.g., Vitrogen, Collagen Corp.).

The asymmetrical molecular structure of collagen permits the formation of rigid gels; highly rigid structures are obtained at 0.1% concentration by UV irradiation or chemical crosslinking with aldehydes (32). These gels are used as biomaterials for vitreous replacements. Pepsin-solubilized collagen forms clear, rigid gels; they are prepared with a 0.2% to 0.4% collagen solution, which consists of unassociated molecules and small fibrils when cooled to ~5°C. As the temperature is raised to 37°C, the collagen molecules aggregate, forming subfibrils that further aggregate to form the gel network (33). The rigidity is then increased by lightly crosslinking with aldehydes.

Optically clear collagen gels have been considered for use in ophthalmic drug delivery. Ocular inserts of succinylated or methylated collagen are patented as soluble

Table 3   Pharmaceutical gels

Applications	Favorable properties
Dental	Highly thixotropic
	Optimal viscosity for filling fissures
	Adherent to enamel surfaces
	Optically clear
	Water soluble
	Orally digestible
Dermatological	Thixotropic
	Good spreadability
	Greaseless (especially for acne preparations)
	Easily removed
	Emollient
	Demulcent (especially for abraded tissue)
	Nonstaining
	Compatible with a number of excipients
	Water soluble *or* miscible
Nasal	Adherent
	Odorless
	Nonirritating
	Water soluble
Ophthalmic	Optically clear
	Sterile
	Mucomimetic
	Lubricating
	Demulcent
	Nonirritating or nonsensitizing
	Water soluble or miscible
Surgical and medical procedures	Lubricating
	Adherent to instrument surfaces
	Maximal contact with mucous membranes
	Nonirritating
Vaginal	Acid stable
	Adherent
	Does not liquify at body temperature
	Slow dissolving
	Lubricating
	Greaseless and nontacky
	Nonirritating

devices for drug delivery (34). Constant, controlled release of pilocarpine hydrochloride was maintained for 5 to 15 days with crosslinked collagen and other collagen-derivative inserts (35). A corneal shield made of non-crosslinked collagen is marketed as Bio-Cor by Bausch & Lomb. This shield is placed over an eye injury and, as collagen slowly dissolves, the cornea is continuously lubricated to promote healing. Collagen implants (Lacri-medics) are also used for relief of dry eye by partially blocking tear removing canals; the implants dissolve within 7 to 10 days. Collagen gels are also used in hemostasis. A lightly crosslinked sterile pad, Instat hemostat (Johnson & Johnson), assists in forming blood clots to arrest bleeding during surgery.

Gelatin

Gelatin is denatured collagen, which is hydrolytically degraded under acid or alkaline conditions to produce Type A or B gelatins, respectively. The amino acid content of acid-processed gelatin is virtually identical to that of collagen, yielding an isoelectric point, pI, between 8 and 9. In contrast, alkaline processing reduces the ratio of amide groups to carboxyl groups, thereby shifting the pI to about 4 or 5.

Gelatin forms elastic gels reversibly by cooling solutions that contain a sufficient concentration. The gel microstructure consists of a three-dimensional network held together by junction zones in which gelatin chains have partly refolded into the triple helix of the parent collagen molecule (36). The physical properties associated with gelatin gels depend on protein concentration, average molecular weight, temperature, pH, and additives (37).

The swelling kinetics of uncrosslinked type B gelatin films in the absence (38) and presence of additives (39) was studied. The water-swelling kinetics of chemically crosslinked matrices (40) were considered for controlling the release of therapeutic agents. Heat-crosslinked gelatin matrices were also examined for drug release (41). Both, the molecular weight between crosslinks, M_c, and the mesh size between crosslinks, ζ, were used to characterize gelatin gel matrices (42) during release of the macromolecular solute dextran. The crosslinking extent and density in gelatin matrices was directly determined by chemical analysis of the uncrosslinked primary amino groups and compared with swelling parameters of crosslinking (10).

Although gelatin has been used by the pharmaceutical industry for mainly producing soft and hard gelatin capsules, some commercial products use a hydrated gel form. The sterile product, H.P. Acthar Gel (Rorer), contains 16% gelatin for sustaining the release of adrenocorticotropic hormone from an intramuscular or subcutaneous injection. A sterile, absorbable gelatin sponge, Gelfoam (UpJohn), which has a lightly crosslinked matrix, is used during surgery to absorb blood and promote clotting. An absorbable gelatin film, Gelfilm Ophthalmic (Upjohn), is available for use in ocular surgery. The ocular implant requires 2 to 5 months for complete absorption.

Polysaccharides

Alginates

Alginic acid is processed from brown seaweed, using a dilute acid, followed by alkalinization with soda ash to yield the water-soluble salt form, sodium alginate. Alginic acid is a linear glycuronoalycan composed of polymannuronic acid blocks (M), polygluuronic acid blocks (G), and mixed blocks of these two uronic acids (MG) (43). The gelling properties and gel microstructure of the various salt forms of alginic acid depend on the M, G, and MG block content. High-M alginates form turbid, weak gels, and high-G alginates form transparent, brittle gels. Gelation depends on the cation type; sodium alginate gels are water-soluble, whereas calcium alginate gels are insoluble, yet swell in water. Many "egg box" junction zones are formed by calcium cations and G blocks to create such rigid gel networks.

Sodium and calcium alginate are used in commercial pharmaceutical formulations. Sodium alginate gels have superior spreading and lubricating properties; they are also nontacky and tasteless, and have emollient qualities. Moreover, sodium alginate is compatible with many compounds such as starch, sodium carboxymethylcellulose, pectin, carrageenan, 25% ethanol, 4% sodium chloride, and most alkali salts (44). Taking advantage of this compatibility and the favorable gel properties, sodium alginate is formulated with sodium carboxymethyl cellulose in the nonirritating, water-soluble lubricating jelly, Ortho Personal Lubricant (Ortho). Calcium alginate is used as a wound dressing for varicose and decubitus ulcers (45), where it forms a hydrophilic gel over the wound by absorbing exudate, which promotes healing. The high rigidities of calcium alginate gels make them suitable for preparing dental impressions and as matrix barriers for controlling drug delivery (46). Theophyline release was studied from granules coated with sodium alginate and calcium lactate through insoluble gel formation (47).

Carrageenan

Carrageenan, a sulfated polysaccharide extracted from red seaweed, may be separated into a number of fractions depending on the species, season, and environment. The three major fractions, lambda-, iota-, and kappa (κ)-carrageenan, contain an alternating sequence of $(1 \rightarrow 4)$-linked (β-D-galactopyranosyl and $(1 \rightarrow 3)$-linked α-D-galactopyranosyl residues, but they differ in the degree and sites of sulfation (48). Of these three fractions, only lambda-carrageenan cannot form gels.

Under optimal ionic strength and polymer concentration, κ-carrageenan forms rigid, thermoreversible gels in the presence of cations. The elastic moduli of these gels depend on the type of cation and follow the Hofmeister series: $Cs^+ > Rb^+ > K^+ \gg Na^+ > Li^+$. The κ-carrageenan gel also undergoes syneresis, the spontaneous liberation of liquid from the matrix. Early models for gelation envisioned multihelical junction zones composed of polysaccharide chains folded into double helices. This model was extended to accommodate cations in that the formation of the helical domains would require mediation by the cations themselves (49). However, other researchers propose (50) an indirect role for cations in which they alter solvent structure around the κ-carrageenan helices, thereby inducing gel formation. Differential scanning calorimetry and isothermal titration calorimetry were used to study mono- and divalent cation binding and induced conformation changes in κ-carrageenan (51).

Gels made with κ-carrageenan and potassium ions have excellent lubricity and emollient properties. Because of such favorable gelling characteristics, these gels are used as vehicles for the topical administration of drugs and as gelling agents in other pharmaceutical preparations. They can also be used in combination with sodium carboxymethylcellulose, which interferes with gel formation resulting in a variety of consistencies and textures. Theophylline and diclofenac sodium release were studied from tablet matrices containing κ-carrageenan and iota-carrageenan with KCl or CaCl$_2$ (52).

Hyaluronic acid

Hyaluronic acid is a linear glycosaminoglycan (an aminopolysaccharide), which is an important component of synovial fluid and the cellular matrix of connective tissue. It comprises a biological gel that supports cells, maintains tissue hydration, and functions as a lubricant and shock absorbent in joints (53). Hyaluronic acid forms transparent, rigid gels at 2% concentration, although they are not as rigid as agar and carrageenan gels. The gel microstructure is constructed by entanglement couplings among the long polysaccharide chains, which have molecular weights ranging from about 1×10^6 to 4×10^6 Da, depending on the source of animal tissue.

A 1% viscoelastic jelly of the sodium salt is commercially available as Healon (Kabi Pharmacia), which is widely employed in ophthalmic surgery. Sodium hyaluronate jelly provides a nonirritating viscoelastic medium for separating tissues during surgery and prevents postoperative adhesion formation (53). Investigators in a clinical trial of intraarticular injections of 500–730 kDa sodium hyaluronate (Hyalgan, Sanofi) for osteoarthritis concluded that this treatment might delay the structural progression of the disease (54). When hyaluronic acid was tested as an ophthalmic gel (55), its mucoadhesive properties improved the ocular bioavailability of tropicamide.

Pectins

Pectins are a complex group of polysaccharides, the structures of which vary with plant source. They are heteropolysaccharides that are extracted from apple pomace and citrus fruit rinds and consist mainly of polygalacturonic acids. The degree of esterification determines the gelation process and, hence, the eventual commercial use. High-methoxy (HM) pectin gels in the presence of high concentrations of sucrose at acidic pH. The sucrose dehydrates pectin to a gel. High-methoxy pectins are used in sweet food products such as fruit jams and preserves.

In contrast, low-methoxy (LM) pectins gel in the presence of divalent cations, especially calcium, by the "egg box" mechanism proposed for alginates. Moreover, calcium pectinate gels prepared at neutral pH are heat stable, whereas acidic pH gels are thermoreversible (56). Gel strength depends on the extent of esterification (levels from 30% to 50% are optimal), the distribution of ester groups on the chain, and the average molecular weight. LM pectins have been used traditionally in antidiarrheal formulations with kaolin. HM pectins were evaluated in controlled release matrix formulations (57). Pectin microspheres were reported to improve ophthalmic bioavailability of piroxicam in rabbits compared with commercial piroxicam eye drops (58).

Starch

Starch is the principal polysaccharide of higher plants and can be extracted from a number of sources, including corn, wheat, and potato. Starch granules can be fractionated into two structurally distinct polysaccharides: 30% amylose (linear polymer) and 80% amylopectin (branched polymer). Starch is insoluble in cold water because of extensive hydrogen bonding between polysaccharide chains. However, the hydrogen bonds break at temperatures above the gelatinization range of 60°C to 70°C, allowing the granules to swell. The starch sol can then form a gel on cooling. The type of gel depends on the starch species; corn starch forms opaque, rigid gels, whereas potato starch forms clear, nonrigid gels (59).

The microstructure of starch gels is an example of a matrix strengthened by filler. Heating causes the amylopectin granules to become swollen and porous, whereas the linear amylose chains dissolve. As the solution cools, amylose sets into a gel matrix that threads through the porous amylopectin granules, thereby producing a reinforced gel (60).

Aqueous starch solutions exhibit retrogradation in which crystalline aggregates form spontaneously over time with Brownian movement. As the solution ages, it becomes opalescent, followed by the gradual precipitation of starch. Starch gels are also unstable because of the formation of crystalline aggregates; however, they undergo syneresis. The amylose fraction is responsible for these instabilities; amylose chains are linear, enabling them to become parallel in order to form aggregates. Starch has been used extensively as a pharmaceutical excipient in tablets, serving as a filler, binder, and disintegrant. Starch gels have found limited use as skin emollients. Starch has been examined as a mucoadhesive in microparticles to improve protein uptake across the nasal mucosa (61).

Table 4 Miscellaneous polysaccharide gelling agents and their uses

Agent	Notes	Product or experimental use	Ref.
Agar	Soluble at > 90°C	Molecular structure	(62)
	Rigid gel from ~0.1%	Bulk laxative	(63)
	Multihelical juntion zones	Rectal administration of insulin	(64)
		Suppository base with NaCMC	(65)
Gellan gum	Good optical clarity	Timoptic-XE (Gelrite; Merck)	
	Forms gels with cations	In situ gelling polymer for ophthalmic delivery	(66)
Glycyrrhiza	Gels are pseudoplastic and thixotropic	Enhanced colon calcitonin absorption	(67)
	Efficient bitter taste masker	Vehicle for antiviral idoxuridine	(68)
Guar gum	Liquifaction at <pH 7		(69)
	Nonionic	Sustained release of quinidine sulfate	(70)
	Binds free water to eliminate syneresis	Colon specific drug carrier	(71)
Tragacanth gum	Acid stable (pH ~ 2)		(72)
	Restore vaginal acidity	Aci-Jel (Ortho)	
	Gel vehicle	Ephedrine sulfate jelly, USP	

Miscellaneous carbohydrates

Table 4 lists less frequently used agents and a few notes about their properties. Also listed are products or experimental uses and references.

Semisynthetic Polymers (Cellulose Derivatives)

Carboxymethylcellulose, sodium

Sodium carboxymethylcellulose (NaCMC) is a carboxymethyl ether of cellulose, the ubiquitous polysaccharide composing the fibrous tissue of plants. The hydroxyl groups on the 2-glucopyranose residues of cellulose are replaced by carboxymethyl groups; the number of replacements is known as the degree of substitution DS. Both the DS and polymer chain length determine the solubility, viscosity, and gel strength of NaCMC. It dissolves in water and mixtures of water with the lower alcohols and glycerin. Aqueous gels are stable from pH 2 to 10 but susceptible to microbial growth.

The microstructure of NaCMC gels was examined on freeze-fractured samples with a transmission electron microscope (73). A fine, quasi-crystalline structure consisting of filaments with thicknesses of 2 to 3 nm was identified. These filaments are microaggregates of individual polymer chains. The rigidity of NaCMC gels can be increased by adding multivalent cations such as Al^{3+} or Fe^{2+}, resulting in ionic bridges between the cations and ionized carboxyl groups (74). These gels are stable indefinitely.

Because of its acid stability, NaCMC is suitable for therapeutic vaginal gels. The base of Ortho-Gynol contraceptive jelly (Ortho) is formulated with NaCMC, water, and propylene glycol and adjusted to pH 4.5 with acetic acid. NaCMC also composes the gel base of Glutose (Paddock), which contains 40% dextrose and is used to treat hypoglycemia. In a study of NaCMC gels as the vehicle for a recombinant human platelet-derived growth factor for treatment of non healing diabetic ulcers, the gel vehicle alone was reported to have a higher healing rate compared to good wound care alone (75).

Hydroxypropyl cellulose

Hydroxypropyl cellulose is produced by substituting propylene oxide for hydroxyl groups on alkalized cellulose. This cellulosic derivative is soluble in cold water and many polar organic solvents such as methanol, ethanol, isopropanol, and propylene glycol (76). The alcohol solubility increases with increasing degrees of hydroxypropyl substitution. Aqueous preparations of hydroxypropyl cellulose are susceptible to hydrolysis (acid unstable); therefore, a pH of 6 to 8 provides optimum stability. Photodegradation and limited biological degradation may also occur.

Hydroxypropyl cellulose gels on heating and forms thermoreversible gels. The pharmaceutical gel products containing hydroxypropyl cellulose take advantage of its compatibility with alcohol. The microviscosity of hydroxypropyl cellulose gels was evaluated for prediction of drug diffusion rates (77). Examples of commercial products with alcoholic and hydroalcoholic gel bases are given in Table 5.

Table 5 Pharmaceutical gel products containing hydroxypropyl cellulose or hydroxypropyl methylcellulose

Brand name	Manufacturer	Therapeutic agent; activity	Alcohol content (%)
Hydroxypropyl cellulose			
Compound W Gel	Whitehall	Salicylic acid; keratolytic	67.5
DuoPlant Gel	Schering-Plough	Salicylic acid; keratolytic	57.6
Erygel	Herbert	Erythromycin; antibiotic for acne	92
Hydrisalic Gel	Pedinol	Salicylic acid; keratolytic	100
Keralyt Gel	Summers	Salicylic acid; keratolytic	19.4
Lacrisert Insert	Merck & Co.	Hydroxypropyl cellulose; lubricant	0
Retin-A Gel	Ortho	Retinoic acid; antiacne	90
Hydroxypropyl methylcellulose			
ArthriCare Triple-Medicated Gel	Commerce	Methyl salicylate; menthol, methyl nicotinate; liniment	
Persa-Gel W	Ortho Derm	Benzoyl peroxide; antibacterial	
Xylocaine Jelly	Astra	Lidocaine HCl; anesthetic	

Hydroxypropyl methylcellulose

Hydroxypropyl methylcellulose (HPMC) is produced similarly to hydroxypropyl cellulose except that methyl chloride is included in the reaction. The composition of the substituted hydroxyl groups ranges from 3% to 12% hydroxypropyl and from 19% to 30% methyl. HPMC is soluble in cold water and the polyethylene glycols up to 600 Da, but, in contrast to hydroxypropyl cellulose, HPMC is not soluble in alcohol. It is also less susceptible to hydrolysis, and is stable from pH 3 to 11.

Aqueous gels are formed on heating; the gel point ranges from 50°C to 90°C, depending on the grade (78). Addition of small amounts of water-miscible solvent, such as ethanol and the glycols, raises the gel point. Examples of HPMC-based pharmaceutical gels that contain only water are included in Table 3. The good lubricating and adherent qualities of HPMC gels are exploited in Xylocaine 2% Jelly (Astra), which is used to minimize discomfort associated with medical procedures. A 2% solution (80 kDa) is commercially available as an ophthalmic surgical aid (OcuCoat; Storz). The influence of indomethacin, propranolol HCl, and tetracycline HCl was studied on the properties and swelling characteristics of matrix gels containing hydroxypropyl methylcellulose and methylcellulose (79).

Methylcellulose

Methylcellulose is a cellulose ether in which methyl groups have been substituted for hydroxyl groups on the 2-glucopyranose residues. It is soluble in cold water at low methoxy contents; increased substitution increases the solubility in hydroalcoholic and alcoholic solutions (80).

Aqueous solutions of methylcellulose gel on heating, whereby micelle-like junction zones form throughout the network. Gel strength and gelling temperature depend on the concentration, degrees of substitution, and average molecular weight. The gelling temperature can be lowered by adding sugar or most electrolytes, which reduce polymer hydration.

High viscosity grades of methylcellulose are used in pharmaceutical gels. The gels are demulcent and have good surfactant properties, which permit easy spreading on body tissues. Therefore, methylcellulose gels are used as dressings for burned tissue because they minimize water loss and are easily removed. The high viscosity grades are used in ophthalmic preparations such as Murocel artificial tears (Bausch & Lomb) and Neo-Synephrine viscous solution (Sanofi Winthrop). Other pharmaceutical applications include the bulk-forming laxative, Citrucel (SK-Beecham), and lubricating jellies for surgical and medical procedures. A methylcellulose gel was investigated for topical administration of tetracycline HCl (81). The bioadhesive properties of 3% methylcellulose gels on slowing mucociliary clearance were examined using a rate model (82).

Synthetic Polymers

Carbomer

Carbomer is a synthetic polyacrylic acid resin, which is copolymerized with about 0.75 to 2% polyalkylsucrose (83). This is the reason why aqueous dispersions of carbomer must be protected against microbial growth. Carbomer is a high molecular weight polymer that contains carboxylic acid groups on about two thirds of its repeat units. Gels are formed on neutralization between pH 5 and 10 with metal hydroxides or amines such as diisopropanolamine and triethanolamine. Neutralization expands the long chains of carbomer by charge repulsion to produce an entangled gel network. Because electrostatic repulsion plays a critical role in forming a gel, viscosity and gel strength depend on both pH and salt content.

The molecular size of carbomer is important in determining gel properties and applications. Carbomer 934 and 940, with average molecular weights of 3×10^6 and 4×10^6 Da, respectively, are most commonly used by the pharmaceutical industry. Both grades have favorable rheological properties for topical applications; the gels undergo plastic flow (84) and have temperature-stable viscosities (85). The gels can be formulated with large quantities of alcohol, but the alcohol dehydrates the polymer network and lowers the viscosity. Ostrenga et al. conducted a systematic investigation of propylene glycol/water vehicles gelled with 1% carbomer to optimize percutaneous absorption of fluocinolone acetonide and fluocinonide (86). These investigators showed under specified conditions that an increasing partition coefficient of the steroid between the vehicle and isopropyl myristate increased the uptake of drug into the skin. These studies laid the ground for commercial use of such gels for a range of steroids.

Carbomer is also compatible with dimethyl sulfoxide. The veterinary product, Domoso (Syntex Veterinary Labs), is a topical gel consisting of carbomer 934 and 90% dimethyl sulfoxide. Carbomer 940 gels exhibit superior optical clarity compared with 934 gels (87), and can be used in ophthalmic preparations. However, only carbomer 934 is approved for internal use. The mucoadhesive properties of carbomer were studied with triamcinolone acetonide (88), with acyclovir (89, 90) and to improve protein uptake across the nasal mucosa (61). Pharmaceutical gel products containing carbomer in their formulations are listed in Table 6. All are dermatological gels except for Anbesol Gel (Whitehall) and Pilopine HS (Alcon).

Poloxamer

Poloxamer is the generic name for a series of block copolymers that are composed of one polypropylene oxide block sandwiched between polyethylene oxide blocks. For example, poloxamer 188 can be written as $(PEO)_{75}$-$(PPO)_{30}$-$(PEO)_{75}$. The poloxamers serve as high molecular weight surfactants because the PEO blocks are hydrophilic, whereas the PPO blocks are hydrophobic.

At relatively high concentrations (>20%), poloxamers form thermoreversible gels; however, they gel on heating rather than cooling The amphiphilic nature supports the

Table 6 Pharmaceutical gel products containing carbomer

Brand name	Manufacturer	Therapeutic agent; activity
Carbomer 934		
Anbesol Gel	Whitehall	Benzocaine, anesthetic; antiseptic
Cleocin T Gel	Upjohn	Clindamycin; antibiotic for acne
Persa-Gel W	Ortho	Benzoyl peroxide; antibacterial
Therapeutic Mineral Ice Gel	Bristol-Meyers	Menthol; liniment
Ben-Gay Vanishing Scent Gel	Pfizer	Menthol, camphor; liniment
Sportsman Ice Gel	Thompson	Menthol; liniment
Carbomer 940		
Benzac W	Galderma	Benzoyl peroxide; antibacterial
Benzagel	Dermik	Benzoyl peroxide; antibacterial
Benzamycin	Dermik	Erythromycin, benzoyl peroxide; antibiotic, antibacterial
Desquam-X 5	Westwood Squibb	Benzoyl peroxide; antibacterial
Double Ice ArthriCare Gel	Commerce	Menthol, camphor, liniment
Estar Gel	Westwood Squibb	Coal tar; antipsoriosis
Flex-all 454 Gel	Chattam	Menthol, methyl salicyliate; liniment
Lidex Gel	Syntex	Fluocinonide; anti-inflammatory
Ordor Free ArthriCare Rub	Commerce	Menthol, methyl nicotinate, capsaicin; liniment
Persa-Gel	Ortho Derm	Benzoyl peroxide; antibacterial
Pilopine HS	Alcon	Pilocarpine HCl; miotic
PrameGel	GenDerm	Pramoxine HCl; antipruitic
Topicort Gel	Hoecht Marion Roussell	Desoximetasone; anti-inflammatory

gelling mechanism of poloxamers, where micelle-like junction zones form at or above room temperature. The junction zones consist of large populations of micelle-like structures, which apparently form a viscous, liquid crystalline phase (91, 92). Poloxamers can also form gels in dilute hydroalcoholic solutions.

Poloxamer gels have many characteristics favorable for use as artificial skin, which is helpful in treating third-degree burns. The gels are nontoxic, enhance healing by controlling water, heat, and electrolyte loss, and provide detergent activity on wound debris (93). Because of poloxamer's inverted thermoreversibility, cool solutions can be poured onto damaged tissue, forming gels when warmed to body temperature. The gels are easily removed by rinsing with cool water.

Poloxamer gels mimic mucus and are optically clear, which makes them suitable for ophthalmic drug delivery. A poloxamer gel formulation containing pilocarpine showed improved bioavailability over an aqueous solution of the drug (94). Release kinetics of lidocaine (91), diclofenac (95), and hydrocortisone (95) from topical poloxamer gels were also assessed. Subcutaneous injection of insulin loaded poloxamer gels prolonged the hypoglycemic effect of insulin in rats (95). Commercial topical gels include AquaTar (Allergan Herbert), a poloxamer-407 base that contains coal tar, and Benzac W (Galderma), a blend of poloxamer-182 and carbomer-940 gels, that contains benzoyl peroxide.

Polyacrylamide

Polyacrylamide (PAAm) is a hydrophilic polymer that absorbs and retains large volumes of water. However, aqueous solutions of PAAm, especially the high molecular weight species, undergo physical aging, which results in a decrease in viscosity. PAAm is soluble in hydrophilic nonaqueous liquids such as glycerol, but insoluble in methanol and ethanol.

Polyacrylamide forms water-based gels at concentrations around 4% w/v, which exhibit pseudoplastic behavior. A PAAm ophthalmic gel containing pilocarpine was compared with other gel vehicles; the ocular bioavailability for the PAAm gel was three times greater than that of the aqueous control solution (97). The kinetics of ibuprofen release for crosslinked PAAm gels was studied (98). A kinetic model was proposed for swelling induced loading of insulin into crosslinked PAAm gels (99).

Polyvinyl alcohol

Polyvinyl alcohol (PVA) is a hydrophilic, synthetic polymer that is prepared indirectly by hydrolyzing polyvinyl acetate. It cannot be produced by direct polymerization of vinyl alcohol because the monomer is unstable (100). The chemical structure of PVA is simple, consisting of a carbon-chain backbone with alternating hydroxyl groups; it favors the formation of crystalline aggregates in solutions, gels, and solids. PVA is soluble in water, glycerin, and mixtures of water with the lower alcohols; however, it can be precipitated from aqueous solutions with sulfates and phosphates. The gelation of PVA occurs in more concentrated solutions; the gel point of 10% PVA in water is around 14°C (101). In general, gel strength depends on the degree of crystallinity of a particular sample.

Polyvinyl alcohol is used in ophthalmic preparations, serving as a mucus mimicking (mucomimetic) agent in artificial-tear formulations such as Liquifilm Tears and Liquifilm Forte (Allergan). Physically crosslinked PVA hydrogels, prepared by low-temperature crystallization, were tested as vehicles for the rectal administration of indomethacin (102). Chemically crosslinked PVA hydrogels have been considered for soft contact lenses. Both, the molecular weight between crosslinks, M_c, and the mesh size between crosslinks, ζ, were used to characterize a covalently crosslinked polyvinyl alcohol gel (8) during evaluation of bovine serum albumin (BSA) release. PVA hydrogel nanoparticles loaded with albumin into poly-lactic/glycolic acid microspheres released albumin up to two months (103). The release of water-soluble pseudo-ephedrine was studied from compressed swellable-soluble PVA matrices (104).

Inorganic Substances

Aluminum hydroxide

Aluminum hydroxide forms a two-phase gel consisting of a network of discrete solid particles in water. Aluminum hydroxide gels are soluble in acidic and extremely basic media, and are compatible with many additives, including glycerin, saccharin, and some preservatives (105).

The aluminum hydroxide gel exhibits thixotropic behavior. In addition, gel stability is enhanced by polyols such as mannitol and sorbitol (106). However, unlike other gels, aluminum hydroxide gels do not have demulcent properties; they are used mainly as an oral antacid preparations.

Smectite clays

Bentonite and hectorite clays consist primarily of hydrated aluminum and magnesium silicates, respectively. Bentonite is recognized for its swelling capacity; one gram can absorb up to 11 ml of water. A commonly used smectite clay is aluminum magnesium silicate (Veegum, R.T. Vanderbilt Co.). These clays have plate-like particles, 1 to 2 μm in size, that form well-ordered gel mesophases spontaneously on contact with water. The gels are formed at about 5% concentration, and are presumably stabilized by opposite electrostatic charges between particle edges and faces (21). Therefore, these smectite gels are incompatible with strong electrolytes, and in particular with di- and trivalent cations. The gels also exhibit plastic flow; they have static yield values and are thixotropic.

Laponite clay also belongs to the smectite class, but is a synthetic gelling agent. Like bentonite, laponite swells considerably in water—but only a 2% concentration is needed to form a gel. Laponite does not contain impurities, which is an advantage over the natural clays; however, some electrolyte must be included in the water to support the gel microstructure (107).

Smectite clays are used by the pharmaceutical industry as mainly suspending and thickening agents. Because of the net negative charge of these clays, cationic drugs can be adsorbed by an ion-exchange mechanism. Release of metronidazole from bentonite complexes was inhibited at acidic pH, but increased significantly at pH 7 (108). Simple gels containing hectorite and gelatin were investigated for rectally administrating insulin to rabbits (109). Finally, the iontophoretic transdermal transport of calcium from a paste of calcium-enriched bentonite was studied using excised pig skin (110).

REFERENCES

1. *Webster's Seventh New Collegiate Dictionary*; Merriam: Springfield, MA, 1971.
2. Flory, P.J. Discuss. Faraday Soc. **1974**, *57*, 7.
3. *The United States Pharmacopeia 24/The National Formulary 19*; Pharmacopeial Convention: Rockville, MD, 2000; 2111–2112.
4. Peppas, N.A. *Hydrogels in Medicine and Pharmacy*; CRC Press: Boca Raton, FL, 1987; I.
5. Peppas, N.A. *Hydrogels in Medicine and Pharmacy*; CRC Press: Boca Raton, FL, 1987; II.
6. Peppas, N.A. *Hydrogels in Medicine and Pharmacy*; Peppas, N.A., Ed.; CRC Press: Boca Raton, FL, 1987; III.
7. Alger, M.S.M. *Polymer Science Dictionary*; Elsevier Applied Science: London, 1989; 69.
8. Gander, B.; Gurny, R.; Doelker, E.; Peppas, N.A. Pharm. Res **1989**, *6*, 578–584.
9. Bray, J.C.; Merrill, E.W. J. Appl. Polym. Sci. **1973**, *17*, 3779–3794.
10. Ofner, C.M., III; Bubnis, B.A. Pharm. Res. **1992**, *13*, 1821–1827.
11. Bryce, T.A.; McKinnon, A.A.; Morris, E.R.; Rees, D.A.; Thom, D. Discuss. Faraday Soc. **1974**, *67*, 331.
12. Rees, D.A. Adv. Carbohydr. Chem. Biochem. **1969**, *24*, 267.
13. deButts, E.H.; Hudy, J.A.; Elliot, J.H. Ind. Eng. Chem. **1957**, *49*, 94.
14. Nagy, M. Colloid Polym. Sci. **1985**, *263*, 245.
15. Vadnere, M.; Amidon, G.; Lindenbaum, S.; Haslam, J.L. Int. J. Pharm. **1984**, *32*, 207.
16. Grant, G.T.; Morris, E.R.; Rees, D.A.; Smith, P.J.C.; Thom, D. FE.B.S. Lett. **1973**, *32*, 1.
17. Noble, O.; Turquois, T.; Taravel, F.R. Carbohydr. Polym. **1990**, *12*, 203.
18. Laurent, T.C. *Chemistry and Molecular Biology of the Intercellular Matrix*; Balazs, E.A., Ed.; Academic Press: New York, 1970; 2, 703.
19. Tanaka, F. Macromolecules **1990**, *23*, 3790.
20. van Olphen, H. *An Introduction to Clay Colloid Chemistry*; Interface Publishers: New York, 1963; 67–68.
21. Schott, H. J. Colloid Interface Sci. **1968**, *26*, 133–139.
22. Barry, M.D.; Rowe, R.C. Int. J. Pharm **1989**, *53*, 139.
23. Tiemessen, H.L.G.M.; Bodde', H.E.; van Mourik, C.; Junginger, H.E. Progr. Colloid Polym. Sci. **1988**, *77*, 131.
24. Clark, A.H.; Ross-Murphy, S.B. Adv. Polym. Sci. **1987**, *83*, 57.
25. Eldridge, J.E.; Ferry, J.D. J. Phys. Chem. **1954**, *58*, 975.
26. Florence, A.T.; Atwood, D. *Physicochemical Principles of Pharmacy*; Chapman and Hall: New York, 282.
27. Florence, A.T.; Atwood, D. *Physicochemical Principles of Pharmacy*; Chapman and Hall: New York, 285.
28. Gibbs, D.A.; Merrill, E.W.; Smith, K.A.; Balazs, E.A. Biopolymers. **1968**, *6*, 777.
29. Barry, B.W. *Dermatological Formulations: Percutaneous Absorption*; Marcel Dekker, Inc.: New York, 1983.
30. Schott, H. Rheology. *Remington: The Science and Practice of Pharmacy*; Gennaro, A.R., Ed.; Mack: Easton, PA, 1995.
31. *The United States Pharmacopeia 24/The National Formulary 19*; Pharmacopeial Convention: Rockville, MD, 2000; 2049.
32. Stenzel, K.H.; Miyata, T.; Rubin, A.L. Annu. Rev. Biophys. Bioeng. **1974**, *3*, 255.
33. Wallace, D.G.; Condell, R.A.; Donovan, J.W.; Paivinen, A.; Rhee, W.M.; Wade, S.B. Biopolymers. **1986**, *25*, 1875.
34. Miyata, T; Rubin, A.L.; Stenzel, K.H.; Dunn, M.W. U.S. Patent. 4,164,559, 1979
35. Vasanthra, R.; Sehgal, P.K.; Rao, K.P. Int. J. Pharm. **1988**, *47*, 95.
36. Veis, A. *Macromolecular Chemistry of Gelatin*; Academic Press: New York, 1964.
37. Ward, A.G.; Courts, A. *The Science and Technology of Gelatin*; Academic Press: New York, 1977.
38. Ofner, C.M., III; Schott, H. J. Pharm. Sci. **1986**, *75*, 790–796.
39. Ofner, C.M., III; Schott, H. J. Pharm. Sci. **1987**, *76*, 715–723.
40. Klech, C.M.; Li, X. J. Pharm. Sci. **1990**, *79*, 999.
41. Welz, M.M.; Ofner, C.M., III. J. Pharm. Sci. **1992**, *81*, 85–90.
42. Mwangi, J.W. *Ph.D. Dissertation*; University of the Sciences in Philadelphia: 2001.
43. Morris, V.J. Gelation of Polysaccharides. *Functional Properties of Food Macromolecules*; Mitchell, J.R.,

Ledward, D.A., Eds.; Elsevier Applied Science: London, 1986, 123.

44. Cottrell, I.W.; Kovacs, P. Algin. *Food Colloids*; Graham, H.D., Ed.; AVI: Westport, CT, 1977; 450.
45. Thomas, S. Pharm. J. **1985**, *235*, 188.
46. Julian, T.N.; Radehaugh, G.W.; Wisniewski, S.J. J. Contr. Release **1988**, *7*, 165.
47. Kaneko, K.; Kanada, K.; Oouchi, K.; Saito, N.; Ozeiki, T. Arch. Pract. Pharm. **1999**, *59*, 8–16.
48. Kennedy, J.F.; White, C.A. *Bioactive Carbohydrates in Chemistry, Biochemistry, and Biology*; Ellis Horwood: Chichester, UK, 1983; 163.
49. Morris, E.R.; Rees, D.A.; Robinson, G.R. J. Mol. Biol. **1980**, *138*, 349.
50. Morris, V.J.; Chilvers, G.R. Carbohydr. Polym. **1983**, *3*, 129.
51. Winstead, D.A. *Ph.D. Dissertation*; Philadelphia College of Pharmacy and Science: 1997.
52. Picker, K.M. Drug Dev. Ind. Pharm. **1999**, *25*, 339–346.
53. Balazs, E.A.; Band, P. Cosrnet. Toilet. **1984**, *99*, 65.
54. Listrat, V.; Ayral, X.; Patarnello, F.; Bonvarlet, J.P.; Simonnet, J.; Amor, B.; Dougados, M. Osteoarthr. Cartilige **1997**, *5*, 153–60.
55. Saettone, M.F.; Chetoni, P.; Torracca, M.T.; Burgalassi, S.; Giannaccini, B. Int. J. Pharm. **1989**, *51*, 203.
56. Gidley, M.J.; Morris, E.R.; Murray, E.J.; Powell, D.A.; Rees, D.A. IBJM **1980**, *2*, 332.
57. Sungthongjeen, S.; Pitaksuteepong, T.; Somsiri, A.; Sriamornsak, P. Drug Dev. Ind. Pharm. **1999**, *25*, 1271–1276.
58. Giunchedi, P.; Conte, U.; Chetoni, P.; Saettone, M.F. Eur. J. Pharm. Sci. **1999**, *9*, 1–7.
59. Heckman, E. Starch and its Modifications for the Food Industry. *Food Colloids*; Graham, H.D., Ed.; AVI: Westport, CT, 1977; 478.
60. Rink, S.G.; Stainsby, G. Prog. Food Nutr. Sci. **1982**, *6*, 323.
61. Witschi, C.; Mrsny, R. J., Pharm. Res. **1999**, *16*, 382–390.
62. Foord, S.A. *Ph.D. Dissertation*; University of Bristol:, 1980.
63. Franz, G. Adv. Polym. Sci. **1986**, *76*, 3.
64. Losse, G.; Muller, F.; Fischer, S.; Wunderlich, G.; Hacker, E. Pharmazie **1989**, *44*, 331.
65. Singh, K.K.; Deshpande, S.G.; Baichwal, M.R. Indian Drugs **1994**, *31*, 149–154.
66. Rozier, A.; Mazuel, C.; Grove, J.; Plazonnet, B. Int. J. Pharm. **1989**, *57*, 163.
67. Imai, T.; Sakai, M.; Ohtake, H.; Azuma, H.; Otagiri, M. Pharm. Res. **1999**, *16*, 80–89.
68. Segal, R.; Pisanty, S. J. Clin. Pharm. Therm. **1987**, *12*, 165.
69. Goldstein, A.M.; Alter, E.N. Guar Gum. In *Industrial Gums*; Whistler, R.L., Ed.; Academic Press: New York, 1959, 338.
70. Bamba, M.; Puisieux, F.; Marty, J.P.; Carstensen, J.T. Int. J. Pharm. **1979**, *2*, 307.
71. Gliko-Kabir, I.; Yagen, B.; Penhasi, A.; Rubinstein, A. Pharm. Res. **1998**, *15*, 1019–1025.
72. Meer, W.A. Plant Hydrocolloids. *Food Colloids*; Graham, H.D., Ed.; AVI: Westport, CT, 1977; 527.
73. Mullet, T.; Hakert, H.; Eckert, T. Colloid Polym. Sci. **1989**, *267*, 230.
74. Greminger, G.K.; Savage, A.B. Methylcellulose and its Derivative. *Industrial Gums*; Whistler, R.L., Ed.; Academic Press: New York, 1959; 665.

75. The Effect of Sodium Carboxymethylcellulose Gel in Patients with Nonhealing Lower Extremity Diabetic Ulcers, American College of Surgeons, Chicago, IL October, 13, 1997
76. Kibbe, A.H. *Handbook of Pharmaceutical Excipients*; American Pharmaceutical Association and the Pharmaceutical Press (London): Washington, DC, 2000; 244–248.
77. Alvarez-Lorenzo, C.; Gomez-Amoza, J.L.; Martinez-Pacheco, R.; Souto, C.; Concheiro, A. Int. J. Pharm. **1999**, *180*, 91–103.
78. Kibbe, A.H. *Handbook of Pharmaceutical Excipients*; American Pharmaceutical Association and the Pharmaceutical Press (London): Washington, DC, 2000; 252–255.
79. Mitchell, K.; Ford, J.L.; Armstrong, D.J.; Elliot, P.N.; Rostron, C. Int. J. Pharm. **1993**, *100*, 165–173.
80. Greminger, G.K.; Savage, A.B. Methylcellulose and its Derivative. *Industrial Gums*; Whistler, A.L., Ed.; Academic Press: New York, 959, 579.
81. Kubis, A.; Dybek, K.; Krutul, H. Pharmazie **1987**, *42*, 519.
82. Zhou, M.; Donovan, M.D. Int. J. Pharm. **1996**, *135*, 115–125.
83. Kibbe, A.H. *Handbook of Pharmaceutical Excipients*; American Pharmaceutical Association and the Pharmaceutical Press (London): Washington, DC, 2000; 79–82.
84. Barry, B.W.; Meyer, M.C. Int. J. Pharm. **1979**, *2*, 1.
85. Penn, L.E. Gel Dosage Forms: Theory, Formulation, and Processing. *Topical Drug Delivery Formulations*; Osborne, D.W., Amann, A.H., Eds.; Marcel Dekker, Inc.: New York, 1990; 381–338.
86. Ostrenga, J.; Steinmetz, C.; Poulsen, B. J. Pharm. Sci 60, 1175–1179.
87. Lochhead, R.Y.; Hemker, W.J.; Castarieda, J.Y. Cosmet Toilet. **1987**, *120*, 89.
88. Shin, S.C.; Kim, J.Y.; Oh, I.J. Drug Dev. Ind. Pharm. **2000**, *26*, 307–312.
89. Rossi, S.; Bonferoni, M.C.; Ferrari, F.; Caramella, C. Pharm. Dev. Tech. **1999**, *4*, 55–63.
90. Bonferoni, M.C.; Rossi, S.; Ferrari, F.; Caramella, C. Pharm., Dev. Tech. **1999**, *4*, 45–53.
91. Chen-Chow, P.C.; Frank, S.G. Int. J. Pharn. **1981**, *8*, 89.
92. Attwood, D.; Collett, J.H.; Tait, C.J. Int. J. Pharm. **1985**, *26*, 25.
93. Nalbandian, R.M.; Henry, R.L.; Balko, K.W.; Adams, D.V.; Neuman, N.R. J. Biomed. Mater. Res. **1987**, *6*, 1135.
94. Miller, S.C.; Donovan, M.D. Int. J. Pharm. **1982**, *12*, 147.
95. Tomida, H.; Shinohara, M.; Kuwada, N.; Kiryu, S. Acta Pharm. Suec. **1987**, *24*, 263.
96. Barichello, J.M.; Morishita, M.; Takamyam, K.; Nagai., T. Int. J. Pharm. **1999**, *184*, 189–198.
97. Saettone, M.F.; Giannaccini, B.; Guiducci, A.; Savigni, P. Int. J. Pharm. **1986**, *31*, 261.
98. Hussain, M.D.; Rogers, J.A.; Mehvar, R.; Vucathala, G.K. Drug Dev. Ind. Pharm. **1999**, *25*, 265–271.
99. Chen, L.L. Pharm. Dev. Tech. **1998**, *3*, 241–249.
100. Molyneus, P. *Water-Soluble Synthetic Polymers and Behavior*; CRC Press: Boca Raton, FL, 1983; I, 122.
101. Pritchard, J.G. *Polyvinyl Alcohol: Basic Properties and Uses*; MacDonald Technical and Scientific: London, 1970.

102. Morimoto, K.; Nagaysau, A.; Fukanoki, S.; Morisaka, K.;
      Hyon, S.; Ikada, Y. Pharm. Res. **1989**, *6*, 338.
103. Wang, N.; Wu, X.S.; Li, J.L. Pharm. Res. **1999**, *16*,
      1430–1435.
104. Quintanar-Guerrero, D.; Ganem-Quintanatar, D.; Ray-
      goza-Trejo, D.; Doelker, E. Drug Dev. Ind. Pharm. **1999**,
      25, 169–175.
105. Nairn, J.G. Solutions, Emulsions, Suspensions, and Ex-
      tracts. *Remington: The Science and Practice of Pharmacy*;
      Gennaro, A.R., Ed.; Mack: Easton PA, 2000, 1515–1518.
106. Shah, D.N.; White, J.L.; Hem, S.L. J. Pharm Sci. **1981**, *70*,
      1101.
107. Neumann, B.S.; Sansom, K.G. J. Soc. Cosm. Chem. **1970**,
      21, 237.
108. Shrivastava, R.; Jain, S.R.; Frank, S.G. J. Pharm. Sci.
      1985, *74*, 214.
109. Ritschel, W.A.; Ritschel, G.B.; Sathyan, G. Res.
      Commun. Pathol. Pharmacol. **1988**, *62*, 103.
110. Szan, A.; Papp, L. J. Control. Rel. **1998**, *56*, 239–247.

BIBLIOGRAPHY

Drug Facts and Comparisons. In *Facts and Comparisons*; St.
   Louis MO, 2000.
Graham, H.D. *Food Colloids*; AVI: Westport, CT, 1977.
Kennedy, I.F.; White, C.A. *Bioactive Carbohydrates in
   Chemistry, Biochemistry, and Biology*; Ellis Horwood
   Limited: Chichester UK, 1983.
Kibbe, A.H. *Handbook of Pharmaceutical Excipients*; American
   Pharmaceutical Association and The Pharmaceutical Press
   (London): Washington DC, 2000.
Mitchell, J.R.; Ledward, D.A. *Functional Properties of Food
   Macromolecules*; Elsevier Applied Science: London, 1986.
Physicians' Desk Reference for Nonprescription Drugs; Medical
   Economics Company Inc. Oradell NJ, 1998.
Physicians' Desk Reference; Medical Economics Company:
   Oradell NJ, 2001.

GENERIC DRUGS AND GENERIC EQUIVALENCY

Arthur H. Kibbe

Wilkes University, Wilkes-Barre, Pennsylvania

G

INTRODUCTION

All drugs that are approved for sale generally carry at least two names. The drugs are given a proprietary or trade name given by the company that first develops them. These companies often are referred to as the innovator company. The drug is assigned a nonproprietary or generic name, which is agreed to by the WHO International Nonproprietary Nomenclature (INN) Committee and the U.S. Adopted Names Council (USAN). A new drug is usually first marketed with some patent protection and at a price that, at a minimum, recoups the cost of development over the remaining life of the patent or other exclusivity arrangement. Eventually, protection from competition is lost to other pharmaceutical companies, often companies or divisions of companies that specialize in marketing off-patent drugs. These companies or divisions are called generic companies. They can apply to the appropriate regulatory body such as the Food and Drug Administration (FDA) for permission to market the same active ingredient under its nonproprietary or generic name. The generic manufacturer is not required to do a complete clinical trial to prove effectiveness and safety because that has already been well established for the drug. However, it is required to show that the new drug product is equivalent to the original drug product. For the purposes of this article, we define the drug as the chemical that has the pharmacological effect and the drug product as a dosage form that contains the drug and other ingredients or excipients that allow the formulation of the dosage form. There is a large economic incentive for the development of generic drug products, especially for highly successful drug products. The pharmaceutical company that first brought the product to market maintains the price at the original level or higher to continue the cash flow into the company. This allows the other companies to develop a formulation of the drug and to win approval to market with the knowledge that, even at a fraction of the selling price of the innovator's product, the company can make a good profit. Some innovators defend their market share by arguing quality and reliability. The FDA must act as an impartial arbitrator of this debate. The debate is clearly about money, but is argued in a scientific forum. The key question is, "Are we

sure that the two products, if used in the same way in the same patient, will yield the same result." If a drug product is subject to this debate, the innovator always says "no" and the second and subsequent manufacturers always say "yes." In the United States, the FDA sets the standards against which the question is resolved, and scientists take sides usually on the issue of "are the current FDA standards good enough." If the FDA gives an "A" rating to a drug product, it is in effect telling the prescriber that the drug product will yield the same therapeutic and side-effects profile as the innovator drug product. The Orange Book specifies the equivalence rating from the FDA. Almost all generic drug products currently marketed are rated A; the FDA has not approved a generic without an A rating in decades. Finally, the consumer pays the price, either in the unnecessarily high cost of drugs if unnecessary studies are performed and generic competition delayed or in risky drug substitution if the FDA is too relaxed in its standards. The tests required by the FDA have changed over the years. They have become more proscriptive and are based on sound statistical grounds. The FDA has also increased the level of oversight of the pharmaceutical companies that manufacture generic equivalents of innovator products. Thus, the regulatory process has become more stringent, and the level of assurance that the public has that a generic product is both safe and effective has gone up. The FDA has often stated that there are no known therapeutic failures from switching among products that have been ruled as equivalent by the FDA.

LEGISLATIVE AND REGULATORY HISTORY

In the early 1970s, most states had antisubstitution laws that required the dispensing of the innovator product when the prescriber wrote for a drug by trade name. Most physicians had learned only the trade name of the drug product, and these laws ensured that generic substitution would be at a minimum (1). The American Pharmaceutical Association (APhA) along with other groups pushed for the repeal of these laws and opened the way for the growth of the generic industry. The lack of bioequivalence data available at that time led to the formation of the Generic Drug Bureau within the Food and Drug Administration. As a result of the efforts of that group, the FDA produced a book, *Approved Drug Products With Therapeutic Equivalence Evaluations*, in the late 1960s. This became known as the Orange Book because of the cover color. The book has been published annually with monthly updates. The contents are now available on the FDA Website (2).

In 1984, the Drug Price Competition and Patent Term Restoration Act was passed. This act, also known as the Waxman–Hatch Bill of 1984, encouraged the development of new innovative drugs by established procedures, extended patent rights, and facilitated the FDA approval process for generic drugs (3). To address the first goal, the law created a mechanism to extend the period of patent protection for manufacturers of innovative new drugs generally ensuring at least 5 years of market exclusivity after approval. To address the second goal, the law established an Abbreviated New Drug Application (ANDA) for applications after 1962. Drugs chemically equivalent to those previously approved by a full application process need only be proven bioequivalent, not clinically equivalent. Depending on the drug, proof of bioequivalence can involve in vitro dissolution studies, in vivo single-dose bioavailability studies, in vivo multidose bioavailability studies, or a combination of these. However, in vitro dissolution studies alone are not adequate proof of bioequivalence for purposes of an ANDA.

SCIENTIFIC BASIS FOR GENERIC DRUG PRODUCT EQUIVALENCY: BIOAVAILABLITY–BIOEQUIVALENCY

The goal of the testing of generic products is not to establish the clinical usefulness of the drug but only to ensure that the generic product or new formulation has the same relative bioavailability as or is bioequivalent to the innovator product.

Bioavailablity has been defined as a measure of the rate and extent of absorption of a drug into the systemic circulation after administration of a dosage form. An intravenous i.v. dose is considered by definition to be 100% bioavailable. All other routes of administration will produce a total bioavailability less than or equal to that of the i.v. dose. Thus, only a drug that is completely absorbed into the systemic circulation can have the extent of bioavailability equal to the dose stated on the label. In addition to the extent of absorption, the rate of absorption

plays a key role when evaluating the potential therapeutic impact of a particular dosage form. Knowledge of the time to onset of drug action, which is directly related to rate of absorption, is a significant concern, especially in acute clinical situations such as asthma attack, hyperglycemic shock, and pain.

The bioavailability of drugs from specific dosage forms is affected by the nature of the inactive ingredients or pharmaceutical excipients and the process used in its formulation. (For additional information, see Bioavailability of Drugs and Bioequivalency in this Encyclopedia.) When comparing similar dosage forms from different manufacturers or different lots from the same manufacturer, it is most useful to determine the relative bioavailability of the two products or lots. Some scientists have attempted to establish an in vitro test that could successfully predict in vivo bioavailability. However, to date, none has been developed.

Pharmacokinetics means the application of kinetics to drugs. It can be defined as the study of the time course and fate of drugs in the body. Teorell is often given credit for the origin of pharmacokinetics with his publications, *Kinetics of Distribution of Substances Administered to the Body* (4, 5). This science is the theoretical support for the use of bioequvalency testing to establish therapeutic equivalence among dosage forms of the same drug. The first approach to a pharmacokinetic understanding of drugs in the body, called compartment analysis, considered the body as a group of compartments through which the drug must pass. The compartment itself does not exist but represents the average of many processes that give rise to the observed phenomenon. The size of the imaginary compartment can be calculated and is useful in understanding the process of absorption, distribution, and elimination or metabolism of the drug. Regardless of the model used, a plot of the plasma concentration of the drug versus time yields a curve that can be described by a polyexponential equation. The area under that concentration–time curve (AUC) is directly related to the amount of drug absorbed. The time to reach peak concentration and the peak concentration itself are related to both the dose and the rate of absorption.

An important limitation of compartment analysis is that it cannot be applied universally to any drug. A simpler approach that is useful in the case of bioequavalency testing is the model independent method. It is based on statistical-moment theory. This approach uses the mean residence time (MRT) as a measure of a statistical half-life of the drug in the body. The MRT can be calculated by dividing the area under the first-moment curve (AUMC) by the area under the plasma curve (AUC) (6).

(See other articles in this Encyclopedia for more detailed discussion of these subjects.)

MEASUREMENT OF RELATIVE BIOAVAILABILITY OR BIOEQUIVALENCY

Drug products often undergo bioavailability testing in the early stages of development. Changes in formulation necessitated by results of clinical trials or stability testing or changes in the availability of excipients or changes in suppliers of excipients often require that the manufacturer perform a relative bioavalability or bioequivalency test to ensure that subsequent lots of a product will yield the same amount of active ingredient at the same rate as was possible in earlier formulations.

Bioequivalency studies are usually performed on young, healthy, male adult volunteers under controlled dietary conditions and fixed activity levels. This is because the goal of the study is not to establish the clinical usefulness of the drug but only to ensure that the two formulations have the same relative bioavailability or are bioequivalent.

Key Parameters

When assessing bioequivalence, the following three parameters that characterize the plasma or blood concentration–time profile of the administered drug are usually measured:

1. Peak height, C_{max}, represents the highest concentration of the drug in the systemic circulation;
2. Time to peak, t_{max}, represents the time for peak height to occur after the drug was administered;
3. Area under the curve, AUC, represents the total integrated area under the concentration–time curve.

The first two parameters are indicators of absorption rate, whereas the third is directly proportional to the extent of drug absorbed into the systemic circulation from the dosage form. Figure 1 is an example of a concentration–time curve for a single dose of drug to a subject.

Although it is theoretically possible to determine the rate and extent of absorption of a drug by measurement of the rate and extent of the appearance of the drug in the urine, this is not considered as reliable a method for evaluation of a drug product's bioequivalency as are blood level data. Thus, the studies commonly performed to demonstrate bioequivalence fall into two catagouries: single-dose and multidose or steady-state studies. There are advantages and disadvantages to each. Single-dose studies are less expensive and expose healthy volunteers

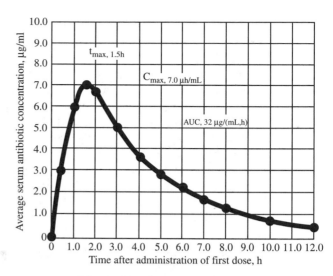

Fig. 1 Blood concentration curve.

to less drug during the course of the study. However, these studies require more sensitive analytical methods and have higher subject-to-subject variability. In both cases, a cross-over study design is used to control for sequence effects. The study is designed to control for or take into account as many variables as possible. The subjects are randomly assigned to groups. Blood samples are obtained from each subject before dosing and at fixed time intervals after dosing. Currently, the data are then analyzed using appropriate statistical ANOVA. The results must meet FDA guidelines for mean and 90% confidence interval for each of the three key parameters. For oral solid dosage forms, the FDA requires that for a product to be considered bioequivalent, the ratio of the parameter for the two products, together with their 90% confidence interval, must fall between 0.8 and 1.25, using log-transformed data. This, in effect, means that drug products that differ by more than 10% in their rate and extent of absorption will not be approved as generic equivalents.

CURRENT SCIENTIFIC ISSUES

Two issues have been raised recently with regard to the approval of generic drugs. The first has to do with the issue of "Narrow Therapeutic Index Drugs," and the second has to do with the use of individual bioequivalence in place of average bioequivalence. The former concern has been addressed in detail by Drs. Benet and Goyan (7). They concluded that narrow-therapeutic-range drugs were the least likely to have therapeutic failures among generic drugs, with proof of bioequivalency. The use of average bioequivalence data is under attack. This is because of the concern that there might be a significant subject–by-product interaction. Regulatory agencies now assume that this is not the case (8). The advantage of using individual bioequivalence studies is the reassurance that if subject/product interactions do occur, the study design would control for them, and a more statistically valid measure of the rate and extent of absorption of the drug from the two product would be determined. Some of the disadvantages associated with shifting from average to individual bioequivalence testing are cost, numbers of subjects needed, and diversity of the study population required. [See other articles that address the impact of the new metrics on the reliability and cost of the performance of bioequivalence testing (9–12).]

THE CHANGING POLITICAL ECONOMY OF GENERIC DRUGS

The modern generic drug industry in the United States really only dates from the passage of the Waxman–Hatch Act in 1984. Within 5 years of passage, generic drugs captured 40% of the market for prescriptions written inthe United States. Since that time, the generic drug market share has stablized between 40 and 50% of the prescriptions written. However, the dollars paid for generic drugs are only 10% of the total sales of drugs in the United States. That statistic alone tells us that the consumer receives enormous benefit from the substitution of therapeutically equivalent generic drugs when available.

A horrendous scandal hit the industry in the late 1980s, wherein firms representing 75% of the production of the generic industry pled guilty to one or more criminal charges involving filing false applications with the FDA, paying illegal gratuities to FDA personnel, and/or related crimes to gain an unfair competitive advantage in the emerging marketplace. Surprisingly, this scandal produced only a small delay in the market share march of generic drugs and only a temporary loss of consumer confidence in generic products.

The scandal was tied to a phenomenon that still dominates the business strategies of generic drug firms to this day: the need to obtain approval to manufacture and distribute before other firms enter the market. Because of the "commodity" nature of the business and the relative ease of entry into the industry, firms devote most of their resources and managerial talent to obtaining first or second approvals from the FDA for their products. Once a generic

drug has four or more competitors, it is no longer profitable for additional generic companies to enter the market.

Generic drug manufacturers typically will continue to manufacture drugs that produce little or no profit because large purchasers that are their prime customers (chain drugs stores, buying groups for smaller community pharmacies, etc.) prefer to buy from companies that can supply most of the common generic drugs. For example, if a generic drug firm no longer produces amoxicillin because it can make more money by shifting its antibiotic production facilities to, for example, a cephalosporin drug for which it has less competition, a large chain may chose to buy its entire generic antibiotic line from another company that supplies both.

The profitable generic drug companies are profitable because they have found a strategy to maintain some control over the price of their products. In the early years (1984–1988), the best way to get "first approval" from the FDA apparently was to be first to file, to get assays or bioquivalence studies done on difficult to duplicate drugs, or to find some way to get an expedited approval from inside the agency. Unfortunately, this sometime involved payoffs to FDA review chemists (those FDA experts assigned the task of evaluating biostudy results, the crucial piece of a generic drug application, remained remarkably free of the scandal). More often, it involved submitting false information to the FDA (including, in a few cases, false biostudies). Many generic drug firms did not survive the scandal, and others survived only after the previous management and ownership were purged from the firms.

For a short period, it was believed that the profitable segment of the business involved not production but distribution. After all, if commodity prices approach marginal cost and the marginal cost of manufacturing drugs is minimal, but the price to the consumer remains significantly more than marginal, there must be middlemen somewhere making the money. Clearly, those middlemen were not in the retail pharmacy where profits continued to be squeezed. Distributors were thought to be the new profit centers. But a funny thing happened on the way to that particular bank… .

Consumers became outraged at the rapid increase in the price of pharmaceuticals as the innovator companies (and some generic firms) rushed to raise prices and as generic drug company after generic drug company was pushed out of the industry in the wake of investigations by a Congressional committee and a federal grand jury. Second, the Administration, in response to public concern about the cost of pharmaceuticals, pressured the pharmaceutical industry and forced lower prices and significant rebates to the federal and state government programs that paid for drugs. Wholesale distributors of all drugs subject to the federal rebates suffered.

Finally, the firms that thought they could profit most from the scandal entered the market. These were innovator firms, many of which had already played a significant role in the distribution of generics. Ultimately, the profit margins from generic drug sales were not sufficient to carry the overhead of the branded companies, and most left the market or returned to their distributor role. Even in the case of the firms manufacturing and marketing generic versions of their own branded products, giving them significant advantage over the remaining pure generic firms in developing and filing of the ANDAs with the FDA and the added advantage of relatively less scrutiny from the scandal-rocked agency, most had exited the marketed by the end of the decade.

Some innovator firms entered the generic drug market so that they could have a product line consistent with their new business strategy: disease state management. This strategy, a function of the rise of HMOs and the return of the concept of scarcity to prescription drug dispensing, was intended to involve the development of a continuum of drug therapies for the treatment of a specific illness (diabetes, depression, etc.), wherein the patient would be tried on the older, less-expensive drug first and, if it did not work, the next most cost-effective drug would be administered and so on until the least cost-effective drug would be the treatment of last resort. Unfortunately, the branded companies that selected this strategy found themselves competing with doctors, hospitals, and insurance companies for control of the treatment regime of individual patients, a losing proposition for the entity with the least amount of information about and access to the individual patient.

Another factor in reducing prices of all drugs that had some form of competition was the rise of the HMO and its pharmaceutical watchdog, the pharmacy benefit manager (PBM). These PBMs create a formulary of approved drugs (drugs for which they would reimburse partially or fully) based on bids from competing companies.

Much of the public's confusion regarding generic drugs arose from a practice of the PBMs to pressure doctors to substitute different chemical entities in the same therapeutic class for the prescribed medicine. Such a switch is called a theraputic substitution as opposed to the switching among manufacturers of therapeutically equivalent drugs (generics and the innovator drug or other FDA "AB"-rated substitutes). Therapeutic substitution involves a switch to a different drug, whereas generic substitution involves a switch to the same drug from a different manufacturer. If a patient is switched between FDA "AB"-rated drugs, the FDA offers the assurance that they can expect the same therapeutic and side–effect profile as the brand drug or another "AB"-rated generic drug. The FDA offers no such assurance if the switch occurs among different drugs, even if they are in the same therapeutic class. For example, aspirin and Tylenol may be equally effective in the treatment of headache, but the FDA makes no such certification, whereas it makes exactly that certification for Bayer aspirin and Safeway aspirin.

The dominance of the HMO (and related organizations) and their PBMs (and related organization types) served to accelerate the substitution of generic drugs at the turn of the 21st century. However, even that pressure could not slow the re-emergence of a high rate of price increase, greater than consumer or comparable wholesale prices as a whole, in prescription drugs. Innovator companies learned that establishing very high prices for "breakthorough" drugs could more than compensate for the loss of patent protection on a highly profitable drug.

Furthermore, the United States is the only developed country in the world that has chosen not to explicitly control the price of any drug product and has used its market power as a huge buyer relatively sparingly. Consequently, U.S. prices for drug products still under patent are usually substantially above those charged anywhere else in the world. Generic prices approach cost except for those few generics that have managed to eliminate or limit for a specific period competition from other generics.

Those generic drug firms that prospered in this restrictive price environment all had one or more niche drugs that were immune from corrosive price competition. Some companies mastered a manufacturing process that produced bioequivalent medicine that the innovator itself found difficult to master lot to lot. Others took advantage of certain exclusivity provisions in the law for those that challenged a product patent in court, ostensibly to cover the cost of litigation. In other cases, the settlement of those cases provided some form of licensing or distribution rights that permitted the sale of a generic product while the patent was still valid. Finally, a fortunate firm might find itself in possession of the exclusive right to purchase the raw material from the only source available to generic drug manufacturers.

All generic drug firms capable of generating the necessary cash to develop and market new drugs are moving toward that lucrative market. For the time being, the United States has chosen to use the market mechanism as its only important control on drug prices. Generics are the competition, and competition is our only real form of price control.

According to the Congressional Budget Office (CBO), consumers saved $8–10 billion in 1994 because of the use of generic drugs. In that same 1998 report, CBO cited the Waxman–Hatch Act, generic substitution laws passed by the states, and government health programs as seminal events leading to the acceptance of generic drugs and the resulting savings.

REFERENCES

1. Knoben, J.E.; Scott, G.R.; Tonelli, R.J. Overview of the FDA Publication Approved Drug Products with Therapeutic Equivalence Evaluations. Am. J. Hosp. Pharm. **1990**, *47* (12), 2696–2700.
2. Food and Drug Administration. *Approved Drug Products with Therapeutic Equivalence Evaluations*; http://www.fda.gov/cder/ob/ FDA: Rockville; Available from the Government Printing Office: Washington, DC, 2000.
3. Weaver, L.C. Drug Cost Containment—The Case for Generics: Situation in the U.S.A. J. Soc. Admi. Pharm. **1989**, *6* (1), 9–13.
4. Teorell, T. Kinetics of Distribution of Substances Administered to the Body. I. The Extravascular Modes of Administration. Archives Internationales de Pharmacodynamie et de Therapie. **1937**, *57*, 205–225.
5. Teorell, T. Kinetics of Distribution of Substances Administered to the Body. II. The Intravascular Mode of Administration. Archives Internationales de Pharmacodynamie et de Therapie. 1937, *57*, 226–240.
6. Yamaoka, K.; Nakagawa, T.; Uno, T. Statistical Moments in Pharmacokinetics. J. Pharmacokinet. Biopharm. **1978**, *6* (6), 547–558.
7. Benet, L.Z.; Goyan, J.E. Bioequivalence and Narrow Therapeutic Index Drugs. Pharmacotherapy **1995**, *15* (4), 433–440.
8. Patnaik, R.N.; Lesko, L.J.; Chen, M.L. Individual Bioequivalence. New Concepts in the Statistical Assessment of Bioequivalence Metrics. FDA Individual Bioequivalence Working Group. Clin. Pharmacokine. **1997**, *33* (1), 1–6.
9. Midha, K.K.; Rawson, M.J.; Hubbard, J.W. Individual and Average Bioequivalence of Highly Variable Drugs and Drug Products. J. Pharm. Sci. **1997**, *86* (11), 1193–1197.
10. Snikeris, F.; Tingey, H.B. A Two-Step Method for Assessing Bioequivalence. Drug Inf. J. **1994**, *28* (3), 709–722.
11. Holder, D.J.; Hsuan, F. A Moment-Based Criterion for Determining Individual Bioequivalence. Drug Inf. J. **1995**, *29* (3), 965–979.
12. Mohandoss, E.; Chow, S.C.; Ki, F.Y. Application of Williams' Design for Bioequivalence Trials. Drug Inf. J. **1995**, *29* (3), 1029–1038.

GERIATRIC DOSING AND DOSAGE FORMS

Cheryl A. Wiens
University of Alberta, Edmonton, Alberta, Canada

Carol A. Borynec
University Hospital, Edmonton, Alberta, Canada

DEMOGRAPHICS

The word *geriatric* refers to individuals who are over age 65 years. This has been described as the most heterogeneous population because it constitutes fit, physiologically healthy patients to extremely frail, debilitated patients in long-term care facilities (LTCF).

Currently, greater than 12% of the population in the United States (1) is aged 65 years and over. This population is prescribed approximately one-third of all prescription medications (2). On average, geriatric patients use four to five medications, and greater than 50% use over-the-counter (OTC) medications. The use of medications is even higher in the LTCF population.

The elderly are also more likely to suffer from chronic disease and multiple disease states and therefore receive long-term treatment with medications. Considering the high medication utilization of geriatric patients, it is pertinent to focus on geriatric dosing and dosage forms.

PHYSIOLOGIC CHANGES WITH AGING

Although development of disease is not considered normal with aging, there are a number of physiological changes which can predispose the elderly to developing illness (Table 1). Many of the age-related physiological changes have been reviewed previously (3, 4). Because of the physiological changes that occur with the aging process, there are changes in the pharmacokinetics and pharmacodynamics of medications.

PHARMACOKINETICS

Pharmacokinetics refers to how the body handles medications. As the body changes with age, its ability to absorb, distribute, and break down drugs can change significantly. Unfortunately, in some cases, it is difficult to predict how significantly aging will affect some people, thus, dosing changes alone cannot be based solely on age. Pharmacokinetics can be broken down into four processes: 1) absorption (of the medication through the gastrointestinal tract, a mucous membrane, or the skin); 2) distribution (of the medication throughout the body); 3) metabolism (most often through the liver); and 4) elimination (most often through the kidneys).

Absorption

There appears to be little change in absorption of medications in the elderly (3, 5, 6). Dry skin may decrease absorption of topically applied medications. A decrease in stomach acid secretion may affect absorption of certain medications when given orally; however, this is not consistent for all geriatric patients. Other changes that may contribute to altered absorption may include dietary changes, a decrease in salivary secretion, or use of dentures (3). Absorption is generally dependent on the concomitant disease states of the patient (3). For example, if a patient had congestive heart failure, with significant congestion of the gastrointestinal (GI) tract, then less medication and nutrients would be absorbed through the GI tract. The decreased absorption is not related to age but results from concomitant systemic or GI diseases.

Distribution

Physiological changes owing to the aging process will result in an increase in lipid mass and a decrease in lean body mass (3, 5, 6). Fat-soluble medications may distribute more widely and remain in the body longer in an elderly patient, whereas water-soluble medications have a smaller volume of distribution because of decreased lean mass.

Distribution of medications is also determined by protein binding in the serum (6, 7). The most common protein is albumin, which binds predominantly acidic drugs such as phenytoin. Another common protein is α-1 acid glycoprotein, an acute-phase reactant, which has a higher affinity for basic drugs such as lidocaine. The most

Table 1 Age-related physiological changes in the elderly

Organ system	Change
Body composition	↓ lean body mass ↑ body fat ↓ body water
Cardiovascular	↓ cardiac output ↓ stress response (β-response blunted)
Central nervous system	↓ peripheral conduction velocity ↓ weight, volume of brain
Endocrine	↓ hormonal secretions menopausal changes ↑ incidence diabetes, thyroid atrophy
Gastrointestinal	↓ secretions ↓ rate of stomach emptying ↓ rate of intestinal transit time ↓ liver volume and blood flow
Genitourinary	Atrophy vagina, prostate
Immune	↓ cell-mediated immunity
Pulmonary	↓ elasticity, chest wall compliance ↓ alveolar surface
Renal	↓ nephrons ↓ creatinine clearance ↓ renal blood flow ↓ glomular filtration rate (GFR)
Sensory changes	↓ accommodation of lens of eye
Skeletal	↓ skeletal bone mass
Skin and hair	↓ hydration of skin ↓ in dermal thickness

↓ Indicates decrease; ↑ indicates increase.

important consideration for protein levels when considering drug distribution is to take into account the health status of the individual. An elderly patient may experience only a small decline in protein levels owing simply to age. However, chronic inflammatory disease states may significantly increase the levels of α-1 acid glycoprotein, thereby decreasing the free level of medication in the blood stream. When considering albumin, it is important to take into account chronic disease states and nutritional status. Poor nutritional intake will result in a lower level of albumin and, therefore, a higher free level of drug. In most cases a higher free level of drug does not result in a clinically significant response (because the liver most often compensates for the increased drug levels and simply metabolizes the excess levels with hepatic reserve); however, this may be quite important for medications with a narrow therapeutic index. Medications such as warfarin require very careful monitoring to maintain the International Normalized Ratio (INR) within a very narrow

therapeutic range. In this case, if warfarin increases even slightly, the response could be far greater than expected.

Second, tissue protein binding of medication can affect drug disposition in the elderly patient. For example, amiodarone binds strongly to tissue proteins, which greatly increases its volume of distribution. In the elderly or chronically ill patient, tissue proteins may change or decline, which can also affect the serum levels of medications.

Finally, free drug levels may be affected by interaction with other medications, which may cause displacement of a drug off the protein. Considering that the elderly are taking more medications, they are more likely to experience protein-displacement drug interactions. However, protein-displacement interactions are not considered as clinically significant as metabolism interactions.

Metabolism

Liver blood flow decreases with age, but overall it does not appear to affect the metabolizing capacity of the hepatocytes. Medications that are dependent on liver blood flow for break down may have a somewhat delayed metabolism (3, 5, 6). There is some decline in phase I metabolism but not necessarily in phase II metabolism (5). Phase I metabolism involves the oxidation/reduction reactions commonly needed to metabolize medications. Phase II reactions, including conjugation reactions, appear to remain grossly intact in the elderly. This means that medications that are metabolized by phase II metabolism are preferred over agents that require phase I metabolism. In elderly patients who appear frail or suffer from chronic disease, both phase I and phase II metabolisms may show a decline. However, age alone does not appear to cause a decline in phase II metabolism. It is important to consider the chronic disease states or lifestyle factors, such as diet, smoking, and ethanol intake, in predicting the metabolizing capability of a patient (3, 5, 6). Patients who have poor diet and negative lifestyle factors such as cigarette smoking and high consumption of alcohol are less likely to have hepatic metabolizing reserve and are more likely to suffer adverse reactions from medication because of relative overdosing (or incapacity to metabolize a standard dose of medication). Although the elderly may have little change in their metabolizing capacity owing to age only (6) applying the above principles to dosing is recommended.

Elimination

Renal function generally decreases with age (3, 6). It is not possible to predict which patients will not experience a decline in renal function, even though it has been estimated that up to 30% of the elderly have no change in their renal function. The most commonly used nomogram to predict renal function is the Cockroft–Gault equation (8), which factors in age, causing a decline in renal function. Unfortunately, this equation was not originally validated in an elderly, frail, or female population. Furthermore, predicting renal function is most difficult in frail patients. Careful monitoring for response to the medication and side effects is necessary to avoid an excessive dosage. It is also difficult to predict renal function in these clinical situations: malnourished patients who have low muscle mass and, therefore, low serum creatinine; patients who are missing a limb; and individuals who do not have stable renal function (creatinine not having reached steady state).

Medications that are eliminated renally should be given in a reduced dosage or given less frequently than in younger patients. However, the exact dosing cannot be predicted accurately in many subpopulations of the elderly including the very old (>85 years) nor in the frail patients. In these populations, it is appropriate to monitor drug response based on clinical improvement or signs and symptoms of toxicity (3, 5, 6). Monitoring drug levels at steady state may also be necessary.

PHARMACODYNAMICS

Pharmacodynamic changes in the elderly are also documented (5, 9); however, they are not as well-researched or defined as are pharmacokinetic changes. Pharmacodynamics refers to the change in response to the medication. Possible mechanisms include (9):

- Change in receptor density
- Change in receptor affinity and receptor characteristics
- Postreceptor alterations (change in transduction signal coupling or amplification)
- Desensitization of receptors
- Altered negative feedback respons
- Target tissues exhibit intrinsic change

These alterations in homeostatic function can result in significant impairment or adverse consequences if these changes are not accounted for while prescribing certain medications (Table 2).

Changes in Sensitivity

The elderly are more likely to be sensitive to a number of different classes of medication because of changes in pharmacodynamics (5, 9–11). It is very important to monitor and adjust the dosage of certain classes of medications in the elderly owing to their increased or decreased sensitivity (Table 3).

ADVERSE DRUG REACTIONS (ADR) / ADVERSE DRUG EVENT (ADE)

As Lamy (12) has pointed out, there is much debate regarding the definition of an adverse drug reaction (ADR) or an adverse drug event (ADE). An ADR has been defined by the World Health Organization (WHO) as a noxious, unintended effect of a drug that occurs in doses normally used in humans for the diagnosis, prophylaxis, or treatment of disease. An ADR also can be defined as an undesirable effect of drug therapy beyond its anticipated therapeutic effects occurring during clinical use. An ADE is defined as a noxious and unintended patient event caused by a drug (e.g., laboratory abnormalities, symptoms, signs, etc.). In the outpatient geriatric population, approximately 30% will experience an ADR and are responsible for approximately 10–20% of hospital admissions (12–14). In hospitalized patients, the incidence of an ADR or ADE is estimated to be 10–25% (15). Studies have found that the majority of events are avoidable (12), and unfortunately, many patients (estimated to be one-third) do not fully recover from the ADR.

ADRs are also a concern because of the associated costs, primarily related to hospitalization. ADRs increase length of stay and risk of mortality, which overall increase costs of the ADR treatment. The elderly with ADRs also visit their physician more frequently than elderly patients who are not experiencing ADRs (16). The elderly patient may not bring up concerns with healthcare professionals (12) and may go on to accept the ADR as a part of normal treatment. The incidence of ADR therefore may be significantly underreported in the elderly population.

Assessing the risk of ADRs in the elderly can be difficult because most clinical trials exclude the elderly because of comorbidities or age. There is also a bias in prescribing, thus, elderly patients at risk of experiencing adverse effects from a drug may not even be exposed to the medication. This provides an underestimate of the true incidence of ADRs in an entire population who may take the medication (5, 12, 17).

The risk of experiencing an ADR is related to the diagnosis, types of medications prescribed, and the number of drugs used (5, 12–14, 17). The most significant factor is multiple drug use and is related to number of coexisting diseases. When the number of medications is decreased, it has been shown that ADRs also decrease (12). It appears that the number of medications increases the risk of ADR exponentially (14).

It is debatable if age alone is an independent risk factor for ADR; however, the elderly are more susceptible to ADRs because of physiological changes resulting in

Table 2 Altered homeostatic mechanisms in the elderly

Altered function	Mechanism	Examples of drugs
Anticoagulation	Poor hepatic production of coagulation factors Poor dietary intake	Anticoagulants Thrombolytics
Arrhythmias	Cardiac hypersensitivity	Antiarrhythmic medication
Higher cognitive function	Central cholinergic transmission Neuronal loss Receptor downregulation	Central anticholinergics Stimulants β-agonists
Orthostasis	Blunting of β response (no tachycardia) Changes in vascular tree Changes in autonomic nervous system Receptor down regulation	Blood pressure medications Tricyclic antidepressants Antipsychotics Diuretics Sedative hypnotics
Postural control	↓ D2 receptors in the striatum ↑ Risk of sway	
Tardive dyskinesia	Impaired dopamine-synthesizing neurons	Traditional antipsychotics Long-term antipsychotic therapy
Thermoregulation	Poor temperature-regulating mechanisms: ↓ shivering ↓ metabolic rate ↓ vasoconstriction ↓ thirst response ↓ subjective awareness of temperature	Medications affecting awareness, mobility, muscular activity, vasoconstrictor mechanisms CNS medications Phenothiazines Barbiturates Benzodiazepines Tricyclic antidepressants Narcotics Alcohol
Visceral muscle function	Visual disturbances (pupillary autonomic responses) Bladder instability (bladder capacity, detrusor contractions) Intestinal motility decreased	Anticholinergic medications

↓ Indicates decrease; ↑ indicates increase.

Table 3   Medications affected by changes in sensitivity

Medication (class)	Altered effect	Recommendation
ACE-I	Greater sensitivity to BP reduction	Lower initial dose
	Increased risk hyperkalemia	
Antiarrhythmics (class I)	Longer elimination $t_{1/2}$	Lower initial dose
Antiarrhythmics (class III)	Longer elimination $t_{1/2}$	Lower initial dose
Anticholinergics	Increased sensitivity to anticholinergic effects, increased risk confusion	Avoid if possible
		Use lowest initial dose when necessary
Antipsychotics	Greater risk orthostasis and movement disorders	Lower initial dose
	Low potency agents—more likely to cause confusion	
β-blockers	Greater sensitivity to BP reduction	Lower initial dose
Benzodiazepines	Longer elimination $t_{1/2}$ Greater sensitivity to sedating effects	Use shorter-acting hydrophilic agents such as lorazepam, oxazepam
Corticosteroids	Increased sensitivity to GI complications	Lower initial dose
	Increased risk osteoporosis	Minimize duration of therapy if possible
Digoxin	Decreased volume of distribution	Lower loading dose
		Lower maintenance dose
Diuretics	↓ responsiveness owing to decline in renal function	Enhanced monitoring of renal function, electrolytes
NSAIDs	Greater risk of GI complications	Used only after acetaminophen for OA
		Recommended with GI-protective agent or use a COX-II inhibitor
Opioids	Increased sensitivity to effect	Lower initial dose
SSRIs	Longer elimination $t_{1/2}$	Avoid using fluoxetine
Tricyclic antidepressants	Longer elimination $t_{1/2}$	Preference for desipramine, nortriptyline (better tolerated secondary amines)
	Greater sensitivity to anticholinergic effects, arrhythmic effects	
Warfarin	Increased sensitivity to anticoagulant effect	Lower initial dose

ACE-I, indicates angiotensin-converting enzyme inhibitor; SSRI, selective serotonin receptor inhibitor; NSAID, nonsteroidal anti-inflammatory drug; OA, osteoarthritis.

altered pharmacokinetics or pharmacodynamics. Some studies have shown that when controlling for confounders such as clinical status of the patient, number of medications, and length of hospital stay, age alone does not predict ADRs (12, 17).

It is important to note that withdrawal of medications may also lead to ADR (18). Certain settings (e.g., LTCF) encourage prescribers to remove medications, some of which may have been used by the patient for many years. If the withdrawal of therapy is not appropriate or is done too quickly, this may cause ADR for the patient (18, 19).

The most common drugs involved in ADRs are cardiovascular medications, aspirin, NSAIDs, and psychotropic agents. However, it should be noted that these are also the most commonly used medications in the elderly (14).

The prevention of ADRs in the elderly has been inadequately studied. Considering that the majority of ADRs are type A (dose-related) it would appear that most ADRs in the elderly could be prevented. Additional study on this subject is necessary to determine the most effective interventions in decreasing the incidence of ADRs in the elderly. A review by Atkin (14) has addressed studies that suggest improvements such as better history-taking and record-keeping by physicians to minimize the number of medications used by patients. Other suggestions include requesting that patients always bring their medications to medical appointments and using medications that would be considered lower risk in this population.

There are a number of different ways to assess and identify an ADE. Listed below are a number of tables that will assist in interpreting signs or symptoms that may indeed be an adverse drug event. Table 4 identifies disease states that may contribute to similar symptoms that may be misdiagnosed as an ADE. Other syndromes that are most commonly associated with toxicity or side effects from specific medications are shown in Table 5. Finally, medication classes that most commonly causes ADEs in the elderly are presented in Table 6.

Falls

Falls are common in the elderly and are often multifactorial (20–22). There is a concern about patients who fall because the complications are significant. Complications include fractures, soft tissue injuries, immobilization and hospital-acquired illness, institutionalization, and even death from additional complications such as pneumonia (20). It is difficult to determine the percentage of patients who fall because many falls do not result in injury and are never reported.

The cost involving treatment of falls is staggering (21, 22), including costs for hospitalization and acute

care, rehabilitation, and institutionalization, if necessary. It has been estimated that falls cost $12.6 billion in lifetime expenses for persons older than 65 years of age. There is also a tremendous emotional impact on the patients, causing many patients to lose their sense of security and to remain housebound.

Although certain illnesses contribute to falls, medications have been shown to cause falls independent of other factors. The most commonly offending drugs are benzodiazepines because they have been shown to increase falls and hip fractures (23). An association between the dose (the higher the dose, the more likely the fall), duration of use, and type of benzodiazepine (e.g., long-acting medications) has also been reported. Other classes of medications that increase the risk of falls include tricyclic antidepressants, SSRIs, and opioid analgesics (23, 24).

It may be entirely appropriate to continue using these medications if they are prescribed. To ensure safe drug use, patients should be cautioned about the risk of falling and encouraged to use extra precautions. High-risk medication should be administered only when needed, rather than on a scheduled basis, because this will hopefully decrease the overall dose. In the elderly, a short-acting phase II metabolized benzodiazepine such as oxazepam or lorazepam would be preferred if a benzodiazepine is necessary.

Delirium

Drug-induced changes in cognition are common and disturbing ADRs for both the patient and the patient's family or caregiver. Delirium is commonly reported on hospital admission (approximately 10–15% of elderly patients meet criteria for diagnosis of delirium) (25, 26). There is also a significant occurrence of delirium in elderly patients undergoing various types of surgery, including general surgery open heart surgery and hip fracture repair (may be as high as 50%) (25, 26). The outcome after diagnosis of delirium is poor. At 1 month, the mortality has been shown to be as high as 14%, and at 6 months mortality is 22%. If the patient survives, change in cognitive symptoms may last for 3 months postdischarge. Furthermore, these patients are at an increased risk for other complications, including prolonged hospital stay, functional decline, and institutionalization.

Medications may cause, or at least exacerbate, delirium in many patients. Polypharmacy has been shown to be a risk factor for delirium. There are a number of different types of medications that may cause delirium. Many have anticholinergic properties, whereas others have a yet-unknown mechanism for causing delirium (Table 4). Patients who present with acute changes in mental status

Table 4 Presenting symptoms and associated adverse drug events (ADE)

Symptom	Underlying condition	Drug cause of ADE
Disturbed mental status/delirium	Hypoglycemia	Anticholinergic medications and/or properties
	Hypothyroidism	Antipsychotics
	B12 deficiency	Antihistamines
	Uremia	Antiparkinsonian agents
		Antispasmodics
		Ophthalmic preparations
		OTC sleep/allergy medications
		Tricyclic antidepressants
		Other medications
		Analgesics/NSAIDs
		Anticonvulsants
		Corticosteroids (high dose)
		Digoxin
		H2 blockers
		Insulin
		Muscle relaxants
		Narcotics
		Psychotropics (anxiolytic, antidepressant, antipsychotic)
		Sedative/hypnotic
		Sulfonylurea
Depression	Hypercalcemia	Hypnotics
	Hypo-hyperthyroidism	Amiodarone
		Lipid-soluble β-blockers
Fatigue	CHFGI bleed	Diuretics β-blockers
	Anemia	Hypnotics
	Hypothyroidism	Muscle relaxants
Falls/syncope	Structural CNS lesion	Antiarrhythmics
	Dehydration	Levodopa
	Hypokalemia	Diuretics
	Arrhythmias	Antihypertensives
		TCA
		Sedatives
		Antipsychotics
		Hypoglycemics
		Alcohol

or delirium must be evaluated medically and should include a review of their medications. Typically, all medications should be discontinued and restarted only if considered life-saving at the time. Long-term chronic medications should be held because it is important to resolve delirium and attempt to identify which medications may be the offending agent (25–27).

Drug–Drug Interactions

Drug interactions are very common in the elderly, attributable in part to the high number of medications prescribed in this population. Drug interactions are considered one type of adverse drug event and have been found to increase with the number of medications prescribed (28). Drug interactions are also a common cause of hospital admission (29).

The elderly are particularly susceptible to interactions because of the changes in physiology, multiple physician prescribing, increased use of OTC medications, nonadherence to complex regimens, and multiple disease states that complicate the handling of medications.

Medication interactions have been found to be poorly monitored. Medications are often necessary, and

Table 5 Common adverse effects

Adverse effect	Possible medications
Anticholinergic effects	Antihistamines
Delirium	Tricyclic antidepressants
Dry mouth	Medications for urge incontinence
Constipation	
Urinary retention	
Tachycardia	
Disturbed vision	
Blurring	See anticholinergic effects
Dry eyes	Glaucoma medications
	Ocular lubricants
Extrapyramidal effects	Antipsychotics
Tremor	Antiemetic (metoclopramide)
Pseudoparkinsonism	
Akathisia	
Sedation	Antipsychotics
	Sedative/hypnotics
	Tricyclic antidepressants
	Muscle relaxants
Orthostatic hypotension	Antihypertensives
	Diuretics
	Levodopa
	Tricyclic antidepressants

Table 6 Medication classes commonly affecting mobility in the elderly

Medication class	Mobility ADE
Antihypertensives	Postural hypotension
Antipsychotics	Postural hypotension
	Sedation
	Extrapyramidal effects
	Falls
Narcotics	Sedation
	Confusion
	↓ coordination (falls)
Sedative/hypnotics	Sedation
	Weakness
	Confusion
	↓ coordination (falls)
Tricyclic antidepressants	Postural hypotension
	Sedation
	Arrhythmias
	Falls

↓ Indicates decrease.

interactions can be handled in a manner in which the patient does not experience adverse effects and yet receives the benefit of appropriate medications.

There are various types of drug interactions. One classification is pharmacokinetic or pharmacodynamic interactions. Pharmacokinetic interactions describe an interaction with absorption, metabolism, or elimination. Medications can also displace each other through competitive protein binding. Many pharmacokinetic interactions result through competition or interaction at the cytochrome enzyme system called the CYP450 system (28). Numerous isozymes, or subtypes, have been discovered. Each isozyme is responsible for metabolizing specific medications. These isozymes may be inhibited or induced by certain disease states or by other medications. Pharmacodynamic interactions refer to additive or antagonistic activity or action of one medication on another. The study of pharmacokinetic interactions is often done in younger, healthy patients and may not reflect what commonly occurs in an elderly patient. It may also be difficult to predict the extent of the interaction; however, some studies have resulted in specific recommendations on how to adjust the dose of interacting medications.

Table 7 contains a list of drug classes and clinically significant drug interactions. This is not a comprehensive list, and the reader is referred to the appropriate chapter dealing with pharmacokinetic drug interactions.

Drug–Food Interactions

Table 8 lists commonly used drugs and potential food interactions. This is not a comprehensive list, but rather highlights many of the clinically significant food–drug interactions (30).

Recent concerns with food products include grapefruit juice, which has been shown interact with many different medications through the CYP450 3A4 isoenzyme. This may increase the levels of medication such as cyclosporine, dihydropyridine calcium channel blockers, midazolam, triazolam, and astemizole (31).

DRUG MANAGEMENT PROBLEMS IN THE ELDERLY

Adherence

Traditionally called compliance, the concept of not taking medication properly is now called nonadherence. However, these words are often used interchangeably. The documented rates range from 25 to 50% in the elderly (32). Intentional nondadherence, or consciously making a decision to not take the medications as prescribed, involves not taking the medication at all or using only

G

(Continued)

Table 7 Drug–drug interactions of commonly used medications in the elderly

Drug	Interacting drug	Mechanism/effect	Management
Analgesics			
NSAIDs	Warfarin	Increased risk of bleeding	Avoid use of NSAIDs while using warfarin
	Corticosteroids	Increased fluid retention; increased risk of GI bleeding	Avoid use of NSAIDs while using corticosteroids; use selective COX-II inhibitors if necessary
Opioids	Alcohol	Increased risk of CNS depression; respiratory depression	Avoid use of multiple CNS depressants; decrease doses of CNS depressants when used concomitantly
	Antipsychotics		
	TCA		
	Sedative/hypnotics		
Acetylcholinesterase inhibitors			
Acetylcholinesterase inhibitors (A.Ch.E.-I) (donepezil, tacrine, rivastigmine)	Phenothiazine antipsychotics; tricyclic antidepressants; anticholinergic medications	Antagonize acetylcholine increasing effect of A.Ch.E.-I	Avoid use of anticholinergics when using A.Ch.E.-I
	Bethanechol	Additive cholinergic side effects (e.g., nausea, abdominal cramping)	Avoid use of bethanechol with A.Ch.E.-I
	Succinylcholine	Exaggerated muscle relaxation	Discontinue A.Ch.E.-I before surgery
	Ketoconazole	Inhibited metabolism of donepezil	Monitor for donepezil toxicity; dose reduction not empirically necessary
	Quinidine		
Donepezil			
Tacrine	Fluvoxamine	Decreased metabolism of tacrine leading to increased levels of tacrine	Avoid use of interacting medications; monitor for signs of toxicity of tacrine
	Cimetidine		
	Quinolones		
	Theophylline	Inhibition of theophylline metabolism	Decrease dose of theophylline while using tacrine
Antibiotics			
Aminoglycosides	Diuretics	Increased risk of dehydration, renal impairment	Monitor renal function, hydration closely
	Cisplatin	Increased risk of nephrotoxicity	Monitor renal function closely
	Vancomycin		
Quinolones	Iron supplements antacids (aluminum-calcium-or magnesium-containing)	Impair absorption of quinolone	Avoid taking quinolone within 2 h of these medications
Ciprofloxacin	Theophylline	Reduced clearance of theophylline and caffeine; increased risk of CNS toxicity	Decrease dose of theophylline; avoid caffeine intake
	Caffeine		
Sulfonamides	Warfarin	Displacement of medications from protein binding sites; transient increase in drug levels and toxicity	Monitor for toxicity of displaced medications
	Sulfonylurea		
	Phenytoin		
	Methotrexate		

Table 7 Drug–drug interactions of commonly used medications in the elderly (*Continued*)

Drug	Interacting drug	Mechanism/effect	Management
Isoniazid (INH)	Phenytoin Carbamazepine	Inhibition of metabolism— increased toxicity of anticonvulsants	Monitor levels of anticonvulsants during INH therapy
	Ethanol	Increased risk of hepatotoxicity	Avoid use of ethanol during INH treatment
Anticonvulsants			
Phenytoin	Amiodarone Cimetidine Fluoxetine Fluconazole Ketoconazole	Increased level of phenytoin	Monitor for phenytoin toxicity; reduce dose as needed
	Carbamazepine Rifampin Theophylline	Decreased level of phenytoin	Increase dose of phenytoin to reach therapeutic blood level
Carbamazepine	Isoniazid	Increased risk of hepatotoxicity	Monitor hepatic function closely while using this combination
	Erythromycin Cimetidine Diltiazem	Increased levels, toxicity of carbamazepine	Monitor toxicity of carbamazepine; dosage may require reduction
	Phenytoin Phenobarbitone Theophylline	Decreased levels of carbamazepine	Increase dose of carbamazepine as necessary
Gabapentin	Antacids (aluminum- or magnesium-based)	Decreased levels of gabapentin	Do not administer antacids within 2 h of gabapentin
Valproic acid	Carbamazepine	Decreased level of valproic acid; enzyme induction	Increase dose of valproic acid as needed
	Aspirin	Increased free level of valproic acid—risk of valproic acid toxicity	Monitor valproic acid toxicity over time—if toxicity continues, consider decreasing dose
	Rifampin	Decreased clearance of valproic acid	Decrease dose of valproic acid while taking rifampin
Antidepressants			
SSRI (citamlopram, fluvoxamine, fluoxetine, sertraline, paroxetine)	Monoamine oxidase inhibitors (MAO-I)	Increased toxicity of MAO-I (e.g., seizures, confusion, hyperpyrexia)	Avoid combination of SSRI and MAO-I
Fluoxetine	Tricyclic antidepressant (TCA)	Increased toxicity of TCA	Avoid combination of SSRI and TCA
	Diazepam	Increased levels of diazepam Increased effect of diazepam	Avoid diazepam use if possible in the elderly; decrease dose if used with fluoxetine
	Trazodone	Increased levels of trazodone	Start with smallest dose of trazodone; decrease dose of trazodone if necessary

(*Continued*)

(*Continued*)

Table 7 Drug–drug interactions of commonly used medications in the elderly (*Continued*)

Drug	Interacting drug	Mechanism/effect	Management
Sertraline	No clinically significant interactions		
Fluvoxamine	Astemizole	Increased levels of astemizole; increased risk of cardiac arrhythmia	Avoid use of astemizole with fluvoxamine; use alternate antihistamine
	Benzodiazepines (triazolam, alprazolam)	Increased levels of benzodiazepine	Decrease dose of benzodiazepines
	Theophylline, caffeine	Increased levels of theophylline or caffeine	Decrease dose of theophylline by approximately 1/3; avoid caffeine intake
	Warfarin	Increased effect of warfarin; increased risk of bleeding	Monitor INR; decrease dose of warfarin if necessary
Paroxetine	Phenytoin	Decreased effect of phenytoin	Monitor phenytoin; increased dose may be necessary
Citalopram	Cimetidine	Increased levels of citalopram	Monitor for side effects of citalopram; reduce dose if necessary
	Azole (e.g., fluconazole, ketoconazole) and erythromycin	Increased levels of citalopram	Monitor for side effects of citalopram during course of antibiotics
Nefazodone	Benzodiazepines (alprazolam, triazolam, midazolam)	Increased levels of benzodiazepines	Decrease dose (50–75%) of benzodiazepines
Bupropion	Levodopa	Increased effect from levodopa	Monitor for Levodopa toxicity; dose of Levodopa should be reduced if necessary
	Anticonvulsants	If anticonvulsant is used to control seizure disorder, bupropion may increase risk of seizures	Avoid use of bupropion in patients with history of seizure disorder
Venlafaxine	MAO-I	Increased risk of toxicity	Avoid use of MAO-I while taking venlafaxine
Mirtazapine	No clinically significant interactions		
TCA	Anticholinergic agents (e.g., antihistamines, low-potency neuroleptics)	Enhanced anticholinergic response	Avoid anticholinergic TCAs (use desipramine, nortriptyline when TCA is necessary); avoid combination with other anticholinergic agents
Cardiovascular			
Antihypertensives	NSAIDs	Decreased renal function, fluid retention; increased BP	Avoid use of NSAIDs if possible; use minimal dose when necessary
	Vasodilators (e.g., nitroglycerin)	Additive drop in BP; risk of orthostasis and falls	Lower BP to goal only; use nonpharm techniques to prevent falls
ACE-I	K+ sparing diuretics; K+ supplements	Increased K+ retention; risk of cardiac arrhythmias	Monitor K+; avoid K+-sparing diuretics while on ACE-I
Digoxin	Amiodarone	Increased level of digoxin	Lower dose of digoxin; smaller dose of amiodarone
Amiodarone	Diuretics	Hypokalemia, digoxin toxicity	Monitor K+; supplement when necessary
	Warfarin	Increased levels of warfarin, potentiation of anticoagulant	Monitor INR; decrease warfarin dose
	Digoxin	Digoxin levels increased; increased risk of digoxin toxicity	Monitor digoxin levels, signs/symptoms of toxicity; decrease digoxin dosing

Table 7 Drug–drug interactions of commonly used medications in the elderly (*Continued*)

Drug	Interacting drug	Mechanism/effect	Management
	Quinidine	Increased (free) levels of quinidine	Decrease dose of quinidine by 30–50%
	Procainamide	Increased levels of procainamide	Decrease dose of procainamide by 30% when starting amiodarone
	Phenytoin	Increased levels of phenytoin	Monitor phenytoin levels and s/s of toxicity; decrease phenytoin dosing if necessary
Diuretics	NSAID/aspirin	Decreased fluid removal, minimized response of BP lowering effect	Avoid NSAID use if possible in the elderly
	Lithium	Competition for lithium elimination; increased lithium levels	Avoid use of diuretics while using lithium; lower dose of lithium if necessary
Warfarin	Amiodarone	Increased anticoagulant effect	Lower dose of warfarin (titrate to goal INR)
	NSAIDs/aspirin	Increased risk of bleeding	Minimize NSAID use while on warfarin
	Estrogen supplements	Pharmacodynamic interaction; procoagulant effect of estrogen	Increased dose of warfarin may be needed; estrogens contraindicated in patient with coagulation disorder
	Antibiotics (e.g., cotrimoxazole, ciprofloxacin, fluconazole, ketoconazole)	Increased levels, effect of warfarin	Monitor INR carefully during course of antibiotics; reduce dose of warfarin if necessary
Endocrinology			
Thyroid supplements	Calcium supplements Sucralfate Cholestyramine Colestipol Iron supplements Aluminum hydroxide	Decreased bioavailability of L-thyroxine	Take thyroid supplement on an empty stomach
	Amiodarone	Alteration in L-thyroxine requirements (may ↑ or ↓)	Monitor thyroid function and adjust L-thyroxine as necessary
Sulfonylurea (e.g., glyburide, glipazide)	β-blockers	May block hypoglycemic responses	Use cardioselective β-blockers (e.g., metoprolol, atenolol); patient education to monitor for sweating
	Fluconazole High-dose salicylates Sulfonamides	Enhanced hypoglycemic response	Monitor for signs/symptoms of hypoglycemia; manipulate diet or reduce dose of sulfonylurea
Metformin	Contrast dye	Lacticacidosis and organ failure	Avoid use of contrast dye while on metformin; avoid renally toxic medications while on metformin
	Cimetidine	Decreased elimination, increased levels of metformin	Avoid use of cimetidine while taking metformin; consider using ranitidine or famotidine
Gastrointestinal			
Cimetidine	Carbamazepine Diazepam Glipizide Phenytoin Theophylline TCA Warfarin	Inhibition of metabolism	Avoid use of cimetidine if possible; use ranitidine or famotidine

(*Continued*)

Table 7 Drug–drug interactions of commonly used medications in the elderly (*Continued*)

Drug	Interacting drug	Mechanism/effect	Management
Proton pump inhibitors	Digoxin Itraconazole Iron salts Ketoconazole	Decreased absorption of medications that are pH-dependent	Monitor response to medication; increase in dose may be necessary
Metoclopramide	Dopamine replacement Parkinson's disease medications	Antagonism of dopamine by metoclopramide	Avoid use of metoclopramide in patients with Parkinson's disease
	Anticholinergics Narcotics	Medications that slow GI motility antagonize the effect of metoclopramide	Avoid use of antagonistic medications
Neuroleptics			
Neuroleptics	Antiparkinson's medications	Neuroleptics may exacerbate or cause Parkinsonian movements	Avoid use of neuroleptics (except clozapine) in Parkinson's patients
	Antihypertensives	Increased risk of orthostasis, hypotension	Monitor BP in patients; reduce dosage of medications as necessary to prevent falls, dizziness
Haloperidol	Carbamazepine	Increase metabolism, decreased effectiveness of haloperidol	Increase haloperidol dose as necessary
Respiratory			
Theophylline	Phenytoin Rifampin Carbamazepine	Decrease serum levels of theophylline	Increase theophylline dosing as needed
	Allopurinol Cimetidine Ciprofloxacin Erythromycin	Increase serum levels of theophylline	Decrease theophylline dosing to prevent toxicity
Corticosteroids	Antidiabetic medications	Increased hyperglycemia from steroids; loss of control of blood glucose levels	Monitor serum glucose closely; increase hypoglycemic medications or add insulin as necessary
	NSAIDs	Increased GI intolerance; risk of GI bleeding	Avoid use of concomitant therapy if possible
	Amphotericin B loop diuretics	Increased risk of hypokalemia	Monitor K$^+$ and replace as necessary

ACE-I, indicates angiotensin converting-enzyme inhibitor; BP, blood pressure; CNS, central nervous system; GI, gastrointestinal; INR, international normalization ratio; K+, potassium; NSAID, nonsteroidal anti-inflammatory drug; SSRI, selective serotonin receptor inhibitor; TCA, tricyclic antidepressant.

Table 8 Clinically significant drug and food interactions in the elderly

Class of drug	Interaction	Clinical significance	Recommendation
Anti-infectives Antibacterials			
Azithromycin	Food decreases absorption	May lower concentration of antibiotic by >50%	Space medication and food at least 2 h apart
Erythromycin	Food decreases absorption; food may decrease some GI upset	Most patients have GI complaints and may prefer to take erythromycin with food; however, this may lead to decreased absorption	Space medication and food 2 h apart if patient can tolerate; if GI complaints, take erythromycin with small snack
Fluoroquinolones (e.g., ciprofloxacin)	Dairy products, iron, multivalent cations decrease absorption of fluoroquinolones	Quinolones ineffective because of chelation	Administer medication at least 2 h apart from any foods
Metronidazole	Alcohol-containing products may cause a disulfiram-like reaction	Nausea, vomiting, vasodilation may be experienced by patients	Avoid all alcohol-containing products while taking metronidazole
Penicillins (oral)	Food decreases absorption	May lower concentration of antibiotic	Space medication and food at least 2 h apart
Tetracyclines	Dairy products, iron, multivalent cations decrease absorption of tetracycline	Tetracycline ineffective because of chelation	Administer medication at least 2 h apart from any foods containing cations
Antifungals			
Griseofulvin	High-fat meal increases absorption	If medication given without a fatty meal, griseofulvin ineffective	Administer with fatty foods
Ketoconazole	Possible insulin-sparing effect	Patient may experience lower blood glucose concentrations on the same insulin dose	Monitor for decreased insulin requirements
	Interference with vitamin D and steroid metabolism	Osteomalacia may develop if long-term administration of ketoconazole is used hypoparathyroidism has developed	Ensure adequate vitamin D and calcium intake Monitor calcium and phosphorus levels if ketoconazole is used long-term
Antituberculars			
Isoniazid	May decrease pyridoxine (vitamin B6); food may decrease absorption of isoniazid	Peripheral neuropathy may develop; decreased absorption of isoniazid may lead to therapeutic failure	Supplement individuals with vitamin B6 50 mg daily; administer isoniazid at least 2 h apart from any foods
Rifampin	May decrease effect of vitamin D	Individuals may be predisposed to osteomalacia	Ensure adequate vitamin D and calcium intake during long-term therapy

(Continued)

(Continued)

Table 8 Clinically significant drug and food interactions in the elderly (*Continued*)

Class of drug	Interaction	Clinical significance	Recommendation
Anticoagulants Warfarin	Vitamin K—green leafy vegetables and green tea antagonize warfarin	Large amounts vitamin K can decrease INR leading to therapeutic failure of warfarin	Avoid excessive consumption of green leafy vegetables; do not alter diet once anticoagulation with warfarin is stabilized
Anticonvulsants Phenytoin	Reduced levels of vitamin D due to increased metabolism of active vitamin D metabolites	Osteomalacia and rickets have been reported with long-term anticonvulsant therapy; additional risk factors for these conditions (e.g., poor sunlight exposure) increases risk	Ensure adequate supplementation of vitamin D, 400 IU daily
	Administering medication with enteral feeds binds phenytoin	Enteral feeds can significantly lower absorption of phenytoin	Hold enteral feeds for minimum of 1 h while administering phenytoin
	Decrease in folate concentrations	Long-term therapy may put patients at risk of folate deficiency	Close monitoring of gingival hyperplasia and megaloblastic anemia if patient is using long-term phenytoin therapy; consider supplementing folate starting at 1 mg daily for prevention
Antidepressants MAO-I (e.g., isocarboxazid, phenelzine, tranylcypromine)	Tyramine-containing foods lead to excessive sympathetic stimulation	Hypertensive crisis can develop	Avoid aged, fermented, pickled, or smoked foods
Tricyclic antidepressants (e.g., amitriptyline, desipramine, nortriptyline, etc.)	Medications inhibit breakdown of food because of decreased saliva production; food in general may cause xerostomia	May cause difficulty in swallowing food	Suck on sugarless hard candy, ice chips, or chew sugarless gum
Antihistamines Chlorpheniramine, dimenhydrinate, diphenhydramine, etc.	Medications inhibit breakdown of food because of decreased saliva production; food in general may cause	May cause difficulty in swallowing food	Suck on sugarless hard candy, ice chips, or chew sugarless gum
Autonomic medications Ephedrine, pseudoephedrine, amphetamines	Caffeine may cause increased nervousness and insomnia	Most significant if taken before bedtime	Minimize daily caffeine intake while using stimulating medications

Table 8 Clinically significant drug and food interactions in the elderly (*Continued*)

Class of drug	Interaction	Clinical significance	Recommendation
Cardiovascular medications			
ACE-I (e.g., lisinopril, enalapril, ramipril, etc.)	Salt substitutes containing potassium	Potassium-containing substitutes and an ACE-I can result in hyperkalemia	Avoid potassium-containing salt substitutes
Captopril	Food decreases absorption of captopril	Taking with food may minimize blood pressure-lowering effects	Space medication and food 2 h apart or take at the same time every day
	Zinc deficiency with high-dose, long-term use	Most pronounced in individuals receiving at least 150 mg daily; taste impairment a marker of zinc deficiency	Monitor for taste impairment; zinc supplementation has not been definitively shown to be of benefit
Digoxin	High-fiber, high-pectin foods delay and decrease absorption	May minimize the benefit of digoxin	Avoid administering digoxin with high-fiber foods; administer at the same time every day
Potassium-sparing diuretics (e.g., triamterene)	Potassium-containing salt substitutes may lead to additive effect of increased potassium	Excessive amounts of potassium may lead to cardiac arrhythmias	Avoid potassium-containing salt substitutes
Corticosteroids			
Hydrocortisone, prednisone, methyprednisolone	Decreased glucose tolerance with carbohydrates	Rapid, small elevation in blood glucose can be seen. Glucose levels do not normalize until steroid therapy is discontinued	Monitor blood glucose levels in persons with diabetes
	Triglycerides and cholesterol may increase	Long-term use may accelerate atherosclerotic processes	Monitor patients at risk of heart disease or elevated cholesterol/triglyceride levels on long-term steroid therapy
Diabetes medications			
Insulin	Possible insulin sparing effect with ketoconazole	Patient may experience lower blood glucose concentrations on the same insulin dose	Monitor for decreased insulin requirements
Metformin	Interaction with the absorption of vitamin B12	Patient may experience vitamin B12 deficiency	Monitor levels closely in patients predisposed to vitamin B12 deficiency
Gastrointestinal medications			
Misoprostol	Increases GI motility, nausea, distress if taken on empty stomach	Taken without food can dramatically increase GI side effects	Take with food

(*Continued*)

Table 8 Clinically significant drug and food interactions in the elderly (*Continued*)

Class of drug	Interaction	Clinical significance	Recommendation
Sucralfate	Food (protein) decreases binding of sucralfate to gastric mucosa	Ineffective binding leads to lack of protection for gastric ulcers	Give sucralfate at least 1 h before meals to allow adequate binding to the gastric mucosa
Lipid lowering medications			
Cholestyramine	Binds iron, folic acid, essential fatty acids, vitamin A	Cholestyramine can significantly lower absorption of nutrients	Consider vitamin supplementation and monitor iron status for long-term use of cholestyramine
	Calcium absorption may be impaired	Long-term use of cholestyramine may increase risk of osteoporosis	Ensure adequate calcium, vitamin D intake by spacing supplements at least 2 h from administration of cholestyramine
Lovastatin	Improved absorption if given with food	If taken on an empty stomach lipid-lowering effect may be minimized	Take with evening meal or snack to maximize absorption of lovastatin
Pulmonary medications			
Theophylline time-release	High-fat meals—rate of absorption can be affected	Elevated theophylline levels may result, possibly causing tachycardia, palpitations, irritability, and tremor	Avoid administering medication with high-fat foods, altering diet while on the medication, or take 1 h before eating
Pain medications			
NSAID (e.g., ibuprofen, naproxen, piroxicam)	Gastric irritation may occur from direct GI contact or through systemic mechanisms (i.e., irritation may occur with suppositories or enteric coated products)	Severe gastric irritation may occur if taken on an empty stomach	Take with food to minimize gastric irritation
Parkinson's medications			
Anticholinergic medications (e.g., benztropine, procyclidine)	Medications inhibit breakdown of food because of decreased saliva production; food in general may cause xerostomia	May cause difficulty in swallowing food	Suck on sugarless hard candy, ice chips, or chew sugarless gum
Levodopa	Competition for absorption with protein	Minimize or nullify benefit of levodopa	Space medication and food 2 h apart or administer with nonprotein meal
Psychiatric medications			
Lithium	Sodium and lithium compete for reabsorption/elimination	Altering sodium intake may alter lithium level	Do not change diet once lithium is stabilized

the amount believed necessary. Causes of intentional or unintentional nonadherence include medication regimens that are difficult to fit into the patient's lifestyle, unwanted effects, expensive medications, or patient's inability to self-administer the product (33, 34). Most important, if patients do not believe they need the medication, they will be less likely to take the prescription.

Risks for nonadherence have been studied, and some of the findings include the complexity of dosing schedule (e.g., four times daily versus once daily dosing); frequent changes in medication; substitution of medication (therapeutic or generic); multiple medications; unpleasant side effects; difficulty in opening containers; cost; difficult routes of administration; inadequate patient education/understanding; and cognitive, visual, or physical function impairment (31, 33, 34). Patients who already have vision or mobility problems may become noncompliant when some of the factors noted above are added to their existing challenges with medication management.

Factors that have been linked to improving adherence include a belief that the medication is important, a belief that it is effective, and regularly attending the same medical clinic and pharmacy (34).

A number of studies have also tried to determine indicators of poor self-medication management. Some of these indicators are cognitive impairment (MMSE <24), physical dependency (Katz $\geq$ 1), and poor self-reported medication management (35).

When prescribing medications for the elderly, it is important to consider physical disability, visual impairment, the shape or color of medications (ability to differentiate), and the belief system of the patient (35, 36). It would be beneficial to have healthcare professionals review the technique of using certain devices and to discuss the use of compliance aids.

Various compliance aids have been studied in an attempt to increase adherence to prescribed regimens (36–38). These aids include alarm clock devices, blister packing, calendar packaging, and more. Some providers feel they greatly assist patients who otherwise would become confused or could not manage multiple medications on their own, which would increase their risk of an adverse event or nonadherence. It has also been argued that these aids can be difficult to use, and the patients who benefit most are often those who would likely manage well without any aids. There are studies providing support for both views, and the subject requires additional study.

It is important to consider that even with compliance aids, the patients must receive appropriate counseling and instruction on how to manage the devices properly (37, 38). The aids must also be recommended and agreed to by the patient for them to be of use. For example, if a patient feels they have lost some of their independence by having to use blister packaging, they are still not likely to become compliant. However, if the patient has agreed that an aid would be helpful and save them time, they are more likely to appreciate the additional assistance and will use the product to increase adherence. Patient preference, agreement, and education are still the most important factors in improving adherence. Additional factors that must be considered are the medication effects. If a patient discontinues a prescription because of side effects, packaging the medications into a compliance aid will not improve adherence. Before a compliance aid is considered, the reason for nonadherence must be carefully reviewed (39) because an aid may not be necessary at all and may offend patients if they think the provider feels they are becoming cognitively impaired.

Polypharmacy

When translated, polypharmacy simply means multiple medications. However, the clinical interpretation of this term usually refers to the use of multiple medications in an inappropriate, illogical, or harmful manner to the patient.

It is expected that the elderly have a higher incidence of chronic disease and will be prescribed more medications to manage their diseases. It is very easy to quickly reach a state of polypharmacy. Risk factors include multiple doctors, diseases, and pharmacies (40). Patients often present with a variety of complaints but may lack a diagnosis, triggering the prescription of medications that are used to manage the complaints that do not resolve the illness. Patients also use numerous nonprescription medications, which may go unmonitored and yet have the potential to interact with prescribed medicines. Patients seeing multiple doctors is often a concern because specialists may not take into consideration other prescribed medications before ordering new drugs for the patient. Similarly, some physicians may not be aware that their patients are seeing other doctors, causing difficulty in monitoring prescriptions in these of patients.

Although it is somewhat controversial, certain personality traits in elderly patients may predispose them to using more medications (36, 40). Elderly patients and their physicians may also be reluctant to discontinue medications. Often, patients with these views feel it is necessary to use medications and to obtain more prescriptions each time they visit a physician. This may also tie in with the attitudes of healthcare providers, who may be pressured to prescribe more medications for the patient. Finally, polypharmacy may be common in the elderly because they often borrow medication from family or friends, sometimes because of lack of education about the risks of inappropriate medication use.

Tablet Splitting

Tablet splitting is common in the elderly population (41) often because of cost-savings and the production of larger dosage strengths to meet the needs of younger patients. The prescriber may feel that the patient requires much less medication than a typical dose and consequently prescribes a dose that the patient must split. This is done frequently with medications that are adjusted throughout the course of treatment, such as warfarin for anti-coagulation. Tablet splitting is also common when titrating medications that cannot be started in full doses because of intolerance. A common example of this is the use of β-blockers post-MI when only small doses are tolerated at the onset, but when the goal is to reach a much higher dose.

This topic has been studied only in a small number of studies and often focuses on younger subjects (42). The process of tablet splitting is also not generalizable to the elderly population because the muscle strength, fatigue, and duration of time to split are often measured in young patients doing repetitive tablet-splitting tasks, which does not reflect the typical scenario in an elderly patient's home.

Underutilization/Undertreatment

Both undertreatment and underutilization of medications are common problems in the elderly. It is often a result of stereotyping by healthcare professionals, lack of education of managing medications in the elderly, and lack of research (4). Examples include treatment of hypertension, prescribing hormone therapy, osteoporosis, treating MI, lipid management, pain management, and depression.

DETERMINING MEDICATION APPROPRIATENESS IN THE ELDERLY

There have been many attempts to characterize and quantify the "appropriateness" of medications in the elderly. The first such scale was developed by Hanlon and is called the Medication Appropriateness Index (43). It has been used most frequently in the Veterans Affairs population in the United States.

Beers et al. (44) developed a list of medications that were considered inappropriate in a nursing home population. Their most recent list further describes appropriate doses of medications that should be used in the elderly (44). For example, digoxin is suggested to be given at 0.125 mg daily because most elderly patients either

become toxic or do not require higher doses for efficacy. Other lists have been developed (11) and updated (10). These lists are generally considered guidelines and should be used with professional judgment when prescribing and managing dosing in the elderly. Other tools have also been studied and are being developed. A review of different instruments has been written by Shelton et al. (45).

DOSAGE FORMS

Geriatric patients are able to use any type of dosage form available; none are contraindicated based on age alone. The most frequently used dosage form in the elderly is the oral route; however, other dosage forms may be used based on disease state. For example, chronic obstructive pulmonary disease is common in the elderly, and the route of choice for administration of medications is by inhalation. Therefore, this population frequently uses inhalers. Another common dosage form used in geriatric patients is eyedrops. Dosage forms requiring hand strength or coordination may be difficult to administer in some geriatric patients with certain conditions such as arthritis, weakness after a stroke, dementia, or other impairments. The challenges with each of these dosage forms are presented later.

Inhalers

Lung diseases such as COPD and asthma are common in the elderly population. The cornerstone of treatment of these conditions is to use medications administered by inhaler, using either a turbuhaler, nebulizer, metered-dose inhaler (MDI), diskhaler, or other breath-activated device. These devices often require good eyesight, hand–eye coordination, hand strength to depress the MDI, and intact cognition to manage the device. Age itself has been found to be a predictor of poor technique; however, other studies (46) found that other disease states that increase with age are more significant predictors of success in using MDIs. A patient with poor hand strength, such as a patient with rheumatoid or osteoarthritis, may have difficulty managing the inhalers. Patients who are blind or have decreased vision may also have difficulty organizing their inhalers in the proper order or manipulating any of the devices. Cognitive decline is also more common in elderly patients and tends to increase with age. This has been found to be a determinant of poor technique when using inhalers (46). It is important for healthcare professionals to assess the ability of patients to use inhalation devices before they are prescribed. Repeated counseling and education are necessary to maintain good technique and appropriate use of these devices in the elderly population (38, 46, 47).

Eye Drops

Disease states frequently requiring medication such as eye drops are common in the elderly. Many elderly patients also use nonprescription natural tear replacement products for lubrication. It is therefore common to have elderly patients using eye drops, even though there are many challenges and difficulties in administering medication by this route. The majority of patients, when asked, admit to having difficulty administering eye drops (48). There is difficulty in raising arms above one's head, which can result from limited range of motion secondary to arthritis or deconditioning. It is also necessary to be in the supine position or to tilt one's head far back to keep the drops in the eye. This is often difficult for patients because of neck osteoarthritis or stiffness. It is also very challenging to aim the drops accurately. A number of devices have been studied, but none make compression of the drops easier (48). It is often difficult for patients to compress the bottle to release the drops, and some patients do not use correct technique and expel more than the required amount of drops. Some of the reasons for difficulty in administering drops are similar to those listed above for difficulty with actuating MDIs. Most of the devices appear to help improve aim only, which is just one part of the problem for elderly patients. Difficulty with eye drops commonly results in treatment failure as patients become nonadherent or administer drops incorrectly and receive less benefit than could be expected. It is important to review technique and to prescribe appropriate compliance aids to make administration easier for patients because often, there are no other options but to use eye drops for ophthalmic conditions.

CONCLUSION

Considering the diversity and challenges in dealing with the geriatric population, it is important to be aware of the physiological changes that occur with aging and the complications that can arise when these changes are not considered when dosing medications. It is also important to be aware of the potential problems that can arise in treating geriatric patients with multiple disease states because they are more likely to experience adverse events and to have more drug-related problems such as nonadherence. Although each patient should be managed individually, there are important principles that should be considered when working with geriatric patients to optimize the dosing and dosage forms used in this population.

REFERENCES

1. U.S. Census Bureau, U.S.A. Statistics in Brief—Population and Vital Statistics. http://www.census.gov/statab/www/part1.html (accessed July 26, 2000).
2. Ostrom, J.F.; Hammarlund, E.R.; Christensen, D.B. Medication Usage in an Elderly Population, Med. Care. 1985; 23, 157–164.
3. Lamy, P.P. Comparative Pharmacokinetic Changes and Drug Therapy in an Older Population, J. Am. Geriatr. Soc. 1982, 30 (11 Suppl.), S11–S19.
4. Hanlon, J.T.; Ruby, C.M.; Shelton, P.S.; Pulliam, C.C. Geriatrics. Pharmacotherapy and Pathophysiologic Approach, 4th Ed.; DiPiro, J.T., Talbert, R.L., Yee, G.C., Matzke, G.R., Wells, B.G., Posey, L.M., Eds.; Appleton & Lange: Stamford, CT, 1999; 52–61.
5. Montamat, S.C.; Cusack, B.J.; Vestal, R.E. Management of Drug Therapy in the Elderly. New Engl. J. Med. 1989, 321 (5), 303–309.
6. Parker, B.M.; Cusack, B.J.; Vestal, R.E. Pharmacokinetic Optimisation of Drug Therapy in Elderly Patients. Drugs Aging 1995, 7 (1), 10–18.
7. Grandison, M.K.; Boudinot, F.D. Age-Related Changes in Protein Binding of Drugs. Clin. Pharmacokinet. 2000, 38 (3), 271–290.
8. Cockroft, D.W.; Gault, M.H. Prediction of Creatinine Clearance from Serum Creatinine. Nephron 1976, 16, 31–41.
9. Swift, C.G. Pharmacodynamics: Changes in Homeostatic Mechanisms, Receptor and Target Organ Sensitivity in the Elderly. Br. Med. Bull. 1990, 46 (1), 36–52.
10. Beers, M.H. Explicit Criteria for Determining Potentially Inappropriate Medication Use by the Elderly. Arch. Intern. Med. 1998, 157, 1531–1536.
11. McLeod, P.J.; Huang, A.R.; Tamblyn, R.M.; Gayton, D.C. Defining Inappropriate Practices in Prescribing for Elderly People: A National Consensus Panel. Can. Med. Assoc. J. 1997, 156 (3), 385–391.
12. Lamy, Peter P. Adverse Drug Effects. Clin. Geriatr. Med. 1990, 6 (2), 293–307.
13. Hanlon, J.T.; Schmader, K.E.; Koronkowski, M.J.; Weinberger, M.; Landsman, P.B.; Samsa, G.P.; Lewis, I.K. Adverse Drug Events in High Risk Older Outpatients. J. Am. Griat. Soc. 1997, 45, 945–948.
14. Atkin, P.A.; Veitch, P.C.; Veitch, E.M.; Ogle, S.J. The Epidemiology of Serious Adverse Drug Reactions Among the Elderly. Drugs Aging 1999, 14 (2), 141–152.
15. Lazarou, J.; Pomeranz, B.H.; Corey, P.N. Incidence of Adverse Drug Reactions in Hospitalized Patients, a Meta-Analysis of Prospective Studies. J. Am. Med. Assoc. 1998, 279, 1200–1205.
16. Veehof, L.J.G.; Stewart, R.E.; Meyboom-de Jong, B.; Haaijer-Ruskamp, F.M. Adverse Drug Reactions and Polypharmacy in the Elderly in General Practice. Eur. J. Clin. Pharmacol. 1999, 55, 533–536.
17. Beyth, R.J.; Shorr, R.I. Epidemiology of Adverse Drug Reactions in the Elderly by Drug Class. Drugs Aging 1999, 14 (3), 231–239.
18. Gerety, M.B.; Cornell, J.E.; Plichta, D.T.; Eimer, M. Adverse Events Related to Drugs and Drug Withdrawal in Nursing Home Residents. J. Am. Geriatr. Soc. 1993, 41, 1326–1332.

19. Graves, T.; Hanlon, J.T.; Schmader, K.E.; Landsman, P.B.; Samsa, G.P.; Pieper, C.F.; Weinberger, M. Adverse Events after Discontinuing Medications in Elderly Outpatients. Arch. Intern. Med. **1997**, *157*, 2205–2210.
20. Cumming, R.G. Epidemiology of Medication-Related Falls and Fractures in the Elderly. Drugs Aging **1998**, *12* (1), 43–53.
21. Monane, M.; Avorn, J. Medications and Falls. Clin. Geriatr. Med. **1996**, *12* (4), 847–858.
22. King, M.B.; Tinetti, M.E. Falls in Community-Dwelling Older Persons. J. Am. Geriatr. Soc. **1995**, *43*, 1146–1154.
23. Leipzig, R.M.; Cumming, R.G.; Tinetti, M.E. Drugs and Falls in Older People—A Systematic Review and Meta-Analysis, I. Psychotropic Drugs. J. Am. Geriatr. Soc. **1999**, *47*, 30–39.
24. Leipzig, R.M.; Cumming, R.G.; Tinetti, M.E. Drugs and Falls in Older People—A Systematic Review and Meta-Analysis, II Cardiac and Analgesic Drugs. J. Am. Geriatr. Soc. **1999**, *47*, 40–59.
25. Inouye, S.K. Delirium in Hospitalized Older Patients. Clin. Geriatr. Med. **1998**, *14* (4), 745–764.
26. Flacker, J.M.; Marcantonio, E.R. Delirium in the Elderly. Drugs Aging **1998**, *13* (2), 119–130.
27. Moore, A.R.; O-Keeffe, S.T. Drug-Induced Cognitive Impairment in the Elderly. Drugs Aging **1999**, *15* (1), 15–28.
28. Seymour, R.M.; Routledge, P.A. Important Drug–Drug Interactions in the Elderly. Drugs Aging **1998**, *12* (6), 485–494.
29. Doucet, J.; Chassagne, P.; Trivalle, C.; Landrin, I.; Pauty, M.D.; Kadri, N.; Menard, J.F.; Bercoff, E. Drug–Drug Interactions Related to Hospital Admissions in Older Adults—A Prospective Study of 1000 Patients. J. Am. Geriatr. Soc. **1996**, *44*, 944–948.
30. Thomas, J.A.; Burns, R.A. Important Drug-Nutrient Interactions in the Elderly. Drugs Aging **1998**, *13* (3), 199–209.
31. Fuhr, U. Drug Interactions with Grapefruit Juice Extent, Probable Mechanism and Clinical Relevance. Drug Safety **1998**, *18* (4), 251–272.
32. Morrow, D.; Leirer, V.; Sheikh, J. Adherence and Medication Instructions Review and Recommendations. J. Am. Geriatr. Soc. **1988**, *36*, 1147–1160.
33. Conn, V.; Taylor, S.G.; Stineman, A. Medication Management by Recently Hospitalized Older Adults. J. Community Health Nurs. **1992**, *9* (1), 1–11.
34. Stewart, S.; Pearson, S. Uncovering a Multitude of Sins: Medication Management in the Home Post Acute Hospitalisation Among the Chronically Ill. Aust. NZ J. Med. **1999**, *29* (2), 220–227.
35. Ruscin, J.M.; Semla, T.P. Assessment of Medication Management Skills in Older Outpatients. Ann. Pharmacother. **1996**, *30*, 1083–1088.
36. Thwaites, J.H. Practical Aspects of Drug Treatment in Elderly Patients with Mobility Problems. Drugs Aging **1999**, *14* (2), 105–114.
37. Cramer, J.A. Optimizing Long-Term Patient Compliance. Neurology **1995**, *45* (Suppl 1), S25–S28.
38. Sexton, J.; Gokani, R. Pharmaceutical Packaging and the Elderly. Pharm. J. **1997**, *259*, 697–700.
39. Weintraub, M. Compliance in the Elderly. Clin. Geriatr. Med. **1990**, *6* (2), 445–452.
40. Stewart, R.B.; Cooper, J.W. Polypharmacy in the Aged Practical Solutions. Drugs Aging **1994**, *4* (6), 449–461.
41. Rochon, P.A.; Clark, J.P.; Gurwitz, J.H. Challenges of Prescribing Low-Dose Drug Therapy for Older People. Can. Med. Assoc. J. **1999**, *160* (7), 1029–1031.
42. McDevitt, J.T.; Gurst, A.H.; Chen, Y. Accuracy of Tablet Splitting. Pharmacotherapy **1998**, *18* (1), 193–197.
43. Hanlon, J.T.; Schmader, K.E.; Samsa, G.P.; Weinberger, M.; Uttech, K.M.; Lewis, I.K.; Cohen, H.J.; Feussner, J.R. A Method for Assessing Drug Therapy Appropriateness. J. Clin. Epidemiol. **1992**, *45* (10), 1045–1051.
44. Beers, M.H.; Ouslander, J.G.; Rollingher, I.; Reuben, D.B.; Brooks, J.; Beck, J.C. Explicit Criteria for Determining Inappropriate Medication Use in Nursing Home Residents. Arch. Intern. Med. **1991**, *151*, 1825–1832.
45. Shelton, P.S.; Fritsch, M.; Scott, M.A. Assessing Medication Appropriateness in the Elderly: A Review of Available Measures. Drugs Aging **2000**, *16* (6), 437–450.
46. Gray, S.L.; Williams, D.M.; Pulliam, C.C.; Sirgo, M.A.; Bishop, A.L.; Donohue, J.F. Characteristics Predicting Incorrect Metered-Dose Inhaler Technique in Older Subjects. Arch. Intern. Med. **1996**, *156*, 984–988.
47. Daniels, S.; Meuleman, J. Importance of Assessment of Metered-Dose Inhaler Technique in the Elderly. J. Am. Geriatr. Soc. **1994**, *42*, 82–84.
48. Winfield, A.J.; Jessiman, D.; Williams, A.; Esakowitz, L. A Study of the Causes of Non-Compliance by Patients Prescribed Eyedrops. Br. J. Ophthalmol. **1990**, *74* (8), 477–480.
49. Kane, R.L.; Ouslander, J.G.; Abrass, I.B. *Essentials of Clinical Geriatrics*, 4th Ed.; McGraw-Hill: New York, 1999.
50. Swonger, A.K.; Burbank, P.M. *Drug Therapy and the Elderly*; Jones and Bartlett Publishers: Boston, 1995.
51. Luisi, A.F.; Owens, N.J.; Hume, A.L. Drugs and the Elderly. *Reichel's Care of the Elderly Clinical Aspects of Aging,*; 5th Ed.; Gallo, J.J., Busby-Whitehead, J., Rabins, P.V., Silliman, R.A., Murphy, J.B., Reichel, W., Eds.; Lippincott Williams & Wilkins: Baltimore, 1999; 59–87, Chap. 5.
52. Beyth, R.J.; Shorr, R.I. Medication Use. *Practice of Geriatrics*, 3rd Ed.; Duthie, E.H., Jr., Katz, P.R., Eds.; W.B. Saunders Company: Philadelphia, 1998; 38–47, Chap. 5.
53. Avorn, J.; Gurwitz, J.H. Principles of Pharmacology. *Geriatric Medicine*, 3rd Ed.; Cassel, C.K., Cohen, H.J., Larson, E.B., Meier, D.E., Resnick, N.M., Rubenstein, L.Z., Sorenson, L.B., Eds.; Springer: New York, 1997, 755–770, Chap. 5.
54. Schwartz, J.B. Clinical Pharmacology. *Principles of Geriatric Medicine and Gerontology*, 4th Ed.; Hazzard, W.R., Blass, J.P., Ettinger, W.H., Jr., Halter, J.B., Ouslander, J.G., Eds.; McGraw-Hill: New York, 1999; 303–331, Chap. 5.
55. Abrams, W.B.; Beers, M.H.; Berkow, R. *The Merck Manual of Geriatrics*, 3rd Ed.; Merck & Co. Inc.: Whitehouse Station: New Jersey, 2000.
56. Hansten, P.D.; Horn, J.R.; Koda-Kimble, M.A.; Young, L.Y. *Hansten & Horn's Managing Clinically Important Drug Interactions*; Applied Therapeutics Inc.: Vancouver, Washington, 1998.
57. Delafuente, J.C.; Stewart, R. *Therapeutics in the Elderly*, 3rd Ed.; Williams & Wilkins: Baltimore, 2000.
58. Kinirons, M.T.; Crome, P. Clinical Pharmacokinetic Considerations in the Elderly—An Update. Clin. Pharmacokinet. **1997**, *33* (4), 302–312.

GLASS AS A PACKAGING MATERIAL FOR PHARMACEUTICALS

Claudia C. Okeke
United States Pharmacopeia, Rockville, Maryland

INTRODUCTION

Glass has been used for over 6000 years, dating to ancient times. Through the years and with more knowledge of its technology, glass has become the most widely used drug packaging material. The origin of the first synthetic glass is unknown; however, Egyptians were known to mold figurines from sand and silicon dioxide (1). The American Heritage dictionary defines glass as a large class of materials with highly variable mechanical and optical properties that solidify from the molten state without crystallization, that are typically based on silicon dioxide, boric oxide, aluminum oxide, or phosphorous pentoxide, that are generally transparent or translucent, and that are regarded physically as supercooled liquids rather than fine liquids (2).

ASTM defines glass as an inorganic product of fusion that has cooled to a rigid condition without crystallizing (3). ASTM further states that glass is typically hard and brittle and has a conchoidal fracture. Glass may be colorless or colored. It is transparent but may be made opaque or translucent (3). Glass is noncrystalline and is amorphous in structure and may be formed from both organic and inorganic materials.

Glass is manufactured at very high temperatures, and at very hot temperatures, it has the properties of a viscous liquid. With the properties of a viscous liquid, hot glass can be formed into many commonly used forms with precision and accuracy. As a result of its noncrystalline nature, it affords a unique transparent property that is maintained because it does not crystallize upon cooling.

There are a variety of uses of glass, one use being a pharmaceutical packaging material. Glass is favored over other types of packaging material because its transparent property enables it to provide good visualization of contained material. Another good quality of glass is its excellent resistance to attack by most liquids, and, therefore, it resists interaction with contained products. It is also totally impermeable to gases, and it can be sterilized with any appropriate process. Glass, when properly colored, also provides protection of a product from light.

GLASS COMPOSITION

There are two glass compositions generally used—soda-lime and borosilicate. The soda–lime compositions are used for ordinary tableware, food, and beverage products, and window glass, among many others. Borosilicate glass is not widely used, but it is more durable and heat-resistant than soda-lime glass. This glass is used for laboratory and scientific glassware, and heat-resistant cookware, among many others. Borosilicate glass affords properties that make it a preferred composition for certain pharmaceutical containers. Glass composition will be discussed in detail below (4).

GLASS MANUFACTURE AND COMPOSITION

Raw Materials

Silicon dioxide (SiO_2) also known as silica, is the principal constituent of glass. Glass is made by melting its ingredients at very high temperatures, such as 1550°C. Because the melting point of silica alone is so high, and, therefore, commercially difficult to melt and form into containers, other oxides are added to silica to lower the melting point and make it easier to fabricate and use commercially (5). These oxides include sodium oxide (Na_2O); aluminum oxide (Al_2O_3); potassium oxide (K_2O); boron oxide (B_2O_3); and calcium oxide (CaO). The addition of one or more of these oxides reduces the melt viscosity for fabrication purposes. Other materials may be added to change a color, facilitate melting, or for other reasons. Sodium and potassium oxides are obtained as the product of chemical processing of naturally occurring materials, and an abundant source is the brines of Searles Lake in California. Sodium is primarily added to silica to lower the melting temperature and aid in the removal of gas bubbles in a reasonable time. Potassium oxide is used in smaller amounts. All of these additives change the properties of silica in such a way that the resulting glass is less resistant to attack by aqueous solutions. Other additives such as calcium oxide, magnesium oxide, and aluminum oxide are also used in various amounts to affect the properties of the glass. Silica has a very low coefficient of thermal expansion, and the addition of an alkali such as sodium oxide increases the thermal expansion.

When fluxing action is needed during melting and glass with high thermal expansion is undesirable, boric oxide is added forming borosilicate glasses, which have lower thermal expansion and improved resistance to attack by aqueous solutions because of lower sodium oxide contents.

Conditions necessary for glass formation may be deduced from either geometric or bond strength considerations. Silica sand deposit is available in all parts of the world. Silica sand is mined by hydraulic dredging, and any impurities are eliminated through further processing. One impurity, iron oxide, may be present, and, if present, may affect the final color of the glass (4). There are other oxides that are potential glass formers and may be used in glass formation: GeO_2, P_2O_5, As_2O_5, P_2O_3, As_2O_3, Sb_2O_3, V_2O_5, Sb_2O_5, Nb_2O_5, and Ta_2O_5 (6). Pharmaceutical containers may require amber glass to provide protection for light-sensitive pharmaceutical products. Amber glass is available in both soda-lime and borosilicate. The amber glasses have negligible transmission in ultraviolet (UV) and near UV regions and, hence, provide the required protection. In these cases, glass is interacted with iron oxide to provide amber color.

For pharmaceutical products that undergo sterilization by means of ionizing radiation, cerium oxide of about 1% or less is added to the glass formulation. This is because ionizing radiation type sterilization [dosages as high as 20–30 kGy (2 to 3 Mrad)] affects ordinary glass by darkening the glass and, thus, inhibits the final inspection of the glass products.

The mechanism by which ionization radiation acts on glass is by dislodging the electrons in the glass structure (usually intermediate density and low cost glasses) to form color centers and creating changes to the multivalent ions in such a way that they absorb visible. The result is a formation of neutral atoms such as sodium that can agglomerate into colloid-like configurations. Cerium oxide, which is multivalent when added to the formulation, counteracts the darkening effect of radiation by capturing these free electrons and minimizing the deleterious effects without adding color to the glass (4).

All raw materials used to formulate a glass composition should be characterized using certain specifications of particle size, distribution, overall purity, and specific impurity content. It is necessary to match the particle size of the raw materials as much as possible to allow trouble-free melting.

Also classified as a raw material is cullet. Cullet is a scrap glass of desired composition, which results from scrap generated during forming operations and kept strictly segregated by composition. Cullet is then recycled through the melting process. The use of cullet conserves raw materials and aids in the melting process. A typical diagram illustrating the process in glass manufacturing is shown in Fig. 1 (1).

FORMULATION—BATCH MIXING, CHARGING, AND MELTING

In a typical factory, a batch formulation is developed that provides the desired glass composition when melted. The raw materials are stored in large capacity silos. Depending on the type of plant facility, the raw material may be proportioned and mixed by a computer programmed with the batch formulation. The computer functions to control the automatic material transport system, weighing equipment, withdrawing the correct amount the raw materials from the perspective silos, and discharging them into a large mixing vessel. After mixing for the desired time, the batch is discharged into cans of mixed batch. These cans are transported to the charging end of the melting furnace. Complete records are maintained for the weighing, mixing, and transportation of batch materials to the furnace.

Usually, when the intimately mixed batch is charged into the hot furnace, a series of melting, dissolution, volatilization, and redox reactions occur between the materials in a certain order and at the appropriate temperature (7). At the furnace, the batch contents are discharged through a screw feeder into the furnace, with temperatures capable of exceeding 1700°C. The batch floats on the surface of the glass already in the furnace and gradually melts into the desired glass composition. The temperature of the furnace is necessary to facilitate melting and producing glass of the desired homogeneity in a commercially acceptable time. The glass is allowed to stay in the furnace until a satisfactory homogeneous product is formed, after which the temperature is lowered at the discharge end to achieve a glass viscosity that allows the desired forming operations to take place.

In most cases, the glass made cannot be characterized by a batch or lot designation but only by the date and time of withdrawal from the furnace. This is because the glass-melting process is a continuous process, even though the glass materials are charged in discrete amounts. The residence time in the furnace permits extensive mixing to occur and, therefore, erases all identity of the batch from individual cans (4).

Devitrification is the uncontrolled formation of crystals in glass during melting, forming, or secondary processing. The optical properties, mechanical strength, and some-

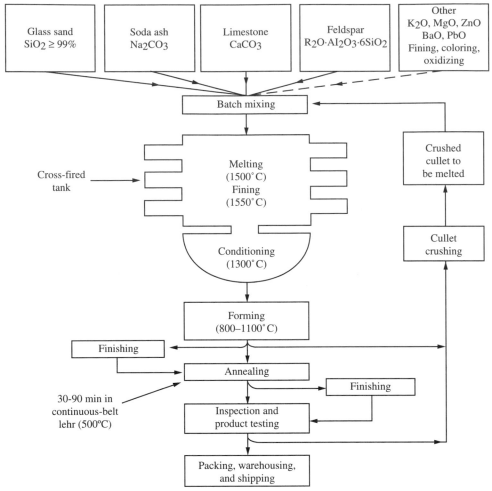

Fig. 1 Glass manufacture. Temperatures used may vary depending on the type of glass. (From Ref. 1).

times the chemical durability of the glass can be adversely affected by devitrification. These unwanted crystals grow homogeneously within the glass or heterogeneously at the air-glass or refracting-glass interface. Devitrification occurs mainly in glasses where the optimum temperatures for maximum nucleation rate and for maximum growth rate nearly coincide. If these glasses are held too long in this critical temperature range or are cooled too slowly through it, the glass starts to crystallize. For soda-lime glasses, the crystal phase, devitrite, forms between 850–900°C. However, since the glass is already quite viscous, the critical temperature range is short, and divitrification is not much of a problem (1–3).

QUALITY OF A GLASS PRODUCT

Following a successful product fabrication, there are some qualities to observe, one of which is total homogeneity of

product. Most glass manufacturers try to ensure that composition of the glass is homogeneous throughout. However, gas bubbles that did not escape the body of glass while in the furnace may cause a nonhomogeneous composition to exist.

Glass bubbles in manufacturing result from chemical reactions that take place during melting. Glass bubbles evolve due to the following: 1) because of gas formation from decomposition of the carbonates or sulfates or both; 2) from air trapped between the grains of the fine-grained batch materials; 3) from water evolved from the hydrated batch materials; and 4) from the change in oxidation state of some of the batch materials, such as red lead. However, with enough time in the furnace, the air bubbles escape the melt by rising slowly to the top. In some cases, the gas bubbles may be withdrawn with glass from the furnace. These bubbles are called seeds or blisters. They are not desirable and may be a cause for rejection of the final glass product, depending on the size and extent. When the surface of a glass final product is broken by the bubble, it is considered a functional defect. However, if the bubble is surrounded by glass, it is considered a cosmetic defect, and while generally it may not be hazardous, it may still be rejected.

Cord is another attribute in glass formation that is not desirable and should be prevented. Cords are formed when glass is not stirred properly at appropriate places in the furnace. It is referred to as the act of improper homogenization. Typically, in this case, glass melting occurs at a very high temperature, and some constituents vaporize from the surface glass and form regions of viscous glass. When small amounts of this glass mix into the body of the melt, they appear as very narrow and long inhomogeneous regions, referred to as cord (4).

Batch segregation, melt segregation, volatilization, and temperature fluctuations, as well as refractory corrosion from tank-lining material, cause stria or cord formation as well. These can also be prevented by melt homogenization and vigorous fining action. The homogeneity leading to cord formation can be removed by diffusion and flow and by vigorous fining, along with convection current mixing process before the glass is cooled. Homogeneity can also be improved by mechanical and static mixers that continuously shear the glass.

The bubble and cord defects that occur during the melting process are the two most commonly encountered. Melting defects should be held to a minimum as much as possible.

Fining is the physical and chemical process of removing glass bubbles (seeds and blisters) from the molten glass melt. Typically, fining agents that react at higher temperatures than are needed for melting are used. Some examples of fining agents are sulfates and sodium-potassium nitrates in combination with arsenic or antimony trioxides. Arsenic trioxide is used for melting glasses at higher temperatures, e.g., 1450–1500°C, whereas antimony is used for lower melting glasses at 1300–1400°C. As glasses cool, oxygen bubbles are removed by the reaction with arsenic or antimony trioxide to form pentoxide (1).

Gas may be evolved from a typical amber soda-lime glass batch, and fining agents are usually employed to resolve the problem (8). A typical batch mixture for amber soda-lime container glass is shown in Table 1.

QUALITY CONTROL IN BATCHING AND MELTING

Producing glass containers for parenteral products requires strict control of all process aspects, starting with raw materials and ending with the testing of glass as a material and as containers or parts of medical devices. The objectives of a quality-control program should be to maintain glass produced within physical and chemical specifications and to prevent off-specification material from reaching the pharmaceutical manufacturer.

Normal practice is to make sure that the raw material meets desired specifications and maintains its integrity during loading and shipping. There are physical as well as chemical requirements associated with each raw material, and these requirements are met by controlling for desired behavior during batching and melting and by the desired properties of the final glass product. The chemical impurity content is usually dictated by the desired attributes of the glass container. For example, raw materials of low iron content are used in order to provide a virtually colorless final product. Raw materials of low sulfur content (in the case of borosilicates) are used to minimize gas bubble formation during melting. Substances that would be harmful if extracted from the glass during terminal sterilization and subsequent storage (e.g., lead or arsenic) should be absent (4).

Most raw material suppliers provide certificates of analysis for the material they provide, and the information is checked by further testing on receipt. Records of performance of raw materials are maintained. The vendor's production facilities are usually inspected to ensure that mixing of raw materials of different grades cannot occur during loading and shipping. Ideally, this is a desirable situation and should be the goal of quality-oriented raw material suppliers and the glass manufacturers.

Scrap glass, or cullet, is also considered a raw material. Proper handling of cullet to prevent mixing of compositions and contamination by foreign materials requires constant attention and is just as important as preventing contamination of a raw material received from outside the plant.

Special considerations should be applied to ensure that all glass batch formulations are prepared by qualified technologists. The formulation for each composition is given in a batch sheet, which specifies the glass type, melting tank, date issued, amounts of raw materials, total batch weight, and weight of glass expected from the batch. In some companies, batch sheets are under the strict control of the glass-technology department, and each sheet denoting a change requires approval by several levels of department management. Changes are made primarily to manage the cullet supply, which can vary. Batch sheets usually provide a continuous time record of a given composition melted in a given furnace, and the batch sheets are supplied to the department responsible for actual

Table 1 Typical batch mixture for amber soda-lime container glass

Batch materials	Weight (kg)	Oxides supplied (kg)					
		SiO_2	Al_2O_3	CaO	Na_2O	FeO	LOI[a](kg)
Sand, SiO_2	300	299.3	0.2	—	—	0.03	0.5
Soda ash, Na_2CO_3	100	—	—	—	58.3	—	41.7
Aragonite, $CaCO_3$[b]	90	—	—	49.0	—	0.02	40.7
Feldspar, $SiO_2 \cdot Al_2O_3$ mineral[c]	40	26.4	7.6	0.4	1.3	0.03	0.1
Salt cake, NaCl	4	—	—	—	2.1	—	1.9
Powdered coal[d]	9	—	—	—	—	—	9
Iron pyrites, FeS_2	1.4					0.84	0.6
Cullet	460	333.7	9.2	48.8	67.2	1.03	0.1
Total	1004.4	659.4	17.0	98.2	128.9	1.95	94.6
Yield of glass, (kg), and wt% oxides present	909.8	72.48	1.87	10.79	14.17	0.21	

[a]Loss on ignition. Generally, the oxides of carbon and sulfur (plus some chlorine, depending on the fining agent) volatilize during melting.
[b]Also 0.2 kg MgO or 0.02 wt%.
[c]Also 4.1kg K_2O or 0.45 wt%.
[d]Used primarily to reduce the Fe_2O_3 to FeO to give the characteristic amber color, although the redox state of the glass melt also influences the fining reactions.
(From Ref. 8.)

weighing and mixing of the raw materials. In most companies, batching and mixing operations are usually under computer control, involving automated weighing, mixing, and conveying operations. Great care is to be exercised in entering the batch formulations into the computer, with continual checking for accuracy.

The next step is the testing of the glass produced. The testing program may be based on the following: 1) glasses are melted in large furnaces in a continuous operation, and the chemical and physical properties of any glass are dependent on one another; 2) continuous melting in large furnaces does not create abrupt compositional changes as might be experienced with discrete batch melting; 3) changes take place slowly in the furnace because of the size and volume of glass contained; therefore, periodic sampling and testing is a necessary production control. Measurement of selected physical properties serves to determine the values of all other relevant physical properties and also serves to define the chemical composition (4).

Samples of glass can be obtained daily from every producing position and subjected to a variety of tests. Each test is performed sufficiently often to ensure product quality. The following properties are determined:

- Seal stress
- Softening (viscosity) point
- Annealing and strain points
- Density
- Light transmission
- Chemical durability
- Chemical analysis

For most manufacturers, seal stress is determined on a daily basis and is a primary indicator of any shift in glass composition. Typically, a sample of daily production is flame-sealed or fused to a reference glass of the same composition having the desired target properties. Any deviation in composition is reflected in the generation of stress in the seal area. The physical property inferred from this test is thermal expansion, which is highly sensitive to changes in alkali content that, in turn, influence the chemical durability. If the test results show sufficient deviation from internal specifications, corrective action is initiated by issuing a slightly modified batch sheet. The effects of the corrective action should be observed in the next day's production.

The other tests mentioned may be performed in time intervals ranging from weekly to biweekly and monthly. The results of all these tests provide a framework describing glass quality on an ongoing basis. Thus, if the daily seal stress and the weekly viscosity points and biweekly chemical durability tests are satisfactory, the monthly chemical analysis will be right on target. It also follows that glass produced at any time, although not specifically tested for durability, will, in fact, be satisfactory if the other tests are satisfactory. In addition, an interlocking database can be used to certify to the pharmaceutical manufacturer that glass produced at any time meets specified requirements.

Process of Forming Pharmaceutical Containers

Pharmaceutical containers can be made by a blow-molding process and by a glass rod or tube-shaping process. Commonly, the large-volume parenterals of 100 ml or more are made by a blow-molding process, whereas small-volume parenterals of 100 ml or less are made by the tube-shaping process.

Although for the purpose of this section, discussion will be limited to pharmaceutical containers, molten glass can be formed in all kinds of shapes and sizes, such as bottles, jars, etc. Molten glass is either molded, drawn, rolled, or quenched, depending on the desired shape and use.

Blow-Molding Process

The blow-molding process uses hot glass as it leaves the furnace. The glass must be at the correct temperature and viscosity for forming to be successful. This process describes a typical blow-molding process. At the exit end of the furnace, the glass flows through an orifice in the bottom of the furnace section called the feeder. A pair of cooled blades cuts the glass stream into discrete chunks called gobs. The gobs contain the correct volume of glass to make one container. The gob is delivered into blank molds where it is settled with compressed air and, ultimately, forced to conform to the interior shape of a cast-iron mold that represents the bottle. This preformed (cast-iron mold shape) stage is obtained with a counter-blow of compressed air. The formed bottle is inverted and transferred into the blow mold where it is further finished by blowing. The mold is hinged so that it opens and allows the removal of the bottle. The bottle is sent through a controlled cooling process, known as annealing, which allows the bottle to cool down to room temperature in a stress-free condition. A press-and-blow machine, such as the Hartford-Empire machine, is an example of a blow machine used for making articles such as drinking glasses. A typical process of blow-and-blow machine is shown in Fig. 2.

Blow-molded containers can be made in clear glass or glass that has been colored for protection of the product from light. In comparison to the tubing process which will be discussed later, the walls of blown containers are usually thicker than those of the tubing process, and, hence, blow–process containers have greater impact strength. However, containers made from tubing process have more uniform distribution of glass in the walls. This may be critical, depending on its intended use, and may impact on optical-inspection equipment. Blow process containers also have thicker bottoms, and this could affect heat transfer during lyophilization.

Tubing Process

The Danner process is a common method used for glass tubing, which is a mechanical process. There is also the hand drawn process described below. Glass tubing can be made with a precisely controlled outside diameter (OD) and wall thickness. There is an upper size limit of about 40-mm OD, which is not a limitation on the tubing-forming process, but on the subsequent forming operations used to make containers. In the hand drawn process, about 15 m of 140-mm OD, 2-mm wall thickness tubing can be made on one draw by a gaffer and two helpers. Gathers of glass up to 30–35 kg can be made with bubble in their center at the end of the blow pipe. This is rotated in place by the gaffer, and rotated and stretched out by one of the helpers walking away from it. The size and the diameter of the tubing is a function of the helper's walking speed and is further controlled by a second helper that cools the tubing by fanning at specified times. Up to 150 m of the much smaller diameter thermometer tubing can be made in this manner from one gather (1, 4, 9).

In the Danner process, a continuous stream of glass, of the proper temperature, flows slowly and controllably onto a rotating mandrel, which is an inclined cylinder made of refractory ceramic materials or of platinum alloy. Glass tubing is drawn off the end of the mandrel, which is tapered, while air blowing through the mandrel helps to maintain tubing dimensions. This air is pressurized to keep the tubing from collapsing toward the end. The glass temperature controls the diameter and the wall thickness of the tubing, the inflating air pressure, and the rate of withdrawal of glass from the cylinder. A schematic representation of the Danner process is shown in Fig. 3.

When tubing has cooled sufficiently, it is cut into lengths convenient to handle and is used as feed stock for the container-forming process. Hairpin cords of inhomogeneity and volatilization from the surface are capable of occurring during the tubing process. The tubing process can be used to make ampuls, vials, syringe barrels, cartridges, and a variety of containers used in medication delivery (4).

Another type of tubing process is the Vello process. In the Vello process, the molten glass passes down through an annulus between a horizontal ring and a vertical bell. The moving stream connects to a nearly horizontal runway, and as in the Danner process, it is drawn off at a suitable rate for dimensional specification and stability. The Vello process forms tubing faster because the glass is cooled more quickly to the appropriate forming viscosity in a stationary forehearth of the desired dimension. However, the Vello

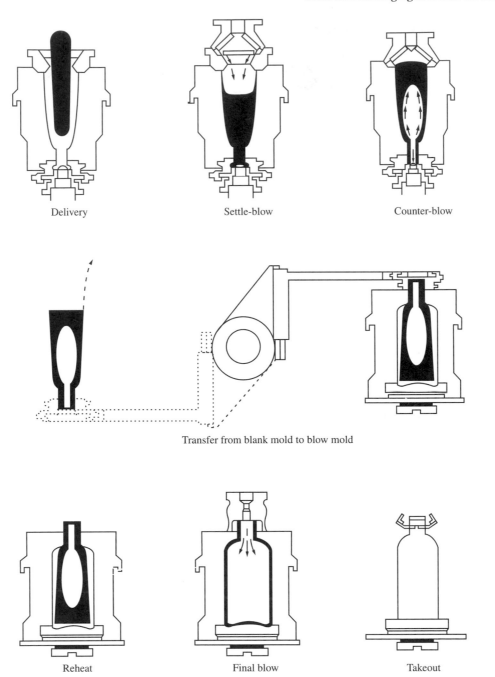

Delivery   Settle-blow   Counter-blow

Transfer from blank mold to blow mold

Reheat   Final blow   Takeout

Fig. 2 The H.E. IS blow-and-blow machine (9). The gob is delivered into a blank mold, settled with compressed air, and then preformed with a counter-blow. The parison or preform is then inverted and transferred into the blow mold where it is finished by blowing. (From Ref. 9.)

process is more difficult to operate and is most suitable for longer production runs having few size changes (1).

In comparison to sized molded containers from the blow-molded process, tubing process containers are made lighter in weight and provide more precisely controlled dimensions than blow-molded containers. The walls and bottom thickness are more uniform, and, hence, are more suited for use in automatic inspection Systems. Clear and light resistant glass compositions can be used in the tubing process.

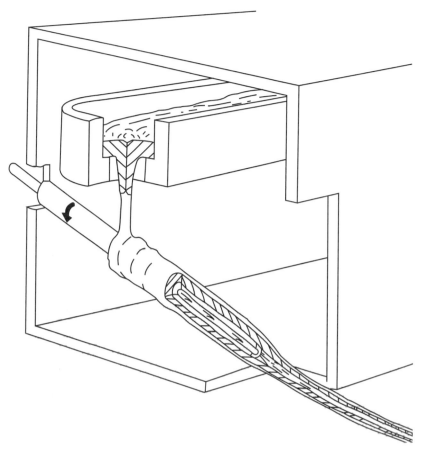

Fig. 3 The Danner process for manufacture of tubing.

GLASS COMPOSITION, PROPERTIES, AND CLASSIFICATION

As mentioned earlier, the focus in this article is on soda-lime-silica glasses and borosilicate glasses.

Soda-Lime-Silica Glasses

These compositions are for glass for every day use. The batch materials for soda-lime glasses are easily available at reasonably moderate cost. These materials readily meet at moderate temperatures. These glasses have a relatively high thermal expansion coefficient and only moderate resistance to attack by a contained product.

The actual compositions of soda-lime are usually more complex than the term soda-lime suggests. As mentioned earlier, these glasses may contain MgO, Al_2O_3, BaO, or K_2O and various colorants, in addition to Na_2O, CaO, and SiO_2. Alumina increases the durability of soda-lime glasses, whereas MgO prevents devitrification. Soda-lime glasses account for 90% of all glass produced and are used

for containers, flat glass, pressed and blown ware, and some types of lighting products (1).

In soda-lime glasses, the amber color is developed by the interaction of iron oxide and a small amount of sulfur (a few tenths of a percent), in the presence of a reducing agent during melting. As such, soda-lime amber glasses are called reduced ambers. Typical compositions of soda-lime and borosilicate glasses are presented in Table 2 (4).

Borosilicate Glasses

Borosilicate glasses are developed to meet more stringent requirements than soda-lime glasses. Because of their composition, these glasses require higher melting temperatures and more costly batch materials. As a result, these glasses are more expensive than soda-lime glasses.

Borosilicate glasses are also known as heat-resistant glasses because they have a lower coefficient of thermal expansion than soda-lime glasses and, hence, are more resistant to fracture from rapid temperature changes (thermal-shock resistance). Borosilicate glasses are used widely as laboratory apparatus, chemical process piping and drain lines, and for baking and cooking dishes in the home. Borosilicates have excellent resistance to chemical attack, and this augments their use as laboratory apparatus and in packaging of pharmaceuticals as containers. The fluxing action of the boron facilitates melting by weakening the network. This is due to the presence of plenar three coordinate boron, which weakens the silicate network at high temperature. Borosilicates are divided into two groups based on the coefficient of thermal expansion.

In borosilicate glasses, the amber color is developed through interaction between iron oxide and titanium oxide or iron oxide and maganese oxide. Reducing agents are not used in borosilicate glasses for color development. Borosilicate ambers are called oxidized ambers.

PROPERTIES OF GLASS

Rheology, the melting, forming, annealing procedures, and limitations of use at high temperature, is determined by the viscosity of the glass. Viscosity is measured between 10(13) and 10 Pa.5 [10(14) and 100 P]. Also, viscosity of glasses is compared qualitatively. The addition of modifiers to a glass can alter the viscosity at certain temperatures. At low temperature, the effects of a modifier on viscosity are controlled by its coordination number. Modifiers with high coordination numbers tend to increase low temperature viscosity due to packing restraints (1).

ASTM provides definition for the procedures and selected reference points discussed in this chapter. Some frequently used reference points are annealing points and strain points. Below are presented some of the ASTM (3):

- *Annealing*: a controlled cooling process for glass designed to reduce residual stress to a commercially acceptable level and to modify structure.
- *Annealing Point (A.P.)*: that temperature corresponding either to a specific rate of elongation of a glass fiber when measured by Test Method C336 or a specific rate of midpoint deflection of a glass beam when measured by Test Method C598. At the annealing point of glass, internal stresses are substantially relieved in a matter of minutes.
- *Annealing Range*: the range of glass temperature in which stress in glass can be relieved at a commercially practical rate. For purposes of comparing glasses, the annealing range is assumed to correspond with the temperature between the A.P. and the strain point (St.P.).
- *Strain Point (St.P.)*: that temperature corresponding to a specific rate of elongation of a glass fiber when measured by Test Method C336 or a specific rate of midpoint deflection of a glass beam when measured by Test Method C598.
- *Softening Point (S.P.)*: that temperature at which a glass fiber of uniform diameter elongates at a specific rate under its own weight when measured by Test Method C338. The viscosity at the softening point depends on

Table 2 Typical compositions and thermal expansions of soda-lime and borosilicate pharmaceutical glasses

| Weight % | Soda-Lime | | | Borosilicate | | | | | |
| | Blow molded | | Tubing | Blow molded | | | Tubing | | |
	Clear	Amber	Clear	Clear	Amber	Clear	Clear	Amber
SiO_2	73.0	71.9	67.7	67.8	66.7	80.4	72.0	69.2
B_2O_3	—	—	1.5	13.6	9.5	12.9	11.4	10.4
Al_2O_3	0.8	1.9	2.8	5.8	5.3	2.6	6.8	5.4
CaO	10.7	10.6	5.7	1.1	1.8	<0.05	0.5	0.4
MgO	0.4	0.8	3.9	<0.1	<0.1	<0.05	0.2	0.3
BaO	—	—	2.0	2.4	1.2	—	—	2.1
Na_2O	13.5	14.1	15.6	8.3	7.4	4.0	6.4	6.0
K_2O	0.3	0.3	0.6	0.8	1.0	—	2.4	2.3
TiO_2	—	—	—	—	—	—	—	2.8
Fe_2O_3	—	0.3	—	—	1.3	—	—	1.0
MnO	—	—	—	—	6.0	—	—	—
Thermal expansion, cm/cm/°C, 0–300°C	88	90	93	56	59	33	55	54

(From Ref. 4.)

the density and surface tension. For example, for a glass of density 2.5 g/cm^3 and surface tension 300 dynes/cm, the softening point temperature corresponds to a viscosity of $10^{6.6}$ Pa·s.

Discussion

At the strain point, internal stresses are substantially relieved in a matter of hours (3).

The Margules Viscometer, a calibrated instrument that measures the force exerted by molten glass on a rotating spindle can be used to measure viscosity. Glass is usually melted and fined at viscosities between 5 and 50 Pa·s (50–500 P). However, the forming and final viscosity requirements may differ. Hard glasses usually have a high softening point whereas soft glasses have a lower softening point. The length of a glass (i.e., long or short) can be used to explain the differences between the strain point and the softening point of glass. A long glass usually has a large difference between the strain point and the softening point, meaning that it solidifies slower than a short glass as the temperature decreases (1).

The temperature required for glass to form into useable shapes is usually above 1000°C for borosilicates and less than 1000°C for soda-lime. The annealing process is very effective in relieving the residual stresses contained in formed glass (10). The temperature range for proper stress-relief annealing of borosilicate is 600–650°C and less for soda-lime. These forming stresses are relieved within minutes at these temperatures, and a subsequent slow cooling to room temperature retains the stress-free state.

Thermal Expansion

The value of thermal expansion is important in determining how a glass container survives sudden changes in temperature, that is, thermal shock resistance. The thermal expansion of a glass determines the range of materials to which it can safely be sealed. The thermal expansion characteristic indicates how much change in dimension (e.g., length) the article undergoes upon a change in temperature. The change in dimension in turn determines the stress generated in the glass. The ability of a glass as a heat exchanger thermal barrier and its ease of melting and forming depend on its heat-transfer properties and emmissivity. In most cases, glass expands when heated and contracts when cooled. If the thermal cycle is slow enough, there is no hysteresis effect. The slope of linear expansion vs. temperature is known as the thermal expansion coefficient, α, which is virtually constant between 0 and 300°C for most glasses. However, as the temperature of the glass rises to near the set point (strain

point +5°C), the thermal expansion increases more rapidly. Glasses used to the extreme limits are vulnerable to thermal shock, and tests should be made before adapting the final design for any use.

For soda-lime glasses, when expansion is high, the stress is high, and the probability of fracture is greatly increased. Borosilicate glasses have lower coefficients of expansion than soda-lime compositions and, hence, can withstand larger temperature changes without fracture. This is important in processes where relatively rapid temperature changes occurs such as in dry-heat sterilization and lypholization, among other processes.

Stresses caused by steady-state thermal gradients may or may not cause failure, depending on the degree of constraint imposed by some parts of the item upon others or by external mounting. Thermal stress resistance (face-to-face temperature differentials) that causes tensile stress is observed in some types of glasses. When glass is suddenly cooled, as by the removal from a hot oven, tensile stresses are introduced in the surfaces and compensating compressional stresses in the interior. On the other hand, sudden heating leads to surface compression and internal tension. In both cases, stresses are temporary and disappear once temperature uniformity is reached. Also, because glass fractures only in tension, usually at the surface, the temporary stresses from sudden cooling are much more damaging than those from sudden heating, assuming all surfaces are heated and cooled at the same time. Thermal shock endurance is generally determined by empirical testing because the strength of glass is greater under momentary stress than under prolonged load. Resistance to breakage can be determined by heating the ware to some appropriate temperature then plunging it into cold water. For example, a resistance of 150°C means that no breakage occurred on heating to 150°C and plunging the glass into water at 15°C. A much higher value of thermal shock can be recorded when other cooling media such as air or oil are used (1).

The thermal shock that a container receives as its temperature is lowered depends on the temperature differential and the time required to reach the lowest temperature. Glass as a material can withstand very low temperatures, but sufficient time must be allowed to reach the low temperature in order to avoid breakage. Although it might seem that thick glass walls withstand thermal shock better because of higher strength, the fact is that thin walls resist thermal shock better because temperature change is accommodated more rapidly, lessening the stress created by the temperature differential (4).

The thermal expansion coefficient depends on the glass composition. It is usually assumed that the lower the expansion the better, but this is not necessarily true. It is true, if soda-lime glass with an expansion of about 90 is compared to borosilicates with expansion coefficients of 33–55. However, there is little to choose from between borosilicates in this range of expansion values. Glasses with expansion coefficients in this range perform satisfactorily under most circumstances. If the application requires cooling rates higher than normally experienced, the lowest expansion glass is of course the choice.

GLASS CONTAINER CHARACTERISTICS: COMPARISON OF BLOW-MOLDING AND TUBING PROCESS

As described earlier, some containers are made from tubing and some by the blow-molding process. Containers made from tubing have a maximum capacity of about 50 ml and a 40-mm OD. Blow molding is more suitable for larger sizes and is used for containers greater than 100 ml in volume. This flexibility in size causes great variation in wall and bottom thickness and weight (4).

Tubing used for containers is produced with closely held dimensions, including wall thickness, wall uniformity, cross section, and straightness. Because these dimensional attributes are strictly controlled, smaller volume containers can be made to much better dimensional precision and accuracy. At the same time, containers made from tubing are likely to exhibit different glass defects than blow-molded containers, mainly because of the kind of defects associated with the manufacture of tubing. Gas bubble inclusions, for example in blow-molded bottles, have a spherical or ovoidal shape, whereas those made from tubing have "air line" gas bubbles that have been stretched out during the forming of the tubing.

Another distinction between the two types of containers is the interior surface composition. For glass to be readily formed, it must be heated to a sufficiently high temperature. Because of this, the more volatile glass constituents tend to escape the surface and condense in cooler regions. This effect is minimal in blow molding, because every part of the forming process leads to lower temperatures, reducing the tendency to vaporize. Containers from tubing, on the other hand, are formed by reheating tubing in specific regions of a tubing length. The result is that some parts of a vial, for example, experience very high temperatures, whereas other parts are barely above room temperature. A typical example of this is the forming of the vial bottom. The glass temperatures required cause vaporization of sodium and boron oxides, together with some chlorides; these compounds condense on the interior vial sidewall, just above the bottom. These so-called

forming deposits or "bloom" can be removed by revaporization during the annealing step, or if this process is incomplete, by washing later.

A special discussion of tubing containers for lyophilization is warranted because a proper design embodies a combination of container and product characteristics that should be taken into account. Blow-molded bottles for lyophilization, although subject to some manufacturing control, cannot be made as uniquely as tubing containers. The same design considerations apply but are under much less control.

The following considerations have been found to be important in the design and use of containers for lyophilization:

- Product characteristics
- Amount of fill
- Thermal shock
- Glass composition
- Container wall thickness
- Container contours
- Container surface damage

The great variability in products to be lyophilized implies that there will be behavior variations in these products as they freeze. Any glass container considered for use should be evaluated with the actual product, rather than trying to simulate product behavior with test solutions.

The result of product freezing and thawing is internal pressure generation. If the container is overfilled, excessive pressure can result with subsequent container breakage. Fills of less than 50% of the container volume are recommended, with an optimum of about 35%.

The contour of the container is important in resisting the forces encountered during product freezing and in ensuring adequate heat transfer through the bottom. There should be as gradual a transition as practicable between the sidewall and the bottom, to reduce the stress concentration effect caused by this angle. A sharp, re-entrant angle between the sidewall and bottom is the worst condition. In addition, a flat bottom with a little "push up" in the center is best for heat transfer. This condition is in concert with a gradual transition in the heel region; both conditions improve performance.

Everything mentioned above as factors for satisfactory performance can be negatively affected by damage to the surface of the container. The container must be as free as possible of scratches, scuffs, impact damage, etc., if the design criteria are to be effective. Maintaining a damage-free glass surface is also a requirement of the filling line, where contact with sharp metal objects should be minimized. The factors discussed above demonstrate that other factors are of importance beside low glass thermal expansion, usually the first and sometimes the only criterion considered (4).

Chemical Property—Durability

ASTM defines chemical durability as:

> the lasting quality (both physical and chemical) of a glass surface. It is frequently evaluated, after prolonged weathering or storing, in terms of chemical and physical changes in the glass surface, or in terms of changes in the contents of a vessel (3).

One of the main reasons for using glass compared to other containers or packaging material is due to its resistance to chemical corrosion. The chemical durability of a glass varies from highly soluble to highly durable, depending on its composition and the solvent used. Glass used in packaging parenteral products and in direct contact with parenteral liquids or solids must have good chemical durability. Analysis are usually based on measurements of weight loss, changes in surface quality of the glass or finished container, or analysis of solutions that were in contact with a glass. A method of determining the durability of a glass is by subjecting grains of uniform size distribution to accelerated attack by high purity water at a temperature characteristic of terminal steam sterilization. In addition, glass compositions can be directly compared with respect to their resistance to attack by aqueous solutions because glass grain are prepared and sized uniformly. These processes will establish the intrinsic durability of the glass. However, the presence of other factors, such as glass constituents that may condense on the surface during high temperature forming process or other volatile deposits, can reduce or improve the durability.

When glass is attacked by water under accelerated test conditions, the pH of the solution increases as a result of an ion exchange process between the alkali (primarily sodium) content of the glass and the hydrogen ions in solution. The higher the pH, the less durable the glass. At large increases in pH, there are high effects on the contained parenteral product and there is an accelerated attack on glass. The extent of pH change can then be determined by titration of attacking solution with diluted acid. Glasses are rated based on the volume of diluted acid required to neutralize the extracted alkali. Additionally, the extent of attack can be determined by the analysis of the solution for specific constituents, including sodium buron, aluminum, calcium, and silicon. The amount of acid required to neutralize the extract solution will correlate with the amount of specific glass constituents found in the solution by direct analysis. The most durable glass will require smaller volumes of acid and lower concentration of the constituents in solution.

These observations apply generally to both glass grain tests and container tests, except that the acid volumes and constituent concentration are much lower when testing containers because of a much lower glass surface-to-solution volume ratio.

The reaction of acids with glass may be either a leaching process or a complete dissolution process. Acids such as hydrofluoric acid attack silica glasses by dissolving the silica network. Other acids such as hydrochloric acid or nitric acid may react by dissolving certain glasses. However, the reaction mechanism is by selective extraction of alkali and the substitution of protons in a diffusion controlled process.

The reaction of bases with most silicate glasses produces dissolution rates when tested in 5% NaOH solution at 95°C. The mechanism also involves a complete dissolution process as that described for acid. Weaker alkaline solutions may both leach and dissolve and sometimes show greater dependence on glass composition. And, in the case of strong alkali solutions, the rate of attack doubles for each 10 K increase in temperature or each increase in pH unit. Usually higher alkali durability glasses are used for laboratory wares.

Also, as stated earlier, the attack of water, is related to the leaching mechanism described for acid. Low alkali, high alumina, or borosilicate glasses generally have high water durability. Weathering of glass is the result of the action of water, carbon dioxide, and other constituents. Water initially is absorbed by the glass and then exchanged for alkalies that form alkali salt solutions and, if left in contact with glass, may cause additional damage. As a result, weathering resistance may not correlate with acid durability. Test methods to accelerate the weathering process are designed in chambers at 50°C and 98% rh.

A comparison of the chemical durability of soda-lime glasses and borosilicate glasses show that borosilicates are far more durable than soda-limes, requiring from 10 to 20× less acid to neutralize solutions in glass-grain tests. This is due to the significantly lower alkali content of the borosilicates. The same result applies when comparing containers made from borosilicates and soda-lime. Thus, when product-container interactions must be limited, as in the case of parenterals, the compositions of choice are the borosilicates.

SPECIAL TREATMENTS

Special treatments include treatments to the container after it has been formed into its final shape. These processes can be performed before or after the annealing process. The processes discussed here are concerned with printing and "sulfur" treatment to improve the chemical durability of the interior container surface.

Printing Treatment (4)

The printing of pharmaceutical containers may involve either applying the printed information as a step in the manufacture of the container or applying of labels as the filled container is processed by the pharmaceutical manufacturer. The printing of information on the container while still in the hands of the glass manufacturer is significant. A number of issues are connected with this, one of which is the strict accountability by the glass producer for containers printed with information on drug type, lot number, etc. Stringent safeguards must be employed during printing to ensure the integrity of the container lots.

Material for printing on glass can include ceramic glazes, epoxy formulations cured by heat, and ultraviolet curing formulations. The latter two are applied after annealing, as the temperatures applied would destroy these materials. Ceramic glazes are applied before the annealing step and have properties such that the annealing temperatures are sufficient to fire on the glaze.

Ceramic glazes provide the most durable type of printing. They are vitreous or glass-like in nature, and form a strong bond with the glass substrate. Ceramic glazes are chemically the most durable. They provide the greatest resistance to abrasion and the highest hardness. However, the glaze and the glass have to be carefully matched. A great disparity in the thermal expansions of the two materials causes problems. The glaze should have a greater expansion than the underlying glass so that as the container cools from the fining process, the glass container develops compressive stress at the glaze–glass interface, rather than tensile stress. Glass is much stronger in compression than in tension. The glaze develops fine cracks or a crazed appearance during cooling, but the underlying glass will not be significantly damaged.

Ceramic glazes are used in ampuls to introduce a controlled-break site. A band of paint is applied at the constriction of the ampule where controlled breakage is desired, so the contents can be withdrawn. The band is used to make Colorbreak ampuls, and its function is to act as a stress concentrator when bending stress is applied to the ampul to break off the stem for product withdrawal. Very consistent ampul break forces are achieved by the use of ceramic bands.

Interior Surface Treatments (4)

Sometimes forming deposits become fused onto the glass surface and are difficult to remove, in effect compromising the durability of the interior surface. These effects are overcome by chemical neutralization of these deposits through surface treatment processes. At the same time, the intrinsic ability of a glass surface to withstand attack by aggressive products is also improved. Thus, there is a two-fold benefit in treatment processes for containers made from tubing: to remove the residual forming deposits and to improve the basic durability of the glass surface. These benefits are derived concurrently during treatment. Blow-molded containers, although not subject to the forming deposit problem, can also benefit from surface treatment.

If an aggressive product of pH 8 and above is to be packaged in a borosilicate container, surface treatment is required. Otherwise, the glass is attacked by the product, resulting in contamination by both soluble and insoluble reaction products. The latter are manifested by entities variously called flakes, shimmers, etc. These flakes are essentially silica that has been stripped off the surface by the attack on the glass. Their presence is direct evidence of excessive attack. Proper surface treatment enhances resistance to attack and results in a glass container that can contain products of pH 8 and higher without being damaged.

The basis of all treatment processes is the removal of alkali from the glass surface, resulting in improved resistance to attack by aqueous solutions. Alkali or sodium removal accomplishes this by greatly hindering the ion exchange process responsible for glass attack. Exchange of sodium ions in the glass for hydrogen ions in solution results in a pH rise in the solution; this can accelerate attack on the basic glass structure. If hydrogen ions cannot readily leave the solution because there are very few labile sodium ions with which to exchange, there will be little pH rise and, hence, little attack.

A common means of removing surface sodium is by reaction with sulfur dioxide in the presence of oxygen or by reaction with sulfur trioxide. The reaction product is sodium sulfate.

Surface treatment of blow-molded containers consists of several stages. As the freshly formed bottle leaves the mold and before it enters the annealing lehr or oven, it is still high in temperature. The bottle is filled with one or several of the following gaseous mixtures: sulfur trioxide, sulfur dioxide and oxygen, or 1,1-difluoroethane. If only moderate treatment is desired, one step suffices. The reaction of these gases with surface sodium starts immediately because of the glass temperature and continues as the bottle enters the annealing process at its elevated temperatures. The reaction product of sodium sulfate is clearly seen in the cool bottle as a whitish haze on the inside surface just prior to packing into cartons. It is easily removed by subsequent washing processes. Blow-molded bottles treated by both of these steps can achieve high durability. These two methods, however, are restricted to large containers with relatively wide openings. Smaller containers made from tubing with much more restricted entry must be handled in a different way.

The effective treatment of containers made from tubing is a much more crucial issue because of the adverse effects of residual forming deposits and because the high pH products are usually packaged in small volume ampuls and vials made from tubing. The same basic treatment scheme is used, that of reacting the surface sodium with a sulfur compound at elevated temperatures. A 3% ammonium sulfate solution is injected into the container just prior to entering the annealing lehr; the volume injected is several tenths of a milliliter. The ammonium sulfate decomposes during the annealing process, with temperatures of 600–650°C being typical. The solution is thought to decompose, resulting in the formation of sulfuric acid vapors or possibly sulfur trioxide, which react with the surface sodium and any residual forming deposits, giving the characteristic sodium sulfate haze.

Containers given an effective surface treatment show a pronounced improvement in chemical inertness. Products packaged in such containers remain unaffected for long periods of time. The improvement of the inside surface, resulting from the surface treatment, is permanent and is not destroyed even by repeated autoclaving.

An additional reason for sulfur treating the interior surface of bottles is to improve the durability of soda-lime glass bottles. Normally, the surface inertness of soda-lime glass does not approach that of borosilicate. Sulfur treatment of a soda-lime surface can improve this situation to the point where products not normally considered for soda-lime containers can be packaged in them. The reason for choosing a treated soda-lime bottle for a mild product rather than a borosilicate bottle is based on economics, as soda-lime bottles are less expensive than borosilicate. It should be noted that this approach is used primarily for blow-molded bottles. There is compendial recognition and control of this, using treated soda-lime bottles in this way. Suffice it to say for the present that these bottles are known as Type-II bottles, according to the *United States Pharmacopeia* (USP). The *USP* and other methods of test and classification of glass for pharmaceutical products are discussed later.

Putting aside the question of testing and classifying Type-II bottles for the moment, it is of interest to consider test methods that determine the effectiveness of interior surface treatment of borosilicate containers made from tubing. It was stated earlier that a measure of durability, or inertness, is the pH rise of a contained solution. There are several commonly used ways of determining this. These methods are based on the pH rise of a water solution in the container after it has been autoclaved at 121°C for 60 min. The pH rise can be evaluated by titrating the solution with dilute acid in the presence of an indicator to a neutral end point. Another way is to include an indicator in the original water fill, autoclave, and observe the color change indicative of pH change. An example of this method uses bromothymol blue indicator adjusted to an initial pH of 5.8–6. The color of the indicator after autoclaving is compared to a series of standards having a range of pH up to at least 7.5 and the pH rise estimated. The autoclave cycle time and temperature used for these tests is that of the *Water Attack Test* as set forth in the *USP* described later in this chapter.

A solution autoclaved in a well-treated container consumes very small amounts of dilute acid upon titration or shows very small pH rise by color change of the indicator. Actual values of acid required, or pH rise, depend on various factors, including container size, as it controls the interior surface area-to-solution volume ratio (4).

Classification of Glass and Glass Containers—Compendial Perspective

The chemical specifications of glassware was first contained in *USP XII* in which specifications of glassware as containers for injections were provided. In subsequent revisions changes appeared and definitions of four types of glassware are described in *USP XIX* (11, 12).

Glass containers for pharmaceutical use are glass articles in direct contact with pharmaceutical preparation. In addition to the *USP*, the *European Pharmacopoeia (EP)* and other pharmacopeias have grouped glass containers suitable for packaging pharmacopeial preparations into the four different classifications specified in *USP XIX* up to *USP 24* (13). The classes are based on the degree of chemical or hydrolytic resistance of these glasses to water attack. The degree of attack is determined by the amount of alkali released from the glass under the influence of the attacking medium under conditions specified. The quantity of alkali used is extremely small in some cases. These tests designs and glass classification are described from *USP 24–NF 19* under section ⟨661⟩ *Containers* (13). These tests are designed to be conducted in areas relatively free from fumes and excessive dust.

Glass Types

The *USP* and *EP* have provided similar classifications that are summarized below.

Type I glass containers

Type I glass containers are comprised of a borosilicate glass with about 80% SiO_2 and 10% B_2O_3 and smaller amounts of Al_2O_3 and Na_2O. It is inert and has the lowest coefficient of thermal expansion. It is least likely to crack when a sudden temperature differential occurs. It is commonly used to make ampuls and vials for parenteral use. It is used for solutions that can dissolve basic oxides to cause an increase in pH that could alter the efficacy or potency of the drug (5).

USP describes Type I glass as:
Highly resistant borosilicate glass, and usually used for packaging acidic and neutral parenteral preparations. Also, where stability data demonstrates their suitability, Type I are used for alkaline parenteral preparations (13).

EP describes Type I glass as:
Neutral glass with high hydrolytic resistance due to the chemical composition of the glass itself. Type I are suitable for all preparations whether or not for parenteral use and for human blood and blood components (14).

Type II glass

A dealkalized form of soda-lime glass with higher levels of Na_2O and CaO. It is less resistant to leaching than Type I but more than Type III. However, to make Type II and other types more resistant to leaching, the surface can be treated with SO_2 to convert surface oxides present to soluble salts that are then washed off. This surface treatment is effective for containers used once and those repeatedly exposed to heat. Type II has a lower melting point than Type I and, therefore, is easier to fabricate. It has a higher coefficient of thermal expansion, and is used in solutions that can be buffered to maintain a pH below 7 (5).

[*USP*] Soda-lime glass that is suitably dealkalized and is used for packaging acidic and neutral parenteral preparations, and also where stability data demonstrates their suitability, is used for alkaline parenteral preparations (13).

[*EP*] Soda-lime silica glass with high hydrolytic resistance resulting from suitable treatment of the surface. These containers are suitable for acidic and neutral, aqueous preparations for parenteral use (14).

Type III glass

A soda-lime glass containing same amount of sodium and oxide levels as in Type II but contains more leachable oxides of other elements. And because of its high reactivity, it is used to package anhydrous liquids and other dry products (5).

[*USP*] These are soda-lime glass containers that are usually not used for parenteral preparations, except where suitable sensitivity test data indicates that Type III is satisfactory for the parenteral preparations that are packaged therein (13).

[*EP*] These are soda-lime glasses with only moderate hydrolytic resistance. They are suitable for nonaqueous preparations for parenteral use, for powders for parenteral use, and for preparations not for parenteral use (14).

Type IV or NP glass

[*USP*] These are general purpose soda-lime glass. They are intended for packaging nonparenteral articles, i.e., those intended for oral or topical use (13).

[*EP*] These are soda-lime silica glass with low hydrolytic resistance. These are suitable for solid preparations that are not for parenteral use and for some liquid or semi-solid preparations that are not for parenteral use (14).

Tests

These glass containers for pharmaceutical use have to comply with relevant tests such as tests for hydrolytic resistance for *EP* (14), and tests chemical resistance for *USP* (13). The test procedure and methods are slightly different for each of the pharmacopeias. However, this article will emphasize the test procedure provided in the *USP 24–NF 19*.

For the four types of glasses, there are designated relevant test types and expected limits. These are provided in Table 3.

USP has provided procedure and test requirements for three types of tests. These are the *Powdered Glass Test*, the *Water Attack* test, and the *Arsenic* test. These tests,

Table 3 USP glass types, test type, and limits

Glass type	Test type	Limits	
		Size[a] (ml)	ml of 0.020 N Acid
I	Powdered glass	All	1.0
II	Water attack	100 or less	0.7
		Over 100	
III	Powdered glass	All	8.5
NP	Powdered glass	All	15.0

[a]Size indicates the overflow capacity of the container.
(Courtesy of *USP 24–NF19* © USP.)

Apparatus, and Reagents for the tests are described below (13).

Apparatus used for these tests[a]

Autoclave: An autoclave capable of maintaining a temperature of 121 ± 2.0°C, equipped with a thermometer, a pressure gauge, a vent cock, and a rack adequate to accommodate at least 12 test containers above the water level is used.

Mortar and pestle: A hardened-steel mortar and pestle, made according to the specifications in the accompanying illustration.

Other equipment: Sieves, about 20.3-cm (8-inch), made of stainless steel including the Nos. 20, 40, and 50 sieves, along with the pan and cover (see *Openings of Standard Sieves* ⟨811⟩), 250-ml conical flasks made of resistant glass aged as specified, a 900-g (2-lb) hammer, a permanent magnet, a desiccator, and an adequate volumetric apparatus are used.

Reagents used for these tests[b]

High-purity water: The water used in these tests has a conductivity at 25°C, as measured in an in-line cell just prior to dispensing, of not greater than 0.15 μs per cm (6.67 Megohm-cm). There must also be an assurance that this water is not contaminated by copper or its products (e.g., copper pipes, stills, or receivers). The water may be prepared by passing distilled water through a deionizer cartridge packed with a mixed bed of nuclear-grade resin, then through a cellulose ester membrane having openings not exceeding 0.45 μm. Do not use copper tubing. Flush the discharge lines before water is dispensed into test vessels. When the low conductivity specification can no longer be met, replace the deionizer cartridge.

Methyl red solution: Dissolve 24 mg of methyl red sodium in purified water to make 100 ml. If necessary,

neutralize the solution with 0.02 N sodium hydroxide or acidify it with 0.02 N sulfuric acid so that the titration of 100 ml of High-purity water, containing 5 drops of indicator, does not require more than 0.020 ml of 0.020 N sodium hydroxide to effect the color change of the indicator, which should occur at a pH of 5.6 (13).

Powdered glass test for Types I, II, and NP glasses[c]

Rinse thoroughly with purified water six or more containers selected at random, and dry them with a current of clean, dry air. Crush the containers into fragments about 25 mm in size, divide about 100 g of the coarsely crushed glass into three approximately equal portions, and place one of the portions in the special mortar. With the pestle in place, crush the glass further by striking three or four blows with the hammer. Nest the sieves, and empty the mortar into the No. 20 sieve. Repeat the operation on each of the two remaining portions of glass, emptying the mortar each time into the No. 20 sieve. Shake the sieves for a short time, then remove the glass from the Nos. 20 and 40 sieves, and again crush and sieve as before. Repeat again this crushing and sieving operation. Empty the receiving pan, reassemble the nest of sieves, and shake by mechanical means for 5 min or by hand for an equivalent length of time. Transfer the portion retained on the No. 50 sieve, which should weigh in excess of 10 g, to a closed container, and store in a desiccator until used for the test.

Spread the specimen on a piece of glazed paper, and pass a magnet through it to remove particles of iron that may be introduced during the crushing. Transfer the specimen to a 250-ml conical flask of resistant glass, and wash it with six 30-ml portions of acetone, swirling each time for about 30 s and carefully decanting the acetone. After washing, the specimen should be free from agglomerations of glass powder, and the surface of the grains should be practically free from adhering fine particles. Dry the flask and contents

[a]From *USP 24–NF 19*, © USP.
[b]From *USP 24–NF 19*, © USP.
[c]From *USP 24–NF 19*, © USP.

for 20 min at 140°C, transfer the grains to a weighing bottle, and cool in a desiccator. Use the test specimen within 48 h after drying.

Procedure

Transfer 10.0 g of the prepared specimen, accurately weighed, to a 250-ml conical flask that has been digested (aged) previously with High-purity water in a bath at 90°C for at least 24 h or at 121°C for 1 h. Add 50.0 ml of High-purity water to this flask and to one similarly prepared to provide a blank. Cap all flasks with borosilicate glass beakers that previously have been treated as described for the flasks and that are of such size that the bottoms of the beakers fit snugly down on the top rims of the ontainers. Place the containers in the autoclave, and close it securely, leaving the vent cock open. Heat until steam issues vigorously from the vent cock, and continue heating for 10 min. Close the vent cock, and adjust the temperature to 121°C, taking 19–23min to reach the desired temperature. Hold the temperature at 121 ± 2.0°C for 30 min, counting from the time this temperature is reached. Reduce the heat so that the autoclave cools and comes to atmospheric pressure in 38–46 min, being vented as necessary to prevent the formation of a vacuum. Cool the flask at once in running water, decant the water from the flask into a suitably cleansed vessel, and wash the residual powdered glass with four 15-ml portions of High-purity water, adding the decanted washings to the main portion. Add 5 drops of Methyl Red Solution, and titrate immediately with 0.020 N sulfuric acid. If the volume of titrating solution is expected to be less than 10 ml, use a microburet. Record the volume of 0.020 N sulfuric acid used to neutralize the extract from 10 g of the prepared specimen of glass, corrected for a blank. The volume does not exceed that indicated in Table 1 for the type of glass concerned (13).

Water attack at 121°C for Type II glasses[d]

Rinse thoroughly twice 3 or more containers, selected at random, with high-purity water.

Procedure: Fill each container to 90% of its overflow capacity with High-purity water, and proceed as directed for *Procedure* under *Powdered Glass Test*, beginning with "Cap all flasks," except that the time of autoclaving shall be 60 min instead of 30 min, and ending with "to prevent the formation of a vacuum." Empty the contents from 1 or more containers into a 100-ml graduated cylinder, combining, in the case of smaller containers, the contents of several containers to obtain a volume of 100 ml. Place the pooled specimen in a 250-ml conical flask of resistant

[d]From *USP 24–NF 19*, © USP.

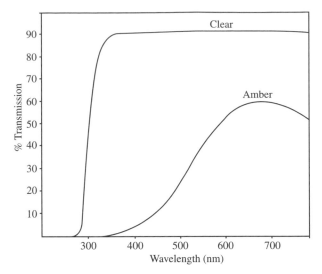

Fig. 4 Typical light transmission of clear and amber borosilicates.

glass, add 5 drops of Methyl Red Solution, and titrate, while warm, with 0.020 N sulfuric acid. Complete the titration within 60 min after opening the autoclave. Record the volume of 0.020 N sulfuric acid used, corrected for a blank obtained by titrating 100 ml of High-purity water at the same temperature and with the same amount of indicator. The volume does not exceed that indicated in Table 1 for the type of glass concerned (13).

Arsenic test[d]

For the *Test Preparation*, 35 ml of the water from one Type I glass container or, in the case of smaller containers, 35 ml of the combined contents of several Type I glass containers, are used and prepared as directed for *Procedure* under *Water Attack at 121°C* and the procedure described for *Arsenic* test in *USP 24–NF 19* general chapter <211> *Arsenic* is then followed. The limit provided for this test is 0.1 ppm.

Light transmission test[d]

In addition to the above-mentioned tests, compendial limits are provided for light transmission for colored light protecting glass containers. These containers intended to provide protection from light or supplied as "light Resistant" are expected to meet the requirements for *Light transmission* in this section. Light Transmission characteristics of typical clear and amber borosilicates are shown in Fig. 4.

In this test, a spectrophotometer of suitable sensitivity is used to a cut section of the glass container. The transmittance of the section is measured, and the observed light transmission is not expected to exceed the limits provided in Table 4.

Table 4   Limits for glass types I, II, and III

	Maximum percentage of light transmission at any wavelength between 2990 and 450 nm	
Normal size (in ml)	Flame-sealed containers	Closure-sealed containers
1	50	25
2	45	20
5	40	15
10	35	13
20	30	12
50	15	10

(From *USP 24–NF 19*, © USP.)

These methods of testing glass are basically similar to other compendial limits and other standards on glass such as those in International Organization for Standardization (ISO), German DIN, and the ASTM. The expected limit and test result expectations and procedures may vary for each standard of compendial method.

There are differences in testing glass as a container compared to glass as a material (glass-grain tests). The glass surface area-to-solution volume ratio is higher in grain tests, resulting in higher concentrations of glass constituents in solution after autoclaving. This facilitates solution analysis and differentiation between glasses. The other major difference is the presence of forming deposits, in the case of containers made from tubing, which influences test results. Blow-molded container test results are not affected by deposits.

SUMMARY

Glass as a packaging material has many advantages. Glass provides:

- Total impermeability to gaseous environmental contaminants
- Total impermeability to loss of essential volatile ingredients by diffusion through the container walls
- Excellent clarity and attractive sparkle
- Ease of cleaning and sterilizing with heat
- Resistance to attack by all liquids except HF and other caustic products
- A variety of shapes and it can accept a wide variety of closure types
- Ease of filling, closing, unscrambling, labeling, and cartoning
- Good compressional strength to allow efficient storage, especially allowing cartons of glass to be stacked high in warehouse
- Ease of hot-filling

Glass has disadvantages that include:

- Breakage—when it breaks, it shatters into numerous sharp fragments
- Weight—with a density of 2–2.5 g/ml, along with brittle character thick container walls, they become quite heavy
- Cost—in some cases, they are very expensive because of their weight and the type of fabrication involved (5)

REFERENCES

1. Boyd, D.C.; Danielson, P.S.; Thompson, D.A. Glass. *Encyclopedia of Chemical Technology*; Kroschwitz, J.I., Howe-Grant, M., Eds.; John Wiley, Inc.: New York, 1994; 12, 555–623.
2. Glass *The American Heritage Dictionary*, 2nd College Ed.; Houghton Mifflin Company: Boston, MA, 1991; 561.
3. ASTM Standard C162-88, Standard Definitions of Terms Relating to Glass and Glass Product. *Annual Book of ASTM Standards*; 1999; 15.02, 1–14.
4. Abendroth, R.P. Glass as a Packaging Material for Pharmaceuticals. *Encyclopedia of Pharmaceutical Technology*; Swarbrick, J., Boylan, J.C., Eds.; Marcel Dekker, Inc.: New York, 1993; 7, 79–100.
5. Jenkins, W.A.; Osburn, K.R. Packaging Drugs and Pharmaceuticals, Drug Packaging Materials. *Cooperation with Institute of Packaging Professionals*; Technomic Publishing Co.: Lancaster, PA, 1993; 99–102.
6. Goldschmidt, V.M. J. Soc. Glass Technol. **1927**, *11*, 337.
7. Woolley, F.E. *Engine Red Materials Handbook*; ASM International: Bilthoven, The Netherlands, 1991; 4, 386–393.
8. Spinosa, W.C.; Stephen, P.M.; Schorr, J.R. *Review of Literature on Control Technology Which Abates Air Pollution and Conserves Energy in Glass Melting Furnaces*; Nov 11, EPA-600/2-77-005,/2-76-269,/2-76-032b Corning, Inc.: Battelle, Columbus, OH, 1977.
9. Giegerich, W.; Trier, W. *Glass Machine Construction and Operation of Machines for the Forming of Hot Glass*; Kreidl, N.J., Ed.; Springer-Verlag: Berlin, 1969.
10. Pincus, A.G.; Holmes, T.R. *Annealing and Strengthening of Glass Industry*; Magazines for Industry, Inc.: New York, 1977.
11. *Containers for Injection, USP XII*; United States Pharmacopeia: Rockville, MD, 1942; 567–576.
12. *Containers, USP XIX*; United States Pharmacopeia: Rockville, MD, 1975; 643–647.
13. *Containers <661>, USP 24–NF 19*; United States Pharmacopeia: Rockville, MD, 2000; 1930–1935.
14. *Containers*; European Pharmacopoeia, Council of Europe: 67075 Strasbourgh Cedex France, 1997; 172–185.

GOOD CLINICAL PRACTICES (GCP)—AN OVERVIEW

Richard A. Guarino

Oxford Pharmaceutical Resources, Inc., Totowa, New Jersey

BACKGROUND

The Good Clinical Practice (GCP) regulations section in the Code of Federal Regulations (CFR) (21 CFR 312) (1) outlines the respective responsibilities of the clinical investigator, the drug sponsor, and the clinical study monitor involved in investigational new product development. These obligations, along with each participant's moral and ethical responsibilities for the safety of subjects who participate in clinical studies, comprise the essence of GCPs. GCPs have long been the norm for the investigator, as written in the 1572 Form (2); however, the first proposed regulations pertaining to investigator, sponsor, and monitor were first circulated in 1977 and 1978. In 1987, 10 years later, GCPs were published as final regulations in the CFR. Today, investigators, sponsors, and monitors are obligated by law to follow these GCPs.

To conduct clinical research that meets the requirements of the FDA for new product approval, it is essential to understand GCP regulations and their subsequent impact on the clinical development process of drugs, devices, and biologics.

The 1987, Investigational New Drug (IND), regulations specified within the current CFR identify (more clearly than in previously proposed GCP guidelines) the delegation of responsibilities in the conduct of clinical trials. Not only do investigators have a key responsibility in assessing patients' efficacy and safety response to new drugs, devices, or biologics, but the sponsor and monitor also have equal responsibility for the patients' safety and welfare. The key players who are obligated under GCP regulations are described below and will be referenced throughout this article:

Investigator. An investigator is the individual who conducts a clinical investigation (i.e., under whose immediate direction the drug is administered or dispensed to the subject). If an investigation involves many physicians at a particular institution, one physician is designated as the Prinicple Investigator (PI) and they are the responsible leader of the team of investigators. The subinvestigator is any other individual member of that team as identified by the PI. These individuals are usually licensed physicians or individuals working under a licensed physician (3).

Sponsor/Investigator. A sponsor/investigator is an individual who both initiates and conducts an investigation (i.e., under whose immediate direction the investigational drug is administered or dispensed). This category refers mostly to physician investigators who are conducting clinical research under an investigator IND (4).

Sponsor. A sponsor is an individual or organization that takes responsibility for and initiates a clinical investigation. This may be an individual, pharmaceutical company, governmental agency, academic institution, or a private or other organization (5).

Monitor. A monitor is the person selected by the sponsor who is qualified by training experience to facilitate and oversee the progress of the investigation (6).

INVESTIGATOR OBLIGATIONS

In 21 CFR 312.53 (7), the regulations deal with the descriptive information provided on form FDA 1572, the Statement of Investigator form. Also included in 21 CFR 312.53 are the selection requirements for clinical investigators. Previously, to conduct studies designated as Phases 1 and 2, investigators were required to complete a Statement of Investigator form FDA 1572; investigators conducting studies designated as phase 3 or phase 4 completed a different Statement of Investigator form, which was known as form FDA 1573. As a result of the IND rewrite regulations, form FDA 1573 is no longer used for any clinical studies. At present, for Phases 1–4, only the Statement of Investigator form FDA 1572 is required. This document states the obligations of investigators conducting clinical research. In addition to the general information on the 1572, new information includes the following: the name and address of any clinical laboratory facility, the address of the Institutional Review Board (IRB) (8) responsible for the review and approval of the protocol, the patient consent form, and the individual investigators participating in the study. This document also states that the sponsor is charged with the responsibility of selecting qualified investigators, who are defined as those who are capable of conducting the study by virtue of their training and experience. By using the phrase "training and experience," the FDA means that clinical investigators conducting a study of a particular disease should have enough experience in that clinical specialty to observe correctly the signs, symptoms, and progress of the disease being treated with a new investigational drug. For example, if a new drug is designed for an Obstetrics/Gynecology practice, a pediatrician would not be expected to have the expertise to assess this drug, nor would a cardiologist have expertise in evaluating a gastrointestinal drug.

Investigators are defined as those who have signed and completed form FDA 1572 or sub- or coinvestigators listed on that form, who are considered to have the academic and experiential qualifications for participating in the clinical program.

The "fine print" on the reverse side of form FDA 1572 is a written agreement whereby the investigators assure the sponsor that they will conduct the study in accordance with the appropriate study plan (i.e., the protocol) (9) and will observe the GCP tenets. Implicit in this agreement is the fact that the Investigator will have obtained signed Informed Consent (IC) (10) forms from patients or subjects participating in the clinical research under their jurisdiction. Form 1572 also charges the investigator with the reporting of adverse experiences that occur during the investigation and provides assurance that the investigator has read and understood the investigator's brochure. In addition, he or she assures that all individuals participating in the supervision of any clinical study, under the direction of the investigator, are aware of their responsibilities. Once form 1572 has been signed by the investigator, he or she further assures compliance with the requirements of providing study materials, protocols, and other pertinent information to an authorized IRB for review. This information, along with a curriculum vitae, should be provided along with the assurance that the investigational plan set forth in the study protocol will be complied with.

To summarize, the primary responsibilities of investigators in clinical trials are the ethical and moral obligations to all the participating patients and subjects in the study. Investigators must provide a measure of safety for each participant in the study so that the patient is protected ethically and morally from any endangerment that might occur during a trial using an investigational drug. After the investigator's responsibilities are outlined and he or she has signed form FDA 1572, any additional information from the sponsor that might be necessary should be requested and any concerns regarding procedures should be raised. An investigator is responsible for: 1) ensuring that an investigation is conducted according to the signed investigator statement, the investigational plan, and applicable regulations; and 2) for protecting the rights, safety, and welfare of subjects participating in a clinical investigation on any unapproved product. Also, the investigators must maintain complete control and accountability of the experimental products under investigation. An investigator shall obtain the informed consent of each human subject to whom the drug is administered and shall administer the drug only to subjects under the investigator's supervision or under the supervision of a subinvestigator responsible to the investigator. The investigator shall not supply the investigational drug to any person not participating in the clinical program.

The investigators are required to maintain adequate records of the disposition of the experimental medications, including dates, quantity, and use by subjects (11). If the investigation is terminated, suspended, discontinued, or completed, the investigator shall account for and return the unused supplies to the sponsor, or otherwise provide written documentation for disposition of the unused supplies of the drug. An investigator is required to maintain accurate case histories designed to record all observations and other pertinent data on each individual treated with the investigational drug. (Usually, this is accomplished by completing case report forms and maintaining medical records).

All investigators shall retain records of all subjects enlisted in investigational trials for 2 years after a new drug application (NDA) is approved for the indication for which the drug is being investigated. If no application is to be filed or if the application is not approved for such indication, records must be maintained 2 years after the investigation is discontinued or the IND is closed and the FDA has notified the sponsor of the status of the application (12).

The investigator shall furnish all reports to the sponsor of the drug. The sponsor is responsible for collecting and evaluating the results obtained. The sponsor also is required to submit annual reports to the FDA on the progress of the clinical investigations.

Investigators shall promptly report to the sponsor any adverse effect that may reasonably be regarded as caused by, or probably caused by, the investigational drug. If the adverse effect is serious (13) the investigator shall report the adverse effect immediately. (See chapter on ADR reporting.)

An investigator shall provide the sponsor with an adequate report shortly after completion of the investigator's participation in the study.

OTHER INVESTIGATOR RESPONSIBILITIES

The investigator must assure that an IRB complies with the regulations established in the CFR and that the IRB is responsible for the initial and continuing review and approval of the proposed clinical study. The investigator must also assure that he or she will promptly report all changes in the research activity and all unanticipated problems involving risk to human subjects Adverse Reactions (ADRs) or others to the IRB. In addition, the investigator will not make any changes in the research protocol without IRB approval, except where necessary to eliminate apparent immediate hazards to human subjects.

An investigator will on request from any properly authorized officer or employee of the FDA, at reasonable times, permit such officer or employee to have access to, copy, and verify any records or reports made by the investigator. The investigator is not required to divulge subject names, unless the records of particular individuals require a more detailed study of the cases or unless there is reason to believe that the records do not represent actual case studies or do not represent actual results obtained.

SPONSOR OBLIGATIONS

The sponsor's primary responsibility is clearly delineated in 21 CFR 312.50 (14) and ensures that clinical studies are conducted in compliance with FDA regulations. The sponsor is responsible for selecting qualified investigators and for providing them with the information they need to conduct an investigation in accordance with the published regulations. Usually, the sponsor accomplishes this task by supplying the potential investigator with an investigator's brochure and a protocol of the clinical investigation on the agent to be investigated. An investigator's brochure (15) contains all information from nonclinical studies and reports and any previous human efficacy and safety study reports that reflect previous experiences of patients of the investigational agent.

Of primary interest in the obligations is the option of a sponsor to transfer total or partial responsibility for the conduct of a clinical study to a Contract Research Organization (CRO) (16). During the last decade, CROs have played a significant role in new drug development. However, CROs who contract with sponsor companies are obligated under the same GCP regulations as defined in this chapter. A CRO may be the sponsor or the monitor with equal obligations as defined in 21 CFR 312. The current regulations noted in 21 CFR 312.52 (17) are specific and require that any transfer, whether in total or in part, be described in writing and agreed to by both parties. The FDA states that any obligations not specifically described by the sponsor in the written transfer of responsibilities will be considered as not transferred to the CRO; the liability for these undefined responsibilities, therefore, remains with the sponsor. The FDA further requires the CRO (once any transfer of responsibilities has been made by the sponsor) to comply with all applicable regulations and notes that the CRO is subject to the same regulatory actions as a sponsor if a CRO does not satisfy FDA regulations in the fulfillment of its contracted duties. As a result of these regulations, it is possible for a CRO to act on behalf of a sponsor once this legal transfer of obligations has been completed. Although the CRO must assure complete compliance with the responsibilities assigned, it remains the sponsor's responsibility to ensure the quality and integrity of data generated under the supervision of a CRO. In this situation, the sponsor would be expected to act as a quality assurance (18) auditor of the data, even though assignment for the conduct of a study has been delegated to the CRO. It is important to note the following: that any such transfer shall be described in writing; if not all obligations are transferred, the description of the specific obligations being assumed by the CRO must be clearly stated. Any obligation not covered by the written description shall be deemed not to have been transferred. The regulations also charge the sponsor with responsibility for the inventory and control of the drug. Only investigators participating in a clinical trial may receive and have access to investigational drug and materials.

SPONSOR AND MONITOR OBLIGATIONS

One of the most important responsibilities of the sponsor is to monitor the progress of every clinical investigation conducted under its direction (21 CFR 312.56) (19). A monitor's obligations, under the auspices of the sponsor, are to ensure that the deficiencies created during the conduct of clinical investigations are corrected or justified by the investigator and that the investigator adheres to the investigational plan. The appointed monitors for any clinical investigation conducted under a sponsor's IND have an obligation to assure that an investigator is complying with the signed Form FDA 1572 and the general investigational plan and that the clinical protocol is being followed. If an investigator does not correct his or her errors and mistakes and no improvement is noted in the progress of the study, the monitor shall promptly secure compliance or discontinue shipment of the investigational new drug to the investigator and end the investigator's participation in the clinical program. In addition the monitors, while monitoring the progress of a clinical investigation, must evaluate the evidence relating to safety and effectiveness. At the same time, sponsors shall make such reports to the FDA regarding information relevant to the safety of the drug, as they are required to do under section 312.32 (20) of the FDA regulations.

When a monitor reports an adverse effect to a sponsor during an investigational study, it is the sponsor's obligation to determine whether there is an unreasonable and significant risk to the subject or patient (21). At that time, the sponsor must determine if the investigational study is to be discontinued. Important among the procedures of reporting adverse effects is the sponsor's obligation to the FDA, the IRB, and to all investigators who, at any time, participate in clinical studies and who are prescribing the experimental drug. Subsequent to this, the sponsor should furnish the FDA with a full report of the sponsor's actions and shall determine whether or not to discontinue the investigation. If the decision to discontinue is made, based on the seriousness of the ADRs reported, the studies should be terminated as soon as possible and no later than 7 days after making the decision.

It is important to understand that the obligations of monitors include the responsibility for assuring that all records and data recorded on case report forms reflect valid data gathered by the investigator and that they coincide with corresponding medical and hospital records of the candidate participating in the investigational study. Detailed auditing and documentation assure the sponsor that the monitor is overseeing the clinical data collected by the investigator and that GCPs are being followed (22). One misconception of many monitors who audit clinical investigations is that their only task is to assure correct entry of data. In fact, it is of extreme importance among the monitor's obligations to note any adverse effects or any deviations in laboratory values that could signify a safety problem to investigational study subjects. This is especially true in large multiclinic studies, in which many centers are conducting investigational studies following the same protocol and many monitors are auditing data. If any abnormal reactions or laboratory deviations are noted

from center to center, the monitors should compare observations and assess an accumulative percentage of occurrence of these deviations. At times, a sporadic, apparently minor deviation can turn out to be a significant deviation when calculated across all centers. If monitors are astute, they can often prevent recurrence of adverse events that might jeopardize the safety of the subjects participating in investigational drug studies.

Another responsibility of the monitor is to assure maintenance of accurate records showing the receipt, shipment, or other disposition of the investigational drug (23). These records are required to include, as appropriate, the name of the investigator to whom the drug is shipped, the date, the quantity, and the batch number of each shipment. The monitor/sponsor shall also assure the return of all unused supplies of the investigational drug from each investigator whose participation in the investigation is discontinued or terminated. The sponsor may authorize an alternative disposition of unused supplies of the investigational drug, provided this alternative disposition does not expose humans to risks. Although the overall responsibilities are assigned to sponsors, it is the monitors' underlying responsibility for drug accountability.

In turn, the investigators, during experimental research, are also responsible for record retention similar to that of the sponsor. They are required to maintain adequate records of the disposition of the drug, including dates, quantity, and use by the subjects or patients. The investigator is also obligated, if he or she is terminated, suspended, or discontinued or if he or she has completed a study, to return all unused supplies of the drug to the sponsor or otherwise provide documentation of how the unused supplies of the drug were disposed. (It is recommended always to return the unused study medication to the sponsor). An investigator is required to prepare and maintain adequate and accurate case histories (designed to record all observations and other data pertinent to the investigation) on each individual treated with the investigational drug. The monitor should assure that all the previous procedures are adhered to and reported in a timely fashion.

An often-neglected investigator responsibility is the requirement to submit periodic reports to the sponsor. An investigator should be prepared to provide the sponsor with progress reports. These should include an update of the ongoing investigational trial. Annual reports to the FDA on the progress of the clinical investigations are required to be submitted by the sponsor. These reports contain information based on the investigators' progress reports (24). Safety reports are another issue. An investigator should promptly report to the sponsor any adverse events that may reasonably be regarded as caused by or likely caused by the investigational drug. Alarming adverse events (i.e., severe adverse reactions that jeopardize a patient's safety in any way) must be reported immediately by the investigator to the sponsor (25). Lastly, when an investigator has completed or terminated an investigational study, a final report shall be provided to the sponsor. This comprehensive report should be submitted to the sponsor shortly after completion of an investigator's participation in the investigation. The report summarizes the final observations of the study and any adverse events that occurred during the course of the clinical investigation. Monitors should also be responsible for encouraging investigators to complete and submit all the reports listed above. Constant follow-up may be necessary by the monitor if these investigator responsibilities are to be fulfilled. In most cases, the clinical monitor usually will provide the investigator with these reports.

Legal repercussions can occur from any neglect of the obligations by investigators, sponsors, or monitors. The CFR stipulates in 21 CFR 312.58 (26) that the FDA can inspect the sponsor's records or reports on request from any properly authorized officer or employee of the FDA. These inspections normally occur at reasonable times and permit the FDA to have access to copy and verify any records and reports relating to a clinical investigation conducted under an IND. On written request by the FDA, the sponsor may be asked to submit the records, reports, or copies of them to the FDA. Under these regulations, the sponsor is also obligated to discontinue shipments of the drug to any investigator who has failed to maintain or make available records or reports of the investigation. Subsequently, an investigator may, on request from any properly authorized officer or employee of the FDA, at reasonable times, permit such an officer or employee to have access to or copy and verify any records or reports made by the investigator. The investigator is not required to divulge subject or patient names unless the records of particular individuals require a more detailed study of the cases.

GCP NONCOMPLIANCE

What are the consequences if an investigator has repeatedly or deliberately either failed to comply with these GCP requirements or has submitted false information in any report to the sponsor (27)? Initially, the Center for Drug Evaluation and Research (CDER) or the Center for Biologics Evaluation and Research (CBER) will furnish the investigator with written notice of the matter complained of and offer the investigator an opportunity to explain the matter in writing or at the option of the investigator, grant an informal conference. If the explanation offered by the investigator is not accepted by the CDER or the CBER, the investigator will then be given an opportunity for a regulatory hearing. At this hearing, the issue of whether the investigator is entitled to receive investigational drugs will be addressed. After evaluating all available information, including any explanation presented by the investigator, the FDA commissioner determines whether the investigator has repeatedly or deliberately failed to comply with the GCP requirements or has deliberately or repeatedly submitted false information to the sponsor in any required report. The commissioner will then notify the investigator and the sponsor of any investigation in which the investigator has been named as a participant that the investigator is not entitled to receive investigational drugs. The investigation can not be terminated without reasonable cause as set forth by the commissioner and committee. Sponsor can also suspend shipment of drugs to the investigator for noncompliance to the protocol. If there is reasonable cause for this action, the investigator becomes subject to further investigation for each IND and each approved application submitted to the FDA containing data reported by this investigator. Therefore, every investigational study conducted by this investigator will be examined to determine whether the investigator has submitted unreliable data. Other investigations that are conducted under the same protocol will be temporarily put on hold. Conversely, the commissioner may determine, after eliminating the unreliable data by the investigator, that the remaining data justify continuing other of the same investigations at other sites. However, if a danger to the public health exists, the commissioner will terminate the IND immediately; the sponsor will be notified and will have an opportunity for a regulatory hearing before the FDA on the question of whether the IND should be reinstated. If the commissioner determines that the data submitted are unreliable and that the data submitted by the investigator cannot be justified, the commissioner will proceed to withdraw approval of the drug product in accordance with the provisions of the Food and Drug Cosmetic Act (FD&C). As a result, an investigator who has been deemed to be ineligible to receive investigational drugs will be blacklisted and unable to participate in any experimental studies. The investigator may be reinstated when the commissioner determines that the investigator has presented adequate assurances that the investigator will use investigational drugs in compliance with FDA regulations.

In conclusion, before an investigator accepts the responsibilities to conduct a clinical investigation with an IND drug, he or she must be aware of the legal obligations he or she has agreed to when form FDA 1572 is signed. Investigators must comply with the protocol and the rules, regulations, and guidelines of GCPs.

Investigators must realize that they are subject to a federal offense and can jeopardize their reputation and, ultimately, their ability to conduct further clinical research. Investigators must know that the precise collection of data is mandatory in the conduct of clinical research. Research must be designed to assess the efficacy of the product and, above all, to assure that the safety of the patient remains the primary concern.

Sponsors' and monitors' responsibilities in complying with GCPs are also subject to serious repercussions under 21CFR 312.58. FDA inspectors are allowed to examine sponsors' files and the interventions of monitors' site visits to assure that GCP compliance was executed. Case report forms and clinical results are subjected to the same scrutiny that are applied to the investigators' responsibilities. If during an FDA inspection discrepancies are found in any form among the investigator, sponsor, and, when appropriate, the CRO (i.e., its documents), all three parties will be held responsible, and the IND will be placed on hold until the findings are resolved.

Investigators', sponsors', and monitors' obligations must be fulfilled by complying with GCP rules and regulations. Sponsors' and monitors' consistent and persistent managing roles are vital in assuring that each person involved in conducting clinical studies meet his or her legal obligations. The success of any clinical program will depend on the cooperation, understanding, and compliance of this triad working together. With this agreement of responsibilities and a well-organized clinical plan, the results can only conclude valid data in support of a new drug application.

REFERENCES

1. *Code of Federal Regulations,* Title 21, Part 312, (annually).
2. Guarino, R.A. The Investigational New Drug Application and the Investigator's Brochure. *New Drug Approval Process*, 3rd Ed.; Marcel Dekker, Inc.: New York, 2000; 100, 74–75.
3. Guarino, R.A. Obligations of the Investigator, Sponsor, and Monitor. *New Drug Approval Process*, 3rd Ed.; Marcel Dekker, Inc.: New York, 2000; 100, 326.
4. Guarino, R.A. The Investigational New Drug Application and the Investigator's Brochure. *New Drug Approval Process*, 3rd Ed.; Marcel Dekker, Inc.: New York, 2000; 100, 56.
5. Guarino, R.A. Obligations of the Investigator, Sponsor, and Monitor. *New Drug Approval Process*, 3rd Ed.; Marcel Dekker, Inc.: New York, 2000; 100, 329.
6. Guarino, R.A. Obligations of the Investigator, Sponsor, and Monitor. *New Drug Approval Process*, 3rd Ed.; Marcel Dekker, Inc.: New York, 2000; 100, 330.
7. *Code of Federal Regulations,* Title 21, Part 312.53, (annually).
8. Guarino, R.A. Institutional Review Board/Independent Ethics Committee and Informed Consent. Protecting Subjects Throughout the Clinical Research Process. *New Drug Approval Process*, 3rd Ed.; Marcel Dekker, Inc.: New York, 2000; 100, 271.
9. Guarino, R.A. Clinical Research Protocols. *New Drug Approval Process*, 3rd Ed.; Marcel Dekker, Inc.: New York, 2000; 100, 219.
10. Guarino, R.A. Institutional Review Board/Independent Ethics Committee and Informed Consent: Protecting Subjects Throughout the Clinical Research Process. *New Drug Approval Process*, 3rd Ed. Marcel Dekker, Inc.: New York, 2000; 100, 278.
11. Guarino, R.A. Obligations of the Investigator, Sponsor, and Monitor. *New Drug Approval Process*, 3rd Ed.; Marcel Dekker, Inc.: New York, 2000; 100, 328.
12. Guarino, R.A. Obligations of the Investigator, Sponsor, and Monitor. *New Drug Approval Process*, 3rd Ed.; Marcel Dekker, Inc.: New York, 2000; 100, 328.
13. Guarino, R.A. Adverse Reactions and Interactions of Drugs. *New Drug Approval Process*, 3rd Ed.; Marcel Dekker, Inc.: New York, 2000; 100, 247.
14. *Code of Federal Regulations*, Title 21, Part 312.50, (annually).
15. Guarino, R.A. The Investigational New Drug Application and the Investigator's Brochure. *New Drug Approval Process*, 3rd Ed.; Marcel Dekker, Inc.: New York, 2000; 100, 86.
16. Guarino, R.A. Working with a CRO. *New Drug Approval Process*, 3rd Ed.; Marcel Dekker, Inc.; New York, 2000; 100, 439.
17. *Code of Federal Regulations* Title 21, Part 312.52, (annually).
18. Guarino, R.A. Quality Assurance. *New Drug Approval Process*, 3rd Ed.; Marcel Dekker, Inc.: New York, 2000; 100, 349.
19. *Code of Federal Regulations,* Title 21, Part 312.56, (annually).
20. *Code of Federal Regulations,* Title 21, Part 312.32, (annually).
21. Guarino, R.A. Adverse Reactions and Interactions of Drugs. *New Drug Approval Process*, 3rd Ed.; Marcel Dekker, Inc.: New York, 2000; 100, 262–263.
22. Guarino, R.A. Obligations of the Investigator, Sponsor, and Monitor. *New Drug Approval Process*, 3rd Ed.; Marcel Dekker, Inc.: New York, 2000; 100, 330–334.
23. Guarino, R.A. Obligations of the Investigator, Sponsor, and Monitor. *New Drug Approval Process*, 3rd Ed.; Marcel Dekker, Inc.: New York, 2000; 100, 331.
24. Guarino, R.A. Obligations of the Investigator, Sponsor, and Monitor. *New Drug Approval Process*, 3rd Ed.; Marcel Dekker, Inc.: New York, 2000; 100, 332.
25. Guarino, R.A. Adverse Reactions and Interactions of Drugs. *New Drug Approval Process*, 3rd Ed.; Marcel Dekker, Inc.: New York, 2000; 100, 260.

26. *Code of Federal Regulations*, Title 21, Part 312.58, (annually).

27. Guarino, R.A. Obligations of the Investigator, Sponsor, and Monitor. *New Drug Approval Process*, 3rd Ed.; Marcel Dekker, Inc.: New York, 2000; 100, 332–333.

28. Guarino, R.A. Clinical Research: The Obligations of the Investigator, Sponsor, and Monitor. Drug Info. J. **1978**, *12* (3), 157.

29. Guarino, R.A.; Cox, B.S. *Practice and Application of Good Clinical Practices*; Cooperation with St. John's University: New York, Oct 1982; The American Federation for Clinical Research Eastern Section.

30. Guarino, R.A. *Practice and Application of Good Clinical Practices. Concepts and Strategies in New Drug Development*; Clinical Pharmacology and Therapeutic Series Praeger Publishers: New York, 1983; 4.

31. Guarino, R.A. *Role of the MD in Protocol Design*; Applied Clinical Trials Conference and Exhibition: Reston, VA, 1993.

32. Guarino, R.A. *Clinical Study Conduct/Procedures*; Drug Information Association Meeting: Chicago, IL, July 1993.

33. Stuart, J.P. *Clinical Trials. A Practical Approach*; John Wiley & Sons: New York, 1983.

34. MacKintosh, D.R.; Zepp, V.J. GCP Responsibilities of Principal Investigators: Beyond the 1572. Appl. Clin. Trials **Nov. 1996**, 32–40.

35. MacKintosh, D.R.; Zepp, V.J. Source Documentation: A Key to GCP Compliance in Clinical Trials. Appl. Clin. Trials **Mar. 1996**, 42–46.

36. Souza, K.; Small, R.D. The use of Total Quality Management Principles in Placing and Monitoring Clinical Trials. Drug Info. J. **1995**, *29*, 695–703.

GOOD LABORATORY PRACTICE (GLP)—AN OVERVIEW

Nigel J. Dent

Country Consultancy Ltd., Northamptonshire, United Kingdom

OVERVIEW

The Good Laboratory Practice Guidelines (GLP) have been in existence for nonclinical safety studies since 1976 (1–8). They have progressed through various transitional phases to become guidelines in some countries and regulatory/statutory instruments in others.

The current document is the Organisation for Economic Co-operation and Development (OECD) Principles of GLP (9) and is currently accepted as the industry standard. This was reviewed and published in January 1997 (10, 11) but must be used in conjunction with the appropriate Scientific Guidelines for the scientific side of the study, i.e., the OECD Toxicology Guidelines etc. (12). This sets out to cover all nonclinical safety studies and gives guidance as to how these studies should be conducted in conjunction with the appropriate regulatory toxicology guidelines and, on that basis, when encompassed in the various Directives of the European Union (EU) (13) or in other Memorandum of Understanding, allow data generated under this program to be mutually accepted by other OECD countries. One must not forget, however, the other equally important Guidelines and Regulations of other countries, such as those of the U.S. Food and Drug Administration (FDA) (14) and the U.S. Environmental Protection Agency (EPA) (15–20), and similar organizations in Japan (21). All have basically similar rules and, being members of the OECD, data generated to the OECD principles will generally be accepted in the United States and Japan. The EPA regulations used to be quite different and were applied to agrochemical and pesticide products. However, having been revised recently, they have been brought in line with the documents of other agencies.

The guidelines themselves, with the exception of those in countries where they are featured as regulations, are, as stated, guidelines to the conduct of the study and aim to cover compliance with the GLP principles but in no way do they dictate how the science will be performed.

It must be remembered that compliance is monitored by adherence to GLP, whereas the regulatory authority and the receiving authority of the dossier when submitted for the application of a marketing permit or similar document review the science.

OBJECTIVE OF THE GUIDELINES

The general objective of the guidelines originates in the very early 1970s, when one pharmaceutical company in particular and a contract research organization (CRO) generated data that, when submitted to the FDA, gave them cause for concern in the accuracy of the data presented and, in certain instances, the honesty of the submission.

At that time, a full review of companies and institutions conducting nonclinical safety studies (toxicology) was undertaken by the FDA (22) and although, in general, the industry was found to be credible, one company (Industrial Biotest) was found to be generating extremely poor-quality data, in many instances, in a fraudulent manner. This, therefore, caused the FDA to put together and implement the GLPs (23, 24).

Over the next 10 years, many countries introduced similar good-practices guidelines. The EU (25) in general produced its guidelines and eventually, despite the fact that the world was operating according to similar principles, a standard document was produced by the OECD in the early 1980s and became the industry standard. The reason this was of benefit to the whole industry was because this now precluded the fact that every submitting company would have to be inspected by each relevant monitoring authority and, when implemented into several directives and legal statutes (26, 27) within the OECD (particularly in the United Kingdom) (28), this allowed data generated by one company to be accepted by several receiving authorities without further inspection.

The objective of the GLPs is to ensure that a standard approach is undertaken covering traceability and accountability and, while still allowing freedom for the scientists, to impose certain restrictions on the generation of data and the experimental work.

It must be remembered that GLP is merely common sense in a formal environment. The key phrases that are currently seen in a GLP environment include good documentation, good training, maintenance and calibration of all equipment, the archiving and storing of data in a formal and retrievable manner, and the use of high-quality, validated equipment and accredited test systems (animals).

This in general is merely good science, and the GLPs have further enhanced this by the addition of an independent Quality Assurance Unit (QAU) and a study director/principal investigator who jointly controls and oversees the project and involves the management in putting together adequate resources and assuming overall responsibility for the study.

This can be seen as good science, with several slight enhancements. The details of these individual subjects are addressed later in this article.

WHO DOES IT AFFECT?

Any company or institution performing nonclinical safety studies for the submission of data for a new chemical entity; a new biological, immunological, pesticide, veterinary or agrochemical product; or, for that matter, a similar product that will eventually appear in the marketplace and be consumed by the general public must adhere to GLP in the conduct of their nonclinical safety study experimentation.

Within a company, every person from senior management to the junior technician is bound by these GLPs and must exhibit clear understanding and training in these practices.

To ensure that the practices are followed, a regulatory inspection takes place on a 2-year basis in most countries, and the objective of this is to review, as an independent group, how these good practices are being followed. Certification or a guarantee that the company is operating according to these standards is the benchmark standard. This is also addressed later in this article.

As we move into the twenty-first century, it is quite apparent that the industry will shrink as mergers and acquisitions (29–33) take place, and, with this, the emergence of the now familiar CRO will become ever more popular in the conduct of nonclinical safety studies. It is, therefore, very important that, in this area, the sponsor has the assurance that these facilities are operating not only to the highest standard of science but also in compliance with GLP and that, as a subcontractor, the data they generate will be equally accepted as if the data were generated by the company itself.

WHY HAVE IT?

In general terms, for companies conducting nonclinical safety studies (34), it is, a regulatory requirement, and without this certificate or certification of compliance, data will generally not be accepted by the receiving/regulatory authorities.

However, one should not embark on the process of obtaining or working to GLP with this sole aim in mind. It should be used as an ongoing improving and quality standard for the laboratory.

In fact, it is the author's experience over the past 5 years, that many companies have gone far beyond the requirements of GLP compliance (35) and that the overall concept of good scientific design and good science has been superseded by the desire merely to obtain compliance. It is quite often seen that an extremely poor quality scientific study has been conducted in complete compliance with GLP. It has been seen on several occasions in a laboratory, for example, where the refrigerator has been located far from its permitted limits; where the temperature has been diligently recorded, signed, and dated as required by GLP, but where no attempt has been made to either document the excursions outside the accepted range or to rectify the problem. The operative was merely under the impression that as long as temperature is recorded, this is GLP despite the damage that excursions outside the temperature range may have caused to any investigational product stored in the refrigerator.

Over the years, those scientists who have worked according to the principles of GLP now readily admit without any prompting that they are unsure how they conducted scientific studies before the advent of these good practices. The ability to reconstruct studies, to work to a standard format across several differing laboratories or countries, and to be able to prove beyond reasonable doubt that these were the values obtained and the results submitted.

Certainly, data with a GLP compliance statement are being accepted more readily by the receiving authorities, which has led to fewer repeated studies. This, in turn, is helping to achieve the aim of all scientists in reducing the use of animals.

From a company's point of view, working according to the principles of GLP shows that it has an attitude that is both ethical and moral to the production of scientific data with products that will eventually enter the human food chain or be of benefit to mankind.

HOW IS IT ENFORCED?

In the OECD countries, for at least 14 years, an Inspectorate has been set up, varying in inspector numbers from several hundred in the United States to one or two in countries not conducting a great deal of scientific nonclinical research. All countries, however, have a regulatory group that, in some instances, also acts as the receiving authority for the review of data, and reports to the GLP Monitoring Authority. This regulatory group visits on a 2-year basis or, in Germany, a 4-year basis, those companies that have claimed compliance and will then be on a rolling program of review (36).

Unlike its role in many areas of regulatory compliance, it is still the responsibility of the sponsoring company to claim compliance from the Monitoring Authority. This claim is made for a particular company, laboratory, and/or series of tests. From the date of compliance when a letter is written to the Monitoring Authority, data generated from then are assumed by that company to be in compliance with GLP. This claim in then verified in a visit from the regulatory inspector. The inspection may be performed by one or two persons for 1 to 5 days. At the end of the inspection, an exit meeting is held, and the company is usually given an indication of its performance. Noncompliance points are noted in writing and discussed, and a report is then prepared. In view of the findings, three levels of compliance can be obtained:

1. Sufficient deviations have been seen to question the integrity of the data and, therefore, a complete rejection of the claim of compliance is made, with a revisit necessary.
2. Minor points of compliance have been seen that can be handled in a specified period in which case, the laboratory is placed under the category, of pending compliance.
3. Very minor points of compliance have been seen, which, when addressed in writing by the management in a 1-month period with supportive paperwork, etc., lead to the company being given a Statement of Compliance, a Certificate of Compliance, or an indication that the laboratory is in compliance. It depends on the specific country whether a Certificate of Compliance is given. If a certificate is given, it generally states that on the particular day that the inspection took place, the laboratory was found to be in compliance with the OECD Principles of GLP. Also, the address of the facility is given as well as a listing of areas in which compliance has been confirmed. This could be stated as *analytical support facilities*, *acute toxicology*, *mutagenicity*, or similar designations.

Naturally, the benchmark standard is either the OECD Guidelines or similar standards in Japan or the United States. The Inspectorate carries out inspections against these documents. It could be said that often it is merely a review of the procedure and an opinion of compliance given by the inspector versus the interpretation of the individual conducting the experimental work. To try to overcome this criticism and to ensure that all inspectors work according to a standard format, over the past 4 years, the OECD has instituted a series of mutual joint visits (MJVs) (37).

The process of an MJV is that a company is inspected by its local inspector and that the inspector is accompanied by inspectors from two other countries as observers. At the conclusion of the inspection, the company is given their findings by its local inspector and, outside that meeting, a review of the performance of the inspector with positive and negative points is given by the two observing inspectors. To ensure continuity, one of these three inspectors would then be on the next MJV.

In the past, Memorandums of Understanding (MoUs) (38) have been instituted between certain major countries, such as Japan and the UK, the United States and Japan or Canada, etc. However, these have generally fallen into nonuse for a variety of reasons, especially in Europe, where it is now, or has been for some time, not possible for a country to negotiate directly with another country. Brussels, however, being the center of the European Community, has to carry out that discussion with a proposed partner in another country. As such, at the time of producing this overview, very few MoUs are currently in force.

WHAT IS GLP?

As noted in the Overview, GLP is a series of guidelines that cover the conduct and data production for nonclinical safety studies.

The OECD covers a series of activities and personnel. Responsibilities, training, quality assurance (QA), standard operating procedures (SOPs), study plans and study reports, data production and recording, equipment maintenance and calibration, computers and validation, test systems and test substances, and archiving are the primary areas covered by the GLPs.

A very brief overview of each of these areas is given hereafter.

Responsibilities

The prime players in a GLP scenario would be the management, the sponsor, the study director, the principal investigator, and the QA.

In a hierarchical structure, management would be totally responsible for the conduct of the work and for the assurance that resources have been made available and that an active role is played by these people in overseeing the conduct of scientific research.

The sponsor is the company that places a contract with a CRO or requests from within a company that work in another department be undertaken. The sponsor is the person who is supplying the money and the request for the work.

The study director is the prime player and is ultimately responsible for the production of the study plan, the conduct of the study, and the overseeing or production of the final report. Naturally, a large amount of delegation may take place; however, this must always be in writing, and the overall responsibility for the conduct of the study; the daily contact with the study staff; the prevention of recording of problems and the assurance that the study has been conducted in line with the study plan, the GLP, and the scientific guidelines solely belongs to this individual.

The Principal Investigator is the next in line of responsibility after the Study Director in a multisite study. For example, they could be the person seen in a field study situation where the crop-spraying, for example, may be undertaken at a place remote from the GLP designated site where the study director works. The principal investigator is therefore the person responsible initially for that portion of the work, although under the direct control of the study director. It may also be that, within a company, work is subcontracted to the Analytical Department, for example, for the analysis of formulated material. The person responsible for this particular aspect of the scientific work is the principal investigator, who is involved in the study plan and responsible to the study director. Another typical scenario is work conducted in a CRO under the control of the study director, where samples of plasma are taken for toxicokinetics, for example, and these samples analyzed by the sponsor. The sponsor's analyst, therefore, may well be designated the principal investigator.

Quality assurance

This is an independent group that does not become involved in the conduct of the study but merely reviews the data, experimental work, and documents produced to ensure compliance with the SOPs, the study plans, and GLP. Other activities such as training and assistance in interpreting GLPs, etc., may be the responsibility of the QAU. (For more information, see the following section in this article or Section II, 1.4 pp. 17–19 of the OECD GLPs.)

Training and recording

It is the responsibility of the management to ensure that training takes place and the responsibility of the Study Director to assure that the individuals conducting the work are adequately trained and have adequate records. At a minimum, there must be a CV, a training record, and a very clear job description. Specifically, with regard to a study director, there must be explicit details of how the study director position can be met and the responsibilities of that individual in carrying out the relevant duties.

There should be procedures detailing how the training will take place; recording of the training must be made on a regular basis, the records must be stored in archives and regularly updated, and a complete and historical review of the trainee's activities, previous training, and ability to conduct the work according to GLP must be documented. (See the OECD Principles, Section I, 2a–d.)

Quality Assurance

This function, as has already been stated, is an independent review. The responsibilities here start with a review of the study plan and continue through the review of the study in the in-life phase, data audits, and the final study report audit.

In addition to these, systems audits and process audits can be undertaken.

The aim of QA is to assure the management that compliance with GLP is maintained throughout the entire study, that the data integrity is maintained, and that compliance with the SOPs and the study plan is adhered to by all experimental study staff. The study audit is a specific audit of the study in direct relation to the study plan. A systems audit, however, rather than proceeding in a vertical line, takes a horizontal line across all studies and would include such tasks as archiving, training, SOPs, general computer validation, animal house operation, and management activities. These are but a few areas that would constitute a systems audit but, hopefully, gives an idea of the type of activities across studies that would be audited.

Process audits, on the other hand, have specifically been addressed in the revised 1997 GLPs, and these are basically aimed at auditing short-term studies of a repetitive nature, generally undertaken by similar teams of people. Here, that the system is working and that parts of the process are reviewed over a quoted period in the QA SOP are assured. The aim is to ensure that all critical aspects of this process are reviewed through different studies over a period of time. This, then, does not necessitate QA review of all short-term studies on every occasion, nor does it require the review of such areas as analytical analysis on a batch-by-batch basis or the analysis of hematology or biochemistry samples each time these come up for analysis.

QA itself is required to produce SOPs that clearly detail operation, method of selection of critical phases, and studies and to report its results to the management.

After every audit, a report is produced that is then discussed with the study director and circulated to the management with the overall agreement from the study director relating to the audit findings and their explanation of the resolution. (For an in-depth review of QA, see Principles of GLP, Section II, 2.1–2.2, p. 20.)

Standard Operating Procedures (SOPs)

These generally have been likened to a complete documented history of the entire aspect of conducting nonsafety studies. Any activity needs to be described in one of these documents. There may be a compilation of activities, or they may address single items such as the calibration and use of an electronic balance. They must be produced by the individual most familiar with the task, agreed on by the management, and countersigned by a person senior to the author.

Once produced, SOPs must be reviewed on a regular basis, (approximately every 2 years) and any changes to these procedures must be made in writing, with the agreement of all parties and circulated to each owner or user of the SOP. The SOP itself must be filed in the archive and additional copies produced. An SOP management system must be set up, whereby a responsible person knows the whereabouts of all SOPs and can retrieve and replace them with amended or superseded revisions and can make sure that they are reviewed regularly and disposed of when no longer required.

The SOP must appear immediately in the area adjacent to the workplace to be readily available to all persons. Frequently, SOPs are the basis of training, and most companies now have SOP-based training schemes. The content and receipt of the SOP should be acknowledged immediately on receipt and a training program set up whereby confirmation of the understanding and the ability to perform the duties stated in the SOP is documented in the appropriate training record.

SOPs should be adequately controlled to prevent unauthorized photocopying, which may lead to the possibilities of a superseded copy not being administered to the known recipients. Someone making an illegal photocopy would not be on the distribution list and, therefore, would not always receive updated versions, with the possibility that an outdated method could be used.

The requirement for archiving historical copies is one of the key attributes of GLP in that traceability can be seen as originating at the archive. The dates and historical record of the SOPs can prove irrevocably that a particular action was the method in use at the time.

SOPs can be paper-based or electronic. The trend toward electronic record-keeping is becoming more common in laboratories. The only requirement made by the inspectorate is that accurate, controlled copies are available on the electronic media and that prevention of copying or unauthorized changing are built into the SOP system. (See GLP Principles Section II, 7, p. 24.)

Study Plans and Reports

Before any study can be undertaken satisfactorily, a study plan must be produced. The study plan is merely an indication of all of the activities that will take place, resources required, time frames, and objectives. The study plan can be likened to a road map that, when given to all the participants, will allow them to start at the beginning and to proceed through the various mazes to the final completion point indicated by the study report. The one golden rule in GLP is one study plan, one study director, and one report.

The study report itself is a mirror image of all the headings in the study plan and serves to confirm that the objectives of the study have been met and that the results and discussions of the data presented give an indication of the outcome of the particular experimental work.

Both the study plan and the report are audited by QA, and each study plan and report are generally determined by the company's format.

Typical headings must be given in both documents. (These can be found in Section II, 8.1–8.3, pp. 25–27 and 9.1–9.2, p. 28, of the OECD Principles of GLP.)

Data

Raw data, or source data, are generally considered the first records made, either electronically in computer-readable form, or records created the first time that the "pen hits the paper."

These should be original signed and dated recordings that may be on any type of media. Cases in which media such as heat-sensitive paper contain the result, should be photocopied in the event of deterioration over a time.

Electronic data can be regarded as the disk, CD-ROM, or similar media provided that this material, when reintroduced to the computer and the software, can generate the images stored on the disk or electronic media in a 100% readable form.

There are many types of electronic media, machines, and source data or raw data within the toxicological environment. However, ironically, the most common storage media and the most common raw data are paper.

Paper and its storage partner, microfilm, have been around for many years, and their stability and reproducibility are well known. Other electronic media, however, do not have the same capability of reproduction known over a long period, and, thus, most industries and companies prefer paper.

In regard to the data they should be recorded promptly, legibly, and signed and dated, and any corrections should be made in a format to allow the original record to be seen, the change described and justified where applicable, and the change signed and dated by the individual making the revision. This procedure, whether on paper or via computer, should have the same standards. With use of the computer, an audit trail is necessary to identify the change and the person making it, along with the reason.

Equipment

As can be imagined, equipment in a toxicological study may be varied, simple, or complex. As such, it is difficult to describe each individual type of equipment in this limited space.

GLP requires that equipment be maintained, calibrated, and generally demonstrated as fit for use.

Equipment such as high-pressure liquid chromatography (HPLC) should have system-suitability checks, installation qualifications, and operational qualifications performed at a minimum.

Other equipment such as centrifuges and balances should be maintained and calibrated and, with regard to the latter, regular checks should be made with known, standardized, regularly calibrated weights. These should be placed on the balance with a frequency to guarantee that data from the machine are accurate. Even if the balance is an electronic calibrating balance, regular manual check weights should be applied.

Each piece of equipment should have a log book that gives a historical record of its use, breakdown, repair, and service. Generally, it is acceptable that these log books be placed by the equipment generating critical data to be presented in the final report.

All equipment should be clearly identified as to the time that it started producing raw data for experimental use and, when no longer required, the equipment should be removed from the laboratory or suitably labeled "not for GLP use."

The calibration and validation of equipment have been addressed extensively but, equipment that can be shown as "fit for use," within the GLP environment is generally acceptable to most regulatory inspectors. (For additional information on the GLP requirements for equipment, see Principles, Section II, 4, p. 22.)

Computers

Over the past few years, computers have played a very important role in many aspects of toxicology. The general trend in the industry and particularly from the Inspectorate is to ensure that they are fully validated.

Validation, however, means different things to different people. Some companies and their Information Technology Group (ITG) will dismantle the computer and its software components, reconfigure them, test them, and then reinstall them. Others will take a more realistic approach and work on the basis that the computer was brought in for a specific task and, is considered validated provided that task is completed with the aid of the computer in a reproducible and acceptable manner.

However, in the most simplistic form, validation could be covered by "evidence that the computer will perform the task for which it was purchased and, more importantly, continue to perform that task for the foreseeable future." In other words, as with other equipment, is the computer fit for purpose?

Several documents have been written from a regulatory standpoint, the most useful being Monograph 10 of the OECD Principles, *Application of GLP to Computer Systems* (39). Many books are available and vary in detail and content to cover everything that one would wish to know about computers, but were afraid to ask, down to the simple documentation giving the essentials for validation and providing a disk with the SOPs to comply with GLP! Several examples are listed in the References (40–42).

The prime concern of the Inspectorate is that the user responsible for performing the validation and producing the report is in control of the equipment and can ensure and prove the integrity of the data when entered into the computer and regenerated in some other form.

It is generally accepted in the industry that acceptance testing is perfectly satisfactory for most computers and assures that the computer, when installed on company premises, will perform the function for which it was purchased. However, each computer must be viewed in the role it will play in the company and suitable testing must be conducted to ensure that the data and integrity are of the highest quality and that total control over output is maintained.

As with all equipment, computer maintenance and calibration records are of paramount importance. If in-house software programs are produced, they are tested and validated, and the source code is made available. One of the key elements required in the computer record-keeping is that of change control and password protection and training. (See GLP Principles Section II, 7(b), p. 25.)

One very important rule is that *the electronic signatures rule* (43), and it must be observed when data are signed off electronically. This FDA requirement became effective August 20th, 1997, and covers all data for which signatures are made electronically and requires that the FDA is officially notified.

Test Systems

This really is a slightly complex name for what is generally considered the animal subject. Test system, however, has been utilized because in many instances in toxicology, GLP now applies to such subjects as ground water, soil, insects such as earthworms and honey bees, and microorganisms such as daphnia and, therefore, the use of the word *animal* is not always applicable.

The main criteria are that the origin of the test system is known with its breeding history, where applicable, that these are purchased from well-known and, if possible, accredited suppliers, and that the quarantine period is observed to ensure that test systems are of high quality and fit for use.

Care, husbandry, intermediate sacrifice if the test system is found to be "in extremis," and humane sacrifice before necropsy are essentials for the test system. Separate housing among species and experimentation is critical, and all aspects of manipulation of the animal from clinical observations, dosing, and special tests such as electro-cardiogram (ECG) need to be well documented and outlined in SOPs.

Animal husbandry itself, the animal room, and the animal room diary giving an indication of exactly what occurred in the room and to the animal are essential items of documentation. Unique identification is also of paramount importance with the animals, cages, and the location of the cages.

Full and documented history of heating and ventilation are required and, in barrier-maintained rooms, signed and dated records of positive to negative pressures are to be kept. These records should also reference any malfunction and its rectification. Furthermore, *excursions outside the permitted range* must be documented, and the effect on the study and data integrity must be identified and addressed by the study director in the final report. (Additional information is available in the GLP Principles, Section, II, 3.2, p. 21.)

Test Substance

In most instances, the test substance can be the new chemical entity (NCE) or an existing product; a comparator, pharmaceutical, veterinary, or agrochemical product; or even a device. Knowledge of the composition, characterization, stability, and other physiochemical properties is essential. Stability, however, may be determined as the short-term studies progress, with the proviso that the overall stability is known, along with full characterization, by the time long-term toxicity studies are carried out. Stability testing may well be carried out in parallel as long as the stability of the active ingredient and formulated product is known sufficiently to allow for control of the dosing to be done within the period of stability known at that time.

One of the key elements of test substance control is accountability. A record of the amount received for toxicity testing should be accurately recorded, and 100% accountability of that product throughout the life of the testing is an essential element of GLP.

Again, formulation of the product is required to be covered in detail, and, in many companies, the elements of GLP are the benchmark standards when dealing with test substance. Use of the test substance in the animal facility, the maintenance of homogenity of suspensions, the mixing of the product in feed, and the testing of the product are all essential. This is one particular area in which within the toxicology testing area, support functions such as analytical studies then come under GLP. These functions will be required to test formulations and feedstuffs, etc. to ensure that the correct amount of the active ingredient is present as determined by the study plan for the various dosing groups. This requires that a validated method be available before any work is carried out, with the ability to analyze samples of the formulated product or plasma samples for toxicokinetics as the study progresses.

It is required that a reserve or retention sample of the active ingredient is retained. This should be retained for as long as it affords reasonable testing and within the expiry period determined by the analytical facility. It is also required that a retention sample be retained for studies that are not considered to be short term. This is one particular area in which revision of the GLPs is sometime not well-thought through. Originally, it had been stated that reserve samples should be taken for studies exceeding 4 weeks. This was subsequently revised to specify "studies that are not considered to be short-term." The glossary in the GLPs defines a short-term study as "a study of short duration with repetitive processes." This, one must admit, does not give a lot of guidance!

(See additional information on systems in GLP Section II, 3.3, p. 21 and 6.1–6.2, p. 23.)

Archives

Having addressed all the various aspects of the study, one can see that much documentation, tissues, slides, and wax blocks could well be accumulating. The requirement is to store this material for "a period of time." Again, very little guidance is given in the GLP, and one is referred to the national guidelines for the storage of data. However, it is of great importance that this material is maintained in good condition in a retrievable format for at least 15 years for or 2 years past the availability of "the product," whichever is longer.

Generally, companies themselves are maintaining that material for far longer, or for 2 years past the availability of the product.

All the material must be retained in a secure location for easy access, under the responsibility of a management-designated archivist and deputy. The security aspect of the archive should preclude damage from outside sources, fire, water, rodents, etc.

The entire aspect of archiving is basically one of common sense, and guidance on how to archive these materials can be obtained from government agencies that store personnel records or from libraries. [Additional information on archiving is available in GLPs under Section II, 3.4, p. 22 and 10, p. 29 and in the British Standard for Archiving (44).]

HOW CAN COMPLIANCE BE MAINTAINED WITHIN A FACILITY?

Compliance, having been granted after an inspection, should be monitored on a daily basis. However, it is the author's opinion that many companies standards of compliance relax after the initial certificate has been granted only to find that, 2 years later, for example, an enormous rush 1 month before an announced inspection is required to generate the appropriate documentation and to update the system. It is suggested that QC reviews be carried out on a regular basis to ensure that points likely to detract from the overall compliance are reviewed regularly and that project meetings be held where QA is invited to give a précis of the regular points seen during audits so that these can be addressed and rationalized.

Training and retraining, along with an awareness of the requirement to comply with GLP, are of immense importance. New equipment, major SOP revisions, and transfer of technicians or scientists among departments are always good signs that additional training be carried out. It must be remembered that GLP is team work. It is no good considering that there are the scientists and technicians on the one hand and, QA on the other. There is also no point in considering that whatever

happens and however little QC is carried out, QA will discover all the mistakes in the final report and review. Remember, it is not QA's problem; that department's role is to ensure that compliance has been maintained; QC and data-checking are the responsibilities of every member of the staff team.

Improvement targets should be set in line with quality-control manuals used in other accreditation systems. It is always a good point to review internally and on a regular basis: 1) problems that have been encountered in experimentation; 2) audit findings; 3) ways to improve work by looking at new systems and reviewing SOPs to ensure that these are current; and 4) and areas where improvements can be made.

An example can be taken from the accreditation systems (45), in which, in addition to QA audits, departments become involved in self-inspection. Each department can identify a QA representative whose daily responsibility is to review compliance issues, to look at the overall quality policy of the company, and to ensure that between QA audits, self-inspection is performed and that a departmental review is made of these findings with action points and a time plan identified.

The primary impetus for the maintenance of compliance, however, is the regular external inspection by the Inspectorate. In addition, it is now becoming frequent for independent consultants to be brought in to do preregulatory inspections. Whichever way one views the system, whether through consultation or by assigning a department to perform inspections in one area and to conduct audits in another, the regular review of compliance should be maintained.

When using CROs, the whole aspect of auditing takes on a different light. Here, subcontracting is usually performed because of internal pressures, shortage of space, or lack of in-house expertise. Dealing with CROs is no different than setting up an in-house GLP system. The CRO should be regarded as an extension of the facility in which the sponsor is conducting its own research.

PITFALLS AND BENEFITS

In conclusion, it is worthwhile to address the pitfalls and benefits of operating according to the principles of GLP.

A pitfall could be seen as a restriction on the scientist against performing free research. It could also be seen as an intrusion by an independent body looking at why problems occur and at the sorts of problems that occur and carrying out regular reviews with senior management about these problems. Costs will increase because of time pressures and the necessity of involving third-party reviews. The recording of data will now be subject to more QC, more required approvals, extra costs, and, generally, more data presented. Time must be taken to write and review SOPs. This in itself can be a very costly exercise; the author knows of one company that, having spent more than 6 months writing its SOPs, classed them as capital pieces of equipment and put a value of $5500 on that volume.

Other companies and personnel may encounter similar pitfalls. The list is not intended to be exhaustive but merely to indicate areas in which additional time, money, and resources will be allocated. However, on the positive side, benefits can be seen immediately.

In talking to many people who have operated under the GLP system for the past 20 years, it is generally heard that the system allows for a better standard of research, less repeated work, the ability to have full accountability and traceability of everything within the experimental phase, and the knowledge that all documentation produced at the end of the study is now safe and secure in the archive and can be readily accessed for regulatory review or inspection.

Fewer studies are being repeated, and, therefore, the immediate benefit is the lowering of subject usage.

The fact that data, when generated with a certificate or a compliance statement, will now be accepted by all OECD member countries means that once the study is completed and the regulatory submission made, the time for acceptance several countries (if submissions are made in a multistate procedure) will be reduced dramatically.

Finally, it is considered that the initial bureaucratic straitjacket of GLP when thrust on the international research community in 1976 has rapidly turned full circle and now is seen as the quality standard to which all companies in all countries want to aspire.

From that point of view, all nonclinical safety studies, when conducted according to the principles of GLP and adequately addressing science as well as compliance, can achieve a very high success rate both in the outcome of the science and in the acceptance of data for a regulatory submission.

REFERENCES

1. U.S. Food and Drug Administration (FDA), Nonclinical Laboratory Studies. Proposed Regulations for Good Laboratory Practice Regulations. Proposed Rule, Federal Register, 1976; 41, 51206–51228.
2. U.S. Food and Drug Administration (FDA), Nonclinical Laboratory Studies. Good Laboratory Practice Regulations. Final Rule, Federal Register, 1978; 43, 59986–60020.
3. U.S. Food and Drug Administration (FDA), Good Laboratory Practice for Nonclinical Laboratory Studies: Amendment of Good Laboratory Practice Regulations. Amendment, Federal Register, 1980; 45, 24865.
4. U.S. Food and Drug Administration (FDA), Good Laboratory Practice Regulations. Proposed Rule, Federal Register, 1984; 49, 43530–43537.
5. U.S. Food and Drug Administration (FDA), Good Laboratory Practice Regulations. Final Rule, Federal Register, 1987; 52, 33768–33782.
6. U.S. Food and Drug Administration (FDA), Good Laboratory Practice Regulations. Minor Amendments. Final Rule, Federal Register, 1989; 54, 15923–15924.
7. U.S. Food and Drug Administration (FDA), Good Laboratory Practice Regulations. Removal of Examples of Methods of Animal Identification. Final Rule, Federal Register, 1991; 56, 32088.
8. U.S. Food and Drug Administration (FDA), Good Laboratory Practice Regulations. Technical Amendment, Federal Register, 1994; 59, 13200.
9. OECD Series on Principles of Good Laboratory Practice and Compliance Monitoring, ENV/MC/CHEM (98)17, As revised in 1997. http://www.oecd.org.ehs/ehsmono.
10. Dent, N.J. Comparison Between the Principles of GLP 1992 as Defined in Monograph 45 and the Draft Revision of the Principles of GLP As Published by OECD on 6th January 1997. Qual. Assurance J. **1997**, *2*, 7–12.
11. Dent, N.J. European Regulatory Compliance Issues: Good Research Practices. J. Am. Coll. Toxicol. **1994**, *13* (1), 79–85.
12. *OECD Guidelines for the Testing of Chemicals*; OECD: Paris, 1993.
13. Directives EEC/87/18, EEC/9, EEC/88/320. Official J. European Commun. **1992**.
14. U.S. Food and Drug Administration, Good Laboratory Practice for Nonclinical Laboratory Studies: Title 21, Part 58, Code of Federal Regulations, FDA, 1993.
15. U.S. Environmental Protection Agency (EPA), Pesticide Programs: Good Laboratory Practice Standards. Final Rule, Federal Register, 1993; 48, 53946–53969.
16. U.S. Environmental Protection Agency (EPA), Toxic Substance Control: Good Laboratory Practice Standards. Final Rule, Federal Register, 1993; 48, 53922–53944.
17. U.S. Environmental Protection Agency (EPA), Toxic Substance Control Act (TSCA): Good Laboratory Practice Standards. Final Rule, Federal Register, 1989; 54, 34034–34050.
18. U.S. Environmental Protection Agency (EPA), Federal Insecticide, Fungicide and Rodenticide Act (FIFRA): Good Laboratory Practice Standards. Final Rule, Federal Register, 1989; 54, 34052–34074.
19. Good Laboratory Practice Standards (FIFRA), EPA. Federal Register 1993; Title 40, Part 160, Code of Federal Regulations, Final Rule revised as of July 1.
20. Good Laboratory Practice Standards (TSCA), EPA. Federal Register 1993, Title 40, Part 792, Code of Federal Regulations, Final Rule revised as of July 1.
21. Shillam, K.W. GLP Legislation 16-29. *Good Laboratory and Clinical Practices: Techniques for the QA Professional*; Carson, P.A., Dent, N.J., Eds.; GLP Regulations Management Briefings—Post Conference Report. U.S. Food and Drug Administration: Rockville, MA, 1979.

22. Lepore, P.D. Overall Responsibilities for GLP 29-39. *Good Laboratory and Clinical Practices: Techniques for the QA Professional*; Carson, P.A., Dent, N.J., Eds.

23. Lepore, P.D. *Good Laboratory Practice Regulations: Questions and Answers*; Available through FDA FOI, FDA, (HFI-35): Rockville, MA, 1979.

24. Lepore, P.D. *Good Laboratory Practice Regulations: Questions and Answers*; Available through FDA FOI, FDA, (HFI-35): Rockville, MA, 1981.

25. Broad, R.D.; Dent, N.J. An Introduction to Good Laboratory Practice 3–16. *Good Laboratory and Clinical Practices: Techniques for the QA Professional*; Carson, P.A., Dent, N.J., Eds.

26. Commission Directive 1999/11/EC of 8th March 1999. Official J. European Commun. **1999**, L77/8 23.03.99.

27. Commission Directive 1999/12/EC of 8th March 1999. Official J. European Commun. **1999**, L77/8 23.03.99.

28. Good Laboratory Practice Regulations 1999. Statutory Instrument 1999 No. 3106. http://www.hmso.go.uk/si/si1999/19993106.htm.

29. Dominated by the Urge to Merge. Scrip Magazine **January 1999**, *46*.

30. A Strategic Approach to R&D Outsourcing. Scrip Magazine **July/August 1999**, *29*.

31. R&D Trends Gives Clues to Future. Scrip Magazine **July/August 1999**, *17*.

32. How Much of a Threat is Virtual Pharma? Scrip Magazine **November 1999**, *41*.

33. The Right Treatment for the Right Patient. Scrip Magazine **January 2000**, *11*.

34. OECD Glossary. OECD Series on Principles of Good Laboratory Practice and Compliance Monitoring. ENV/MC/CHEM(98)17. As revised in 1997. http://www.oecd.org.chs/ehsmono.

35. Dent, N.J. Forget Compliance and Concentrate on Science. Qual. Assurance J. **1998**, *3*, 103–108.

36. Personal Communication from OECD.

37. Personal Communication from OECD.

38. Personal Communication from OECD.

39. OECD GLP Consensus Document on the Application of the Principles of GLP to Computerised Systems. Environment Monograph (10), 116, OECD Series on Principles of Good Laboratory Practice and Compliance Monitoring. ENV/MC/CHEM(98)17. As revised in 1997. http://www.oecd.org.ehs/ehsmono.

40. *Computerized Data Systems for Non-Clinical Safety Assessment-Current Concepts and QA*; The Drug Information Association: Maple Glen, PA.

41. Double, M.E.; McKendry, M. *Computer Validation Compliance—A QA Perspective*; Interpharm Press: Buffalo Grove, IL.

42. Chamberlain, R. *Computer Systems Validation for Pharmaceutical and Medical Device Industries*; Interpharm Press: Buffalo Grove, IL.

43. U.S. Food and Drug Administration, Electronic Records; Electronic Signatures; Final Rule, Federal Register, 1997; 62, 13429–13466.

44. Lawrence, R.G. Archives 155-171. *Good Laboratory and Clinical Practices: Techniques for the QA Professional*; Carson, P.A., Dent, N.J., Eds.; 155–171.

45. Piton, A. Quality Assurance: The Present and Future Role of International Standardization. *Implementing International Good Practices—GAPs, GCPs, GLPs, GMPs*; Dent, N.J., Ed.; 251–265.

46. Kracht, W.R. Implementing the ISO 9000 Quality Standards in a GMP or GLP Environment. *Implementing International Good Practices—GAPs, GCPs, GLPs, GMPs*; Dent, N.J., Ed.; 267–277.

BIBLIOGRAPHY

Carson, P.A., Dent, N.J., Eds.; *Good Laboratory and Clinical Practices—Techniques for the Quality Assurance Professional*; Butterworth.

Compliance Programme Manual. http://www.fda.gov.ora.cpgm.default.htm.

Dent, N.J. *Implementing International Good Practices—GAPs, GCPs, GLPs, GMPs*; Interpharm Press Inc.: Buffalo Grove, IL USA, 1993.

EPA Homepage. http://www.epa.gov.

EuropeanQuality. http://www.euroqual.org.

GALPs.http://www.epa.gov/doc/irm_galp.

GLPRegulations Questions and Answers. http://www.fda.gov/cder/guidance/index.htm.

Good Research Practices—A Practical Guide to the Implementation of the GXPs.

GoodLaboratory Practice on Line. http://www.glpguru.com.

International Organization for Standardization. http://www.iso.ch.

OECDHomepage. http://www.oecd.org.

Title 21 Code of Federal Regulations Part 58. http://www.access.gpo.gov/nara/cfr/index.html.

U.S.Federal Register–Environmental Issues. http://www.epa.gov.fedrgstr.

GOOD MANUFACTURING PRACTICES (GMP)—AN OVERVIEW[a]

G

Ira R. Berry

Duramed Pharmaceuticals, Inc., Somerset, New Jersey

INTRODUCTION

The Current Good Manufacturing Practice (cGMP) regulations for finished pharmaceuticals that have been promulgated by the U.S. Food and Drug Administration (FDA) have been a subject of active discussion since they were first published with the passage of the Kefauver–Harris Drug Amendments in 1962 (1, 2). GMPs were intended to establish minimum manufacturing and control practices for the pharmaceutical industry and focus on what needed to be done rather than how it should be done. Failure to comply with the current Good Manufacturing Practice regulations as set forth in the "Code of Federal Regulations," 21 CFR Parts 210 and 211 (3), constitutes adulteration of a drug that is entered into interstate commerce and is therefore subject to regulatory action. These requirements apply to human and animal drugs. The regulations in Part 210 are introductory in nature; Part 211 contains the more detailed and descriptive regulations and which will be discussed in this chapter.

In the late 1970s, the FDA organized a task force to study the GMPs. Revised GMPs were published in September 1978, and became official in March 1979. At that time, the FDA also considered establishing more specific GMP regulations for products such as small-volume parenterals, medicinal gases and drug substances, to supplement the existing umbrella regulations.

Today, separate GMPs are in effect for biologics and foods but have not yet been promulgated for small-volume parenterals, medicinal gases or drug substances. In attempting to create regulations for specific products, the FDA concluded that it would be better to first issue guidances and guidelines rather than to revise regulations. Thus, what is put forth in 21 CFR Part 211 is supplemented with a number of guidances, guidelines and Compliance Policy Guides (4–11). There remain some differences, however, between guidances and guidelines from the Center for Biologics Evaluation and Research (CBER), the Center for Drug Evaluation and Research (CDER), and the Compliance Policy Guides, sometimes leaving a firm's

cGMP status subject to the interpretation of a field investigator.

Based on the amount of time needed to promulgate a revision of the regulations, it is understandable that it is preferable to work with guidances, guidelines, and compliance policy guides. Current GMPs are supposed to be, as their title indicates, a description of the current manufacturing and control practices that are acceptable for a pharmaceutical company selling products in the United States. Although these cGMPs are not enforced in some foreign countries, an FDA inspection in a foreign country, based on current GMPs, can be the key to importing and marketing a product in the United States.

The FDA is required to inspect a firm every 2 years for compliance to cGMPs. With the advent of programs such as the new drug preapproval inspection program implemented in 1990, inspections may be more frequent and have expanded into areas not previously investigated regularly by the FDA, such as clinical manufacturing. An unsatisfactory inspection can delay approval of new products and lead to further regulatory action by the FDA, such as seizure and injunction, for existing products. The penalties can apply to the individual or both the firm and individuals.

The GMPs as set forth in 21 CFR Part 211 also have been applied to drug substances and clinical products. Guidelines and guidances have been issued to describe the FDA interpretation of 21 CFR Part 211 pertaining to drug substances and the production of investigational drugs and reinforce the agency's understanding that cGMPs are applicable (12, 13). The FDA has reinforced the connection between registration of drugs and the manufacture of active pharmaceutical ingredients by the issuance of guides to industry (14–16). Recently, the FDA has issued for comment a draft guidance for "Good Manufacturing Practice for the Manufacturing, Processing, and Holding of an Active Pharmaceutical Ingredient" (17). Finalization of these draft cGMP principles is being written into a guideline that is being coordinated through the International Conference on Harmonization of Technical Requirements for the Registration of Pharmaceuticals for Human Use (ICH) toward publication of a guidance for active pharmaceutical ingredients that will be standardized

---

[a]Revised from Ref. 1.

and followed by manufacturers in the United States, Europe, and Japan (18). As a sidenote, active pharmaceutical ingredients have also been called drug substances and bulk pharmaceutical chemicals.

The "Status of Current Good Manufacturing Practice Regulations for Finished Pharmaceuticals" is as follows:

Section 210.1(a) The regulations set forth in this part and in parts 211 through 226 of this chapter contain the minimum current good manufacturing practice for methods to be used in, and the facilities or controls to be used for, the manufacture, processing, packing, or holding of a drug to assure that such drug meets the requirements of the act as to safety, and has the identity and strength and meets the quality and purity characteristics that it purports or is represented to possess.

(b) The failure to comply with any regulation set forth in this part and in parts 211 through 226 of this chapter in the manufacture, processing, packing, or holding of a drug shall render such drug to be adulterated under section 501(a)(2)(B) of the act and such drug, as well as the person who is responsible for the failure to comply, shall be subject to regulatory action.

The "Applicability of Current Good Manufacturing Practice Regulations for Finished Pharmaceuticals" is as follows:

Section 210.2(a) The regulations in this part and in parts 211 through 226 of this chapter as they may pertain to a drug and in parts 600 through 680 of this chapter as they may pertain to a biological product for human use, shall be considered to supplement, not supersede, each other, unless the regulations explicitly provide otherwise. In the event that it is impossible to comply with all applicable regulations in these parts, the regulations specifically applicable to the drug in question shall supersede the more general.

(b) If a person engages in only some operations subject to the regulations in this part and in parts 211 through 226 and parts 600 through 680 of this chapter, and not in others, that person need only comply with those regulations applicable to the operations in which he or she is engaged.

This article reviews Part 211, Current Good Manufacturing Practice for Finished Pharmaceuticals. Title 21, Parts 600 through 680 for biological products, supplement but do not supersede the regulations in this part, unless the regulations explicitly provide otherwise. The focus of Good Manufacturing Practice for all products is on a quality control unit that has the responsibility and authority to approve or reject all components, drug product containers, closures, in-process materials, finished product, and production and control documentation. "Quality Control Unit" refers to any person or organizational element designated by the firm to be responsible for the duties relating to quality control. Specific subparts of Part 211 are summarized and described later.

This article is not intended to reproduce the complete GMPs, but certain parts are excerpted for emphasis.

SUBPART A: GENERAL PROVISIONS

This subpart reinforces Part 210, which is an introduction to the more detailed and specific practices described in Part 211. It establishes the scope of GMP and carries forth the definition of terms in Part 210.

SUBPART B: ORGANIZATION AND PERSONNEL

Section 211.22: Responsibilities of Quality Control Unit

(a) There shall be a quality control unit that shall have the responsibility and authority to approve or reject all components, drug product containers, closures, in-process materials, packaging material, labeling, and drug products, and the authority to review production records to assure that no errors have occurred or, if errors have occurred, that they have been fully investigated. The quality control unit shall be responsible for approving or rejecting drug products manufactured, processed, packed, or held under contract by another company.

(b) Adequate laboratory facilities for the testing and approval (or rejection) of components, drug product containers, closures, packaging materials, in-process materials, and drug products shall be available to the quality control unit.

(c) The quality control unit shall have the responsibility for approving or rejecting all procedures or specifications impacting on the identity, strength, quality, and purity of the drug product.

(d) The responsibilities and procedures applicable to the quality control unit shall be in writing; such written procedures shall be followed.

The intent of this subpart is to ensure that there is a group within the organization that can review and judge the acceptability of procedures used to produce pharmaceutical products on an independent basis, as well as judging the products themselves, before they are entered into interstate commerce. The FDA has emphasized separation of the quality control unit from production (organizationally). In addition, the FDA considers the organizational level to which the quality control unit reports very important.

From a legal perspective, the chief executive officer (CEO) or president of a firm is considered the most responsible official and thereby becomes the most liable. Therefore, he is subject to criminal prosecution should the organization be found to violate the Food, Drug and Cosmetic (FDC) Act. One of the most serious infractions is fraud, that is, the intent to mislead the FDA. Hence, it is incumbent on the CEO to have well-qualified personnel in the organization and an organizational structure that reinforces quality.

Section 211.25:
Personnel Qualifications

This section emphasizes the training of personnel both in cGMP and in their specific responsibilities with regard to manufacturing, processing, packing or holding of a drug product and functions to provide assurance that the drug product has the safety, identity, strength, quality, and purity that it purports or is represented to possess. This section also requires that there be a sufficient number of qualified personnel.

(a) Each person engaged in the manufacture, processing, packing, or holding of a drug product shall have education, training, and experience, or any combination thereof, to enable that person to perform the assigned functions. Training shall be in the particular operations that the employee performs and in current good manufacturing practice (including the current good manufacturing practice regulations in this chapter and written procedures required by these regulations) as they relate to the employee's functions. Training in current good manufacturing practice shall be conducted by qualified individuals on a continuing basis and with sufficient frequency to assure that employees remain familiar with cGMP requirements applicable to them.

(b) Each person responsible for supervising the manufacture, processing, packing, or holding of a drug product shall have the education, training, and experience, or any combination thereof, to perform assigned functions in such a manner as to provide assurance that the drug product has the safety, identity, strength, quality, and purity that it purports or is represented to possess.

(c) There shall be an adequate number of qualified personnel to perform and supervise the manufacture, processing, packing, or holding of each drug product.

This section makes it clear that the quality control unit is not the only group responsible for the quality of products and conformance with GMP. Because the quality of a product must be "built in," control (at the manufacturing level) of raw materials and process control are important.

SUBPART C:
BUILDINGS AND FACILITIES

This section requires that the buildings and facilities are adequate, provide specifically defined areas for certain operations and are designed to prevent mix-ups. Included are design and construction features; lighting; ventilation, air filtration, air heating and cooling; plumbing; sewage and refuse disposal; washing and toilet facilities; sanitation; and maintenance. Lighting, ventilation, air filtration, and air heating and cooling must be adequate. Again, the word adequate is used frequently. This is where an individual investigator's and firm's interpretations can differ.

This section also requires written procedures associated with sanitation and that the facilities should be maintained in a good state of repair. Although it may seem obvious that maintenance should be performed regularly, it can happen that preventative maintenance programs compete with production requirements for attention; however, an in-depth preventative maintenance program should be in place.

SUBPART D:
EQUIPMENT

This section addresses equipment design, size, and location, as well as construction, cleaning and maintenance. Similar to the requirements for buildings and facilities, it is necessary to provide appropriate equipment for the manufacture of a product and ensure that the equipment material of construction is not reactive, additive, or absorptive. In the 1978 version of the GMPs, requirements for equipment cleaning and use logs, as well as written procedures for equipment cleaning and maintenance were added. These requirements aid in the investigation and solution of problems by identifying batches that may also be implicated in a particular problem.

This section also covers the use of automatic, mechanical, or electronic equipment. Additional information relating to compliance with this section can be found in Compliance Policy Guides 7132a.07 (5), 7132a.08 (6), 7132a.11 (8), 7132a.12 (9), and 7132a.15 (10). Compliance Policy Guide 7132a.15 interprets Section 211.68 (b) as requiring maintenance of the program as part of the validation package for computer systems. Reliance on validated computer systems in place of several manual checks has become widely accepted.

SUBPART E:
CONTROL OF COMPONENTS
AND DRUG PRODUCT CONTAINERS
AND CLOSURES

This section relates to the receipt, identification, storage, handling, sampling, testing, and approval or rejection of components and drug product containers and closures, and the requirements for written procedures for each. It also covers the use of approved materials, retesting of approved material, and prevention of use of rejected materials. Although the requirements of this section indicate that each lot be appropriately identified as to its status and that materials in different statuses be stored separately, the implementation of computerized warehouses has made it possible to eliminate status labels and physical separation of quarantined and approved materials. Rejected materials are usually handled separately. These practices are not to imply that a computerized system can be used without appropriate assurance of controls.

The current GMP requirement that materials must be tested or examined for all specifications and released prior to use is in conflict with the philosophy of vendor certification, which is based on a consistent, reliable record of good quality. Only vendors with well-controlled processes and a good record of acceptable batches qualify for such a program. Thus, a material could be put into use based on the quality record of the supplier (vendor), even if testing is only for identification [211.84(d) (2)].

This section also requires the use of oldest approved stock first, retesting of approved stock "as appropriate," and controls for drug product containers and closures. It prohibits use of rejected components and drug product containers and closures.

SUBPART F:
PRODUCTION AND PROCESS CONTROLS

This section focuses again on the need for written procedures and formal authorization by the quality control unit for any deviation from written procedures. Areas covered are addition of components; calculation of yield; equipment identification; sampling and testing of in-process materials and drug products; time limitations on production; control of microbiological contamination; and reprocessing.

Many drug companies are using electronic means of verifying component names or item codes, receiving and control numbers, weights, or measures, and even the verification of component addition to a batch. There is a range of acceptability on the part of the FDA of electronic means of verification and batch documentation; however, the validation of such systems must be performed to accept electronic means of identification and verification.

The process controls required in this section should be based on process capabilities rather than conforming with a checklist based on the regulations. This would mean that tests not typically used for a particular dosage form may be appropriate, whereas other more commonly used tests may be without any value. This not only depends on the validation of the process but also equipment and process qualification. In addition, the need for microbiological controls can be greatly reduced by knowing whether a product supports microbial growth and whether the environment in the production area is maintained at a sufficiently low bioburden. Clearly, certain products require close attention to the production environment because of the ingredients and the end use.

Many firms use the so-called clean-zone concept, in which the restrictions on personnel entering a production area and the required protective clothing are based on the nature of a product—whether the product is prone to the growth of microbes or whether it is required to be sterile. Even for products not required to be sterile or that are not supportive of microbial growth, this concept controls the production environment through reduction of bioburden.

Reprocessing frequently receives considerable attention from the FDA. Over the years, reprocessing appears to have decreased, not only because of FDA pressures, but also because more products and processes are being validated and better controls are being exercised during production. At times, however, there is the need to reprocess, but it requires authorization of the quality control unit.

For a product covered by a New Drug Application (NDA) or Abbreviated New Drug Application (ANDA), provision for reprocessing must be included in the approved registration document. Although it is not always possible in the filing of an NDA or ANDA to foresee all reasons why a product may need to be reprocessed, a procedure for reprocessing can be evaluated and included in the registration document. If not included in the approved registration document, the regulations require submission of a supplemental application and prior approval in order to market a reprocessed batch.

To some people, batch or lot yield may seem to be more of a business concern rather than a regulatory or technical matter. However, GMPs require that yield tolerances be established and that yields outside of the tolerances be investigated. The need for an investigation is to determine that yields outside of normal limits can be an indication of problems during production that would not be evident with routine testing. A minor deviation may be relatively insignificant and could simply mean that the yield tolerances need to be reevaluated, a procedure that should be followed periodically.

It may seem that the identification of equipment in the processing record is also a superfluous burden. If several pieces of equipment have been shown to be used interchangeably, one might question the reason for this additional documentation; however, when a problem arises, it is necessary to know exactly which equipment was used. It may be possible to trace this back by reviewing equipment cleaning and use logs, but the investigation is simplified by having this information in the batch record. Recording variable batch information concerning the equipment, such as tablet compressing speeds, is also necessary.

SUBPART G:
PACKAGING AND LABELING CONTROLS

This subpart covers one of the aspects of pharmaceutical production that has received much attention because of recalls, including an increase in recalls related to labeling errors or product mix-ups associated with the packaging and labeling operation. Specific requirements identified in this section recently include the following.

Section 211.122:
Materials Examination and Usage Criteria

(f) Use of gang-printed labeling for different drug products, or different strengths or net contents of the same drug product, is prohibited unless the labeling from gang-printed sheets is adequately differentiated by size, shape, or color.

(g) If cut labeling is used, packaging, and labeling operations shall include one of the following special control procedures:

1. Dedication of labeling and packaging lines to each different strength of each different drug product;
2. Use of appropriate electronic or electromechanical equipment to conduct a 100% examination for correct labeling during or after completion of finishing operations; or
3. Use of visual inspection to conduct a 100% examination for correct labeling during or after completion of finishing operations for hand-applied labeling. Such examination shall be performed by one person and independently verified by a second person.

(h) Printing devices on, or associated with, manufacturing lines used to imprint labeling upon the drug product unit label or case shall be monitored to assure that all imprinting conforms to the print specified in the batch production record.

Section 211.125:
Labeling Issuance

Section 211.125 has been amended by revising paragraph (c) to read as follows:

(c) Procedures shall be utilized to reconcile the quantities of labeling issued, used and returned, and shall require evaluation of discrepancies found between the quantity of drug product finished and the quantity of labeling issued when such discrepancies are outside narrow preset limits based on historical operating data. Such discrepancies shall be investigated in accordance with Section 211.192. Label reconciliation is waived for cut or roll labeling if a 100% examination for correct labeling is performed in accordance with Section 211.122(g)(2).

Section 211.130:
Packaging and Labeling Operations

Section 211.130 has been amended by redesignating paragraphs (b), (c), and (d) as paragraphs (c), (d), and (e), respectively, and by adding a new paragraph (b) to read as follows:

(b) Identification and handling of filled drug product containers that are set aside and held in unlabeled condition for future labeling operations to preclude mislabeling of individual containers, lots, or portions of lots. Identification need not be applied to each individual container but shall be sufficient to determine name, strength, quantity of contents, and lot or control number of each container.

These requirements reflect an increased use of electronic means to ensure correct labeling and tight controls on the practice of filling containers that will be labeled at a later date. A time-consuming operation required in the current GMPs is associated with the reconciliation of labels. The recalls and associated investigations demonstrate that unless 100% account-ability can be achieved in the reconciliation process, there will not be an effective means of ensuring correct labeling.

Section 211.132 was revised on February 2, 1989, to describe tamper-resistant packaging and labeling require-ments for over-the-counter (OTC) human drug products. Compliance Policy Guide 7132a.17 (11) was issued in 1992 to describe the standardized tamper-resistant packaging requirements. This section also covers infor-mation concerning requests for packaging and labeling exemptions. It allows changes in packaging and labeling to comply with the requirements for OTC products subject to approved NDAs to be implemented prior to FDA approval as provided for in Section 314.70(c). Manufacturing changes to provide for sealed capsules require prior FDA approval under Section 314.70(b).

Section 211.132 states that none of the requirements for "special packaging" (child-resistant packaging), as defined in Section 310.3 (1) and required under the Poison Prevention Packaging Act of 1970, are affected.

Subpart G also covers drug product inspection and expiration dating. The expiration date that is required in Section 211.137 relates to stability studies performed on the drug product described in 21 CFR 211.166. It requires that expiration dates be related to storage conditions stated on the product labeling.

Furthermore, the programs established are to use stability-indicating methods, under controlled conditions, in the marketed container–closure system and on an adequate number of batches to determine the appropriate expiration date. The FDA has issued guidelines on stability testing which outline in more detail the requirement to establish a stability program to determine and support the expiration date of a product (4a, 4b, 7). A new draft guidance for stability testing was published by the FDA in 1998 (19), and discussions with comments to finalize this guidance are still continuing.

SUBPART H: HOLDING AND DISTRIBUTION

This section covers warehousing and distribution and the procedures required for the quarantine of drug products before release by the quality control unit, storage of drug products under appropriate conditions, procedures to ensure use of the oldest approved stock first, and a system for documenting the distribution of each lot of drug product. This is another area where computerized systems are being used extensively. During inspections, the FDA review includes evaluation of the validation of any computerized systems and controls.

SUBPART I: LABORATORY CONTROLS

This entire section refers to the requirements covering the testing of drug products and their components prior to release for distribution. It also covers stability testing and special testing, including testing for penicillin, if a reasonable possibility exists that a nonpenicillin drug product has been exposed to cross-contamination with penicillin and laboratory animals. Additional information can be found in the Good Laboratory Practices, 21 CFR 58.

Reserve samples arc required to be maintained for active ingredients and drug products. These specific requirements are elucidated in 211.170. The section on reserve samples also requires that a visual inspection of reserve samples of drug products be conducted at least once a year for evidence of deterioration.

Fundamental to the testing requirements is the need for validated methods with established and documented accuracy, sensitivity, specificity, and reproducibility. It is also necessary to have meaningful sampling and testing plans that meet statistical quality control criteria. Judgments made with regard to sampling procedures should be based on the quality of the process control or the reliability of the vendor who supplies a raw material, drug substance, or packaging component.

SUBPART J: RECORDS AND REPORTS

This section details the records and reports required to be maintained for pharmaceutical drug products, their components, and the equipment used in the processing of a drug product. Through these records, the entire history of a batch can be traced. The records cover equipment cleaning and use logs; component, container, closure, and labeling records; master production and control records and production record review; laboratory records; distribution records; and complaint files. Because this amount of recordkeeping can be voluminous, Section 211.180(d) allows for microfilm, microfiche, or other accurate reproductions of the original records for storage. Many firms are using the electronic generation of batch and analytical records. It is important to be able to retrieve all of the above records easily during an FDA inspection. Electronic methods must be supplemented with proper procedures to ensure that the records do not deteriorate over a period of time and can be retrieved when the computer systems used to generate the records have been revised or replaced.

This section also requires a master production and control record for each product, from which the batch production and control records are generated. These records must include complete instructions concerning the manufacture of a batch and precautions to be followed. Prior to the commercial distribution of a drug product into interstate commerce, all executed production and control records must be reviewed. If there is a discrepancy or a failure of any batch or any of its components to meet specifications, there must be an investigation and a written report of the findings. The investigation are to extend to other batches of the same or other drug products that may have been associated with the out of specification batch or discrepancy.

Another part of this section covers complaint files, which are reviewed regularly during FDA inspections. In fact, a complaint file review may be the sole reason for an inspection if the FDA receives a complaint directly from a pharmacist, which may be a cause for concern. Sometimes the FDA will visit a firm to follow up on a complaint, even though the firm may not have been informed by the complainant. In the event that a complaint is received by a firm, it should be evaluated and a response sent to the complainant. It may be necessary also to conduct an investigation and prompt further action regarding the product or batch in the marketplace.

SUBPART K:
RETURNED AND SALVAGED
DRUG PRODUCTS

This section requires that extensive records be maintained on returned drug products including ultimate disposition.

Again, if the reason that a drug product is returned implicates other batches, an investigation is to be conducted in accordance with 211.192. Drug product salvaging is not allowed for drug products that have been subjected to improper storage conditions. If there is a question as to whether drug products have been subjected to such conditions, they may be salvaged only if there is evidence from laboratory tests that all applicable standards of identity, strength, quality, and purity have been met. In addition, evidence is required from the inspection of the premises that the drug products and associated packaging were not subjected to improper storage conditions as a result of a disaster or accident. Understandably, the value of the material to be salvaged is taken into consideration when such rigorous requirements exist for salvaging.

CONCLUSION

Compliance with cGMP requires that responsible employees in a firm be knowledgeable about the practices that other firms follow in order to comply. FDA investigators visit many firms and find a broad picture of current manufacturing and control practices. Thus, Current Good Manufacturing Practices are "state of the art," constantly changing. To be in regulatory compliance, a firm must review their procedures and systems regularly and revise them as necessary.

REFERENCES

1. Vickory, H.; Nally, L. Good Manufacturing Practices: An Overview. *Encyclopedia of Pharmaceutical Technology*; Marcel Dekker, Inc.: New York, 1993; 7, 109–120.

2. Berry, I.R., Nash, R.A., Eds. *Pharmaceutical Process Validation*; Marcel Dekker, Inc.: New York, 1993.

3. *Code of Federal Regulations*; Title 21, Parts 210 and 211, U.S. Government Printing Office: Washington, DC, 1999.

4. *Compliance Policy Guides*, Requirements for Expiration Dating and Stability Testing (1995). 7132a.04.

5. *Compliance Policy Guides*; Computerized Drug Processing; Input/Output Checking, 1987; 7132a.07.

6. *Compliance Policy Guides*; Computerized Drug Processing; Identification of "Persons" on Batch Production and Control Records, 1987; 7132a.08.

7. *Compliance Policy Guides*; Lack of Expiration Date or Stability Data, 1995; 7132a.10.

8. *Compliance Policy Guides*; Computerized Drug Processing; CGMP Applicability to Hardware and Software, 1987; 7132a.11.

9. *Compliance Policy Guides*; Computerized Drug Processing; Vendor Responsibility, 1987; 7132a.12.

10. *Compliance Policy Guides*; Computerized Drug Processing; Source Code for Process Control Application Programs, 1987; 7132a.15.

11. Tamper-Resistant Packaging Requirements for Certain Over-the-Counter (OTC) Human Drug Products. 1992, 7132a.17.

12. Berry, I.R.; Harpaz, D., Eds.; *Validation of Bulk Pharmaceutical Chemicals*, 1st Ed.; Interpharm Press: Buffalo Grove, IL, 1997.

13. Berry, I.R.;, Harpaz, D. Eds.; *Validation of Active Pharmaceutical Ingredients*, 2nd Ed.; Interpharm Press: Englewood, CO, 2000.

14. *Guide to Inspections of Bulk Pharmaceutical Chemicals*; U.S. Government Printing Office: Washington, DC, 1991.

15. *Guide to Inspections of Sterile Drug Substance Manufacturers*; U.S. Government Printing Office: Washington, DC, 1994.

16. *Guide to Inspections of Foreign Pharmaceutical Manufacturers*; U.S. Government Printing Office: Washington, DC, 1996.

17. *Guidance for Industry: Manufacturing, Processing, or Holding Active Pharmaceutical Ingredients*; U.S. Department of Health and Human Services: Rockville, MD, 1998.

18. ICH Good Manufacturing Practice Guide for Active Pharmaceutical Ingredients Draft, International Conference on Harmonization of Technical Requirements for the Registration of Pharmaceuticals for Human Use, London, UK, 2000.

19. Stability Testing of Drug Substances and Drug Products. *Compliance Policy Guides*; Draft Guidance U.S. Department of Health and Human Services: Rockville, MD, 1998.

HARMONIZATION OF PHARMACOPEIAL STANDARDS

Lee T. Grady
Jerome A. Halperin
United States Pharmacopeia, Rockville, Maryland

INTRODUCTION

The USP and NF[a] standards of strength, quality, purity, and packaging and labeling are recognized by the U.S. Federal Food, Drug, and Cosmetic Act and Amendments since 1906. These requirements are enforced by the Food and Drug Administration (FDA), a party in the harmonization of requirements for drugs.

Although originally founded as an organization to standardize medicines in the United States, the USP and its products and services are now known and utilized throughout the world. In today's transitional and global economy for pharmaceuticals, the USP has a strong international presence and influence. Economic forces are driving major trading parties to affiliate to reduce trade barriers. Integral to this process is harmonization of requirements, regulations, and standards governing the approval and marketing of drugs, devices, etc., by governments. The mission of the USP is to promote the public health through establishing and disseminating legally recognized standards of quality and information for the use of medicines and related articles by health care professionals, patients, and consumers.

This mission is not limited to the United States. Almost from its beginning in 1820, the USP has been aware of and part of international initiatives affecting pharmacopeial standards and their use by governments and professional organizations to control drug quality. That early commitment to internationalism has now grown to formal, on-going projects of harmonization with the pharmacopeias of Europe and Japan and agreements with pharmacopeias of Argentina, Brazil, and Mexico. International programs in drug information exist with a number of multinational organizations, foreign governments, and professional groups.

Harmonization is wanted strongly for the role of pharmacopeias in product registration exercises. That is, product development can proceed as is, without the later repeating of studies or testing to support registration in other than the original region. The primary beneficiaries, thus, are international companies. But harmonization has an independent value in facilitating international commerce in existing products, especially excipients.

Globalization

Twenty years ago, the vast majority of all drug substances and finished dosage forms used in the United States were prepared in the United States. For various reasons before globalization, the United States lost synthetic chemical operations due to stringent environmental requirements. Also, some manufacturing was lost because of inducements of low taxes by other governments to pharmaceutical manufacturers to relocate to their countries. Neither of these factors is the same as globalization. Globalization may be the single most important, historical *worldwide* trend at this time. The entire structure of international commerce and the allocation of capital and expertise are features of globalization. In this regard, the pharmaceutical industry is not particularly different from any other industry. Today's development of drugs or biological products may occur in the United States, Europe, or a combination of nations, and no one nation can be pointed to as to the innovator of a particular drug. Also, international companies would prefer to market the minimum number of formulations worldwide. But product registration of formulations is a very complex area, and the pharmacopoeias are one evidence of the fact that different formulations may require different test methods. The end point of harmonization must be monographs that are acceptable to the registration authorities in different regions. Differences in pharmacopeial standards could be seized upon to create technical barriers to trade.

---

[a]Throughout this article, the abbreviation USP, when used alone, signifies the United States Pharmacopeial Convention, Inc. The abbreviation *USP* in italics and followed by Roman numerals signifies a particular revision of the *United States Pharmacopeia*. The abbreviation USP–NF signifies the *United States Pharmacopeia–National Formulary*, two books in a single binding.

Table 1   List of Interpharmacopeial Open Conferences

Conference	Location	Date
Joint Pharmacopeial Open Conference on International Harmonization of Excipient Standards	Orlando, Florida, U.S.A.	January to February 1991
Interpharmacopeial Open Conference on Harmonization of Biotechnology-derived Products Standards	Verona, Italy	April 1993
Second Joint Pharmacopeial Open Conference on International Harmonization of Excipient Standards	St. Petersburg, Florida, U.S.A.	January to February 1994
Joint Pharmacopeial Open Conference on Sterility/Preservatives	Barcelona, Spain	February 1996
International Harmonization—General Monographs on Dosage Forms and Pharmacotechnological Test Methods	Seville, Spain	October 1998

Alternative Methods

The three regional pharmacopeias—the *USP*, the *European Pharmacopoeia (EP)*, and the *Japanese Pharmacopoeia (J)* allow an individual laboratory, able to do the official method, to validate an alternative method of analysis. The latter is chosen usually for speed, convenience, or economy but also to incorporate an existing database when a new or revised pharmacopeial method is adopted. Under those provisions, a laboratory can validate a method from another pharmacopeia, thereby avoiding duplication of routine work. In all three cases, only the official method could be used in compliance or contest. One point of harmonization is to avoid even the more remote instances of duplicative testing, in addition to international product registration.

There should be support at both the national and international community levels for pharmacopeial harmonization. There should be support both for harmonization of excipients and for harmonization of common general tests and assays. In doing so, one should prefer meaningful standards, not the lowest common denominator or the most stringent. Complicating the International Conference on Harmonization 1 was the attempt to be entirely consistent with the concept of forward harmonization.

Major support for pharmacopeial harmonization would come from increased cooperation and contribution to pharmacopeias on all the nonharmonization work. Harmonization takes away scarce resources from pharmacopeias, and there are other constituencies of the pharmacopoeias to be served. This is an obvious consequence of the fact that pharmacopeial standards apply to products already in the marketplace, both brand name and generic.

Harmonization has three essential values. The first is the facilitation of international commerce. The second is the facilitation of product registration processes in multiple nations. The third is to reduce duplicative testing costs. The facilitation of registration is for any new molecular entity—a onetime event for each country; whereas for the facilitation of international commerce and reduction, the duplicative testing remains throughout the lifetime of the product.

Pharmacopeial harmonization is challenging. The fact is that differences exist because of the different histories of the pharmacopeias. There are many factors. The most obvious are: content, language, legalities, speed, and the audiences for the standards. The *USP* applies also to the practice of pharmacy, both in a community pharmacy and hospital, and, thus, the standards set are appropriate to those environments.

There is an obverse to harmony and that is disharmony. An example of disharmony is the need to repeat tests using rabbits for pyrogen where testing for bacterial endotoxin is otherwise prescribed. This represents the most extreme disharmony of methods. But there is a greater disharmony; i.e., reaching different conclusions whether to pass/fail the specimen. In this case, the quality control professionals must make a judgment whether or not this material can be sold in one or more regions. Functionally equivalent to harmonization is the absence of disharmony. Because of a difference in policy, pharmacopeias may differ on adoption of a test. If certain tests are considered necessary by one pharmacopeia in order to protect the consumer, then it is appropriate for that pharmacopeia to adopt the test without reference to any other region.

Reference Standards

Most discussions of harmonization revolve around excipients or general tests and assays. But the performance of even a harmonized method using different reference standards is not an optimal situation. In fact, harmonization of reference standards preceded many of the harmonization efforts of the last 10 years. Pharmacopeias and the World Health Organization (WHO) have, in the past, shared bulk materials to create their individual reference standards. Where a drug exists as a highly purified crystal, then the difference in pharmacopeial reference standards is administrative and legal in that no difference in results in laboratories is to be seen. This is not the case with mixtures, such as an antibiotic reference standard, which may be established based on different microbiological assays. Hormone records were part of the very earliest reference standard programs.

Biotechnology-derived products have led to renewed interest in establishing reference standards based on the same bulk of material. Thus, a single formulation, assay, and reference standard may be the fact world-wide. This situation can become complex, such as with insulin, where both biotechnology-derived insulin and animal-source insulin are in the marketplace at the same time.

HISTORY OF HARMONIZATION

One of the earliest references to USP's commitment to international harmonization may be found in the historical introduction to the 3rd revision (1) of the *USP* (1851): "The new Dublin and London Pharmacopoeias were compared with our own, with a view of introducing uniformity wherever more important considerations did not seem to forbid the requisite modifications." Note that uniformity for its own sake was not the sine qua non.

Awareness of the Committee of Revision in 1851 of the importance of keeping the *Pharmacopeia* up-to-date may have been enhanced because of the enactment of the Drug Import Act in 1848, which mandated that drugs imported into the United States had to meet the standards of the country of origin and had to comply with the standards of the *USP* or one of the major European pharmacopeias. The U.S. Customs Service

established laboratories at major port cities and analyzed the imported drugs according to the declared standard. Ties to European medicine remained strong due to Americans traveling to foreign countries for study.

Harmonization of pharmacopeial standards as a practical matter began at the International Congresses of Pharmacy between 1865 and 1910 (2), but the first formal attempt can be traced to 1902. USP President Horatio C. Wood, M.D. and Frederick M. Power, Ph.D., an American chemist of the Wellcome Chemical Research Laboratories of London, were appointed by the U.S. Secretary of State as delegates to represent the U.S. government at the *International Conference for the Unification of the Formulae for Heroic Medicines*, a conference of 19 countries from Europe and North America (3). The second conference occurred in 1918; the third, in 1925, was attended by 31 countries from all continents except Asia and Australia, and was drafted a new "International Convention," which came in force in 1929. It revised the 1902 agreements on 77 "heroic" medicines and introduced the concept of maximum dose. It also requested that the League of Nations create a permanent secretariat of pharmacopeias (4). Andrew G. DuMez, Ph.D., represented the USP, and was officially appointed by the U.S. Public Health Service to represent the United States at this conference (4, 5). An expert committee of the League of Nations planned a third conference for 1938, but it was never convened because of World War II (2).

Other attempts to exchange information among committees for revision of pharmacopeias were attempted through the International Congresses of Pharmacy. Joseph B. Remington, Ph.D., Chairman of the USP Committee of Revision, attending the 1913 conference in The Hague as a delegate of the American Pharmaceutical Association, introduced a resolution to establish an International Bureau of Information to provide information to pharmacopeial revision committees in every country and to operate a testing laboratory. Remington was named to a committee to implement the plan as put forth by Prof. Alexander T. Schirch of Berne, Switzerland (6).

Latin America

Seeking to establish dialogues with Central and South America, the USP, in 1905, responded to a request for a Spanish edition of the *Pharmacopeia* by contracting with Dr. Jose Guillermo Diaz, Dean and Professor of the College of Pharmacy of the University of Havana, Cuba. Support for this project may have come from a resolution adopted by the Second International Sanitary Convention of the American Republics in 1905, which read in part (3): "Resolved, that a translation of this *United States Pharmacopeia* into the Spanish language would prove of great benefit to the medical profession and pharmacists in each of the republics represented in this Convention."

The Spanish edition of *USP VIII* was published in 1908. It was adopted by Cuba, Puerto Rico, and the Philippines. Addressing the Convention of 1910, Joaquin Bernardo Calvo, representing Costa Rica, stated (3): "offering to our physicians and pharmacists who do not speak English the *Pharmacopeia* of the United States translated into Spanish; it is one of the most useful works of its kind, if not the most useful, among those published up to the present date." Spanish editions continued to be published through *USP XV* in 1955. The Spanish edition of *USP XI* was adopted as the official pharmacopeia first by Costa Rica.

In his report to the Convention of 1960, however, Secretary Adley B. Nichols stated (7): "The distribution picture of the *USP* in Spanish has not been satisfactory for some time, and this is especially the case with *USP XV*. In no country is there a marked demand for the translation. Apparently the English language is sufficiently widely known today to permit the use of the readily available English edition." Perhaps the best summary of why the USP produced a Spanish edition of the pharmacopeia can be found in the words of Dr. Charles H. LaWall, Chairman of the Committee of Revision: "The publication of the Spanish edition can never be considered financially advantageous to the Convention, but it should be continued as a patriotic duty and in recognition of the in-use of the book in the Spanish-speaking American countries."

The *USP* again published in Spanish in 1995, with semiannual supplements since then. This was now possible through "machine translation." The situation today is mixed, but the English version maintains its importance in Latin America.

MODERN FORUMS FOR HARMONIZATION OF DRUG QUALITY STANDARDS

Forums for harmonization emerged immediately after a USP Open Conference in May of 1989 in Williamsburg, Virginia (8). It was concluded there that a thrust should be made toward harmonizing excipients and, possibly, test methods. This position was laid before two international meetings in 1989. The first in Strasbourg,

France, in June of that year, celebrated the 25th anniversary of the *EP* (9). The second, in September, in Tokyo, Japan, sponsored by the Pharmaceutical Manufacturers Associations of Tokyo and Osaka, focused on a theme of drug quality and the role of the pharmacopeias in the year 2000 (10). At both of these well-attended conferences, the representatives of the industry spoke of the need for harmonization of standards among the pharmacopeias representing the major drug discovery and drug manufacturing areas of the world—the United States, Europe, and Japan—to facilitate international commerce in pharmaceuticals.

The areas of pharmacopeial standards most frequently cited at those meetings as in need of harmonization were pharmaceutical excipients and analytical tests and assays. Excipients posed the greatest barrier to commerce as a result of a patchwork of standards in the *USP*, *EP*, and *JP* for a small universe of substances and many natural products of animal, mineral, and vegetable origin that are shared throughout the world. Standards for these common substances reflect cultural, scientific, and temporal differences in how and when these standards were established and last revised. Similarly, differences in tests and assays among the three compendia frequently resulted in situations where meeting the standards of a pharmacopeia in one sector would not predict meeting the standards for that same substance in another sector. That is, testing for the same parameter by another method, often resulting in extra expenditures for capital equipment for laboratories, as well as extra time and resources for conducting the tests and in maintaining trained analysts for different procedures.

PHARMACOPEIAL DISCUSSION GROUP

Founded in Tokyo in September 1989 as the "Quadripartite Group," the Pharmacopeial Discussion Group (PDG) was originally composed of representatives of the BP, EP, JP, and USP. The current group includes members from the EP, JP, and USP. At its first meeting at the USP headquarters in Rockville, MD, in March 1990, important agreements were reached:

- To meet twice yearly in a small group consisting of the senior staff executive and scientific officers of each pharmacopeia.
- To implement the concept of forward harmonization, which was agreed in Tokyo (10). *Forward harmonization* has three characteristics: a preference for the selection of methods that would be acceptable well into

the future; retaining of any standard meaningful to an individual pharmacopeia; and unilateral progress not inhibited by trying to have every new advance occur simultaneously in every pharmacopeia.

- To include two additional concepts of harmonization: *prospective*—to avoid conflicts among pharmacopeial standards before they occur, and *retrospective*—to resolve conflicts among existing pharmacopeial standards.
- To solicit advice from the pharmaceutical industry and government regulatory agencies on candidate articles for harmonization and their relative priorities.
- To convene open international pharmacopeial conferences.

Articulating the three concepts for harmonization was particularly important. Prospective and retrospective concepts clarify the distinction between work required to avoid conflict when establishing standards for pharmacopeial articles (for which standards do not exist or where few standards exist among the pharmacopeias), from work required to reconcile differences among well-established standards for articles that may have been in the pharmacopeias for considerable time. Prospective harmonization was inaugurated for biotechnology-derived products. Retrospective harmonization focused on pharmaceutical excipients and analytical tests and methods. Forward harmonization expresses a philosophy and environment for harmonization consistent with advances in pharmaceutical analysis.

Establishing a process for harmonization requires recognizing that each pharmacopeia is a sovereign entity, and has certain authorities and obligations derived from the legislation or treaty that created it that harmonization processes must recognize. Complicating the process was the realization that, different from anything that had been attempted before, a forward-moving process was being devised involving the revision systems of three pharmacopeias, each having evolved in different cultures and histories over periods ranging now from 30–180 years, resulting in profound differences in pharmacopeial policies.

Importantly, this was a voluntary effort; there was no legislative or treaty mandate to harmonize. In fact, no organization can compel harmonization. Complicating the process are the differences worldwide trend among the times for appearance of a first monograph, revision publication schedules, public notice and comment opportunities, and updating provisions. The ideal system would allow closely concurrent, if not simultaneous, actions by each pharmacopeia. The realities of level of funding, publication, and acceptance procedures, however, fall short of ideal. As a matter of fact, harmonization takes

resources away from all other pharmacopeial programs because no specified support is received.

The first attempt at soliciting advice for pharmacopeial priorities was the joint issuance of a letter in May 1990 by the USP in English, by the EP in English and French, and by the JP in Japanese (11). It went to the regulatory agencies and pharmaceutical industry associations in the countries and regions served by each of the pharmacopeias. Reflecting the sentiments of the speakers at the 1989 conferences, the letter was devoted to pharmaceutical excipients and asked only three questions: 1) Which excipients have been a source of problem or delay? 2) Has it been necessary to repeat stability or bioavailability studies because of differences in standards for excipients? 3) What are candidates for the top 10 excipients for harmonization? It also asked respondents to identify those specifications, tests, and assays in the monographs for these excipients that are most important to be harmonized.

Responses were returned from individual pharmaceutical companies through their industry associations and the regulatory agencies in the respective sectors. The complete response was compiled by the USP, and a list of the top-10 excipients was developed as the focal point for initial harmonization efforts, after review by each pharmacopeia. The idea of a "*lead*," subsequently called the *coordinating pharmacopeia*, was adopted, which would take leadership for the revision of the monographs for the excipients for which it had volunteered. The initial list of assignments included: magnesium stearate, microcrystalline cellulose, lactose, starch, cellulose derivatives, sucrose, povidone, stearic acid, calcium phosphate, and polyethylene glycol (12).

The three pharmacopeias have periodicals in which the respective publics are informed of any proposed changes or additional standards (13). Standards do not get out of synchronization through ignorance, because the other two pharmacopeias are familiar with upcoming harmonization-related text in each other's periodicals. And the industry by and large subscribes to all three periodicals and, therefore, should be kept abreast of developments in harmonization. The disconnect arises out of the working speeds and legal procedures of each.

Prospective harmonization is particularly successful when dealing with biotechnology-derived products (14, 15). That is because there are only a couple of manufacturers involved. There should be no reason for the pharmacopeias to arrive at different standards proposed for any particular medicine. This is in stark contrast to the situation where there are multiple manufacturers of drugs no longer covered by patent protection. There is no possibility of harmonization of the some 4000 monographs for individual substances and preparations.

The USP must pay strict attention to the legal situation in the United States. Here, one cannot write "lock-out specifications," thereby keeping somebody out of the business of pharmaceuticals. The other two pharmacopeias, confronted with the same situation, came to the same place in due course, but not at the speed that the USP demonstrates in avoiding any possibility of lock-out specifications. Where there is a valid medical or pharmaceutical reason for specifications that lock out competitors, then the pharmacopeia will set such standards.

One expression frequently heard is to "essentially harmonize." To essentially harmonize is the practical limit of what is possible. It is necessary to rate harmonization on a scale from 0 to 100% harmonized. But in passing judgment, an old expression pertains: "Where you sit is where you stand." The USP's scale for harmonization takes the point of view of a laboratory supervisor who schedules work, training, and capital goods purchases. This would seem to be the point of view that is of most practical value. To assign a quantitative characterization, one must make judgments as to the significance of differences. A completely harmonized requirement would use the same method and establish the same limits. Another, slightly less harmonized requirement would use the same method, but two pharmacopeias would have different limits where one set of limits is nested within the other. If those limits are not nested, then there is a degree of disharmony. Summaries of the overall state of excipient harmony, both from the PDG list and of 200 excipients that appear in *NF* and elsewhere, have appeared in *Pharmacopeial Forum* (16).

The reason a scale for harmonization is necessary is the fact that each pharmacopeial monograph may contain some 10 requirements, and individual monographs will be harmonized on perhaps 7, 8, or even all 10 of those requirements. So where 8 requirements out of 10 are harmonized, it is reported as an 80% harmonized monograph (16).

The goal of harmonization is to bring the policies, standards, monograph specifications, analytical methods, and acceptance criteria of pharmacopeias into agreement. We recognize such unity may not always be achievable. Where unity cannot be achieved, harmonization means agreement based upon objective comparability and a clear statement of any differences. The goal, therefore, is harmony, not unison.

INTERPHARMACOPEIAL OPEN CONFERENCES

Copresented by the BP, EP, JP, and USP, the first Interpharmacopeial Open Conference on Standards for Excipients was convened in Orlando, Florida, from January 30 to February 1, 1991. Attended by 165 participants, representation included 11 countries, 59 pharmaceutical or excipient manufacturers or suppliers, 3 regulatory agencies (FDA, EEC, and HPB), and 7 pharmacopeias (the copresenters and the French, Italian, and Spanish Pharmacopeias) (17). In preparation for this conference, the USP convened open meetings on magnesium stearate and lactose, attended by almost every major manufacturer from Europe and the USP.

The conference endorsed the goals of the pharmacopeias to improve and harmonize standards for existing excipients, to focus on testing methods and address specifications after test methods had been agreed upon, and to develop functionality tests, including particle size, surface area, and density.

Implementation of the open conference recommendations led to a change in configuration of the membership in the pharmacopeial harmonization process. Whereas the BP had been an independent member of the Quadripartite Group from its inception, implementation of harmonization of standards and tests for excipients was recognized as a regional matter under the aegis of the EP, and the BP's independent membership in the process ended. The resulting group of the USP, JP, and EP became known as the PDG and has continued its efforts in tripartite configuration.

A second Joint Pharmacopeial Open Conference on International Harmonization of Excipients was held in St. Petersburg, Florida, in January, 1994 (18). Major progress was achieved and established the principle that conferences were the key component of harmonization. Progress on pharmacopeial harmonization was reported at the International Conference on Harmonization in Brussels in November 1991, and activity of the PDG to fulfill its goals is high. Several tangible and important milestones have been reached. First and most important is the recognition by the JP of its need to develop a vehicle for public notice and comment for pharmacopeial revision, and the essentiality of such a vehicle to the communication process. Recognizing that need, the JP reached a decision to publish the *Japanese Pharmacopoeial Forum* (JPF) on a quarterly basis. The first edition in January 1992 (11) included proposals for the revision of magnesium stearate and lactose monographs. Notable also is the fact that matters in JPF relating to international harmonization are printed in English, whereas domestic revision matters appear in Japanese.

A second milestone was a letter by the PDG in May 1992 soliciting further candidates, beyond excipients. Responses to that inquiry focused primarily on tests and assays. Replies were ranked by order of priority. The priority of excipients was expanded to the top 25, based on further analysis of responses. The lists of combined assignments and priorities for pharmacopeial harmonization appeared in the forum publications of the pharmacopeias (12, 13).

JP took another step toward harmonization by announcing that it would implement an annual supplement program to update the *JP* between editions, beginning with an October 1993 supplement to *JP XII* (11).

Refinement of the process of pharmacopeial harmonization occurs ongoing (see Fig. 1 and Appendix which details the process as of December 1999). Accommodating the revision processes, time requirements, and publication schedules of three revision systems and nine publications proved infeasible as initially envisioned. It required continual adjustment as issues reach stages in revision that had not been foreseen or did not fit within existing systems. Also complicating progress was that, although the USP in 1980 established the first expert group that focused on excipients (Subcommittee on Pharmaceutic Ingredients), the other pharmacopeias did not have task groups readily at hand devoted specifically to excipients.

Experience gained by harmonizing the first of the excipients (lactose and magnesium stearate) showed that, because so many parties are affected and multiple expert groups must be convened, forward, retrospective harmonization is intrinsically a multiyear process.

TESTS AND STANDARDS

Impurities in Excipients

Limit tests have a long standing in pharmacopeias. For some (heavy metals is an example), the sensitivity of the method was the basis for the standard. Modern limits in the *USP–NF* are toxicity based. There is divergence in harmonization because of toxicity-based rather than method-based standards. The modern basis avoids the exclusion of safe products from the marketplace, whereas the older approach could lead to lock-out specifications considered technical barriers to trade.

Biotechnology-Related Standards

Implementation of prospective harmonization began formally with a second conference on standards for biotechnology-derived products. The conference was attended by about 150 scientists and regulators from 20 countries. With participation by experts on pharmaceutical revision bodies from each of the three pharmacopeias, the conference produced a series of recommendations relating to informational chapters, general chapters on tests and assays, and group and individual monographs for selected biotechnology-derived human drugs and biologics (14).

The introduction of biotechnology-derived products presented a decisive moment (15): an opportunity to avoid conflicting standards through the commitment of the pharmacopeias to the process of harmonization for pharmacopeial standards for an emerging technology. Included in this opportunity are the practical values obtained from common reference standard materials.

The complexity of the technology, in concert with medical conditions, and clinical environments, and the desire for instant globalization of return on investment call for facilitation and avoidance of ambiguities by uniform standards worldwide.

Biotechnology-derived drugs are of mutual interest to the USP and the International Conference on Harmonization on Drug Quality (ICH-Q6). The relationship is uncertain between compendial standards and the development and approval of biotechnology-derived drugs by regulatory agencies. The *USP* contains many general chapters (i.e., "horizontal standards" such as stability, injections, and bacterial endotoxins), which are cited extensively by the biotechnology industry, and an informational chapter on biotechnology-derived products that explains terminology and facilitates communication.

Status of Interpharmacopeial Harmonization

Supplements to *USP24–NF19* contain updates of an informational chapter by this name. It lists all of the projects undertaken by the PDG. Appendixes list the projects as of January 2000, and identify the coordinating pharmacopeia. However, these do not report the official status of each project because this changes with each supplement.

Because revision programs work on different schedules, one should compare only the current texts of two or more pharmacopeias whenever divergence of mandatory requirements is an issue. The official pharmacopeial texts should be compared.

Harmonization proposals do not have official status. The work of the PDG is finished at Stage 5B. The progress of the harmonization projects can and should be verified in the most recent number of the periodicals: *Pharmacopeial Forum, Japanese Pharmacopoeial Forum*, and *Pharmeuropa*. For standards in force in *USP24–NF19*, see also the latest supplement or Interim Revision Announcement.

Equivalence

Tests and assays of the EP and the JP that have been elaborated through the PDG Procedure are considered as equivalent to *USP–NF*, except as noted in Chapter ⟨1196⟩ entitled *Status of Interpharmacopeial Harmonization* found in supplements to *USP24–NF19*. Because the legal status of each may not be at the same stage, a precautionary check should be made to support any plans or actions.

Equivalence is attributed to those monographs, tests, or assays that have arrived at Stage 5B. The nature and reason for divergences are expected to be described in the three pharmacopeial periodicals. Only those stated exceptions are considered nonequivalent.

INTERNATIONAL CONFERENCE ON HARMONIZATION

Founded in 1990, the International Conference on Harmonization (ICH) is comprised of the pharmacopeial manufacturers associations in Europe (EFPIA), Japan (JPMA), the United States (PMA), and the drug regulatory agencies in Europe (EEC), Japan (MHW), and the United States (FDA), with the International Federation of Pharmaceutical Manufacturers Association (IFPMA) serving as secretariat. Pharmacopeias are not members of the ICH, where membership is reserved for three PMAs and three regulatory agencies. Invited observers include Canada, WHO, and the European Free Trade Association (EFTA).

With expert working groups in the areas of drug efficacy, drug safety, and drug quality, the ICH is the foremost opportunity for harmonization among the leading drug regulatory and manufacturing groups in the world. The ICH Expert Working Group on Drug Quality (EWG-Q) includes the topic Q4, "Pharmacopeias."

The pharmacopeias have worked with the ICH process to facilitate the international environment of pharmaceutical research and product registration. On the other hand, the additional situation for compendia is that the standards that they have published now apply to all of the products already marketed. In that case, a company has testing history in their quality control (QC) departments. The QC departments are the most conservative elements within the pharmaceutical industry—an attribute necessary to their task. QC departments are reluctant to change methods when they feel that their products are properly represented by their current suite of tests. Thus, there is resultant tension between trying to develop harmonized standards that facilitates one area of activity in the world of pharmaceuticals and not disturbing a satisfactory marketplace. A vast amount of progress has been made in harmonization of pharmacopeial methods.

At the first biennial meeting of the ICH in Brussels in November 1991, the United States, Japanese, and European Pharmacopeias presented papers relating to progress being made in the harmonization of pharmacopeial standards for excipients (19). Other topics, such as stability, validation, impurities, and biotechnology, were established. The pharmacopeias are involved in all these issues. In fact, *USP* general chapters served as background for harmonization for some of these topics.

The ICH Steering Committee responded favorably to a request by USP for *observer status*, recognizing it as a nongovernment, nonindustry body with official status under U.S. statutes. Now, each of the three pharmacopeias can participate in EWG-Q activities and in ICH biennial meetings as independent bodies.

Stability is a key quality concern that is addressed in various ways by pharmacopeial standards. It was also the first subject for which the EWG-Q developed a guideline. The USP has redefined the concept of *Controlled Room Temperature* in terms of a Mean Kinetic Temperature of 25°C, which is identical with the long-term storage temperature promoted by ICH. Furthermore, ICH has advised against including recommended storage label statements that could conflict with United States, or other regions' practices. Thus, the USP standards and the ICH guideline agree on this overarching concern for the stability of pharmaceuticals. The USP actively participated in achieving this desirable outcome.

Validation of analytical procedures is intrinsic to both new drug approval and compendial revision.The *USP* had already established an informational chapter, ⟨1225⟩ entitled *Validation of Compendial Methods* before the international harmonization effort began— a joint effort among the Pharmaceutical Research Manufacturers Association, the FDA, and the *USP*. It was useful in the work of the EWG-Q to prepare a document on validation of analytical procedures that concentrated on the submission of a new drug to the reviewing authorities. Later, in response to demands of users, the ICH document was expanded to more readily meet the scope of *USP* ⟨1225⟩. Differences that arose were resolved, thereby securing the harmonized situation. The emergent ICH document and the *USP* chapter are harmonized in breadth and detail in such a way that the vocabularies of validation and the underlying analytical strategies are in concert.

A recommendation by the PDG to establish a harmonized procedure for stability to light was taken up by the EWG with Japanese participants responsible for a first draft of a guideline. A harmonized procedure emerged, again for the purpose of new drug approval.

Impurities are of many kinds, and, therefore, the issues for harmonization are numerous. Everyone concerned agrees that toxic impurities must be controlled at very low levels, and the analytical difficulties in measuring low levels limit choice. It follows that harmonization of methods is straightforward, once the objectives of analysis are laid out. Both, the USP and ICH limit measurement to impurities at or above 0.1%, which is of practical significance in everyday commerce in bulk pharmaceutical chemicals. In addition, the ICH guideline refers to the pharmacopeial limits on toxic impurities, such as heavy metals. Thus, on all critical issues, there is no conflict between the ICH guideline for new chemical entities and established USP impurity policies, which apply to hundreds of drugs already on the market. The USP further identifies as signal impurities those that are distinctly informative of the purification or decomposition of a drug substance. The remaining impurities are considered in nonspecific categories of ordinary impurities and a labeling requirement for other impurities and are limited to 2% total. ICH sets no such ceiling limit. These policies do not require disclosure of proprietary synthesis or purification details, yet they accomplish the necessary task of limiting bias, thereby assuring meaningfulness of tests and assays. But here ICH guidelines demand identification of each impurity and of individual limits, requiring detailed lot-to-lot bookkeeping on all impurities. Impurities in excess of 0.1% are to be "qualified" (i.e., toxicity considered); USP policy requires notification to USP of any known toxic impurities.

For some years, the USP had a requirement on organic volatile impurities. When the EP was adopting a similar requirement, it was clear that toxicologists on different sides of the ocean would come to different conclusions as to appropriate limits on solvents. At the request of the pharmacopeias, this topic was taken up by (EWG-Q). The effort was successful, and a guideline on residual solvents emerged. Relative to the existing USP limits, it was necessary to revise some upward and others downward, but none to any great extent. This new effort was 15 years subsequent to the initial exercise. However, there remains an unresolved solvent and that is benzene.

Specifications Documents

The ICH–EWG–Q produced two guidelines, Q6A and Q6B, dealing with specifications to support a new drug registration. Biotechnology-related specifications are treated by Q6B, and all others that were previously the subject of EWG-Q guidelines are treated by Q6A. Pharmacopcial methods are intrinsic to these guidelines.

ICH–EWG-Q developed a list of 12 general chapters (tests and assays) that were deemed critical to new product registration and urged the PDG to concentrate on prompt harmonization (see Appendix III). One of these, *Antimicrobial Preservatives Effectiveness*, was dropped in 1999 when nonharmonizability was clear because of differences in the essence of utilization of the same microbiological procedure. Of the 11 remaining chapters, all but two (*Microbial Limits of Non-sterile Articles* and *Dose Uniformity*) were harmonized with regard to scientific content by the end of 1999; only the necessary publication sequences were unfinished.

The Q6A and Q6B documents were preceded by the North American Conference on Specifications. In all cases, no method selection, scope of application, or overall policy (dissolution, impurities, particulate matter, etc.) is at odds with USP—a remarkable situation in view of the breadth of the topics covered. The main difference was and is the proportion of active ingredient in a formulation that triggers choice of determination of content or of weight to establish uniformity of dosage units.

Concordance

In the future, harmonization could be accelerated by reference to laboratory data, rather than by trying to achieve harmonized texts, tests, or assays that establish the same attribute of an article (i.e., water by titration vs. loss on drying). Inherent in this allowance is the assumption that concordant methods can be shown to yield comparable outcomes with regard to acceptable identification, strength, quality, purity, bioavailability, or labeling in the context of the monograph of a recognized article. In the event of a dispute, however, only the result obtained by the procedure given in the appropriate pharmacopeia is conclusive.

This concordance rests on the probable presumption of good manufacturing practices in production and control, now a reasonable presumption in today's international environment.

The use of concordant methods does not necessarily require identical reagents, procedures, or measurements. Official procedures of pharmacopeias, per se, require no validation, but validation of the applicability of official procedures to each preparation (formulation) is to be presumed (e.g., the presence of interfering ingredients).

Concordance would facilitate international commerce in official articles by allowing the reduction of duplicative testing or delay in national product registration or approval proceedings. No provision of the USP General Notices is abrogated, and the allowance, therein, for alternative methods is not foreclosed by a monograph citation to the concordance.

As stated in the General Notices, an article is recognized in *USP–NF* when a monograph for the article is published in it. Each monograph contains standards that define an acceptable article, and gives tests and assays and other specifications designed to demonstrate that the article is acceptable. Monographs and their interpretation are subject to the provisions of the General Notices and general chapters. The tests and assays required in a single monograph are intertwined, therefore, and may further state any necessary variation from the designated general chapters or the General Notices. That is, pharmacopeial monographs define interdependent attributes, each drawn in light of other monograph requirements and the General Notices and must be viewed in total. Consequently, allowances for concordance would only be utilized when supported by an initial verification through duplicate testing of the same specimens and evidence that both methods were validated.

APPENDIX I: WORKING PROCEDURES OF THE PDG

Stage 1: Identification

PDG identifies subjects to be harmonized and nominates a coordinating pharmacpoeia for each subject.

Stage 2: Investigation

The coordinating pharmacopeia for a subject to be harmonized collects the information on the existing specifications in the three pharmacopeias, on the grades of products marketed, and on the potential analytical methods. For new products or new methodologies, existing information in the scientific literature or from manufacturers is collected and analyzed. The coordinating pharmacopeia prepares a draft monograph or chapter, accompanied by a report giving the rationale for the proposal, with validation data where appropriate and available. Stage 2 ends with the proposal draft, which is mentioned in this procedure as the Stage 3 draft. The Stage 3 draft, accompanied by supporting comments or data that explain the reasons for each test method or limit proposed, is sent by the coordinating pharmacopeia to the secretariats of the other two pharmacopeias.

Stage 3: Proposal

The three pharmacopeias publish the Stage 3 draft in the next available issue of their forums, in the style provided by the coordinating pharmacopeia. If necessary, questions are addressed to the readers of the forums when specific issues require their advice, information, or data. In *Pharmeuropa* and the *Japanese Pharmacopoeial Forum*, the Stage 3 draft is published in a specific section entitled *International Harmonization*. In the *Pharmacopeial Forum (USP)*, the Stage 3 draft is published in the *Pharmacopeial Previews* section. The draft is published in its entirety. The corresponding secretariats may have to add information needed for the understanding of implementation of the texts, e.g., the addition of the description of an analytical method or of reagents that did not exist in the pharmacopoeia. Comments by readers of these forum resulting from this preliminary survey are to be sent to their respective pharmacopeial secretariat, preferably within 4 months of publication. The period for public review and comment should not exceed 6 months, however. Each pharmacopeia analyzes the comments received and submits its consolidated comments to the coordinating pharmacopeia within 2 months of the end of the public review/comment period. The coordinating pharmacopeia reviews the comments received and prepares a harmonized document (Stage 4 draft) accompanied by a commentary discussing comments received regarding the previous text and providing reasons for action taken in response to those comments. The Stage 4 draft together with the commentary is sent to the secretariats of the other pharmacopeias (end of Stage 3).

Stage 4: Official Inquiry

The Stage 4 draft is published in the *forum* of each pharmacopeia, with the style adapted to that of the pharmacopeia concerned. In *Pharmeuropa* and the *Japanese Pharmacopoeial Forum*, the Stage 4 draft together with the commentary is published in a specific section entitled *International Harmonization*. In *Pharmacopeial Forum*, the Stage 4 draft is published in the *In-Process Revision* section. Comments regarding this draft are to be sent by readers of the forum to their respective pharmacopeial secretariat, preferably within 4 months and at most within 6 months of publication in the forum. Each pharmacopeia analyzes the information received and submits its consolidated comments to the coordinating pharmacopeia within 2 months of the end of the review/comment period. The coordinating pharmacopeia reviews the comments received and prepares a draft harmonized document (Stage 5A draft), accompanied by a commentary discussing comments received regarding the previous text and providing reasons for action taken in response to those comments. The Stage 5A draft, together with the commentary, is sent to the secretariats of the other two PDG members (end of Stage 4).

Stage 5: Consensus

a. *Provisional.* The stage 5A draft is reviewed and commented on by the other two pharmacopeias within 4 months of receipt. The three pharmacopeias shall do their utmost to reach full agreement at this stage, with a view to reaching a final consensus. If the consensus is reached, a Stage 5B draft is developed. In those rare instances where consensus is not reached or where novel, unanticipated serious issues are identified by any of the parties and need to be considered, depending on the complexity and gravity of the issues, more than one mechanism for resolution may be adopted. This includes the coordinating pharmacopeia call for a meeting of experts from the three pharmacopoeias to search for a consensus. This group prepares a modified 5A document (5A-2) that will be published in the three forums for public comments. These are then reviewed by the group of experts that finalized the consensus document (5B).

b. *Final.* When consensus has been reached, the Stage 5B draft (consensus document) is sent by the coordinating pharmacopeia to the other pharmacopeias for final sign-off.

Note: The last two stages of the implementation of the "harmonized" chapters and monographs take place individually, according to the procedures established by each pharmacopeial organization.

Stage 6: Adoption

The document is submitted for adoption to the organization responsible for each pharmacopeia. Each pharmacopeia incorporates the harmonized draft according to its procedure. If necessary, the Stage 5B draft can be adopted, with specific amendments identified as such, corresponding to a general policy in the territory of the pharmacopeia in question. The monographs may, therefore, be harmonized, without being identical in every respect. Adopted texts are published by the pharmacopeias in the Supplements or, where applicable, in a new edition/revision. If a consensus has not been reached at Stage 5A, the pharmacopeias prepare together an article on divergences to be published by all three pharmacopeias in the respective forums.

Stage 7: Date of Implementation

The pharmacopeias will inform each other of the date of implementation in the particular region.

APPENDIX II: EXCIPIENT HARMONIZATION

Excipient	Coordinating pharmacopoeia
Alcohol	EP
Benzyl alcohols	EP
Dehydrated alcohol	EP
Calcium disodium edetate	JP
Calcium phosphate, dibasic	JP
Calcium phosphate, dibasic (anhydrous)	JP
Carboxymethylcellulose, calcium	USP
Carboxymethylcellulose, sodium	USP
Carboxymethylcellulose, sodium (cross-linked)	USP
Cellulose (microcrystalline)	USP
Cellulose (powdered)	USP
Cellulose acetate	USP
Cellulose acetate phthalate	USP
Citric acid (anhydrous)	EP
Citric acid (monohydrate)	EP
Crospovidone	EP
Ethylcellulose	EP
Hydroxyethylcellulose	EP
Hydroxypropylcellulose	USP
Hydroxypropylcellulose (low-substituted)	USP
Hydroxypropylmethylcellulose	JP
Hydroxypropylmethylcellulose phthalate	USP
Lactose (anhydrous)	USP
Lactose (monohydrate)	USP
Magnesium stearate	USP
Methylcellulose	JP
Methyl parahydroxybenzoate	EP
Petrolatum	USP
White Petrolatum	USP
Polyethylene glycol	USP
Polysorbate 80	EP
Povidone	JP
Saccharin, calcium[a]	USP
Saccharin (free)	USP
Saccharin, sodium	USP
Silicon dioxide	JP
Silicon dioxide (colloidal)	JP
Sodium chloride	EP
Sodium starch glycolate	USP
Starch, corn (maize)	USP
Starch, potato	EP
Starch, rice	EP
Starch, wheat	EP
Stearic acid	EP
Sucrose	EP
Talc	EP
Titanium dioxide	JP
Ethyl parahydroxybenzoate	EP
Propyl parahydroxybenzoate	EP
Butyl parahydroxybenzoate	EP
Glycerol	USP

[a] The JP declines to participate in harmonization, so the USP and EP will harmonize bilaterally.

Note: PDG affirmed that harmonization was not to be undertaken in view of the different drinking waters standards elaborated by various governments. See the monograph for Purified Water.

APPENDIX III: STATUS OF GENERAL TESTS AND ASSAYS

	Coordinating pharmacopeia	ICH-Q6 lists
Dissolution[a]	EP/USP	*
Disintegration	EP/USP	*
Dose uniformity[b]	JP/USP	*
Color and clarity	EP	*
Extractable volume	EP	*
Heavy metals	USP	*
Particulate matter	EP	*
Residue on ignition—sulfated ash	JP	*
Sterility	EP	*
Bacterial endotoxin	JP	*
Microbial contamination	EP	*
Preservative effectiveness[c]	EP	*
Particle size distribution estimation by analytical sieving	USP	*
Inhalations	EP	
Bulk density and tapped density	EP	
Optical microscopy—powder fineness	USP	
Powder flowability	USP	
Specific surface area	EP	
Tablet friability	USP	

[a]Apparatuses 1, 2, and 4 are harmonized. Not all apparatuses appear in other pharmacopeias, and decision rules are harmonized. Approach to selection of media is not harmonized and may not be a valid subject in view of population and formulation differences.
[b]Includes content uniformity and weight variation.
[c]In view of two-test nature of an otherwise highly similar procedure used in different modes in US and Europe, this is nonharmonizable on test times and decision values.

REFERENCES

1. The United States Pharmacopeial Convention, Inc. *The United States Pharmacopeia*; 3rd rev., Lippincott, Grambo and Co.: Philadelphia, 1851.

2. Proceedings of the First International Conference on Harmonization. D'Arcy, P.F., Harron, D.W.G., Eds.; Queen's University of Belfast: 1992; 135–182.

3. The United States Pharmacopeial Convention, Inc. *Abstract of the Proceedings of the National Convention of 1910 for Revising the Pharmacopeia*; Washington, D.C., 1910.

4. The U.S. Pharmacopeial Convention, Inc. *Abstract of the Proceedings of the United States Pharmacopeial Convention of 1930*; Washington, D.C., 1931.

5. Anderson, L. *Unpublished manuscript. USP history*; 1906–1929; 55–56.

6. The United States Pharmacopeial Convention, Inc. *Abstract of the Proceedings of the Decennial Meeting, The United States Pharmacopeial Convention 1940*; Washington, D.C., 1941.

7. The United States Pharmacopeial Convention, Inc. *Abstract of the Proceedings of the Decennial Meeting, The United States Pharmacopeial Convention 1960*; Washington, D.C., 1961.

8. The United States Pharmacopeial Convention, Inc., Proceedings of the USP Open Conference of Revision Issues. Rockville, MD, 1989.

9. Proceedings of the 20th Anniversary of the European Pharmacopoeia. Pharmeuropa **1990**, *2* (1), 266–268.

10. PMA of Tokyo and Osaka, Conference on International Harmonization of Pharmaceutical Quality-Vision of Pharmacopoeia in the 21st Century. PMA: Tokyo, 1990.

11. Society for the Japanese Pharmacopoeia. Jap. Pharmacop. Forum **1992**, *1* (1), 20–29.

12. Pharmacop. Forum **1993**, *19* (4), 5849.

13. Pharmeuropa **1993**, *5* (2), 65.

14. Proceedings of Interpharmacopeial Open Conference on Standards for Biotechnology-Derived Products, Pharmeuropa, 1993 Special Edition

15. Dabbah, R.; Grady, L.T. Curr. Opin. Biotechnol. **1998**, *9*, 307–311.

16. Cecil, T.L.; Paul, W.L.; Grady, L.T. Update of the Degree of Harmonization Survey of Excipient Monographs. Pharmacop. Forum **1997**, *23* (2), 3895–3902.

17. The United States Pharmacopeial Convention, Inc., Proceedings of the Joint Pharmacopeial Open Conference on International Harmonization of Excipient Standards. First Conference: Rockville, MD, 1991.

18. Ibid **1994**, SecondConference.

19. Proceedings of The First International Conference on Harmonization, Brussels, 1991.

20. Proceedings of The Second International Conference on Harmonization, Orlando, FL, 1993.

21. Proceedings of The Third International Conference on Harmonization, Yokohama, 1995.

22. Proceedings of The Fourth International Conference on Harmonization, Brussels, 1997.

HEALTH CARE SYSTEMS: OUTSIDE THE UNITED STATES

Albert I. Wertheimer

Temple University, Philadelphia, Pennsylvania

Sheldon X. Kong

Merck & Co. Inc., Whitehouse Station, New Jersey

INTRODUCTION

It is quite fascinating how the organization, structure, and financing of health care services can be so very diverse in different countries around the world. One might think that leaders and policymakers would be aware of each other's national health systems and, by emulating the best features, that they would tend to move toward harmonization and greater similarity.

Actually, this assumptions is false. National health care systems vary widely and are more related to variables in each country (1). In fact, the health system in a given country is a mirror of how that society functions at large. Health care delivery systems must be compatible with the: 1) *economic system*: socialist, capitalist, or mixed; 2) *political system*: major or minor role of degree of government centralization; 3) *wealth of the country*: use of primary care facilities, access to specialists and tertiary care facilities; 4) *traditions and conventions as seen in their history*—fundamental, visible things are difficult to change; 5) *geography*: whether the majority of the population is located in a few metropolitan areas, with the remainder scattered in rural areas, or whether the population is spread over hundreds of islands; 6) *infrastructure*: roads, communication systems, and air service; and 7) *extent of and belief in high technology* (2).

There are other factors as well: the system from a previous colonial power, extent of literacy and education, and relationships with outside countries, to name a few.

BACKGROUND

The remainder of this article examines the health care delivery systems in six very different countries. Even though Canada and the United States are similar countries with a shared border and language and with open communication, their health care delivery systems could not be any more different. Each side of the border is aware of what happens on the other side, however, a series of complex and powerful forces keep them moving in their own directions.

We look at six countries very briefly in this article to highlight the incredibly diverse approaches to health service organization and financing. In essence, most health systems fit into one of the following models:

1. State ownership and control—The best examples are the British National Health Service and the Swedish system in which clinics, hospitals, and most service providers are owned and operated by the government (3).
2. State health insurance program—Here, the government is the sole or major payer. However, some of the facilities and resources are in nongovernment hands. This is the case in much of Europe (4).
3. Mixed systems—This is seen in much of Asia and Central America and usually where there is a small wealthy class and a massive lower class. The lower class receives care from public facilities, and the small upper class uses private-sector, fee-for-service, and self-paid care.

    Other scenarios fit into this category as well. The United States has several independent health care systems including the military, veterans, Medicaid (a federal program for the medically indigent), Medicare (a federal insurance program for those 65 years of age and older), private-sector for-profit, and not-for-profit clinics, hospital chains, managed-care organizations, religious, prison health, and university teaching facilities (5).
4. Exclusively private sector—This category is shrinking as nations realize that health maintenance and disease prevention/wellness are important to their national goals of strength and productivity. Switzerland would still fit into this category, where most health care resources are in private hands (6).

Encyclopedia of Pharmaceutical Technology

SPECIMEN NATIONAL SYSTEMS

Canada

Organization

Canada uses a national health service, which provides medical services and hospital care to its entire population. The individual provincial governments operate health plans that conform to national legislation but can differ in various aspects. This "Medicare" program guarantees comprehensiveness, universal access, portability, and public administration (7).

Health Canada is the national, federal health agency; however, the operation of health service provision is delegated to the provincial governments, which control virtually 100% of Canada's hospitals. There is a gatekeeper primary health care system, with GPs (general practitioners) or primary care family doctors serving as the entry point. Access to specialists, diagnostic testing, hospitals, and others is through the GP. Individual citizens have the freedom to choose their own doctors, 95% of whom are self-employed in private practice. The provincial government pays these doctors on a fee-for-service basis.

The individual provincial governments offer different supplemental benefits not covered by the national Medicare program, such as drugs, dental care, and vision care to the poor, elderly, and other specific groups. Supplemental benefits for the typical, employed, and nonelderly person come from the purchase of supplemental health insurance from private sources (8).

Pharmaceuticals

Canada created the Patented Medicine Prices Review Board (PMPRB) in 1987 to guarantee that pharmaceutical products would not have excessive prices in Canada. The board reviews prescribed and over-the-counter (OTC) prices and publishes annual guidelines for manufacturers. Compliance with PMPRB guidelines is voluntary; however, since 1993, the board has the authority to reduce excessive prices and return the excess amount to the government, and to punish the manufacturer.

The PMPRB compares prices in Canada with those in seven industrialized nations (France, Germany, Italy, Sweden, Switzerland, the United Kingdom, and the United States) to ensure that Canadian prices are in line with those of comparable countries. There is some controversy that existing drug products are well-controlled regarding prices, but that such is not the case with newly introduced pharmaceuticals.

Further controls exist at the provincial level at which each province maintains a published formulary of drugs that are reimbursable along with the reimbursement level. Quebec, observers perceive, lists nearly all new drug products, whereas Ontario appears to be slow to list newly approved products. Each province has additional control mechanisms. Ontario requires the first generic drug to be at least 40% less costly than the branded originator product. Some components of the reference price system are seen in British Columbia and Newfoundland.

There is growing harmonization among the provinces; however, there is still no national, standardized, and interchangeable list of drugs for ambulatory care use. In hospitals, drugs that are administered are paid for by Medicare. Each province has interesting and different features in its drug benefit plan.

The Prince Edward Island plan pays for seniors; welfare recipients; nursing home patients; and those with rheumatic fever, diabetes, tuberculosis, multiple sclerosis, AIDS, and several other conditions. New Brunswick has an annual copayment cap for seniors and for organ transplant recipients and for selected other patient categories. A copayment is set at approximately $9 (Canadian) but is waived for some groups in Quebec, along with an annual copay ceiling of $750.

Other interesting features of the Canadian system include its 1998 mutual recognition agreement with the EU, prohibition of prescription drug advertising to consumers, a 20-year patent exclusivity period, and the establishment of the PMPRB to ensure fair pricing of medications (9, 10).

Republic of South Africa

Organization

The Republic of South Africa (RSA) has a most diverse health care environment, with world-class practice and facilities in wealthy urban areas and some of the most primitive care in poor remote villages, with a vast array between these extremes. Primary care is now the focus of the ANC government in an effort to correct years of neglect and undemocratic practices under the earlier apartheid-oriented regimes. Public health services are being brought to the Black townships as rapidly as resources permit (11).

However, there are virtually no funds for new drugs against HIV infection in patients, a problem most prevalent in the RSA. To maximize the value of its drugs budget, the RSA has enacted legislation to create an Essential Drugs List for the public sector, along with generic substitution authority, the removal of some pharmacists' unique professional privileges, and legislation permitting the parallel importation of pharmaceutical products already registered in the RSA. Obviously, this conserves resources, stretching them for more patients, but this angers the RSA and multinational pharma firms.

South Africa is still the wealthiest country in Africa, with a (1997) GDP at approximately $130 billion. It must be noted, though, that aggregate numbers hide massive racial differences. It is improving, but the standard of living for Blacks is yet only slightly better than it is in neighboring countries, whereas whites enjoy a standard of living similar to that found in North America or Western Europe. An unemployment rate of over 30% (mostly among Blacks) exacerbates the fiscal situation (12).

Routine immunizations for children, conforming to the World Health Organization (WHO) recommended schedule is the governmental policy, but it is not yet accomplished in all regions. Infectious diseases including HIV remain a serious challenge. Planning and budgeting for resource allocation are difficult because accurate census figures do not exist. Total health expenditures appear to be in the area of $300 per person per year, and it is estimated that the private sector accounts for greater than 50% of total expenditures.

Public-sector expenditures emphasize primary care, lately, at the expense of tertiary care facilities. Private-sector spending is primarily through private "medical schemes." These are nonprofit organizations supported by employer associations and employees. There are slightly fewer than 200 of these schemes, providing insurance and care payment for nearly 3 million workers and their 5 million dependents (of a total estimated RSA population of 40 million). The largest area of medical scheme expenditure is for medicines, which causes the pressures on pharmaceutical pricing addressed below. After drugs, the next largest expenditures are for private hospitals, medical specialists, general practitioners, and dentists (13).

The RSA Department of Health (DOH) has totally restructured the previous apartheid system of racial and provincial health systems into a coordinated national health program operated through health regions and local health districts. Still, there are major differences in knowledge, education, expectations, and wealth within different subpopulations (14, 15).

Pharmaceuticals

Until recently, manufacturers were free to establish their desired price for a drug. Wholesalers and retailers added what they chose to reach the retail selling price for medications. In 1997, a proposed scheme of prices extending to the retailer was agreed on, but resistance was met from the Pharmaceutical Manufacturers Association(PMA). In the

legislation, a pricing board composed of members selected by the Minister of Health would establish prices for each product and a maximum selling price. Public-sector primary care drugs are reimbursed 100% by the government. Hospital care outpatient drugs can have copayments. The Essential Drugs List would be the core of what is to be available at public facilities, but there appears to be a long way to go before most of these agents will be regularly available on a consistent basis at primary care centers or at public hospitals (13).

The parallel importation of RSA-registered drugs available at lower prices abroad is the basis for PMA litigation against the Drug Legislation of 1997. In addition to the price-setting committee, DOH efforts to encourage the use of generic drugs has proven to be a source of conflict. Other features of the new legislation bar dispensing samples or making bonus payments to dispensers of medicines; the creation of a Code of Ethics for pharmaceutical marketing; and a series of safety regulations, dealing primarily with limiting practice to fully qualified and licensed professionals.

There is a fast lane for new drug approvals if the product is already in at least one of the following jurisdictions: the United Kingdom, Canada, United States, Sweden, or Australia. Approxmately 85% (by value) of pharmaceuticals go through the nearly 3,000 community pharmacies. Yet, approxmately 80% of the population rely on the public sector for drugs, received through clinics, hospitals, primary care posts, or military facilities. Although there is a 20-year patent period of exclusivity/ protection, the parallel imports option effectively defeats this protection.

It will be interesting to see how the access to drugs, price controls, and quality improvement forces will interact and what the actual situation will be in South Africa in the coming years, especially as the country complies with intellectual property and World Trade Organization policies and rules (16).

Japan

Organization

After North America and before Western Europe, Japan is the second largest pharmaceutical market in the world. Its population of 126 million spends $70 billion on pharmaceuticals each year. On average, each Japanese resident spends $2000 each year on health care with $550 of that on pharmaceuticals. Perhaps the primary single features of the Japanese market are the above-average proportion of elderly in the population and the higher than usual consumption of drugs. It has been estimated that by the year 2050, nearly 30% of the population will be older than 65 years of age. The high consumption rate is attributed to drugs being injected and/or sold by the physician, a practice used, in part, to increase the total price of an office visit (17).

The primary funding source for health services in Japan is the Social Insurance System (SIS), made up of employee programs that pay for nearly 55% of care. The Medical Service for the Aged program covers another 35% of care. Private expenditures and a very small portion for public health promotion and disease prevention make up the difference. The Ministry of Health and Welfare (MHW) maintains overall responsibility for health care services and functions via a number of bureaus. Numerous sources comment that regulations are difficult to understand and interpret, often overlapping, and that this serves as a barrier to foreign firms desiring to enter a market. Physicians, for example, are authorized to own and operate hospitals, effectively excluding corporate owners or physicians not licensed in Japan (18).

Universal health insurance was established in 1961. Nearly the entire population is covered through the employer plans or through programs for the unemployed, retired, or self-employed. Employees pay 10% of the cost of treatments, up to an annual ceiling, and also pay a portion of their premiums, with their employers.

Pharmaceuticals

The MHW sets prices for reimbursable drugs (those approved for the Social Insurance System). Physicians, clinics, and private hospitals are reimbursed at a price slightly higher than their actual acquisition cost. The government has scheduled annual reductions in the reimbursement prices to reduce this source of additional income to physicians. Patients make copayments of 20%, although for children and low-income elderly the copayment is waived, and recently a plan to eliminate copayments for persons 70 years of age and older was introduced.

The MHW reductions of 5–10% of the prices of existing drug products appear to have had the opposite of the intended impact. Doctors are prescribing more of the newest, high-priced pharmaceuticals that have not had their margins reduced yet, thereby earning a bigger amount from the wider difference between their actual cost and the listed reimbursement amount.

With regard to generic drugs, astute observers believe that the Japanese government wants its R&D-intensive firms to be successful. A regulation requires generics to be priced at not less than 40% of the innovator brand price. It is reasonable to assume that the margins (Yakkasa) for physicians are lower with generic drugs, and that these margins will continue into the future, as will the reference price scheme (19).

There is a Japanese pharmacopeia that sets official standards and diverse government agencies that perform tasks undertaken by an FDA. It is rumored that the Japanese will establish a Western-style FDA in the near future.

One of the most disliked regulations in the view of foreign and multinational pharmaceutical companies is the requirement for duplicative clinical trials with humans in Japan, because those carried out elsewhere are not recognized. Also of interest is the fact that Japan, like Korea and Taiwan, has no separation between prescriber and dispenser of drugs. Called "Bungyo," it is a major source of revenue for doctors and clinics. Fewer than 20% of prescriptions ever reach a pharmacy for dispensing (19).

Good post-marketing surveillance practices (GPMSP) rules have been in place since 1993. Postmarketing experience reports are to be sent to a government agency. Both GPMSP and periodic safety reporting requirements are in place that require a review of the product each year while it is in its re-examination period, immediately after marketing approval. Unlike in the United States, where a new drug application is approved for an indefinite period, in Japan, there is a periodic full reassessment. Such re-evaluations are conducted every 5 years once the initial re-examination period for a drug product has ended.

Drug products are distributed primarily via the 2000 wholesalers, and in addition, there exists a small second channel with drugs going directly to hospitals, GPs, and pharmacies. There are approximately 66,000 pharmacies, most of which are family-owned independents. There are chains as well. However, a growing market for OTCs is found in convenience stores.

Physicians administer and sell drugs to patients as a highly profitable sideline. The incentive is for the physician to use as much of the most costly drug products as possible. There is only a small OTC market, because physicians try to prescribe and dispense as much as is possible. Other than some concern about a drug lag, the pharmaceutical environment in Japan is robust. Periodically, there are calls to separate prescribing and dispensing; however, this is not likely in the near future given the powerful forces backing the status quo (20).

United Kingdom

Organization

With a population of more than 60 million and GDP per capita of more than US $22,000, the United Kingdom is one of the richest nations in the world. It is one of the G7 countries, a member of the European Union, and a member of the Organization for Economic Co-operation and Development (OECD).

In 1996, total health care expenditure in the United Kingdom was approximately 7.0% of the GDP. Public expenditure by the National Health Service (NHS) accounts for most of the health care costs. The NHS was set up after World War II, with the aim of unifying health care services by voluntary and local hospitals. The NHS offers free health services to all U.K. residents, funded through general taxation.

Two of the major characteristics of the U.K. health care system include health authorities responsible for hospital services and GP fundholders responsible for primary care. In 1996, 100 health authorities became operational in England, responsible for the provision of NHS hospital and community health services covering geographic boundaries with populations ranging from 125 thousand to over 1 million. There are four levels of hospital services. At the community level, community hospitals offer basic medical care for the treatment of acute cases and patients requiring convalescent and long-term/terminal care. General practitioners are the key staff here. At the district level, district general hospitals operate the key acute units, serving an average population of a quarter-million. At the regional level, major specialty services such as neurosurgery, open-heart surgery, and radiotherapy are provided. At the national level, highly specialized hospitals provide complex services for parts or for the entire country (21).

GPs are the gatekeepers and fundholders of the health care system. The principle of fundholding is that GPs manage their own budgets. They can obtain a defined range of services from hospitals and manage patients at the GP level whenever possible to reduce costs. In the late 1990s, GPs fundholders were organized into Primary Care Groups (PCGs). These networks of GPs cover wide geographic areas with an average population of 100,000. In 1999, there were 481 PCGs in England and Wales, and all have unified budgets (e.g., drugs, hospital care services). With a population of a small to medium-sized HMO in the United States, these PCGs have a very broad influence on patient health care and the selection of drugs through formularies.

Pharmaceuticals

The regulatory authority in the United Kingdom is the Medicines Control Agency (MCA) under the Department of Health. The agency's responsibilities include drug licensing, clinical trials licensing, pharmacovigilance and drug safety, communication and provision of information on medicines, inspection of facilities and enforcement of regulations, and the *British Pharmacopoeia*. The United Kingdom is a reference member state for the European Union mutual recognition procedure. The European Union's pharmaceutical registration system came into

effect for all member countries in 1995. The aim of the EU system is to harmonize pharmaceutical regulations throughout the EU. The centralized registration procedure is handled by the European Medicines Evaluation Agency (EMEA). Authorization through the central registration procedure is immediately valid in all EU member countries. The decentralized procedure relies on the principle of mutual recognition. After registration has been obtained in a member country under the centralized procedure, application may be made for registration in one or more other member countries via the decentralized procedure (21).

The majority of pharmaceuticals are distributed through wholesalers to retail pharmacies, with large pharmacy chains now dominating the market. There are approximately 11,000 community pharmacies in the United Kingdom (21). In recent years, pharmacy services are increasingly available in supermarkets at the expense of local independent pharmacies.

Total expenditure on pharmaceuticals in the United Kingdom amounted to approximately 8650 million pounds in 1999, accounting for approximately 17% of the total health expenditure (21). The NHS covers prescription drugs. However, the government does not reimburse for over-the-counter (OTC) products. The Department of Health indirectly controls pharmaceutical prices. Because the price control scheme is related to profit control, rather than to the prices of individual products, pharmaceuticals are relatively free-priced in the United Kingdom. The government operates a negative list for products that are not reimbursable. The cost of most licensed prescription products is fully reimbursed. However, cost constraints and prescribing budgets mean that GPs will often prescribe a generic when one is available. As a result, new prescription drugs usually have a slower penetration rate in the United Kingdom than in the United States. The recently introduced National Institute for Clinical Excellence (NICE) will add more barriers to the introduction of new pharmaceutical products in the United Kingdom.

National Institute for Clinical Excellence

Funded by the government, the National Institute for Clinical Excellence (NICE) was set up as a Special Health Authority in the United Kingdom in 1999 and, as such, it is a part of the National Health Service (NHS). It was set up to "provide the NHS [patients, health professionals, and the public] with authoritative, robust and reliable guidance on current best practice." Its key functions are "to appraise the clinical benefits and the costs of those [health care] interventions and to make recommendations." Guidance is issued from each appraisal based on the clinical benefits, cost-effectiveness, and total economic impact on the

National Health Service. The government does not have to adhere to the recommendations by the NICE in its guidance and financial payment to health care providers. However, many believe that a negative recommendation from the NICE will have a detrimental impact on the pricing, reimbursement, and sales of the appraised product not only in the United Kingdom but also throughout Europe, Australia, and Canada.

The guidance covers both individual health technologies (including medicines, medical devices, diagnostic techniques, procedures, and health promotion) and the clinical management of specific conditions. The Institute may recommend a technology for general use, for specific indications, or for defined subgroups of patients. Based on the appraisal, a therapeutic intervention (e.g., drug) will be classified into one of three categories: category A, routine use in the NHS; category B, further trials needed; and category C, not recommended for routine use in the NHS.

The NICE has a board reflecting a range of expertise including the clinical professions, patients and user groups, NHS managers, and research bodies. The Board ensures that the NICE conducts its business on behalf of the NHS in the most effective manner. Details of the appraisal process and membership of the Appraisals Committee are available on the NICE Web site (www.nice.org.uk). Because the NICE was new at the time of completion of this article, its impact on the pharmaceutical industry is still not clear.

Germany

Organization

With a population of approximately 82 million in 1998 and a GDP per capita of more than $26,000, Germany is one of the world's largest economies and health care markets. The population enjoys a generally good standard of health with a high degree of public awareness about health-related issues. Life expectancy in Germany is among the highest in the world. In 1997, the life expectancy for males was 74 years and for females 80. Approximately 15.8% of the population were over 65 years in 1997, and it has been projected that by 2020, the number of German inhabitants aged over 60 years will be 28.2% (22).

In 1997, health expenditures in Germany totaled $298 billion, equal to 14.2% of the GDP. The health care system in Germany is decentralized, and health care expenditures are covered by a variety of sources/payers. The statutory insurance system (GKV) represents the biggest proportion of the total care coverage (for almost 50%). Employers, government budget, private households, private insurance, retirement insurance, and accident insurance cover the remaining 50% of the health care expenditures. The largest spending sector is hospital expenditure, representing 34.3% of the total GKV health care expenditures (22).

The federal government has little executive responsibility for the provision of health care in Germany. Its primary responsibility is to provide a regulatory framework within which the individual Länder have to operate. The health ministries of the individual Länder are responsible for implementing the federal legislation, enacting their own legislation, supervising subordinate authorities and the medical profession, hospital planning, and regional administration.

Hospitals in Germany can be classified into three major categories based on ownership: public, nonprofit, and private. In 1997, the public sector operated approximately 40% of general hospitals, and nonprofit organizations operated another 40%. However, the number of privately owned facilities has been increasing steadily over the past decade.

The number of practicing doctors has risen steadily for the past 10 years. More than 70% of the practicing doctors are specialists, with general medicine as the largest specialty. Fewer than 30% of doctors practice without any specialty.

Pharmaceuticals

Germany is a reference member of the EU pharmaceutical registration system. The European Medicines Evaluation Agency (EMEA) handles the centralized registration and the decentralized registration procedures in individual countries. After marketing authorization of a product with a new active substance has been granted in one country, the mutual recognition procedure is compulsory in other member countries. The mutual recognition procedure is also compulsory for line extensions and generic products. Marketing authorization approvals in Germany are valid for 5 years and renewable thereafter in 5 year periods.

Germany is the home of some major multinational pharmaceutical companies such as Aventis, BASF, Bayer, Boehringer Ingelheim, Merck KGaA, and Schering AG. VFA is the research-based manufacturers' association, whereas the Bundesverband de Pharmazeutischen Industrie (BPI) represents small and medium-sized companies. Because North America is the largest pharmaceutical market in the world, many of the VFA pharmaceutical companies locate their key operations in the United States. Exports to Western European countries represent a major source of income for many of the German pharmaceutical companies.

The pharmaceutical market in Germany is one of the largest in the world. Based on drug use per capita, Germany is second only to Japan in the consumption of pharmaceuticals. The principal distribution channels for pharmaceuticals in Germany are public retail pharmacies and hospital pharmacies. In 1998, there were 47,322 pharmacists in Germany, equal to 0.6 pharmacists per thousand population (22). Public (retail) pharmacies employed 96% of all pharmacists in 1998 and they obtained their supplies primarily from wholesalers. Prescribed drugs, including both branded and generic products, can only be dispensed in a pharmacy with a doctor's prescription. The generics market in Germany is one of largest and fastest-growing in Western Europe, representing approximately one-third of the European generics markets. OTC products can be divided into three overlapping categories: prescription OTC medicines, nonprescription OTC medicines, and freely available OTC products that can be sold freely through all retail outlets such as health food stores, supermarkets, and other retail outlets.

Mexico

Organization

Mexico is a federal republic of 31 states and a federal district. The population was officially estimated to be 97.7 million in 1997. GDP per capita was estimated at approximately US $4400 in 1998. As a developing nation, communicable diseases are still one of the major causes of mortality, although chronic and degenerative diseases have become the leading cause of death during the past decade.

One of the major challenges for the government is to address the inadequacies of the Mexican health care system. Approximately 10 million people have virtually no access to regular basic health care services, and another 20 million people have less than adequate access. In 1996, the total health care expenditure in Mexico was equivalent to approximately 4.6% of GDP. Spending by the public sector accounted for approximately 60% in 1996 (23).

There are three sectors in the Mexican health care system: public, social security, and private. The public sector is primarily directed and operated by the Secretariat of Health. The public sector of health services is under the Secretariat of Health and is coordinated by over 200 health districts. The Federal District Department provides health care services to some 3.2 million people in Mexico City. The Mexican Social Security Institute (IMSS) Solidarity program covers another 10 million people in rural areas.

The social security system covers health services for government employees, managed by the Social Insurance Institute of State Employees (ISSSTE), and for private-sector workers, managed by the Mexican Social Security Institute (IMSS). The two agencies operate their own networks of hospitals and clinics and provide similar benefits. Some other smaller social security agencies exist, providing medical services for special groups such as the army, navy, and state oil company personnel.

The private (commercial) sector includes private hospitals, doctor's offices, and practitioners of traditional medicine. Charity organizations such as the Red Cross also play a role in the Mexican health care system.

Pharmaceuticals

The regulatory authority in Mexico is the Dirección General de Control de Insumos para la Salud (DIGECIS). The Health Secretariat issues pharmaceutical registration. Safety and efficacy must be proven by phase III clinical trials in Mexico to register drugs that are new to the Mexican market. All major pharmacopeia (*International Pharmacopoeia, US Pharmacopeia, British Pharmacopoeia, French Pharmacopoeia, Swiss Pharmacopoeia, European Pharmacopoeia*, and *Japanese Pharmacopoeia*) are acceptable in Mexico.

Most domestic producers in Mexico are wholly owned or licensed subsidiaries of multinational pharmaceutical firms. Exports have been growing fast, with other Latin American countries as the major destination markets. However, the United States is the major supplier of pharmaceutical imports in Mexico.

Pharmaceuticals in Mexico are subject to government price control. The private sector accounts for approximately 85% of the pharmaceutical market. Prescription drugs account for the majority of the pharmaceutical market, with antibiotics as one of the largest classes. Because the use of generics is still a relatively new phenomenon, most of the prescribed pharmaceuticals are branded products. OTC products represent approximately one-fifth of the total pharmaceuticals market.

SUMMARY

As presented, these six representative countries use vastly different organizations, financing mechanisms, goals, and provision structures. In fact, few systems around the world are identical because the systems represent the values and priorities and political as well as economic leanings and traditions of that country. If there were one perfect system, we would be seeing migration toward that model. However, because this is not the case, it is reasonable to assume that most of the various systems encountered around the world are at least satisfactory in their foundations and macrolevel characteristics, even if some of the operating details are not always popular (24).

The world is full of interesting additional approaches that a serious student of this subject might wish to explore further. Some of these include the "need clause" used in Norway, where, for example, their FDA had the authority to refuse to accept and review a new drug because Norway already had six benzodiazepines on the market. The FDA deemed that sufficient unless the sponsoring company knew of a new indication or other therapeutic breakthrough from its use. The Swedes bought all of the then-existing community pharmacies in the country in 1970 to rationalize distribution, and service level and to create a monopsonistic body for negotiating with manufacturers in price-setting. The French and others place new drugs into one of several reimbursement categories. Clearly, life-saving drugs are put in the 100% reimbursement (to the patient) category. Most others strive for the 70% reimbursement category; however, if the manufacturer cannot agree on a price satisfactory to the Social Security agency, the product will be placed in a lower reimbursement category, effectively hampering its market success. This is a powerful bargaining chip for the government to contain drug prices.

It will be interesting to watch the future in this area to see how medications previously requiring a doctor's prescription that move to OTC status are handled, and how nutraceuticals, herbals, homeopathic, and naturopathic drugs, without the benefit of rigorous, randomized clinical trial or outcome data are handled as well. Similarly, we can be certain that there will be excitement galore when the nations in Central America and the Middle East decide to control pharmaceuticals and to end the practice of lay-person purchases of virtually any product without the benefit of a physician's order. Separation of pharmacy and physician functions will occur in the Far East in the not too distant future, causing even more excitement or grief.

If logic dictates, we should expect to see in the future a trend to offer incentives for prescribers who use the most cost-beneficial products (bonuses) and disincentives for patients (reimbursement level co-payment differences) and physicians when less than optimal choices are made. Irrespective of whatever does actually occur, it will be most interesting to observe.

REFERENCES

1. Roemer, M.I. *National Health Systems of the World*; Oxford University Press: Oxford, UK, 1993; 2, 61.
2. Fry, J.; Farndale, W.A.J. *International Medical Care*; Washington Square East: Wallingford, PA, 1972; 367.
3. In *OECD Health Systems: Facts and Trends*; OECD: Paris, 1993; 100–161.
4. Hewitt, M. *International Health Statistics*; Office of Technology Assessment, U.S. Congress: Washington, D.C., 1993; 76–86.
5. Elling, R.H. *International Health Perspectives*; Springer: New York, 1977; 4, 17–25.
6. Joseph, S.C.; Koch-Weser, D.; Wallace, N. *Worldwide Overview of Health and Disease*; Springer: New York, 1977; 7–43.
7. Korman, R.A. *Academic Reference Manual: Canadian Health Care Information*; IMS Health: Mississauga, Ontario, 1999; 80–162.
8. *World Pharmaceutical Markets: Canada*; Espicom Business Intelligence: Chichester, UK, May, 1999; 9–48.
9. Alleyne, G.A.O. *Health Statistics from the Americas*; Pan American Health Organization: Washington, DC, 1998; 17–37.
10. Alleyne, G.A.O. *Health in the Americas*; Pan American Health Organization: Washington, DC, 1998; 1, 325–337.
11. Monekosso, G.L. *Eighth Report on the World Health Situation; African Region*; WHO: Brazzaville, 1994; 2, 2–37.
12. Nokagima, H. *Eighth Report on the World Health Situation*; 147–165 Global View: Geneva, 1993; 1, 37–59.
13. *World Pharmaceutical Markets: South Africa*; Espicom Business Intelligence: Chichester, UK, Feb 1999; 3–13.
14. *World Development Report 1993, World Bank*; Jamison, D.T., Ed.; 108–170 Oxford University Press: Oxford, 1993; 3–65.
15. *World Tables 1995*; World Bank: Washington, DC, 1995; 22–66.
16. Basch, P.F. *Textbook of International Health*; Oxford: New York, 1990; 144–326.
17. *Bartholomew's Mini World Factfile*; Harper Collins: London, 1995; 44, 102, 175.
18. *Eighth Report on the World Health Situation: Western Pacific Region*; World Health Organization: Manila, 1993; 7, 79–83.
19. *World Pharmaceutical Markets: Japan*; Espicom Business Intelligence: Chichester, UK, Jan 1999; 10–23.
20. SCRIP: London UK, 1998, 1999, and 2000.
21. *World Pharmaceutical Markets: United Kingdom*; Espicom Business Intelligence: Chichester, UK, Feb 1999; 17–70.
22. *World Pharmaceutical Markets: Germany*; Espicom Business Intelligence: Chichester, UK, Feb 1999.
23. *World Pharmaceutical Markets: Mexico*; Espicom Business Intelligence: Chichester, UK, Feb 1999.
24. Brudon, P. *The World Drug Situation*; WHO: Geneva, 1988; 7–108.

FURTHER READING

Alexander, T.J. *Internal Markets in the Making: Health Systems in Canada, Iceland, and the UK*; OECDF: Paris, 1995.
Saltman, R.B.; Figueras, J.; Sakellarides, C. *Critical Challenges for Health Care Reform in Europe*; Open University Press: Buckingham, UK, 1999.
Schneider, M.; Dennerien, R.K.; Kose, A.; Scholtes, L. *Health Care in the EC Member States*; Elsevier: Amsterdam, 1992.
Spivey, R.N.; Wertheimer, A.I.; Rucker, T.D. *International Pharmaceutical Services*; Haworth: Binghamton, NY, 1992.
The Use of Essential Drugs: 6th Report of the WHO Expert Committee; WHO: Geneva, 1995.
Van de Water, H.; Van Herten, L.M. *Health Policies on Target*; THO Prevention and Health: Leiden, 1998.

HEALTH CARE SYSTEMS: WITHIN THE UNITED STATES

Henri R. Manasse, Jr.

American Society of Health-System Pharmacists, Bethesda, Maryland

INTRODUCTION

A national health care system reflects the social, political, economic, and cultural character of a nation. A nation's historical roots and dominant values shape policies and directions for the organization, quality, financing, and access to health care services. These factors determine who gets what kind of care—at which locations, for what price, and paid by whom.

The distinctive historical antecedents of American cultural and social development have shaped the present health care system. These contexts have led to a health care system that is uniquely American in character and composition. Although the issues currently facing the American health care system bear some similarity to those in other developed, industrialized nations, many of the factors are unique to the United States.

Social values, that is, the collective societal beliefs about the nature of the human being and the structure of a society, play a strong role in the development of national policies. Political and economic decisions rest in large measure on the prevailing values held in a society. Hence, if a predominant social value rests on the notion that all societal members have a right to health care, political and economic policy developments will follow suit. One way of examining these contexts is to look at a spectrum of social values.

Donabedian (1) has proposed that such a spectrum might be considered from two polar positions: libertarianism versus egalitarianism. Dougherty (2) adds the dimensions of utilitarianism and contractarianism. The essence of these taxonomies of social values is that they characterize specific sets of beliefs and values held by a wide array of individuals.

Libertarian philosophical thought places major emphasis on personal achievement and freedom from political intervention. It holds that individuals should be free to exert their rational capacity to evaluate and determine what is good for them. They can then further act on these determinations for themselves from their own personal, fiscal, physical, and human resources. To this view, Dougherty (2) adds:

Because they can think, persons can understand their circumstances and the alternatives available to them. Because they can choose, persons can act to affirm or change their circumstances. Because they can think and choose, persons are free to create their own life plans and the values of which they are made.

It follows then, that predominant libertarian values are deeply entrenched in the notion of the self-made person and that social rewards should only accrue if they are deserved and earned. The role of government is, therefore, limited to those functions that absolutely do not abridge the rights of the individual to exert his or her own will for what he or she believes to be best. Moreover, government's role would be limited to those functions and needs for which individuals could not provide (national defense, negotiation of treaties, etc.).

Egalitarian principles focus on the equal moral standing of all individuals regardless of achievement or station in life. This philosophy also centers on the right to equal opportunity and to the extent possible, to be free from need and want. Thus, egalitarianism (2) can be viewed as follows:

Practically, this means an equal right to a reasonable share of those basic goods and services known to be necessary for a decent human life, including a right to a job, minimum income support, or provision in kind of the goods necessary for life, as well as a right to a range of social and health care services designed to prevent and minimize psychological and physical suffering, disabilities, and premature death.

Egalitarian values place specific demands on government and political policy to construct broad services and support systems so that all members of society are provided with equal opportunity designed to prevent and minimize psychological and physical suffering and disabilities, and to achieve one's life's aims. In this fashion, government would act on the entitlements due to all members of society. Such entitlements might be derived from legal or other forms of social consensus.

This range of social values from libertarianism to egalitarianism holds differing beliefs about equality, justice, opportunity, rights, and the functional responsibilities of government. When this spectrum of social values is held over health, health care, and the administration and financing of health care services, it is not surprising that a vastly different array of designs emerge. Because health and health care are so tightly wound into personal, cultural, and social beliefs, it is not surprising that such a vast array of health care systems and notions about health have emerged across the world.

America's historical foundations have leaned strongly to the libertarian philosophical viewpoint (3). The influence of the "Protestant ethic" from Europe, coupled with the opportunities that a fresh land provided to "become one's own person," are strongly borne out in American society. An unbridled, free-market economy and freedom from governmental intervention in the daily lives of the citizenry are strong values that have been integrated into the American lifestyle and American political economic thought. The notion of "pulling yourself up by your bootstraps" succinctly reflects these dominant social, political, and economic values. Such antecedents are reliable markers for characterizing America's health care system. Consequently, it is a fascinating mosaic of pluralistic approaches. It is a strongly market-driven, industrialized system, which, at the same time, may be described as one of the world's best and one of the world's most troubled systems.

The United States does not have a universal health insurance program characteristic of many developed nations. Nor does it have national health care services like that of the United Kingdom and other nations. Except for those persons in the United States who possess special legal entitlements, the American health care system is largely a private enterprise; in other words, an industrialized system. The providers, payers, and institutions of care represent a rich mixture of private agents, corporations, insurance systems, and governmental agencies. There is not a singular rationalizing source for setting broad-based national policy and direction for the health care system as a whole. Rather, the vast market place of ideas has a variety of options in order to implement any proposal for which someone will pay. Relman has termed this approach "the industrialization of health care" (4).

The role of the national and state governments in the health care system is limited to those entitlement programs that have been legislated into federal or state law or where there is a federal and state partnership. Federal involvement in the provision of health care services began with the U.S. Public Health Service (PHS), an agency of the U.S. government. The PHS was established in 1798 to provide essential health care services to merchant marine personnel and members of the U.S. armed forces. Subsequent federal involvement in the provision of and the payment for health care has incrementally increased to include care for individuals with special entitlements. The latter include veterans of the armed forces, the elderly, indigent people, Native Americans, persons with HIV/AIDS, certain disabled individuals, and qualifying persons with end-stage renal disease. For example, qualified veterans of the armed forces have access to a federal system of hospitals, clinics, and long-term care facilities under the Department of Veterans Affairs (a cabinet-level agency of the executive branch of the federal government). Since 1965, the federal government sponsors Medicare, a health insurance program for the elderly (65 years of age and over and later the disabled). The federal government also cost-shares with participating state governments to provide the Medicaid program (also enacted in 1965). The latter is an insurance program for health services directed toward qualifying indigent people. In Medicare and Medicaid, institutional and individual providers participate as contractors under a set of specific conditions for participation.

State and local (city and county) governments have limited roles in the provision of health care services. State, county, and city health departments are as differently organized and functioning, as there are states, counties, and cities in the United States. These agencies reflect and represent the special needs of the geographic areas and demographic compositions of their respective domains. Hence, the functioning and expanse of services offered by the New York City Department of Health is vastly different from a similar agency in rural Montana.

This unique approach to the application of a health care system must also be examined in light of the diversity of the demography and geography of the United States. Approximately 273 million people inhabit the United States across a geographic expanse of 3.5 million square miles of land. Ranging from the deserts of Nevada to the Rocky Mountains of Colorado and Wyoming to the tropics of Florida and the oceanic seaboards of the east, west, and southern coasts, American geography and topography is expansive (5). Hence, a substantial challenge to the delivery of health care services exists in this array of geographical areas.

The American population is equally diverse and expansive. There are almost 35 million people who are age 65 or older. African Americans constitute 12.8% of the population, Asian and Pacific Islanders 4%, American Indians 0.9%, and Caucasians make up 82% of the population (5). Because the United States is largely a nation of immigrants, there are literally hundreds of additional ethnic groups that are part of the American social fabric. As of March 1997, 25.8 million individuals in the United States were foreign-born, which represents a 30% increase from 1990, when there were 19.8 million foreign-born individuals in the United States. Mexico was the place of origin for 7 million or 28% of the total foreign born population in 1997 (5). During 1996 and 1997, 1.3 million people moved to the United States from abroad, and 92% of those individuals moved to metropolitan areas. Additionally, during this time period, 3 million people left the central cities and 2.8 million moved to the suburbs (6). The health care system of the United States should then be viewed in the following context:

- A diverse spectrum of social values, which have historically pointed more toward libertarianism than egalitarianism
- Limited roles of the federal, state, and local governments in the provision of, and payment for, health care services
- A pluralistic, free-market approach to the provision of health care services
- A geographically diverse and substantive land mass
- A culturally diverse and numerically large population whose characteristics are changing toward more elderly and racial and ethnic heterogeneity

It is critical that the reader be sensitive to these contextual variables to understand the American health care system and how health care policy is shaped and implemented in the United States.

THE ORGANIZATION OF U.S. HEALTH CARE SERVICES

Health care services in the United States are provided by a broad array of facilities, which are financed from a variety of payment sources. As of 1998, there were 6021 hospitals (7), 1,012,582 hospital beds, 33,765,940 admissions, and 241,574,380 inpatient days. In 1998, the average length of stay in community hospitals was 6 days, whereas it was 7.7 days in 1975 (7).

It is also notable that the numbers of hospitals in urban and rural settings are shrinking. In 1993, there were 3012 urban hospitals and 2249 rural, whereas in 1998, there were 2816 urban and 2199 rural hospitals (13). The numbers of public acute care hospitals decreased from 1390 in 1993 to 1260 in 1997 (8). Closure of hospitals and simultaneous reductions in hospital beds has occurred in inner city areas where care is provided for large numbers of indigent patients. Such closures are related to the high costs of care, which are not concomitantly reimbursed by state and federal sources

either because the individuals are not eligible or because payment rates do not cover the costs incurred. Small, isolated rural hospitals are facing similar economic and, hence, survival difficulties. The plight of rural hospitals is of special significance because their survival is often linked to the economic and social survival of a rural community.

While the world's population grows at an annual rate of 1.7%, the population over 65 increases by 2.5% per year. There are just fewer than 600 million people over the age of 60 in the world. Approximately 360 million of the world's over 60 population lives in the developing world, in which 7.5% of the population is elderly. In contrast, 18.3% of the population is elderly in the developed world. The most rapid changes are occurring in some developing countries where an increase of 200–400% in the elderly population is predicted over the next 30 years (9). Because of the growth of the elderly population, there has been an increase in the demand for geriatric and long-term care facilities. Over the next several decades, the elderly's health care consumption in the United States will be approximately $25,000 per person (in 1995 dollars) compared to $9200 in 1995 (10). In this respect, the United States is following the trends exhibited in most developed industrialized countries.

The increased utilization of health care services by the elderly is expected to put additional strains on an already besieged health care system. Increasing the life span, either through preventive measures or through other acts of distributive justice, solves some problems while creating others. This astounding paradox will assuredly complicate the political and social processes of decision making. Equally likely will be the burdens these phenomena add to an already overburdened national economy.

In the last several years, it is the substitutability that has been emphasized, as more and more procedures are performed in outpatient settings. Many services previously performed in the hospital now take place in physician offices. In 1996, there were 734,493,000 visits to the physician, with an average of 3.4 per person (11), and the most frequent principal reason for a visit was a general medical examination, with a total of 54.7 million in 1996. Also in 1996, there were 67.2 million visits to outpatient departments, and 40.3 million inpatient surgery procedures were performed (11). This analysis points to the increasing importance of the ambulatory care setting as a place for rendering care. The relevance of outpatient care will continue to grow as more medical procedures are performed outside hospitals and greater emphasis is placed on preventive care. Outpatient visits in community hospitals alone have advanced from 263,631,000 in 1986 to 301,329,000 in 1990 to 474,193,000 in 1998 (7).

The National Association of Home Care estimates that more than 20,000 providers deliver home care services to approximately 8 million individuals each year (12). According to the Health Care Financing Administration (HCFA), the average number of home health visits a year per Medicaid beneficiary was 80, compared to 27 visits in 1989. Additionally, the number of home health agencies participating in Medicare has increased from almost 5000 in 1988 to over 10,000 in 1997 (13). Care of patients in home settings is likely to expand as data further suggest reduced cost for such care without compromising quality. Technological and scientific developments related to providing sophisticated treatments in the home will also stimulate growth in this sector of health services.

TRENDS IN HEALTH INSURANCE COVERAGE

According to the President's Advisory Commission on Consumer Protection and Quality in the Health Care Industry, there are five trends that summarize the characteristics of health insurance plans of the late 1990s:

- Increased complexity and concentration of health plans
- Increased diversity of health insurance products
- Increased focus on network-based delivery
- Shifting financial structures and incentives between purchasers, health plans, and providers
- The development of clinical infrastructure for utilization management and quality improvement (14)

In response to rapidly increasing health care costs, private insurance companies and employers (who pay the premiums in whole or in part for their employees) have increased their part in implementing cost-containment strategies. A dramatic effort has been the application of business principles to purchasing and vendor selection and payment for and selection of health care providers and institutions of care.

Private employers, the federal government, and state and local governments invest significant financial resources in health care purchasing expenditures. In 1995, private employers contributed $183.8 billion to private health insurance premiums, whereas the federal government spent $11.3 billion on private health insurance premiums, and state and local government spent $47.1 billion (14). In 1995, more than 83% of the insured population was covered by private insurance, whereas about 31% was enrolled in a public program, such as Medicare or Medicaid.

Probably the most significant change in the American health care system in recent years is the development of managed care. In managed care settings, the covering company is responsible for providing services, whereas, at the same time, it is exposed to the financial risks of unanticipated services. Health Maintenance Organizations (HMOs) contract with hospitals and certain physician providers for services within a negotiated schedule of fees. HMOs and other such managed care organizations specify where and by whom care is to be given. The latter is a radical departure from the historically preeminent "freedom of choice" that patients and care providers enjoyed under the traditional indemnity and fee-for-service reimbursement programs. The traditional method of paying for medical services is fee-for-service when the provider charges a fee for each service provided, and the insurer pays all or part of that fee.

Managed care is an umbrella term for HMOs and all health plans that provide health care in return for preset monthly payments and coordinate care in a defined network of primary care physicians and hospitals. A network includes physicians, clinics, health centers, medical group practices, hospitals, and other providers that a health plan selects and contracts with to care for its members. An HMO is an organization that provides health care in return for preset monthly payments. Most HMOs provide care through a network of physicians, hospitals, and other medical professionals that their members must use in order to be covered for that care.

There are a number of different types of HMOs. A staff model HMO is an HMO in which the physicians and other medical professionals are salaried employees, and the clinics or health centers in which they practice are owned by the HMO. A group model HMO is made up of one or more physician group practices that are not owned by the HMO but operate as independent partnerships or professional corporations. The HMO pays the groups at a negotiated rate, and each group is responsible for paying its doctors and other staff as well as covering the cost of hospital care or care from outside specialists. An Independent Practice Association (IPA) generally includes large numbers of individual private practice physicians who are paid either a fee or a fixed amount per patient to take care of the IPA's members. A Preferred Provider Organization is a network of doctors and hospitals that provides care at a lower cost than through traditional insurance. PPO members have more health coverage when they use the PPO's network and pay higher out-of-pocket costs when they receive care outside the PPO network (15).

An integrated health system is a network that provides a coordinated continuum of services and is clinically and fiscally accountable for outcomes. There was a significant growth of integrated health systems during the late 1990s. In 1997, there were 228 integrated systems and, in 1998, there were 266, representing an increase of almost 17% (16). Simultaneously, there has been a disintegration of systems when mergers fail and disassemble. Iglehart comments on how managed care has changed the face of health care:

> Before the emergence of managed care, it was largely physicians, acting individually on behalf of their patients, who decided how most health care dollars were spent. They billed for their services, and third-party insurers usually reimbursed them without asking any questions, because the ultimate payers—employers—demanded no greater accounting. Now, many employers have changed from passive payers to aggressive purchasers and are exerting more influence on payment rates, on where patients are cared for, and on the content of care. Through selective contracting with physicians, stringent review of the use of services, practice protocols, and payment on a fixed, per capita basis, managed-care plans have pressured doctors to furnish fewer services and to improve the coordination and management of care, thereby altering the way in which many physicians treat patients. In striving to balance the conflicts that arise in caring for patients within these constraints, physicians have become "double agents." The ideological tie that long linked many physicians and private executives—a belief in capitalism and free enterprise—has been weakened by the aggressive intervention of business into the practice of medicine through managed care (17).

There has been a recent challenge to the core tenet of managed care that centralized decision making could deliver improved care at a reduced cost. In November 1999, a large health care company decided to allow physicians to choose what care patients need without the insurance company's intervention or approval. This action opens the door to further discussions about how managed care principles are utilized. Regardless of managed care's future course, cost containment measures will be necessary to prevent an explosion of health care costs. The demand for cost containment will need to be weighed against the imperative to insure that patients have access to care. Paul Ellwood, often referred to as the "father of the HMO," believes that there will be a new era in which patients, not employers and government purchasers, will have power (18). Regardless, the weight of political and consumer pressures, along with experience and economic efficiency, will determine the future of managed care.

HEALTH CARE FINANCING

The expenditures for health care in the United States have grown from $51 billion in 1967 (6.3% of GNP) to over $1 trillion in 1997 (14% of GDP).[a] In 1997, on a per capita basis, $4090 was spent on health care (19) and 0.64 per day/capita was spent on prescription drugs (20). This is substantially higher than that of other industrialized nations. When comparing health expenditures in the major industrialized countries comprising the Organization for Economic Cooperation and Development (OECD), for example, dramatic differences in per capita expenditures are noted (21). Such differences also exist in the percentage share of GDP spent on health care (21), and relative growth in health care expenditures over time varies greatly among these countries (21, 22).

The Health Care Finance Administration asserts that national health expenditures are projected to total $2.2 trillion and reach 16.2% of the GDP by 2008. The growth in health spending is projected to average 1.8 percentage points above the growth rate of the GDP for 1998–2008. This differential is higher than recent experience but remains below the historical average for 1960–1997, where growth in health spending exceeded growth in GDP by close to three percentage points. There are a number of factors that contribute to the projected acceleration, including:

- An increase in private health insurance underwriting cycle
- A slower growth in managed care enrollment
- A movement towards less restrictive forms of managed care
- A continued trend toward increased state and federal regulation of health plans

The growth of health care expenditures without a concomitant gain in health status of the population is receiving more and more attention on the governmental and corporate agenda. On the governmental level, an increasing proportion of federal and state budgets is being allocated to health care. In the private sector, corporations and individuals are bearing larger proportions of health care costs. Although no particular percentage of GDP has been determined to be an acceptable or unacceptable expenditure for health care services, the fact is that costs are increasing and the health care sector is gaining an increasing share of the economy. This follows several other interesting trends. During the period of 1961 to 1997,

---

[a] The GNP is the total annual flow of goods and services in a nation's economy. Most industrial countries now use GDP, which measures the value of all goods and services produced within a nation, regardless of the nationality of the procedure.

national health expenditures as a percentage of GNP rose from 5.4% to over 14%. In the same period, dramatic differences occurred in the source of revenues for health care expenditures. The pattern of spending these resources also changed significantly (13).

In 1960, 49% of health care revenues came from out-of-pocket payments from individuals. Out-of-pocket spending is defined as expenditures for coinsurance and deductibles required by insurers, as well as direct payments for services, which are covered by a third party. In 1990, individual consumers spent $144.4 billion directly for out-of-pocket payments for personal health services (23). This accounted for 38% of all personal health spending. In 1998, consumers spent $183.7 billion in out-of-pocket payments, which accounts for 33% of the $558.7 billion in personal health spending (23).

Consumers have spent and continue to spend less of their own personal money for health care services. This decrease in personal spending has been shifted largely to third parties, such as private health insurance, government programs, philanthropic organizations, and other sources. It is evident that the shift away from personal, out-of-pocket health spending has resulted in greater consumption of health care services. This transition reflects the general maxim in health care economics that the consumption of health care services is probably insatiable (24). Moreover, unlike other sectors of the economy and the laws of economics they obey, prices for health care services do not fall with increased consumption or purchasing.

According to Iglehart, the decline in personal spending is "attributed in large part to the growth in health maintenance organizations (HMOs), which traditionally offer broad benefits with only modest out-of-pocket payments. In the past few years, however, most HMO enrollees have had increased cost-sharing requirements, as employers and health plan managers have sought to constrain spending even further. Out-of-pocket payments are still considerably less in an HMO than with indemnity insurance (17)." However, "The overall declines in per capita out-of-pocket spending mask the financial difficulties of many poor people and families. A recent study estimated that Medicare beneficiaries over 65 years of age with incomes below the federal poverty level (in 1997 the level was $7755 for individuals and $9780 for couples) who were also eligible for Medicaid assistance still spent 35% of their incomes on out-of-pocket health care costs. Medicare beneficiaries with incomes below the federal poverty level who did not receive Medicaid assistance spent, on average, half their incomes on out-of-pocket health care costs (17)."

Historically, a lack of public insurance programs created obstacles to health care services. For those who could not afford to pay for private insurance, the costs associated with health care were larger than most could afford. After lengthy debate, the U.S. Congress passed legislation in 1965 that established Medicare and Medicaid. Medicare covers over 95% of the elderly in the United States as well as many individuals who are disabled. Coverage for the disabled began in 1973 and is divided in two parts: 1) hospital insurance and 2) supplementary medical insurance. The total disbursement for Medicare in 1997 was $213.575 billion, and there were 36,460,143 enrollees, of which 32,164,416 were elderly.

The total expenditure for the Medicaid program was $160 billion in 1996. Of the total amount spent in 1996, Medicaid payments for nursing facilities and home health care totaled $40.5 billion for more than 3.6 million recipients. The average cost per recipient in 1996 was $12,300, and almost 45% of the total cost of care for individuals using nursing homes and Medicaid was paid for home health care (13).

Since the enactment of Medicare and Medicaid, there have been various legislative and administrative changes. The Balanced Budget Act of 1997 enacted the most significant changes to Medicare and Medicaid since its inception, including a capped allocation of monetary resources to states and the addition of the Children's Health Insurance Program. The Children's Health Insurance Program set aside $24 billion over 5 years for states to provide health care to over 10 million children who are not eligible for Medicaid.

In 1960, public programs paid for one quarter (24.5%) of all health care spending; by 1988, this share had increased to 42.1%. Together Medicare and Medicaid financed $351 billion in health care services in 1996, which is more than one-third of the nation's total health care bill. Additionally, it represents three-quarters of all public spending on health care. There has been a significant increase in Medicare managed care enrollment—from 3.1 million at the end of 1995 to 6.3 million in 1999, leaving approximately 33 million beneficiaries in a traditional fee-for-service Medicare program.

An area of controversy is the limitation on coverage for prescription drugs. Spending on prescription drugs is the fastest-growing piece of personal health expenditures, amounting to $78.9 billion in 1997. Additionally, spending for prescription drugs has increased at double-digit rates: 10.6% in 1995, 13.2% in 1996, and 14.1% in 1997 (17). The reason for this rapid growth, according to Iglehart, includes: "Broader insurance coverage of prescription drugs, growth in the number of drugs dispensed, more approvals of expensive new drugs by the Food and Drug Administration, and direct advertising of pharmaceutical products to consumers. The use of some new drugs reduces hospital costs, but not enough to offset the increase in expenditures for drugs (17)." In the year 2000, 86% of health care plans will have an annual limit on brand and generic drugs, and there will be increased use of copayments for prescription drugs (25).

The budget cuts imposed by Congress in 1997 to help balance the budget have restricted the fees that caregivers receive for the elderly and disabled. When federal health programs cut funding significantly, as occurred in the Balanced Budget Act of 1997, the resulting cutbacks at the institutional and health-system level trickled down to providers' abilities to provide an acceptable level of service designed to protect patient safety and foster appropriate medication use. Partial restoration of the Balanced Budget Act in 1999 addressed the transition to an outpatient prospective payment system for hospitals, payments to skilled nursing facilities and home health agencies, payments for indirect medical education, and a number of rural health care provisions.

The dramatic shift of third parties (government, private health insurance) toward paying for a greater and greater proportion of personal health care services has led to a paradigm shift in attitudes and actions toward health care financing and cost control. Several approaches have been adopted in the governmental sector to slow the increases in costs and expenditures. The most dramatic of these has been the introduction in 1983 of the prospective payment system (PPS) to curb the growth in hospital costs and expenditures. By imposing prospective limits on Medicare payments to hospitals through a system of reimbursing average costs of specific diagnoses, hospital utilization has decreased dramatically. The average length of stay and admission rates in community hospitals of elderly patients (those covered by Medicare) dropped sharply after the introduction of PPS (13).

Because of cost-containment strategies of both the private and governmental sectors, hospital utilization has declined. This has resulted in a decline in the number of patient beds, the average length of stay, and patient bed census (7). The present predominant view is that hospitalization of any patient, regardless of revenue source, is to be avoided wherever possible. Only those patients for whom hospitalization can be fully justified are admitted.

As much as the financing of America's health care system is a major issue on the policy agenda of the nation, so too is the continuous question about the relationship between the costs and the outcomes of care. As costs increase, the numbers of policy analysts, organizations, and governmental agencies calling for a better definition of the cost-outcome relationship has sharply risen.

Cost-effectiveness and cost-benefit analyses are frequently mentioned in academic and policy-analysis circles. These notions center on careful examination of the costs and their corresponding outputs. Eisenberg (26) defines cost-effectiveness analysis as the measure of the net cost of providing service (expenditures minus savings) as well as the results obtained (e.g., clinical results measured singly or a series of results measured on some scale). Cost–benefit analysis determines whether the cost is worth the benefits by measuring both in the same units (26). Such analyses will be critical, as future policy decisions are made with regard to the collection, allocation, and utilization of finite resources in the health care system for the enhancement of health status of the American people.

Private-sector strategies and governmental plans to curb health care costs have not escaped criticism. Ginsberg, for example, argues that the notion of "for profit" hospital chains has severe limitations with respect to garnering large proportions of market share and, consequently, greater profits (27). He bases this view on the limited amount of private funding available for hospital care. On the other hand, he sees this sector as being able to grow in the area of nursing homes and other businesses related to the care of the elderly.

ACCESS TO HEALTH CARE SERVICES IN THE UNITED STATES

There are three classes of individuals who have open access to and can derive some form of services from America's health care system:

- Those who receive support from governmental sources because of specific entitlements (indigents, elderly, and veterans)
- Those who are provided with basic health insurance coverage from their employers
- Those who choose to cover their expenses from out-of-pocket payments

There are, however, those who have no specific financial support or capacity to pay for health care services and who are not eligible for any type of entitlements. These individuals must rely on some form of charity care or services. In addition, there are those who, for reasons of geographic remoteness or total inability to gain access, have no access to health care services. This group represents a complex, resource-based demand model, which also has an equally complex pattern of health care system and services-utilization requirements.

With increasing health care costs and consequent increases in insurance premium costs, gaining access to health care services without incurring personal costs has become more difficult. Not all services are covered for individuals in the federal Medicare and Medicaid programs. Moreover, there are strict limitations on the extent of services offered in these programs. A similar set of restrictions may be found in private-sector health care coverage strategies. Because few insurance programs and none of the federal programs provide coverage for unlimited long-term care, all but the very rich are at risk of financial ruin.

The health care lexicon includes two new terms to reflect these problems: underinsured and uninsured. The underinsured may include the "working poor," those individuals who have jobs and may be covered by a very limited, if any, health insurance program by their employers. They are likely low wage earners and those receiving incomes at, or slightly above, the poverty level. Typically, they do not qualify for Medicaid entitlements, do not have employer-paid health insurance benefits, and cannot afford (or choose not to purchase) third-party coverage for payment of health care services.

There are no specific policy plans available to finance uninsured and underinsured care. Whether planned as charity care or unplanned as financial loss, the "price tag" for uncompensated care in the United States was $18.5 billion in 1997, which is 6% of the total of hospital expenses (28). This percentage has remained constant since 1984, when the percentage of total expenses for uncompensated care was also 6% (8).

Reduced payments and high levels of uncompensated care have led to the closing of hospital facilities in both urban and rural blighted areas, making access to care even more difficult for some. Whiteis and Salmon (29) refer to this phenomenon as "disinvestment in the public goods." Because privately owned and not-for-profit hospitals and private clinics, pharmacies, and physician's offices must rely on their own financial soundness, any threat to that foundation may lead to closure.

The amount of uncompensated care is magnified in areas where serious social problems exist because health status is directly related to social status. Health status should be examined in broad terms by reviewing morbidity and mortality data available for the whole population. The life expectancy of people who live in the United States has grown by almost 10 years, from 68.5 years in 1936 to 76.1 years in 1996. Women were expected to live to 79.1 years in 1996, whereas the average for men was 73.1 years (11). The leading causes of death in 1996 among people living in the United States were (11):

1. Heart disease (733,361 deaths)
2. Cancer (539,533 deaths)
3. Stroke (169,942 deaths)
4. Pulmonary diseases (108,027 deaths)
5. Accidents (94,948 deaths)
6. Pneumonia and flu (63,727 deaths)
7. Diabetes (61,787 deaths)
8. AIDS (31,130 deaths)
9. Suicide (30,903 deaths)
10. Liver disease (25,047 deaths)

Infant mortality, another measure of the health status of a nation, stated as the number of deaths per live births, was 7.2 per 1000 live births in 1997 compared to 9.9 per 1000 live births for 1988. Overall, these figures are comparable to those of the major, industrialized nations of the world.

Major morbidity in the United States is currently centered on diseases of life style. These morbidities contrast sharply with disease patterns prevalent during the early part of the 20th century. Outside of AIDS and other sexually transmitted diseases, infectious diseases represent a small proportion of prevalent morbidity. Rather, life-style diseases, associated with smoking, poor nutrition, a sedentary life style, alcohol and other chemical consumption, homicides, suicides, and accidents, represent the majority of morbidity in the United States. Significant preventive strategies can markedly reduce the incidence, prevalence, and mortality associated with these health care problems.

Not surprising, in areas with high concentrations of indigent people, there are similarly high concentrations of uninsured individuals requiring intense health care services. These areas exist in both rural and urban settings. Emergency rooms have become a major resource for primary health care services in areas where physician office services or other service providers (clinics) are not available because of location, cost, or quality. Emergency rooms have also become providers of high-intensity care for victims of gun shot wounds, drug overdoses, communicable diseases, and other trauma associated with poor social conditions. Much of the care in emergency rooms is uncompensated because the quality and amount exceed the allowable reimbursement. Some trauma centers in economically blighted areas have been closed (30).

Hospitals in inner cities and blighted rural areas also care for a higher proportion of "at-risk" patients than hospitals in the for-profit sector generally located in more affluent areas (29). In fact, affluent hospitals sometimes "dump" their uncovered patients on charity care and other public hospitals in order to reduce their financial risks. This, however, increases the financial risks of public or charity hospitals. Again, the reimbursement levels under present schemes for large numbers of "at-risk" patients simply do not cover costs; thus, the United States has witnessed hospital closings, particularly in those areas where such loss is most noticeable (30).

American health policy continues to grapple with these issues related to the underinsured and the uninsured (31). A multiple-tiered health care system based on social class and ability to pay is unacceptable in a nation that boasts incomparable riches and political agendas of democracy and rights. Ginsberg (27) notes:

> Despite all our efforts of recent years, then, health care costs continue to increase.... There is undoubtedly waste in the health care system, but no solid proposals have been advanced to recapture the $100 billion, plus or minus, that some believe can be saved. I believe that we will not reshape our national health policy agenda unless and until we achieve a broad consensus on the key issues. Do the American people, for example, desire to ensure access to health care for the entire population? In that case they must agree to pick up a sizable additional tab, which they have thus far avoided.

The issue of quality health care has become an increasing issue of concern in the face of cost constraints and limited access to health care. The *President's Advisory Commission on Consumer Protection and Quality in the Health Care Industry* (32) states that "the purpose of the health care system must be to continuously reduce the impact and burden of illness, injury and disability and to improve the health and functioning of the people of the U.S." According to the Commission, there are basic characteristics of health care that, as a nation, we should strive to achieve. The Commission has created "Guiding Principles for the Consumer Bill of Rights and Responsibilities" for the health care of people in the United States. These include the following:

- All consumers are created equal.
- Quality comes first.
- Preserve what works.
- Costs matter.

THE FUTURE OF HEALTH CARE

Suggestions for broad reform, which address the financial, access, and quality of care issues for America's health care system, have emerged during the past decade. Iglehart emphasizes the irony of the American health care system. He writes (17):

> By many technical standards, U.S. medical care is the best in the world, but leaders in the field declared

recently at a national round table that there is an "urgent need to improve health care quality." The stringency of managed care and a low inflation rate have slowed the growth of medical spending appreciably, but a new government study projects that health care expenditures will soon begin escalating again and will double over the next decade. In short, the American system is a work in progress, driven by a disparate array of interests with two goals that are often in conflict: providing health care to the sick, and generating income for the persons and organizations that assume the financial risk.

The President's Commission (32) outlines areas in which the American health care system could be improved in light of the reality that many individuals receive substandard care and 44.3 million individuals are without health insurance coverage. This commission outlines several types of quality problems including avoidable errors, underutilization of services, overuse of services, and variation in services. Based on the reality of these quality problems, the Commission recommended that the initial set of national aims should include (32):

- Reducing the underlying causes of illness, injury and disability
- Expanding research on new treatments and evidence on effectiveness
- Ensuring the appropriate use of health care services
- Reducing health care errors
- Addressing oversupply and undersupply of health care resources
- Increasing a patient's participation in his or her care

The President's Commission engages a broad consumer advocacy movement in public and private sectors calling for a major reform of the U.S. health care system to improve access to care for more individuals living in America. Consistent with previous patterns, however, these calls have only led to incremental adjustments in policy and slight quality changes in direction. The major problems, for the most part, remain unaffected. Although broad based health care reform efforts have been unsuccessful, market forces and more targeted legislation and regulatory efforts have changed the face of health in the 1990s.

The 1993–94 Clinton health care reform plan, in its ideology, provided an ambitious plan to eliminate the enormous problem of lack of access to health care. It proposed to guarantee comprehensive health benefits for all American citizens and legal residents, regardless of health or employment status. The proposal was unsuccessful due to a number of factors, including its vast scope, the complicated nature of the plan, and an underestimation of the politics involved with radically reforming health care. The failure of the Clinton administration health care reform agenda and the subsequent events to revise the American health care system are important lessons of health-care-system related politics.

Unfortunately, since the failure of the Clinton Administration plan in 1994, the number of uninsured individuals in America has grown. According to the Census Bureau, 44.3 million people are uninsured, comprising about 16.3% of the population. Of those uninsured, 15.4% are under 18 years of age, and the largest percentage is among individuals between 18 and 24 years of age. People of Hispanic origin make up 35.3% of those uninsured and 43% of the total uninsured population are not citizens of the United States (6).

The number of uninsured persons is expected to continue to grow. Proposals for health care reform to combat this problem include President Clinton's proposal for Medicare buy-in proposals for "middle aged" adults and House Majority Leader Dick Armey's (R-TX) proposal for a refundable tax credit to pay for insurance for the uninsured. The 2000 presidential campaign opened the debate for legislation that will improve health care coverage for the uninsured. This public debate on how to enhance access to care will stimulate creative ways to improve the U.S. health care system. However, rhetoric is not enough; it needs to be translated into programs that attack the problem.

The essence of the health care financing dilemma is related to how much a nation wishes to spend, on whom these funds are to be expended, and by what methods a relationship among cost, quality, and outcomes might be determined. In a time when advancing science and technology is flourishing in the health care field, "high tech" medicine will continue to evolve with an ever-increasing price tag. Furthermore, the costs of unanticipated and complex disease problems (e.g., HIV/AIDS) add to the unpredictability of health care system costs. This is all to say that most policy makers understand what needs to be done. They are in a quandary, however, in finding the appropriate and acceptable solution. Hence, it is likely that costs and expenditures will continue to rise (and, thereby, increase the percentage of GNP that will be spent for health care) and that solutions may become even more elusive.

Although some might argue that the available resources for expenditures on health care are ultimately limited, few are able to say exactly where that limit is or should be. In the United States, there has been an expansion of technologies and procedures based on scientific advancements without a concomitant development of a moral and ethical policy for determining who might be best served by such advancements. Rationing of health care services or otherwise limiting access to high cost services, for example, has resulted from political policy rather than from deliberated public policy and rational decision making. This is most notably evidenced in the Medicaid component of the U.S. health care system.

As cost pressures continue to mount, there will likely be a return to having patients pay more of the health care expenditure dollar from their own resources. This will take the form of higher deductibles and co-insurance payments. Perhaps returning the burden of health care financing to the individual will raise the collective consciousness of American society that "there is no such thing as a free lunch" insofar as using and paying for health care services is concerned. Certainly, this phenomenon has occurred in social welfare "reform" in which the programs that have had mixed success have been restructured to "roll" participants off of welfare to work.

On the other hand, there are perhaps no solutions forthcoming on some of the problems represented in the arena of health care financing. As Hardin suggests, there is indeed a class of human problems that have no technical solution (33). In using Hardin's analogies, Hiatt (34) suggests that "nobody would quarrel with the proposition that there is a limit to the resources any society can devote to medical care, and few would question the suggestion that we are approaching such a limit. The dilemma confronting us is how we can place additional stress on the medical commons without bringing ourselves closer to ruin."

CONCLUSION

These are the principal contemporary features of the U.S. health care system. A massive societal structure is at once saviour, behemoth, juggernaut, and question mark. It certainly will be in a constant state of flux and gradual change. It therefore bears constant vigilance and careful guidance by those who derive their livelihoods from it and those who are the beneficiaries of its caring. Most importantly, it will require significant pressure from those who are disenfranchised from it.

REFERENCES

1. Donabedian, A. *Aspects of Medical Care Administration: Specifying Requirements for Health Care*; Harvard University Press: Cambridge, 1973.
2. Dougherty, C.J. *American Health Care: Realities, Rights, and Reforms*; Oxford University Press: New York, 1998.

3. Bella, R.N.; Madsen, R.; Sullivan, W.M.; Swidler, A.; Tipton, S.M. *Habits of the Heart*; Harper & Row: New York, 1985.
4. Relman, A. Reforming the Health Care System. New Engl. J. Med. **1990**, *323* (14), 991–992.
5. www.census.gov (accessed Oct 1999).
6. www.doc.gov (accessed Oct 1999).
7. *American Hospital Association, Hospital Statistics*, Health Forum: Chicago, IL, 2000.
8. *Modern Healthcare*, By the Numbers 1999 Edition (Supplement to Modern Healthcare), July 19, 1999.
9. www.who.gov (accessed Nov 1999).
10. Fuchs, V.R. Health Care for the Elderly: How Much? Who Will Pay for it? Health Aff. **1999**, *18* (1), 11–21.
11. www.cdc.gov/nchs (accessed Oct 1999).
12. www.nahc.org (accessed Dec 1999).
13. www.hcfa.gov (accessed Dec 1999).
14. Quality First: Better Health Care for all Americans. *The President's Advisory Commission on Consumer Protection and Quality in the Health Care Industry*, 45.
15. www.NCQA.org (accessed Oct 1999).
16. Landis, N. Am. J. Health Syst. Pharm. **1999**, *56*, 1392.
17. Iglehart, J. The American Health Care System: Expenditures. New Engl. J. Med. **1999**, *340* (1).
18. New Health Care Model Balances Cost, Quality, Shifts Power to Patients. PR news wire. Nov. 1999.
19. www.hcfa.gov (accessed Oct 1999).
20. www.bea.doc.gov (accessed Oct 1999).
21. Schieber, G.J. Health Expenditures in Major Industrialized Countries, 1960-87. Health Center Financing Review **1990**, *11* (4), 159–167.
22. www.phrma.org (accessed Oct. 1999).
23. Smith, S.; Freeland, M.; Heffler, S.; McKusick, D. Health Tracking: Trends. Health Aff. **1998**, *17* (5), 128–140.
24. Klarman, H.E. *The Economics of Health*; Columbia University Press: New York, 1965.
25. www.hcfa.org (accessed Oct. 1999). Medicare + Choice: Changes for the Year 2000 Executive Summary.
26. Eisenberg, J.M. Clinical Economics: A Guide to the Economic Analysis of Clinical Practice. JAMA **1989**, *262*, 2879–2886.
27. Ginsberg, E.N. For Profit Medicine: A Reassesment. New Engl. J. Medicine **1988**, *319* (12), 757–761.
28. www.aha.org (accessed Nov 1999).
29. Whiteis, D.G.; Salmon, J.W. *The Corporate Transfer of Health Care*; Baywood Publishing Company: Amityville NY, 1990.
30. Christianson, J.B. Institutional Alternatives to the Rural Hospital. Health Care Financing Review **1990**, *11* (3), 87–97.
31. McLennan, K. Care and Cost. *Current Issues in Health Policy*; Westview Press: Boulder CO, 1989.
32. Quality First: Better Health Care for all Americans, The President's Advisory Commission on Consumer Protection and Quality in the Health Care Industry.
33. Hardin, G. The Tragedy of the Commons. Science **1968**, *162*, 1243–1248.
34. Hiatt, H.H. Protecting the Medical Commons: Who is Responsible. NEJM **1975**, *293*, 235–241.
35. Quality First: Better Health Care for All Americans, Final Report to the President of the United States. The President's Advisory Commission on Consumer Protection and Quality in the Health Care Industry.
36. To Err is Human: Building a Safer Health System, Institute of Medicine. National Academy of Sciences, 1999.
37. Kronick, R.; Todd, G. Explaining the Decline in Health Insurance Coverage, 1979–1995. Health Aff. **Mar/April, 1999**, 30–47.
38. Merrill, R.A. Modernizing the FDA. *An Incremental Revolution. Health Affairs*, Mar/April, 1999; 96–111.
39. Robinson, J.C. *The Future of Managed Care Organization. Health Affairs*, Mar/April, 1999; 7–24.
40. Grunback, K. Primary Care in the United States—The Best of Times, The Worst of Times. New Engl. J. Med. **1999**, *341* (26).
41. Smith, B.M. Trends in Health Care Coverage and Financing and their Implications for Policy. New Engl. J. Med. **1997**, *337* (14).
42. Vladeck, B.C. *The Political Economy of Medicare. Health Affairs*, Jan/Feb, 1999; 22–36.

HISTORY OF DOSAGE FORMS AND BASIC PREPARATIONS

Robert A. Buerki
The Ohio State University College of Pharmacy, Columbus, Ohio

Gregory J. Higby
American Institute of the History of Pharmacy, Madison, Wisconsin

INTRODUCTION

The creation and manufacture of dosage forms has been at the center of pharmacy practice for the past thousand years. For American pharmacists of the nineteenth century, *secundem artem*, or the acronym "S.A." in physicians' prescriptions, instructed them to use their special skills "according to the art" of their profession to compound a medicine; it was out of this art, rather than science, that almost all of today's major dosage forms arose. Tablets, capsules, injectables, and oral solutions were all known to pharmacists and physicians a century ago. In addition, there were scores of specialized dosage forms that attempted to meet the medical needs of patients, even if the drugs administered in these doses were ineffective or designed to treat symptoms rather than the underlying disease. The origins of most of these dosage forms are lost in history. For this reason, the authors have elected to forego a contrived narrative tying together the few facts at hand with an equally large amount of speculation about the history of dosage forms. Rather, we have assembled a glossary of terms used in orthodox Western medicine to describe both common and unusual modes of drug administration.

For most of its history, the field of pharmacy was much more concerned with drug preparations than with the resulting dosage forms. Up to the sixteenth century, almost all drugs were derived from plants and were made into preparations that served as the ingredients for medicines; these preparations were called *galenicals*, after the great central figure of Western therapeutics, Claudius Galen of Pergamon (131–201). Strictly speaking, galenicals are pharmaceutical preparations obtained by macerating or percolating crude drugs with alcohol or some other menstruum to remove only the desired principles and leave the inert constituents undissolved. Examples of galenicals include decoctions, extracts, fluidextracts, fluidglycerates, infused oils, infusions, oleoresins, resins, tinctures, and vinegars. The term is used very loosely today to designate any type of simple pharmaceutical preparation, whether it is an extract of a crude drug or a solution of chemicals. Because galenicals were often administered without alteration, the pursuit of new extraction and other preparative techniques sometimes led to developments in dosage forms as well. The goal of medicine preparers since Galen's time has been to create dosage forms that are stable, free from inert material, therapeutically efficacious, and concentrated to facilitate handling and administration.

Tables 1 and 2 provide a comprehensive classification of ancient and modern pharmaceutical preparations recognized in pharmacopeias and other official and unofficial compendia, but do not make the distinction between dosage forms prepared by maceration or percolation (galenicals) and other chemically or physically similar dosage forms. Preparations are divided into liquids and solids. The liquids are further subdivided as: 1) general aqueous solutions and preparations, 2) sweet or viscid aqueous solutions and preparations, 3) general nonaqueous solutions and preparations, 4) alcoholic or ethereal solutions and preparations, 5) oleaginous solutions and preparations, and 6) parenteral solutions and preparations. The solids are subdivided as: 1) medicated solids, 2) medicated particulate solids, 3) medicated solid applications, 4) oral individual dosage forms, and 5) nonoral individual dosage forms. The dosage forms are arranged alphabetically and include Latin titles and synonyms. The historical development of individual dosage forms is traced to about 1950; it was about then that modern pharmaceutical science was applied in depth to the problems of dosage forms, and the term itself gained general currency in the literature of pharmacy.

DOSAGE FORMS AND BASIC PREPARATIONS

Abstracts: Abstracts are powdered extracts of crude drugs prepared by percolating the drug with an appropriate menstruum, reserving a certain portion, evaporating the weak percolate to a thin extract, blending this extract with the reserve portion and lactose, and evaporating the

Table 1   Liquid pharmaceutical preparations

General aqueous solutions and preparations

Acids, diluted	Enemas	Milks	Vapors
Aerosols	Fomentations	Solutions	Vinegars
Baths	Gargles	Solutions, irrigating	Washes
Decoctions	Infusions	Solutions, nasal	Washes, mouth
Douches	Inhalations	Solutions, ophthalmic	Washes, aromatic
Draughts	Insessia	Sprays	
Drops	Juices	Suspensions	

Sweet or viscid aqueous solutions and preparations

Condita	Linctus	Mixtures	Shampoos
Confections	Lohochs	Mucilages	Syrups
Conserves	Lotions	Oxymels	
Honeys	Magmas	Quiddonies	

General nonaqueous solutions and preparations

Fluidglycerates	Glycerites	Paints, medicinal

Alcoholic or ethereal solutions and preparations

Collodions	Elixirs	Juleps	Tinctures
Cordials	Essences	Solutio	Wines
Drops, toothache	Fluidextracts	Spirits	

Oleaginous solutions and preparations

Balsams	Liniments, dental	Oleates	Petroxolins
Emulsions	Oils	Oleoresins	
Liniments	Oils, infused	Oleovitamins	

Parenteral solutions and preparations

Ampuls	Injections	Serums

mixture until dry. The mass is weighed and enough lactose added to make the finished product exactly half the weight of the drug from which it is derived. The resulting product represent twice the strength of the original drug. Although they were convenient for compounding prescriptions, abstracts gained little popularity. Made official in the *United States Pharmacopoeia VI* published in 1880, abstracts were dropped in the next revision (1).

Acetum: See *Vinegars*.

Acids, diluted: Diluted acids are acid preparations, usually 5–10% strength, used for both internal and external medicines. Acids became official with the first *United States Pharmacopoeia* (1820). The term comes from the Latin *acidus* meaning "sharp" or "sour" (2, 3).

Acidum dilutum: See *Acids, diluted*.

Aerosols: Aerosols are a system of finely divided liquid or solid particles dispersed in and surrounded by a gas. The roots of the modern aerosol go back to 1862 and J.D. Lynde, who received a patent for a valve, complete with dip tube, designed to dispense an aerated liquid from a bottle.

In 1899, Helbing and Pertsch added liquefied gases. Patents in the early twentieth century usually were related to spraying perfumes. Aerosol fire extinguishers came into use in the 1930s, and insecticide sprays (bug bombs) appeared during World War II. Introduced in 1947, medical aerosol use increased greatly during the 1950s. In 1952, fewer than half a million such aerosols were produced; by 1963, this figure had risen to almost 40 million (4).

Ampulla: See *Ampuls*.

Ampuls: Ampuls are small, flask-shaped, hermetically sealed glass containers containing a sterile medicinal liquid intended for hypodermic injection, either subcutaneously, intramuscularly, or intravenously. Also, ampul is the class name adopted by the *National Formulary* V (*N.F.*) (1926) for the solutions in these containers. The ampul was invented in 1886 by the French pharmacist Stanislas Limousin (1831–1887) in response to a need by physicians to conserve their stocks of injectable solutions, which were difficult to transport and deteriorated rapidly due to the development of mold. In his classical essay, "Ampoules hypodermiques; nouveau mode de préparation des solutions hyperdermiques," published in *Archives of*

Table 2 Solid pharmaceutical preparations

Medicated solids

Bandages	Electuaries	Lamels	Resins
Cones, medicated	Extracts	Moxa	Silk, oiled
Dressings, medicated	Gums	Papers, medicated	Soaps
Dressings, protective	Inhalants	Papers, waxed	

Medicated particulate solids

Abstracts	Oil sugars	Salts	Teas
Cucufa	Powders	Salts, artificial	Triturations
Insufflations	Precipitates	Salts, effervescent	
Magisteries	Saccharures	Salts, smelling	

Medicated solid applications

Applications	Epithema	Ointments, ophthalmic	Rubifacients
Auristilla	Frontalia	Pastes	Sacculi
Cataplasms	Gelatins	Pencils, medicated	Scutum
Caustics	Gels	Plasma	Spasmadraps
Cements	Glycerogelatins	Plasters	Stypes
Cerates	Inunctions	Plasters, adhesive	Swabs
Cerecloths	Litus	Plasters, blister	Vesicatories
Creams	Mulls	Plasters, porous	
Dentifrices	Ointments	Pomatum	

Oral individual dosage forms

Bacillules	Granules	Pills	Triturates, tablet
Cachets	Masses	Powders, divided	Troches
Capsules	Parvules	Tablets	Wafer envelopes
Capsules, soft	Pastilles	Tablets, hypodermic	Wafers
Dragées	Pearls	Tablets, poison	
Globules	Pellets	Tablets, solution	

Nonoral individual dosage forms

Bougies	Pessaries	Politzer plugs	Suppositories

Pharmacy (1886), Limousin outlined the essential directions for their manufacture:

> These ampoules have the form of a small ovoid balloon. They are terminated by a tapered glass tube, and their capacity is a little greater than one cc.
>
> I sterilize the inside of these small containers, using the method of M. Pasteur, by submitting them in an oven to a temperature of about 200 degrees [Celsius]. I then fill them with the medicated solution, be it by introducing the point of the hot ampoule into the cold liquid, or be it by injecting the hot liquid by means of a small injector at the highest point of the ampoule.
>
> The ampoule being filled, I close it over the oxidation flame by holding the open end of the tube into the uppermost part of the flame.

Although great advances have been made in the techniques and mechanics of ampul production,

Limousin's simple rules capture the basic underlying principles. In the United States, ampuls, or "hermetically sealed containers which are filled with a medicinal liquid in a sterile condition, intended for parenteral use," became official in the *National Formulary V* (1926); that same year, the *United States Pharmacopeia X* included a chapter on sterilization but no monograph for individual ampuls. Iodine Ampuls, N.F., containing Iodine Tincture, *United States Pharmacopeia*, in sealed containers, intended to be broken and the liquid applied topically for the emergency disinfection of cuts or wounds, remained official through the *National Formulary XIII* (1970). The French term *ampoule* came from the Latin *ampulla*, which originally designated an earthen jar container for perfume (2, 4–6).

Antiseptic cottons: See *Dressings, medicated*.

Antiseptic gauzes: See *Dressings, medicated*.

Antiseptic pencils: See *Pencils, medicated*.

Apozemes: See *Decoctions*.

Applicatio: See *Applications*.

Applications: Any preparation for external use (5).

Aqua: See *Waters*.

Artificial salts: See *Salts, artificial*.

Astringent pencils: See *Pencils, medicated*.

Auristilla: Auristilla is a preparation used for medication of the ear canal. The *National Formulary V* (1926) Compound Oil of Hyoscyamus is an illustration of the type, closely resembling the Baumé Tranquille of the French *Codex* (1908) (5).

Bacillula: See *Bacillules*.

Bacillules: Bacillules are rod-shaped lozenges, prepared by massing the lozenge material, rolling it into cylinders or pill pipes, and cutting the cylinders into sections approximately twice the length of the diameter. Licorice lozenges are frequently prepared in this form, a popular example of which was formerly known as Wister's lozenge (see *Troches*) (5).

Bacillum: See *Bougies*.

Balneum: Balneum is a bath for general application (see *Baths*) (5).

Balsams: Balsams are natural solutions of resin in an essential oil, which may also contain benzoic or cinnamic acids. The term has ancient roots in words referring both to spices and to embalming. In premodern times, balsams (*baumé* in French) were any resinous vegetable juices or gums, acquiring their modern meaning in the 1800s. Several official preparations, such as Balsam of Copaiba, do not meet this definition but still carry the name because of their outward similarities with true balsams (1, 7).

Balsamum: See *Balsams*.

Bandages: Bandages are strips or ribbons of muslin gauze or other material employed in surgery for the retention of dressings and for the compression, protection, or support of diseased or injured parts. Bandages may be classified as inelastic, semielastic, elastic, or splint bandages. Inelastic bandages include muslin ribbon or roller bandages, gauze bandages, and water dressing bandages; semielastic bandages include flannel bandages; elastic bandages include rubber, rubberized, or crepe bandages; splint bandages include plaster-of-Paris bandages and crinoline bandages (gauze stiffened with dextrin) or starch bandages (gauze stiffened with starch paste), used to form the base upon which plaster-of-Paris is applied (5).

Baths: The word baths refers to the external application of water to the body, one of the oldest therapeutic techniques. Although some drugs were added, the simple water bath, or balneum, was most common. In the nineteenth century, when the therapeutic application of water was at its peak, baths were divided into hot or vapor (above 36.1°C), warm (29.4–36.1°C), tepid (18.3–29.4°C), and cold (0–18.3°C). The hot bath was a stimulant; the warm bath was soothing; the tepid bath was for treating skin problems; and the cold bath could be used as a stimulant, tonic, or sedative, depending on the administration technique (8).

Blister plasters: See *Plasters, blister*.

Boluses: Boluses are large pills, over 325 mg (5 grains) in weight. The term comes from the Greek *bolos* meaning "lump" (see *Pills*) (2, 5).

Bougia: See *Bougies*.

Bougies: Bougies are instruments or shaped, solid medications for insertion into the urethra or other body cavities. The term comes from the French *bougie*, signifying a thin wax candle named for the Algerian city, Bougie (2, 5).

Buginarium: A nasal bougie (see *Bougies*) (5).

Cachets: Cachets are lenticular or spoon-shaped rimmed disks pressed from rice-flour wafer sheets, used to administer bitter or nauseating drug powders. The powder is deposited in dry concave cachets, and the rims are moistened with water; empty convex cachets are placed on top, sealing the cachets and enveloping the powder. The term "cachet" is from the French *cacher*, "to hide." The *cachet de pain* was invented by the French pharmacist Stanislas Limousin (1831–1887) in 1873 as an improvement over wafers and wafer envelopes. Limousin also developed a perforated board, accommodating three sizes of cachets, a powder measurer, powder funnels, and wooden "wetter and pressers" to speed extemporaneous cachet production by the pharmacist. A popular brand of cachets and cachet apparatus was manufactured around

1885 under the trade name Konseals by the J.M. Grosvenor Company of Boston around 1885. The Konseal apparatus consists of three perforated, nickel-plated metal plates, hinged together to form a cover plate, a base plate, and a shield plate. Saucer-shaped rice-flour Konseals are pressed into the perforations on the cover and base plates, while the shield plate is folded back over to protect the sealing edges of the Konseals in the base plate. The Konseals in the base plate are filled with powdered drug with the help of special funnels and are tamped down with thimble compressors. The shield plate is lifted, and a moistened roller is passed over the edges of the empty Konseals in the cover plate, which is closed over the base plate, sealing the Konseals. The Konseals are made of thinner material than ordinary cachets, and the finished product is less bulky and neater in appearance. Johann Schmidt later introduced rimless Dry Seal Cachets resembling flattened capsules, which were sealed by pressure without moistening (see *Wafers*) (2, 4, 5).

Cachets, dry seal: See *Cachets.*

Caementum: See *Cements.*

Cambric, oiled: See *Silk, oiled.*

Capsula: See *Capsules.*

Capsula amylacea: Starch capsule (see *Cachets*).

Capsula dura: Hard capsule (see *Capsules*).

Capsula gelatina: Gelatin capsule (see *Capsules*).

Capsula mollis: Soft capsule (see *Capsules, soft*).

Capsules: Capsules are telescoping, interconnecting shells of hard gelatin and sugar used for the administration of solids, masses, and liquids. The term comes from the Latin *capsula*, which is the diminutive of *capsa*, meaning "box." Successor to the soft capsules invented by the French pharmacist François Mothes in 1833, the telescoping hard gelatin capsule was invented and patented in 1847 by James Murdoch of London. In the United States, the New York firm of H. Planten manufactured two-part capsules sometime after 1836, but their usefulness was impaired by their poor fit. In 1863, the firm developed jujube paste capsules intended for dispensing powders alone, offering them to the trade before 1870. Another manufacturer, Dundas Dick, experimented in the same direction and secured a patent on cone-shaped capsules in 1865. Twelve years later, inspired by reports from Italy,

the Detroit pharmacist F.A. Hubel made molds of iron wire mounted in blocks of wood, which could be dipped in a gelatin solution. Using pins of different diameters for the body and cap allowed Hubel to produce capsule sections which would telescope into each other, producing a small cylinder closed at both ends—the prototype of the modern hard gelatin capsule. Hubel sold his entire output to Parke, Davis & Co. in 1875, securing the first in a series of patents in 1877. Despite this protection, several small competing firms soon emerged that made capsules for other companies to sell or for their own sales organizations, most of which were consolidated by James Wilkie into the U.S. Capsule Company. Around 1901, this firm and its subsidiary, the M.L. Capsule Company, were purchased by Parke, Davis & Co., which expanded and improved its manufacturing processes under Wilkie's supervision. Wilkie is also credited with introducing phosphorbronze wire for capsule molds, a material superior to iron and one which remained in use until replaced by stainless steel in the 1930s. Capsule manufacturing received its greatest impetus in the 1920s when automatic filling devices were perfected. Pharmacists extemporaneously fill capsules at the prescription counter by "punching" capsule bodies into a smooth layer of medicated powder and filler at a uniform level of compression, replacing the caps, and checking the weight of the filled capsule (see *Capsules, soft*) (2, 9–11).

Capsules, elastic: See *Capsules, soft.*

Capsules, enteric-coated: See *Enteric-coated doses.*

Capsules, gelatin: See *Capsules.*

Capsules, glutoid: See *Enteric-coated doses.*

Capsules, hard: See *Capsules.*

Capsules, soft: Soft capsules are elastic globular shells of gelatin, containing sufficient glycerin to retain permanent flexibility, and intended primarily for the administration of irritating or nauseating oily liquids. They were invented in 1833 by French pharmacist François Mothes; an improved capsule was patented by Mothes and Joseph Dublanc the following year and perfected in 1840 by the court apothecary Adolph Steeger of Bucharest. Soft capsules are easier to swallow than hard capsules and are desirable for administering large volumes of liquids. The original Mothes capsules were hollow globes of soft gelatin with an opening at the top for filling. Once filled, the capsules are sealed with a drop of hot gelatin. In 1846, Giraud introduced olive-shaped elastic capsules with an elongated neck, made by dipping molds into a warm glycerogelatin solution. After drying, the molds were stripped and the capsule necks sealed for future use. Pharmacists cut off the necks of the capsules as needed, filled them with a dropper or syringe, and sealed them with a drop of warm glycerogelatin or the blade of a hot spatula. The first official formula for the manufacture of soft gelatin capsules appeared in the French *Codex Medicamentarius* of 1866 (see *Capsules*) (4, 5, 10, 5, 12).

Capsules, starch: See *Cachets*.

Carbasus: Gauze see *Dressings, medicated*.

Cataplasma: See *Cataplasms*.

Cataplasms: Cataplasms are moist substances intended for external application and are of a consistency as to accommodate themselves accurately to the surface to which they are applied, without being so liquid as to spread over the neighboring parts, or so tenacious as to adhere firmly to the skin. Cornelius Celsus (50–25 B.C.) described early Roman softening ointments or malagma (from the Latin *malasso*, meaning "soften") made by boiling flour in water to make a stiff paste that was admixed with melted gums or wax. The word "cataplasm" derives from two Greek words, *kata*, meaning "down," and *plasso*, meaning "to mold." Modern cataplasms are made by rubbing together glycerin and a dry powder, such as kaolin, to make a very firm mixture. Since cataplasms (or poultices) were commonly used in the United States in domestic practice and made in the home, they were rarely prepared by pharmacists. A kaolin cataplasm became official in the *United States Pharmacopeia VIII* (1905) but was transferred to the *National Formulary IV* in 1916 (2, 4, 5, 13).

Caustic pencils   See *Pencils, medicated*.

Caustics: Caustics are local remedies that destroy life on the part of the body to which they are applied. The term comes from the Greek *kaustikos*, meaning "to burn." The strongest common caustic (*causticum commune acerrimum*) was potassium hydroxide, or caustic potash, used to form issues on the body or to open abscesses. The *United States Dispensatory* (1836) advised that the most convenient mode of employing a caustic to form an issue was:

> To apply to the skin a piece of linen spread with adhesive plaster, having a circular opening in its centre corresponding to the intended size of the issue, and then to rub upon the skin within the opening a piece of the caustic previously moistened

at one end. The application is to be continued until the life of the part is destroyed, when the caustic should be carefully washed off by a wet sponge or wet tow, or neutralized by vinegar.

Caustic potash was sometimes used to remove strictures in the urethra or, in solution, as an application to the spine in treating tetanus. A contemporary caustic, silver nitrate, was described in the seventh century A.D. by Geber; it remains official in the *United States Pharmacopeia* as Fused Silver Nitrate. Christopher Glaser, apothecary to Louis XIV, first prepared it in sticks for use as a caustic (2, 5, 13).

Cements: The 7th edition of the *National Formulary* (1942) listed a formula for a Cement of Zinc Compounds and Eugenol, which was widely used by dentists as a temporary filling. The cement was supposed to exert a sterilizing effect and protect the dentine from further destruction. The formula passed out of the *National Formulary* with its 9th edition (1950) (14).

Cerates: Cerates are unctuous substances for external application as dressings for inflamed surfaces. Derived from the ancient Greek *keroma* (from *keros*, "wax"), cerates are generally made with oil, lard, or petrolatum as a basis, with sufficient wax, paraffin, spermaceti, or resin added to raise the melting point of the oils and fats employed. Cerates should be of such consistency that they may be easily spread at ordinary temperatures upon muslin or a similar material with a spatula and, yet, not so soft as to liquefy and run when applied to the skin. The most widely used cerate was Ceratum Cantharidis, a blistering plaster made of Spanish flies that was official in the *United States Pharmacopeia* and later in the *National Formulary* until 1950 (see *Plasters, blister*) (5).

Ceratum: (See Cerates).

Cerecloths: Cerecloths are an early form of dipped plasters, described by William Salmon in his *Pharmacopoeia Londonensis* (1691), used chiefly to lay upon issues—small ulcers produced by caustics or cutting, the discharge from which was encouraged to fulfill certain therapeutic indications. Also known as spasmadraps or sparadraps (see *Plasters*) (15).

Cereolus: A cereolus is an urethral bougie (see *Bougies*) (5).

Charta: The term comes from the Greek *chartes* or papyrus (see *Papers, powder*) (2).

Charta amylacea: Starch papers (see *Cachets*).

Charta cerata: (see *Papers, waxed*).

Chrisma: A salve (see *Ointments*) (5).

Clysters: See *Enemas*.

Coatings, pill: Rhazes (850–923) used a mucilage of psyllium seed to coat offending pills; a century later, Avicenna (980-1037) introduced silver and gold coatings for pills not merely to mask bad taste but to enhance the supposed medicinal effect. Later, the influential seventeenth-century Parisian physician and pharmacist Jean de Renou recommended that pills with a bitter taste should be gilded and mixed among some powdered spices. Coating pills with gold and silver leaf was commonly practiced in France, other parts of Europe, and the United States until well into the nineteenth century but then fell into disuse. Mohr, Redwood, and Procter's classic *Practical Pharmacy* (1849) reported that foil-coated pills were "still occasionally administered, but much less frequently than formerly." Sugar-coated and gelatin-coated pills had their first acceptance as an indirect consequence of the invention of the gelatin capsule. In 1838, M. Garot, a Parisian pharmacist, coated offending pills with gelatin. A year earlier, the French pharmacist Labelonie had recommended that pills of cubeb and copaiba be covered with sugar, a process that was patented by Adolphe Fortin of Paris in 1837. Over the next several years, other French pharmacists (Deschamps, Bousquet, Mayer, and Roman) secured patents for coating pills with various combinations of sugar, honey, and acacia. By 1862, England's Bernard Proctor could list 45 distinct processes for coating pills with a variety of substances. In the United States, the first manufacture of sugar-coated pills was associated with the patent-medicine industry, probably as early as 1845. New Yorkers Cornelius V. Clickener and Zadoc Porter and a Philadelphia physician named Swayne all claimed to be the "inventor" of the sugar-coated pill but doubtlessly adapted French technology. By 1857, five different sugar-coated patent-medicine pills were available to American pharmacists, but no process was available for pharmacists who wished to sugar-coat pills extemporaneously. About that same time, Henry A. Tilden and William R. Warner independently developed processes for manufacturing sugar-coated pills and began selling them in bulk; in 1866, Warner began manufacture under his own firm name, William R. Warner & Company. That same year, Henry Wathew of Philadelphia developed and patented a prototype of the angled coating pans still employed today.

By the mid-1870s, a variety of small mechanical coating pans were available to American pharmacists, although the quality of the extemporaneous coatings that could be achieved was generally inferior to that of the manufactured variety, which caused pharmacists to relinquish the practice (16–18).

Coatings, tablet: After the introduction and acceptance of the compressed tablet as a dosage form superior to pills, the same techniques that had been employed for sugar-coating pills were adapted to tablets (see *Coatings, pill*). Moreover, compression coating techniques were also introduced by Charles Carter of Philadelphia as early as 1858. In 1896, P.J. Noyes invented an apparatus incorporating a movable die cavity into which the coating material was fed; the powder was compressed to form a coating around the pill or tablet by striking the upper punch with an automatic hammer. The following year, Noyes patented an improved machine that not only applied the coating but also performed the preliminary compression of the tablet. F.J. Stokes received a patent for a similar machine in 1917, although the compression coating of tablets did not become widely adopted until the 1950s (18).

Collodions: Collodions are liquid, external preparations with a base of pyroxylin dissolved in a mixture of alcohol and ethyl oxide or similar solvent. They were used medicinally soon after the discovery of gun cotton by Schoebein in 1846, first as a surgical dressing by Maynard in 1847 (19).

Collodium: See *Collodions*.

Collunarium: See *Solutions, nasal*.

Collutorium: See *Washes, mouth*.

Collyrium: See *Solutions, ophthalmic*.

Compressed pills: See *Tablets*.

Compressed tablets: See *Tablets*.

Condita: Condita are comprised of candied or preserved roots or fruits. They are made by boiling the plant parts until tender, soaking them in hot syrup, and then pouring off the syrup; the procedure was repeated several times, reusing the syrup after boiling it down to a thick consistency. Condita can also be a compound of wine, honey, and spices (often pepper). Condita are also known as confitures or sweetmeats (18, 20).

Cones, medicated: Cones are light, porous hemispherical masses of sucrose and egg albumin, used as a vehicle for homeopathic medications. The cones, also called disks, are designated (in millimeters) according to size by the diameter of the base. The common size (No. 6) should absorb about 2 drops of dispensing alcohol. Cones are medicated by adding a sufficient quantity of the dilution to saturate them and pouring off the excess liquid (5).

Confectio: See *Confections*.

Confections: Confections are saccharine, soft solids, in which one or more medicinal substances are incorporated to provide an agreeable form of administration and a convenient method for preservation. In the thirteenth century, some apothecaries were called *confectionarii* from *confectio* meaning "a composition." Confections are made by adding medicinal ingredients in either the form of a smooth paste, a fine powder, or a liquid to a basis of finely powdered sugar. Confection of Rose and Confection of Senna were official in the *National Formulary* through the 5th edition (1926) (2, 5).

Confitures: See *Condita*.

Conserva: See *Conserves*.

Conserves: Conserves are confections prepared from fresh medicinal agents and refined sugar, beaten into a uniform mass. The *United States Dispensatory* (1836) noted that "as active substances even thus treated undergo some change, and those which lose their virtues by desiccation cannot be long preserved, the few conserves now retained are intended rather as convenient vehicles of other substances, than for separate exhibition." Conserves are also known as preserves (also see *Confections*) (5, 13, 20).

Cordiale: See *Cordials*.

Cordials: Cordials are sweetened alcoholic preparations of high alcoholic content. They are also a tonic medicine formulated to stimulate the heart (5, 20).

Cottons, antiseptic or medicated: See *Dressings, Medicated*.

Creams: Creams are semisolid emulsions, usually medicated, intended for external application. The term "cream" has been used to refer to a wide variety of opaque, soft semisolids or thick liquids intended for external use. The *British Pharmacopoeia* classifies creams as medicated

liquid emulsions consisting of a mixture of anhydrous lanolin, olive oil (or other fixed oil), and lime water; milk of magnesia is often referred to as a cream, and many cosmetic preparations are called creams. Claudius Galen (131–201) prepared the first *unguentum refrigerans* or "cold cream," an ointment containing olive oil, rose oil, white wax, and a small quantity of water. This was a prototype for other cosmetic ointments introduced by Johann Mesue, Jr., in the thirteenth century. A modern version, consisting of almond oil, spermaceti, white wax, and rose water, passed into the *United States Pharmacopeia* as "Rose Water Ointment" or "Galen's Cerate." Pharmaceutical creams became official with the introduction of the formula for a "Sun Cream" in the *National Formulary VIII* (1946), a product designed to prevent sunburn but permit tanning. Cosmetic creams, which are usually not medicated, include preparations classified as all-purpose creams, baby creams, barrier creams, bleaching creams, cleansing (or rolling) creams, cold (or fatty) creams, foundation (or vanishing) creams, hair creams, and hand creams (4, 5, 21).

Cremor: See *Creams*.

Cucufa: Cucufa is a cap, dusted on the inside with medicinal powder, which is applied to the head to strengthen the brain (22).

Curatio: See *Dressings, medicated*.

Decoctions: Decoctions are a solution of vegetable drugs, obtained by boiling the substances in water; they are also known as apozemes (8).

Decoctum: See *Decoctions*.

Dental liniments: See *Liniments, dental*.

Dental wax: *See Drops, toothache*.

Dentifrices: Dentifrices are powders, pastes, washes, or medicated soaps used for cleaning the teeth. Dentifrices are usually flavored with aromatic oils, frequently contain soap, almost always some form of chalk, and are applied with a toothbrush. The *National Formulary* carried official formulas for a liquid dentifrice through its 5th edition (1926) and a powder dentifrice through its 11th edition (1960) (5).

Dentifricium: See *Dentifrices*.

Dentilimentum: See *Liniments, dental*.

Dermatologic pastes: See *Pastes*.

Diluted acids: See *Acids, diluted*.

Disks: See *Cones, medicated*.

Dispensing tablets: See *Tablets, solution*.

Douches: Douches are a column of fluid, of a certain nature and temperature, allowed to fall on a part of the body. Air can also be a used as a douche (20).

Dragées: Dragées are candied or preserved roots and fruits described by the Arab Najm ad-dyn Mahmoud in the eighth century and reintroduced in the eighteenth century by the famous French pharmacist Moyse Charas (see *Confitures*). By the middle of the nineteenth century, the term was extended to include a type of sugar-coated pill formed by repeatedly shaking slightly moistened, tiny 6-mg (1/10 grain) sugar granules (or nonpareils) in a basin of finely powdered drug mixed with sugar. After a sufficient number of layers had been built up, the dragées would receive a final coating of sugar or copal and tolu balsam, a painstaking process described by Ernest Agnew in the *American Journal of Pharmacy* (1870) (see *granules*) (18, 23).

Draughts: Draughts are liquid medicines usually prepared to be taken in a single dose or "draught." Draughts are also known as potions (5).

Dressings, medicated: Medicated dressings are external applications resembling ointments in consistency but remaining semisolid at body temperature. Paraffin Dressing, formerly official in the *National Formulary VI* (1936), was employed as an air-excluding, soft, pliable, analgesic, splint-like covering for surfaces denuded by burns. A wide range of materials have been used as coverings or protectives to apply heat or medicaments to a diseased or injured part, to prevent wound infection, and to absorb and prevent decomposition of wound discharges. Antiseptic or Medicated Cottons include borated cotton, iodoform cotton, iodized cotton, and styptic cotton; Antiseptic or Medicated Gauzes include borated gauze, corrosive sublimate gauze, carbolated gauze, iodoform gauze, and picric acid gauze; Antiseptic or Medicated Lints include borated lint; Cellulose Waddings or wood wools include moss, peat, sawdust, jute, and oakum or marine lint. See the *British Pharmaceutical Codex* (1924) for representative formulas (also see *Bandages* and *Dressings, protective*) (5, 24).

Dressings, protective: Protective dressings are comprised of a wide range of materials employed as wound coverings, either to shield the parts from external infection or to prevent the escape of fluids contained in the dressing. Protective dressings are also used as a covering for poultices and for the retention of heat. Common protective dressings include oiled silk, oiled muslin or cambric, waxed paper, gutta percha tissue, rubber dams, mackintosh or jaconet, and rubber sheeting (5).

Drops: Drops are pharmaceutical mixtures meant to be given in small amounts. Before the twentieth century, the term applied to solutions used in small quantities expressed in "drops." These were commonly strong medicines "dropped" into water, such as Vinegar of Opium or "black drop." In modern pharmacy, the term became more associated with the need to get a medicine into an appropriately small amount of vehicle for application to the eye (ophthalmic), ear (otic), or passages of the nose (nasal). As a dosage unit, the drop is troublesome because it can vary greatly in size, depending on the size of the dropper orifice and the surface tension of the liquid. The *United States Pharmacopeia IX* (1910) set the official dropper at 20 drops per gram of water at 15°C ± 10% (3, 20).

Drops, ear: See *Drops*.

Drops, eye: See *Drops*.

Drops, nose: See *Drops*.

Drops, toothache: Drops for toothache are comprised of a solution of phenol in oil of cinnamon and methyl salicylate. The solution entered the *National Formulary V* (1926). A mixture of phenol, creosote, or volatile oils dissolved in paraffin, with a few filaments of cotton added, and molded into sticks constitutes Dental Wax (5).

Ductum: See *Douches*.

Dry seal cachets: See *Cachets*.

Ear drops: See *Drops*.

Eclectus: See *Linctus*.

Eclegma: See *Lohoch*.

Effervescent salts: See *Salts, effervescent*.

Elaeosacchara: See *Oil sugars*.

Elastic capsules: See *Capsules, soft*.

Electuaries: Electuaries are confections prepared from dried medicinal agents, especially powders, combined with syrup or honey in order to render them pleasant to the taste and convenient for internal use. The *United States Dispensatory* (1836) noted that electuaries "should not be so soft ... as to allow the ingredients to separate, nor so firm ... as to prevent them from being swallowed without mastication." French writers recommend using brown sugar syrup to prepare electuaries, because it is less apt to crystallize than that made from refined sugar. The term comes from the Greek words *ek*, meaning "out," and *leichein*, "to lick" (2, 13) (see *Confections*).

Electuarium: See *Confections*.

Elixirs: Sweetened, hydroalcoholic, flavored liquid medicines, which became popular in mid-nineteenth-century America. The word is derived apparently from the Arabic *al-iksir*, which is an Arabic form of the Greek, *xirion*. Originally the term meant "dry powder." Elixirs came into medicine through their connection with alchemy. Elixir Rubrum, one of the most renowned alchemical compounds, could supposedly turn mercury to gold or prolong life. The term was picked up by followers of Paracelsus (1493–1541) and became applied to liquid preparations. European elixirs were generally bitter. One of the first American elixirs was Cordial Elixir of Quinine (ca. 1838), made by John T. Heinitsh of Lancaster, Pennsylvania. After the Civil War an "elixir craze" began, which led to scores of companies competing for business. As much as any other development, the "craze" led to the publication of the first *National Formulary* in 1888 (25, 26).

Embrocatio: See *Liniments*.

Emplastrum: See *Plasters*.

Emulsions: Emulsions are a preparation consisting of two immiscible liquids, usually water and oil, one of which is dispersed as small globules in the other. Before the late seventeenth century, the term only applied to natural emulsions, such as ground almonds and water, which resembled milk. In 1674, a physician named Grew reported the preparation of oils and egg yolk to the Royal Society of Great Britain. In the 1700s, other emulsions were made with acacia, honey, tragacanth, and other natural emulsifying agents. In the 1800s, the wet-gum (ca. 1850) and dry-gum (ca. 1870) methods were established as standard preparation techniques. Interest in medicinal emulsions peaked in the early to mid-twentieth century with the development of several new emulsifying agents. Originally listed under "Mixtures" in the *United States Pharmacopeia*, they are a separate entry in the 7th revision (1890) (4).

Emulsum: See *Emulsions*.

Enemas: Enemas are injections of liquid, either plain or containing drugs, into the rectum and colon to empty the lower intestine or to introduce food or medicine for therapeutic purposes. Enemas are one of the most ancient and widely used methods of introducing therapeutic substances into the body. The origins of use are lost in prehistory, but written records in Egypt before 1000 B.C. describe enemas being used to both cleanse the bowel and administer medicines. These early enemas consisted of three parts: a vehicle (usually water, beer, or milk), an emollient (usually oil or honey), and a medicinal substance. The Greek historian Herodotus (fifth century B.C.) attributed the general good health of the Egyptians to their use of enemas and claimed they had achieved their expertise through their experiences with injecting embalming fluids via the anus. Pliny (first century A.D.), however, argued that the Egyptians had learned to administer enemas by watching the ibis use its curved bill to inject itself with Nile River water as a purge. Hippocrates recommended enemas to treat fevers and constipation. Other authors of antiquity, such as Galen and Oribasius, wrote at length about what substances could be introduced via enemas. Enema apparatus was first described in detail by Arabian physicians of the eleventh and twelfth centuries. Albulcasis described a device made of an anal tube or funnel attached to a bag made from an animal bladder or sheep skin. The metal piston syringe came into use in the 1400s and supplanted these clumsy bags. The enema syringe soon became the object of much medical ingenuity, particularly in France. In 1480, Louis XI suffered a severe stroke and recovered, giving credit to the enemas he had received, beginning a 400-year period of fascination with the enema among the French, who refined the syringe apparatus. Molière referred to enemas repeatedly in his works, and Ambrose Paré devised a syringe instrument about 1580 that allowed enema self-administration. During the seventeenth century, other special apparatus were designed to allow administrations of tobacco smoke via enemas. The Dutch anatomist Regner de Graaf completed the first book-length study of enemas in 1668. In the mid-eighteenth century, gum rubber began to be used in enema apparatus, replacing skin bags. In 1820, John Read developed a two-way syringe with ball valves (the first modern stomach pump), which was also used for enemas. Spring-loaded syringes and other advances followed, but by the late nineteenth century the dangers of improper enema use became apparent, especially the consequences of high-pressure administration. By the mid-twentieth century, enemas were again administered with simple funnels and gravity, a reflection of their prehistoric origin. Enemas are also known as clysters or glysters (27, 28).

Enteric-coated capsules: See *Enteric-coated doses*.

Enteric-coated doses: Enteric-coated doses are dosage forms that have been coated or chemically treated to prevent disintegration in the stomach but which disintegrate in the intestinal tract. Enteric coating is employed when the medicinal substances would be decomposed or rendered inactive by gastric enzymes or when they would irritate the gastric mucosa. The *Pacific Medical and Surgical Journal* (1867) noted that collodion protects pills from dissolving in the stomach, but gastric insolubility as a basis for medication is generally credited to the German dermatologist Paul Unna, who introduced keratin-coated pills in 1884; Ceppi introduced salol as an enteric coating in 1891. Glutoid capsules are a special form of enteric coating prepared by subjecting soft or hard gelatin capsules to the action of formaldehyde until they become insoluble in the stomach but not in the intestine. The hardening process was developed in Switzerland by Weyland in 1895 and patented by Hausmann in Germany that same year. Pharmacists have extemporaneously coated capsules, pills, and tablets with salol, keratin, casein, and shellac, or with a mixture of *n*-butyl stearate, carnauba wax, and stearic acid to create enteric coatings. Early patented enteric coatings included keratin (Pohl, Germany, 1885), fat-covered capsules enclosed in membranous sacs (Webb and Webb, Great Britain, 1906), and benzoin-coated capsules (Horigan, 1928). Later patented coatings utilized cellulose nitrate and acetate (Volwiler, 1928), cellulose esters and ethers with saponifiable organic compounds (Glaessner, Austria, 1931), ammoniacal bleached shellac (Wruble, 1933), stearic acid, carnauba wax, petrolatum, elm bark, and agar (Miller, 1935, and Worton, 1938), and abietic, oleic, and benzoic acids with methyl abietate (Eldred, 1937). Since 1940, research on enteric coatings has focused on the synthesis of resinous polymers, which are insoluble in acids, such as cellulose acetate phthalate (Hiatt, 1940) and a glycerol-stearic acid-phthalic anhydride ester (Volweiler and Moore, 1940) (4, 5, 12, 17).

Enteric-coated pills: See *Enteric-coated doses*.

Enteric-coated tablets: See *Enteric-coated doses*.

Epispastics: Epispastics are local remedies, the application of which produce a serous discharge beneath the cuticle, forming a blister. Epispastics are also known as vesicatories (13).

Epithema: Epithema consists or topical applications other than ointments or plasters. Liquid epithema include fomentations, soft epithema include cataplasms, and dry epithema include bags filled with dried drugs (20).

Escharotica: See *Caustics*.

Escharotics: Caustic applications (see *Caustics*) (5).

Essences: The term essences sometimes refers to a volatile oil or to a simple tincture; most often, the term is used interchangeably with spirits (20).

Essencia: See *Essences*.

Extracta: See *Extracts*.

Extracts: Extracts are either pasty or semisolid masses or dry, solid, or powdered products prepared by exhausting drugs with appropriate solvents, carefully evaporating the products to fixed standards. An extract is intended to preserve the useful constituents of a drug in a concentrated, relatively uniform, permanent condition, and in a form suitable for medication. The *Edinburgh Pharmacopoeia* (1817) and *Dublin Pharmacopoeia* (1826) distinguish between extracts prepared from infusions, decoctions, or tinctures, and those prepared from the expressed juices of plants, calling the latter *succi spissati* or inspissated juices. Three forms of extracts are recognized: semiliquid or those of syrupy consistency; plastic masses known as pilular or solid extracts; and dry powders known as powdered extracts (4, 5, 13).

Extractum: See *Extracts*.

Eye Drops: See *Drops*.

Eye Washes: See *Solutions, ophthalmic*.

Fluidextracts: zzFluidextracts are concentrated liquid preparations representing the therapeutically active principles of vegetable drugs. They are formulated in such a way that the activity of one gram of the drug is contained in one milliliter of the fluidextract. They are generally prepared by some form of percolation, using alcohol in the menstruum. Fluidextracts first became official in 1850 when five were entered in the *United States Pharmacopoeia* by their heyday in the late nineteenth century, almost 100 were official. Joseph Remington called fluidextracts "American preparations," because they were developed by such native pharmaceutical scientists as William Procter, Jr., and Edward Squibb. Fluidextracts were perhaps the ultimate galenical class because of their permanence, concentrated form, and uniform relationship between the strength of the extract and the drug it contained. With the dominance of synthetic chemical drugs in the twentieth century, fluidextracts all but disappeared, except for those used for flavoring purposes (1, 19, 29).

Fluidextractum: See *Fluidextracts*.

Fluidglycerates: Fluidglycerates are a class of fluidextracts in which a mixture of glycerin and water is used as the primary menstruum during percolation instead of alcohol and water. The preparation of these extracts was suggested by Beringer in 1908. They were briefly official from the 5th–7th editions of the *National Formulary* (1926–1942) (3).

Fluidglyceratum: See *Fluidglycerates*.

Fomentations: Fomentations consists of an external application of cloths dampened with hot water or a medicinal decoction. Narcotic drugs were sometimes used. Dry fomentations were heated bricks wrapped in cloth and applied externally (5, 20).

Fomentum: See *Fomentations*.

Fotus: See *Fomentations*.

Frontalia: Medicines applied to the forehead (20).

Gargarisma: See *Gargles*.

Gargles: A gargle is a liquid medicine intended to be retained in the mouth and placed in contact with the back of the throat by throwing back the head and agitated by air released from the larynx (20).

Gauzes, antiseptic or medicated: See *Dressings, medicated*.

Gelatin capsules: See *Capsules*.

Gelatina: See *Gelatins*.

Gelatins: Gelatins are semisolid gelatinous preparations for internal or external use (5).

Gelatum: See *Gels*.

Gels: Gels are semisolid organic or inorganic colloids rich in liquid, consisting of hydrated threads or granules of the dispersed phase intimately associated with the dispersion medium. Although Francesco Selmi studied inorganic colloids in the 1840s, modern colloid science began in 1861 with the work of Thomas Graham, who investigated diffusion and dialysis and introduced such terms as colloid, glue, sol, gel, peptization, and syneresis. In the early 1900s, Freundlick introduced the terms *lyophilic* and *lyophobic* to describe colloids in which the dispersed phase has a high or a low affinity, respectively, for the dispersion medium. In 1950, Weiser divided gels into inorganic gels, which include gelatinous precipitates (such as Milk of Magnesia) and inorganic jellies (such as Bentonite Magma), organic gels or jellies (such as Pectin Paste), and crystalline or amorphous jellylike networks in which both solid and liquid phases are continuous (see *Magmas*) (4).

Globules: Globules are spheres of sugar (see *Pills*). They can also be round or oval glycerogelatin capsules (see *Pearls*) (5).

Glutoid capsules: See *Capsules, glutoid*.

Glycerinum: See *Glycerites*.

Glycerites: Glycerites are solutions of medicinal substances in glycerin introduced in the 5th revision of the *United States Pharmacopoeia* (1873). Glycerites afford a rapid and simple method of making aqueous solutions of phenol, tannic acid, tar, and other substances that are not otherwise easily soluble. This class of preparations is called glycerins in Great Britain (4, 5).

Glyceritum: See *Glycerites*.

Glycerogelatins: Glycerogelatins are soft, medicated masses, usually molded into the form of blocks, which melt at body temperature and have as a base a mixture of gelatin, glycerin, and water; Glycerated Gelatin United States Pharmacopoeia is generally used as a base. At the time of application, the blocks are melted, and the liquid applied to the skin with a soft brush. Four glycerogelatins were introduced into the 3rd edition of the *National Formulary* (1906), and a general formula remained official through the 8th edition (1946). Under the title *Gelatinum*, the *British Pharmaceutical Codex* (1922) included preparations that were either similar to glycerogelatins, that more closely resembled dermatologic pastes, or that were intended for internal administration and called jellies (4, 5).

Glycerogelatinum: See *Glycerogelatins*.

Glysters: See *Enemas*.

Gossypium: Cotton (see *Dressings, medicated*).

Granula: Granular effervescent salts (see *Salts, effervescent*).

Granules: Granules are small spheres of sugar pellets that are saturated with liquid medication before being swallowed. They can also be very small pills of 0.06 g or less, sometimes called parvules, made by slightly moistening sugar granules (or nonpareils) with a syrup in which an active ingredient has been dissolved. Granules containing 1 mg of powerful medications, such as arsenious acid or aconite, found favor among physicians in Europe, particularly in Italy, because they provided powerful drugs in small, precise doses (see *Dragées*; also see *Pills*) (4, 23).

Gums: Gums are mucilaginous, amorphous, transparent, or translucent glucosidal principles of plants used internally (as demulcents or expectorants), externally (as emollients or protectives), or for their emulsifying action. Three distinctive types of gums are recognized: arabin, which is completely soluble in water; bassorin and cerasin, which are partially soluble or swell in contact with water; and mucilages and pectins, which swell to form jellies. Many gums are complex mixtures of several of these types (5).

Guttae: See *Drops*.

Hard capsules: See *Capsules*.

Haustus: See *Draughts*.

Homeopathic: *tinctures*:   See *Tinctures*.

Homeopathic: *triturations*:   See *Triturations*.

Honeys: Preparations with honey as the vehicle (8).

Infused oils: See *Oils, infused*.

Infusions: Infusions are aqueous solutions obtained by soaking vegetable drugs in cold or hot (not boiling) water (8).

Infusum: See *Infusions*.

Inhalants: Inhalants are products consisting of finely powdered or liquid drugs that are carried into the respiratory passages by the use of powder blowers or low-pressure aerosol containers holding a suspension of the drug in a liquefied propellant. A dry inhalation is a product consisting of finely powdered drugs that are carried into the respiratory passages with the help of special devices. Inhalants can also refer to drugs or a combination of drugs which, by virtue of their high vapor pressure, can be carried by an air current into the nasal passages where they exert their effect. In the latter form of inhalant, the drug is absorbed on fibrous material and enclosed in an inhaler—a plastic or metal tube fitted with a cap to prevent loss of medicament when not in use. The patient removes the cap, inserts the nasal tip into a nostril, and breathes the air drawn through the inhaler to obtain the drug (4).

Inhalatio: See *Inhalations*.

Inhalations: Inhalations are medicinal agents administered by breathing in gases and vapors. A wide variety of techniques and purposes fall under this category. The isolation of pure gases by Priestley, Scheele, and others in the late eighteenth century motivated Thomas Beddoes to found the Pneumatic Institute (1798) in England to treat lung diseases. The gases used for inhalation therapy included oxygen, nitrous oxide, and ether. Gases were applied as surgical anesthesia in the 1840s largely through the efforts of the Americans Crawford Long, Horace Wells, and W.T.G. Morton; their innovations were the first great contributions to medical science by citizens of the United States. The therapeutic use of gases continued throughout the nineteenth century, especially for the treatment of tuberculosis. During this period, devices were designed to vaporize liquid drugs with steam for the treatment of lung disorders. The first apparatus developed to atomize medicinals, made by Berson in 1860, was a combination inhaler and atomizer operated by steam that was generated by heating water in a closed vessel. These devices were quite popular for home use, and their modern counterparts remain a part of home health care. The term *inhalation* has also been applied to preparations more properly called inhalants, such as Compound Eucalyptus Inhalation, or sprays, such as

Epinephrine Inhalation (see *Inhalants and sprays*) (24, 30, 31).

Inhalations, dry: See *Inhalants*.

Injectio: See *Injections*.

Injections: Injections are sterile solutions or suspensions used for administering pharmaceutical preparations by intravenous, subcutaneous, intramuscular, and intraspinal injection. The term *injections* is also the class name adopted by the 5th edition of the *National Formulary* (1926) for solutions in ampuls intended for hypodermic injection. Although ancient humans may have invented the concept of introducing drugs through punctures in the skin by attempting to recreate the effects of venomous snake and insect bites through the use of poisoned arrows, perhaps the first introduction of medication through the skin for medicinal purposes was inoculation for smallpox. Human inoculation with the smallpox virus by pricking the body with needles dipped in pus from an active case of the disease was practiced for centuries among people of the Orient but was only introduced into Western medicine about 1717. In 1796, Edward Jenner (1749–1823) performed his first vaccination with material from a cowpox sore. In 1657, Sir Christopher Wren was the first to inject a drug intravenously, a practice successfully adopted by the English practitioner Johan D. Major in 1662 under the title "chirurgica infusoria." Physicians experimented with the injection of water, opium, arsenic, cinnamon, oil of sulfur, and other substances with limited and often fatal results. Injections of purging medicines, such as jalap resins, were particularly popular in the treatment of syphilis. Nevertheless, the successful utilization of intravenous injection awaited the proof of the germ theory of disease and the discovery of sterile methods by Pasteur, Koch, Lister, and others in the latter half of the nineteenth century; the introduction of the hypodermic syringe, which was suggested by Charles G. Pravez of Lyons in 1853, popularized by Alexander Wood of Edinburgh and Charles Hunter of London in 1855–1858, and improved by Luer in 1894; and the invention of the ampul by Stanislas Limousin in 1886. A committee of the Royal Medical and Chirurgical Society of London gave approval to hypodermic injections in 1867, the same year the *British Pharmacopoeia* published a monograph for the first official injection, *Injectio Morphinae Hypodermica*. No attempt was made to sterilize these solutions, but E.R. Squibb (1873) and others recommended that parenteral solutions could be preserved by the addition

of small amounts of carbolic acid, salicylic acid, chloroform, or camphor. At about the same time (1875), John Tindall developed the process of sterilization by discontinuous heating, which bears his name. Nevertheless, hypodermic routes of administration were slow to gain widespread recognition, for physicians became increasingly aware of fevers and other toxic symptoms following the use of crudely prepared injections. Ehrlich's introduction of hypodermic injections of salvarsan for syphilis (1910) provided the strongest impetus for the development of parenteral administration, stimulating a series of rapid advancements in technique. In 1911, Martindale and Wynn discussed the pharmaceutical manipulation of salvarsan, emphasizing sterilization and aseptic techniques. That same year, Hort and Penfold applied the term *pyrogens* to describe substances that cause a febrile reaction upon injection. They found that distilled water sealed in sterile containers gave rise to toxic symptoms, whereas freshly distilled water caused no reaction; later that same year, Wechselmann showed that febrile reactions could be eliminated if solutions were made from sterile distilled water. Seibert confirmed these findings in 1923, noting that poorly constructed stills could produce pyrogenic distilled water. In 1930, Rademaker formulated a rigid set of aseptic precautions and rules, governing the preparation of parenteral fluids, which are still valid today, and setting the stage for modern intravenous medicines. Injections are also known as parenterals (4, 5, 24, 32–33).

Insessia: Insessia refers to a vapor bath, usually administered by having the patient sit on a perforated chair, beneath which is placed a large container filled with hot water or a hot decoction of a plant drug (20).

Insufflatio: See *Insufflations*.

Insufflations: Insufflations are powders used for blowing into the nose, preferably by means of one of the various kinds of powder blowers or insufflators made for the purpose. They may also be applied directly in the way in which snuff is usually taken. Also, a snuff. The term comes from the Latin *insufflare* meaning "to breath into" or "to blow into" (2, 5).

Inunctions: Inunctions are ointments applied with friction, intended for local application and quick absorption. The term was formerly applied to preparations consisting of wool fat in which mercury or other medicinal agents were incorporated. A Compound Menthol Inunction (retitled Compound Menthol Ointment in 1936) remained official in the *National Formulary* until 1960 (5, 24).

Inunctum: See *Inunctions*.

Irrigating solutions: See *Solutions, irrigating*.

Irrigatio: See *Solutions, irrigating*.

Jellies: See *Gels*.

Juices: Juices are liquids obtained by expression from the fresh parts of plants. The *British Pharmaceutical Codex* (1949) contained monographs for the juices of garlic, lemon, and taraxacum. In the United States, Cherry Juice remained official through the 16th edition of the *National Formulary* (1985) as a flavoring agent (4).

Juices, inspissated: Extracts prepared from the expressed juices of plants (see *Extracts*).

Juleps: A julep is a sweet drink, usually a demulcent, acidulous, or mucilaginous mixture. Much more popular in Europe than in the United States, a typical julep of the late nineteenth century (*mistura gummosa*) contained 10 parts acacia triturated with 30 parts syrup of acacia, 100 parts water, and 10 parts orange flower water (3, 20).

Konseals: Konseals is a trade name for the brand of cachets and cachet apparatus manufactured by the J.M. Grosvenor Company of Boston about 1885, originally introduced as "Morstadt's cachets" by Karl Morstadt of Prague (see *Cachets*) (5).

Lamella: See *Lamels*.

Lamels: Lamels are small disks, about 3 mm in diameter, cut or stamped from thin films of glycerinated gelatin, containing definite quantities of various medicaments used in ophthalmology. Lamels, or eye disks, are applied with a camel's-hair brush to the inner surface of the lower eyelid, where they are immediately dissolved in the lachrymal fluid. Four lamels were official in the *British Pharmacopoeia* until 1953 (24).

Lavatio: See *Washes, mouth*.

Ligamentum: See *Bandages*.

Linctus: A linctus is a thick viscid liquid that must be licked from a spoon or licorice stick, from the Latin *lingere*, "to lick" (see *Lohochs*) (5).

Liniments: Liniments are external preparations of a consistency thicker than water, but thinner than ointments, usually applied to the skin with a gentle rubbing of the hands. Liniments are among the oldest of dosage forms, along with related forms, such as plasters and ointments. The term came to its present use about 1600. Drying liniments are preparations which dry when smeared on the skin, forming a medicated film removable by water (5, 8, 19).

Liniments, dental: Dental liniments were introduced in the *National Formulary V* (1926) through cooperation between dental and pharmaceutical authorities; these concentrated, often poisonous liniments, were designed to be rubbed into the gums (5, 19).

Liniments, drying: See *Liniments*.

Linimentum: See *Liniments*.

Linimentum: exsiccantum: Drying liniment (see *Liniments*).

Lints, antiseptic or medicated: See *Dressings, medicated*.

Linteum: Lint (See *Dressings, medicated*).

Liquor: See *Solutions*.

Litus: A litus is fluid preparation applied with a brush (see *Paints, medicinal*) (5).

Lohochs: Lohochs are thick syrupy medicines, usually used to fight a cough, to be sipped slowly or licked, sometimes called a looch. If in the latter dosage form, it is usually called a linctus (5).

Looch: See *Lohochs*.

Lotio: See *Lotions*.

Lotions: Lotions are fluid preparations, usually containing suspended insoluble material and applied externally. They are different from liniments by being aqueous, rather than oleaginous or alcoholic in nature. Lotions were official in the first *National Formulary* (1888). In the mid-nineteenth century, lotions were often applied by wetting linen and placing on the affected area (1, 20).

Lozenges: See *Troches*.

Magisteries: Certain precipitates from saline solutions bore this title, but it was usually applied to secret remedies (20).

Magmas: In modern pharmacy, the term magma means an aqueous preparation containing precipitated inorganic material in a fine state of subdivision. *Magma Bismuthi* and *Magma Magnesiae* (milk of magnesia) were the first official magmas in the *United States Pharmacopeia IX* (1916). In the nineteenth century and previous eras, this term referred to the residue obtained after expressing organic substances to extract their fluid parts, usually referred to as a marc (19, 20).

Massa: See *Masses*.

Masses: Masses are plastic, semisolid pharmaceutical preparations composed of active medicinal substances combined with a diluent or filler and an excipient, capable of being shaped into pills with little or no further treatment. The three essential requirements of a pill mass are: adhesiveness (the mass must be sufficiently adhesive to retain its shape and yet be soft enough to be worked by the fingers or suitable apparatus into the desired form); firmness (the mass must possess sufficient firmness to permit the pills to retain their shape); and plasticity (a natural result of the proper degree of adhesiveness and firmness). Two masses appear to have survived the changes in modern medicine: Mass of Mercury (or Blue Mass), a cholagogic preparation last official in the *National Formulary IX* (1950), and Ferrous Carbonate Mass (or Vallet's Mass), a hematinic last official in the *National Formulary X* (1955) (4, 5, 24).

Medicated cottons: See *Dressings, medicated*.

Medicated dressings: See *Dressings, medicated*.

Medicated gauzes: See *Dressings, medicated*.

Medicated oils: See *Oils*.

Medicated paints: See *Paints, medicated*.

Medicated papers: See *Papers, medicated*.

Medicated pencils: See *Pencils, medicated*.

Mel: See *Honeys*.

Mellita: See *Honeys*.

Milks: Historically, the term *milk* has been applied generally to any liquid that possesses the outward appearance of milk, such as milk of magnesia. Legend holds that the class of beauty preparations called toilet milks may have arisen from Cleopatra and her milk baths. The modern milks are oil-in-water emulsions, named for their appearance and use as additives to baths. Moreover, actual milk was used and modified, especially with the addition of malt, as a medicinal beverage. Fermented Milk, or kumyss, is fresh cow's milk, to which sugar and yeast are added for fermentation. Fermented milk was official in the 3rd through the 5th edition of the *National Formulary* (1906–1926). Humanized Milk was a combination of cow's milk and fresh cream, plus Humanizing Milk Powder, which contained a small amount of Compound Pancreatic Powder and lactose, made official in *National Formulary III* (1906) (7, 34).

Mistura: See *Mixtures*.

Mixtures: Mixtures are aqueous preparations for internal use containing insoluble, nonfatty substances. They differ from emulsions in containing no fat and from liniments in being used internally. Both mixtures and emulsions were originally grouped under *Mistura* in the *United States Pharmacopoeia*; in the 7th revision (1890), emulsions were given separate recognition. Examples include Compound Mixture of Opium and Glycyrrhiza (Brown Mixture), Carminative Mixture (Dalby's Carminitive), Mixture of Copaiba (Lafayette Mixture), Mixture of Copaiba and Opium (Chapman's Mixture), Mixture of Magnesia, Asafetida, and Opium (Dewees' Carminative), Oleobalsamic Mixture (Hoffman's Balsam), Compound Mixture of Opium and Chloroform (Squibb's Diarrhoea Mixture), and Expectorant Mixture (Stokes' Expectorant) (3, 5).

Mouth washes: See *Washes, mouth*.

Moxa: Moxa are cones of combustible matter used for cauterization by burning (see *Cones*). Moxibustion, the burning of moxa, was an ancient method of counter-irritation or cautery arising out of China. Small cones of combustible organic material (originally *Artimesia moxa* or common mugwort) were placed on certain areas of the skin, ignited, and allowed to burn down, leaving a blister. Moxa entered Western medicine in the seventeenth century as a treatment for gout but fell into disuse a century later along with other forms of cautery (5, 28).

Mucilages: Mucilages are viscid preparations made by dissolving or suspending gummy substances in water.

The term comes from the Latin *mucus*. The gummy substances, if natural, are carbohydrates obtained from the exudates of trees or shrubs. Gums have been used since ancient Egypt. Hippocratic works (ca. 400 B.C.) mention acacia. Mucilage of Acacia was official in the first *United States Pharmacopoeia* (1820), with Mucilage of Tragacanth becoming official in the 1st revision (1830). Both have been used as thickening agents or to prevent the creaming of emulsions (2, 19).

Mucilago: See *Mucilages*.

Mulla: See *Mulls*.

Mulls: Mulls are ointments of high fusion points, containing the desired medicinal agent, and spread on soft muslin or mull in a manner similar to that of ordinary spread plasters. The most suitable base for preparing mulls is a mixture of suet and lard, with the occasional addition of wax or lead oleate plaster. Mulls are prepared extemporaneously by tacking unsized mull over a sheet of moistened parchment paper and spreading a melted, partially cooled ointment over the mull with a broad, flat bristle brush and smoothing the surface with two warmed elastic spatulas. When cooled, the mull is covered with waxed paper and rolled into a cylinder for dispensing. Salicylic Acid Mull, Salicylated Creosote Mull, Corrosive Mercuric Chloride Mull, and Zinc Mull were last official in the *National Formulary V* (1926) (5).

Muslin, oiled: See *Silk, oiled*.

Nasal solutions: See *Solutions, nasal*.

Nebula: See *Sprays*.

Nodulus: Nodulus is an abbreviation for *nodulus uterinus*, a form of uterine bougie.

Nose drops: See *Drops*.

Oculentum: See *Ointments, ophthalmic*.

Odontalgicum: See *Toothache drops*.

Oil sugars: Mixtures of sugar with fixed and volatile oils, rendering the oils miscible to water to an certain extent, offered as a convenient mode of administering medicines to children. The *National Formulary* offered a general formula for 2% oil sugars through its 7th edition (1946) (5, 13).

Oiled silk: See *Silk, oiled*.

Oils: Any liquid that greases; i.e., leaves, when dropped on a cloth, a stain which water does not wash out; this stain makes paper translucent. If a solid substance exhibits similar properties, it is called a fat. Oils are called volatile or fixed, according to whether this stain disappears on warming or is permanent because of the nonvolatility of the oil. A few medicated oils, such as Phenolated Oil N.F. and Phosphorated Oil N.F., were briefly official (3, 31).

Oils, infused: Oleaginous preparations for external use made by macerating a drug with alcohol and ammonia water, and digesting the mixture with sesame oil at 60–70°C until the alcohol and ammonia water have evaporated. The most common, Infused Oil of Hyoscyamus, was used to make Compound Oil of Hyoscyamus. This preparation was popular in France for the treatment of earache under the name *baumé tranquille* (3).

Ointments: Semisolid preparations intended for application to the skin with or without inunction. In addition to serving as vehicles for the topical application of medicinal substances, ointments may also serve as emollients for the skin and as protectives to prevent contact of the skin surface with aqueous solutions and skin irritants. Ointments are made by fusion, incorporation, or chemical reaction. Ancient humans attributed special powers to the fats of animals and humans, and their mixtures with resins, waxes, powdered herbs, and minerals represent one of the earliest dosage forms employed. A greaseless ointment, consisting of hartshorn beaten up with incense and flour and mixed with sweet ale appears in the Ebers papyrus (1500 B.C.). The Greeks did not distinguish between liquid or semisolid preparations used for an ointment, but rather according to use or ingredients. For example, *malagma* were softening ointments, whereas *keroma* were wax ointments, the predecessor of the later cerates. Plant mucilages, balsams, and oils mixed with wax were also classified as ointments. Galen's rose water ointment (or cold cream) was an early departure (second century A.D.) from the entirely fatty type of preparation (see *Creams*). By the thirteenth century, pharmacists distinguished between *olea* or oils (liquid oily ointments), *emplastra* or plasters (masses sticking firmly to the skin), and *unguenta* or ointments (semisolid smears), a concept that remained unchanged for nearly 500 years. The first *United States Pharmacopoeia* (1820) recognized lard as the chief ingredient of the first official ointments, which were rendered to the consistency of butter by the addition of suet, wax, or spermaceti. By the middle of the nineteenth century, however, natural ointment bases began to be replaced by artificial bases, introduced with special regard to the purposes they were to serve. Schacht introduced Glycerite of Starch in 1858, a translucent jelly prepared by heating glycerin and starch in certain proportions to a certain temperature, and W.A. Miller introduced Petrolatum in 1873 as "Cosmolin and Paraffin Ointment," both of which preparations were adopted by the *United States Pharmacopeia* in 1880. In 1885, the pharmacologist Oscar Liebreich rediscovered the therapeutic value of wool fat, the *oesypus* of the ancient Greeks, which he called lanolin; it was recognized by the *Pharmacopeia* in 1893. Later, the Russian chemist Lifschuetz discovered that the emulsification power of lanolin depended upon the free alcohols he had isolated as a group (1895–1898). In 1907, the dermatologist Paul G. Unna introduced eucerin, a new ointment base consisting of 1 part of Lifschuetz's alcohols, 20 parts of paraffin ointment, and 20 parts of water, the forerunner of the American "Aquaphor." Between 1920 and 1944, hydrogenated oils, sulfated and sulfonated hydrogenated oils, as well as stearic acid, sodium stearate, self-emulsifying glyceryl stearate mixtures, polymers of glycols (such as polyethylene glycol 4000), and esters of these glycols (such as polyethylene glycol monostearate) became important, followed by such modern bases as Plastibase, attapulgite, Veegum, guar gum, Carbopol, and the silicones, which were introduced between 1945 and 1959 (4, 5, 24).

Ointments, ophthalmic: Sterile ointments designed for application to the eyelids. Petrolatum, petrolatum-mineral oil, and petrolatum-anhydrous lanolin bases are often used in ophthalmic ointments because of their low irritating potential. Finely powdered, sterile active ingredients are aseptically incorporated into a sterile base, using sterile utensils, and dispensed in sterile ophthalmic-tipped tubes to reduce the possibility of contamination (4).

Ointments, softening: See *Cataplasms*.

Oleates: Usually liquid preparations made by dissolving alkaloids in oleic acid. Oleate of Mercury, however, is an ointment-like product of mercuric oxide in oleic acid. Oleic acid was named by the pharmacist Chevreul after olives (2, 5).

Oleinata: See *Oleates*.

Oleatum: See *Oleates*.

Oleoresina: See *Oleoresins*.

Oleoresins: Extracts of plant drugs prepared by percolation using a selective solvent (usually ether or acetone),

followed by complete removal of the solvent by evaporation. The term first arose in the 1820s (Buchner and Peschier), and the oleoresins first appeared in the *United States Pharmacopeia* of 1860 through the efforts of William Procter, Jr. (19).

Oleosacchara: See *Oil sugars*.

Oleovitamins: Preparations using fish liver oil, fish liver oil diluted with an edible vegetable oil, or a solution of vitamin concentrate in fish liver oil or in an edible vegetable oil. Oleovitamins were created during World War II to fill a therapeutic gap created by the interruption in cod liver oil supplies. The class became official in the second supplement to the *United States Pharmacopeia XI* (1942) as a source of vitamins A and D (31).

Oleum: See *Oils*.

Oleum infusum: See *Oils, infused*.

Ophthalmic ointments: See *Ointments, ophthalmic*.

Ophthalmic solutions: See *Solutions, ophthalmic*.

Orbicules: Spherical globules of sugar (see *Pills*) (5).

Oxymels: Acid-honey preparations containing acetic acid or vinegar (see *Honeys*) (4).

Paints, medicinal: Liquid medicinal preparations possessing antiseptic, caustic, soothing, or stimulating properties, usually applied by means of a brush. Paints intended to remain in contact with a specified surface are usually prepared with collodion, glycerin, glycerin and water, egg albumin in alcohol, or gutta percha. Paints intended to be absorbed are prepared with oleic acid or fatty oils. Caustic substances are usually applied dissolved in distilled water, alcohol, or ethereal vehicles, whereas resinous substances, such as benzoin, storax, tolu balsam, or sandarac dissolved in ether, are employed as bases for medicated varnishes, and used for application to the skin and raw mucous surfaces (5).

Papers, medicated: Preparations intended primarily for external application, either by saturating paper with medicinal substances or by applying the latter to the surface of the paper by the addition of some adhesive liquid. Potassium Nitrate Paper remained official in the *National Formulary* through its 5th edition (1926), but the most widely used paper is Mustard Paper, commonly called mustard plaster, a mixture of powdered black mustard and a solution of rubber spread on paper, cotton cloth, or other fabric, which remained official in the *National Formulary* through its eleventh edition (1960). Mustard poultices or cataplasms were formerly called sinapisms, after the botanical name for black mustard, *Sinapis nigra,* and were described in the *United States Dispensatory* (1836) as

> Powerfully rubefacient... usually becoming insupportably painful in less than an hour... . As a general rule, the poultice should be removed when the patient complains much of the pain; and in cases of insensibility should not, unless greatly diluted, be allowed to remain longer than one, or at most two hours, as violent inflammation, followed by obstinate ulceration, is apt to occur.

Home-made mustard plasters (equal parts of mustard and flour, moistened with tepid water to form a paste and applied to the skin in a muslin bag) still play a role in folk medicine (5, 13, 24).

Papers, powder: See *Powders, divided.*

Papers, waxed: Parchment-like paper treated with melted wax or paraffin used largely as an economical substitute for more expensive protective dressings (see *Dressings, protective*) (5).

Parenterals: See *Injections.*

Parogenum: See *Petroxolins.*

Parvula: See *Parvules.*

Parvules: Small sugar-coated pills, of 0.06 g or less, sometimes incorrectly called granules. (also see *Granules*) (4, 5).

Pasta: See *Pastes.*

Pasta dermatologica: Dermatologic pastes (see *Pastes*).

Pastes: Ointment-like mixtures of starch, dextrin, zinc oxide, sulfur, calcium carbonate, or other medicinal substances made into a smooth paste with glycerin, soft soap, petrolatum, lard, or other fats, and medicated with antiseptic or astringent agents, designed for external use. Early pastes, such as *Pasta Glycyrrhizae* and *Pasta Althaeae*, were internal preparations, most of which were of gum-like consistency. The modern pastes were introduced by the noted dermatologists Paul G. Unna

and Oskar Lassar around 1900. Dermatologic Pastes normally contain a higher proportion of powdered material than that included in ointments and are less greasy but more absorptive than other preparations for external application. The *British Pharmaceutical Codex* groups Witch Hazel Cream, Vanishing Cream, Tannic Acid Jelly, Catheter Lubricant, and a wide assortment of "medicated preparations for external application, employed principally as antiseptic, caustic, cooling, protective or soothing dressings" under the title "Pastes." Pastes entered the *National Formulary III* in 1906 (4, 5, 24).

Pastes, dermatologic: See *Pastes.*

Pastilles: A form of lozenge, particularly those which are chocolate flavored (see *Lozenges*); also, combustible cones of aromatic drugs used for fumigation (see *Cones*). The term came into English usage around 1650 from the French *pastille*, which was derived from the Latin *pastillus*, meaning "little loaf" (2, 5).

Pastillus: See *Pastilles* and *Cones*.

Pearls: Round or oval capsules made by enclosing liquids, solids, or tablets in a shell of glycerogelatin material. Pearls are less elastic than soft capsules and contain no air space, the glycerogelatin shell being completely filled with the medicinal substance. Pharmacists made pearls extemporaneously by laying a softened sheet of glycerogelatin over a warmed molding plate containing a specified number of semicircular (or other shaped) depressions. The sheet was covered with a measured quantity of medicinal liquid, and the liquid with a second sheet of glycerogelatin to exclude air. The whole assembly was covered with a matching molding plate, and compressed with a mechanical press to form the pearls, an exacting and time-consuming process requiring special apparatus. This process has been superseded in industry by a continuous automated process in which a liquid is injected between two ribbons of gelatin while passing between revolving dies (also see *Capsules, soft*) (4, 5).

Pelleta: See *Pellets.*

Pellets: Small spheres of sucrose saturated with an alcoholic tincture, primarily used in homeopathic medicine. Pellets are made in different sizes, designated according to the diameter of ten pellets measured in millimeters. *Remington's Practice of Pharmacy* (1926) states that pellets "should be made of the purest materials, should be perfectly white and odorless and able to withstand all the tests prescribed for sucrose or cane sugar" (also see *Globules*) (5, 24).

Pencils, antiseptic: See *Pencils, medicated*.

Pencils, astringent: (See *Pencils, medicated*).

Pencils, caustic: (See *Pencils, medicated*).

Pencils, medicated: Cylinders used in dermatologic practice to apply medicinal agents directly to the skin. The medicinal agent is incorporated into a paste consisting of starch, dextrin, tragacanth, and sucrose with sufficient water to form a plastic mass, which is rolled into cylinders about 5 mm in diameter, cut into sections about 5 cm long, dried on parchment paper at room temperature, and wrapped in tinfoil. Medicated pencils intended as a caustic application, such as sticks of silver nitrate, are sometimes referred to as escharotica. Salicylic Acid Pencils, the last official medicated pencils, appeared in the *National Formulary V* (1926); also known as Antiseptic, Astringent, Caustic, Salve, or Styptic Pencils (5).

Pencils, salve: See *Pencils, medicated*.

Pencils, styptic: See *Pencils, medicated*.

Perles: See *Pearls*.

Pessaries: Medicated vaginal suppositories, globular or oviform in shape, weighing between 4 g (if made from oil of theobroma or cocoa butter) and 10 g (if made from glycerated gelatin). The term derives from a Greek word describing the small stones used for playing the game of draughts (5, 35).

Pessarium: See *Pessaries*.

Pessum: See *Pessaries*.

Petroxolins: Fluid preparations for external use with a base of liquid petrolatum and ammonium oleate. The preparations became official in the 6th edition of the *National Formulary* (1936) (3).

Pigmentum: See *Paints, medicinal*.

Pill coatings: See *Coatings, pill*.

Pills: Small, solid masses of a globular, ovoid, or lenticular shape intended for oral administration. Pills are

prepared by incorporating medicinal agents with other materials to form a cohesive, plastic mass, which is divided into the requisite number of portions, each of which is formed into the desired shape. Pills usually range in weight from 0.10 to 0.30 g. Exceptionally large pills of 0.60 g or more are referred to as boluses; very small sugar-coated pills of 0.06 g or less are known as parvules or granules; pellets, globules, or orbicules are small spheres of sugar saturated with an alcoholic tincture, largely used in homeopathic medicine. When the pill came into use in ancient Mesopotamia and Egypt, it offered for the first time a definite dose corresponding with a desired therapeutic action. The Greeks named the little balls of medicine *katapotia* ("something to be swallowed"), later Latinized to *catapotium*; by the first century A.D., the term *pilula* came into use In Rome. Pills persisted as a major dosage form for a remarkably long period of time. For example, over half of the prescriptions dispensed at a Charlestown, Massachusetts, pharmacy during the years 1872–1875 were for pills. Moreover, certain combinations of drugs persisted for thousands of years in pill form. The Pills of Rufus, for example, were originally a *hiera* (bitter powder) made into pill form by the Arabs and popularized by Avicenna (980–1033); a modern version, Pills of Aloe and Mastic, were last official in the 8th revision of the *United States Pharmacopeia* (1905) (4, 5, 36–37).

Pills, compressed: See *Tablets*.

Pills, enteric-coated: See *Enteric-coated doses*.

Pilula: See *Pills*.

Pilula comprimata: Compressed pills (see *Pills*).

Pilula enterica: Enteric-coated pills (see *Pills*).

Pilules: See *Pellets*.

Plasma: Nonfatty unctuous preparations (5).

Plasters: Substances intended for external application, made of such materials and of such consistency as to adhere to the skin. Adhesive plasters afford protection and mechanical support, whereas medicated plasters furnish an occlusive and macerating action, bringing the medication into close contact with the skin; when spread on perforated cloth, the product is called a porous plaster. Plasters are among the most ancient of all pharmaceuticals. Primitive humans may have used plasters of mud and leaves to help heal wounds or relieve pain. The Ebers papyrus (1500 B.C.)

describes several plasters and poultices for treating burns, and the Greeks assigned a special place within their temples where plasters were prepared. Indeed, the word plaster is derived from the Greek *emplastron* meaning "to smear on" or "to mold on." The famous diachylon plaster, made from oil, litharge, and certain plant juices was compiled by Menecrates, physician of the Emperor Tiberius about 39 A.D. and passed on in verse form to Claudius Galen (131–201), who developed a number of practical formulas for plasters and procedures for their preparation which endured for centuries. A modern version of diachylon plaster survived as Lead Oleate Plaster (or Lead Plaster) in the *United States Pharmacopeia* and later in the *National Formulary* through its 8th edition (1946). Originally, plasters were spread directly on the affected part of the body; by the sixteenth century, plaster material was being spread on linen or leather or dipped. In 1514, Giovanni da Vigo popularized spread plasters called sparadraps or spasmadraps; in 1691, William Salmon described dipped cerecloths in his *Pharmacopoeia Londonensis*. Plasters were spread with the aid of an offset spatula or plaster iron heated by means of a spirit lamp, an arduous and time-consuming process which exhausted the patience of pharmacists who struggled trying to keep the refractory plaster masses warm and malleable. Although Elisha Perkins of Baltimore is credited with obtaining the first American patent for a manufactured plaster (1830), John C. De La Cour of Camden, New Jersey, is generally credited as among the earliest producers of machine-spread adhesive plasters (1836), one of the first commercially prepared dosage forms manufactured in the United States. In 1852, an English apothecary named Mather patented a method of spreading plasters on leather by the use of heated rollers, producing a thinner and more uniform product, leading Edward Parrish to observe in his classic text, *American Pharmacy* (1856), that "the spreading of plasters which was formerly an important part of the business of the apothecary has now ... been monopolized by manufacturers who bring machinery to their aid." The only plaster which still finds significant use today is Salicylic Acid Plaster, United States Pharmacopeia—the common corn plaster (also see *Plasters, adhesive*, and *Plasters, porous*) (4, 5, 15, 24, 38).

Plasters, adhesive: A mixture of rubber, resins, and waxes, with a filler of absorbent powder, such as zinc oxide, orris root, or starch, mechanically mixed and spread on cotton cloth. Early adhesive plasters were composed of resin and litharge or diachylon spread on calico, muslin, or linen. In 1843, B.C. Rowland of Liverpool, England, reported on an "India Rubber Court Plaster" made by dissolving India rubber in naphtha or turpentine and spreading the liquefied rubber on silk or satin. Two years later, Horace Day and William Shecut of New York City patented a combination of India rubber and gums as a plaster mass. In 1852, Benjamin Nickels of Surrey, England, patented an "elastic plaster" combining adhesive material on an elastic fiber. In 1863, Joshua Melvin of Lowell, Massachusetts, patented the manufacture of adhesive plaster in roll or cylindrical form. By the early twentieth century, two types of rubber-based adhesive plasters emerged: surgeons' adhesive plaster, a plain yellow-colored mass, and zinc oxide adhesive plaster, a white mass containing zinc oxide. Modern adhesive plasters, consisting of vinyl resin, plasticizers, and other chemical additives have an excellent ability to remain adhered under severe conditions of moisture and heat, and rarely cause skin irritation. Adhesive plaster remained official through the 19th revision of the *United States Pharmacopeia* (1975) (also see *Plasters* and *Plasters, porous*) (5, 15, 24).

Plasters, Blister: Plasters designed to produce inflammation, blisters, or issues (running sores). Many blistering agents were used to prepare blister plasters, but the potent and powerful cantharides (or Spanish flies), was the most widely applied. It was used internally by the ancients, who were well aware that it produced hematuria even when applied externally. Aretaeus introduced an external preparation of cantharides as a blistering agent in the second century to the shaved head to relieve headache. This treatment was also used for epilepsy and vertigo, and persisted through the centuries, but only after the patient had been given milk to drink for 3 days to protect the bladder from injury. "In many constitutions the strangury will ensue, especially where the discharge of serous juice is too great," an English textbook on materia medica advised in 1730. "But, however it be, such applications are necessary when a patient proves delirious, as frequently happens in high fevers." A century later, the *United States Dispensatory* (1836), in discussing the use of Cerate of Cantharides, "the common blistering plaster of the shops," remarked that

> When the full operation of the flies is desirable, and the object is to produce a permanent effect, the application should be continued for twelve hours... . It should then be removed, and followed by a bread and milk poultice, or some other emollient dressing, under which the cuticle rises, and a full blister is usually produced. By this management the patient will escape strangury, and the blister will very quickly heal after the discharge of the serum.

Elisha Perkins of Baltimore obtained a patent in 1830 for an apparatus to prepare blister plasters. George W. Carpenter of Philadelphia sold and recommended Perkin's blister cloth in 1831 as "a very convenient article for the country physician, being ready spread for immediate use." *Ceratum Cantharides* was official in the *United States Pharmacopeia* and, later, in the *National Formulary* until 1950 (13, 15, 28).

Plasters, porous: Adhesive plasters spread on perforated cloth. Sir William Butts, royal physician to Henry VIII, devised a "spasmadrap or dypped plaster" which was to be poked "full of smalle hoolys." In 1845, Horace Day and William Shecut of New York City patented a rubber-based "porous plaster" rendered full of minute holes to "allow the free escape of the perspiration." In 1854, Somerville Scott Alison of London patented a porous or "perforated Lambskin... prepared according to the process called chamois curing." The porosity is considered a mechanical advantage in that it prevents the plaster from slipping from the point of application, each opening serving as a stop. Porous plasters are also far more comfortable than the nonporous variety, which they have superseded (also see *Plasters* and *Plasters, adhesive*) (5, 15).

Politzer plugs: Greased pellets of cotton about the size of a coriander seed with a thread attached, for insertion into the ear as a protective. The pellets were named after Adam Politzer (1835-1920), an Austrian otologist (1, 2).

Pomatum: Fats saturated with odorous principles (5).

Potio: See *Draughts*.

Potions: See *Draughts*.

Potus: See *Draughts*.

Poultices: Originally spelled "pultes" in sixteenth-century England, the term came from the Latin *puls or pultes* meaning "a pottage of meal" (also see *Cataplasms*) (2).

Powder papers: See *Papers, divided*.

Powders: Intimate mixtures of dry, powdered medicinal substances reduced to a fine powder by the processes of comminution and trituration. Bulk powders are divided into two categories: simple, consisting of one substance, and compound, consisting of two or more powders mixed together. One of the most ancient compound powders was *hiera picra* ("sacred bitters"), a mixture of aloe and canella introduced about 500 B.C. as a laxative, the prototype of a

large number of bitter powders containing aloe as the principal ingredient and bearing the general title *Hiera*. This powder was listed in various pharmacopoeias and was last recognized in the 4th edition of the *National Formulary* (official until 1926). Powders were designed originally as a convenient mode of administrating hard vegetable drugs such as roots, barks, and woods; powders were also found to be convenient for the dispensing of insoluble chemical compounds such as calomel, bismuth salts, mercury, and chalk. Famous compound powders of the past include: Compound Powder of Glycyrrhiza, a variant of Compound Senna Powder recognized by the first *London Pharmacopoeia* (1618); Powder of Ipecac and Opium, or Dover's Powders, introduced by the English physician Thomas Dover as *Pulvis Diaphoreticus* in the early eighteenth century; Aromatic Powder of Chalk, a simplified version of a complex confection devised by Sir Walter Raleigh during his imprisonment and introduced into the *London Pharmacopoeia* of 1721 as *Confectio Raleighana*; and Antimonial Powder, patented in 1747 as Dr. James's Fever Powder. The *United States Dispensatory* (1836) noted that "the form of powder is convenient for the exhibition of substances which are not given in very large doses, are not very disagreeable to the taste, have no corrosive property, and do not deliquesce rapidly on exposure." Today, drugs not available in capsule or tablet form can still be conveniently administered in powdered form by placing them on the back of the tongue and swallowing them with water. Flavored powders are particularly useful for children who might have difficulty swallowing a tablet or capsule (also see *Powders, divided*) (4, 5, 13, 24).

Powders, divided: Intimate mixtures of dry, powdered medicinal substances intended for oral administration, divided into single doses, each of which is folded into a small sheet of glassine paper. One of the oldest of dosage forms, divided powders have largely been replaced by capsules or tablets. Nevertheless, the preparation of powders permits the drugs to be reduced to a very fine state of subdivision, a physical condition which frequently intensifies their therapeutic activity, a factor in increasing the efficacy of homeopathic triturations, calomel and sodium bicarbonate mixtures, and Dover's Powder (Powder of Ipecac and Opium). Divided powders also furnish a convenient means for administering drugs that are not excessively bitter, nauseous, or otherwise offensive to the taste. One of the most durable divided powders is Seidlitz Powders, a saline cathartic originated and patented by Thomas Savory in 1815. Savory claimed that the powders owed their value to the mineral properties of the Seidlitz spring in Germany, which contains magnesium sulfate. The powders consist of sodium bicarbonate (wrapped in blue paper) and tartaric acid and potassium and sodium tartrate (wrapped in white paper), each of which are dissolved separately in water and then mixed. The formula was exposed in a book of recipes for patent medicines published by the Philadelphia College of Pharmacy in 1824, and remained official as Compound Effervescent Powders in the *United States Pharmacopeia*, and later in the *National Formulary* through its 12th edition (1965); also known as *Powder papers* (5).

Precipitates: Drugs prepared by separating particles from a previously clear liquid by physical or chemical means. Precipitation usually occurs when a hot saturated solution of an amorphous substance is allowed to cool or when a liquid in which the dissolved substance is insoluble is added to its solution. Pharmacists formerly used the process of precipitation as a convenient method of obtaining solid substances in fine particles (precipitated calcium carbonate), to purify solids (precipitated calcium phosphate), or to prepare mercury salts. White precipitate (ammoniated mercury) was first described by Beguin in 1632, a soluble double chloride of mercury and ammonium known to the alchemists as *sal alembroth* and *sal sapientiae*, respectively. Red precipitate (red mercuric oxide) was known to alchemists as *hydragyrum precipitatum per se* or "precipitate per se"; yellow precipitate is a synonym for yellow mercuric oxide (5, 24).

Preserves: See *Conserves*.

Protective dressings: See *Dressings, protective*.

Pulvis: See *Powders*.

Quiddonies: Preparations with a vehicle of thick, quince-flavored syrup (also see *Syrups*) (39).

Resina: See *Resins*.

Resins: Solid preparations consisting chiefly of the resinous principles from vegetable bodies. The officially prepared resins differ from alcoholic extracts in that the latter contain all of the alcohol-soluble principles in the drugs, whereas the resins contain only the alcohol-soluble principles that are insoluble in water. The term probably arose from the Greek *rheos*, "to flow," referring perhaps to the flow of pine resin commonly observed (2, 5).

Rotula: Globules or orbicules (see *Pills*) (5).

Rubificients: Local remedies which produce redness and inflammation of the skin. The word comes from two Latin words: *ruber*, meaning "red," and *facio*, meaning "to make" (2, 13).

Saccharures: Preparations made by saturating sucrose with a tincture, drying it, and grinding the mixture to a powder (5).

Saccelli amylacea: See *Wafer envelopes*.

Sacculi: Abbreviation for *sacculi medicinales*, or "bags of drugs" (20).

Sal: See *Salts*.

Sal effervescens: See *Salts, effervescent*.

Sal factitium: See *Salts, artificial*.

Salts: Compounds formed by the union of acids and bases, by the action of alkalies upon metals, or by the direct union of elements. The term is often incorporated in the common name of salts used as pharmaceuticals: bitter salts, epsom salt, or Seidlitz salt (magnesium sulfate), preparing salt (sodium stannate), Preston's salts (ammonium chloride), Rochelle salt or Seignette's salt (potassium and ammonium tartrate), salt of Mars (ferrous sulfate), salt of Saturn (lead acetate), salt of tartar (potassium carbonate), salt of tin (stannous chloride), salt of wisdom (mercury bichloride and ammonium chloride), sore-throat salt (fused potassium nitrate), vinegar salts (calcium acetate), and vomiting salt (zinc sulfate). The term is also applied to some acids, such as salt of lemon or sour salt (citric acid), salt of sorrel (oxalic acid), and spirit of salt (muriatic acid) (5, 13).

Salts, artificial: A mixture of the more important chemical salts naturally present in several of the well-known mineral springs of Europe. "These are properly labeled artificial," notes *Remington's Practice of Pharmacy* (1926), "and if used to prepare effervescent salts or mineral waters they should be sold only as an imitation of the genuine" (5).

Salts, effervescent: Granular effervescent salts were formerly made by mixing dry powders with dry tartaric acid and sodium bicarbonate and moistening the mixture with strong alcohol. The pasty mass was passed through a sieve, and the granules dried quickly in a hot room, sifted, and filled into bottles, which were hermetically sealed to prevent the access of moisture. This method was greatly improved upon by mixing the powders in a flat enameled dish and heating in an oven to about 100°C or by heating the mixture in a deep jacketed kettle or in a pill-coating pan, heated, as it revolves, by a gas flame. When the mixture becomes moist, it is manipulated with a wooden spatula to make it uniform in consistency, and rubbed through a coarse tinned iron sieve; the granules obtained are dried slowly at a low heat in an oven (5).

Salts, smelling: Ammonia-based preparations used as a restorative in "hysterical syncope" (fainting). Dry smelling salts (or vinaigrettes) are composed of ammonium chloride and potassium carbonate, perfumed with lavender; liquid smelling salts are composed of ammonium carbonate dissolved in stronger ammonia water and alcohol, and perfumed with oils; solidified smelling salts are similar preparations solidified with stearic acid (5).

Salve pencils: See *Pencils, medicated.*

Salves: This term probably arose from the Anglo-Saxon *sealf* or the German *salbe*, both meaning "ointment" (see *Ointments*) (2).

Scutum: Abbreviation for *scutum stomachicum*, a large plaster, applied to the breast or stomach (20).

Semicupia: A half-bath, used interchangeably with Insessia (20).

Sericum oleatum: See *Silk, oiled.*

Serums: Serum therapy came into prominence in the 1890s when Emil von Behring (1854–1917) extended Pasteur's theory of attenuated viruses. Behring demonstrated that the serum of animals immunized against attenuated diphtheria toxins can be used as a preventive or therapeutic inoculation against diphtheria in other animals through a specific neutralization of the toxin of the disease. In 1894, Behring began to produce his new antitoxic serum on a grand scale; it soon became recognized as the specific treatment for diphtheria. Antisera act by combining with the toxin in the blood of the patient, rendering it inert. Scarlet fever, tetanus, erysipelas, botulism, and gas gangrene have been successfully treated by antitoxic serums prepared in this manner. Antibacterial serum is produced by injection of an animal with successive doses of bacteria. The immune substances thus formed act by enhancing phagocytosis, destroying the bacteria. Pneumonia, streptococcic infection, and spinal meningitis have been aided by the use of this type of serum. Mixed serum

contains both antitoxic and antibacterial immune bodies; the serum used to treat scarlet fever is of this type (3, 40).

Shampoos: A wash for the hair or soap for hair washing. The term comes from the Hindustani word *tshampa*, meaning "to squeeze" or "to press," probably associated with hot oriental baths (2).

Silk, oiled: A thin, very soft, and pliable protective dressing made of fine silk, coated with a flexible linseed-oil varnish. Oiled Silk is available in semitransparent or opaque form, made by the addition of talc or starch in the final coating. Oiled Muslin or Oiled Cambric is similar to oiled silk, except that the basic fabric is of glazed cotton; it is thicker and heavier and consequently less pliable than oiled silk (see *Dressings, protective*) (5).

Sinapismus: See *Plasters, blister.*

Sindon oleata: Oiled muslin or Oiled cambric (see *Silk, oiled*).

Snuffs: See *Insufflations.*

Soaps: A class of chemical substances which are metal salts of fatty acids. Pliny (first century A.D) records that the ancient Romans learned the preparation of soap from Nordic tribes, who used a pomade prepared from goat fat and the calcined ashes of beechwood. *Sapo*, the Latin word for soap, is derived from the Nordic *sepe*. The chemistry of soaps was elucidated in the early nineteenth century by French chemist M.E. Chevreul (1786–1889). Soaps may be divided into two classes: soluble soaps (or detergent or cleansing soaps), which are compounds of fatty acids with alkali metals, particularly sodium and potassium; and insoluble soaps, which are compounds of fatty acids and metals of any other group, such as Lead Oleate Plaster or Lime Liniment, a calcium soap of linseed oil. Soluble soaps include Hard Soap (or Castile Soap), prepared from olive oil and sodium hydroxide, official through the 11th edition of the *National Formulary* (1960), and Soft Soap (or Green Soap), prepared from linseed oil, glycerin, and dekanormal solutions of sodium and potassium hydroxide; the latter continues to hold official status (4, 5).

Soft capsules: See *Capsules, soft.*

Solutio: Dental preparations official only in the 5th edition of the *National Formulary* (1926), consisting of a solution of a resinous material dissolved in chloroform (3).

Solution tablets: See *Tablets, solution.*

Solutions: Liquid preparations that contain one or more substances dissolved in a solvent and, by reason of their ingredients or method of preparation, do not fall into some other category of preparation. From the seventeenth century on, the term *liquor* denoted liquid solutions. By the early twentieth century, liquor usually referred to aqueous solutions of nonvolatile substances. For example, Solution of Magnesium Citrate, *United States Pharmacopeia*, had the Latin title *Liquor Magnesii Citratis*. Beginning with the *United States Pharmacopeia XVI* and the *National Formulary XI* (1960), the term liquor was dropped and solutions were listed by their active ingredient or ingredients (19).

Solutions, irrigating: A preparation to be applied continuously by means of a special device for the purpose, as in the treatment of wounds with Dakin's solution (5).

Solutions, nasal: Solutions of drugs for instilling in the nose rather than spraying are generally a modern development. The first nasal solutions were formulated with menthol and thymol dissolved in light mineral oil. Later isotonic aqueous solutions were designed as drops (3).

Solutions, ophthalmic: Originally called collyria, ophthalmic solutions arose from the eye washes of the ancient world. Early preparations were not the sterile, buffered solutions of today. The term collyrium comes from the Greek *kollurion*, which Hippocrates used to designate fatty suppositories for gynecological purposes. They were formed into sticks, from which a paste was made with a liquid. Eventually, more liquid was added and the paste thinned to a lotion. This lotion was used as an eye wash, and term came to be used exclusively for this type of preparation. Remington's formula for a collyrium of 260 mg (4 grains) of sodium borate in 30 mL (1 oz) of camphor water was a standard from 1886 into the mid-twentieth century (2, 41).

Sovella: See *Tablets, solution*.

Spasmadraps: Pieces of linen or other cloth dipped in or spread with a medicinal plaster, popularized in 1514 by Giovanni da Vigo (1460–1525), physician to Pope Julius II. From the Latin *spasma* meaning "healing powder" and the French *drap* meaning "cloth." Also known as sparadraps or cerecloths (see *Plasters*) (15).

Species: See *Teas*.

Spirits: Solutions of volatile substances (usually volatile oils) in alcohol. Some editions of the *National Formulary*

stated that "spirits of volatile oils" contained 6.5% of the volatile oil, but that figure was later rejected as too low. Although used internally, several spirits were used medicinally by inhalation or as flavorings (4, 31).

Spiritus: See *Spirits*.

Sprays: Medicated liquids prepared for dispersal by atomizers or nebulizers, usually on external surface or mucous membranes of the respiratory tract. In the *United States Pharmacopoeia*, sprays were called *inhalatio*; the *National Formulary* referred to them as *nebulae*. Sprays of the early twentieth century were formulated with aromatics dissolved in light mineral oil. As injuries from inhaled oils became apparent, especially among children, these sprays were displaced by buffered aqueous solutions (1, 31).

Starch capsules: See *Cachets*.

Steam: See *Vapors*.

Steatina: A salve mull (see *Mulls*) (5).

Stilus dissolubilis: Dissolving pencils (see *Pencils, medicated*). Pencils containing a caustic or an astringent (5).

Stilus medicatus: See *Pencils, medicated*.

Stilus unguentis: Salve pencils, cooling, antiseptic, or astringent (see *Pencils, medicated*) (5).

Stupa: See *Stypes*.

Stypes: Cloths wrung out of hot water and sprinkled with a counterirritant (2).

Styptic pencils: See *Pencils, medicated*.

Succus: See *Juices*.

Succus spissatus: Condensed juice (see *Extracts*).

Sugar plums: See *Condita*.

Suppositories: Conical or ovoid medicated solids intended for insertion into one of the several orifices of the body, excluding the mouth. Suppository use has been known as early as 2600 B.C., and was recommended in the works of Hippocrates (ca. 400 B.C.). The term derives from the Latin *suppositus*, meaning "to place under." Premodern suppositories were made by hand using soap or other semisolid fatty substances as the main vehicles. They were not commonly used until the seventeenth and eighteenth centuries and did not become popular until the mid-nineteenth century and the advent of cocoa butter as vehicle. In 1766, Antoine Baumé described a suppository mold which used liquefied cocoa butter. This technique was popularized in America by Alfred B. Taylor about 1852 using paper cones as molds. Metal molds were introduced about 1860, although many pharmacists continued to form suppositories by hand without heat. Cold compression of cocoa butter was made possible through the introduction of metal suppository presses about 1868, although the first popular compression mold was not introduced until 1879. After 1870, mixtures of glycerin and gelatin came to be used as vehicles for suppositories, beginning a quest for the perfect vehicle that continues to the present (2, 19, 42).

Suppositorium: See *Suppositories*.

Suspensio: See *Suspensions*.

Suspensions: Heterogeneous systems containing coarsely dispersed material that settles. A wide variety of pharmaceutical preparations have been used as suspensions, for example, White Lotion, Magma of Bismuth, and Compound Mixture of Opium and Glycyrrhiza (Brown Mixture). In addition, several official ointments are suspensions of solids in a semisolid base. A large number of suspensions are categorized as mixtures in the *United States Pharmacopeia* and the *National Formulary* (19).

Swabs: Ampuls containing Iodine Tincture, *United States Pharmacopeia*, covered with gauze or other absorbent material, and used for first-aid treatment. Iodine Swabs, later called Iodine Ampuls, were official in the *National Formulary* through its 13th edition (1970). When iodine tincture is required for first aid, the tip of the ampul is broken and the gauze absorbs the iodine and provides a means of applying it directly to the wound. Some Iodine Ampuls are in the form of fine capillary tubes, which are broken when needed and the tincture applied directly (24).

Sweetmeats: See *Condita*.

Syrups: A nearly saturated aqueous solution of sugar (usually sucrose) with or without medicinal or flavoring ingredients. Syrups are usually divided into flavored, containing a fruit or aromatic substance for a pleasant taste, and medicated, containing a drug. Simple Syrup,

United States Pharmacopeia was commonly used in the preparation of pill masses and other mixtures (3, 8, 19).

Syrupus: See *Syrups*.

Tabella: See *Tablets*.

Tablet Triturates: See *Triturates, tablet*.

Tablets: Dosage forms prepared by molding or compressing medicinal substances in dies. Tablets vary widely in shape, the most common form being discoid, and range from 0.06 to 0.60 g in weight. Jean de Renou applied the Latin word *tabella* to a special type of troche in 1608; Burroughs Wellcome & Company coined the term "tablet" in 1878 to refer to its brand of compressed pills; the term is derived from the French *tablette*, meaning "shelf" and the Latin *tabula*, meaning "board." In 1843, the English apothecary William Brockedon patented a device for compressing medicinal agents commonly employed in pills and lozenges without the use of liquid adhesive agents; the resulting product was known as compressed pills. The Philadelphia druggist Jacob Dunton invented a similar device in 1864, marketing his own compressed pills in 1869; Joseph Remington devised a similar machine in 1875 to allow the retail druggist to "manufacture his own medication called for on prescription." Each of these devices consisted of a compression cylinder and lower die (to hold the medicinal substance) as well as an upper die which was struck with a mallet to compress the material. More reliable compression was achieved by using the screw devices invented by Germany's Professor Rosenthal (1874) and perfected by Austria's Carl Engler (1907). Another advancement was the lever device introduced by Philadelphia's Bennett L. Smedley (1879). The first rotary tablet machine was developed in 1872 by Henry Bower, an employee of the Philadelphia drug manufacturer John Wyeth; two years later, Joseph A. McFerran received a patent for the first fully automatic tablet machine (2, 4, 43).

Tabletta: See *Tablets*.

Tablets, compressed: See *Tablets*.

Tablets, dispensing: See *Tablets, solution*.

Tablets, enteric-coated: See *Enteric-coated doses*.

Tablets, hypodermic: Molded tablet triturates intended to be dissolved in water to make a solution to be injected parenterally. The usual weight of hypodermic tablets is about 0.03 g, which distinguishes them from ordinary tablet triturates that weigh about 0.06 g. Formerly prepared extemporaneously by pharmacists, modern compressed hypodermic tablets are not intended to be sterile, although they are manufactured under strict conditions as a precaution against contamination (see *Triturates, tablet*) (4).

Tablets, molded: See *Triturates, tablet.*

Tablets, poison: Tablets of mercury bichloride in an angular, not discoid shape, blue in color, each having the word "POISON" and the skull-and-crossbones design distinctly stamped upon it. A unique one-product classification, poison tablets (or *Toxitabellae*) first became official in the *United States Pharmacopoeia IX* (1916), and two strengths remained official in the *National Formulary* through its 10th edition (1950); the larger tablets remained official through the 12th edition (1965). Diluted in a solution of 1:1000 concentration, mercury bichloride is an antiseptic used chiefly for the disinfection of inanimate objects and the unabraded skin (4, 5, 24).

Tablets, solution: Molded or compressed tablets containing large amounts of potent substances not intended for administration, but rather as a convenience in dispensing; also known as Dispensing Tablets. To lessen the risk of their being dispensed by mistake for other tablets, dispensing tablets are always of angular rather than discoid shape. They are usually scored to facilitate division into more or less accurate fractions. Also tablets to be dissolved in water for external use (4).

Teas: Coarsely powdered mixtures of dried herbs intended for medicinal teas or poultices; also known as Species. The *National Formulary* recognized an Emollient Species, used as a cataplasm; a Laxative Species (St. Germain Tea); and a Pectoral Species (Breast Tea) for a "catarrhal condition of the respiratory tract" through its 5th edition (1926). Similar teas from home-grown herbs persist as common household remedies. True tea from China was introduced to England by Christopher Borough in 1379. The English word probably comes from the Dutch *thee* (2, 5, 24).

Tinctura: See *Tinctures.*

Tinctures: Alcoholic or hydroalcoholic solutions of drugs, usually of plant origins. The term comes from the Latin *tingere*, "to dye or soak in color." Tinctures, as alcoholic solutions, entered medical practice in the thirteenth century through the efforts of Raymond Lull and Arnald of Villanova. Paracelsus (1493–1541) was a strong advocate for tinctures; inasmuch as he was controversial, his advocacy probably discouraged their incorporation into compendia until the 1700s. In the 1800s, wine remained the prime hydroalcoholic vehicle in the United States. After the turn of the century, however, tinctures (and elixirs) displaced those wines because of their wide variation in strength. Moreover, prohibition impeded their widespread use. As galenicals declined throughout the twentieth century, tinctures lingered on as an official class, mainly as flavorings, for example, Tincture of Orange Peel. Homeopathic Tinctures are generally prepared by long maceration of freshly dried succulent plants or their parts in alcohol, the completed tincture being made to represent one part of the dry crude material in each ten parts of the completed preparation (2, 5, 19).

Tinctures, homeopathic: See *Tinctures.*

Tincture triturations, homeopathic: See *Triturations.*

Toothache drops: See *Drops, toothache.*

Toxitabella: See *Tablets, poison.*

Triturates, tablet: Small, disk-like masses of medicinal powders prepared by forcing a moistened tablet mass into a die by manual pressure and allowing them to dry and harden. The basis of tablet triturates is usually a mixture of lactose and sucrose in a 5:1 ratio, moistened with a volatile liquid such as alcohol. Tablet triturates were introduced in New York in 1878 by Dr. Robert W. Fuller as a palatable and convenient means of administering potent drugs by mouth. Fuller's original triturates consisted of triturations of metallic, mineral, and vegetable matter, mixed into a paste with alcohol or water, and molded into the desired shape. In 1882, Fuller described a perforated, hard rubber tablet triturate mold with a corresponding pegged plate, which was practically identical to those available today. Tablet triturates served the purposes of homeopathic physicians well and undoubtedly helped to further the use of homeopathic doses. Twentieth-century pharmacists also prepared hypodermic tablets (used for preparing hypodermic injections) utilizing the technique. Today, tablet triturates and hypodermic tablets are formed by compression and are termed molded tablets (4, 5, 43).

Trituratio: See *Triturations.*

Triturations: Dilutions of potent powdered drugs prepared by intimately mixing them with a suitable diluent, usually lactose, in a definite proportion by weight, usually 10%, used as a dispensing aid. Such poisonous substances as strychnine sulfate, arsenic, mercury bichloride, and atropine are much more accurately dispensed using this technique, the pharmacist weighing a multiple of the prescribed drug in a triturated form. Homeopathic triturations were formerly prepared by triturating one part of a drug into 99 parts of lactose over a period of at least one hour; homeopathic tincture triturations were prepared by mixing 10 mL of a homeopathic "strong tincture" with 10 g of lactose and triturating the mixture gently until dry. Although such powdered triturations were being replaced by commercially prepared tablet triturates by the mid-1920s, a general formula for triturations, specifying geometric dilution, remained official in the *United States Pharmacopeia* through its 14th revision (1950) (5).

Triturations, homeopathic: See *Triturations*.

Trituraations, tincture: See *Triturations*.

Troches: Solid dosage forms in the form of small disks, cylinders, or tablets, intended to be placed in the mouth and allowed to dissolve or disintegrate slowly. The term is derived from the Greek *trochos*, meaning "round" or "circular." They were subsequently called *pastils* in French and lozenges in English. One of the earliest troches (500 B.C.) was *terra sigillata*, or sealed earth, a product composed of clay from the island of Lemnos and goat's blood, rolled and cut into disks and impressed with a seal; by the Middle Ages, a variety of troche presses were employed. In 1856, Edward Parrish described an apparatus for rolling and cutting troches consisting of a rolling-board, wooden roller, and cutting punch. During the next two decades, F.L. Slocum (1879), F.E. Harrison (1880), Wallace Procter (1894), and nearly a dozen others patented similar machines. The 4th edition of the *National Formulary* (1916) featured nine formulas for troches; by the mid-1930s, troches were being replaced by tablets: the 6th edition (1936) featured only Troches of Elm. Modern troches consist of powdered drugs bound with sugar and tragacanth or incorporated into a hard candy or glycerogelatin base (2–4).

Trochiscus: See *Troches*.

Unguenta extensa: See *Mulls*.

Unguentum: See *Ointments*.

Vapor siccus: See *Inhalations, dry*.

Vapors: Steam, plain or medicated, generated by the use of steam or boiling water or by the use of a specially constructed apparatus (5).

Vesicatories: Local remedies, the application of which produces a serous discharge beneath the skin, forming a blister. Also known as epispastics (13).

Vials: See *Ampuls*.

Vinaigrettes: See *Salts, smelling*.

Vinegars: Infusions or solutions of drugs in vinegar or acetic acid; one of the oldest methods of drug preparation. Ancients knew that vinegar was often a better solvent than water and a preservative as well. The first preparation listed in the first *United States Pharmacopeia* (1820) was *Acetum Opii*, or Vinegar of Opium. The English word derives from the French *vin*, "wine," and *aigre*, "sour" (2, 8, 19).

Vinum: See *Wines*.

Wafer capsules: See *Cachets*.

Wafer envelopes: Preformed envelopes of rice flour used to administer bitter or nauseating drugs. Developed by Johann Schmidt as *saccelli amylacei*, wafer envelopes marked an improvement of convenience over wafer sheets. Pharmacists often furnished empty wafer envelopes to their patients, who transferred doses to them from prepared powder papers (see *Wafers*) (5).

Wafers: Flat sheets of rice flour used to administer nauseating drugs. When dry, wafer sheets are nonadhesive, stiff, somewhat brittle, and slightly thicker than ordinary cardboard. Powders are administered by floating a piece of wafer sheet upon water until it becomes thoroughly softened, passing a tablespoon underneath and lifting it out, and depositing the powder in the center and folding over the corners to thoroughly enclose the powder. If water is poured into the spoon, the concealed powder can be swallowed without any disagreeable taste being perceived. Wafer sheets are made by pouring a mixture of rice flour and water upon hot greased plates or rolling it between two hot, polished, revolving cylinders (5).

Washes: Aqueous preparations designed to cleanse specific parts of the body. Examples include enemas, eye drops, mouth washes, and nasal washes. General washes made official include Alkaline Aromatic Solution N.F. and Antiseptic Solution N.F. (31).

Washes, eye: See *Solutions, ophthalmic*.

Washes, mouth: Hydroalcoholic solutions of soap flavored with essential oils for cleansing the oral cavity; they became first official in the *National Formulary V* (1926) (31).

Waters, aromatic: Saturated solutions usually of volatile oils or similar substances in distilled water. Aromatic waters such as rose water were used in antiquity. Distilled waters containing volatile oils reached their therapeutic peak in the early sixteenth century. Although their therapeutic use declined in modern times, they continued to be used as flavorings. Hamamelis water (witch hazel) has lingered on as an aftershave and astringent (19).

Wax, dental   See *Drops, toothache*.

Waxed papers: See *Papers, waxed*.

Wines: Alcoholic liquids prepared from drugs by the process of solution, maceration, or percolation, differing from tinctures only in that wine is used as a solvent or menstruum instead of various strengths of alcohol; one of the oldest liquid preparations, since the alcoholic content of the wine improved its solvent characteristics in many cases. The *National Formulary IV* (1916) recognized 15 wines, but the passage of Prohibition convinced the revisors to drop red and white wine, as well as all medicated wines, from that compendium (3).

REFERENCES

1. Arny, H.V. *Principles of Pharmacy*; W. B. Saunders Company: Philadelphia, 1918.
2. Wain, H. *The Story Behind the Word*; Charles C. Thomas: Springfield IL, 1958.
3. Arny, H.V. *Principles of Pharmacy*; With the Collaboration of Robert P. Fischelis W.B. Saunders Company: Philadelphia, 1937.
4. *American Pharmacy: An Introduction to Pharmaceutical Technics and Dosage Forms*; Sprowls, J.B., Jr., Lyman, R.A., Eds.; J. B. Lippincott Company: Philadelphia, 1966.
5. Cook, E.F.; LaWall, C.H. *Remington's Practice of Pharmacy*; J. B. Lippincott Company: Philadelphia, 1926.
6. Bender, G.A. *Great Moments in Pharmacy: The Stories and Paintings in the Series A History of Pharmacy in Pictures by Parke, Davis & Company*; Northwood Institute Press: Detroit, 1966.
7. *Kremers Files for the History of Pharmacy [A Topical Reference Collection]*; School of Pharmacy, University of Wisconsin-Madison.
8. Wood, H.C.; Remington, J.; Sadtler, S. *The Dispensatory of the United States of America*; J. B. Lippincott Company: Philadelphia, 1886.
9. Urdang, G. The Invention of Gelatin Capsules. Pharm. Arch. **1943**, *14* (4), 58–59.
10. Alpers, W.C. Gelatine Capsules: 1. History of the Capsule; 2. Filling the Capsule with Powders or Pill Mass. Proc. Am. Pharm. Assoc. **1896**, *44*, 175–185.
11. Stadler, L.B. Innovations in Dosage Forms: The Gelatin Capsule. J. Am. Pharm. Assoc. (Pract. Pharm. Ed.) **1959**, *20* (12), 723–724.
12. DuMez, A.G. A Contribution to the History of the Development of the Enteric Capsule. J. Am. Pharm. Assoc. **1921**, *10* (5), 372–376.
13. Wood, G.B.; Bache, F. *The Dispensatory of the United States of America*; Grigg & Elliott: Philadelphia, 1836.
14. Wood, H.C.; Osol, A. *The Dispensatory of the United States of America*; J. B. Lippincott Company: Philadelphia, 1943.
15. Griffenhagen, G. The Lost Art of Plaster Spreading. Am. Prof. Pharmacist **1957**, *23* (2), 139–143.
16. Kremers, E.; Urdang, G. *History of Pharmacy: A Guide and a Survey*; J. B. Lippincott: Philadelphia, 1940.
17. Thompson, H.O.; Lee, C.O. History, Literature, and Theory of Enteric Coatings. J. Am. Pharm. Assoc. (Sci. Ed.) **1945**, *34* (5), 135–138.
18. Sonnedecker, G.; Griffenhagen, G. A History of Sugar Coated Pills and Tablets. I. Invention and Acceptance. J. Am. Pharm. Assoc. (Pract. Pharm. Ed.) **1957**, *18* (8), 486–488, II. Methods and Equipment. *J. Am. Pharm. Assoc. (Pract. Pharm. Ed.)*, **1957**, *18* (9), (1957) 553–555.
19. *American Pharmacy: Fundamental Principles and Practices*; Lyman, R.A., Ed.; J. B. Lippincott Company: Philadelphia, 1945.
20. *Medical Lexicon: A Dictionary of Medical Science*; Dunglison, R., Ed.; Enlarged and Thoroughly Revised by Robley Dunglison Henry C. Lea: Philadelphia, 1874.
21. Harry, R.G. *Modern Cosmeticology: The Principles and Products of Modern Cosmetics*; Revised by J. B. Wilkinson in Cooperation with R. Clark, E. Green, and T. P. McLaughlin Chemical Publishing Company, Inc.: New York, 1962; I.
22. Lémery, N. *Pharmacopée Universelle*; P. Gossey: Paris, 1729.
23. Agnew, E. Medical Dragées and Granules. Am. J. Pharm. **1870**, *42* (3), 270–272.
24. *Remington's Practice of Pharmacy*; Martin, E.W., Cook, E.F., Leuallen, E.E., Osol, A., Tice, L.F., Van Meter, C.T., Eds.; Mack Publishing Company: Easton, PA, 1961.
25. Lloyd, J.U. *Elixirs and Flavoring Extracts: Their History, Formulae, and Methods of Preparation*; William Wood & Company: New York, 1892.
26. Higby, G.J. *One Hundred Years of the National Formulary*; American Institute of the History of Pharmacy: Madison, WI, 1989.
27. Taber, C.W. *Taber's Cyclopedic Medical Dictionary*; F. A. Davis Company: Philadelphia, 1961.
28. Brockbank, W. *Ancient Therapeutic Arts: The Fitzpatrick Lectures Delivered in 1950 and 1951 at the Royal College of Physicians*; William Heinemann Medical Books, Ltd. London, 1954.

29. Remington, J.P. *The Practice of Pharmacy*; J. B. Lippincott Company: Philadelphia, 1905.

30. Davis, A.B. The Development of Anesthesia. Am. Sci. **1982**, *70* (5), 522–528.

31. Cook, E.F.; Martin, E.W. *Remington's Practice of Pharmacy*; Mack Publishing Company: Easton, PA, 1951.

32. Griffenhagen, G.B. The History of Parenteral Medication. Bull. Parenter. Drug Assoc. **1962**, *16* (2), 12–19.

33. Groves, M.J. *Parenteral Products: The Preparation and Quality Control of Products for Injection*; William Heinemann Medical Books, Ltd. London, 1962.

34. Toilet Milks. Chemist Druggist **1937**, *127* (2998), 89.

35. Griffenhagen, G. Tools of the Apothecary: 4. Suppository Molds. J. Am. Pharm. Assoc. (Pract. Pharm. Ed.) **1956**, *17* (6), 402–403.

36. Griffenhagen, G. Tools of the Apothecary: 5. Pill Tiles and Spatulas. J. Am. Pharm. Assoc. (Pract. Pharm. Ed.) **1956**, *17* (7), 464–465.

FURTHER READING

Adrian, L.A. *Étude historique sur les Extraits Pharmaceutiques cont. la Description des div. Procédés et Appareils...*; Paris, 1889.

An Account of the Rise and Attempts of a Way to Convey Liquors Immediately into the Mass of Blood. Philos. Transac. **1665**, *1* (December 4).

Ansel, H.C. *Introduction to Pharmaceutical Dosage Forms*; Lea & Fegiber: Philadelphia, 1981.

Barach, A.L. Symposium —Inhalation Therapy: Historical Background. Anesthesiology **1962**, *23* (4).

Bartholow, R. *Manual of Hypodermic Medication*; Lippincott: Philadelphia, 1869.

Boberg, E.J. *Gelatin Capsules*; University of Wisconsin, 1912.

Boston Society for Medical Improvement. *Report of a Committee... on the Alleged Dangers Which Accompany the Inhalation of the Vapor of Sulphuric Ether*; David Clapp: Boston, 1861.

Bringhurst, F. On Pill Machines. Proc. Am. Pharm. Assoc. **1867**, *15*.

Brockbank, W. The Ancient Art of Enema Administration. *Ancient Therapeutic Arts: The Fitzpatrick Lectures Delivered in 1950 and 1951 at the Royal College of Physicians*; William Heinemann Medical Books, Ltd. London, 1954.

Brockbank, W.; Corbett, O.R. De Graaf's 'Tractatus De Clysteribus.'. J. Hist. Med. **1954**, *9* (2).

Brockbank, W. The Less Ancient Art of Intravenous Injection of Drugs. In *Ancient Therapeutic Arts: The Fitzpatrick Lectures Delivered in 1950 and 1951 at the Royal College of Physicians*; William Heinemann Medical Books, Ltd.: London, 1954.

Brockbank, W. *Ancient Therapeutic Arts: The Fitzpatrick Lectures Delivered in 1950 and 1951 at the Royal College of Physicians*; William Heinemann Medical Books, Ltd.: London, 1954.

Brown, H.M. The Beginnings of Intravenous Medication. Ann. Med. Hist. **1917**, *1* (2).

Buess, H. *Die Historischen Grundlagen der Intravenösen Injektion. Ein Beitrag zur Medizingeschichte der 17. Jahrhunderts*; H. R. Sauerländer & Co. Aarau Switzerland, 1946.

Burrin, P.L. Innovations in Dosage Forms: Some Unique Dosage Forms. J. Am. Pharm. Assoc. (Pract. Pharm. Ed.) **1959**, *20* (12).

Caujolle, F. Vegetable Essences in French Pharmacopoeia. Indian Pharm. **1954**, *10* (3).

Collard, E. Il Y a Pommade Et Pommade. Rev. d'Hist. Pharm. **1962**, *50* (172).

Crellin, J.K.; Scott, J.R. Pharmaceutical History and Its Sources in the Wellcome Collections: III. Fluid Medicines, Prescription Reform and Posology 1700–1900. Med. Hist. **1970**, *14* (2).

Cyr, G.N. Innovations in Dosage Forms: Innovations in Percolation. J. Am. Pharm. Assoc. (Pract. Pharm. Ed.) **1959**, *20* (12).

Diepgen, P. *Das Analzäpfchen in der Geschichte der Therapie*; Stuttgart, 1953.

Dobler, F. Die Tinctura Bei Theophrastus Paracelsus. Experimentalle Überprüfung Seiner Haupttinkturen. Band 13. *Die Vorträge der Hauptversammlung der Internationalen Gesellschaft fur Geschichte der Pharmazie*, 1958.

Dragstedt, C.A. Intravenous Injections. Am. Prof. Pharm. **1948**, *14* (2).

Dutton, W.F. *Intravenous Therapy*; F. A. Davis Co.: Philadelphia, 1924.

Eisenberg, L. History of Inhalation Therapy Equipment. Int. Anesthes. Clin. **1966**, *4* (3).

Ellis, E.T. A New Method of Making Suppositories. Am. J. Pharm. **1879**, *51* (4).

England, J.W. An Historical Note on the Official Rosin Cerates. J. Am. Pharm. Assoc. **1933**, *22* (11).

Evans, A.J.; Train, D.A. *A Bibliography of the Tabletting of Medicinal Substances*; The Pharmaceutical Press: London, 1963.

Evolution of the Hypodermic Syringe and Other Instruments for Parenteral Therapy. Chem. Drug **1953**, *159* (3824).

Fairthorne, R.F. On the Preparation of Suppositories. Am. J. Pharm. **1871**, *43* (10).

Feinstein, K. *Thoretische und praktische Untersuchungen ueber das Perkolationsverfahren nebst einem Ueberblick uber dessen Entwicklung*; Zurich, 1936.

First Rotary Tablet Press Traced to Wyeth, 1872. Pulse of Pharmacy [Wyeth] **1959**, *13* (1).

Foote, P. *Tablets*; Bulletin of the University of Wisconsin, Serial No. 1566, Madison, 1928.

Friedenwald, J.; Morrison, S. The History of the Enema With Some Notes on Related Procedures: Part I. Bull. Hist. Med. **1940**, *8* (1), 68–114, Part II, *ibid.*, *8* (2), **1940**.

Furst, P.T.; Coe, M.D. Ritual Enemas. Nat. Hist. **1977**, *86* (3).

Garrison, F.H. *An Introduction to the History of Medicine*; W. B. Saunders Company: Philadelphia, 1929.

Goodman, H. The Hypodermic Syringe: The Early History With Notes on the Forgotten Anatomical Instrument. Med. Times (N.Y.) **1956**, *84* (6).

Griffenhagen, G. Tools of the Apothecary: 6. Pill Machines. J. Am. Pharm. Assoc. (Pract. Pharm. Ed.) **1956**, *17* (8).

Griffenhagen, G. A History and Evolution of the Suppository Mold. Am. J. Pharm. **1953**, *125* (3).

Griffenhagen, G. Tools of the Apothecary: 10. Lozenges, Tablets, and Capsules. J. Am. Pharm. Assoc. (Pract. Pharm. Ed.) **1956**, *17* (12).

Guitard, E.-H. L 'emplâtre. Rev. d'Hist. Pharm. **1960**, *48* (167).

H

Halsband, R. New Light on Lady Mary Wortley Montagu's Contribution to Inoculation. J. Hist. Med. **1953**, *8* (4).

Hamarneh, S. At the Smithsonian–Exhibits on Pharmaceutical Dosage Forms. J. Am. Pharm. Assoc. **1962**, NS2 (8).

Hamarneh, S. Early Arabic Pharmaceutical Instruments. J. Am. Pharm. Assoc. (Pract. Pharm. Ed.) **1960**, *21* (2).

Harrop, J. Monograph on Fluid Extracts. *Solid Extracts and Oleoresins*; Columbus OH, 1895.

Hehre, F.W. Early Events in the Development of Inhalation Therapy. Conn. Med. J. **1958**, *22* (11).

Heizer, R.F. The Use of the Enema Among the Aboriginal American Indians. Ciba Symp **1944**, *5* (11).

Helfand, W.H.; Cowen, D.L. Evolution of Pharmaceutical Oral Dosage Forms. Pharm. Hist. **1983**, *25* (1).

Hoff, E.C.; Hoff, P.M. The Life and Times of Richard Lower, Physiologist and Physician, 1631–1691. Bull. Inst. Hist. Med. **1936**, *4* (7).

Holland, M.O. Collyria . Am. Prof. Pharmacist **1938**, *4* (6).

Howard, JonesN. A Critical Study of the Origins and Early Development of Hypodermic Medication. J. Hist. Med. **1947**, *2* (2).

Jonas, A.S. The History of Plaster of Paris Bandages. Surg. Gynec. Obstet. **1956**, *102* (2).

Kane, H.H. *The Hypodermic Injection of Morphia, Its History, Advantages and Dangers*; New York, 1880.

Kebler, L.F. The Tablet Industry—Its Evolution and Present Status; the Composition of Tablets and Methods of Analysis. J. Am. Pharm. Assoc. **1914**, *3* (6).

Kebler, L.F.; ibid. **1914**, *3* (7).

Kebler, L.F.; ibid. **1914**, *3* (8).

Kilmer, F.B. Manufacture of Medicinal Plasters. Am. J. Pharm. **1910**, *82* (9).

Kirkby, W. The Story of the Pill from the Days of the Ebers Papyrus to Recent Times. Chem. Drug. **1939**, *130* (Special Issue).

Kratzenstein, C.G. *Abhandlung von dem Nutzen der Electricität in der Arznuwissenschaft*; (facsimile, c. 1978): Halle, 1744–1745.

Krüger, M. *Zur Geschichte der Elixiere, Essenzen und Tinkturen*; Bd. 10, *Veröffentlichungen aus dem Pharmaziegeschichtlichen Seminar* der Technischen Hoschule: Braunschweig, 1968.

Krüger, M. *Zur Geschichte der Elixiere, Essenzen, und Tinkturen*; Bd. 10, Veröffentlichungen aus dem Pharmaziegeschichtlichen Seminar...: Braunschweig, 1968.

Lee, C.O. Emulsions. University of Wisconsin: 1930.

Leigh, J.M. The Evolution of Oxygen Therapy Apparatus. Anaesthesia **1974**, *29* (4).

Lémery, N. *Pharmacopée Universelle*; P. Gossey: Paris, 1729.

Lieberman, W. The History of the Enema. Ciba Symp **1944**, *5* (11).

Lieberman, W. Notes and Literary References to the Clyster. ibid. **1944**, *5* (11).

Lieberman, W. A Chronology of the Enema. ibid. **1944**, *5* (11), 1712.

Lillico, J. The Use of Enemata by Primitive Peoples. Ann. Med Hist. (Third Series) **1941**, *3* (1).

Lloyd, J.U. *Elixirs, Their History, Formulae and Methods of Preparations, Including Practical Processes for Making the Popular Elixirs of the Present Day and Those Which Have Been Officinal in the Old Pharmacopoeias, with a Resume of Unofficinal Elixirs from the Days of Paracelsus*; Cincinnati, 1883.

Lloyd, J.U. The Chapman Suppository Mold. Proc. Am. Pharm. Assoc. **1902**, *50*.

Mattison, R.V. On Suppository Molds. Proc. Am. Pharm. Assoc. **1875**, *23*.

Manufacturing Industries of the Drug Trade: Planten's American Medical Capsulery and Laboratory, 1836–1896. Pharm. Era **1896**, *16* (27).

Mendelsohn, S. A Short History of Elixirs. Manuf. Chem. **1952**, *23* (12).

Meredith, D.T. Innovations in Dosage Forms: Friable Pills and Escaps. J. Am. Pharm. Assoc. (Pract. Pharm. Ed.) **1959**, *20* (12).

Moeller, H.W. Innovations in Dosage Forms: The Story of Lozenges. J. Am. Pharm. Assoc. (Pract. Pharm. Ed.) **1959**, *20* (12).

Mohr, F.; Redwood, T.; Procter, W., Jr. *Practical Pharmacy: The Arrangements, Apparatus and Manipulations of the Pharmaceutical Shop and Laboratory*; Lea and Blanchard: Philadelphia, 1849.

Morton, W.J. *The Invention of Anaesthetic Inhalation*; Appleton: New York, 1880.

Nielsen, H. *Ancient Ophthalmological Agents*. A Pharmaco-historical Study of the Collyria and Seals for Collyria Used During Roman Antiquity, as well as of the Most Frequent Components of the Collyria. In *Acta Historica Scientiarum Naturalium et Medicinalium*; Odense University Press: Odense Denmark, 1974; 31.

On a New Suppository Mold. Am. J. Pharm. **1867**, *49* (2).

Paris, J.A. *Pharmacologia; or the History of Medicinal Substances*; F. & R. Lockwood: New York, 1822.

Parrish, E. *Introduction to Practical Pharmacy*; Blanchard and Lea: Philadelphia, 1856.

Parrish, E.; Bakes, W.C. Fancy and Fashion in Pharmacy: Suppositories. Am. J. Pharm. **1861**, *28* (1).

Penn, H.P. The Geoffrey Kaye Museum Collection of Portable Ether Inhalers. Anaesth. Intensive Care **1975**, *3* (4).

Petit, P. Vers Un Renouveau Des Préparations Magistrales Grâce à La Formation Continue. Le Pharmacien De France No. 12 (June, 1974), P. 569, Through. Rev. d'Hist. Pharm. **1975**, *63* (227).

Randone, M.; Ponte, P.L. Un Metodo Di Cura Del '700: Le Pillole Di Mercurio Di Agostino Belloste. Minerva Med **1967**, *58* (77, Suppl.).

Remington, J.P. On An Improved Pill Press. Am. J. Pharm. **1876**, *48* (3).

Remington, J.P. *The Practice of Pharmacy: A Treatise on the Modes of Making and Dispensing Officinal, Unofficinal, and Extemporaneous Preparations, with Descriptions of Their Properties, Uses, and Doses. Intended as as Hand-book for Pharmacists and Physicians and a Text-book for Students*; et seq J. B. Lippincott Company: Philadelphia, 1887.

Richtmann, W.O. *Bibliography of Aromatic Waters*; Chronologic, 1809 to 1900: Milwaukee, 1902.

Rodman, R.W. The Gilded Pill. J. Am. Pharm. Assoc. (Pract. Pharm. Ed.) **1943**, *4* (7).

Runne, H. Die Entwicklung Der Praktischen Pharmazie in Den Letzten Vierhundert Jahren. Arch. Pharm. **1931**, *269*.

Rusek, V. Vyvoj Injekcni Formy Leciv. I. Ceskoslovenská Farmacie [Prague] **1960**, *9* (10), II. [on technology] *12* (1), (1963). (In Czech, with English and German abstracts.)

Scheel, P.; Dieffenbach, J.F. *Die Transfusion des Blutes und die Einsprützung der Arzneyen in die Adern. Historisch und in*

Rucksicht auf die practische Heilkunde bearbeitet; (Reprinted 1972) F. Brummer: Copenhagen, Berlin, 1802/1803–1828.

Seel, E. Ueber Arzneitabletten. Pharm. Zenthalle **1906**, *47* (43).

Siedler, P. sterile Ampuls. *Die chemischen Arzneimittel der letzten 113 Jahre...*; Bornträger: Berlin, 1914.

Siedler, P. Gelatine Capsules. *Die chemischen Arzneimittel der letzten 113 Jahre...*; Berlin, 1914.

Simpson, J.A.; Weiner, E.S.C. *The Oxford English Dictionary*; Clarendon Press: Oxford; Oxford University Press: New York, 1989.

Sullivan, W.N. The Coupling of Science and Technology in the Early Development of the World War II Aerosol Bomb. Mil. Med. **1971**, *136* (2).

Taylor, A.B. Suppositories . Am. J. Pharm. **1852**, *24* (3).

The Means of Fumigating Infected Chambers, Etc. *The Family and Ship Medicine Chest Companion: Being a Compendium of Domestic Medicine ...*; Philadelphia, 1851.

Thomas, K.B. The Early Use of Chloroform; with Some Notes on Certain Apparatus Designed for its Delivery. Anaesthesia **1971**, *26* (3).

Thomas, K.B. An Ether Vaporiser of 1847. Anaesthesia **1968**, *23* (4).

Thompson, C.J.S. The Pomander, a Link in the History of Preventive Medicine. d'Hist. Med. ,2e Congres. International (also appeared as a separate, Evreux, 1922).

Tui, C. Practical Aspects of Pyrogen Problems. J. Am. Pharm. Assoc. (Pract. Pharm., Ed.) **1944**, *5* (2).

Urdang, G. Compressed Tablets [Historically Considered]. What's New [Abbott] **1943**, (76).

Van Itallie, P.H. Innovations in Dosage Forms: Pioneers of Tablet-Making. J. Am. Pharm. Assoc. (Pract. Pharm., Ed.) **1959**, *20* (12).

Van, I.; tallie, H. History of Syringes and Injection Therapy. S. D. J. Med. Pharm. **1965**, *18* (1).

Weiser, H.B. Gels I: Gelatinous Precipitates and Jellies of Inorganic Substances and Gels II: Organic Jellies. In *A Textbook of Colloidal Chemistry*; John Wiley & Sons, Inc.: New York, 1949.

Wood, J.R. *Tablet Manufacture, Its History, Pharmacy and Practice*; Lippincott: Philadelphia, 1906.

Wright, S.P. On Suppositories. Am. J. Pharm. **1870**, *42* (3).

Zekert, O.F. Zur Geschichte Der Extrakte. Pharm. Monatsh. **1923**, *4* (3).

HOMOGENIZATION AND HOMOGENIZERS

Venkatesh Naini
Barr Laboratories, Inc., Pomona, New York

Shailesh K. Singh
Wyeth-Ayerst Research, Peral River, New York

INTRODUCTION

Homogenization encompasses techniques of emulsification of one liquid into another, dispersing solid particles uniformly in a product, and disrupting cell membranes. Traditionally, homogenizers have been used in the pharmaceutical industry for emulsification. However, they are finding increasing applications in the manufacture of liposomes (1), nanosuspensions (2), solid–lipid nanoparticles (3), tablet coating dispersions (4), micro-encapsulation (5), and in cell disruption for harvesting therapeutic proteins in cell cultures (6).

Pharmaceutical emulsions are generally classified as oil-in-water (o/w) or water-in-oil (w/o) systems, where the first component represents the dispersed phase, although more complex systems are feasible. The first step in the process of emulsification involves application of mechanical energy (homogenization) to break up the dispersed phase and form a stable emulsion. Homogenization is also used for particle size reduction in pharmaceutical suspensions. Important factors controlling the formation of pharmaceutical emulsions and dispersions are mechanical and/or formulation related. Mechanical forces during homogenization cause droplet or particle size reduction by shear, turbulence, impact, and cavitation (7). Shear is caused by elongation and subsequent breakup of droplets, due to acceleration of a liquid. Cavitation is caused by an intense pressure drop, leading to formation of vapor bubbles in the liquid, which implode causing shock waves in the fluid. This leads to disruption of droplets, particles, and cell membranes. Homogenizers, available from different manufacturers operate using a combination of these forces (8).

This review will focus on commonly used homogenizers in the pharmaceutical industry viz. high-pressure homogenizer, rotor-stator homogenizer, microfluidizer, and ultrasonic homogenizer.

HIGH-PRESSURE HOMOGENIZATION

Auguste Gaulin introduced the first high-pressure homogenizer in 1900 for homogenizing milk (9). The basic high-pressure homogenizer consists of a positive displacement pump attached to a homogenizing valve assembly (Fig. 1). The pump forces liquid into the valve area at a high pressure. As the product is forced through the adjustable gap (D), its velocity increases tremendously with a corresponding decrease in pressure. The emerging product then impinges on the impact ring (C). This sudden change in energy causes increased turbulence, shear, and/or cavitation, resulting in droplet size reduction and uniform dispersion of particles. High-pressure homogenizers are used in emulsification (10–12), preparation of microparticles and nanodispersions (13–16), liposomes (1, 17, 18), and in cell disruption (6, 19). A laboratory scale model of the high-pressure homogenizer is shown in Fig. 2. For emulsion processing a single-stage or two-stage valve assembly can be used, where 10% of the total pressure is applied at the second stage. Another commonly used approach is the multiple-pass homogenization, if a very narrow particle size distribution is needed. This can be achieved by using a series of homogenizers or processing several discrete passes through the same machine.

Several factors affect the final emulsion formulation obtained using high-pressure homogenization. More importantly the level and type of surfactant (11, 12), level of the oily phase, and homogenization process parameters, such as pressure, number of cycles, or discrete passes through the homogenizer, play a significant role. Pandolfe studied the effect of several of these factors and found that the premix condition (prior to homogenization), emulsifier concentration, and energy input by the homogenizer, significantly affected the quality of the final emulsion (11). The effect of increasing homogenizing pressure on emulsions with

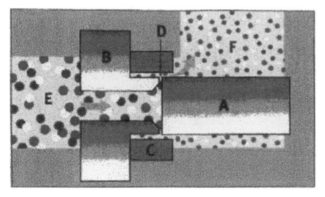

Fig. 1 Homogenizing valve assembly in a high-pressure homogenizer. (With permission: APV Homogenizer Group, Wilmington, MA.)

different levels of oily phase, in poor premix (turbine stirrer at 1000 rpm) and good premix (prehomogenized at 500 psi) samples, is shown in Fig. 3. Although droplet size reduction is seen at all conditions, more effective

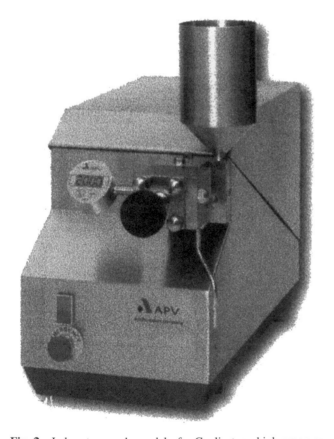

Fig. 2 Laboratory scale model of a Gaulin type high-pressure homogenizer. (With permission: APV Homogenizer Group, Wilmington, MA.)

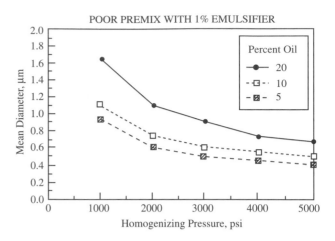

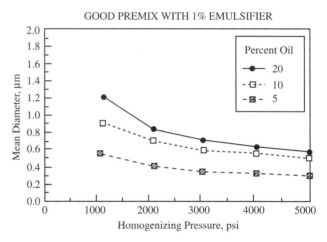

Fig. 3 Mean droplet diameter versus homogenizer pressure for emulsions with 1% emulsifier and 5%, 10%, or 20% oily phase. (Adapted from Ref. 11.)

formulations can be obtained by using the lowest amount of oily phase at the highest homogenization pressure with a properly premixed dispersion. It was also concluded that increasing homogenization pressure could effectively reduce the amount of emulsifier required in a formulation. Because of its efficient droplet size reduction, high-pressure homogenization can be used for preparing parenteral fat emulsions (10). Here the requirement is that number of droplets or particles above 1 μm should be limited and no particle should be larger than 5 μm.

Calvor and Muller (13) used high-pressure homogenization and a novel method to prepare biodegradable microparticles of poly(D,L-lactide) (PLA) and poly (D,L-lactide-co-glycolide) (PLGA). They heated the drug–polymer-containing suspensions above the glass transition temperature (T_g) of the polymer, followed by high-pressure homogenization. Above the T_g of the

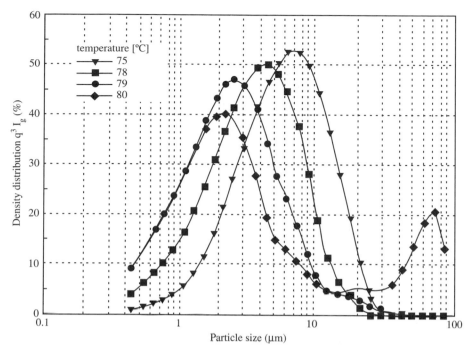

Fig. 4 Volume size distribution of poly(D,L-lactide-*co*-glycolide) particles at a homogenization temperature of 75°C (▼), 78°C (■), 79°C (◆) and 80°C (●). (Adapted from Ref. 13.)

polymer, the viscosity of the dispersed phase was lowered leading to efficient droplet size reduction by homogenization. Fig. 4 shows the effect of homogenization temperature on particle size reduction in PLGA ($T_g \sim 40°C$) containing systems. Traditionally, Gaulin-type homogenizers are known to uniformly disperse and breakup particle agglomerates. Actual breakup of primary particles in the suspension was considered highly unlikely. However, more recently, high-pressure homogenization was successfully employed to prepare nanosuspensions of poorly soluble drugs, starting from micron-sized material (14). Some factors controlling size reduction of drug particles during homogenization include, gap width in the homogenizer, particle shape and size in the feed material, and fragility of drug crystals. Nanosuspensions have promising applications in injectable formulations of poorly soluble drugs or reformulating solution parenterals, which contain toxicologically less favorable excipients. They can also be used to enhance saturation solubility and bioadhesive properties of drugs in the GIT, leading to better bioavailability following oral administration (2). Due to the abrasive nature of suspended drug particles, erosion of contact surfaces and heavy-metal contamination is a major concern during high-pressure homogenization. A study by Krause and coworkers

found that heavy-metal contamination was minimal (<1 ppm) in nanosuspensions after being homogenized at 1500 bar for 50 cycles (20).

Liposomes are phospholipid vesicles containing an aqueous compartment surrounded by one or more bilayers (1). They are finding increasing application as carriers for small molecule drugs, controlled release and targeting of protein and peptide therapeutics, and as immunological adjuvants in vaccines (17). Due to the realization that liposomes need to be produced on a large-scale, high-pressure homogenizers are well suited for industrial production under aseptic conditions. The effects of shear and cavitation during homogenization usually form small unilamellar vesicles (SUVs). The number of passages through the homogenizer and pressure used affects the vesicle sizes (17, 18). For a certain combination of lipid and water, increasing homogenization pressure produces smaller and narrower (decreasing polydispersity) vesicles with an optimum diameter. Any further increase in the number of passes results in broader size distributions due to coalescence (17). Bachmann and coworkers, used a continuously operating high-pressure homogenizer to scale-up production of liposomes using the "one-step" method, where SUVs are prepared from powdered lipid and aqueous drug solution (18). Encapsulation efficiency and entrapped aqueous volume of the vesicles are

Table 1 Encapsulation efficiency and entrapped volumes of vesicles prepared using a high-pressure homogenizer

Number of cycles	40 MPa		Homogenizing pressure (70 MPa)	
	Encapsulation efficiency (%)	Aqueous volume entrapped (l/mol)	Encapsulation efficiency (%)	Aqueous volume entrapped (l/mol)
1	11.8	0.91	11.6	0.89
5	10.4	0.80	9.0	0.69
10	8.0	0.62	7.5	0.58
20	7.6	0.58	6.1	0.47

(From Ref. 18.)

summarized in Table 1. Liposomes prepared with phosphatidylcholine fraction of soybean lecithin (SPC) were homogenized at 40 MPa or 70 MPa, with the higher pressure producing much smaller vesicles. However, extensive recirculation decreased these differences after several passes through the homogenizer. In addition, encapsulation efficiencies decreased at higher pressures and repetitive processing (Table 1).

Recent advances in biotechnology have produced several new protein drugs from mammalian and bacterial cell cultures. High-pressure homogenization is widely used to harvest intracellular proteins and enzymes of interest in cell cultures (6, 19). Lander et al. conducted a mechanistic study of cell disruption caused by homogenization (19). Shear and cavitation were found to play an important role in cell membrane disruption and release of intracellular contents. High-pressure homogenizers for cell disruption applications use special valve assemblies for efficient rupture of cell walls (6). Other process parameters to consider during cell disruption are viscosity of the cell suspension, flow rate, and number of passes through the homogenizer.

MICROFLUIDIZATION

The microfluidizer is a high-pressure homogenizer that works, on a different principle. The pre-homogenized liquid is forced through an interaction chamber using a high-pressure pump. The interaction chamber consists of ceramic microchannels, which cause the liquid feed to split into two streams. These streams are then recombined at very high velocities producing forces of shear, impact, and cavitation, which cause droplet or particle-size reduction in emulsions and suspensions. A complete description of the operation of the microfluidizer is summarized in US Patent 4,533,254 (21). A schematic diagram of the microfluidizer process is shown in Fig. 5. These homogenizers are commercially available from Microfluidics Corporation (Newton, MA). Microfluidizers are capable of handling emulsions (21–23), artificial blood (24, 25), suspensions (26), and liposomes (27–30). A microfluidizer that can operate at process pressures of up to 40,000 psi is shown in Fig. 6.

Because of their efficient droplet size reduction and ease of scale-up, microfluidizers are frequently used to prepare parenteral feeding emulsions (22, 23). Droplet diameters were directly related to the process pressure used, number of passes through the microfluidizer, and concentrations of emulsifier and oily phase in the emulsion (22). Reduction in droplet size of a 10% emulsion as a function of number of passes through the microfluidizer is shown in Fig. 7 (22). When the homogenizer was operated at its maximum operating pressure of 10,000 psi, droplet diameters decreased from 380 nm for a single pass to a plateau of 250 nm after four cycles, with further processing having no significant effect. Lidgate et al. used a microfluidizer to prepare an o/w parenteral emulsion for use as a vaccine adjuvant and compared its stability to emulsions prepared by other methods (23). Stress tests to induce creaming were used to test emulsions produced by various techniques. Microfluidization produced a superior parenteral emulsion compared to a homogenizer mixer. Stability correlated well with increasing number of microfluidizer cycles used to process the emulsion (23).

The microfluidizer has distinct advantages over conventional milling processes in particle size reduction of pharmaceutical suspensions. Absence of heavy-metal contaminants due to surface erosion and easy scale-up to production were observed when using the microfluidizer

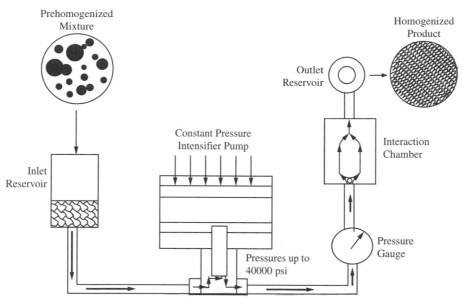

Fig. 5 Microfluidizer processor flow diagram. (Microfluidics Corporation, Newton, MA.)

for preparing radiopaque suspensions (25). Several reports deal with scaled up production of liposomes using the microfluidizer (28–30). In one study, liposome dispersions with relatively high lipid concentrations (400 μmol/ml) could be processed to narrow size distributions using the microfluidizer (26). In addition, a US Patent (4,776,991) describes the large-scale production of liposome encapsulated hemoglobin for use as a blood substitute (30). Liposomes produced with high-pressure homogenizers usually result in small unilamellar vesicles (SUVs). Their main disadvantages are low encapsulation efficiency and tendency to leak their contents more often than multilamellar vesicles (MLVs). Sorgi and Huang used the microfluidizer to prepare cationic liposomes, where the active component is not encapsulated, but forms

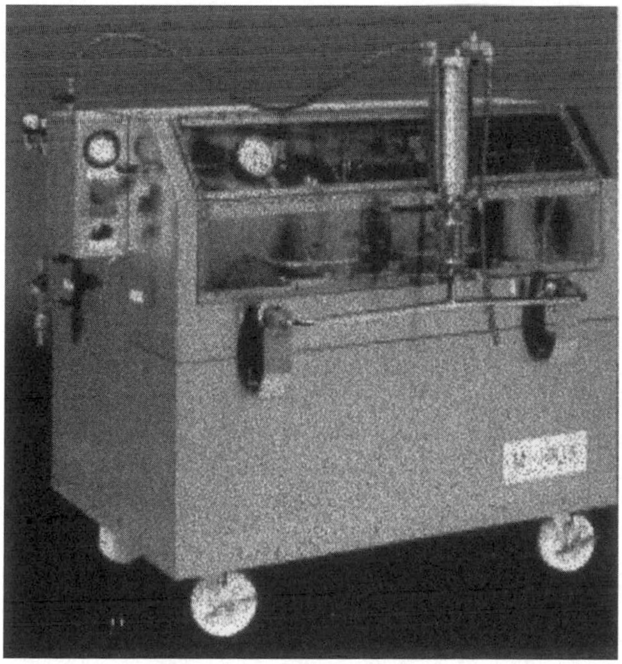

Fig. 6 The M-140K Microfluidizer processor. (Microfluidics Corporation, Newton, MA.)

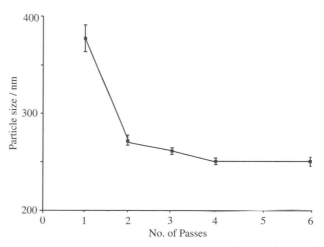

Fig. 7 Emulsion droplet size versus number of passes through the microfluidizer for a 10% oily phase emulsion processed at 10,000 psi. (Adapted from Ref. 22.)

a complex with the liposome using charge interaction (29). The microfluidizer was well suited for preparation and scale-up of cationic liposomes of a plasmid DNA, which was successfully used in gene therapy clinical trials (29).

ROTOR-STATOR HOMOGENIZATION

The rotor-stator homogenizer is one of the most commonly used pieces of equipment in the pharmaceutical industry. Although they have limited capability in achieving very fine droplets or particles, rotor-stator mixers are capable of handling liquids at much higher viscosities, compared to high-pressure homogenizer and the microfluidizer. A rotor-stator homogenizer consists of an impeller in close tolerance to a stationary housing, which restricts the flow of liquid caused by the impeller movement. Shear and impact comminute particles and droplets caught between the rotor and stator (5, 31). The colloid mill is an extreme example of the rotor-stator homogenizer, where the gap between the rotating truncated cone (rotor) and its housing (stator) is adjustable. However, the colloid mill suffers from disadvantages like generation of excessive heat and incorporation of air in the finished product. Various geometries and configurations of the mixing head in the rotor/stator design are available from different manufacturers (8). They can be used in the batch mode and continuous, or "in-line," mode. An "in-line" rotor/stator homogenizer is depicted in Fig. 8. Parameters affecting final product quality in rotor/stator homogenization are homogenization intensity, residence time of product in the shearing field, viscosity of the dispersed and continuous phases, surfactant concentration, rotor/stator design,

volume of the mixer, and volume ratio of the two phases (5, 31).

Djakovic and coworkers, studied several factors such as homogenization time, emulsifier concentration, and homogenization intensity to determine optimal parameters for emulsification, using a rotor-stator homogenizer (32). Mean droplet diameter and polydispersity were used as measures of final product quality. For constant homogenization intensity (rpm) and mixing time, droplet size and polydispersity decreased with increasing emulsifier concentration before reaching an optimum level (32). Maa and Hsu (5) compared the batch mode and a flow-through apparatus, using rotor/stator homogenization for microencapsulation. Emulsion droplets obtained using the flow-through method were consistently higher than the batch mode. Since emulsification is effected by residence time of liquid in the shearing field, the flow-through method induced lower shear compared to the batch mode. However, using effective recirculation in the flow-through mode can overcome this problem (31).

ULTRASONIC HOMOGENIZATION

Sonication emulsifies primarily by cavitation. An ultrasonic homogenizer consists of a generator, converter, and horn tip (8, 31). The converter consists of a piezoelectric quartz crystal, which transforms electrical energy into high intensity vibrations and transmits them to the horn tip immersed in the liquid. Droplet size reduction occurs

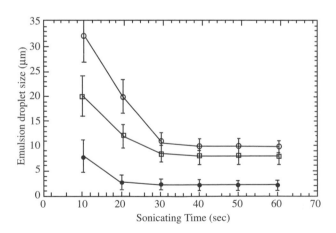

Fig. 9 Effect of sonication time on emulsion droplet size for 0.4 g/ml of poly(methyl methacrylate)/methylene chloride solution in 6% of polyvinyl alcohol (PVA) solution at a volume ratio of 15:2 (ml/ml) sonicated at 20% (○), 50% (□), and 100% (●) of full power. (Adapted from Ref. 31.)

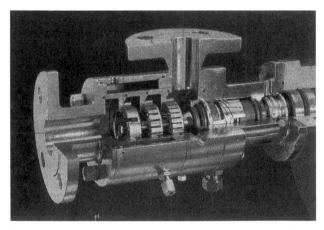

Fig. 8 An in-line rotor/stator homogenizer. (IKA Works, Wilmington, NC.)

Table 2 List of homogenization euipment spplied by various manufacturers

Type of homogenizer	Model (manufacturer)	Mode of operation (Batch/continuous)	Operating parameters	Capacity	Applications
High-pressure	APV Model 2000 (APV Homogenizers)	Laboratory scale; batch or continuous	Maximum pressure: 30000 psi	Batch (100 ml) Continuous (11 L/h)	Emulsions, nanodispersions, liposomes, ointments, cell disruption, vaccines, parenteralemulsions
	Gaulin and Rannie Models (APV Homogenizers)	Production scale; batch or continuous	Maximum pressure: 21750 psi	Up to 50000 L/h	
	Ariete Model NS8315 (Niro Soavi)	Production scale; batch or continuous	Pressure range: 2000–15000 psi	8000–50000 L/h	
Microfluidizer	M-110Y (Microfluidics)	Laboratory scale; batch or continuous	Pressure range: 3000–23000 psi	Batch (>60 ml) Continuous (250–600 ml/min)	Dispersions, emulsions, cell disruption, encapsulation, liposomes, vaccines, parenteralemulsions
	M-140K (Microfluidics)	Laboratory scale; batch or continuous	Pressure range: 8000–40,000 psi	Batch (1000 ml) Continuous (500 ml/min)	
	M-210EH (Microfluidics)	Production scale; batch or continuous	Pressure range: 2500–30,000 psi	Batch (3.8 L) Continuous (5.7 L/min)	
Rotor-stator	Silverson Model GX25	Production scale; batch	Maximum rpm: 3600	2400 L (low viscosity) 400 L (high viscosity)	Emulsions dispersions, pastes, creams, lotions
	Ultra-Turrax UTL (IKA Works, Inc.)	Production scale; continuous	Maximum rpm: 6000	3500 L/h	
Ultrasonic	Microson XL2007 (Misonix, Inc.)	Laboratory scale; batch	Power: 100 W; Frequency: 22.5 kHz	<50 ml	Emulsions, dispersions, cell disruption
	Flocell 800D (Misonix, Inc.)	Production scale; continuous	Power: 475 W Frequency: 20 kHz	With booster horn 40 L/min	

mainly by intense shock waves generated in close proximity to the tip. For large-scale applications, ultrasonic homogenizers can be used in the continuous mode with a flow-cell (33). In general, droplet size reduction in ultrasonic homogenizers is affected by sonication intensity, viscosity of the mixture, emulsifier concentration, and time of sonication (31, 34). Fig. 9 shows the effect of increasing sonication power on emulsion droplet size in liquid–liquid emulsification (31). Higher sonicating power resulted in smaller emulsion droplets. At all power levels the droplet size reduced dramatically, initially followed by a leveling-off phase. Sonication is comparable to rotor-stator homogenization if sufficient power is used. However, as liquid viscosity increases, rotor-stator homogenization is more efficient due to shear effects (31).

EQUIPMENT CONSIDERATIONS

A variety of homogenizers capable of performing a range of processes are available. Important considerations during formulation development include the feasibility and availability of pilot and production scale equipment, which can reproduce the same results. A sampling of homogenizers available from selected manufacturers is given in Table 2. High-pressure homogenizers and microfluidizers are available in a wide range of capabilities ranging from bench-top models to production equipment capable of handling large amounts of material. These homogenizers are limited in their handling of high viscosity fluids compared to rotor-stator homogenizers, which are designed to handle even thick pastes and creams. However, particle size reduction is more efficiently carried out using high-pressure homogenizers and microfluidizers. Ultrasonic homogenizers are also capable of handling large volumes by using the continuous or flow-through approach. However higher intensities are needed to cause cavitation and droplet reduction in high viscosity fluids. As indicated in Table 2, high-pressure homogenizers and microfluidizers can be easily adapted for batch or continuous processing. Rotor-stator homogenizers are available either as batch processors or in-line dispersers, which can be used continuously or by recirculating the product.

REFERENCES

1. Brandl, M.M.; Bachmann, D.; Drechsler, M. Liposome Preparation Using High-Pressure Homogenizers. *Liposome Technology*, 2nd Ed.; Gregoriadis, G., Ed.; CRC Press: Boca Raton, 1993; 1, 49–65.
2. Muller, R.H.; Peters, K. Nanosuspensions for the Formulation of Poorly Soluble Drugs I. Preparation by a Size Reduction Technique. Int. J. Pharm. **1998**, *160*, 229–237.
3. Muller, R.H.; Mehnert, W.; Lucks, J.-S.; Schwarz, C.; Muhlen, A.; Weyhers, H.; Freitas, C.; Ruhl, D. Solid Lipid Nanoparticles (SLN)—An Alternative Colloidal Carrier System for Controlled Drug Delivery. Eur. J. Pharm. Biopharm. **1995**, *41* (1), 62–69.
4. Bodmeier, R.; Chen, H. Hydrolysis of Cellulose Acetate Butyrate Pseudolatexes Prepared by a Solvent Evaporation—Microfluidization Method. Drug Dev. Ind. Pharm. **1993**, *19* (5), 521–530.
5. Maa, Y-H.; Hsu, C.C. Liquid–Liquid Emulsification by Rotor/Stator Homogenization. J. Control. Release **1996**, *38*, 219–228.
6. Pandolfe, W.D. *Cell Disruption by Homogenization;* APV Homogenizers: Wilmington, MA, 1996; 1–20.
7. Walstra, P. Formation of Emulsions. *Encyclopedia of Emulsion Technology: Basic Theory*; Becher, P., Ed.; Marcel Dekker, Inc.: New York, 1979; 1, 58–128.
8. Scott, R.R. A Practical Guide to Equipment Selection and Operating Techniques. *Pharmaceutical Disperse Systems*; Lieberman, H.A., Rieger, M.M., Banker, G.S., Eds.; Marcel Dekker, Inc.: New York, 1989; 2, 1–71.
9. Ed. *Processing of Emulsions and Dispersions by Homogenization;* APV Homogenizers: Wilmington, MA, 1996; 1–23.
10. Bock, T.K.; Lucks, J.-S.; Kleinbudde, P.; Muller, R.H.; Muller, B.W. High Pressure Homogenization of Parenteral Fat Emulsions—Influence of Process Parameters on Emulsion Quality. Eur. J. Pharm. Biopharm. **1994**, *40* (3), 157–160.
11. Pandolfe, W.D. Effect of Premix Condition, Surfactant Concentration, and Oil Level on the Formation of Oil-in-Water Emulsions by Homogenization. J. Dispersion Sci. Tech. **1995**, *16* (7), 633–650.
12. Daniels, R.; Schulz, M.B. Hydroxypropylmethylcellulose (HPMC) As Emulsifier for Submicron Emulsions: Influence of Molecular Weight and Substitution Type on Droplet Size After High-Pressure Homogenization. Eur. J. Pharm. Biopharm. **2000**, *49*, 231–236.
13. Calvor, A.; Muller, B.W. Production of Microparticles by High-Pressure Homogenization. Pharm. Dev. Tech. **1998**, *3* (3), 297–305.
14. Grau, M.J.; Kayser, O.; Muller, R.H. Nanosuspensions of Poorly Soluble Drugs—Reproducibility of Small Scale Production. Int. J. Pharm. **2000**, *196*, 155–157.
15. Liedtke, S.; Wissing, S.; Muller, R.H.; Mader, K. Influence of High Pressure Homogenization Equipment on Nanodispersions Characteristics. Int. J. Pharm. **2000**, *196*, 183–185.
16. Lamprecht, A.; Ubrich, N.; Perez, M.H.; Lehr, C.-M.; Hoffman, M.; Maincent, P. Influences of Process Parameters on Nanoparticle Preparation Performed by a Double Emulsion Pressure Homogenization Technique. Int. J. Pharm. **2000**, *196*, 177–182.
17. Brandl, M.; Bachmann, D.; Drechler, M.; Bauer, K.H. Preparation by a New High Pressure Homogenizer Gaulin Micron Lab 40. Drug Dev. Ind. Pharm. **1990**, *16* (14), 2167–2191.

18. Bachmann, D.; Brandl, M.; Gregoriadis, G. Preparation of Liposomes Using a Mini-Lab 8.30 H High-Pressure Homogenizer. Int. J. Pharm. **1993**, *91*, 69–74.
19. Lander, R.; Manger, W.; Scouloudis, M.; Ku, A.; Davis, C.; Lee, A. Gaulin Homogenization: A Mechanistic Study. Biotechnol. Prog. **2000**, *16*, 80–85.
20. Krause, K.P.; Kayser, O.; Mader, K.; Gust, R.; Muller, R.H. Heavy Metal Contamination of Nanosuspensions Produced by High-Pressure Homogenization. Int. J. Pharm. **2000**, *196*, 169–172.
21. Cook, E.J.; Lagace, A.P. Apparatus for Forming Emulsions. US Patent 4,533,254, Aug 6, 1985.
22. Washington, C.; Davis, S.S. The Production of Parenteral Feeding Emulsions by Microfluidizer. Int. J. Pharm. **1988**, *44*, 169–176.
23. Lidgate, D.M.; Fu, R.C.; Fleitman, J.S. Using a Microfluidizer to Manufacture Parenteral Emulsions. Biopharm. **1989**, *10*, 28–33.
24. Zheng, S.; Zheng, Y.; Beissinger, R.L.; Wasan, R.T.; McCormick, D.L. Hemoglobin Multiple Emulsion as an Oxygen Delivery System. Biochim. Biophys. Acta. **1993**, *1158*, 65–74.
25. Zheng, S.; Beissinger, R.L.; Wasan, D.T.; Sehgal, L.R.; Rosen, A.L. Oxygen Carrying Multiple Emulsions. US Patent 5,438,041, Aug 1 1995.
26. Illig, K.J.; Mueller, R.L.; Ostrander, K.D.; Swanson, J.R. Use of Microfluidizer for Preparation of Pharmaceutical Suspensions. Pharm. Tech. **1996**, *10*, 78–88.
27. Talsma, H.; Ozer, A.Y.; van Bloois, L.; Crommelin, D.J.A. The Size Reduction of Liposomes with a High Pressure Homogenizer (Microfluidizer®). Characterization of Prepared Dispersions and Comparison with Conventional Methods. Drug Dev. Ind. Pharm. **1989**, *15* (2), 197–202.
28. Vemuri, S.; Yu, C.; Wangsatorntanakun, V.; Roosdorp, N. Large-Scale Production of Liposomes Using a Microfluidizer. Drug Dev. Ind. Pharm. **1990**, *16* (15), 2243–2256.
29. Sorgi, F.L.; Huang, L. Large Scale Production of DC-Chol Cationic Liposomes by Microfluidization. Int. J. Pharm. **1996**, *144*, 131–139.
30. Farmer, M.C.; Beissinger, R.L. Scaled-up Production of Liposome-Encapsulated Hemoglobin. US Patent 4,776,991, Oct 11, 1988
31. Maa, Y.-H.; Hsu, C.C. Performance of Sonication and Microfluidization for Liquid–Liquid Emulsification. Pharm. Dev. Tech. **1999**, *4* (2), 233–240.
32. Djakovic, L.M.; Dokic, P.P.; Sefer, I.B. Mathematical and Experimental Essentials of the Emulsification Process: Optimal Parameters Determination. J. Disp. Sci. Tech. **1989**, *10* (1), 59–76.
33. *Continuous Ultrasonic Processing Cell*; Misonix Corporation: Farmingdale, NY, 1998.
34. Higgins, D.M.; Skauen, D.M. Influence of Power on Quality of Emulsions Prepared by Ultrasound. J. Pharm. Sci. **1972**, *61* (10), 1567–1570.

HOT-MELT EXTRUSION TECHNOLOGY

Michael Repka

The University of Mississippi, University, Mississippi

John J. Koleng, Jr.
Feng Zhang
Jim W. McGinity

The University of Texas at Austin, Austin, Texas

INTRODUCTION

Hot-melt extrusion is one of the most widely applied processing techniques in the plastics industry. Joseph Brama invented the extrusion process for the manufacturing of lead pipes at the end of the eighteenth century. However, hot-melt extrusion was not applied in the plastics' industry until the mid-nineteenth century, when it was first introduced into a wire insulation polymer coating process. Today, hot-melt extrusion is not only widely applied in the production of polymeric articles but also in polymer production and compounding. Currently, more than half of all plastic products, including plastic bags, sheets, and pipes, are manufactured by this process (1).

For pharmaceutical systems, several research groups have recently demonstrated that the hot-melt extrusion technique is a viable method to prepare granules, sustained release tablets, and transdermal and transmucosal drug delivery systems. Molten thermoplastic polymers during the extrusion process can function as "thermal binders and/or drug release retardants" once they exit the extruder and solidify. For film processing, a polymer can be shaped into a film via the heating process rather than through the traditional solvent-cast technique.

For pharmaceutical applications, hot-melt extrusion offers many advantages over traditional processing techniques. The advantages are as follows: 1) neither solvents nor water are used in this process; 2) fewer processing steps are needed, and, thus, time-consuming drying steps are eliminated; 3) there are no requirements on the compressibility of the active ingredients, and the entire procedure is simple, continuous, and efficient; 4) the intense mixing and agitation during processing cause suspended drug particles to de-aggregate in the molten polymer, resulting in a more uniform dispersion of fine particles; and 5) the bioavailability of the drug substance could be improved when it is dispersed at the molecular level in hot-melt extruded dosage forms. To produce the pharmaceutical dosage forms via hot-melt extrusion, a pharmaceutical grade polymer must be selected that can be processed at a relatively low temperature due to the thermal sensitivity of most drugs. All components must be thermally stable at the processing temperature during the short duration of the heating process.

PROCESS AND EQUIPMENT

Hot-melt extrusion equipment consists of an extruder, downstream auxiliary equipment, and other monitoring tools used for performance and product quality evaluation (2). The extruder is typically composed of a feeding hopper, barrel, screw, die, screw driving unit, and a heating/cooling device. A diagram of a typical extruder is shown in Fig. 1. Downstream equipment is used to collect the extrudates prior to further processing. Monitoring devices on the equipment include temperature gauges, a screw speed controller, an extrusion torque monitor, and pressure gauges.

During the hot-melt extrusion process, different zones of the barrel are preset to specific temperatures before the extrusion process. A blend of the thermoplastic polymers and other processing aids is then fed into the barrel of the extruder through the hopper. The materials are transferred inside the heated barrel by a rotating screw. Temperatures at different sections of the barrel are normally controlled by electrical heating bands, and the temperature is monitored by thermocouples. The materials inside the barrel are heated mainly by the heat generated due to the shearing effect of the rotating screw and the heat conducted from the heated barrel. The molten mass is eventually pumped through the die, which is attached to the end of the barrel. The extrudates are then subject to further processing by auxiliary downstream devices.

During a continuous extrusion process, the feed stock is required to have good flow properties inside the hopper.

Encyclopedia of Pharmaceutical Technology

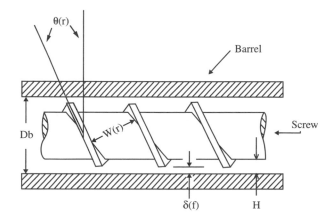

Fig. 1 Schematic diagram of a single-screw extruder. (From Ref. 11.)

For the material to demonstrate good flow, the angle between the side wall of the feeding hopper and a horizontal line needs to be larger than the angle of repose of the feed stock. In the case of cohesive materials or for very fine powders, the feed stock tends to form a solid bridge at the throat of the hopper, resulting in erratic powder flow. For these situations, a force-feeding device is sometime used.

The design of the extrusion screw has a significant influence on the efficiency of the hot-melt extrusion process. The function of the screw is to transfer the material inside the barrel and then to mix, to compress, and to melt the polymeric materials and to pump the molten mass through the die. Several parameters are used to define the geometrical features of the screw (Fig. 2).

Most screws are made from stainless steel that is surface-coated to withstand friction and potential surface erosion and decay that may occur during the extrusion process. Based on the geometrical design and the function of the screw at each section, an extruder is generally divided into three zones: feeding section, melting or compression section, and metering section, as seen in Fig. 1. Only single-screw extruders were used during the early days of this technology. Twin-screw extruders were invented in the late 1930s. The two screws can either rotate in the same direction (co-rotating extruder) or in the opposite direction (counter-rotating screw). Twin-screw extruders possess many advantages when compared to single-screw extruders, such as easier material feed, more intensive mixing, less tendency to overheat the materials, and a shorter residence time.

The purpose of the feeding section is to compact and to transfer the feed stock into the barrel of the machine. The channel depth (Fig. 2) is normally greatest in this section.

The performance of the feeding section depends on the external friction coefficient of the feed stock at the surface of the screw and barrel. The friction at the inner surface of the barrel is the driving force for the material feed, whereas the friction at the surface of the screw restricts the forward motion of the material. A high friction coefficient in the barrel and a low friction coefficient at the screw surface would contribute to a more efficient transfer of the materials in the feed section. Other properties of the feed stock, such as bulk density, particle size, particle shape, and material compactability, can also have an impact on the performance of the feeding section. The transfer of the

Fig. 2 Geometrical diagram of an extruder screw: 1) diameter of the barrel (Db): inside diameter of the barrel; 2) channel depth (H): distance from screw roots to barrel inner surface; 3) flight clearance (δ_f): the distance in between the flight and the barrel inner surface; 4) channel width ($W(r)$): distance in between two neighboring flights; and 5) helix angle (θr): angle formed in between the flight and the direction perpendicular to the screw axis.

material should be efficient in order to maintain an increase in pressure in the compression zone and the metering zone. The pressure rise in these zones should be high enough to provide an efficient output rate of the extrudate. It is also possible to finetune the barrel temperature at the feeding section in order to optimize the friction at the surface of the barrel. Inconsistent material feed may result in a "surge" phenomenon that will cause cyclical variations in the output rate, head pressure, and product quality.

The polymer will begin to melt once the material enters the compression section of the extruder. The temperature of the melting section is normally set at 30–60°C above the glass transition temperature of amorphous polymers or the melting point of a semicrystalline polymer.

Under typical processing conditions, polymer melts behave as pseudoplastic fluids. The viscosity of a pesudoplastic fluid is shear rate dependent and is described by the following power law (Eq. 1):

$$\%1\eta = K \times \gamma^{n-1} \tag{1}$$

where η represents the viscosity of the polymer melt; γ is the shear rate imposed on the polymer; K depends on the properties of the polymer and is an exponential function of the temperature; n is a constant (in the range of 0.25–0.9 for the polymer melt) and depends only on the properties of the polymer.

A minimum temperature of the barrel must be reached in order to extrude the polymer. Otherwise, the shear torque on the screw may overload the capacity of the driving unit due to the high viscosity of the polymer melt. The dependence of polymer melt viscosity on the temperature at a given shear rate follows the Arrhenius equation (Eq. 2):

$$\%2\eta = K' \times \eta^{Ea/RT} \tag{2}$$

In Eq. 2, K' is a constant, depending on the structure and the molecular weight of the polymer; Ea is the activation energy of the polymer for the flow process, and it is a constant for the same type of polymer; R is the gas constant; and T is the temperature in degrees Kelvin.

The heat conducted from the barrel contributes to the melting process. However, most of the heat is generated from viscous heat dissipation due to the shearing of the polymer melt. Viscous heat generation is a process of transforming the mechanical energy into the thermal energy of the polymer melt. The rate of heat generation per unit volume due to the viscous heat dissipation is calculated from Eq. 3:

$$\%3E = m \times \gamma^{n+1} \tag{3}$$

where m is a constant, γ represents the shear rate, and n is the power law constant (3).

The efficiency of the melting process depends on the properties of the polymer and the geometrical design of the extruder. Generally, the melting process of polymers of low viscosities and high thermal conductivities is a more efficient process. Changes in the screw design are sometimes warranted to improve the melting process. A solidified plastic or polymer component may block the channel if the melting step is insufficient. This could also result in a "surge" of the extrudate.

Thermoplastic polymers primarily exist in a molten state in the metering section. The output rate of the extrudate is highly dependent on the channel depth and the length of the metering section of the screw. The metering section has a shallow channel. Similar to the feeding section, the relative motion between the stationary barrel and the rotating screw metering section results in a velocity vector in the down channel direction, are known as "drag flow." However, the flow of the polymer melt down in the channel is restricted due to a pressure build-up in the die. This decrease in output rate of the polymer melt due to this pressure is called "pressure flow." The total flow rate is the difference between the "pressure flow" and the "drag flow" (5).

The die is attached to the end of the barrel. The geometrical design of the die will control the physical shape of the molten extrudate. The cross section of the extrudate increases due to swelling as the molten mass exits the die. Due to its viscoelastic properties, the polymer melt is able to recover some of the deformation imposed by the screw inside the barrel during the extrusion. This is referred to as "die swelling."

Hot-melt extrusion processing conditions depend on the chemical stability and physical properties of the thermal polymer such as molecular weight, glass transition temperature, and the melting point (in the case of a semicrystalline polymer). During the melt extrusion process, polymers are subjected to a mechanical shear stress imposed by the rotating screw and thermal stress due to the relatively high processing temperature. Under these stresses, polymeric materials may undergo physical chain scission, chemical depolymerization, or thermal degradation. Techniques, such as differential scanning calorimetry and gel permeation chromatography, are widely used to monitor the stability of the polymer under the melt extrusion process. In order to improve the stability of the polymer during the extrusion process, plasticizers, antioxidants, and other additives are often included in the formulation.

Different types of downstream processing equipment are necessary for the hot-melt extrusion process. For extruded film preparations, chill rolls are used to cool down and control the film temperature before it is taken up by the roller. The thickness of the film can also be controlled by adjusting the rotating speed of the chill rolls. Control of the chill roll temperature also influences the properties of the film. When the extrudate is in a rod shape, it can be chilled through a water bath or a cooling air tunnel and cut into granules by a pelletizer.

MATERIALS USED IN HOT-MELT EXTRUSION

The materials used in the production of hot-melt extruded dosage forms must meet the same levels of purity and safety as those used in traditional dosage forms. Most of the compounds used in the production of hot-melt extruded pharmaceuticals have been used in the production of other solid dosage forms such as tablets, pellets, and transdermals. The materials used in hot-melt extruded products must possess some degree of thermal stability in addition to acceptable physical and chemical stability. The thermal stability of each individual compound and the composite mixture should be sufficient to withstand the production process.

Hot-melt extruded dosage forms are complex mixtures of active medicaments and functional excipients. The functional excipients may be broadly classified as matrix carriers, release modifying agents, bulking agents, and miscellaneous additives. The selection and use of various excipients can impart specific properties to hot-melt extruded pharmaceuticals in a manner similar to those in traditional dosage forms.

The properties of the active drug substance often limit the formulation and preparation options available to the pharmaceutical scientist in the development of an acceptable dosage form. Hot-melt extrusion offers many benefits over traditional processing techniques. This is a relatively new technique to the pharmaceutical industry. The process is anhydrous, thus avoiding any potential drug degradation from hydrolysis following the addition of aqueous or hydroalcoholic granulating media. In addition, poorly compactable materials can be incorporated into tablets produced by cutting an extruded rod, thus eliminating any potential tableting problems seen in traditional compressed dosage forms. As an initial assessment, the thermal, chemical, and physical properties of the drug substance must be characterized. Depending on the unique properties of the drug substance and the other excipients in the formulation, the drug may be present as undissolved particles, a solid solution, or a combination in the final dosage form. The state of the drug in the dosage form may have a profound impact on the processability and stability of the product.

In addition to thermal degradation, the active compound may interfere with the functionality of the other components in the formulation. Oxprenolol hydrochloride was shown to melt under the hot-melt extrusion processing conditions, thus decreasing the viscosity of the extrudate to yield a material with poor handling properties (6). In similar work preparing dosage forms by injection molding, Cuff and Raouf (7) reported that fenoprofen calcium inhibited the hardening of a PEG–MCC matrix, thus resulting in an unusable product. Lidocaine was shown to effectively lower the Tg of Eudragit® E/HDPE films (8), and hydrocortisone demonstrated a time-dependent lowering of the glass transition temperature of hydroxypropylcellulose (HPC) films (9). These changes may be beneficial, as in the last two examples, or detrimental, as in the first two examples.

As mentioned previously, the drug may be present in one of several forms in the final product. The advantages and disadvantages of each form have been discussed in both injection molding (7) and melt extrusion (10) systems. Solid dispersion systems may be more stable and more easily processed than solid solution systems, but solid solution systems may be produced that are transparent and have increased bioavailability of poorly soluble compounds. Figs. 3 and 4 show the X-ray diffraction patterns for a polymer film containing lidocaine. The absence of the lidocaine peaks in the extruded samples, and the reported decrease in polymer T_g in these systems confirms that the drug exists in a solid solution within the film matrix.

In hot-melt extruded drug delivery systems, the active compound is embedded in a carrier formulation comprised of one or more meltable substances and other functional excipients. The meltable substances may be polymeric materials (6–12) or low melting point waxes (13, 14). The selection of an appropriate carrier compound is important in the formulation and design of a hot-melt extruded dosage form. The properties of the carrier material often dictate the processing conditions necessary for the production of the dosage unit, and the physical and chemical properties of the carrier often modulate the release of the active compound from the final dosage form. Table 1 lists some of the properties of various carrier compounds used in the production of hot-melt extruded dosage forms.

The use of polymeric carriers usually requires the incorporation of a plasticizer into the formulation in order to improve the processing conditions during the manufacturing of the extruded dosage form or to improve the physical and mechanical properties of the final product. The choice of a suitable plasticizer will depend on many factors, such as plasticizer-polymer compatibility and plasticizer stability. Triacetin (6), citrate esters (8, 9), and low molecular weight polyethylene glycols (6, 9, 12) have been investigated as plasticizers in hot-melt extruded systems. As mentioned previously, certain drug compounds were reported to function as plasticizers in different hot-melt extruded systems (6, 8, 9). The plasticizer functions to reduce the glass transition temperature T_g of the polymer and to reduce the processing temperatures necessary for production. The reduction in polymer T_g is dependent upon the plasticizer type and level. Fig. 5 demonstrates the effectiveness of various plasticizers in lowering the T_g of hydroxypropylcellulose films. The reduction in processing temperatures may improve the stability profile of the active compound (9) and/or the polymeric carrier (6, 12). Plasticizers also reduce the shear forces needed to extrude a polymer, thus improving the processing of certain high molecular weight polymers (9, 12). Table 2 demonstrates the profound influence on the incorporation of PEG 3350 into hot-melt extruded tablets containing PEO (MW 1,000,000) and

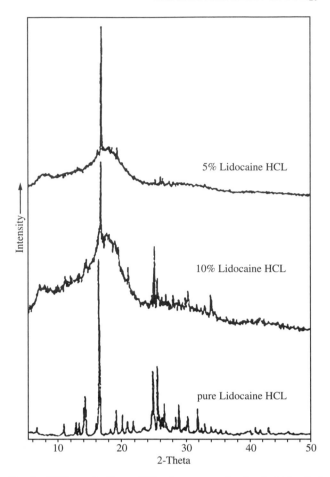

Fig. 4 Wide angle X-ray diffraction scans of a physical blend of Eudragit E100 with 5 and 10% lidocaine HCL compared with lidocaine HCL crystals. (From Ref. 8.)

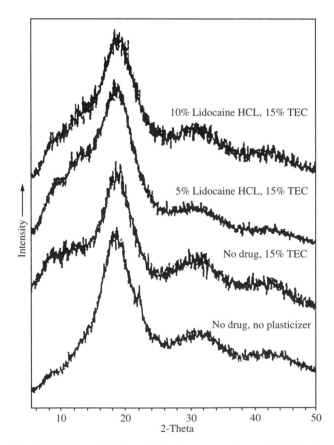

Fig. 3 Wide angle X-ray diffraction scans of extruded Eudragit E films showing the effect of plasticizer and drug on the packing of polymer film. (From Ref. 8.)

chlorpheniramine maleate. The incorporation of PEG 3350 into the carrier matrix reduces the temperatures necessary for processing and prevents the degradation of the polymer as noted by an equivalent molecular weight. The stability of a plasticized polymethacrylate system has been reported where the residual monomer content only increased 0.003% following extrusion using triacetin (6). Ethyl cellulose was also reported to be fairly stable following processing (11).

The thermochemical stability and volatility of the plasticizer during processing and storage must also be taken into consideration (9, 15–17). Table 3 illustrates these factors. Repka and McGinity demonstrated that the amount of plasticizer remaining in hot-melt extruded films over time was a function of the plasticizer type. The amount of plasticizer recovered in these films was compared to the initial theoretical amount added in all formulations. HPC films containing polyethylene glycol 400 and 8000 (PEG 400, PEG 8000), triethyl citrate (TEC)

Table 1 Properties of selected carriers used in the design and production of hot-melt extruded dosage forms

Chemical name	Trade name	Molecular weight range (s)	Melting point range (s)	Glass transition temperature	Reference
Polymeric carriers					
Ethylcellulose	Ethocel® Aqualon® EC	N-7 to N-100 based on viscosity	Decomposes at >190°C	130–133°C	6, 41
Hydroxypropyl cellulose	Klucel®	80,000–1,150,000	Chars at 260–275°C	Softens at 130°C	9, 42
Polyethylene glycol	Carbowax®	1000–20,000	37–63°C	−17°C for MW 6000	7, 15, 43
Polyethylene oxide	Polyox® WSR	100,000–7,000,000	65–80°C	−40 to −60°C	4, 44
Polymethacrylates	Eudragit® RSPM Eduragit® E	>100,000	—	52°C 40°C	6, 8, 44
Chemical name	Melting point Rage	Saponification Value	Reference		
Non-polymeric carriers					
Carnuba Wax	81–86°C	78–95	13, 14, 45		

and acetyltributyl citrate (ATBC) were tested at these two conditions: 25°C/0% RH and 25°C/50% RH for 1-week (initial), 3-month, and 6-month testing intervals. As can be seen from the results, both the citrate esters had a minimal loss at both testing conditions for the duration of the study. The most stable plasticizer for this 6-month study was PEG 8000. However, the lower molecular weight PEG had the greatest loss of any of the other three plasticizers investigated. At the more rigorous testing conditions of 25°C/50% RH, only 63% PEG 400 was detected in the HPC films for the duration of the study. These results indicate the tendency of PEG 400, and potentially other plasticizers, to evaporate or degrade under hot-melt extrusion processing and storage. It is also evident that these findings for PEG 400 explain changes upon mechanical testing of PEG 400-incorporated HPC films (9).

Plasticizers may also be incorporated into hot-melt extruded dosage forms to improve the physical–mechanical properties of the final dosage form. In transdermal films, the addition of a plasticizer to the polymer matrix can improve the film's flexibility (8, 9). Plasticizers may also influence the product's tensile strength and elastic modulus. In addition to the plasticizer's effect on the performance of hot-melt extruded polymer systems, the thermal history of the material may impact the properties of the final dosage form. The properties of high molecular weight polymers often depend upon the processing and storage conditions experienced prior to incorporation into the final dosage forms. Exposure to heat and/or moisture may influence the stability and processing of different batches of polymeric materials. There have been several reports on the influence of heating and cooling on the physical and chemical properties of PEG-containing systems (16–21).

For systems employing nonpolymeric carrier materials, similar concerns must be addressed. The compatibility between the active substance and carrier should be addressed. The incorporation of a low-melting point compound into a low-melting point wax may result in the formation of a eutectic mixture or a reduction in the melting point of the material that may prevent the formation of a solid dosage form. The production of granules using carnauba wax has been reported (13, 14). The granules contained diclofenac sodium and could be produced at temperatures less than the reported melting point of the wax material. The use of waxes and wax-based materials may be advantageous due to their reported chemical inertness (13).

The drug release rate from hot-melt extruded dosage forms is highly dependent upon the characteristics of the carrier material. Most of the materials reported for use in hot-melt extruded dosage forms are water insoluble (6, 11, 13, 14) or have slow hydrating or gelling rates (9, 12). To improve or to modulate drug release from these systems, functional excipients may be added. Depending upon the physical and chemical properties of these additional excipients, various release profiles may be achieved. Follonier and coworkers (11) investigated a variety of compounds in several polymeric systems using diltiazem hydrochloride as a model compound. The additives were incorporated into the formulation in an effort to increase the drug release rate by increasing the porosity of the pellet during dissolution. Viscosity inducing agents were incorporated

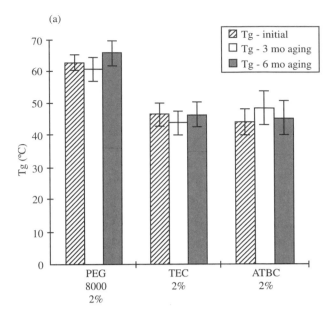

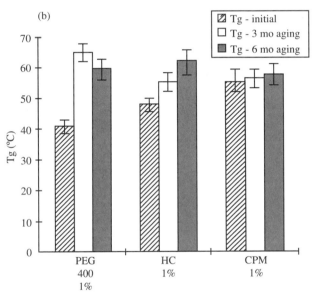

Fig. 5 (a) Glass transition temperatures of HPC films containing PEG 8000 2%, TEC 2%, and ATBC 2% at 1 week, 3 months, and 6 months; (b) Glass transition temperatures of HPC films containing PEG 400 1%, HC 1%, and CPM 1% at 1 week, 3 months, and 6 months. (From Ref. 9.)

in the polymer matrix to limit the burst effect often seen with matrix systems. The use of ionic or pH-dependent polymers in the carrier matrix may allow for zero-order drug release or pH-dependent drug delivery. Swelling agents, such as AcDiSol® and Explotab were also investigated as a method to modulate drug release. In contrast, it has been demonstrated that Explotab could be used as a "super-absorbent" in HPC hot-melt

extruded films to facilitate moisture or exudate uptake in wound care applications (22). A similar approach of drug release modification was applied to wax containing systems (13, 14). Hydroxypropylcellulose, Eudragit L, and sodium chloride were incorporated into diclofenac sodium/carnauba wax matrices. Increasing the content of the cellulose derivative or methacrylic acid copolymer resulted in a substantial increase in the release of diclofenac sodium. The release of diclofenac sodium from hydroxypropyl cellulose/wax matrices was less pH dependent than the system containing wax/Eudragit L because the methacrylic acid copolymer is insoluble in water or in solutions with pH < 6. The effect of sodium chloride was less pronounced and was attributed to the negligible swelling effect of this material.

The properties of poly(vinyl acetate) as a carrier for theophylline from matrix dosage forms prepared by hot-melt extrusion has been investigated (23). The influence of granule size and drug loading level on the drug release properties was studied. The thermal stability of poly(vinyl acetate) was also investigated. In this study, Zhang and McGinity ground the rod shaped extrudates and then compressed them into tablets with various combinations of microcrystalline cellulose. The influence of granule size on the release rate of theophylline from the compressed tablets containing the hot-melt extruded granules is seen in Fig. 6. As the size of hot-melt extruded theophylline/PVAc granules was increased, there was a significant decrease in the release rate of the theophylline. Because the drug was released from the matrix by a diffusion mechanism, the decrease in the drug release rate from the tablets containing larger granules was concluded to be a result of a longer diffusion pathway. The influence of theophylline loading on the release properties of these tablets containing extruded granules is shown in Fig. 7. The PVAc was demonstrated to have a high solids carrying capacity when processed by hot-melt extrusion. It is important to note that a powder blend containing 50% theophylline could be readily processed utilizing this hot-melt technique.

These same investigators studied the stability of PVAc to shear stress using a Plasticorder® rheometer (23). As shown in Fig. 8, the initial peak indicated the heating process of the added PVAc. The torque gradually decreased as the temperature of the polymer melt in the chamber was increased. No further change in the torque was observed after the initial heating step. This finding confirmed that PVAc was not susceptible to degradation by either thermal or shearing stress under the processing conditions.

Other materials may also be included in the formulation of hot-melt extruded dosage forms. These miscellaneous compounds include embodying agents and antioxidants.

Table 2 Stability of polyethylene oxide (MW 1,000,000) in hot-melt extruded tablet formulations containing 6 wt% chlorpheniramine maleate processed at different temperatures

Formulation	PEO (wt%)	PEG 3350 (wt%)	Zone 1 temperature	Zone 2 temperature	Die temperature	Weight average MW	Standard deviation
1	94	0	100°C	115°C	130°C	710,000	50,000
2	54	40	70°C	75°C	85°C	900,000	100,000
Pure polymer	100	—	—	—	—	920,000	80,000

(From Ref. 12.)

Table 3 Stability of plasticizers in hot-melt extruded HPC films processed at 180°C as a function of storage conditions ($n = 6$)

Plasticizer type	%Theoretical (25°C/ 0% RH)			% Theoretical (25°C/ 50% RH)		
	1 wk	3 mon	6 mon	1 wk	3 mon	6 mon
TEC	94.4 (1.83)	93.6 (0.77)	92.3 (1.20)	94.1 (2.21)	93.1 (1.97)	92.8 (2.33)
ATBC	92.8 (2.11)	91.4 (1.65)	90.0 (1.77)	91.5 (1.36)	90.1 (2.87)	88.3 (2.53)
PEG 8000	97.3 (0.38)	97.1 (1.36)	96.6 (0.34)	97.1 (0.56)	96.5 (1.73)	96.6 (1.43)
PEG 400	88.7 (3.15)	79.1 (3.82)	74.3 (2.67)	86.1 (2.18)	66.5 (2.08)	63.0 (1.98)

Standard deviation denoted in parentheses.
(From Ref. 17.)

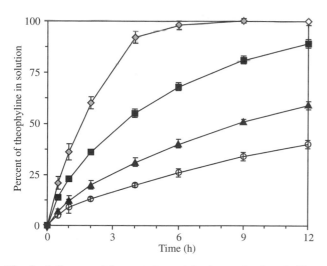

Fig. 6 Influence of the granule particle size on the theophylline release properties of the tablets containing hot-melt extruded granules ($n = 3$). Tablets: 20% extruded granules (Formula 3: 25% theophylline, 2% PEG, and 73% PVAc), 79.5% Avicel® PH 200, and 0.5% magnesium stearate (◆) Less than 125 μm; (■) 180–212 μm; (▲) 300–425 μm; (○) 500–600 μm. (From Ref. 23.)

Cuff and Raouf (7) reported the incorporation of microcrystalline cellulose into PEG 8000 matrices in order to improve the formulation viscosity and plasticity of the resulting tablets formed by injection molding. Excessive temperatures needed to process unplasticized or underplasticized cellulose-based polymers (i.e., hydroxypropyl-cellulose or ethyl cellulose) may lead to polymer oxidation. One manufacturer of these materials recommends the incorporation of an antioxidant, such as butylated hydroxytoluene or ascorbic acid, into formulations containing low molecular weight hydroxypropylcellulose (24). Similarly, a combination of an antioxidant, light absorber, and acid acceptor is recommended for systems employing ethyl cellulose (25). Poly(ethlyene oxide) films have been reported to be protected from free radical and oxidative degradation by the incorporation of an antioxidant (26).

The materials used in the production of hot-melt extruded dosage forms are the same pharmaceutical compounds used in the production of more traditional systems. Thermal stability of the individual compounds is a prerequisite for the process, although the short

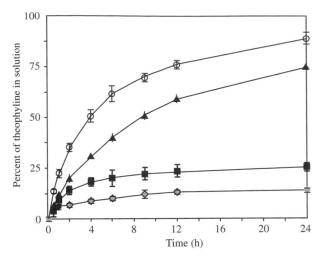

Fig. 7 Influence of drug loading levels on theophylline release properties of the tablets containing hot-melt extruded granules ($n = 3$). Tablets: 20%, 300–425 μm extruded granules (Formule 1–4: theophylline, 2% PEG and PVAc qs to 100%), 79.5% Avicel PH 200, and 0.5% magnesium stearate. (♦) 5% loading; (■) 15% loading; (▲) 25% loading; (○) 50% loading. (From Ref. 23.)

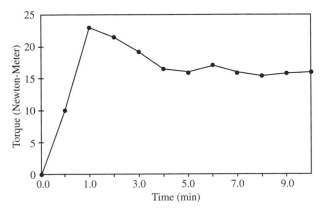

Fig. 8 Heat and shear stability of poly(vinyl acetate) monitored via Plasi-corder rheometer. (From Ref. 23.)

processing times encountered in this process may not limit all thermolabile compounds. The incorporation of plasticizers may lower the processing temperatures encountered in hot-melt extrusion, thus reducing drug and carrier degradation. Drug release from these systems can be modulated by the incorporation of various functional excipients. The dissolution rate of the active compound can be increased or decreased depending on the properties of the rate-modifying agent. For systems that display oxidative or free radical degradation during processing or storage, the addition of antioxidants, acid acceptors, and/or light absorbers may be warranted.

APPLICATIONS

For over two decades, the value of "continuous processing" in the pharmaceutical industry has been recognized. The potential of automation, reduction of capital investment, and the reduction in labor costs has made hot-melt extrusion worthy of consideration (27).

Conventional extrusion/spheronization is a significant process in obtaining controlled release pellets, as are solution/suspension techniques (28, 29). The quality of these pellets or granules is important, as was recognized by Gamlen et al. (10) and Lindberg et al. in the mid-1980s (30, 31). However, control of porosity, content uniformity, consistent pellet size distribution, as well as achieving a true continuous process, were not easily attained. Pellet technology has advanced in the 1990s with the advent of new processing equipment. Such developments have given the pharmaceutical scientist numerous opportunities to apply scientific principles to the design of novel dosage forms.

Until recently, hot-melt extrusion had not received much attention in the pharmaceutical literature. Pellets comprising cellulose acetate phthalate were prepared using a rudimentary ram extruder in 1969 and studied for dissolution rates in relation to pellet geometry (32). More recently, production of matrices based on polyethylene and polycaprolactone were investigated using extruders of laboratory scale (33, 34). Mank et al. reported in 1989 and 1990 on the extrusion of a number of thermoplastic polymers to produce sustained release pellets (35, 36). A melt-extrusion process for manufacturing matrix drug delivery systems was reported by Sprockel and coworkers (37). As one can see, a review of the pharmaceutical scientific literature does not elucidate many applications for hot-melt extrusion in this field.

Follonier and coworkers in 1994 investigated the possibility of using hot-melt extrusion technology to produce sustained-release pellets (6). Fig. 9 exhibits the ram extruder used in their investigations. Again, it was the researchers' goal to provide a product in a simple, single, and continuous manner. Thermal degradation was recognized as a limitation of this hot-melt process. Diltiazem hydrochloride, a relatively stable, freely soluble drug, was incorporated into their polymer-based pellets for sustained-release capsules. Prior to formulation, polymers and plasticizers were selected to optimize the possibility of a successful product. In this report, ethyl cellulose (EC), cellulose acetate butyrate (CAB), poly(ethyl acrylate/methyl-methacrylate/trimethyl ammonio ethyl methacrylate chloride) (Eudragit RSPM), and poly(ethylene-co-vinyl acetate) (EVAC) were the polymers utilized. Plasticizers used included triacetin and

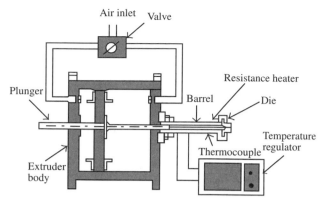

Fig. 9 Schematic diagram of a laboratory ram extruder. (From Ref. 6.)

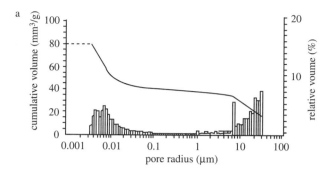

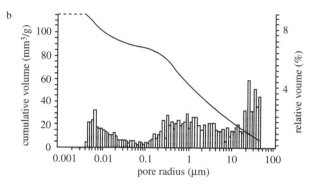

Fig. 10 Mercury infusion curves and pore size distributions of Eudragit RSPM (a) and Elvaxr 40W (b) based pellets containing diltiazem hydrochloride. (From Ref. 6.)

diethyl phthalate. The porosity of the formulations was assessed by mercury porosimetry. Pellets that were produced exhibited a rather smooth surface and low porosity, as demonstrated in Fig. 10. The in vitro release of diltiazem was biphasic, with the CAB and EVAC pellets giving the slowest release rate, as seen in Fig. 11, 12. They also found that the stability of Eudragit RSPM was adequate for extrusion at a temperature of 130°C. Not surprisingly, the type and percent of plasticizer used, drying time of the polymers, extrusion temperatures, and plasticization times varied with each formulation. In a latter study, Follonier et al. examined different parameters influencing the release of diltiazem hydrochloride from hot-melt extruded pellets (11). These parameters included polymer type, drug/polymer ratio, and pellet size. The authors also incorporated various polymer excipients into the pellet formulations to vary the drug release rate, such as croscarmellose sodium (Ac-Di-Sol®) and sodium starch glycolate (Explotab). These pellets could be applicable for incorporation into hard gelatin capsules. With optimization of techniques and formulations, it is apparent that hot-melt extrusion of these and other sustained-release pellets is a viable drug delivery technology.

Currently, the most frequent means of producing thin films for transdermal/transmucosal drug delivery and wound care is via film casting from organic or aqueous solvents (8). However, it is recognized that there are numerous problems with these types of films. For example, Gutierrez-Rocca and McGinity showed that physical aging of both aqueous- and solvent-cast acrylic films resulted in a decrease in elongation or elasticity and an increase in the tensile strength. The changes in the mechanical properties were related to a relaxation of the polymer chains toward a state of equilibrium (16). Also, it has been demonstrated that the type and level of

plasticizers, curing time, and temperatures will have a significant effect on the dissolution rate of drugs from films formed from aqueous dispersions (38–40).

Aitken-Nichol and coworkers investigated the viability of hot-melt extrusion technology in 1996 for the production of thin, flexible, acrylic films for topical drug

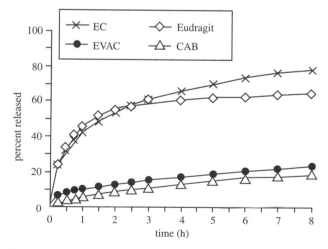

Fig. 11 Release profiles of diltiazem hydrochloride from extruded pellets based on various polymers (polymer/drug ratio: 1:1; size: 2 × 2 mm). (From Ref. 6.)

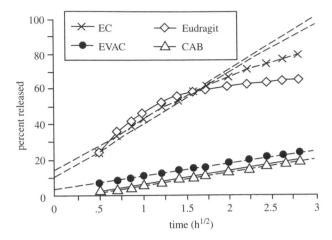

Fig. 12 Diltiazem hydrochloride released (%) as a function of the square root of time and calculated regression lines (—). (From Ref. 6.)

delivery (8). One of the advantages that the researchers pointed out was that the manufacturing process is not restricted by solvent concerns. Although a truly continuous operating mode was not utilized in this investigation, the potential for one definitely exists. The investigators compared a cast film with various extruded films. The data in Table 4 illustrate the effects of types and levels of plasticizers and model drugs used in this study on the glass transition temperature (T_g) and the mechanical properties of high density polyethylene (HDPE) and Eudragit E-100 extruded films. Eudragit E-100 was the primary thermoplastic polymer extruded. The authors found that

hot-melt extrusion was a viable technology for the production of free films of this acrylic resin. Although triethyl citrate was an acceptable plasticizer for this polymer, these researchers showed that lidocaine HCl was also able to plasticize the acrylic films. The authors concluded that the differences in the dissolution and ductile properties between cast films and extruded films were due to the amount of drug dissolved in the polymer. The dissolution rate of lidocaine HCl was affected by the drug loading, in contrast to the solvent-cast films tested.

Transdermal and transmucosal drug delivery systems are frequently produced by films cast from organic or aqueous solvents. Repka and coworkers discussed the numerous disadvantages accompanying these techniques, including long processing times, environmental concerns, and excessive costs (9). Hot-melt extrusion technology was used by these researches to produce HPC films utilizing a Killion extruder. Various plasticizers and two model drugs were incorporated into the HPC films. The influence of these plasticizers and drugs on the physical–mechanical properties of the films was investigated. The authors observed that a pure HPC film could not be produced without the incorporation of a plasticizer due to the high stress exhibited in the extruder. The results in Table 5 illustrate the effects of a number of conventional plasticizers and two model drugs on the three mechanical properties of HPC films. With the exception of PEG 400, all plasticizers investigated demonstrated adequate stability for the duration of the study. PEG 400, although initially exhibiting excellent plasticizer qualities for the HPC films, was found to be unstable in all parameters

Table 4 Mechanical properties of Eudragit E100 films containing diphenhydramine HCL (DPH) and lidocaine HCL (L-HCL)

Polymer	Plasticizer	Drug	T_g (°C)	d-spacing (Å)	Peak stress(c) σ (kg/cm²)	Elongation at break ε (%)
E100	none	none	40	4.76	N/A	N/A
E100-Ex	15% TEC	none	18	4.92	13.4	59.3
E100-Ex	12% triacetin	none	25	4.76	29	47.9
E100-Ex	15% TEC	5% DPH	20	N/A	12.9	53.5
E100-Cast	15% TEC	5% L-HCL	20	5.03	3.65	549
E100-Ex	15% TEC	5% L-HCL	21	4.79	9.88	218
E100-Ex	15% TEC	10% L-HCL	10.5	4.80	2.47	376.8
HDPE-E100	none	5% L-HCL	35[a]	4.76[b]	77.7[c]	110.0[c]
1:1—Ex					3.0[d]	3.0[d]
Ex—Extruded						

[a] T_{neck} at 111°C
[b] Crystalline peaks at 4.1, 3.60, and 2.49-Å.
[c] Tested in the direction of orientation.
[d] Tested perpendicular to orientation.
(From Ref. 8.)

Table 5 Influence of plasticizers and drugs on tensile strength (TS), percent elongation (%E), and Young's modulus (YM) of HPC extruded films stored at 25°C

	TS (initial)	TS (3 mon)	TS (6 mon)
PEG 8000 2%	13.7 (1.1)	13.2 (1.3)	12.2 (0.7)
TEC 2%	17.2 (1.7)	18.9 (1.1)	20.8 (0.7)
ATBC 2%	26.1 (2.6)	19.2 (1.5)	19.6 (1.4)
PEG 400 1%	37.6 (3.5)	29.9 (2.7)	27.9 (2.1)
HC 1%	26.7 (2.7)	33.0 (2.7)	34.1 (3.8)
CPM 1%	32.7 (3.4)	32.9 (3.1)	30.8 (1.8)
	%E (initial)	**%E (3 mon)**	**%E (6 mon)**
PEG 8000 2%	5.01 (0.4)	4.45 (0.6)	4.39 (0.7)
TEC 2%	5.29 (0.4)	5.37 (0.4)	5.08 (0.6)
ATBC 2%	6.02 (0.6)	6.13 (0.5)	6.40 (0.7)
PEG 400 1%	6.62 (0.6)	5.25 (0.6)	5.05 (0.5)
HC 1%	5.40 (0.4)	4.82 (0.4)	4.55 (0.4)
CPM 1%	5.26 (0.4)	5.03 (0.7)	4.87 (0.7)
	YM (initial)	**YM (3 mon)**	**YM (6 mon)**
PEG 8000 2%	4.25 (0.2)	4.31 (0.6)	4.21 (0.4)
TEC 2%	4.43 (0.3)	4.11 (0.4)	4.09 (0.4)
ATBC 2%	4.75 (0.6)	3.09 (0.5)	3.19 (0.4)
PEG 400 1%	4.05 (0.3)	7.13 (0.3)	6.15 (0.6)
HC 1%	6.57 (0.3)	7.98 (0.3)	8.60 (0.3)
CPM 1%	5.38 (0.3)	4.44 (0.4)	4.64 (0.3)

Standard Deviations denoted in parenthesis; $n = 6$.
(From Ref. 9.)

tested. The influence of processing temperature and storage time on the two model drugs was investigated and is outlined in Table 6. Besides the fact that CPM proved to be an excellent plasticizer for HPC, providing mechanically stability for the hot-melt extruded film, it also proved to be chemically stable for up to 12 months. In addition, it was demonstrated by differential scanning calorimetry that CPM was fully dissolved in the HPC film

Table 6 Influence of processing temperature and storage at 25°C on percentage of chlorpheniramine maleate (CPM) and hydrocortisone (HC) remaining in HPC extruded films ($n = 6$)

(°C)	CPM (1 wk)	CPM (6 mon)	CPM (12 mon)
170	98.6 (1.6)	98.5 (1.9)	98.4 (1.9)
180	98.5 (1.9)	98.5 (2.1)	98.1 (2.4)
190	98.1 (2.2)	97.6 (2.7)	97.3 (2.5)
200	97.9 (2.3)	97.7 (2.2)	97.6 (2.3)
(°C)	**HC (1 wk)**	**HC (6 mon)**	**HC (12 mon)**
170	93.9 (2.3)	92.4 (3.0)	91.4 (2.4)
180	87.7 (2.2)	83.1 (2.8)	79.9 (2.2)
190	75.9 (3.2)	70.7 (2.7)	71.6 (2.4)
200	70.2 (3.8)	68.8 (3.3)	62.9 (3.1)

Standard deviations denoted in parenthesis.
(From Ref. 9.)

up to the 10% level (Fig. 13) (17). As can be seen, CPM is amorphous within the HPC film thus, a solid solution exists. Hydrocortisone was shown to be a good plasticizer comparable to that of the conventional plasticizers studied however, the chemical stability of HC incorporated into the HPC films was demonstrated to be a function of processing temperature and residence time in the extruder.

Repka et al. (9) also found an inverse relationship during film testing. All extruded films exhibited a marked decrease in tensile strength, in contrast to a large increase in percent elongation, when testing was performed perpendicular to flow vs. in-the-direction of flow, as seen in Fig. 14. This is in contrast to the findings of Aitken-Nichol et al. (8). These researchers reported a 25- to 35-fold increase in both tensile strength and percent elongation in a high density polyethylene/Eudragit E100 (50:50 polymer ratio containing 5% lidocaine HCl) extruded film when tested in the direction of orientation versus perpendicular to orientation (15). The differences between the findings in the two studies, however, may be explained by the poor compatibility of the two polymers. Such mechanical property differences illustrate the importance of "flow orientation" when designing delivery systems or wound care applications utilizing extruded films.

Vitamin E TPGS NF (D-α-tocopheryl polyethylene glycol 1000 succinate) has been utilized for numerous applications in pharmaceutical dosage forms. Its chemical structure contains both a lipophilic and a hydrophilic moiety, making it similar to a conventional surface-active agent. Due to TPGS's unique properties as a solubilizer,

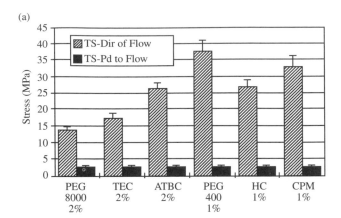

(a)

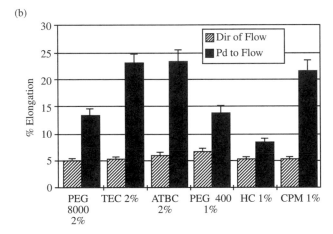

(b)

Fig. 14 (a) Tensile strength of HPC films containing various plasticizers and drugs tested in direction of flow and perpendicular to flow; (b) Percent elongation of HPC films containing various plasticizers and drugs tested in direction of flow and perpendicular to flow. (From Ref. 9.)

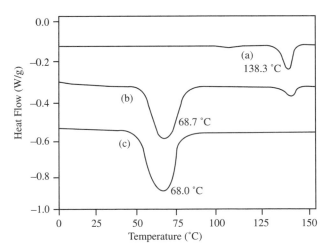

Fig. 13 Differential scanning calorimetry profiles of hot-melt extruded films containing chlorpheniramine maleate and hydroxypropylcellulose: (a) chlorpheniramine maleate (CPM); (b) 10% CPM and 90% HPC (Klucel HF) physical mix; and (c) 10% CPM and 90% HPC (Klucel HF) extruded film. (From Ref. 17.)

absorption enhancer, and a potential controlled drug release vehicle, transdermal and transmucosal applications have been shown to be possible via hot-melt extrusion technology (41). Repka and McGinity prepared films containing hydroxypropylcellulose and polyethylene oxide (PEO) using a Randcastle extruder (Model # 750) with and without Vitamin E TPGS as an additive. As can be seen from Fig. 15, the addition of 1, 3, and 5% TPGS, respectively, decreased the glass transition temperature of the extruded films containing either a 50:50 or 80:20 ratio of HPC to PEO in an almost linear fashion. The presence of 3% Vitamin E TPGS lowered the T_g over 11°C when compared to the HPC/PEO 50:50 blend film without TPGS, thus functioning as a plasticizer. The films containing 3% Vitamin E TPGS had similar mechanical properties to that of the films containing 3% PEG 400 and a three-fold increase in percent elongation when compared to the films containing TEC 3% and ATBC 3%. In addition,

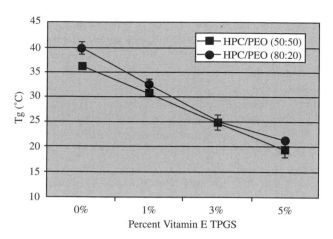

Fig. 15 Glass transition temperatures of films containing different levels of Vitamin E TPGS incorporated into two formulations of HPC/PEO hot-melt extruded films ($n = 4$). (From Ref. 41.)

the Vitamin E TPGS facilitated the processing of the HPC/PEO films by decreasing the barrel pressure, drive amps, and torque of the extruder equipment (Table 7). The unique properties of Vitamin E TPGS can function to promote more applications and opportunities in wound care and in transdermal and transmucosal drug delivery.

Another application of hot-melt extrusion was described by Zhang and McGinity (12). These researchers investigated the properties of polyethylene oxide (PEO) as a drug carrier and studied the release mechanism of chlorpheniramine maleate (CPM) from matrix tablets. In these extruded tablets, PEG 3350 was included as a plasticizer to facilitate processing. In this study, the stability of the primary extruded polymer, PEO, as a function of processing temperature was reported (Table 2). Again, polymer type, temperature, and residence time in the extruder was shown to be of great importance. These authors also reported that the drug, polymer, and other ingredients must be stable at the elevated processing

temperature during the approximately 2 min that the powder blend is processed through the equipment. In addition, the researchers showed that additional mixing of the components occurred in the barrel of the extruder, because the content uniformity of the extruded tablets was within 99.0–101.0% of the theoretical content. The profiles in Fig. 16 illustrate the influence of PEG 3350 on the release of CPM from the extruded matrix tablets. It can be seen that as the percent of PEG 3350 increases, the release rate of CPM increases. Polyethylene glycol is composed of the same structural unit as PEO but has a lower molecular weight than PEO. Thus, PEG 3350 hydrated and dissolved faster than the PEO. The hydration and dissolution rates of the entire matrix system were, thus, accelerated due to the presence of the plasticizer. The influence of drug loading on the release of CPM is shown in Fig. 17. When the drug content was increased from 6 to 12%, no change in the percentage of drug release with respect to time was observed. There was only a slight increase when the drug loading reached 20%. This study conveys the reproducibility of dissolution data for the tablets produced by hot-melt extrusion.

A bioadhesive hot-melt extruded film for intraoral drug delivery and the processing thereof has been patented (42,43). Applications of these films may be utilized in transmucosal drug delivery or even transdermal systems. The films may be produced separately and layered after extrusion, or in some cases, a multilayered system may be extruded in one continuous process. Currently on the market is an extruded film device that is utilized as a denture adhesive. This system includes thermoplastic polymers that have a bioadhesive quality when the film is wetted. Before application and wetting, however, this thin film may be held in one's hand and shaped or cut. This device is again produced by a one-step, continuous process using hot-melt extrusion technology.

A polymeric film that possesses inherent bioadhesive properties has the added benefit of simplifying the dosage

Table 7 Processing conditions for hot-melt extruded films containing a 50:50 ratio of hydroxypropylcellulose to polyethylene oxide with vitamin E TPGS as an additive ($n = 4$)

Vitamin E TPGS (%)	Melt temparature (°C)	Pressure (psi)	Drive amps	Torque (N.m)	Screw speed
0	180	>3000	>4.00	overload	25
0	190	2100	3.84	40	40
1	180	1800	3.06	33	40
3	180	1500	2.61	28	40
5	180	1100	2.07	21	40

(From Ref. 17.)

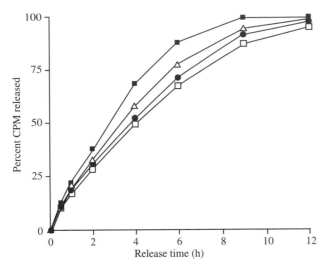

Fig. 16 Influence of polyethylene glycol (3350) on the release of chlorpheniramine maleate from matrix tablets using USP method II at 37°C and 100 rpm in 900 ml purified water: □, 6% CPM, 0% PEG (3,350) and 94% PEO (1.0 m); ●, 6% CPM, 0% PEG (3,350) and 88% PEO (1.0 m); △, 6% CPM, 20% PEG (3,350) and 74% PEO (1.0 m); and ■, 6% CPM, 40% PEG (3,350) and 54% PEO (1.0 m). (From Ref. 12.)

form design and reducing the preparation cost, due to the elimination of the adhesive layer in the system. It is desirable for the film to have adequate adhesion strength so that desirable retention at the application site can be

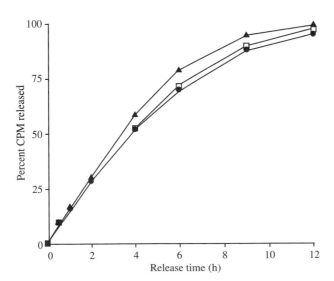

Fig. 17 Influence of drug loading on the release of chlorpheniramine maleate from matrix tablets using USP method II at 37°C and 100 rpm in 900 ml purified water during the first 6 h: ●, 6% CPM, 94% PEO (1.0 m); □, 12% CPM, 88% PEO (1.0 m); and ▲, 20% CPM, 80% PEO (1.0 m). (From Ref. 12.)

achieved. Bioadhesion, however, has been a difficult phenomenon to measure. The test method itself can be problematic as well as the specific property being measured. Physical-mechanical And bioadhesive characteristics are important parameters in the product development of films, for transdermal, transmucosal, and wound care applications. Repka and McGinity conducted bioadhesion testing of hot-melt extruded HPC films, with various additives in human subjects, utilizing a Chatillon testing apparatus (17, 22). Fig. 18 shows a schematic of the equipment used for this testing. Also illustrated is an example of a force deflection profile obtained from bioadhesion experiments in this study (Fig. 19). These researchers found that the force of adhesion, elongation at adhesive failure, and modulus of adhesion are a function of the type of additive in the extruded film. Fig. 20 shows the force of adhesion of the hot-melt extruded films tested. It can be seen that the force of adhesion was highest for the films containing carbomer 971P (Carbopol® 971P) and a polycarbophil (Noveon AA-1®). This study demonstrates that a single layer HPC film may be produced with the bioadhesive incorporated into the matrix, thus eliminating a separate "adhesive layer" and simplifying the process of transdermal and transmucosal delivery systems.

Miyagawa, Sato, and coworkers studied the controlled-release and mechanism of release of diclofenac in studies conducted in 1996 and 1997 (13, 14). These researchers utilized a twin-screw compounding extruder to prepare wax matrix granules composed of carnauba wax, the model drug, and other rate controlling agents. Their first investigation showed that a wax matrix with high mechanical strength could be obtained even at temperatures lower than the melting point of the wax. Dissolution release profiles of diclofenac from the wax matrix granules were strongly influenced by the formulation of the

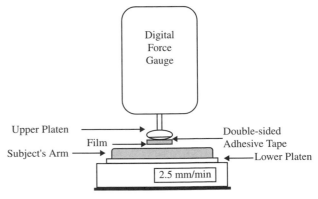

Fig. 18 Schematic of the Chatillon apparatus used to perform butt bioadhesion experiments in vivo in human subjects. (From Ref. 22.)

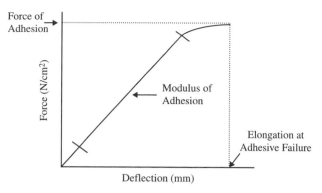

Fig. 19 Example of a force-deflection profile obtained from a butt bioadhesion experiment utilizing hot-melt extruded films in vivo using a Chatillon digital force gauge attached to a motorized test stand. (From Ref. 22.)

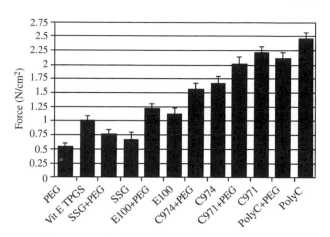

Fig. 20 Force of adhesion of hydroxypropylcellulose hot-melt extruded films containing various polymer additives (12 subjects, $n = 6$). (From Ref. 17.)

granules. The rate-controlling additives that were varied in the formulations included hydroxypropylcellulose, methacrylic acid copolymer (Eudragit L-100), and sodium chloride. The authors emphasized the advantages of using the twin-screw extruder for wax matrix tablets, such as the utilization of low temperatures, high kneading and dispersing ability, and low residence time of materials in the extruder. The investigators concluded in the second study (14) that the selection of rate-controlling agents based on their physicochemical properties, i.e., solubility and swelling characteristics, had a significant impact on the properties of wax matrix granules prepared from this extrusion process.

Koleng and McGinity (44) utilized hot-melt extrusion technology for the preparation of rapid release granules. In this investigation, a hot-melt extrusion process was used to granulate acetaminophen and filler excipients with low molecular weight poly(ethylene glycol)s. The resultant granules were then combined with additional excipients (disintegrant and lubricant) and compressed into tablet compacts. Table 8 lists the release characteristics of the bulk granules and tablets produced from hot-melt extruded granules for formulations containing 15–25% polyethylene glycol 6000. The granules displayed improved drug release compared to the tablets. Tablets containing 15% poly(ethylene glycol) released greater than 80% of the incorporated acetaminophen after 30 min, as required for acetaminophen tablets in the USP 23.

SUMMARY

Although a relatively new technology in the pharmaceutical industry, hot-melt extrusion has been visualized and employed to revolutionize the production of many different dosage forms and systems. It has demonstrated to be applicable to immediate release and sustained release dosage forms including granules, pellets, and tablets. It has

Table 8 Release of acetaminophen from hot-melt extruded granules and tablets prepared from hot-melt extruded granules containing poly(ethylene glycol) 6000 as a thermal binder in 900 ml of 50 mM phosphate buffer (pH 5.8) at 37°C and a paddle speed of 50 rpm

Time (min)	15% PEG 6000		20% PEG 6000		25% PEG 6000}	
	Granules (%)	Tablets (%)	Granules (%)	Tablets (%)	Granules (%)	Tablets (%)
5	85.0	18.1	77.1	15.5	79.3	17.4
15	95.5	53.0	99.0	45.3	94.2	35.8
30	98.5	91.4	100.0	77.7	100.0	65.5
45	99.2	95.9	—	95.1	—	86.2
60	100.0	100.0	—	100.0	—	97.8

also been shown to provide numerous advantages in the production of thin films for both drug delivery and wound care applications. New chemical entities that demonstrate a low bioavailability due to solubility issues are prime candidates for hot-melt technologies. These drugs and pharmaceutical devices encompass both prescription products and over-the-counter medications. Hot-melt extrusion technologies may offer numerous advantages over traditional methods. Shorter and more efficient processing times to the final product, environmental advantages due to elimination of solvents in processing (including the possibility of recycling), and increased efficiency of drug delivery to the patient make hot-melt extrusion an exciting challenge for the pharmaceutical scientist.

REFERENCES

1. Kaufman, H.S.; Falcetta, J.J. Introduction to Polymer Science and Technology. *An SPE Textbook*; John Wiley & Sons: New York, 1997.
2. Kruder, G.A. *Encyclopedia of Chemical Technology*; John Wiley & Sons: New York, 1996.
3. Rauwendaal, C. *Polymer Extrusion*; Hanser/Gardner Publications: Cincinnati OH, 1994.
4. Nielsen, L.E. *Polymer Rheology*; Marcel Dekker, Inc.: New York, 1977.
5. Tadmor, Z.; Klein, I. *Engineering Principles of Plasticating Extrusion*; Van Nostrand Reinhold Company: New York, 1970.
6. Follonier, N.; Doelker, E.; Cole, E.T. Evaluation of Hot-Melt Extrusion as a New Technique for the Production of Polymer-Based Pellets for Sustained Release Capsules Containing High Loading of Freely Soluble Drugs. Drug Dev. Ind. Pharm. **1994**, *20* (8), 1323–1339.
7. Cuff, G.; Raouf, F. A Preliminary Evaluation of Injection Molding as a Technology to Produce Tablets. Pharm. Tech. **June, 1998**,97–106.
8. Aitken-Nichol, C.; Zhang, F.; McGinity, J.W. Hot-Melt Extrusion of Acrylic Films. Pharm. Res. **1996**, *13*, 804–808.
9. Repka, M.A.; Gerding, T.G.; Repka, S.L.; McGinity, J.W. Influence of Plasticizers and Drugs on the Physical-Mechanical Properties of Hydroxypropylcellulose Films Prepared by Hot-Melt Extrusion. Drug Dev. Ind. Pharm. **1999**, *25* (5), 627–635.
10. Grünhagen, H.H.; Müller, O. Melt Extrusion Technology. Pharm. Manu. Int. **1995**, *1*, 167–170.
11. Follonier, N.; Doelker, E.; Cole, E.T. Various Ways of Modulating the Release of Diltiazem Hydrochloride from Hot-Melt Extruded Sustained Release Pellets Prepared Using Polymeric Materials. J. Controlled Release **1995**, *36*, 243–250.
12. Zhang, F.; McGinity, J.W. Properties of Sustained Release Tablets Prepared by Hot-Melt Extrusion. Pharm. Dev. Tech. **1998**, *4* (2), 241–250.
13. Miyagawa, Y.; Okabe, T.; Yamaguchi, Y.; Miyajima, M.; Sunada, H. Controlled-Release of Diclofenac Sodium from Wax Matrix Granule. Int. J. Pharm. **1996**, *138*, 215–254.
14. Sato, H.; Miyagawa, Y.; Okabe, T. Dissolution Mechanism of Diclofenac Sodium from Wax Matrix Granules. J. Pharm. Sci. **1997**, *86*, 929–934.
15. Price, J.C. Polyethylene Glycol. *Handbook of Pharmaceutical Excipients*; Wade, A., Weller, P.J., Eds.; American Pharmaceutical Association: Washington DC, 1994; 355–361.
16. Gutierrez-Rocca, J.C.; McGinity, J.W. Influence of Aging on the Physical–Mechanical Properties of Acrylic Resin Films Cast from Aqueous Dispersions and Organic Solutions. Drug Dev. Ind. Pharm **1993**, *19*, 315–332.
17. Repka, M.A. *Physical–Mechanical and Chemical Properties of Topical Films Produced by Hot-Melt Extrusion*; The University of Texas at Austin: Austin Texas, 2000.
18. Lin, C.; Cham, T. Compression Behavior and Tensile Strength of Heat-Treated Polyethylene Glycols. Int. J. Pharm. **1995**, *118*, 169–179.
19. Craig, D.Q.M.; Newton, J.M. Characterisation of Polyethylene Glycols Using Differential Scanning Calorimetry. Int. J. Pharm. **1994**, *74*, 33–41.
20. McGinity, J.W.; Maincent, P.; Steinfink, H. Crystallinity and Dissolution Rate of Tolbutamide Solid Dispersions Prepared by the Melt Method. J. Pharm. Sci. **1984**, *73*, 1441–1444.
21. Fassihi, A.R.; Davies, P.J.; Parker, M.S. Effect of Punch Pressure on the Survival of Fungal Spores During the Preparation of Tablets from Contaminated Raw Materials. Zbl. Pharm. **1997**, *116*, 1267–1271.
22. Repka, M.A.; McGinity, J.W. Physical–Mechanical, Moisture Absorption and Bioadhesive Properties of Hydroxypropylcellulose Hot-Melt Extruded Films. Biomaterials **2000**, *21* (14), 1509–1517.
23. Zhang, F.; McGinity, J.W. Properties of Hot-Melt Extruded Theophylline Tablets Containing Poly (vinyl Acetate). Drug Dev. Ind. Pharm. **2000**, *29* (6), 938–948.
24. Klucel® Hydroxypropylcellulose; Physical and Chemical Properties. *Technical Bulletin*; Hercules, Inc.: Wilmington DE, 1997.
25. Aqualon® Ethylcellulose (EC); Physical and Chemical Properties. *Technical Bulletin*; Hercules, Inc.: Wilmington DE, 1996.
26. Bailey, F.E.; Koleske, J.V. *Poly(ethylene oxide)*; Academic Press: New York, 1976.
27. Gamlen, M. Continuous Extrusion Using a Raker Perkins MP50 (Multipurpose) Extruder. Drug Dev. Ind. Pharm. **1986**, *12*, 1701–1713.
28. Reynolds, A.; Manf. Chem. **1970**, *41*, 40–44.
29. Harris, M.R.; Ghebre-Sellassie, I. Aqueous Polymeric Coating for Modified Release Oral Dosage Forms. *Aqueous Polymeric Coatings For Pharmaceutical Dosage Forms*; McGinity, J.W., Ed.; Marcel Dekker, Inc.: New York, 1997; 79.
30. Lindberg, N.O.; Tufvesson, C.; Olbjer, L. Extrusion of an Effervescent Granulation with a Twin Screw Extruder, Baker Perkins MPF 50 D. Drug Dev. Ind. Pharm. **1987**, *13*, 1891–1913.
31. Lindberg, N.O.; Tufvesson, C.; Holm, P.; Olbjer, L. Extrusion of an Effervescent Granulation with a Twin Screw Extruder, Baker Perkins MPF 50 D. Influence on

Intragranular Porosity and Liquid Saturation. Drug Dev. Ind. Pharm. **1998**, *14*, 1791–1798.

32. Rippie, E.G.; Johnson, J.R. Regulation of Dissolution Rate by Pellet Geometry. J. Pharm. Sci. **1969**, *58*, 428–431.

33. Shivanand, P.; Hussain, A.S.; Sprockel, D.L. Factors Affecting Release of KCl from Melt Extruded Polyethylene Disks. Pharm. Res. **1991**, *8*, S–192.

34. Prapaitrakul, W.; Sprockel, D.L.; Shivanand, P.; Sen, M. Development of a Drug Delivery System Through Melt Extrusion. *Abstracts of the 4th AAPS, Pharm. Res*; Atlanta, GA; 6, S98.

35. Mank, R.; Kala, H.; Richter, M. Darstellung Wirkstoffhaltiger Extrusionformlinge Auf Der Basis Von Thermoplasten., Teil 1, Untersuchungen Zur Wirkstoffliberation. Pharmazie **1989**, *44*, 773–776.

36. Mank, R.; Kala, H.; Richter, M. Darstellung Wirkstoffhaltiger Extrusionformlinge Auf Der Basis Von Thermoplasten., Teil 2, Untersuchungen Zur Optimierung Der Wirkstofffreigabe. Pharmazie **1990**, *45*, 592–593.

37. Sprockel, O.; Sen, M.; Shivanand, P.; Prapaitrakul, W. A Melt-Extrusion Process for Manufacturing Matrix Drug Delivery Systems. Int. J. Pharm. **1997**, *155*, 191–199.

38. Steuernagel, C.R. Latex Emulsions for Controlled Drug Delivery. *Aqueous Polymeric Coatings For Pharmaceutical Dosage Forms*; McGinity, J.W., Ed.; Marcel Dekker, Inc.: New York, 1989.

39. Factors Affecting Drug Release from Sustained-Release Film-Coated Pellets Using Acrylic Aqueous Dispersions 6th International Conference on Pharmaceutical Technology, Paris, France, June 2–4, 1992.

40. Schmidt, P.C.; Niemann, F. The MiniWiD-Coater. III. Effect of Application Temperature on the Dissolution Profile of Sustained-Release Theophylline Pellets Coated with Eudragit RS 30 D. Drug Dev. Ind. Pharm. **1993**, *19*, 1603–1612.

41. Repka, M.A.; McGinity, J.W. Influence of Vitamin E TPGS on the Properties of Hydrophilic Films Produced by Hot-Melt Extrusion. Int. J. Pharm. **2000**, *202* (1–2), 63–70.

42. Schiraldi, M.T.; Perl, M.M.; Rubin, H. Bioadhesive Extruded Film for Intra-Oral Drug Delivery and Process. US Patent 4,713,243, December 15, 1987.

43. Schiraldi, M.T.; Perl, M.M.; Rubin, H. Bioadhesive Extruded Film for Intra-oral Drug Delivery and Process. US Patent RE33,093, October 17, 1989.

44. McGinity, J.W.; Koleng, J.J. Preparation and Evaluation of Rapid-Release Granules Using a Novel Hot-Melt Extrusion Technique, Abstracts of the 16th Pharmaceutical Technology Conference, Athens Greece, 1997; 2 153.

45. Dahl, T.C. Ethylcellulose. *Handbook of Pharmaceutical Excipients*; Wade, A., Weller, P.J., Eds.; American Pharmaceutical Association: Washington DC, 1994; 186–190.

46. Harwood, R.J.; Johnson, J.L. Hydroxypropylcellulose. In *Handbook of Pharmaceutical Excipients*; Wade, A., Weller, P.J. Eds.; American Pharmaceutical Association: Washington DC, 1994; 223–228.

47. Braun, D.B.; DeLong, D.J. Polyethers (Ethylene Oxide Polymers). *Encyclopedia of Chemical Technology*; Kirk-Othmer, Ed.; John Wiley & Sons, Inc.: New York; 1982; 616–632.

48. Shukla, A.J. Polymethacrylates. *Handbook of Pharmaceutical Excipients*; Wade, A., Weller, P.J., Eds.; American Pharmaceutical Association: Washington DC, 1994; 362–366.

49. Kobayashi, N.H. Carnauba Wax. *Handbook of Pharmaceutical Excipients*; Wade, A., Weller, P.J., Eds.; American Pharmaceutical Association: Washington DC, 1994; 552–553.

HYDROLYSIS OF DRUGS

Kenneth A. Connors

University of Wisconsin-Madison, Madison, Wisconsin

Jason M. LePree

Boehringer Ingelheim Pharmaceuticals, Ridgefield, Connecticut

INTRODUCTION

The term "hydrolysis" describes a chemical reaction in which a chemical bond is split (lysis) via the addition of water. This reaction is one of the most important routes of drug decomposition, as it occurs frequently in active ingredients and excipients of pharmaceutical dosage forms. A search of the scientific literature, performed with a popular electronic database and using the combination of keywords "hydrolysis" and "drugs," yielded over 3300 articles from January 1989 to September 1999. A more selective analysis of a collection of stability data on 91 drugs (1) shows that 70 of these undergo hydrolytic degradation reactions. Of these, 61% can be classified as reactions of carboxylic acid derivatives, 4.3% of phosphoric acid derivatives, 20% of carbonyl derivatives, and 14.3% are nucleophilic displacements, often on the aliphatic carbon. These classes are discussed in the subsequent sections of this chapter.

HYDROLYTIC REACTIONS AND MECHANISMS

Carboxylic Acid Derivatives

Some drugs contain an acyl group, RCO^- in the compound RCOX, where X is called the leaving group. The most important types of acyl or carboxylic compounds, also called carboxylic acid derivatives are given in Table 1. The characteristic reaction of acyl compounds involves cleavage of the C—X bond. The net result of the attack of a nucleophile Y^- on an acyl compound is cleavage of the C—X bond and formation of the C—Y bond; these reactions, shown in Eq. 1, are, therefore, called acyl transfers.

$$R-\overset{\overset{\displaystyle O}{\|}}{C}-X + Y^- \longrightarrow R-\overset{\overset{\displaystyle O}{\|}}{C}-Y + X^- \tag{1}$$

In a hydrolysis, H_2O (or OH^-) is the attacking nucleophile, and hydrolysis of a carboxylic acid derivative is an acyl transfer to water, as in Eq. 2.

$$R-\overset{\overset{\displaystyle O}{\|}}{C}-X + HOH \rightleftharpoons R-\overset{\overset{\displaystyle O}{\|}}{C}-OH + HX \tag{2}$$

An important example of acyl transfer reactions is ester hydrolysis, where two sites of bond cleavage, both leading to the same product, are possible. The possibilities, shown in structure **1**, are denoted acyl–oxygen fission (Ac) and alkyl–oxygen fission (Al).

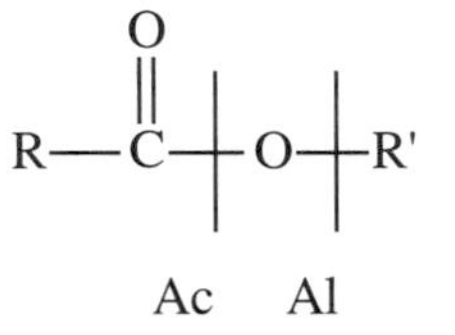

$$R-\overset{\overset{\displaystyle O}{\|}}{C}\!+\!O\!+\!R'$$

Ac   Al

1

Alkyl–oxygen fission constitutes a nucleophilic substitution on carbon, shown in Eq. 3.

$$R'CH2-OCOR + Y^- \longrightarrow R'CH_2 - Y + RCOO^- \tag{3}$$

Al

Several experimental methods have been devised to establish the type of cleavage in ester hydrolysis; in nearly all cases, it is found to be acyl–oxygen cleavage via nucleophilic attack on the carboxyl group. Ester reaction mechanisms are often discussed in terms introduced by Ingold (2), who classified the type of bond fission (Ac or Al), the reaction molecularity (1 or 2), and the ionic form of the substrate (A for the conjugate acid $RC(OH)OR^+$ and B for the conjugate base RCOOR). Ingold's classification is shown in Table 2.

For the bimolecular reaction with Ac cleavage, two reasonable mechanisms have been suggested. The first is a direct displacement analogous to the S_N2 mechanism of aliphatic nucleophilic substitution. This route is shown in Eq. 4; structure **2** is the transition state (‡), although it is

Table 1 Carboxylic acid derivatives

Structure	Chemical class	Comments
O‖ RC—Cl	Acid chloride	
O‖ O‖ RC—OCR	Acid anhydride	
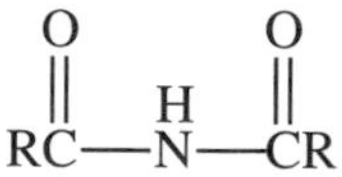 O‖ H O‖ RC—N—CR	Imide	May also be cyclic and may be substituted
RCH——CO \ | (CH$_2$)$_n$—NH	Lactam	May be substituted
RCH——CO \ | (CH$_2$)$_n$—O	Lactone	
O‖ RC—OH	Carboxylic acid	
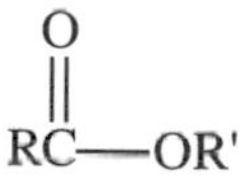 O‖ RC—OR'	Ester	Aliphatic or aromatic, depending on R'
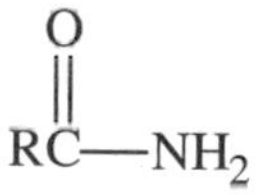 O‖ RC—NH$_2$	Amide	Unsubstituted as shown or substituted by replacement of H
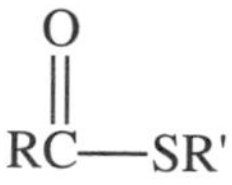 O‖ RC—SR'	Thiol ester	

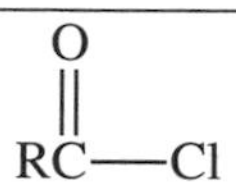

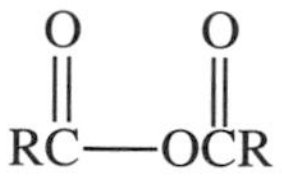

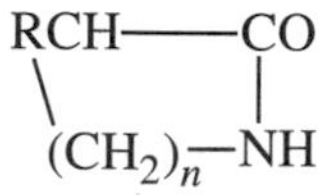

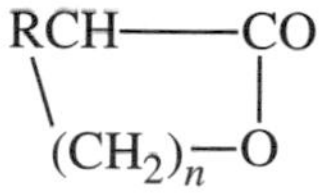

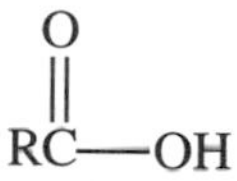

oversimplified because it does not incorporate electronic redistribution of the carbon–oxygen ‡ double bond.

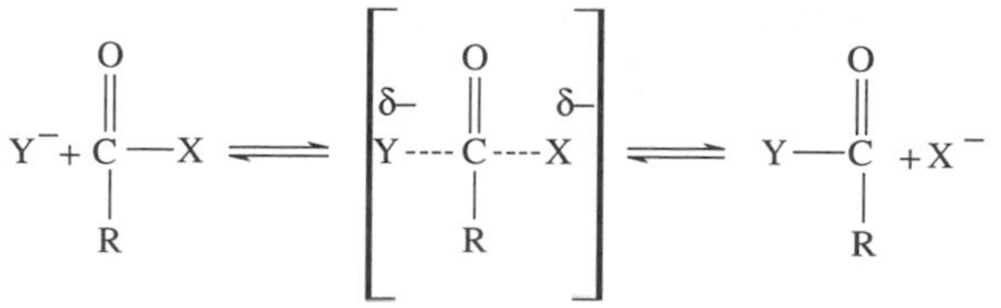

$$Y^- + \overset{O}{\underset{R}{C}} - X \rightleftharpoons \left[\overset{O}{\underset{R}{{}^{\delta-}Y\cdots C\cdots X^{\delta-}}} \right] \rightleftharpoons Y - \overset{O}{\underset{R}{C}} + X^- \quad (4)$$

2

The second mechanism is the two-step addition–elimination pathway shown in Eq. 5; it invokes the

formation, by nucleophilic addition to the carboxyl group, of tetrahedral intermediate, **3**.

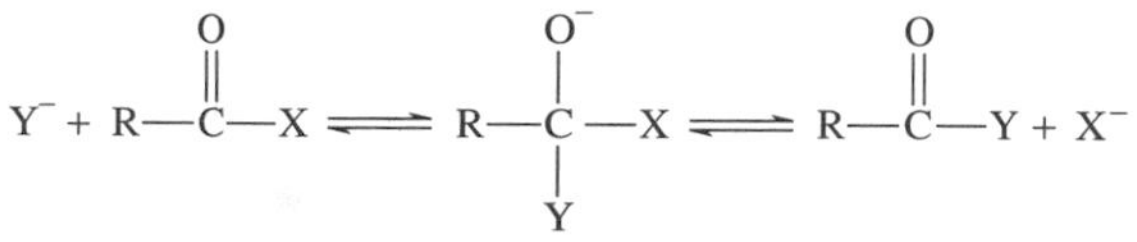

$$Y^- + R - \overset{O}{C} - X \rightleftharpoons R - \overset{O^-}{\underset{Y}{C}} - X \rightleftharpoons R - \overset{O}{C} - Y + X^- \quad (5)$$

3

In 1951, Bender provided the first diagnostic test of mechanism for these reactions (3). The alkaline hydrolysis of several benzoate esters, a B$_{Ac}$2 reaction, was studied with

Table 2 Classification of ester hydrolysis reactions

Conjugate form	Type of fission	
	Acyl	Alkyl
Acid	$A_{Ac}1$	A_{Al} (S_N1)
	$A_{Ac}2$	$A_{Al}2$ (unknown)
Base	$B_{Ac}1$ (unknown)	$B_{Al}1$ (S_N1)
	$B_{Ac}2$	$B_{Al}2$ (S_N2)

esters enriched in ^{18}O at the carbonyl oxygen. If the S_N2 mechanism in Eq. 6 is operative, no ^{18}O exchange with the solvent during hydrolysis would be expected, because the carbonyl oxygen does not engage in any reversible step. The tetrahedral intermediate mechanism, however, provides a route for ^{18}O exchange, concurrent with hydrolysis, by the symmetrical partitioning shown in Eq. 7.

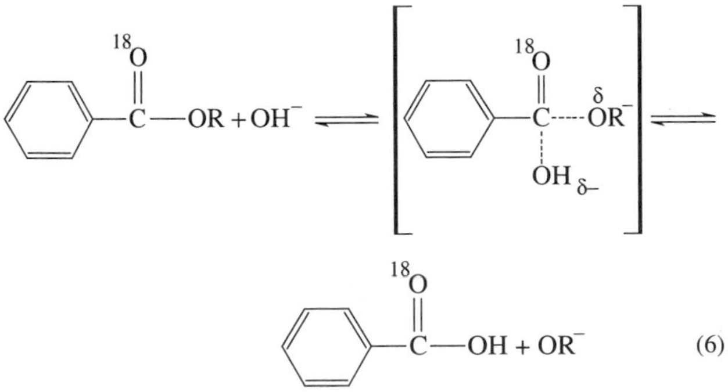

(6)

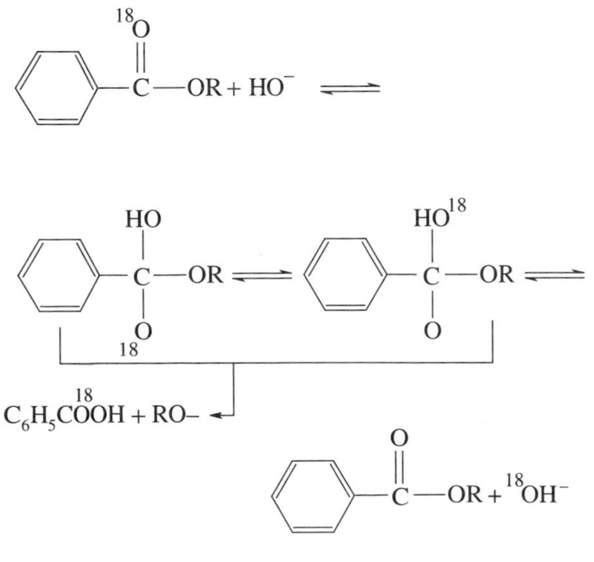

(7)

When ethyl benzoate carbonyl-^{18}O was subjected to alkaline hydrolysis, samples of ester isolated during the progress of the reaction were found to contain less ^{18}O than the initial ester. This demonstration of concurrent oxygen exchange and hydrolysis is strong (though not definitive) evidence for the tetrahedral-intermediate mechanism. In other reactions, evidence of different kinds supports the tetrahedral-intermediate mechanism; for example, the intermediate has been detected spectroscopically in certain instances. In some reactions, it has been possible to identify a change in the rate-determining step as the pH is changed; this observation can be explained only by invoking a two-step reaction mechanism.

The two-step addition–elimination is taken here as a mechanistic description of the hydrolysis reaction. Alkaline ester hydrolysis is the example given in Eq. 8.

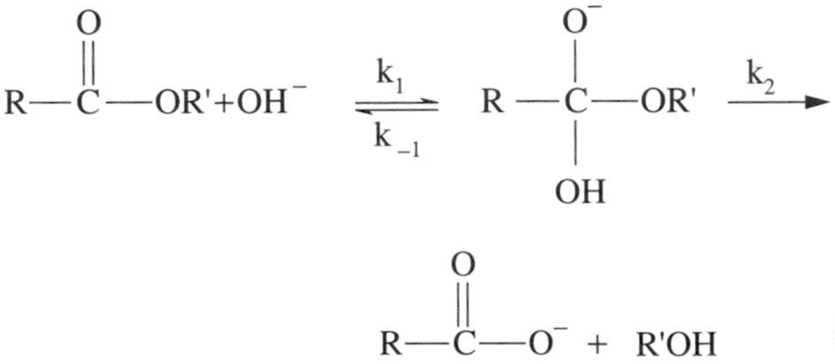

(8)

The differential rate equation for the intermediate (I) is given by Eq. 9.

$$\frac{d[I]}{dt} = k_1\left[OH^-\right][RCOOR] - (k_{-1} + k_2)[I] \qquad (9)$$

Because the intermediate is consumed as rapidly as it is produced, its concentration is invariant over the time course of the reaction, and the steady state approximation can be applied to give Eq. 10.

$$[I] = \frac{k_1[RCOOR][OH^-]}{k_{-1} + k_2} \qquad (10)$$

The rate of ester hydrolysis is $v = k_2[I]$ or as in Eq. 11.

$$v = \frac{k_1[RCOOR][OH^-]}{k_{-1}/k_2 + 1} \qquad (11)$$

The ratio k_{-1}/k_2 describes the "partitioning" of the tetrahedral intermediate between the reactant and the product states. The experimental rate equation is shown in Eq. 12.

$$v = k[RCOOR][OH^-], \qquad (12)$$

where k is the observed second-order rate constant. It follows that Eq. 13 holds that

$$k = \frac{k_1}{(k_{-1}/k_2) + 1} \cdot \qquad (13)$$

If $k_2 \gg k_{-1}$, then $k \cong k_1$ and the first step is the rate-determining step (rds) of the reaction; if $k_2 \ll k_{-1}$, then $k \cong k_1 k_2/k_{-1}$, and the second step (decomposition of the tetrahedral intermediate) is the rds. Eq. 13 provides a basis for the interpretation of structural effects on reactivity. Eq. 8 can be generalized to give Eq. 14

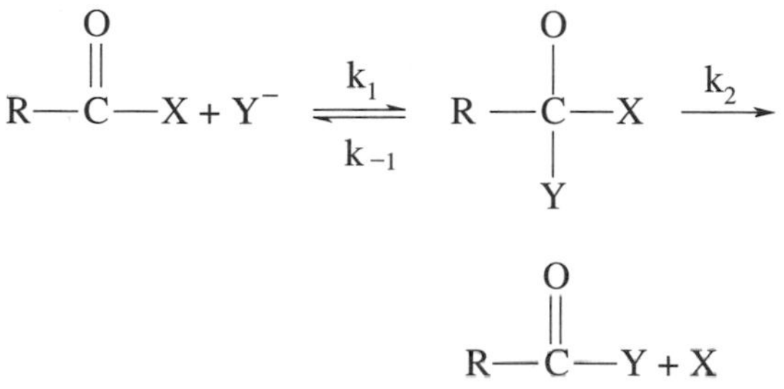

$$(14)$$

Eq. 13 applies to this kinetic scheme. Changes in the structures of R, X, and Y^- affect k through their separate effects on k_1 and k_{-1}/k_2 (4). The carboxyl group is polarized, as shown in structure **4**.

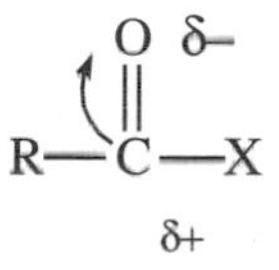

4

Attack by the nucleophile Y^-, which may be OH^- or H_2O in hydrolyses, therefore, takes place at the electron-deficient carboxyl carbon and is aided by electron withdrawal at R and X. Such effects increase k_1, and, hence, k. At the same time, these structural effects influence k_{-1}/k_2. Increased electron withdrawal by R should make it more difficult for both X^- and Y^- to leave the tetrahedral intermediate, resulting in decreases in both k_{-1} and k_2, with little change in the ratio k_{-1}/k_2. Structural changes that increase the electron-withdrawing ability of X, however, tend to decrease k_{-1} and increase k_2, thus decreasing k_{-1}/k_2. The resultant effect on k depends upon the magnitude of k_{-1}/k_2 relative to unity, as in Eq. 13; in most cases, it appears k is dominated by k_1.

The previous discussion can be used to interpret the hydrolytic behavior of a series of compounds that possess the same acyl group but varied leaving groups. For example, the order of hydrolytic reactivity for an amide, an ester, an anhydride, and an acid chloride is:

$$RCOCL > RCOOCR > RCOOR > RCONH_2$$

Such a series exhibits great variations in k_1 and k_{-1}/k_2. The effect on k_1 in this series is a combination of inductive and resonance effects; the latter releases electrons from the leaving group to the acyl group, as indicated in structure **5**.

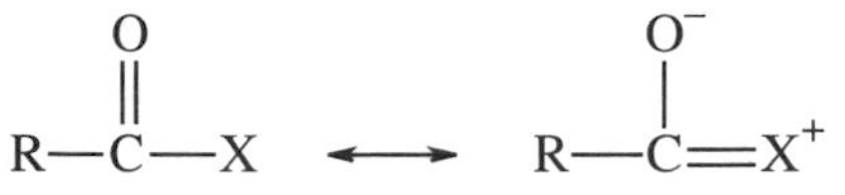

5

These effects make k_1 smaller for amides than for esters, for example. At the same time k_{-1}/k_2 is affected by the ability of the leaving group (its "nucleofugality"). In the reverse of the k_2 step, that is, an attack by the nucleophile X^-, the more basic X^-, the more effective it is as a nucleophile. Hence, the more basic the leaving group X^-, the less effective it is as a leaving group, and the smaller is k_2. The order of increasing basicity of the leaving groups in the above series is $Cl^- < RCO_2^- < RO^- < NH_2^-$, and, therefore, k_2 is smaller for the amide than for the ester and so on. The ratio k_{-1}/k_2 is highest for the amide, and k, the hydrolytic rate constant, is the smallest. Because the basicity of the leaving group can be measured by the pK_a of its conjugate acid, correlations of reactivity (expressed as log k) with the pK_a of the leaving group (for a constant acyl group) are often successful. Thus, aromatic esters (leaving group a phenoxide ion) are more reactive than are aliphatic ester (leaving group an alkoxide ion.)

A very important example of ester hydrolysis of a pharmaceutical is that of the anion of aspirin, **6**, given in Eq. 15

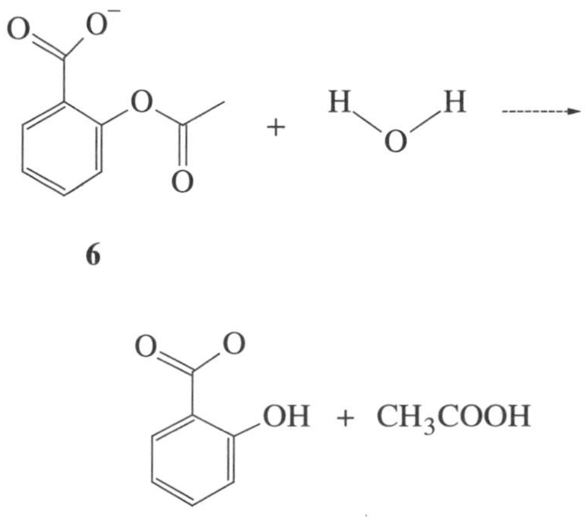

6

$$(15)$$

The marked instability of aspirin is due to two structural features: one, that it is an aromatic ester and, for reasons previously discussed, it is, therefore, more labile than an aliphatic ester and two, the ortho relationship of the acetoxy group to the carboxylate. Owing to this proximity, aspirin is subject to intramolecular catalysis of the ester hydrolysis. The pK_a of aspirin is 3.6, and, therefore, it exists predominately in the anionic form above pH 5. This intramolecularly catalyzed reaction accounts for the hydrolytic instability of aspirin in neutral solutions. Additional pharmaceutical examples of hydrolysis of a lactone (a cyclic ester), an amide, and a lactam (a cyclic amide) are warfarin, acetaminophen, and the penicillins, respectively. Equations for these reactions are given in the first edition of this encyclopedia (5).

Phosphoric acid derivatives can be conveniently discussed with the carboxylic acid derivatives, owing to their similar reaction mechanisms. The structural class is extremely important biologically (6), but few pharmaceutical examples within it exist. For discussions of hydrolytic reactions of the phosphoric acid derivatives, the reader is referred to the first edition of this encyclopedia (5).

Derivatives of Carbonyl Compounds

The characteristic reaction of an acyl (carboxyl) compound RCOX is cleavage of the C—X bond. The reactions of carbonyl compounds, such as aldehydes RCHO and ketones R_2CO, do not involve cleavage of the C—R or C—H bonds. Many drugs are derivatives of carbonyl compounds, though their parentage may not be obvious.

Carbonyl addition reactions take place with bond formation between the carbonyl carbon (which is electrophilic) and the nucleophilic portion of an adding species. The reaction of a reagent with a single dissociable proton can be described by Eq. 16.

$$R-\overset{\overset{\displaystyle O}{\|}}{C}-R + HX \rightleftharpoons \begin{array}{c} R \\ \diagdown \\ C \\ \diagup \diagdown \\ R \quad X \end{array} \overset{OH}{} \quad (16)$$

This is a simple addition. If the reagent has two protons, a two-step addition-elimination occurs, as in Eq. 17.

$$R-\overset{\overset{\displaystyle O}{\|}}{C}-R + H_2X \rightleftharpoons \begin{array}{c} R \quad OH \\ \diagdown \diagup \\ C \\ \diagup \diagdown \\ R \quad XH \end{array} \rightleftharpoons$$

$$R-\overset{\overset{\displaystyle X}{\|}}{C}-R + H_2O \quad (17)$$

Reaction (17) is a condensation reaction. The reverse of a condensation reaction is a hydrolysis of the C—X bond, the process of interest here. This is shown in Eq. 18, where the product of the reaction is a hydrate.

$$R'-\overset{\overset{\displaystyle O}{\|}}{C}-R + H_2O \rightleftharpoons \begin{array}{c} R \quad OH \\ \diagdown \diagup \\ C \\ \diagup \diagdown \\ R' \quad OH \end{array} \quad (18)$$

Carbonyl compounds can form hemiacetals, **7**, which in the presence of acids can form acetals, as shown in Eq. 19, and they are subject to hydrolysis.

$$R-\overset{\overset{\displaystyle O}{\|}}{C}-H + R'OH \rightleftharpoons \underset{\mathbf{7}}{\begin{array}{c} R \quad OH \\ \diagdown \diagup \\ C \\ \diagup \diagdown \\ H \quad OR' \end{array}} \overset{R'OH}{\underset{}{\rightleftharpoons}}$$

$$\begin{array}{c} R \quad OR' \\ \diagdown \diagup \\ C \\ \diagup \diagdown \\ H \quad OR' \end{array} \quad (19)$$

The hydrolysis of acetals (**8**, R_2 = H), ketals, and ortho esters (**8**, R_2 = OR) has been thoroughly investigated (7).

$$\begin{array}{c} R_1 \quad OR \\ \diagdown \diagup \\ C \\ \diagup \diagdown \\ R_2 \quad OR \end{array}$$

8

The overall reaction is given in Eq. 20:

$$\begin{array}{c} R_1 \quad OR \\ \diagdown \diagup \\ C \\ \diagup \diagdown \\ R_2 \quad OR \end{array} + \begin{array}{c} H \quad H \\ \diagdown \diagup \\ O \end{array} \rightleftharpoons$$

$$\begin{array}{c} R_1 \\ \diagdown \\ C=O + 2\ ROH \\ \diagup \\ R_2 \end{array} \quad (20)$$

The pathway, a unimolecular reaction of the conjugate acid (or A1 mechanism), is shown in Eqs. 21–24.

$$
\begin{array}{c}
\underset{R_2}{\overset{R_1}{>}}C\underset{OR}{\overset{OR}{<}} + H^+ \rightleftharpoons \underset{R_2}{\overset{R_1}{>}}C\underset{OR}{\overset{\overset{H}{\underset{|}{O}}R^+}{<}}
\end{array} \qquad (21)
$$

$$
\underset{R_2}{\overset{R_1}{>}}C\underset{OR}{\overset{\overset{H}{\underset{|}{O}}R^+}{<}} \rightleftharpoons \underset{R_2}{\overset{R_1}{>}}\overset{+}{C}{-}OR + ROH \qquad (22)
$$

$$
\underset{R_2}{\overset{R_1}{>}}\overset{+}{C}{-}OR + \underset{H}{\overset{H}{>}}O \rightleftharpoons \underset{R_2}{\overset{R_1}{>}}C\underset{OH}{\overset{\overset{H}{\underset{|}{O}}R^+}{<}} \qquad (23)
$$

$$
\underset{R_2}{\overset{R_1}{>}}C\underset{OH}{\overset{\overset{H}{\underset{|}{O}}R^+}{<}} \rightleftharpoons \underset{R_2}{\overset{R_1}{>}}C{=}OH^+ + ROH \qquad (24)
$$

Much of the interest in acetal chemistry is related to carbohydrates, because polyhydroxyaldehydes exist predominantly as cyclic hemiacetals (8). Digoxin, for example, possesses acetal functions subject to hydrolysis.

The hydrolysis of imines is the reverse of the addition of amines to carbonyls, and the two-step scheme of Eq. 25 applies.

$$
\underset{R_2}{\overset{R_1}{>}}C{=}NR + \underset{H}{\overset{H}{>}}O \rightleftharpoons \underset{R_2}{\overset{R_1}{>}}C\underset{NHR}{\overset{OH}{<}} \rightleftharpoons
$$
$$
\underset{R_2}{\overset{R_1}{>}}C{=}O + \underset{R}{\overset{H}{>}}N{-}H \qquad (25)
$$

The kinetic behavior of this process depends upon the pH of the medium. In the alkaline region, the addition of water is rate-determining, and the reaction probably involves attack of the hydroxide ion on the protonated amine (which is kinetically equivalent to attack by water on the neutral imine), as shown in Eq. 26.

$$
\underset{R_2}{\overset{R_1}{>}}C{=}NRH^+ + OH^- \xrightleftharpoons{\text{slow}} \underset{R_2}{\overset{R_1}{>}}C\underset{NHR}{\overset{OH}{<}} \xrightleftharpoons{\text{fast}}
$$
$$
\underset{R_2}{\overset{R_1}{>}}C{=}O + \underset{R}{\overset{H}{>}}N{-}H \qquad (26)
$$

At a somewhat lower pH, as the fraction of protonated imine increases (typical pK_a values are 6–7) and the concentration of hydroxide decreases, the attack of water on the protonated imine becomes important, as shown in Eq. 27.

$$
\underset{R_2}{\overset{R_1}{>}}C{=}NRH^+ + H_2O \xrightleftharpoons{\text{slow}} \underset{R_2}{\overset{R_1}{>}}C\underset{NRH_2^+}{\overset{OH}{<}} \xrightleftharpoons{\text{fast}}
$$
$$
\underset{R_2}{\overset{R_1}{>}}C{=}O + NRH_3^+ \qquad (27)
$$

The rate becomes briefly pH independent when all of the imine is protonated, but with further decrease in pH, the rate-determining step shifts to loss of amine from the carbinolamine intermediate, as in Eq. 28.

$$
\underset{R_2}{\overset{R_1}{>}}C{=}NRH^+ + H_2O \xrightleftharpoons{\text{slow}} \underset{R_2}{\overset{R_1}{>}}C\underset{NRH_2}{\overset{OH}{<}}
$$
$$
\xrightleftharpoons{-H^+} \underset{R_2}{\overset{R_1}{>}}C\underset{NRH_2^+}{\overset{O^-}{<}}
$$
$$
\Big\Updownarrow \text{slow}
$$
$$
\underset{R_2}{\overset{R_1}{>}}C{=}O + NRH_2 \qquad (28)
$$

The hydrolysis of nitrofurantoin, **9**, an example of the hydrolysis of an imine, is shown in Eq. 29.

$$(29)$$

Nucleophilic Substitution

Several classes of nucleophilic substitution reactions can be distinguished (in addition to similar processes, such as acyl transfer to a nucleophile): substitution on aliphatic carbons, on aromatic carbons, and on elements other than carbon, such as metals in metal-ligand coordination complexes. Of these, substitution on aliphatic carbon is most frequently encountered.

The reaction is of the type shown in Eq. 30

where the nucleophile Y^- may be anionic or neutral. In hydrolysis reactions, the nucleophile is H_2O or OH^-; the hydrolysis of an alkyl halide, given in Eq. 31 is typical:

$$OH^- + C_2H_5Br \longrightarrow C_2H_5OH + Br \qquad (31)$$

In aliphatic nucleophilic substitutions two mechanistic routes have been clearly identified; one is the two-step process shown in Eqs. 32, 33.

$$R{-}X \xrightarrow{\text{slow}} R^+ + X^- \qquad (32)$$

$$R^+ + Y^- \xrightarrow{\text{fast}} R{-}Y \qquad (33)$$

The first step, which is rate-determining, is an ionization to a carbocation intermediate that reacts with the nucleophile in the second step. Because the transition state for the rds includes R-X but not Y^-, the reaction is unimolecular and is labeled S_N1 (substitution nucleophilic

unimolecular). First-order kinetics are observed, with the rate being independent of the nucleophilic identity and concentration.

The second mechanism is a one-step direct displacement reaction, shown in Eq. 34.

$$Y^- + R{-}X \longrightarrow [Y\text{-----}R\text{-----}X]^{\ddagger-} \longrightarrow$$
$$R{-}Y + X^- \qquad (34)$$

This bimolecular process is called the S_N2 mechanism. It yields second-order kinetics, unless the nucleophile is the solvent, in which case apparent first-order kinetics are seen. The species in brackets is the transition state.

The S_N reactions have been very carefully studied (9, 10). The S_N1 mechanism is favored by structural features that lead to stabilization of the carbocation, and, therefore, tertiary aliphatic substrates tend to react via the S_N1 route. Primary substrates react by the S_N2 mechanism. Secondary substrates may react by the S_N1 or S_N2 mechanism, depending the details of the reaction; alternatively, secondary substrates may proceed by a "borderline" mechanism having some features of both S_N1 and S_N2. In solvolyses, the distinguishing characteristic of the S_N2 route is the covalent participation in the rds. The extent of such participation, which is absent in a pure S_N1 reaction, can be estimated by studying solvent effects (11) or the pressure effects (12) on reaction rates.

A pharmaceutical example of a nucleophilic substitution reaction is thiamine hydrochloride, **10**, which is cleaved, as shown in Eq. 35. The cationic moiety can support the electron transfer and is a good leaving group.

$$(35)$$

HYDROLYTIC KINETIC PHENOMENA

In the experimental study and interpretation of hydrolytic reaction rates, many kinetic effects provide opportunities for probing the detailed nature of the reaction or have significant practical consequences on drug stability. The topics of temperature dependence, catalysis and solvent effects, were discussed in the first edition of this encyclopedia (5).

REFERENCES

1. Connors, K.A.; Amidon, G.L.; Stella, V.J. *Chemical Stability of Pharmaceuticals*, 2nd Ed.; Wiley-Interscience: New York, 1986; 1–864.
2. Ingold, C.K. *Structure and Mechanism in Organic Chemistry*; Ch. XIV; Cornell University Press: Ithaca New York, 1953; 751–791.
3. Bender, M.L. Oxygen Exchange as Evidence for the Existence of an Intermediate in Ester Hydrolysis. J. Am. Chem. Soc. **1951**, *73*, 1626–1629.
4. Bender, M.L. Mechanisms of Catalysis of Nucleophilic Reactions of Carboxylic Acid Derivatives. Chem. Revs. **1960**, *60*, 53–113.
5. Connors, K.A. Hydrolysis of Drugs. *Encyclopedia of Pharmaceutical Technology*, 1st Ed.; Marcel Dekker, Inc.: New York, 1993; 8, 1–29.
6. Bruice, T.C.; Benkovic, S. *Bioorganic Chemistry*; W.A. Benjamin: New York, 1966; 2, 1–786.
7. Cordes, E.H. Mechanism in Catalysis for the Hydrolysis of Acetols, Ketols and Ortho Esters. Prog. Phys. Org. Chem. **1967**, *4*, 1–44.
8. Capon, B. Mechanism in Carbohydrate Chemistry. Chem. Revs. **1969**, *69*, 407–498.
9. Ingold, C.K. *Structure and Mechanism in Organic Chemistry*; Ch. VII; Cornell University Press: Ithaca, New York, 1953; 306–418.
10. Bunton, C.A. *Nucleophilic Substitution at a Saturated Carbon Atom*; Elsevier: Amsterdam, 1963; 1–172.
11. Bentley, T.W.; Schleyer, P.V.R. Medium Effects on the Rates and Mechanisms of Solvolytic Reactions. Adv. Phys. Org. Chem. **1977**, *14*, 1–67.
12. Asano, T.; LeNoble, W.J. Activation and Reaction Volumes in Solution. Chem Revs. **1978**, *78*, 407–489.

BIBLIOGRAPHY

Conors, K.A. *Chemical Kinetics: The Study of Reaction Rates in Solution*; VCH: New York, 1990; 1–480.
Jencks, W.P. *Catalysis in Chemistry and Enzymology*; McGraw-Hill: New York, 1969; 1–836.
Maskill, H. *The Physical Basis of Organic Chemistry*; Oxford University Press: London, 1986; 1–490.
Stewart, R. *The Proton: Applications to Organic Chemistry*; Academic Press: Orlando, FL, 1985; 1–234.

IMMUNOASSAY

Stephen G. Schulman
G. J. P. J. Beernink
University of Florida, Gainesville, Florida

INTRODUCTION

Immunoanalytical methods that are based on the selective, reversible binding of small molecules (drugs) or macromolecules by biologically derived antibodies have revolutionized the field of biomedical analysis. Immunoassays have allowed the determination of very small amounts of analytes that were previously unassayable in biological matrices by other techniques. Since the original work on the analysis of insulin by Berson and Yalow (1), immunoassay methods have been developed for the determination of a wide variety of drugs, pesticides, hormones, and biological proteins. Immunoassays are relatively simple procedurally. This has led to the development of many "kit-type" immunoassay systems that are used routinely for home diagnostics.

Antibodies that are used as reagents in immunoassays are, in general, molecules of the immunoglobulin G (IgG) type. They are produced by white blood cells in response to foreign substances introduced in mammalian species. Millions of years of vertebrate evolution have developed immunoglobulins into exquisitely discriminating devices capable of recognizing subtle differences between molecules; for example, a mouse can generate millions of different immunoglobulin specificities. These immunoglobulins combine specifically with the substances (antigens) that elicited their formation. This then triggers processes by which the foreign antigens are cleared from the organism, which is the ultimate goal of the immune process (2).

These molecules are heterogeneous, bifunctional glycoproteins in which the variable amino acid sequence in the polypeptide component provides its biologic activity. This polypeptide component is made up of two heavy or H chains (50,000 Da) and two light or L chains (20,000 Da), held together by disulfide bonds. The two binding sites of the antibody molecule appear to reside on the NH_2 terminal ends of the polypeptide chains (3). Antibodies produced by injection of foreign antigens into a host animal are structurally heterogeneous and respond to different aspects of the same antigen with different binding strengths and specificities. If the antibody-producing blood cell can be isolated in a pure cell culture, however, only one particular antibody structure will be produced (4). Antibodies harvested from pure cell cultures are referred to as monoclonal antibodies, are homogeneous and react with only one or a few closely related antigens. The antibody producing cells which can be grown in culture are produced by cell fusion techniques and provide superior antibodies for use in immunoassays because of their identical specificities and binding strengths. Antigens must have molecular weights in excess of 10^4 Da in order to evoke antibody production. However, small molecules, such as drugs, can be bound to macromolecular carriers and some of the antibodies produced from these will respond to the drug (hapten).

All immunoassay procedures take advantage of the specific reactions between antibodies and antigens. They involve measurement, directly or indirectly, of the extent of binding between antibodies (reagents) and antigens (analytes). Labels are used in conjunction with the antigens or antibodies so that the concentrations of molecular species can be measured instrumentally. Labels are entities that impart some measurable signal, such as radioactivity, fluorescence, chemiluminescence, on electrochemical or enzyme activity to the antibody or antigen to which it is attached. The determination of the extent of antibody binding requires measurements of the amounts of labeled antigen or antibody in the complexed (bound) and in the free forms. This is generally expressed as the bound/free (b/f) concentration ratio, which is related to the concentration of analyte (5). The measured signal can be either directly or inversely proportional to the b/f ratio depending on the chemistry of the system used. There are two ways to determine the amount of antigen present: one using a limited amount of reagent (competitive assays), the other using an excess amount of reagent (noncompetitive assays).

The competitive assay uses a limited amount of antibody, which is insufficient to bind all of the antigen. The antigen competes with a fixed amount of labeled antigen for the limited number of antibody binding sites. From the proportion of bound (or free) labeled antigen, the concentration of unlabeled antigen can be determined.

The noncompetitive assay uses an excess of antibody. Different approaches to detect the bound antigen have been developed, the most common use an antibody, in excess, coupled to a solid phase. The bound antigen is then detected with a second antibody labeled in a way that aids detection (e.g., radioactive, fluorophore, etc.). The amount of antigen in the sample is then directly proportional to the amount of labeled antibody captured on the solid phase.

Both assays require differentiation of bound label from free label. This can be achieved by two methods: heterogeneous assay or homogeneous assay. Heterogeneous assay separates bound label from free label using a means of removing the antibody. Homogenous assay compares the signal of the label when antigen is bound to antibody compared to when the antigen is free.

RADIOLABELED IMMUNOASSAYS

The earliest (1) immunoassays made use of radioactively labeled antigens or antibodies. These analytes are referred to as radiolabeled immunoassays. Antibody binding sites are extremely specific and to retain this specifity the best option would be to replace a nonradioactive isotope in the tracer molecule by its radioisotope (e.g., replace hydrogen by ^{3}H). However when the substitution is made in a part of the molecule away from the antibody binding site, the choice of radioisotope can be governed by other considerations, such as half-life, availability, high activity, and radiochemical purity.

The most common radioactive label is ^{125}I, which is bound to antibodies and antigens by a variety of techniques including chloramine-T, iodogen, or lacto-peroxidase iodination. Iodination with ^{125}I is the preferred radiolabeling technique because the isotope is a γ-emitter, inexpensive, can be easily detected, has an appropriate half-life for most analytical purposes, and can be obtained in preparations with high specific activity. Problems occasionally associated with radio iodination include loss of immunoreactivity due to the size of the label or chemical alteration of reagents due to the high energy of decay (6). Use of beta-emitting isotopes (^{14}C and ^{3}H) may resolve these problems, but require more complicated scintillation counting for label measurement.

Labeled Antigen Radioimmunoassays

Labeled antigen radioimmunoassays involve competition between a labeled antigen and an unlabeled antigen (analyte) for a limited number of antibody-combining sites as shown in the following reactions:

$$Ag^{*}-Ab + Ag \rightleftharpoons Ag-Ab + Ag^{*}$$

where Ag^{*} is labeled reagent antigen, Ag is analyte antigen, and Ab is antibody against Ag.

The Ag^{*} and Ab are analytical reagents with concentrations fixed so that when a sample containing Ag is added, competition between Ag and Ag^{*} for Ab binding sites occurs. Increasing concentrations of Ag result in a lesser degree of binding of Ag^{*} and the measurement of radioactivity of the binding or free fraction can be used to determine the amount of Ag present in a sample.

Determination of the distribution of Ag^{*} between the antibody-bound and free fractions, in radioimmunoassay procedures, requires a separation step which isolates Ag^{*} from Ag^{*}—Ab. Once separated, measurement of the radioactivity of the label in one or both the fractions provides a signal that is approximately exponentially related to the concentration of unlabeled antigen. The graphical relationship can have either a positive or a negative slope depending on whether the antibody-bound or free fraction is measured. The exact shape of the calibration curve however, is dependent on the antibody-binding equilibrium constant (7).

A variety of methods has been applied to the separation of bound and free Ag^{*}. These include precipitation, solid phase attachment, capillary electrophoresis, chromatography, and microfiltration. Originally, precipitation and solid-phase extraction were the most common types of separations techniques. However the ease of automation of capillary electrophoresis and flow-injection analysis (chromatography) makes these two techniques very interesting.

Precipitation

Precipitation techniques can be categorized into two general classes, nonspecific and specific. The nonspecific separations involve the addition of a salt or solvent that decreases the solubility of the antigen–antibody complex under conditions that do not affect the free-labeled antigen. After addition, the immune complexes can be precipitated by centrifugation and the radioactivity in either the supernatant solution or the precipitate can be measured. Examples of precipitation reagents used in immunoassays include alcohol, ammonium sulfate, polyethylene, and dioxane. Care must be taken to avoid coprecipitation of the unbound label.

Specific precipitation is a technique that has been devised to overcome some of the problems associated with nonspecific techniques. In this approach, a second antibody (Ab'), specific to the analytical antibody is added in excess to cause precipitation of the primary antigen–antibody complex as shown below:

$$Ag^*\text{–}Ab + Ab' \rightleftharpoons [Ag^*\text{–}Ab]Ab'$$

The method has been termed the double-antibody technique and can be used for a wide variety of analytes (8). The double antibody techniques generally require more time because the second antibody reaction can require days to reach equilibrium. The speed of precipitation clearly depends on the concentration of the second antibody. Polyethylene glycol has been used as a cosolvent to increase the precipitation rate.

Solid phase techniques

Many early immunoassays used solid phases to separate the labeled antigen from the complex by differential adsorption of the former. Examples of the solid phases uses are dextran-coated charcoal, ion-exchange resins, and cellulose powder. Once the labeled antigen has been adsorbed, the bound, labeled antigen could be decanted to allow the measurement of the radioactivity of the bound and/or free-labeled materials separately. Because of problems with nonspecific adsorption and errors due to stripping of the labeled antigen from the solid, these types of separations have been largely replaced by those employing solid phases in which the reagent is covalently bound to the solid, as for example, in the solid phase attachment of a specific antibody (Ab^{SP}), which binds labeled and unlabeled antigen competitively as shown below:

$$Ab^{SP}\text{–}Ag^* + Ag \rightleftharpoons Ab^{SP}\text{–}Ag + Ag^*$$

The solid phase to which the antibody is bound can be either suspended in solution, on particles such as cellulose, agarose, or dextran beads or can be attached to the surface of a test tube or a microtiter plate. The stationary solid phases eliminate the centrifugation step that is necessary with the suspended beads although plastic solid phases have a limited capacity of binding proteins.

Capillary electrophoresis

This technique has proven to be a powerful separation technique for the separation of macromolecules, such as antibodies, for two reasons: the near flat plug flow profile and the small diffusion constant of the antibodies. These characteristics eliminate band broadening. With both superior separation power and high detection sensitivity, capillary electrophoresis (CE) can separate free Ab and Ag

from bound Ab and Ag rapidly and is suitable for immunoassays. CE can combine immunologic recognition with on-line quantitation, microscale analysis, and automatic instrumentation to offer unique advantages for immunoassays. In immunoassays CE can be coupled to all of the existing CE detection techniques from UV and laser induced fluorescence (LIF) to mass spectrometry (MS). CE coupled to LIF has been applied to the determination of a variety of compounds including therapeutic drugs, peptides, and antibodies (9).

Flow-injection analysis

This technique introduces a sample into a flow of reagents. The reaction proceeds during transport in a reactor, after which the product is measured downstream in a detector. By combining immunoassays with flow-injection analysis (FIA), the long incubation times usually associated with heterogeneous assays become irrelevant, since FIA exploits nonequilibrium conditions. The washing steps are performed automatically by the continuous flow of buffer. Besides the irrelevance of incubation times, another advantage over normal immunoassays is that the reactor can be used several times because regeneration by using a suitable agent (e.g., glycine HCl) is possible. Sequential injections can be used to deliver reagents, substrate (if necessary), and regeneration agents to the immunoreactor. Many different assays using electrochemical, fluorescent and chemiluminescent detection have been developed.

Labeled Antibody Radioimmunoassays (Immunoradiometric Assays)

The problem of binding proteins to solid phases can be avoided by employing a solid phase antigen (Ag^{SP}) and a labeled antibody (Ab^*) as shown in the following reactions:

$$Ag^{SP} + Ab^* \rightleftharpoons Ab^*\text{–}Ag^{SP}$$

$$Ag + Ab^* \rightleftharpoons Ab^*\text{–}Ag$$

Where the unlabeled antigen (the analyte) competes for antibody binding sites with the solid phase antigen. This approach may have some difficulties caused by the requirement for purification of the immunospecific antibody. Because monoclonal antibodies are produced as essentially immunospecifically pure populations, they are ideal for labeled antibody techniques.

Another approach that utilizes labeled antibodies is the so-called "sandwich technique" (10). In this method, the analyte antigen is bound both by an antibody that is attached to a solid phase (Ab^{SP}) and a labeled antibody as follows:

$$Ab^{SP} + Ag + Ab^* \rightleftharpoons Ab^{SP}\text{–}Ag\text{–}Ab^*$$

The reaction is noncompetitive and thus, the concentration of unlabeled antigen has a direct relationship with the amount of label bound in the complex. The sandwich radioimmunoassays are both sensitive and convenient but are limited to analytes which are, at least, bivalent; i.e., antigens that can provide at least two sites for antibody attachment. Also, highly purified antibodies are required for the sandwich technique.

ENZYME IMMUNOASSAYS

Early work demonstrated the use of enzymes coupled to antibodies or antigens as reagents in immunoassay. Enzyme activity can be measured in a variety of ways, each with certain advantages, which makes a variety of enzymes good labeling substances. Most assay methods are based on spectroscopic properties derived from an enzymatically transformed substrate. These methods are colorimetry, flurorometry, luminometry, and electrometry.

The development of enzyme immunoassays was pioneered in 1972 by Engvall and Perlmann (11) and by Van Weemen and Schuurs (12) and is translated into a wide variety of enzyme-based systems used both in research and in routine analysis with sensitivities approaching those of radioimmunoassays. Enzyme immunoassays (EIAs) can be divided into two major classes, homogeneous and heterogeneous.

Homogeneous Enzyme Immunoassays

Homogeneous immunoassay (HOIA) does not require physical separation of the free and antibody-bound antigen because the measured physical signal derived form the antibody-bound, labeled material may be significantly different from that of the unbound entity. There may be an enhancement or an inhibition of enzyme activity upon binding of the antibody to the antigen. HOIA are simple to perform and automation can be carried out easily (13). Elimination of the separation step avoids a major source of imprecision in the assay. However selectivity may be compromised since interfering substances are not eliminated in the separation step.

HOIA using an enzyme labeled antigen

Rubenstein et al. (14) described a HOIA method for morphine using lysozyme as the enzyme label. The covalent enzyme labeled antigen (Ag^E) competes with sample antigen (Ag) for a limited concentration of antibody (Ab) to form a complex. The resultant complex exhibits very little enzyme activity because of either steric hindrance (14) or allosteric inhibition (15) caused by the bound antibody. In the presence of Ag there is competition for the Ab leaving more Ag^E uncomplexed and free to catalyze the conversion of substrate to product. Thus, the enzyme activity, which can be measured by either the appearance of product (P) or disappearance of substrate (S), is directly proportional to the amount of free antigen in the sample (16).

$$Ab + Ag^E \rightleftharpoons Ab\text{–}Ag^E$$

$$Ab\text{–}Ag^E + Ag \rightleftharpoons Ab\text{–}Ag + Ag^E$$

$$Ag^E + S \longrightarrow P$$

$$Ab\text{–}Ag^E + S \longrightarrow \text{No reaction}$$

HOIAs based on this principle have been developed for a number of therapeutic agents and endogenous compounds using glucose-6-phosphate dehydrogenase (G-6PDH) under the name $EMIT^R$ (Enzyme Mediated Immunoassay Technique). Enzyme activity is conveniently measured by absorption spectroscopy following the production of NADH from NAD which absorbs light strongly at 340 nm. The assay is rapid and sensitive to picomole levels (17).

HOIA using an antigen labeled enzyme modulator

This method is based on stability of an antigen labeled with an enzyme modulator (Ag^M) to modulate the activity of an indicator enzyme. The Ag^M competes with free antigen (Ag) for a limited amount of antibody (Ab). The Ag^M, on binding with Ab, is unable to modulate the activity of the indicator enzyme. As the concentration of analyte increases it competes successfully for binding sites on the antibody, leaving more Ag^M free to complex with indicator enzyme, thereby, modulating its activity (18, 19). A positive modulator will increase while a negative modulator will decrease enzyme activity. Thus, in the case of a positive modulator the enzyme activity will be directly proportional to the concentration of the analyte and for a negative modulator the activity will be inversely proportional to the concentration of the analyte.

$$AgM + Ab \rightleftharpoons AgM{-}Ab$$

$$AgM{-}Ab + Ag \rightleftharpoons Ag{-}Ab + AgM$$

$$AgM + S \longrightarrow P$$

$$AgM{-}Ab + S \longrightarrow \text{No reaction}$$

Based on this principle, practical assays for human serum thyroxine (20) and theophylline (21) have been developed and different distinct classes of modulators have been investigated.

HOIA using an antigen labeled with a fluorogenic enzyme substrate

This method was originally developed by Burd and Wong (22). The antigen is linked to a fluorogenic enzyme substrate ($AgFS$) to form a stable conjugate, which competes with the sample antigen (Ag) for a limited concentration of antibody (Ab). The antigen conjugated substrate is a fluorogenic substrate for the enzyme that reacts only when it is not bound to the Ab. Thus, at high concentrations of sample antigen, more of the $AgFS$ would remain free to act as the substrate for the enzyme and more products would be formed. Thus, fluorescence intensity increases with increasing concentration of the sample antigen.

$$AgFS + Ab \rightleftharpoons AgFS{-}Ab$$

$$AgFS{-}Ab + Ag \rightleftharpoons Ag{-}Ab + AgFS$$

$$AgFS + E \longrightarrow P \text{ (fluorescent)}$$

$$AgFS{-}Ab + E \longrightarrow \text{No reaction}$$

A derivative of umbelliferyl-β-galactoside serves as a fluorogenic substrate for *E. coli* β-galactosidase in this system (23) and solid-phase reagent strips based on this method have been developed (24).

HOIA using cloned enzyme donor immunoassay (CEDIA®)

This technique uses two different inactive enzyme fragments, a large fragment called enzyme acceptor (EA) and a very small fragment called enzyme donor (ED)

(25). Those fragments can associate to give an active enzyme.

In this technique, the antigen is labeled with enzyme donor ($AgED$) capable of contributing to enzyme activation with enzyme acceptor (AD). When the labeled antigen binds to an antibody (Ab), the enzymatic activity is lost. The $AgED$ conjugate competes with sample antigen (Ag) for antibody complex formation. An increase in sample antigen concentration, therefore, leads to increased displacement of $AgED$, leaving more free $AgED$ to associate with EA, resulting in more enzyme activation to form product (P). The enzyme activity is directly proportional to the amount of free sample antigen.

$$AgED + Ab \rightleftharpoons AgED{-}Ab$$

$$AgED{-}Ab + Ag \rightleftharpoons Ag{-}Ab + AgED$$

$$AgED + EA \longrightarrow E$$

$$E + S \longrightarrow P$$

CEDIAs are available for the important relevant therapeutic drugs and most have picomolar detection limits.

Heterogeneous Enzyme Immunoassays

Heterogeneous immunoassays (HEIA) have at least one separation step which allows the differentiation of bound from free material. The enzyme-linked immunosorbent assay (ELISA), is a heterogeneous immunoassay which has been widely used. In this method, either antigen or antibody is immobilized on a solid phase. An essential difference from HOIA is that in HEIA the enzyme label is designed to retain its activity even after its reaction with the antibody. In comparison with RIA, non isotopic HEIA such as enzyme labeled assay has several important advantages, including better reagent shelf life, fewer health hazards and simpler equipment required. HEIA can be divided into the classes of competitive and noncompetitive assays.

Competitive assays

Enzyme-labeled antigen conjugate: In this assay, the enzyme labeled antigen (AgE) competes with sample antigen for a limited amount of antibody which has been immobilized on a solid-phase, for example, polystyrene ($AbSP$). After incubation, the unbound AgE is separated by washing with a detergent solution. The solid phase $AbSP$ containing bound labeled and unlabeled antigen is incubated with a substrate (S) and the product concentration is determined using a colorimeter or fluorimeter.

The enzyme activity or product concentration is inversely proportional to the concentration of sample antigen.

$$Ab^{SP} + Ag^E \rightleftharpoons Ab^{SP}-Ag^E$$

$$Ab^{SP}-Ag^E + Ag \rightleftharpoons Ag^{SP}-Ag + Ag^E$$
$$\text{(Separate)}$$

$$Ab^{SP}-Ag^E + S \longrightarrow P$$

This method is very important for the measurement of low-molecular mass analytes such as steroids or melatonin or drugs such as cocaine (26). The most sensitive of these assays can detect <1 fmol analyte.

Enzyme-labeled antibody: This assay employs labeled antibody (Ab^E) and the antigen is attached to the solid phase (Ag^{SP}). The binding of Ag^{SP} to Ab^E is decreased by the addition of sample Ag.

$$Ab^E + Ag^{SP} \rightleftharpoons Ab^E-Ag^{SP}$$

$$Ab^E-Ag^{SP} + Ag \rightleftharpoons Ag^{SP} + Ab^E-Ag$$
$$\text{(Separate)}$$

$$Ab^E-Ag^{SP} + S \longrightarrow P$$

The enzyme activity is inversely proportional to the concentration of sample Ag. Human IgG at the picomole level has been quantified in less than 1.5 h with this method (27). Estrone-3-glucuronide at the femtomole level has been quantified with this method.

Noncompetitive assays

Enzyme-labeled antigen: In this method, the sample is first incubated with a moderate excess of solid-phase immobilized antibody (Ab^{SP}). After washing, excess enzyme-labeled antigen (Ag^E) is allowed to bind to unreacted Ab^{SP}.

$$Ab^{SP} + Ag \rightleftharpoons Ab^{SP}-Ag$$

$$Ab^{SP} \text{ (unreacted)} + Ag \rightleftharpoons Ab^{SP}-Ag^E$$

$$Ab^{SP}-Ag^E + S \longrightarrow P$$

The concentration of P is inversely proportional to the concentration of standard or test antigen.

Enzyme-labeled antibody: The sample antigen (Ag) is incubated with a moderate excess of enzyme-labeled antibody (Ab^E). The mixture is then added to an excess of immobilized antigen (Ag^{SP}) to remove unreacted Ab^E.

$$Ag + Ab^E \rightleftharpoons Ab^E-Ag$$

$$Ag^{SP} + Ab^E \rightleftharpoons Ab^E-Ag^{SP}$$
$$\text{(Separate)}$$

$$Ab^E-Ag^{SP} + S \longrightarrow P$$

The enzyme activity is inversely proportional to the concentration of sample and the procedure has been used to measure α-fetoprotein (28).

Sandwich or double antibody: This method is used with antigens having multiple antibody binding sites (epitopes). Immobilized unlabeled antibody (Ab^{SP}), in excess, is incubated with sample or antigen. After washing, the antibody–antigen complex is then incubated with an excess of enzyme-labeled antibody (Ab^E) which binds to one or more antigenic sites to form a sandwich type complex.

$$Ab^{SP}-Ag + Ab^E \rightleftharpoons Ab^{SP}-Ag-Ab^E$$

In this case, the concentration of enzyme product is directly proportional to the concentration of sample antigen.

Sandwich type assay is well suited for quantifying antigens with multiple antigenic determinants, such as antibodies, rheumatoid factors, polypeptide hormones, proteins, and hepatitis B surface antigens. The results obtained with sandwich type immunoassays are comparable to those obtained with those using radiolabels in term of precision, convenience and sensitivity. Highly sensitive thyroid-stimulating hormones assays are developed, as well as assays to measure estrogen and estradiol at attomole levels (29).

Avidin–Biotin Systems

An integral necessity of every enzyme immunoassay is the availability of enzyme-labeled antibody or antigen conjugates. The assays discussed in the first part of this article used chemical methods for forming these conjugates. An alternative approach has been widely employed that is based on the avidin–biotin reaction. Avidin is a protein of molecular weight about 60,000 that is found in egg white. It consists of 4 identical subunits. Each subunit binds biotin with an extremely high affinity. A dissociation constant of 10^{-15} corresponding to a dissociation half-life of about 160 days was reported. Hence, from a practical point of view, this binding can be regarded as almost irreversible in nature.

The rationale behind the use of the biotin–avidin system in immunochemistry is that avidin binds biotin substituted structures. Peptides and proteins can be easily biotinylated via their amino groups by using activated biotin-*N*-hydroxysuccinimide.

Reagents for biotinylation of proteins and peptides are commercially available and allow the fast and efficient derivatization of antibodies and enzymes without the loss of enzyme or antibody activity. Several reagents are also available for the biotinylation of sulfhydryl groups aldehydes, nucleic acids and carbohydrates. Hence, in addition to proteins and peptides, a variety of antigens can be labeled with biotin.

Avidin can be coupled to enzymes by covalent binding techniques or by employing the so-called avidin–biotin complex (ABC). In the latter case, a complex between avidin and polybiotinylated enzyme is formed. The ratios of avidin to polybiotinylated enzymes are chosen in such a way that the resulting complex incorporates a number of enzyme molecules, but retains free biotin binding sites for the interaction with biotinylated antibody or antigen structures. A great selection of ABC complexes for a great variety of different enzymes is commercially available. The possibility of easily making biotinylated antibody or antigen structures and the availability of a variety of enzyme-labeled avidin derivatives or complexes facilitates the flexible design of enzyme immunoassays.

The most frequently used assay version uses a primary antibody which is immobilized to a solid support (e.g., the surface of a microtiter plate). In the first step, the antigen (analyte) is added to the wells. After the antigen is bound to the immobilized antibody, the wells are washed and a biotinylated second antibody is added to the tubes. The resulting sandwich between immobilized antibody; antigen and biotinylated antibody is incubated with the ABC complex. After washing, the antibody–antigen–biotinylated antibody–ABC complex is detected by addition of the enzyme substrate. The non competitive nature of this assay in conjunction with the extremely high amplification of the signal by the ABC complex results in an assay (in the femtomole range), that often exceeds the sensitivity of radioimmunoassays.

Competitive immunoassays based on the avidin–biotin approach have also been described. In this case, the antibody is immobilized on microtiter plates. Wells are incubated with a constant concentration of biotinylated antigen in the presence of different concentrations of standards or the sample. After washing, the ABC complex is added. The formed antibody–biotinylated antigen–ABC sandwich is then detected by the addition of enzyme substrate. The immobilized enzyme–activity is inversely proportional to the concentration of analyte in the sample, resulting in a typical sigmoidal calibration curve.

FLUORESCENCE IMMUNOASSAYS

Fluorescence immunoassay (FIA) entails the measurement of the photoexcited fluorescence from an antibody or antigen which participates in an immunochemical binding system, and whose spectral properties vary with the concentration of the analyte. Because few naturally occurring antigens and antibodies have the requisite fluorescent properties, they are usually substituted with fluorescent labels. Fluorescent labels are used in homogeneous and heterogeneous immunoassay systems and may be bound to competing (labeled and unlabeled) antigens; antibodies or solid phases or they may exist in solution as parts of enzyme substrates.

The fluorogenic molecules used to covalently label the antigens or the antibodies to be used in a fluorescence immunoassay are called fluorescent probes or labels. Fluorescent probes are small molecules whose fluorescent properties are altered subsequent to interactions with proteins or other macromolecules.

In quantitative immunoassay using fluorescent labels, there are several chemical and spectroscopic properties that the fluorochrome should possess. The labeled ligand should have a relatively high water solubility because immunoassays are usually carried out in the aqueous environment in which the antibodies are stable. The presence of certain functional groups on the fluorochrome will facilitate its conjugation to the ligand. Derivatives of the fluorochromes containing reactive groups such as acid chlorides, isothiocyanates and diazonium salts can be used for the conjugation of the label to the ligand. A major concern in labeling a ligand with a fluorescent probe is the possibility of altering the specificity of the ligand for its antibody. Consequently the site of the conjugation chosen should provide maximum exposure of functional groups necessary for antibody recognition. In addition, the stability and shelf life are also important considerations.

The spectral characteristics of greatest importance in the selection of a fluorochrome are the molar absorptivity at the selected wavelength of excitation, the quantum yield of fluorescence of the labeled species, the spectral regions of absorption and emission of radiation, and the Stokes' shift. Ideally, the fluorescent label should have an absorption spectrum with a high molar absorptivity in the visible region of the electromagnetic spectrum, well removed from the excitation spectra of proteins and other endogenous interferences normally present in biological fluids. The emission wavelength should also lie well into the visible region with Stokes' shift (displacement of the fluorescence maximum from the longest wavelength absorption maximum) of at least 50 nm. A high quantum yield of fluorescence in the antibody-bound or free labeled ligand is also desirable.

The labels most commonly used are fluorescein isothiocyanate (FITC) and a number of reactive rhodamine dyes. Fluorescein isothiocyanate has a relatively high quantum yield and can be conjugated to drugs and other ligands under fairly mild conditions (30, 31).

Ligand labeling with fluorescent metal chelates has created a versatile class of fluorescent probes. The chelates of rare earth metals have unique emission characteristics in that, upon excitation of aromatic portions of the ligands of the lanthanide complex, the energy of excitation is efficiently transferred to the lanthanide ion. This causes f–f transitions that produce very narrow almost line-like emission bands that permit all of the emitted light to be collected by the detector with narrow emission slits. In addition, the rare earth chelates possess large quantum yields in combination with very large Stokes' shifts. The excitation region of these chelates is fairly broad and these aspects of the lanthanide luminescence permit excellent sensitivity and selectivity by enabling the use of fairly wide bandwidths for excitation and narrow bandwidths for emission. With the proper combination of rare earth chelate and fluorimetric technique, very sensitive immunoassays can be developed that avoid a large number of interferences commonly encountered in the immunoassay process.

Homogeneous Fluorescence Immunoassay

Because of the extreme sensitivity of the quantum yield and spectral position of fluorescence to the microenvironment of the fluorophore, fluorescence immunoassay often lends itself well to homogeneous techniques. The elimination of the necessity of a step for the separation of bound and free ligand represents one of the major advantages of fluorescence immunoassay and provides the opportunity for simple, fast and reliable quantitation. The free and antibody-bound ligands reside in different microenvironments. In the aqueous environment, the free labeled antigen will experience strong polarizing forces as a result of interactions with water molecules. These forces will be exerted to different degrees in the ground and excited states of the labeled antigen because these electronic states have different dipole moments. Also, certain functional groups on the fluorophore may be free to rotate prior to and subsequent to the fluorescent transition in water. In the hydrophobic environment of an antibody binding site, the dielectric strength is low and rotation of functional groups on the fluorophore is severely restricted. The solvation and restricted rotational freedom of the antibody-bound labeled antigen usually cause this species

to fluoresce at shorter wavelengths than the free labeled antigen because the relative stabilization of the excited state of the latter by strong electrostatic and electromeric interactions is much greater than in the bound labeled antigen. Moreover, the weak solvation and restricted rotational freedom of the antibody-bound probe also cause the bound probe to fluoresce more intensely than the free probe because the bound probe is somewhat shielded from internal conversion which competes with fluorescence for deactivation of the excited state.

If the fluorescent emission spectrum of the bound labeled ligand is sufficiently displaced, enhanced or decreased in intensity (quenched) relative to that of the free labeled ligand, the resulting spectroscopic measurements can be used for quantitation without a separation step. Additionally, the techniques previously described in enzyme immunoassays, such as reactant-labeled immunoassay, can form the bases of fluorescent immunoassay. For example the fluorophore, from whose optical properties quantitation is derived, can be generated or consumed in an enzymatic reaction.

Two rather interesting variations on fluorescence immunoassay that do not require the fluorescence spectra of free and bound labeled materials to have different spectral positions have fairly recently become rather popular in clinical analysis. These are fluorescence polarization immunoassay and time-resolved fluorescence immunoassay.

Fluorescence polarization immunoassay (FPIA)

The physical principle underlying fluorescence polarization immunoassay involves the selective elimination of light waves whose electric vectors do not all lie in a single plane. This is accomplished by passing the exciting light through a polarizing filter. The resulting polarized radiation will selectively excite (photoselect) those molecules whose absorption transition moments have a significant component in the plane of the electrical vector of the exciting beam (32). As a result, molecules excited with polarized light will emit radiation that is polarized in the same direction as the exciting light, to a degree inversely related to the amount of Brownian rotation occurring during the interval between absorption and emission of light (33). This means that the photoselected molecules originally excited by polarized light and having fairly small volumes (i.e., free labeled antigen) will have random orientations with respect to the plane of polarization of the exciting light because they will rotate faster than they fluoresce. They therefore, will display very little polarized fluorescence. However, photoselected molecules having very large volumes such as the antibody proteins and their complexes, will rotate at a rate comparable to or slower than the rate at which they fluoresce. Consequently, randomization of fluorescent transitions moments will not occur in these large molecules and substantial fluorescence polarization will be observed.

On binding of an antigen to an antibody there will be a reduction or a restriction in the rotational Brownian motion of the fluorescent label. This will cause considerable polarization of the fluorescence along or perpendicular to the optical axis of the excitation polarizer, depending upon whether the fluorescence transition moment of the molecule is oriented closer to 0 or 90° to the transition moment associated with the absorption band excited. Let us first consider the case where the transition moments for excitation and fluorescence are parallel (or nearly so).

If a second polarizing film (emission polarizer) is placed between the fluorescing sample and the photodetector of the fluorimeter, with its optical axis perpendicular to that of the polarizing film between the lamp and the sample, a much greater fraction of the highly polarized fluorescence from the antibody-labeled ligand will be filtered than would be of the unpolarized fluorescence from the same concentration of free labeled ligand excited under the same conditions. If the optical axes of both polarizers are parallel and the excitation and emission moments of the fluorophore are parallel, or nearly so, the emission polarizer will pass relatively more radiation from the bound labeled ligand than from the free labeled ligand, to the detector, because the unpolarized emission will be dispersed over all angles to the optical axis of the emission polarizer and some will therefore be filtered. Regardless of the orientation of the optical axis of the second polarizer with respect to the first, the fluorescence intensity registered by the detector should, ideally, be the same for unpolarized fluorescence (i.e., that of the free labeled ligand) while, in the case of parallel absorption and fluorescence transition moments, the intensity of the polarized fluorescence, from the bound labeled ligand, measured when the optical axes of the polarizers are parallel ($F_{\parallel}$) should be greater than when the optical axes of the polarizers are perpendicular ($F_{\perp}$). In the case of perpendicular absorption and fluorescence transition moments, for the free labeled ligand $F_{\parallel} = F_{\perp}$ (unpolarized fluorescence) and for the bound labeled ligand $F_{\perp} > F_{\parallel}$ (polarized fluorescence). We now define the degree of polarization as:

$$P = (F_{\parallel} - F_{\perp})/(F_{\parallel} + F_{\perp}) \tag{1}$$

For a free labeled ligand $F_{\parallel} = F_{\perp}$ so that $P = 0$ at all excitation wavelengths. For a bound labeled ligand it is possible to have $+1/2 > P > -1/3$, depending upon the

wavelength of excitation. However, if a system is contrived which originally contains all antibody-bound, labeled ligand, upon addition of the unlabeled ligand the labeled drug will be displaced. The relative increase in unpolarized fluorescence and decrease in polarized fluorescence from the solution will cause a net decrease in P as calculated from its operational definition in Equation (1). If all the labeled ligand were ultimately displaced from the antibody complex, P would fall to zero. Depending on the extent of binding of the labeled ligand, the degree of polarization varies between some non zero value and zero. This permits the construction of a calibration curve of degree of fluorescence polarization versus concentration of unlabeled ligand and permits the execution of a homogeneous immunoassay.

The use of polarized fluorescence for the quantitation of several antigen–antibody reactions is widely used. Two assays of particular interest are those applied to the measurement of serum levels of gentamicin and phenytoin (30, 34, 35). The use of fluorescence polarization as a method for routine drug level determinations is limited by the light energy losses in the polarizing films and the background interferences that result in reduction of sensitivity.

Time-resolved fluoroimmunoassay

All of the fluorimetric techniques, so far considered, have been based on the measurement of the intensity of fluorescence produced under "steady state" conditions. "Steady-state" fluorimetry is derived from the excitation of the sample with a continuous temporal output of exciting radiation. The lamps and their power supplies used in conventional fluorimeters are sources of continuous radiation. After a short period of initial excitation of the sample, a steady state is established in which the rate of excitation of the analyte is equal to the sum of the rates of all processes deactivating the lowest excited singlet state (fluorescence, internal conversion, and intersystem crossing). When the steady state is established, the observed fluorescence intensity becomes time invariant and produces the temporally constant signal which is measured by the photodetector. With the development of modern electro-optics however, it has become possible to excite a potentially fluorescent sample with a thyratron pulsed flash lamp which emits its radiation in bursts of 2–10 ns duration with about 0.2 ms between pulses or with a pulsed laser whose pulses occur with durations upward of a few picoseconds. A fluorescent sample excited with such a pulsed source will not fluoresce continuously. Rather, its fluorescence intensity, excited by a single pulse will decay exponentially until the next pulse again excites the sample. The pulsed source then acts very much as does a mechanical chopper in phosphorimetry. The fluorescence from the sample excited by the pulsed source can be represented, after detection, as a function of time on a fast sampling oscilloscope or on an $x-y$ plotter used in conjuntion with a multichannel pulse analyzer. The former approach is called pulsed-source fluorimetry and the latter, time-correlated single photon counting. In either case, fluorescence with decay times much longer than the lamp pulse characteristics can be treated in the same way that radioactive decay curves are analyzed. A semilogarithmic plot of fluorescence intensity against time will yield a straight line (or a series of intersecting lines if several fluorophores have comparable, but not identical decay times) whose slope is proportional to the decay time and whose vertical axis intercept can be compared with that of a standard solution of the fluorophore for quantitative analysis. If, however, the lamp pulse time and the decay–time of the fluorophore are comparable, the lamp characteristics must be substracted from the observed signal to obtain the fluorophore's decay characteristics. This is usually accomplished by using a computer to solve a deconvolution integral representing the composite temporal characteristics of the lamp and the fluorophore output.

The pulsed-source (time-resolved) method, then effects spectroscopic separation of the emission of several fluorescing species by taking advantage of differences in their decay times rather than their fluorescence intensities. This means that several overlapping fluorescences, such as those of free and antibody-bound ligand can be quantified simultaneously. Lanthanide chelate-labeled antibodies, which have long lifetimes (in the $1 = ms$ to $1 = \mu s$ range) form the basis of a time-resolved FIA, for which instrumentation is commercially available.

Heterogeneous Assays

Most research and development of fluorescence immunoassays, to date, have been concentrated in the area of homogenous assay. Unfortunately, homogeneous assays may not always provide optimum analytical sensitivity. This may be due to the endogenous background fluorescence of proteinaceous materials, Rayleigh and Raman scatter caused by proteins or to the lack of environmental sensitivity of the emission from the fluorescent label. Notwithstanding the speed and simplicity of the homogenous assay procedures, it is occasionally desirable to circumvent these problems by physically separating the antibody–ligand complex from other species in the sample before fluorimetric quantitation.

The separation of the antibody-bound ligands from free ligands and other fluorescing species present in solution can be accomplished by various methods based on the chemical, physical or immunological differences between the free ligand and the antibody–ligand complex and include gel permeation chromatography, chemical precipitation with inorganic salts or organic solvents and double antibody methods as well as the use of a solid phase support to which the antibody is either adsorbed or bonded covalently. In the latter method, the solid material may be paper discs, the walls of test tubes, glass or plastic beads, cross-linked dextrans or agaroses. Once the antibodies are immobilized on the solid support, the labeled and unlabeled ligands are introduced and allowed to compete for available binding sites on the antibody. The bound, labeled fraction is then separated from the free labeled ligand by washing. The labeled ligand complexed to the antibody can then be measured directly, without removal from the solid phase, by a fluorimeter with a front-surface fluorescence attachment (36).

CHEMILUMINESCENCE IMMUNOASSAYS

In all exergonic reactions energy is released. This energy is generally emitted as heat. In some reactions, however, this energy is released as light, a phenomenon known as chemiluminescence. During the course of chemiluminescence reactions, one or more of the resulting products is formed in an electronically excited state. Light is then emitted from the excited molecules by the process of fluorescence. Chemiluminescent reactions are almost invariably oxidation–reduction reactions. A number of compounds that show chemiluminescence of an intensity that is suitable for analytical detection systems or that are catalysts or reagents in chemiluminescent reactions have been investigated to be used in chemiluminescence immunoassays. Among these are synthetic organic compounds (e.g., phthalazinediones, acridinium esters), cofactors in bioluminescent reactions (NAD and ATP) and enzymes (peroxidase, oxidases, kinases, luciferases).

Covalent linking to either the antigen or antibody is carried out by chemical modification of the label (e.g., diazotisation or reaction with isothiocyanate, N-hydroxysuccinimide, hemisuccinate, imidoesters), by chemical modification of antigen or antibody (e.g., by reaction with hemisuccinate, glutaraldehyde), or by conjugation using bifunctional reagents (e.g., mixed anhydride carbodiimide, bis (N-hydroxy succinimides) or azidosuccinimides).

One of the most intensely chemiluminescent compounds is luminol (5-amino-2,3-dihydrophthalazine-1, 4-dione). If the amino group is linked to position 6 of the aromatic ring, the molecule is called isoluminol.

Isoluminol can be easily attached to antibodies or antigens via alkyl spacer groups. Aminobutylethylisoluminol (ABEI) has been shown to be very effective as a chemiluminescence labeling group, since the activity is generally not changed by coupling to low- or high-molecular-weight compounds. It can be easily coupled to activated carboxylic groups of immunologically relevant compounds using the mixed anhydride reaction (37). Proteins such as antibodies can be labeled sufficiently with ABEI through reaction of free amino groups of the proteins with an ABEI-isothiocyanate derivative (38).

The oxidative reactions of luminol and isoluminol derivatives at high pH result in the formation of 3-aminophthalate or 4-aminophthalate and nitrogen via an electronically excited state. The transition from the excited to the ground state induces the emission of light having a wavelength maximum of 425 nm. Quantitation is possible at picomolar or even attomolar levels of the aminophthalhydrazide.

In aprotic solvents, only oxygen and a base are necessary for the oxidation. In protic solvents a catalyst has to be present, in addition. As catalysts, enzymes such as horseradish peroxidase are frequently employed.

Acridinium esters are used also in immunological procedures. They have the advantage that no catalyst is necessary for the luminescence reaction. The solution has to be adjusted to a pH of 6–7 before the oxidant peroxide is added in order to ensure the highest activity.

Direct Chemiluminescence Immunoassays

The above reactions can be used in an immunological assay by coupling the chemiluminescent compound to an antigen or antibody; under the assumption that the immunological and chemiluminescent properties of the derived coupling product are not substantially changed. The approach to coupling chemiluminescent molecules to the required ligand obviously depends on the nature of the two species. When both species are small molecules, conventional synthetic organic chemistry can be used. A problem arises however when one or both molecules are more complex (e.g., proteins). Since the functionality of these molecules is determined by the chemical and physical environment, the range of chemistries that can be used is limited. As an example of direct chemiluminescence immunoassay, antibody might be immobilized onto a solid support and antigen allowed to bind to this antibody. After subsequent washing, a second chemiluminescent-labeled antibody that recognizes a different epitope of the antigen is added. After further washing, the chemiluminescent label is activated and the emitted light is quantified.

Since this assay is based on the sandwich principle, increasing amounts of analyte will produce increased light emission.

A chemiluminescent assay using competitive immunological techniques can be easily designed when chemiluminescent antigens are employed. In this case chemiluminescent antigen and sample compete for immobilized antibodies. Depending on the nature of the reaction antigen, bound and unbound label can also be separated by adsorption onto charcoal.

Indirect (Enzyme-Mediated) Chemiluminescence Immunoassays

An indirect chemiluminescence immunoassay is an assay, with another component than the primary chemiluminescent emitter coupled to the antigen or antibody. This can be a cofactor or a catalyst or even a molecule capable of converting a nonchemiluminescent precursor to a chemiluminescent or potentially chemiluminescent species. Most indirect assays are enzyme mediated.

One widely used enzyme mediated chemiluminescence immunoassay (39) uses the firefly enzyme luciferase that catalyzes the oxidation of D-Luciferin in the presence of ATP. D-luciferin, but not luciferin esters such as phosphates, is oxidized in the presence of the enzyme. An antigen or antibody-enzyme conjugate (e.g., alkaline phosphatase conjugate) is bound to a solid support by an antigen–antibody reaction. The immobilized enzyme enzymatically releases D-luciferin, which subsequently is quantified in a luciferase based luminometric assay, here described for the determination of alkaline phosphatase.

The chemiluminescent signals of luminol derivatives can be enhanced by the addition of firefly luciferin to the reaction mixture using hydrogen peroxide as oxidant and horseradish peroxidase as catalyst (40). This causes prolongation of the light production. Benzothiazoles, such as dehydroluciferin and 6-hydroxybenzothiazole derivatives also enhance the light emission by a factor of about 500 to 1000-fold and show a more constant light emission over time than luminol. A relatively constant emission of light over a period of 15 min has been observed for these derivatives (41). This constant and prolonged light emission pattern simplifies the analytical procedures as multiple reactions can be initiated outside of the luminometer without the necessity of initiating the chemiluminescence reaction in front of the photomultiplier.

Another chemiluminescent enzyme system is based on the use of stabilized dioxetane substrates. Dioxetanes are intermediates in many chemiluminescent reactions. It's possible to synthesize stabilized dioxetanes (phosphatase and β-galactose moieties) that do not spontaneously react. When exposed to the right enzyme (alkaline phosphatase and β-galactosidase, respectively) the dioxetane will be destabilized and spontaneously undergo a chemiluminescence reaction (42).

ELECTROCHEMICAL IMMUNOASSAYS

Electrochemical immunoassays include a wide variety of devices based on the coupling of immunological reactions with electrochemical transduction. All of them involve the immobilization of an immunoreagent component on the surface of the electrode transducer. Electrochemical detection is based on the direct intrinsic redox behavior either of an analyte species or of some reporter molecule. For the detection no expensive equipment is needed, with the measurement of either a simple current or a voltage charge. Different electrochemical detection strategies are used, but amperometric detection is most widely used. Potentiometric and conductometric detection are applied in different assays as well.

For the detection different electrode supports and a great variety of immobilization procedures have been used. Gold electrodes, screen-printed electrodes and carbon materials (such as graphite and glassy carbon) have been frequently used. The sensing phase is constructed onto the surface of the electrode by means of covalent linkage, physical adsorption or membrane entrapping of the specific immunoreagent.

The major advantage of electrochemical immunoassays is the fact that it's based on the use of a nonoptical detection system, which makes it possible to detect signals in the presence of whole blood samples. There are three different ways in which electrochemistry is used in a detection system.

Direct monitoring of the antigen–antibody reaction

This is by far the simplest approach to electrochemical immunoassay, because there is no label needed. There are several methods demonstrated by analyzing simple solutions, however, considerable work will be necessary for detection when sensors are exposed to biological sample matrices.

Using electroactive compounds as labels

In order to be used as an immunoassay label, an electrochemically active compound has to possess suitable electrochemical properties. It has to be soluble in aqueous media and should be stable in solution over a wide pH range. To be detectable, it must allow highly selective electrochemical detection or possess chemical properties to allow selective membranes to be used in the measurement electrode.

One of the advantages of an intrinsically electroactive label is that there is no need for substrate, cofactor or the special incubation steps for an enzyme label. However a consequence is the loss of enzyme signal amplification which increases the demands on detection sensitivity. Human serum albumin has been detected in a competitive heterogeneous assay using indium ions (43).

Using enzymes as amplification labels with the enzyme monitored by measurement of an electro-active product or substrate

The direct detection of electrochemical labels entails problems with sensitivity. For this reason the majority of electrochemical immunoassay development has focused on the measurement of enzyme labels by detection of electroactive products arising from enzyme catalyzed reactions. A wide variety of enzyme labels have been used for electrochemical immunoassays. These include glucose oxidase, glucose-6-phosphate dehydrogenase and alkaline phosphatase (44).

Glucose oxidase catalyses the conversion of glucose to gluconic acid with reduction of oxygen to hydrogen peroxide. In principle, either the consumption of oxygen or the liberation of hydrogen peroxide can be monitored to detect the activity of glucose oxidase. However due to the high background level of oxygen in biological fluids, hydrogen peroxide monitoring is more often used. Other glucose oxidase assays have been used (e.g., ferrocene and 1,4-benzoquinone), where oxygen is replaced by an alternative electron acceptor because of faster reaction rates, lower oxidation potential and the detection system is less sensitive to the levels of oxygen in the sample. A homogenous assay based on ferrocene was developed for digoxin (45).

Glucose-6-phosphate dehydrogenase catalyses the conversion of glucose-6- phosphate to 6-phosphogluconate while reducing NAD^+ to NADH. However the direct electrochemical measurement of NAD(P)H is rather difficult, owing to by a high overvoltage that is required for the electrode reaction and by electrode fouling. By using redox mediators (e.g. quinones, ferrocenes, and phenoxazine) these problems can be overcome. Theophylline, and phenytoin have been detected using glucose-6-hydrogenase.

Alkaline phosphatase is one of the most suitable enzymes for electrochemical immunoassays owing to its high turnover number and broad substrate specificity. Different substrates have been used, but 4-aminophenyl phosphate is most suitable, since the reaction product,

4-aminophenol is easily oxidized without fouling of the electrode surface. Thyroxine-binding globulin, cortisol, and prostatic acid phosphatase have been detected by using alkaline phosphatase.

LIPOSOME IMMUNOASSAYS

Liposomes are formed when phospholipid molecules spontaneously self-assemble in aqueous solution to produce spheres in which an aqueous cavity is enclosed by one or more phospholipid bilayer membranes. This cavity can be used to entrap a variety of materials. For immunoassays, a variety of detectable labels, called markers, have been encapsulated. The markers used range from inorganic salts [e.g., KCl, $K_4Fe(CN)_6$] for electrochemical detection, through widely used fluorescent markers (e.g. calcein, carboxyfluorescein, sulforhodamine B and chelates) to enzymes (e.g., alkaline phosphatase, horseradish peroxidase, and glucose-6-phosphate dehydrogenase). A wide range of detection methods and substrates is available for these enzymes. The amount of the encapsulated molecule is directly related to the amount of antigen. To achieve the lowest limit of detection the amount of encapsulated molecule (marker) should be as high as possible. Fluorescent markers are most commonly used because these markers can be measured easily and very sensitively. Besides these mostly small fluorescent molecules larger molecules, as enzymes and enzyme cofactors are also entrapped. The advantage of using larger molecules is that they tend to leak less through the liposome membrane. Most markers are water soluble, but lipophilic markers (e.g., perylene derivatives) can also be incorporated in liposomes (46). These markers are mainly incorporated in the membrane which eliminates leakage.

The amount of liposome-encapsulated marker has to be related to the amount of antigen, therefore the liposome has to be conjugated to the antigen. This can be done either directly or indirectly. With the direct approach the liposome is bound to the antigen. The indirect approach either uses an antibody or a secondary molecule bound to the liposome.

Homogeneous Liposome Immunoassays

Because of the special structural characteristics of liposomes it's possible to develop adapted schemes exploiting these characteristics. It's essential that the liposomes retain their structural integrity in the presence of lytic agents, which might be present in biological fluids. However most liposome immunoassays use a natural lytic agent, the two most frequently used are complement (47) and mellitin (48).

When foreign cells enter the human body they are captured by antibodies, which attach themselves to the cell membrane surface. Complement binds to these antibodies in a specific order, after which the target cells are lysed. Because the liposome bilayer is structurally similar to the cell wall, complement can be used to completely lyse antibody-bound liposomes. Attention has to be paid to the fact that although complement is specific, some liposomes are susceptible to complement lysis, without being bound to an antibody. Most liposome immunoassays are homogeneous complement-based assays.

Mellitin is also able to lyse liposomes completely, although rather slowly, it is found in bee venom and its biological task is cell destruction. Cytolysin mediated assays use a conjugate of mellitin with the antigen. The conjugate is free and able to lyse the liposomes or bound to an antibody and unable to lyse the liposomes. The activity is thus reversed, proportional to the amount of antibody present in the sample. The disadvantage of mellitin-based assays is that the range of antigens is limited in size, because the presence of a large antigen will inhibit the activity of mellitin. Biotin and digoxin have been analyzed by a homogeneous liposome immunoassay using mellitin as lytic agent.

Homogeneous liposome immunoassays using lytic agents other than complement and mellitin have also been used. Phospholipase C catalyzes the dephosphorylation of phospholipids, which in turn destabilizes the liposome. The assay is based on the inhibition of the lytic activity by an antibody binding to an antigen conjugated to phospholipase C (49). Gentamicin is analyzed by this method.

Assays that use liposomes coated with murine monoclonal antibodies and magnetic particles coated with antimurine monoclonal antibodies, have been developed. Incubation of these two components results in destabilization of the liposome by binding to the magnetic particles. As a result the entrapped marker will be released (50).

Heterogeneous Liposome Immunoassays

Compared to homogeneous assays only a small number of heterogeneous assays have been developed. As all heterogeneous assays, a heterogeneous liposome immunoassay or a liposome immunosorbent assay always use one or more steps to separate the specifically bound liposomes from the free liposomes by washing. After washing lysis of the liposomes can be performed with a detergent which effectively and quickly lyse all liposomes, such as Triton X-100. These assays can be regarded as modifications of enzyme-linked immunoassays.

We have presented in this article a brief overview of existing immunological assays. New drug developments will, in the future, require more versatile and sensitive assays. It can be said with certainty that immunological assays will retain their importance for achieving these goals.

REFERENCES

1. Berson, S.A.; Yalow, R.S. Quantitative Aspects of the Reaction Between Insulin and Insulin-Binding Antibody. J. Clin. Invest. **1959**, *38*, 1996–2016.
2. Male, D.; Champion, B.; Cooke, A. Maturation of the Immune Response. *Advances Immunology*; J. B. Lippincott Co.: Philadelphia, 1987; 10.1.
3. Edelman, G.M.; Gall, W.E. Antibody Problems. Ann. Rev. Biochem. **1969**, *38*, 415–466.
4. Kohler, G.; Milstein, C. Continuous Cultures of Fused Cells Secreting Antibody of Predefined Specificity. Nature **1975**, *256*, 495–497.
5. Campfield, L.A. Mathematical Analysis of Competitive Protein Binding Assays. *Principles of Competitive Protein Binding Assays*; Odell, W., Franchimont, P., Eds.; John Wiley & Sons: New York, 1983; 125–148.
6. Izzo, J.L.; Roncone, A.; Izzo, M.J.; Bale, W.F. Relationship between Degree of Iodination of Insulin and its Biological Electrophoretic and Immunochemical Properties. J. Biol. Chem. **1964**, *239*, 3749–3754.
7. Potts, J.T., Jr; Sherwood, L.M.; O'Riordan, L.L.H.; Aurbach, G.D. Radioimmunoassay of Polypeptide Hormones. Advan. Intern. Med. **1967**, *13*, 183–240.
8. Midgley, A.; Hepburn, M.R. Use of Double Antibody Method to Separate Antibody Bound From Free Ligand in Radioimmunoassay. *Methods in Enzymology: Immuno-chemical Techniques*; Langone, J.J., Ed.; Academic Press: New York, 1980; 74, 266–273.
9. Bao, J.J. Capillary Electrophoretic Immunoassays. J. Chromatogr. B. **1997**, *699*, 463–480.
10. Salmon, S.E.; Smith, B.A. Sandwich Solid Phase Radioimmunoassays for Characterization of Human Immunoglobulins Synthesized In-Vitro. J. Immunol. **1970**, *104*, 665–672.
11. Engrall, E.; Perlman, P. Enzyme – Linkend Immunosorbent Assay (ELISA): Quantitative Assay of Immunoglobulin G. Immunochemistry **1971**, *8*, 871–874.
12. Van Weeman, B.K.; Schuurs, A.H.W.M. Immunoassay Using Antigen-Enzyme Conjugates. FEBS Letter **1971**, *15*, 232–236.
13. Brunk, S.D.; Hadjiioannou, T.P.; Hadjiiannou, S.I.; Malmstadt, H.V. Adaptation of Emit Technique for Serum Phenobarbital and Diphenylhydantoin Assays to Miniature Centrifugal Analyzer. Clin. Chem. **1976**, *22*, 905–907.
14. Rubenstein, K.E.; Schneider, R.S.; Ullman, E.F. Homogeneous Enzyme Immunoassay – New Immunochemical Technique. Biochem. Biophys. Res. Commun. **1972**, *47*, 846–851.
15. Rowley, G.L.; Rubenstein, K.E.; Huisjen, J.; Ullman, E.F. Mechanism by Which Antibodies Inhibit Hapten-Malate Dehydrogenase Conjugates. J. Biol. Chem. **1975**, *250*, 3759–3766.
16. Ngo, T.T. *Enzyme-mediated Immunoassay*; Plenum: New York, 1985.
17. Chang, J.; Gotcher, S.; Gunshaw, J.B. Homogeneous Enzyme-Immunoassay for Theophylline in Serum and Plasma. Clin. Chem **1982**, *28*, 361–367.
18. Ngo, T.T.; Lenhoff, H.M. Enzyme Modulators as Tools for the Development of Homogeneous Enzyme Immunoassays. FEBS Letter **1980**, *116*, 285–288.
19. Ngo, T.T.; Lenhoff, H.M. Antibody Induced Conformational Restriction as Basis for New Separation-Free Enzyme-Immunoassay. Biochem. Biophys. Res. **1983**, *116*, 1097–1103.
20. Finley, P.R.; Williams, R.J.; Lichti, D.A. Evaluation of a New Homogeneous Enzyme-Inhibitor Immunoassay of Serum Thyroxine with Use of a Bichromatic Analyzer. Clin. Chem. **1980**, *26*, 1723–1726.
21. Blecka, L.J.; Shaffar, M.; Dworschack, R. Inhibitor Enzyme Immunoassays for Quantitation of Various Haptens: A Review. *Immunoenzymatic Techniques*; Avrameas, S., Dmet, P., Mosseyeff, R., Feldman, G., Eds.; Elsevier: Amsterdam, 1983; 207.
22. Burd, J.F.; Wong, R.C.; Feeney, J.C.; Carrico, R.C.; Boguslaski, R.C. Homogeneous Reactant-Labeled Fluorescent Immunoassay for Therapeutic Drugs Exemplified by Gentamicin Determination in Human-Serum. Clin. Chem. **1977**, *23*, 1402–1408.
23. Bogulaski, R.C.; Li, T.M.; Benoric, J.L.; Ngo, T.T.; Burd, J.F.; Carrico, R.C. Substrate Labeled Homogeneous Fluorescent Immunoassays for Haptens and Proteins. *Immunoassays: Clinical Laboratory Technique for the 1980's*; Nakamura, R.M., Dito, W.R., Tucker, E.S., III Eds.; Alan Liss: New York, 1980; 45–64.
24. Walter, B.; Greenquist, A.C.; Howard, W.E., III Solid-phase Reagent Strips for Detection of Therapeutic Drugs in Serum by Substrate-Labelled Flourescent Immunoassay. Anal. Chem. **1983**, *55*, 873–878.
25. Engel, W.D.; Khanna, P.K. Cedia In Vitro Diagnostics with a Novel Homogeneous Immunoassay Technology – Current Status and Future Prospects. J. Immunol. Meth. **1992**, *150*, 99–102.
26. Spiehler, V.; Fay, J.; Rogerson, R.; Schorenforfer, D.; Nied Bala, R.S. Enzyme Immunoassay Validation for Qualitative Detection of Cocaine in Sweat. Clin. Chem. **1996**, *42*, 34–38.
27. Halliday, M.I.; Wisdom, G.B. Competitive Enzyme-Immunoassay Using Labelled Antibody. FEBS Letter **1978**, *96*, 298–300.
28. Masseyeff, R. Assay of Tumour-Associates Antigens. Scand. J. Immunol. **1978**, *8* (Suppl. 7), 83–90.
29. Klein, K.O.; Baron, J.; Colli, M.J.; McDonnell, D.P.; Cutter, G.B. Estrogen-Levels in Childhood Determined by Ultrasensitive Recombinant Cell Bioassay. Clin. Invest. **1994**, *94*, 2475–2480.
30. Watson, R.A.A.; Landon, J.; Shaw, E.J.; Smith, D.S. Polarization Fluoro-Immunoassay of Gentamicin. Clin. Chim. Acta. **1976**, *73*, 51–55.

31. Shaw, E.J.; Watson, R.A.A.; Landon, J.; Smith, D.S. Estimation of Serum Gentamicin by Quenching Fluoro-Immunoassay. J. Clin. Path. **1977**, *30*, 526–531.

32. Weber, G. Polarization of the Fluorescence of Macromolecules. Biochem. J. **1952**, *51*, 145–155.

33. Chen, R.F. Extrinsic and Intrinsic Fluorescence of Proteins. *Practical Fluorescence: Theory, Methods and Techniques*; Guilbault, G.G., Ed.; Ch. 12 Marcel Dekker, Inc.: New York, 1973.

34. McGregor, A.R.; Crockall-Grenning, J.O.; Landon, J.; Smith, D.S. Polarization Fluoro-Immunoassay of Phenytoin. Clin. Chim. Acta. **1978**, *83*, 161–166.

35. O'Neal, J.S.; Schulman, S.G. Fluorescence Polarization Immunoassay of Phenytoin Employing a Sulfonamido Derivative of 2-Napththol-8-Sulfonic Acid as a Lablel. Anal. Chem. **1984**, *56*, 2888–2891.

36. Blanchard, G.C.; Gardner, R. Two Immunofluorescent Methods Compared With a Radial Immunodiffusion Method for Measurement of Serum Immunoglobulins. Clin. Chem. **1978**, *24*, 808–814.

37. Kohen, F.; De Boever, J.; Kim, J.B. Recent Advances in Chemiluminescence Based Immunoassays for Steroid-Hormones. J. Steroid Biochem. **1987**, *27*, 71–79.

38. Patel, A.; Campbell, A.K. Homogeneous Immunoassay Based on Chemiluminescence Energy-Transfer. Clin. Chem. **1983**, *29*, 1604–1608.

39. Geiger, R.; Miska, W. Bioluminescence Enhanced Enzyme-Immunoassay: New Ultrasensitive Detection Systems for Enzyme Immunoassays. J. Clin. Chem. Biochem. **1987**, *25*, 31–38.

40. Whitehead, T.P.; Thorpe, G.H.G.; Carter, T.J.N.; Groucutt, C.J.; Kricka, L.J. Enhanced Luminescence Procedure for Sensitive Determination of Peroxidase – Labeled Conjugate in Immunoassay. Nature (London) **1983**, *305*, 158–159.

41. Thorpe, G.H.G.; Moseley, S.B.; Kricka, L.J.; Stott, R.A.; Whitehead, T.P. Enhanced Luminescence Determination of Horseradish Peroxidase Conjugates: Application of Benzothiazole Derivatives as Enhancers in Luminescence Assays on Microtitre Plates. Anal. Chim. Acta. **1985**, *170*, 101.

42. Bronstein, I.; Voyta, J.C.; Thorpe, G.H.G.; Krica, L.J.; Edwards, B. Chemiluminescent Enzyme-Immunoassay of Alpha-Fetoprotein Based on an Adamantyl Dioxetrance Phenyl Phosphate Substrate. Clin. Chem. **1989**, *35*, 1441–1446.

43. Doyle, M.J.; Halsall, H.B.; Heineman, W.R. Enzyme-Linked Immunoasorbent Assay with Electrochemical Detection for Alpha-1-Acid Glycoprotein. Anal. Chem. **1982**, *56*, 2318–2322.

44. Heineman, W.R.; Halsall, H.B. Strategies for Electrochemical Immunoassay. Anal. Chem. **1985**, *12*, 1321–1331.

45. Suzawa, T.; Ikariyama, Y.; Aizawa, M. Multilabeling of Ferrocenes of a Glucose-Oxidase Digoxin Conjugate for the Development of a Homogeneous. Anal. Chem. **1994**, *66*, 3889–3894.

46. Schott, H.; Von Cunow, D.; Langhals, H. Labeling of Liposomes with Intercalating Perylene Fluorescent Dyes. Biochim. Biophys. Acta. **1992**, *1110*, 151–157.

47. Kinsky, S.C. Antibody-Complement Interaction with Lipid Model Membranes. Biochim. Biophys. Acta. **1972**, *265*, 1–23.

48. Litchfield, W.J.; Freytag, J.W.; Adamich, M. Highly Sensitive Immunoassays Based on Use of Liposomes Without Complement. Clin. Chem. **1984**, *30*, 1441–1445.

49. Kim, C.K.; Park, K.M. Liposome Immunoassay (LIA) for Gentamicin Using Phospholipase-C. Immunol. Methods **1994**, *170*, 225–231.

50. Wright, S.E.; Huang, L.; J. Liposome Res. **1992**, *2*, 257–273.

INHALATION, DRY POWDER

**Lynn Van Campen and
Geraldine Venthoye**

Inhale Therapeutic Systems, Inc., San Carlos, California

INTRODUCTION

Drug delivery to the lung has been historically aimed at controlling local respiratory disease where the central airways may be as suitable a target for drug deposition as the deeper lung. With little exception, currently marketed inhalation products provide therapy for asthma, chronic obstructive pulmonary disease (COPD), and bronchitis. More recently, however, there has been significant interest in using the lung, and in particular the deep lung alveolar surface, as a portal to the systemic circulation for drugs not readily administered orally. Therapeutic targets have therefore broadened substantially because pulmonary delivery is recognized for its potential to provide a noninvasive alternative to injection. New delivery systems capable of delivering drug in particles or droplets small enough to reach the peripheral or deep lung are under intense development to meet these new therapeutic targets.

Delivery of drugs to the lung depends on administration by any one of three methods: nebulizer, metered-dose inhaler (MDI), or dry powder inhaler (DPI). The nature of the drug substance and its therapeutic target may dictate which lung-delivery dosage form is more appropriate for the drug. Nebulization, for example, requires that the drug dissolve well in an aqueous medium at a concentration suitable for convenient dosing. Drugs developed as MDIs must dissolve or suspend well in a nonaqueous propellant medium at a concentration appropriate for doses metered in volumes generally less than 100 µl. For DPIs, the physical properties of the drug substance determine the ease with which processing will yield a stable powder that can be effectively aerosolized in milligram quantities by the inhaler device to deliver the proper drug dosage.

Nebulizers

Nebulizers have a long history in pulmonary delivery. Although generally effective, traditional nebulizer systems require lengthy (10–20 min) administration periods during which drug solution is delivered with relative inefficiency using an external power source. More convenient hand-held systems are currently in development and offer the convenience of portability and metered-dose administration (1). Depending on drug solubility and dose, these systems may require multiple actuations to deliver an effective dose.

MDIs

Since the 1970s, MDIs have dominated inhalation delivery, especially in the United States. MDIs are more convenient to use than nebulizers, generally offering 100–300 metered doses per pocket-sized canister. Limitations to the reliability of their therapeutic effectiveness, however, typically arise from the need for the patient to coordinate MDI actuation with breath inhalation (2) and from the deposition of a sometimes significant amount of drug, driven by the propellant blast, to the back of the throat instead of the lung. Then, in the late 1980s, the chlorofluorocarbon (CFC) propellants used in MDIs were identified as agents contributing to the depletion of the ozone layer. This led to industry-wide reformulation efforts still underway to replace CFCs with environmentally more friendly propellants.

DPIs

The technical challenges of MDI reformulation have contributed to a growing interest in the potential of DPI technology for the development of new products that satisfy similar therapeutic, market, and environmental needs.

The DPI device presents medication to the patient as a dry powder in a form that can be inhaled orally for delivery to the target lung tissues. The delivery system should assist in the generation of very fine particulates of medication in a way that enables them to avoid the impaction barriers that normally operate in the lung to prevent the ingress of potentially harmful particles. These barriers include the oropharynx and, for deep lung delivery, the air-conducting bronchi and bronchioles.

Studies have shown that to clear the oropharyngeal impaction barrier (comprising the mouth, throat, and pharynx), particles with aerodynamic diameters smaller than 5 μm are required (3, 4). Only particles with aerodynamic diameters less than 3 μm will reach the terminal bronchi and the alveoli in significant numbers (5). Therefore, the particle diameter required to be produced by the delivery system will depend to a great extent on the intended target lung tissue. Lung deposition is also affected substantially by the specific inhalation dynamics of the patient, which, in turn, are influenced by the delivery device. This article addresses various attributes of the dry powder inhalation product, from intrinsic material properties to final product performance.

More simple in concept than implementation, DPI technology is rapidly expanding to address a broadening therapeutic need as well as market opportunity. Characteristics of the ideal DPI system will include most or all of the following attributes:

- Simple and comfortable to use;
- Compact and economical to produce;
- Highly reproducible fine-particle dosing;
- Reproducible emitted dose;
- Physically and chemically stable powder;
- Minimal extrapulmonary loss of drug, with low oropharyngeal deposition, low device retention, and low exhaled loss;
- Multidose system;
- Powder protected from external environment and can be used in all climates and protected from moist exhaled air;
- Overdose protection; and
- Indicate number of doses delivered and/or remaining.

Outline

Fine particle powders can be produced by various methods such as micronization or spray drying. The physicochemical nature of these fine particles generally defines the stability of the bulk powder, which in turn is critical to the long-term effective performance of the dry powder product. The section *Fine Particles and the Solid State* is an introduction to better understanding the fundamental properties that underlie the behavior of bulk powders. Commentary on the various means of producing fine powders follows in the section *Powder Production: Formulation and Processing*.

Drug containment in DPIs falls into two categories: unit dose, in which the dose is premetered during manufacture, and reservoir, in which the drug dose is metered during dose administration. Some devices store multiple unit doses for convenience. These are addressed in the section *Filling and Packaging*. The next section, *Devices: Forming the Dry Powder Aerosol*, considers the various

means of aerosolizing powder in the context of device design history and functionality. Advantages and disadvantages of different design types are considered.

Performance and Regulatory Requirements describes various ways of characterizing the dry powder aerosols and provides information on product quality performance requirements and how these attributes must be reflected in registration applications.

The Role of DPIs in Therapy briefly addresses factors affecting the therapeutic profiles of drugs delivered by DPI profiles. The article concludes with *DPIs: A Burgeoning Industry*, which surveys the DPI products on the market in 1999 and a selection of those known to be under development. Thoughts on the potential of the DPI dosage form in future therapeutic applications conclude the article.

FINE PARTICLES AND THE SOLID STATE

Crystalline and Amorphous (Glassy) States

Pharmaceutical solids can generally be described as either crystalline or amorphous (or glassy). In fact, the actual solid phase composition of a pharmaceutical formulation is usually characterized by an intermediate composition composed of both crystalline and amorphous character. In a multicomponent system such as a solid formulation comprising drug and excipient(s), certain components or even a single component may be amorphous. Because the amorphous form of a material is always a less stable, higher-energy form than its crystalline counterpart, the distinction between these forms relates to thermodynamic stability of the solid.

Crystalline materials are characterized by a three-dimensional, long-range order that translates into a distinct and unique molecular pattern that can be characterized by X-ray diffraction (XRD) (6). The molecular arrangement of the glassy state resembles that of the liquid state and lacks three-dimensional order. Thus, the classically glassy state has been designated as amorphous, that is, without structure. Pharmaceutical operations commonly used in the manufacture of DPI formulations, such as milling, spray drying, and lyophilization (freeze drying), produce materials possessing amorphous character (7).

Milling of crystalline materials introduces or increases amorphous character as the result of the significant mechanical activation that takes place during the process, including friction, deformation, attrition, and agglomeration (8). The extent of disorder, or amorphous character, introduced by the milling process depends on the behavior of the material and its inherent resistance to the milling-imposed stresses, the amount of energy imposed by the process, and the time scale of energy release. Solid particles formed from the liquid phase, as in spray drying or freeze drying product from solution, are predominantly amorphous materials.

Crystalline materials exhibit a characteristic melting point at which they convert into a liquid form, whereas amorphous materials show no such defined transition. Rather, amorphous materials change on heating from a brittle glassy state to a rubbery state over a narrow temperature range known as the glass transition temperature, or T_g. Orders of magnitude of change in properties such as viscosity and molecular mobility take place near the T_g for amorphous materials; the temperature dependence of these properties near the T_g is typically non-Arrhenius (9). Glassy to rubbery transition is also associated with a stepwise change in the heat capacity. Thus, the T_g of an amorphous material may be determined using a differential scanning calorimeter where a stepwise change in heat flow (corresponding to a change in heat capacity) is observed during sample heating (10). For many hydrophilic drugs and excipients, water acts as a plasticizer, increases molecular mobility, and reduces the glass transition temperature. It is not uncommon for as little as 2–3 wt% water to depress the T_g by 30–40°C. The physical and chemical stability of a glassy material decreases as it approaches the T_g because of that mobility. Thus, the presence of water promotes instability. The rate at which a compound crystallizes from an amorphous state will likewise increase as the temperature of storage approaches T_g and as moisture content is increased (11, 12).

Effect of Physical State on Stability of Dry Powder Formulations

The impact of even subtle changes in physical properties of a DPI formulation can lead to substantial changes in aerosol behavior. Moisture uptake by the hydrophilic components of the formulation can lead to surface dissolution and liquid bridging between particles. This in turn leads to crystal growth, particle fusion, and an increase in particle size, which can result in strongly diminished aerosol performance (13). Powder densification under vibration during unit dose or reservoir filling, as well as product shipping, can also affect the observed aerosol behavior of dry powders.

Because of their greater molecular mobility in the solid state, amorphous systems generally exhibit greater physical and chemical instability at any given temperature compared with their crystalline counterparts. Thus, DPI formulations are desirably prepared in a crystalline state. The low molecular weight of drugs in DPI products currently marketed supports their crystalline nature. Since the late 1980s, there has been increased interest in delivering drugs of biological origin, such as proteins for systemic uptake. These molecules typically do not crystallize and tend to remain amorphous. In freeze-dried and spray-dried biologicals for pulmonary delivery, excipients that act as protectants such as sugars must also remain amorphous to interact with the protein and/or provide a rigid matrix around the protein molecules to restrict and stabilize their motion. As with any amorphous product, physical change can be minimized by storage at temperatures well below the T_g and protection from moisture during handling and storage.

The chemical stability of an amorphous formulation also is usually a function of its storage temperature relative to T_g. The enhanced molecular mobility achieved near the glass transition translates into an increase in translational diffusion-dependent degradation pathways such as aggregation in proteins. It should be recognized that the reaction kinetics near the T_g do not obey Arrhenius kinetics and that extrapolation of the accelerated stability data generated near the T_g to stability at the storage temperature should be viewed with extreme caution. Amorphous materials must be stored well below the glass transition (at least 10°C and typically 40–50°C below T_g) to maintain their physical and chemical stability.

When dealing with partially crystalline materials such as those produced by milling, the impact of water uptake is exaggerated. The amorphous component likely absorbs greater quantities of water than its crystalline counterpart, leading to reduced T_g, increased molecular mobility and both physical and chemical instability.

Bulk Powder Properties

The respirable powders of a DPI cannot be characterized adequately by single particle studies alone; bulk properties must also be assessed because they contribute to ease of manufacture and affect maximal system performance. Primary bulk properties include particle size, particle size distribution, bulk density, and surface area. These properties, along with particle electrostatics, shape, surface morphology, etc., affect secondary bulk powder characteristics such as powder flow, handling, consolidation, and dispersibility.

The characterization and control of primary particle size and the particle size distribution of drug-containing particles are perhaps the most important factors in the design and manufacture of dry powders for inhalation. The size, density, and shape of a particle determine its aerodynamic behavior and therefore its likelihood of depositing in the desired region of the lung. The mean (average) or median (50th percentile) particle size may be based on the number of particles, the mass (or volume) of particles, or even the surface area of particles. The particle size distribution describes the range or frequency of particle sizes occurring in a sample or the width of the particle size distribution in a sample. The variation in these size parameters owing to sampling errors must be considered in characterizing blended powders, powders stored for prolonged periods, or powders that have been mechanically agitated.

Mass median diameter (MMD) is the most common descriptor of primary particle size and may be determined by sieving or centrifugal sedimentation. Volume median diameter, as determined by laser diffraction, may be used as an approximation of MMD provided the particle density is known and does not vary with size and the particle shape is near spherical. The MMD of a powder can be used as a predictor of aerodynamic diameter by:

$$MMAD = MMD \cdot \rho_{true}^{1/2}$$

where MMAD is the mass median aerodynamic diameter, and ρ_{true} is the true density of the particle, usually determined by helium pycnometry. Cohesion/adhesion between particles normally results in the MMAD being larger than predicted. Values of MMAD less than 5 μm are considered necessary to facilitate airborne particle transit past the larynx and deposition within the lung. Powders intended for delivery to the deep lung, such as treatments for asthma or for systemic delivery, require aerodynamic behavior reflected by MMAD values between 1 and 3 μm (14). Particles of MMAD less than approximately 0.5 μm are likely to be exhaled.

Surface area is a bulk powder characteristic directly dependent on particle size distribution, porosity, and morphology. It is commonly determined by nitrogen adsorption, whereby the adsorption isotherm data are fit to a suitable mathematical model from which surface area is derived. If the particle size distribution is sufficiently narrow and the particles are not hollow or porous, the surface area can be used as a measure of change in average particle rugosity or shape. Surface area may be a more sensitive means of monitoring process control during fine particle manufacturing (jet milling or spray drying) than are particle sizing techniques.

Bulk powder density, porosity, and consolidation rate are used as characteristics of powder structure and ease of flow. These properties are typically more difficult to determine for fine respirable powders than for coarse particles owing to the formation of bridging structures caused by high interparticulate interaction. These forces must be overcome by introducing energy, such as ultrasonic vibration or mechanical agitation, to fluidize micron-sized powders in a controllable manner. Carrier-based powder formulations are designed in part to overcome the inherent cohesion of micron-sized particles. In these formulations, the microfine drug adheres to larger carrier particles, improving powder flow and metering capability. For effective delivery, the drug particles must, of course, separate from their carrier on aerosolization and/or inhalation.

Pelletization is often used to improve the flow properties of micron-sized powders. Pelletization converts an ensemble of single particles into larger agglomerates through the formation of weak solid bridges between particles. This process also results in increased bulk powder density (ρ_{bulk}). The solid bridges formed during pelletization may aid powder flow and metering but must be overcome during aerosolization (15).

Bulk powder density must be distinguished clearly from the true density of particles. Bulk powder density is simply the mass of a powder bed divided by its volume. The volume of the powder bed includes the spaces between agglomerates, between primary particles, and the volume of micropores within the particles. These voids within the powder bed volume are collectively the powder porosity. Powder porosity (F) is calculated as:

$$F = (1 - \rho_{true}/\rho_{bulk})$$

The average number of contact points between particles increases as bulk density increases, and the interparticulate forces at these contact points must be overcome to produce a dispersed aerosol cloud. Therefore, a powder of low bulk density may be more easily dispersed as an aerosol than an otherwise identical powder of high bulk density.

However, a powder with low bulk density may be more prone to consolidation than a powder with high bulk density. Powder consolidation can be envisioned as a process of densification or packing of the particles. Consolidation occurs most rapidly during the powder agitation that accompanies powder filling or product shipping; even the imperceptible vibrations a powder experiences during seemingly static storage cause consolidation with time. The rate and extent of consolidation are dependent on particle size distribution and particle shape and can be used to describe the dynamic behavior of powder structures. The extent of powder consolidation, or compressibility, can be evaluated by performing tap density measurements, and using the following relationship:

$$100 \times (\rho_{tap} - \rho_{aerated})/\rho_{tap} = \% \text{ compressibility}$$

where ρ_{tap} is the tapped bulk density, and $\rho_{aerated}$ is the aerated bulk density.

An understanding of the behavior of a powder during the manufacturing process, e.g., during blending, may aid in the identification of an optimal filling and packaging process. Blended powders may also undergo segregation of active particles from carrier particles concurrently with consolidation. Although segregation can lead to poor drug content uniformity, it is in fact desirable in the case of aerosolizing a powder composed of drug blended with a larger particle size carrier.

POWDER PRODUCTION: FORMULATION AND PROCESSING

The primary factor influencing the manufacture of DPI powders is the need to produce material that can penetrate into the lung. The manufacturing of fine particles is challenging, especially with regard to reproducibility. This challenge has resulted in the development of various approaches to the controlled production of fine particles, primarily depending on the nature of the drug. Of the processes described later, micronization and blending and, more recently, spray drying are used most often.

Once manufactured, small particles present another challenge. At small particle diameters, gravity ceases to be the major force exerted on the particles, and instead, interparticle forces become more prominent. The resultant increase in the cohesive and adhesive nature of the particles produces problems such as poor flowability, fillability, and dispersibility. These problems are typically minimized by blending with larger, less cohesive excipient particles such as lactose or pelletization of the individual drug particles. The cohesive nature of particles can be reduced further by modifying the particle surface, the goal of several emerging technologies.

Secondary processing techniques are often employed in powder production to ensure that the stability of the manufactured drug product is ensured. These major technologies are addressed in more detail later.

Formulation

Formulation of dry powders for inhalation must rely on a very short list of excipients to fulfill the customary roles of diluent, stabilizer, solubilizer, processing aid, and property modifier (e.g., flow sustain release agent). Only a few materials are approved in the United States for use in inhalation products, and of those (e.g., propellants, surfactants), many are of little help in dry powder formulation.

Where dose requirements and drug properties allow, drug may be processed in the absence of any excipient, e.g., Astra's Pulmicort Turbuhaler. Most DPIs marketed or under development, however, rely on the addition of lactose as filler and flow enhancer (see *Blending*). Given the proprietary nature of product development, it is not known what additional excipient materials will immerge in the future as safe for inhalation. It is likely, however, that the expansion of inhalation technology to systemic delivery will call for the addition of sugars, buffer salts, and other excipients common to parenteral dosage forms to the list of acceptable inhalation excipients.

Controlled Crystallization or Precipitation

Crystallization, or precipitation, is the process by which particles are produced from solution of the material in a suitable solvent. The level of control over this process determines the physical nature and size of the finished particles. Most pharmaceutical bulk material is produced through crystallization as the final stage of the manufacturing process. The formation of a stable, crystalline material is normally the target of this final step.

In the production of materials for use in DPI products, however, the particle size of the crystallized product is normally too large. Subsequent reduction in particle size is then necessary and can significantly alter the physical nature of the material (16).

Micronization

Micronization is a high-energy particle-size reduction technique that can convert coarse-diameter particles into particles of less than 5 μm in diameter. Different types of equipment can micronize particles, for example, jet or fluid energy mills and ball mills. Although the different equipment have different operating parameters, the fundamental method of reducing the particle size is the same. All techniques involve applying a force on the particle, typically in the form of a collision, either particle–particle or particle–equipment. The force acts at imperfections in the crystal surface, initiating crack propagation through the particle. As the size of the particle decreases, the number of imperfections decreases, thereby making the task of reducing particle size more difficult.

Micronization has been used for the past 50 years to produce small particles for inhalation therapy. However, only in recent years have batch-to-batch reproducibility and stability problems been associated with the technique. Batch-to-batch variations can be caused by morphological differences in starting material; thus, it is critical that a reproducible raw material supply be available. Stability issues typically derive from changes to the varying quantities of amorphous material that are produced by the micronizing process on the surface of the resulting particles (17). This can be minimized through careful control of the micronization process, including processing conditions, batch size, and feed rate, or by the addition of a secondary processing procedure. In addition, micronization can cause decomposition of some materials (18). The issues associated with micronization are forcing many companies to investigate alternative methods of producing small particles.

Blending

The most commonly used method for improving the flowability, fillability, and dispersibility of small cohesive particles is blending the drug with excipient particles, most commonly lactose, of considerably larger particle size. Typically, these large excipient particles are greater than 60 μm, and the small drug particles are less than 5 μm. The objective of the mixing process is to produce an ordered powder in which the small particles attach themselves to the surface of larger "carrier" particles. The challenge is to ensure that the force of adhesion between the drug and carrier is strong enough to withstand segregation during blending and product storage and weak enough to allow separation of the drug particles from the carrier surface on aerosolization (19, 20). During formulation feasibility, the blends are made by mortar and pestle and/or geometric mixing in a tumbling blender. For high-volume production, the process generally involves a high-shear mixer.

The final product performance of a powder blend in a DPI is ultimately dependent on the individual drug and carrier properties as well on the process by which they are blended (21, 22). Small changes in carrier morphology can result in significant variations in the dose received by a patient (16). Again, control of the raw material supply is critical to successful product development. Moreover, secondary processing may be required to ensure that carrier particles behave consistently from batch to batch. Steps that involve transport or storage of the finished blend should be monitored closely to avoid segregation, which occurs when the drug separates from the carrier or when carriers of different sizes separate. Segregation can be minimized by the careful selection of formulation and process equipment. For example, hopper design can play a significant role in minimizing segregation.

Pelletization

Pelletization, which often does not require the use of excipients, may offer an alternative to blending for high-dose therapeutics. The process involves deliberate agglomeration of the fine drug material into less cohesive, larger units (23). Pelletization is usually achieved by vibratory sieving or any process that tumbles powder. All processes require particular attention to time and energy parameters to ensure a consistent product. The resultant pellets must be used in a system capable of deaggregating to an appropriate particle size for aerosol drug delivery (15).

Secondary Processing

As discussed, materials used in dry powder inhalation are predominantly crystalline in nature, with varying degrees of amorphicity. This typically results from the high-energy milling process, which introduces regions of amorphous material within a crystalline material. Occasionally, however, the converse is true. Minimizing any change over time and ensuring that the material is physically stable before final packaging are major formulation challenges. These stability issues tend to be physical in nature, but occasionally chemical changes such as impurity formation also occur.

The technique generally used to minimize the degree of change in crystallinity of the milled product is to eliminate the water or other solvents from the product, usually by packaging the material within a suitable barrier (for example, aluminum foil laminate). Other techniques include the production of a 100% crystalline material, which may eliminate the effects of moisture. This technique, however, may require a secondary production stage of annealing or a quarantine period to allow the product to equilibrate under controlled storage conditions.

The final measure of crystallization effects is assessed by appropriate rigorous stability data [for example, 6 months accelerated stability at 40°C/75% relative humidity (RH)]. This may seem excessive, but measuring the degree of crystallinity is inherently difficult because of low analytical sensitivity (for example, amorphous components below 5 wt%), and pure single-phase standards are difficult to prepare and, subsequently, to measure.

Spray Drying

Spray drying, a process typically used in the production of coarser (up to 500 μm) food, pharmaceutical, and industrial powders, can also be used to prepare microparticulate powders for DPIs (13, 24–26). A typical first step involves creating a solution of the excipients and drug. Dissolving the excipients and drug ensures a uniform distribution of all the excipients and the active drug in the finished powder in contrast to the heterogeneous nature of blended powders. The solution is then atomized and mixed with a drying medium, usually air, or an inert gas if the feed consists of an organic solvent. The solvent is evaporated and removed from the drug solids.

Each spray-dried droplet forms a single particle whose size is determined by the droplet size, the dissolved solids of the feed solution, and the density of the resulting solid particle. For a given formulation and process, both the solid content and density of the powder remain constant within a batch and from batch to batch. Therefore, the distribution of the primary particle size is determined by the droplet size distribution. A narrowly distributed particle size can be achieved with a well-designed atomizer and well-controlled atomizer process parameters.

The droplet has a relatively short residence time (on the order of seconds) in the spray dryer, which minimizes the degradation of heat-sensitive components. In addition, the drug is exposed to a temperature much lower than that at the drying inlet owing to the cooling effect of the solvent evaporation. Control of droplet residence time and the lower temperature defines the amorphous versus crystalline nature of the material.

A spray dryer consists of a feed tank, a rotary or nozzle atomizer, an air heater, a drying chamber, and a cyclone to separate the powder from the air. A rotary atomizer uses centrifugal energy to form the droplet. Pressure nozzle atomizers feed solution to a nozzle under pressure, which forms the droplet. Two fluid nozzles feed solution separately into a nozzle head, which produces high-speed atomizing air that breaks the solution into tiny droplets. Both the feed solution and the drying air are fed into the drying chamber in a standard cocurrent flow (27).

Lyophilization

Lyophilization, although a relatively expensive process, can be a good process for relatively unstable compounds. In lyophilization, the solvent (usually water) is frozen and then removed by sublimation in a vacuum environment. The low temperature maintained during the entire process minimizes thermal degradation of the drug compound.

Typically, the drying process can be divided into primary and secondary phases. During the primary phase, the drug solution is filled into vials and then placed within a temperature-controlled drying chamber. There, the solution is frozen according to physiochemical principles as the shelf temperature is lowered to below freezing. The shelf temperature is subsequently increased but maintained below the freezing point. A vacuum is applied to the chamber to sublimate the solvent. This phase of the drying process extracts the majority of the solvent (50–80%).

During the secondary drying phase, the remainder of the solvent is removed at an elevated but still subfreezing temperature. During freezing, supercooling is necessary to encourage crystallization of the drug compound. The extent to which the compound is supercooled depends on the nature of the compound, the temperature program of the shelf, the heat transfer properties of the container, and the presence of particulates in the solution. The degree of supercooling determines the size of the solvent crystal and, subsequently, the size of the channel formed during primary drying. Consequently, the degree of supercooling affects the rate of sublimation, the rate of secondary drying, and, eventually, the surface area of the finished powder. A goal of secondary drying is to minimize product moisture content.

Therefore, it is most important to select a cooling temperature profile to achieve the desired objective(s). The objective could be simply to achieve a uniform degree of supercooling and freezing or to add an annealing process to allow the solute to crystallize or the ice crystal to grow. The possibility of allowing a long annealing process gives great flexibility to achieve the desired solid-state property for the powder.

The lyophilized cake must then be milled. Compared with particles generated by spray drying, the particle size of milled lyophilized powders generally has a broader distribution than does spray-dried powder, which is formed one particle at a time in a continuous process. Despite the longer processing time necessary to create a dry powder through lyophilization (and the consequent economic implications), this process can provide the formulator with better control of the powder in its solid state.

Supercritical Fluid Technology

Extraction by supercritical fluids, carbon dioxide and propane in particular, is currently being investigated as a means of controlling the size and shape of particles for inhalation. Supercritical fluids are liquids above their critical pressure and temperature (28). Under these conditions, the molecules exhibit the flow, polarity, and solvency properties common of liquids but have the diffusivities and reactivities characteristic of gases.

Precipitation of the particles occurs by two methods involving atomization of a feed: 1) rapid expansion of supercritical solutions containing dissolved drug, and 2) gas antisolvent recrystallization, the supercritical fluid acting as an antisolvent for dissolved drug contained in droplets of another miscible or partially miscible liquid (for example, ethanol, methanol, and acetone).

The second technique, sometimes described as SEDS (solution-enhanced dispersion by supercritical fluids), has been scaled up successfully for an inhalation application to pilot plant manufacture. As with spray drying, this technique is a single-step process. The drug material must show solvency in the cosolvent but complete insolubility in the supercritical carbon dioxide. The resultant solvent-free particles are less cohesive than micronized material as high crystallinity is achieved, leading to decreased charging effects (29). Particle size distributions for these powders are reported to be narrow, with small median aerodynamic diameters (<2.5 μm). In addition, regular particle morphologies are obtained for these thermodynamically stable powders, making them amenable to further processing steps and handling (30).

FILLING AND PACKAGING

The primary consideration when developing systems for packaging dry powders for dose delivery is the goal of delivering the correct drug dosage to the patient. When dealing with drug powders intended for use in DPIs, some basic issues must be considered—specifically, that the drug usually must be delivered in a small volume, which is often difficult to handle owing to small particle size.

The greatest challenge faced in developing packaging systems for dry powders relate to maintaining dispersibility in packaging, which can be affected by compression and electrical charge. Compression of the drug powder, which can be a consequence of excessive handling, can result in an unintended increase in drug concentration. The small drug particles are also vulnerable to alteration in electrical charge, which can result from the motion of particles, against both themselves and the packaging equipment, and from the unintended absorption of water by the drug powder.

Package dose metering can be accomplished by weight or by volume. Dry powders developed for DPIs are formulated to deliver a specific dose of drug per a given unit of drug powder. Drug powders can be packaged either in unit dose or in reservoir systems, each of which has certain advantages (Table 1).

Unit-Dose Systems

Unit-dose systems package drug powders into individual-use packages that contain a known quantity of drug. Patients may use single or multiple units of the drug to obtain a given dose. The greatest advantage of unit-dose systems is that a greater degree of control at the manufacturing level can be maintained. Individual drug doses can be metered by weight or volume. Although metering by weight results in a high degree of accuracy, it is a slow process. Thus, more commonly, unit-dose packaging is metered by volume.

Metering by volume, although offering a reliable means for high-volume production, has disadvantages related to the dispersibility of the drug powder, which in turn can affect the accuracy and precision of the drug dose. Dispersibility can be managed by devising filling processes that optimize powder flow, which will vary by drug compound; by minimizing handling and thereby compression of the drug powder; and by minimizing the relative motion of drug particles against other drug particles and against the filling equipment. Minimizing drug powder motion can reduce electrostatic charging of particles and consequent equipment malfunctions and problems with packaging, which include dose-extraction difficulties and particle dispersion at the time of drug administration.

Unit-dose systems typically rely on blister packaging or capsules to contain the drug until it is dispersed by the delivery device. Blister packages have several advantages over capsules. Those constructed of aluminum are generally impervious to moisture. Inner linings of either polyvinyl chloride or polypropylene create means for sealing the package. Gelatin capsules generally contain approximately 12% water under ambient conditions and thus are a potential source of moisture to powder not equilibrated to ambient relative humidities.

Reservoir Systems

Reservoir systems offer the advantage of variable dosing, generate less waste, are less expensive to manufacture, and are simpler to use than unit-dose systems. Relying on a metering system contained within the delivery device, they

Table 1 Primary packaging for DPI drug formulation

Dosing system	Advantages	Disadvantages
Unit-dose	Simpler, cheaper device, less prone to malfunction	Patient must handle and load individual unit-dose packages into the device before dosing
	Protects powder up to the time when it will be delivered to the patient as an aerosol	Dose titration is limited to dose-quantity available from drug supplier (similar to pills)
Multidose	More convenient for the patient	The device becomes more complex because means to load multiple doses are required
		Also, means for displaying number of doses left are required
		Device may be more prone to malfunction owing to jamming or improper indexing
Reservoir	Multidose and dose titration easy to implement	Powder not generally well protected after reservoir is opened; physical and/or chemical characteristics may deteriorate with time
	Convenient—no separate unit-dose blisters to worry about	Biological contamination may be an issue
		Metering of the dose is carried out by the device, which increases the device complexity; metering often is not adequately controlled because the physical characteristics of the powder are often unknown at the time of dosing

may be less precise in their drug delivery. Because the drug reservoir must be accessed repeatedly, these systems encounter an increased difficulty in maintaining moisture level. Maintaining a highly flowable drug powder in this system may also lead to greater drug formulation challenges.

DEVICES: FORMING THE DRY POWDER AEROSOL

Design Objectives and Constraints

The ultimate goal of all pulmonary delivery devices is to reproducibly deposit the required quantity of drug in the target lung tissues. Many factors influence the selection of a particular DPI design, including the characteristics of the drug to be delivered, its powder formulation, and its associated therapeutic regime. Other factors that must be considered include drug cost, desired dose, market factors, and expected degree of patient compliance.

Drug cost plays an important role in determining the economic feasibility of a device by determining how much of a drug may be lost in administration and routine device use. Drug dose and side effects may determine the reproducibility bounds of particle size and mass of drug delivered that are necessary for effective

therapy. The drug target tissue may determine the importance of achieving a very small particle size; local delivery of drugs to the upper airway may allow for a larger particle size than delivery of particles to the deep lung for systemic absorption. The degree of cohesiveness of the powder particles will determine how much energy the device must transfer to produce a particle of a given size. The therapeutic regime and a range of market factors, such as degree of convenience and cost of other available drugs and/or therapies, may determine how portable or inexpensive the device must be. The anticipated degree of patient compliance may favor some technological solutions over others.

DPIs cannot be considered devices alone but must be considered as components of a larger delivery system, which also includes the formulation of the drug powder, its manufacturing processes, and packaging.

Functional Description

Several DPI designs have been proposed, developed, and successfully marketed in the past 3 decades. Although these devices vary widely in characteristics and operation, they all perform certain basic functions. A DPI must extract the dose from the bulk powder drug package, generate a fine cloud of drug particles by deagglomerating the powder and diluting it with air, and deliver the drug cloud to the patients' airways.

Bulk Powder Drug Package

The first task for a device in delivering a dose is extracting the dose from the drug package. As addressed earlier, two primary alternatives are available: 1) a number of doses may be stored in a powder reservoir, and 2) each dose may be individually packaged as a unit dose. Reservoir systems are inherently multidose. With unit-dose systems, the device may require individual loading of a unit-dose package before inhalation or loading of several unit-dose packages into the device for multidosing.

Energy Sources

Energy input is required to extract the powder from its packaging, generate the fine particle cloud, and dilute it with air. Historically, this energy comes from the patient's inhalation effort (Table 2). In some cases, the energy for extracting/metering the powder comes from the mechanical manipulation of the device by the patient (31, 32). More recent designs use concepts borrowed from the MDI industry or novel approaches involving other technologies.

Uncontrolled vs. on-demand aerosol generation

DPI devices that rely on patient inhalation are inherently on-demand, that is, only when the patient inhales is the aerosol delivered. In contrast, MDIs are inherently uncontrolled, and the patient's breathing maneuver has to be carefully synchronized to the aerosol generation event for effective dosing (Table 3).

DPI devices that rely on sources of energy other than patient inhalation effort may face similar problems as MDIs. Devices may "trigger" the aerosol generation event, which then follows uncontrollably. Alternatively, the delivery of energy to the powder may be modulated by the device and controlled based on monitoring of the patient inhalation maneuver. Table 3 gives some advantages and disadvantages to both approaches.

Homogeneous Powders and Blends

Dry powders must be able to flow readily to leave the capsule or powder reservoir but also must generate a fine aerosol so that the patient can inhale a proper dose. These two requirements are often difficult to achieve simultaneously. Fine powders tend to be cohesive and have poor flow properties. Blending with a carrier phase, pelletization, and other approaches have been used to overcome these limitations. The use of blends and homogeneous powders is compared in Table 4 from a DPI device perspective.

PERFORMANCE AND REGULATORY REQUIREMENTS FOR DPIS

Performance Characterization

Two critical attributes characterize the performance of DPIs: the uniformity of the delivered dose and the aerodynamic assessment of particle size distribution. To determine delivered-dose uniformity, an apparatus capable of quantitatively retaining the delivered dose leaving the device is used. For aerodynamic particle size assessment, a multistage liquid impinger or cascade impactor is used. All aerosol performance testing must be conducted under defined temperature and humidity conditions.

Table 2 Energy sources for delivery

Patient inhalation		Other (air pump, metered propellant, electrical, other)	
Advantages	Disadvantages	Advantages	Disadvantages
No need to coordinate aerosol generation with patient inhalation	Delivery, dispersion performance and thus dose is affected by the patient's ability to inhale at a suitable high flow rate	Decouples aerosol generation from patient ability to perform a correct inhalation maneuver	Adds complexity and cost to the device by increasing the number of subsystems in it
Device is generally very simple in many cases, no moving parts are involved in powder deagglomeration		Allows the extraction and deagglomeration of more cohesive powders because additional energy can be applied in the process	

Performance Specifications

Currently, the United States, European, and British pharmacopoeias specify different requirements for delivered-dose uniformity. Table 5 details these requirements as well as proposed U.S. Food and Drug Administration (FDA) expectations (33). The *Japanese Pharmacopoeia* does not specify a delivered-dose uniformity requirement. Current compendia should be consulted as references.

Of the four pharmacopoeias, the *U.S. Pharmacopeia* (USP) has the strictest requirements for delivered-dose uniformity. Although the *British Pharmacopoeia* (BP) allows the same performance range, the USP defines the range around the label claim, and the BP defines the range around the average value. FDA expectations for delivered-dose uniformity is currently tighter than those specified in all the pharmacopoeias.

The various pharmacopoeias outline appropriate methods for aerodynamic assessment of particle size distribution. The USP defines the size distribution through mass median aerodynamic diameter (MMAD) and geometric standard deviation (GSD). None of the pharmacopoeias specify a requirement for particle size. However, the particle size specifications that are set should be appropriate for the intended use of the product. For example, if the particles are intended to reach the deep lung, the MMAD of particles exiting the device should be less than 5 μm. In general, the smaller the aerosol MMAD, the greater the deposition in the lung.

Two recent trends originating with the FDA may influence the assessment and reporting of aerodynamic particle size distribution. The first is determining the particle size distribution from a single or unit-emitted dose. This may pose an analytical challenge in some cases because the amount of active ingredient in each stage may be present only in trace amounts. The second is setting a drug quantity specification for each stage of the impinger or cascade impactor.

RELEASE AND STABILITY TESTING PARAMETERS

Various dry powder attributes are assessed at release and on stability. These include physical characteristics such as powder appearance, content uniformity, delivered dose uniformity, and particle size distribution. Chemical attributes that may be assessed include drug content, purity, and identity as well as the water content of a powder. Dry powders may also undergo microscopic evaluation for foreign particulate matter, unusual agglomeration, and particle size. Microbial limits also should be examined, including the total aerobic, yeast, and mold counts. The presence of specific pathogens should be ruled out. The dry powders also may be dissolved to test for pH level. In addition, certain compendial requirements for content and delivered-dose uniformity should also be measured.

The USP and *European Pharmacopoeia* (EP) propose that the total aerobic count not exceed 100 CFU/g, that the total yeast count and mold count not exceed 10 CFU/g, and that no specific pathogens be detectable. Specifications for the other attributes should be based on the intended use

Table 3 Control of aerosol generation

Uncontrolled		On-demand	
Advantages	**Disadvantages**	**Advantages**	**Disadvantages**
Device is simpler; no feed-back systems are required to monitor the patient.	More prone to patient misuse	Aerosol is delivered when patient can inhale it most effectively	Device is more complex because feed-back systems (mechanical or electronic) are required
"Violent" aerosol generation processes are allowable, permitting the delivery of large amounts of energy to the powder in a very short period of time	Typically requires the use of a holding chamber to store the aerosol in between generation and patient inhalation, resulting in a larger-size device	Better dose control	Energy delivery to the powder has to be very well-controlled
			Device may be more prone to failure

Table 4 Influence of powder behavior on device design

| Blends (lactose carrier) | | Homogeneous powders | |
Advantages	Disadvantages	Advantages	Disadvantages
Powder can be easily extracted from its packaging	On delivery, coughing and other unpleasant sensations may be induced because the carrier particles deposit in the mouth and throat	Little mouth and throat deposition; patient does not "feel" he/she is inhaling an aerosol	Formulation process becomes a key factor in the development of the product; the properties of the compound to be delivered dominate the performance of the resulting powder
Inclusion of the c arrier phase usually facilitates dispersion	A larger amount of powder needs to be moved and dispersed; in terms of energy requirements, united dispersion may be offset by the increase in payload		

and the historical performance of the product. As with other dosage forms, specifications must be met throughout the intended shelf life of the product.

The International Conference on Harmonization (ICH) has identified stability requirements for room temperature storage and testing intervals. It recommends that dry powders be stored at 25°C and 60% RH for real-time conditions; at 40°C and 75% RH for accelerated conditions; and 30°C and 60% RH if significant change is observed at accelerated conditions. The ICH recommends testing samples every 3 months for the first year, every 6 months for the second year, and yearly thereafter. In addition to these requirements, the FDA suggests a storage condition at 25°C and 75% RH if significant change is observed at the accelerated condition. Six-month data would be required at the time of the New Drug Application (NDA) submission, and the study must cover 1 year.

When an NDA is submitted, the FDA requires that 12 months of data be collected at real-time conditions and 6 months of data be collected under accelerated conditions. If significant change is observed at 6 months for the accelerated condition, 6-month data at the 30°C and 60% RH condition must be submitted, and the study must cover 1 year.

ROLE OF DPIS IN THERAPY

Some direct comparisons of DPI and MDI for the same drug have been made in the interest of developing alternative but comparable products for patients. The therapeutic performance of inhalation delivery systems is as dependent on the patient as it is on the product itself. Therefore, some demonstration of clinical comparability is generally required to support product substitution.

The deposition pattern of the inhaled dry powder aerosol can be strongly influenced by the patient's inhalation dynamics and lung anatomy. At high inhalation flow rates, a given particle will have a greater tendency to impact the back of the throat or to deposit in the upper airways. For those delivery systems requiring high flow to deaggregate the powder particles, deep lung deposition is less accessible. The proliferation of device designs has been in part the result of attempts to minimize dosing variability regardless of source (34).

The target for lung deposition varies depending on the therapy under consideration. In the treatment of asthma by β-adrenergic agonists, the Central airways are generally targeted. On the other hand, therapies intended to treat alveolar disease, chronic obstructive pulmonary disease, or systemic conditions must reach the peripheral regions of the deep lung.

Among the pharmacokinetic advantages offered by delivery to the lung are fast onset of action and lack of first-pass effect. Doses to the lung can prove 10–20 times more effective than oral dosing and for local therapy can result in substantially reduced side effects.

In a study, three different fluticasone propionate products—an MDI and two DPI products, Diskhaler and Diskus—were directly compared in healthy volunteers and patients (35). The systemic drug bioavailability was highest for the MDI, whereas the bioavailability was similar for the two DPIs. The pharmacokinetic results are consistent with the in vitro evaluation in which the MDI gave the highest fine particle dose (FPD), whereas the two

Table 5 Product quality requirements

Pharmacopoeia	First-stage testing ($N = 10$)	Second-stage testing (additional 20)
United States	NMT (Not more than) 1 of 10 outside the range of 75.0–125.0% of label claim None outside the range of 65.0–135.0% of label claim; if 2–3 are outside of 75.0–125.0% and none are outside of 65.0–135.0% proceed to second stage	NMT 3 of 30 outside the range of 75.0–125.0% of label claim; none outside the range of 65.0–135.0% of label claim
British	NMT 1 of 10 outside the range of 75–125% of average value None outside the range of 65–135% of average value; if 2–3 are outside of 75–125% and none are outside of 65–135%, proceed to second stage	NMT 3 of 30 outside the range of 75–125% of average value; none outside the range of 65–135% of average value
European	NMT 1 of 10 outside the range of 65–135% of average value; none outside the range of 50–150% of average value If 2–3 are outside of 65–135% and none are outside of 50–150%, proceed to second stage	NMT 3 of 30 outside the range of 65–135% of average value; none outside the range of 50–150% of average value
FDA, proposed[a]	NMT 1 of 10 outside the range of 80–120% of label claim None outside the range of 75–125% of label claim; if 2–3 are outside of 80–120% and none are outside of 75–125%, proceed to second stage	NMT 3 of 30 outside the range of 80–120% of label claim; none outside the range of 75–125% of label claim
Japan	No delivered-dose uniformity specification	N/A

[a](From Ref. 30.)

Table 6 Earliest dry powder inhalation systems

Year introduced	Name	Manufacturer	Indication	Packaging/ metering	Energy source(s)	Blend
1949	Aerohaler	Abbott	Asthma, COPD	Unit dose; "sifter" cartridge	Mechanical, patient inspiration	No
1971	Spinhaler	Fisons (now Aventis)	Asthma, COPD	Unit dose; hard gelatin capsule	Mechanical, patient inspiration	Yes
1977	Rotahaler	Allen and Hanburys (now Glaxo)	Asthma, COPD	Unit dose; hard gelatin capsule	Mechanical, patient inspiration	Yes
1988	Turbuhaler	Astra	Asthma, COPD	Reservoir	Mechanical, patient inspiration	No
	Diskhaler	Allen and Hanburys (now Glaxo)	Asthma, COPD	Multidose blister	Mechanical, patient inspiration	Yes
	Inhalator	Boehringer–Ingelheim	Asthma, COPD	Unit dose; hard gelatin capsule	Mechanical, patient inspiration	Yes

Table 7 More recent dry powder inhalation systems[a]

Name	Manufacturer	Packaging/metering	Energy source(s)
Pulvinal	Chiesi	Reservoir	Mechanical, patient inspiration
Easyhaler	Orion	Reservoir	Mechanical, patient inspiration
Clickhaler	ML Labs	Reservoir	Mechanical, patient inspiration
Discus	Glaxo	Multidose blister	Mechanical, patient inspiration
Monohaler	Astra	Unit dose	Mechanical, patient inspiration
AIR[b]	Alkermes	Unit dose	Mechanical, patient inspiration
Spiros[b]	Dura	Multidose blisters	Mechanical, not driven by patient inspiration
Inhance™ Pulmonary Delivery System	Inhale	Unit dose	Mechanical, not driven by patient inspiration

[a]This list is not exhaustive. Many other manufacturers, in both the United States and Europe, are also developing dry powder inhalation drug-delivery systems.
[b]In clinical trials; not yet on the market.

DPIs had similar FPD values. It was also reported that in a separate study using healthy volunteers, the pharmacokinetics of a nonchlorofluorocarbon formulation have been shown to be similar to that for the original chlorofluorocarbon formulation for a fluticasone propionate MDI product. Consistent with their similar pharmacokinetic results, the clinical performance of Diskhaler and Diskus is similar in both children and adults (36, 37).

DPIS: A BURGEONING INDUSTRY

The first commercially available DPI system appeared on the market in 1949, developed and marketed by Abbott under the name Aerohaler. Like all pulmonary drug-delivery methods that existed before now, it delivered small molecule compounds (brochodilators or inhaled corticosteroids) to the airway (not necessarily to the deep lung) for the treatment of asthma or chronic obstructive pulmonary disease. Table 6 lists some of the early DPI systems and their basic characteristics.

Table 7 presents some of the newer entrants in the DPI field, most still focusing on local delivery of small molecule drugs to the airway for asthma or COPD but some in clinical trials for systemic delivery of macromolecules such as insulin via the deep lung.

New DPI technologies in development by Inhale Therapeutic Systems and Alkermes are enabling the delivery of macromolecules to the deep lung. Leading this field is Inhale's insulin product, currently in the phase 3 trials with Pfizer. In the next years, it is expected that dry powder inhalation will become a broadly accepted and effective means of delivering a wide variety of therapeutics–antibiotics, analgesics, antibodies, hormones, proteins, and perhaps gene therapeutics. The potential of this technology continues to be explored.

ACKNOWLEDGMENT

We thank D.B. Bennett, S. Duddu, S. Fong, S. Wong, J. Lord, J. Parks, C. Schuler, and S. White for their contributions to this article.

REFERENCES

1. Steed, K.P.; Freund, B.; Zierenberg, B.; Newman, S.P. Proceedings of Drug Delivery to the Lungs VI London UK, 1995; *14–15.*
2. Crompton, G.K. The Adult Patients' Difficulties with Inhalers. Lung **1990,** *659–662.*
3. Stahlhofen, W.; Gebhart, J.; Heyder, J. Experimental Determination of the Regional Deposition of Aerosol Particles in the Human Respiratory Fact. J. Am. Int. Hyg. Assoc. J. **1980,** *41,* 385–398.
4. Byron, P.R. Pulmonary Targeting with Aerosols. Pharm. Tech. **1987,** *11,* 42–56.
5. Wong, D.Y.T.; Wright, P.; Aulton, M.E. Influence of Drug Particle Size on the Performance of Dry Powder Inhalations of Nedocromil Sodium Proceedings of the 14th Pharmaceutical Technology Conference, Barcelona, Spain, 1995; *3,* 86–108.
6. Ford, J.L.; Timmins, P. *Pharmaceutical Thermal Analysis, Techniques And Applications*; Ellis Horwood: Chichester, UK, 1989.
7. Elamin, A. *Effect of Milling and Spray Drying on Water Interactions and Physicochemical Properties of Pharmaceutical Materials*; Uppsala University: Sweden, 1994.
8. Sebhatu, T.; Angberg, M.; Ahlneck, C. Assessment of the Degree of Disorder in Crystalline Solids by Isothermal Microcalorimetry. Int. J. Pharm. **1994,** *104,* 135–144.
9. Oksanen, C.A.; Zografi, G. The Relationship Between the Glass Transition Temperature and Water Vapour Absorption by Polyvinyl Pyrrolidone. Pharm. Res. **1990,** *7,* 654–657.
10. Saleki-Gerhardt, A.; Ahlneck, C.; Zografi, G. Assessment of Disorder in Crystalline Solids. Int. J. Pharm. **1994,** *101,* 237–247.
11. Hancock, B.C.; Zografi, G. The Relationship Between the Glass Transition Temperature and the Water Content of Amorphous Pharmaceutical Solids. Pharm. Res. **1994,** *11,* 471–477.
12. Hancock, B.C.; Shamblin, S.L.; Zografi, G. Molecular Mobility of Amorphous Pharmaceutical Solids below their Glass Transition Temperatures. Pharm. Res. **1995,** *12,* 799–806.
13. Venthoye, M.G. *Characterization of an Amorphus Dry Powder Aerosol System*; Ph.D. Thesis, London University, 1997.
14. Curry, S.H.; Taylor, A.J.; Evans, S. Br. J. Clin. Pharmacol. **1995,** *2,* 267–270.
15. Wetterlin, K.I. Design and Function of the Turbohaler®. *A New Concept in Inhalation Therapy*; Newman, S.P., Moren, F., Crompton, G.K., Eds.; Medicom: Amsterdam, 1987, 85–89.
16. Kassem, N.M. *Generation of Deeply Inspirable Clouds From Dry Powder Mixtures*; Ph.D. Thesis, University of London, 1990.
17. Ward, G.H.; Schultz, R.K. Process-Induced Crystallinity Changes in Albuterol Sulphate and its Effect on Powder Physical Stability. Pharm. Res. **1995,** *12,* 773–779.
18. Rogerson, C. The Design and Production of Microparticles for Inhalation Proceedings of Recent Advances in Dry Powder Inhalers. London, 1996
19. Moren, F. In Vitro and In Vivo Performance of Powder Inhalers, Proceedings of Respiratory Drug Delivery II Interpharm Press: Buffalo Grove, IL, 1990
20. Zanen, P.; Van Spiegel, P.I.; Van der Kolk, H.; Tushnizen, E.; Enthoven, R. The Effect of Inhalation Flow on the Performance of a Dry Powder Inhalation System. Int. J. Pharm. **1992,** *81,* 199–203.
21. Kassem, N.M.; Ho, K.K.L.; Ganderton, D. The Effect of Air Flow and Carrier Size on the Characteristics of an Inspirable Cloud. J. Pharm. Pharmacol. **1989,** *41* (Suppl), 14p.
22. Ganderton, D.; Kassem, N. Dry Powder Inhalers. Advan. Pharm. Sci. **1992,** *6,* 165–191.
23. Bell, J.H. Pelletised Medicament Formulations, Fisons Patent, Application No. 152047, 1975.
24. Vidgren, M.T.; Vidgren, P.A.; Paronen, T.P. Comparison of Physical and Inhalation Properties of Spraydried and Mechanically Micronised Disodium Cromoglycate. Int. J. Pharm. **1987,** *35,* 139–144.
25. Chawla, A. *Spray-Dried Powders For Use In Dry Powder Aerosol Formulation*; Ph.D. Thesis, University of London, 1993.
26. Chawla, A.; Taylor, K.M.G.; Newton, J.M.; Johnson, M.C.R. Production of Spraydried Salbutamol Sylphate for Use in Dry Powder Aerosol Formulation. Int. J. Pharm. **1994,** *108,* 233–240.
27. Masters, K. *Longman Scientific and Technical. Spray Drying Handbook*, 5th Ed.; John Wiley & Sons: New York, 1991.
28. Phillips, E.M.; Stella, V.J. Rapid Expansion from Supercritical Solutions: Application to Pharmaceutical Processes. Int. J. Pharm. **1993,** *94,* 1–10.
29. York, P. Solid-State Properties of Powders in the Formulation and Processing of Solid Dosage Forms. Int. J. Pharm. **1983,** *14,* 1–28.
30. York, P. New Approaches to the Preparation of Particles for Inhalation. Proceedings of Recent Advances in Dry Powder Inhalers. London, 1996.
31. Schultz, R.K.; Miller, N.C.; Smith, D.K.; Ross, D.L. Powder Aerosols with Auxiliary Means of Dispersion. J. Biopharm. Sci. **1992,** *3,* 115–122.

32. Hill, M. Characteristics of An Active Multiple Dose Dry Powder Inhaler, Proceedings of Respiratory Drug Delivery. IV Interpharm Press: Buffalo Grove, IL, 1994; 109–116.

33. Guidance for Industry. *Metered Dose Inhaler (MDI) and Dry Powder Inhaler (DPI) Drug Products, Chemistry, Manufacturing, and Controls Documentation Draft*; U.S. Food and Drug Administration: Department of Health and Human Services: Rockville, MD, October 1998.

34. Timsina, M.P.; Martin, G.P.; Marriott, C.; Ganderton, D.; Yianneskis, M. Drug Delivery to the Respiratory Tract Using Dry Powder Inhalers. Int. J. Pharm. **1994**, *101*, 1–13.

35. Johnson, M. Fluticasone Propionate: Pharmacokinetic and Pharmacodynamic Implications of Different Aerosol Delivery Systems, Respiratory Drug Delivery VI, **May 3–7, 1998,** 61–70

36. Cater, J.I.; Vare, M.; Peters, W.J.; Olsson, B.; Gomez, E. Comparison of the Efficacy of Fluticasone Propionate Given Twice Daily via the Diskus™/Accuhaler™ and the Diskhaler™ in Patients with Asthma. Eur. Resp. J. **1995**, *8*, 427S.

37. Bousquet, J.; Tosserard, B.; Medley, H.V. Double-Blind Parallel Group Study to Compare the Long Term Clinical Efficacy and Safety of Two Different Methods of Administering Inhaled Fluticasone Propionate in Chronic Severe Asthmatic Patients. Eur. Resp. J. **1995**, *8*, 427S.

INHALATION, LIQUIDS

Michael E. Placke
Jeffrey Ding
William C. Zimlich, Jr.
Battelle Pulmonary Therapeutics, Inc., Columbus, Ohio

INTRODUCTION

Using the inhalation route to deliver therapeutic aerosols is a common practice in the treatment of patients with various airway diseases. Drug delivery via inhalation offers many advantages in the administration of pharmaceutical compounds, because the drugs are delivered directly to the site of action. Therefore, the required therapeutic dose for each treatment is lower than if the dose is administrated via oral or parenteral routes. As a consequence, the inhalation route reduces adverse effects due to systemic absorption and intensifies the amount of drug deposited to the targeted tissue. In the U.S. market, bronchodilator, anticholinergic, anti-inflammatory, and corticosteroid drugs are common inhaled dosage forms used for the treatment of respiratory diseases, such as asthma and COPD. Additional drug classes, such as antibiotics, antifungals, and antiviral compounds, are also used or under development for topical delivery via inhalation. Further, new inhaled applications are being developed for the treatment of systemic diseases. These products include both small and macromolecules. Pulmonary delivery of peptides and proteins is a rapidly growing area of inhaled drug delivery, spearheaded by the development of inhaled insulin for treatment of diabetes.

An aerosol is defined in its simplest form as a collection of solid or liquid particles suspended in a gas such as air. Aerosols are two-phase systems consisting of the particulates and the gas in which they are suspended (1). Aerosol science has been studied for many decades in various disciplines, especially related to environmental sciences, to understand the health effects associated with exposure to air pollutants. These activities have improved our understanding of the dynamic behavior of aerosol particles and their relative effects on human health, but also laid the foundation for the pharmaceutical industry to use inhalation of aerosols for therapeutic purposes. Pharmaceutical aerosols deliver therapeutically active drug compounds to the human respiratory tract for local or systemic actions. This dosage form is intended to be inhaled through either the mouth or the nose. The increasing use of inhalation therapy has been mainly driven by the confluence of three factors:

1. Advances in aerosol generation technology, which provide more efficient and controlled delivery of aerosolized pharmaceutical compounds into the human respiratory airway;
2. Advances in biotechnology, with the development of new therapeutic agents that are often difficult to deliver by other routes of administration;
3. A better understanding of the pathophysiology of disease, which allows physicians and scientists to envision a broader range of therapeutic options.

Those involved with the pulmonary delivery of therapeutic agents are challenged in all three areas, especially the first two. We can now develop new therapies, but we must be certain that we can reproducibly deliver those therapeutic agents to the desired site, in the dosage and form in which they will be most effective (2).

The benefit of using the respiratory airways as a route for drug delivery has been increasingly explored over the last 10 years (3). The large surface area of the human respiratory system, sometimes compared to the size of a tennis court (~ 100 m^2), is an attractive target site for pulmonary delivery of drugs intended for absorption into the blood. Drug administration via inhalation has many advantages for the systemic delivery of pharmaceutical compounds such as proteins and peptides, which are often degraded when delivered through the GI tract and avoid the need for repeated injections (4).

Inhaled aerosols also provide high drug concentrations in the respiratory tract. The treatment of airway diseases by aerosol inhalation is beneficial because of intensified localized drug deposition and fewer side effects. Consequently, smaller doses are needed to achieve the therapeutic level in the lungs via inhalation thereby avoiding high systemic levels of the drug. Therefore, inhaled drug aerosols have become the standard clinical approach for managing asthma, respiratory distress syndrome (RDS), chronic obstructive pulmonary disease (COPD), cystic fibrosis, and other respiratory tract diseases (5). Despite

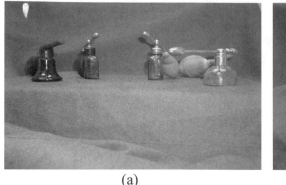 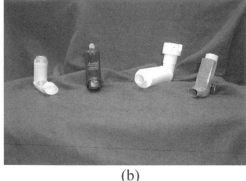

(a)   (b)

Fig. 1 Drug delivery devices. (a) Squeezing bulb nebulizers (courtesy of Bruce McVeety) and (b) pMDIs.

the spectrum of opportunities that now exists for new inhaled therapies, successful development of pulmonary drug products is a challenging task. The problems and barriers are multidisciplinary in nature, perhaps explaining why this field has not accelerated faster (6).

Using aerosolization to administer drugs to the respiratory airway dates back to the early part of the 20th century, when the pneumatic nebulizer was used as a drug delivery device. Fig. 1a shows some examples of the first types of nebulizers used, the simplest of which were powered by squeezing the bulb attached to the device. Fig. 1b shows more modern units such as pMDIs.

The nebulization principle for the squeeze-bulb nebulizers is the same as many conventional nebulizers. Liquid is forced through a small critical orifice. The particle size of aerosol generated from the early squeeze-bulb nebulizers was generally large (due to the inability to accurately machine small holes) and, therefore, largely unsuitable for human inhalation. However, the concept of delivering drug products via inhalation was an important milestone that established the foundation for developing better pulmonary drug delivery technology.

The modern pressurized metered dose inhaler (pMDI) was developed between 1955 and 1956. However, the pMDI had its roots in research carried out many years before (7). During the 1930s and 1940s, the discovery of liquefied propellants (chlorinated-fluorocarbons or freon propellants) such as CFC12, CFC114, CFC11, and CFC22 was a major step in the realization of a portable inhaler. However, the first pMDI was not invented until 1956, when the metering valve used in the device was developed and patented (7).

The invention of the first pMDI by Riker Laboratories (now 3M Pharmaceuticals) was described in detail recently, and was approved by the FDA in March 1956 (8). The Medihaler-Ept™ and Medihaler-Iso™ were launched at the same time. Illustrations from the first brochure of these inhalers are presented in Fig. 2. The Medihaler-Iso was changed to accommodate suspension formulations during 1957. This proved particularly useful for formulating difficult to solubilize drugs, such as many of the steroids later developed for the treatment of asthma. The successful innovation of the pMDI established the foundation for the development of drug delivery via

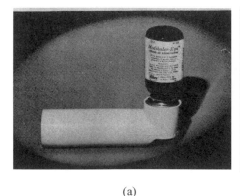 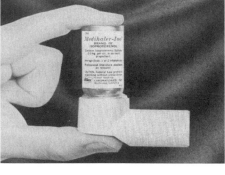

(a)   (b)

Fig. 2 The metered dose inhaler. (a) Medihaler-Ept and (b) Medihaler-Iso. (Courtesy of Charles Thiel.)

respiratory airways and remained the primary small volume nebulizer for the next 40 years.

Successful administration of any pharmaceutical compound to the human respiratory airway requires the generation and delivery of the drug in the form of an suitable for human inhalation. The human airway is a very complex structure that has evolved to serve two purposes: 1) exchanging gases vital to metabolism (O_2 and CO_2) and 2) defending against foreign particulates from entering the lungs. The generation of drug aerosols and their site of deposition in human lungs are dependent on many factors, such as the physical and chemical properties of aerosol particles, the mechanism of action and quality of performance of the drug delivery device, the patient's breathing pattern, and the morphometry of the human lungs. These factors are significant because:

- Aerosol properties, such as particle size distribution, aerosol velocity, and hygroscopicity, affect aerosol deposition in the human lungs. Aerosol size distribution, including mass median aerodynamic diameter (MMAD) and geometric standard deviation (GSD), is one of the most important variables in governing the site of droplet or particle deposition in the lungs (3).
- Device characteristics play an important role in the delivery of pharmaceutical compounds to human lungs. The mechanism by which aerosols are created affect particle size distribution, kinetics of aerosol delivery, and the reproducibility of drug dosing from the delivery device. These factors are key to controlling the delivery of a constant amount of drug aerosol across a diverse patient population.
- The breathing patterns or maneuvers of a patient can also significantly affect the site of aerosol deposition in the human lungs, even of aerosols with similar characteristics (e.g., MMAD and GSD). Aerosol deposition mechanisms in the airway mainly consist of sedimentation, inertial impaction, and diffusion. Pharmaceutical aerosols deposit mainly by sedimentation and impaction. Therefore, aerosols delivered under high velocity conditions, either due to high ballistic velocity produced by the device or due to high patient inspiratory flow rates, result predominantly in deposition due to inertial impaction, markedly enhancing conducting airway deposition. Conversely, deposition in the peripheral lung can be promoted by decreasing the velocity of an aerosol during inhalation. Further, deposition of these particles that reach the deep lung can be enhanced by a postinspiratory pause (i.e., breath-hold), allowing particles to settle more completely.

- Morphometry of the upper and lower airways will also affect the drug deposition in the lungs. Anatomical conditions such as airway size, disease status, and degree of obstruction are different from patient to patient; thus there will be variability in the site of drug deposition between patients.

The inhalation drug delivery devices currently available commercially consist of metered dose inhalers (MDIs), dry powder inhalers (DPIs), and nebulizers. The advantages and disadvantages of those devices have been reviewed extensively in the literature. This article will focus on the inhalation of aerosols generated from liquid systems using either small volume inhalers, or larger home or clinical nebulizers. Aerosols produced in powder form are covered in another chapter. Various drug delivery devices, including those available commercially and those under development, will be discussed in detail, so that the reader will have a better understanding of the advantages and disadvantages of those devices for pulmonary drug delivery. An emphasis will be given to new pulmonary drug delivery device technology in development, and its potential application to deliver pharmaceutical compounds for both local targeting and systemic absorption of drugs intended to act outside the lung. Over the last 10 years, many innovations have occurred in the area of inhalation drug delivery stimulated by advances in aerosol generation technology and the demand created by new biopharmaceuticals.

COMMERCIALLY AVAILABLE PULMONARY DELIVERY TECHNOLOGY

The inhalation drug delivery devices currently available commercially consist of metered dose inhalers (MDIs), dry powder inhalers (DPIs) and nebulizers. The effective performance (or lack thereof) of the inhalation devices is well recognized as being crucial in how effective a pulmonary delivered drug is in the treatment of diseases, both topical and systemic disorders. In order for a drug to be effective by inhalation, the generated aerosol must be of proper size to be deposited in the targeted location. The patient needs to inhale the drug formulation properly, and the drug must be deposited with sufficient quantity at the action site so that it can be absorbed or distributed effectively. The drug delivery devices available commercially have been used widely for the treatment of airway diseases such as asthma and chronic obstructive pulmonary diseases (COPDs). Such treatment is effective mainly because of the wide therapeutic index of the drug compounds. It is useful to review the advantages and disadvantages of current device technologies to provide a better understanding of how the devices are used by patients and what kind of improvements are needed to deliver various drug compounds by inhalation. This article is limited to discussion of devices that generate liquid drug aerosols as solutions, suspensions, and emulsions[a]

There are several ways to categorize drug delivery devices. The inhalation drug delivery devices discussed in this chapter are categorized according to their operating principles or fundamental mechanism of generating aerosols.

Pressure-Driven Devices

Jet nebulizers

The jet nebulizer has been used for many years to treat airway diseases both in the clinical setting and in home use. The jet nebulizer utilizes compressed gas from an air source either from a hospital air line or from a portable compressor to convert the liquid drug solution into small droplets by forcing the liquid through a small hole known as a critical orifice. Atomization occurs as a result of the disruption of the surface tension holding the liquid together by the action of internal and external forces. In the absence of such disruptive forces, surface tension tends to pull the liquid into the form of a sphere, since this has the minimum amount of surface energy (9). The droplets produced by atomization contain many large drops, which will undergo further disruption to form small particles. The particle size of the droplets will depend not only on the kinetic energy used during the nebulization, but also the pore diameter of the critical orifice and on the physical properties of the liquid formulation.

The jet nebulizer is driven by air pressurized typically at 20–40 psi. The compressed air accelerates through a narrow orifice to break the bulk liquid into sheets, jets, films, or streams. Those ligaments are accelerated to a velocity sufficient to impact on baffles or on the nebulizer wall. The outgoing air becomes saturated with water vapors derived from the liquid retained in the nebulizer, and this has two important consequences:

1. The nebulizer is cooled and reaches an equilibrium temperature approximately 10°C below ambient, so that the patient inhales a relatively cool aerosol cloud.
2. The evaporation of water causes the concentration of solutes to increase with time as the vehicle carrier evaporates (10).

[a]Devices producing liquid dry powder aerosols is discussed in *Inhalation, Dry Powder*, page 1529–1544.

Droplet formation: A general theory for the formation of droplets by nebulization has not been fully developed, although the understanding of the nebulization principle has been improved with mathematical modeling. A rigorous mathematical description of droplet formation requires knowledge of distribution of aerodynamic pressure on the droplet surface and the interaction of this pressure with internal forces acting on the droplets. Therefore, before further discussing of the effect of various parameters on the nebulization performance, it is beneficial to consider briefly the various ways in which a single droplet of liquid can break up under the action of aerodynamic forces. Once the droplets are generated using a compressed air source during the primary atomization, unstable droplets experience further disintegration to form smaller particles, which is referred to as "secondary atomization." The formation of a single droplet under the aerodynamic forces exerted by the external sources, together with the internal forces of the liquid formulation, such as surface tension and viscosity, dictate the formation of the droplet. The relationship between these forces was described by Klusener (11), who offered the following equation:

$$P_1 = P_a + P_\sigma = \text{constant} \tag{1}$$

where P_1 is the internal pressure at any point on the droplet surface, P_a is the external aerodynamic pressure due to the compressed air source, and P_σ is the pressure caused by the surface tension. From the equation, it is observed that a droplet can maintain its stability as long as the change in the air pressure, P_a, is balanced by a corresponding change in the pressure caused by surface tension, so that the internal pressure remain constant. When the aerodynamic pressure is greater than the pressure due to surface tension, the external pressure will deform the droplet in order to reduce the pressure by surface tension to maintain the constant internal pressure. This deformation will continue to break up the droplet into smaller particles (9).

For a formulation with low viscosity, such as aqueous formulation, the viscous force is relatively small compared with the surface tension force. Under such relative conditions, a dimensionless parameter can be obtained, as shown in Eq. 2 (8). For a given liquid with low viscosity, the critical condition for the droplet to break up occurs when the aerodynamic force equals the surface tension, expressed as

$$C_D \frac{\pi d^2}{4} 0.5\rho V^2 = \pi d\sigma \tag{2}$$

where C_D is the coefficient of drag, d is the diameter of the droplet, ρ and σ are the density and surface tension of the liquid, respectively. From the above equation one can calculate the maximum stable droplet diameter,

$$d_{\max} = \left(\frac{8\sigma}{C_D \rho V^2}\right) \qquad (3)$$

and the critical velocity at which the droplet will disrupt

$$V_{crit} = \left(\frac{8\sigma}{C_D \rho d}\right)^{0.5} \qquad (4)$$

The equation can also be expressed as the dimensionless parameter called the Weber number, as

$$We_{crit} = \left(\frac{\rho V^2 d}{\sigma}\right)crit = \frac{8}{C_D} \qquad (5)$$

which is the ratio of external aerodynamic force to surface tension force. Using the above equations, the maximum diameter at a particular critical velocity can be estimated. However, it should be noted that the estimated diameter results from only the process of primary atomization. Secondly, atomization will generally decrease and exaggerate the particle size distribution. Additionally, when a droplet impacts a baffle immediately after the primary atomization, the droplet diameter drops sharply. Baffles are used in nebulizer systems to help control the particle size distribution of the droplets so that generated aerosols are within a desired particle size range, usually with mean values that are less than 10 μm and preferably less than 5 μm, for effective deposition in the human lungs.

Effect of physical properties of formulation: The physical properties of the formulation, such as viscosity and surface tension, are important parameters that affect the process of nebulization. Surface tension can be considered as a consolidating influence that attempts to minimize the production of increased surface area, and the liquid viscosity exerts a stabilizing influence by opposing any change in the shape of droplets as they are produced (12). Studies (13) have shown that the droplet size is proportional to the liquid surface tension for low-viscosity liquids, while the density has only a small effect on the droplet size. The effect of viscosity on the droplet size seems to be complex. Research by Searls and Snyder (14) showed that high-viscosity liquids not only have increased nebulization time (decreasing the mass output), but also reduced mean particle size. However, Hinds et al. (15) reported little change in droplet size with viscosity ranged from 17 to over 100 cP using a Laskin aerosol generator operated at 20 psi.

An extensive study was conducted by McCallion et al. (16) investigating the effects of different physicochemical properties on the performance of the jet nebulizer.

Materials with different viscosity and surface tension were nebulized using three different nebulizers, Pari LC (Pari-Werk GmbH, Starnberg, Germany), Sidestream (Medic Aid, Pagham, United Kingdom), and Cirrus (Intersurgical Complete Respiratory Care, Workingham, United Kingdom). However, only data from the Pari LC nebulizer were presented in the paper. The particle size distribution of the aerosols was quantified using laser diffraction, which has been shown by Clack (17) to be a robust and reliable technique having good correlation with in vivo deposition data. Table 1 shows the experimental data for different formulations obtained using the Pari LC jet nebulizer. The mass median diameters were obtained using two nebulization flow rates, 6 and 8 L/min, respectively. The authors concluded that the more viscous fluids tended to produce smaller droplets. Within a specific range of the surface tension, of approximately 70 dyne/cm (70.0–72.9 dyne/cm), the mass median diameter decreased from 3.2 to 2.5 μm as the viscosity increased from 1.0 to about 6.0 centipoise. The same was true for surface tension of approximately 20 dyne/cm: as the viscosity increased, the particle size decreased. The effect of surface tension on particle size distribution was not as clear. However, the authors pointed out that a correlation between surface tension and mass median diameter appeared to exist when the fluid systems were analyzed separately. In glycerol and propylene glycol solutions, surface tension was directly proportional to droplet size, while the converse was true for silicone fluids. A trend was reported for the other two nebulizers tested, but no data were presented (18, 19).

Drug concentration effects: Because of the large volume of air used during nebulization, there is continuous evaporative loss of any solvent, such as water. This phenomenon has been described in several studies (20–23). Theoretically, the increase in drug concentration will continue until the solute concentration in the reservoir reaches the limit of drug solubility, at which point precipitation may occur. In practice, many drugs used in nebulizers (such as bronchodilators) are very hydrophilic, and the nebulizer solutions are formulated at concentrations well below the solubility limit (3), so there is little issue with precipitation. However, this results in changing particle size distribution with variable deposition patterns, and a change in the unit dose given per unit time. Collectively, this produces variable and unpredictable deposited doses for many drug products. The magnitude of the change in solution concentration is difficult to quantitatively predict and depends strongly on the formulation, nebulization condition, and type of nebulizers. Niven (12) has recently derived a mathematical equation based upon the early work by Mercer (21) to

Table 1 Average mass median diameter for fluids nebulized in a Pari LC nebulizer

Fluid	Viscosity (cP)	Surface tension (dyne/cm)	Mass median diameter (μm)	
			6 L/min	8 L/min
Water	1.00	72.8	3.6	3.1
Ethanol	1.19	24.1	3.0	2.5
Glycerol 10%	1.31	72.9	3.1	2.9
Glycerol 25%	2.09	72.2	2.6	2.4
Glycerol 50%	6.03	70.0	2.5	2.0
P. Glycol 10%	1.50	62.0	1.9	1.6
P. Glycol 30%	3.00	52.0	1.6	1.5
P. Glycol 50%	6.50	45.0	1.3	1.2
S.F. 200/0.65 cs	0.49	15.9	3.3	2.9
S.F. 200/1 cs	0.82	7.4	2.4	2.0
S.F. 200/5 cs	4.60	19.7	1.6	1.3
S.F. 200/10 cs	9.40	20.1	1.7	1.7
S.F. 200/20 cs	19.00	20.6	1.7	1.5
S.F. 200/50 cs	48.00	20.8	1.2	1.1
S.F. 200/100 cs	97.00	20.9	1.4	1.4

P. Glycol = Propylene glycol; S.F. = silicon fluid.
(Adapted from Ref. 16.)

describe the relationship of drug concentration in the nebulizer as a function of time. The drug concentration obtained by Mercer (21) was expressed as

$$C(t) = C_0 \left(\frac{V_0}{V_0 - (W + S)Ft} \right)^{(WW+S)} \quad (6)$$

where W and S are the solution output and solvent output per liter of air (ml/L air) respectively as shown in Fig. 3. V_0 is the initial fill volume into the nebulizer, and F is the nebulization flow rate. A more user-friendly version of the equation was derived (12) and expressed in terms of drug mass output that might be of more practical use in predicting drug output from a nebulizer for a range of operation conditions as claimed by the author:

$$M_{out} = M_0 \left[1 - \left(\frac{V}{V_0} \right)^{(WW+S)} \right] \quad (7)$$

where M_0 is the initial amount of drug in the solution, and V is the solution volume at any time, t, expressed as

$$V = V_0 - [W + S]Ft. \quad (8)$$

Newman et al. (24) evaluated the concentration change using four different jet nebulizers, with a gentamicin solution, which is used to treat patients for cystic fibrosis. The types of nebulizers used were the Bird micronebulizer, DeVilbiss 646, Bard Inspiron mini-neb, and Medic-Aid Upmist. All were operated at four different air flow

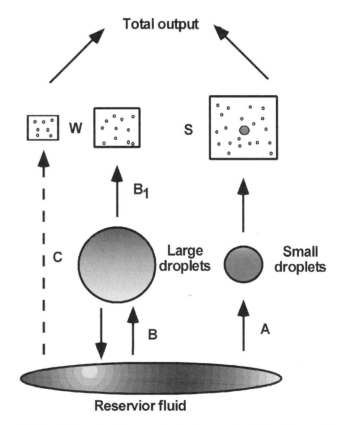

Fig. 3 Schematic diagram of nebulizer output. Droplets small enough will be carried out by air stream (route A), and the large droplets will be either recycled to the nebulizer reservoir (route B) or carried out by the outgoing air stream (route B1). Some of the solvent will be evaporated (route C). (Adapted from Ref. 12.)

rates: 6, 8, 10, and 12 L/min. Nebulization time was defined as 30 s after the last visible release of aerosol. The concentration of the drug solution left in the nebulizers was then measured using an Osmometer. The initial drug concentration was 40 mg/ml for both fill volumes. Table 2 shows the final concentration of gentamicin solution at different nebulization flow rates.

It was found that the ratio of final to initial drug concentration ranged from 1.35 to 1.70 for the 2 ml fill volume, and from 1.45 to 1.96 for the 4 ml fill volume. The ratio did not vary significantly between the four different nebulization flow rates, but was significantly higher ($p <$ 0.01) for the 4 ml fill volume than for the 2 ml fill volume, indicating that the larger volume allowed more time to concentrate the reservoir drug solution. The same phenomenon was observed using a albuterol solution, and the drug concentration increased after the nebulization (25). It was also found that the concentration ratio decreased with the increase in solution fill volume, which is different from the results shown in Table 2. However the discrepancy may result from the different nebulization sources, where dry oxygen versus an electric powered air compressor were used in the experiment (25).

Temperature effects: It is well known that the nebulizer solution cools during nebulization, because a large amount of compressed air is used to generate aerosol particles (20, 21). The temperature of the nebulizer solution decreases several degrees (5–10°C) due to the evaporation of solvent in the solution during the first several minutes of nebulization until a new heat balance is established. Some cooling of the solution in the nebulizer due to adiabatic expansion of the compressed air source may be absorbed by the thermal energy released by break-

up and impact of the liquid (26). The magnitude of temperature change in the nebulization solution depends on many factors, such as heat capacity, properties of nebulizer material, ambient conditions, and the humidity and temperature of the compressed air. Fig. 4 shows the change in solution temperature as a function of nebulization time (20). Four different types of nebulizers were used together with different air compressors to aerosolize a sodium chloride solution. The solutions in the nebulizers were initially at ambient temperatures (approximately of 23°C).

Different nebulizers had different temperature reduction profiles, depending on the compressed air flow rate applied during the nebulization, as pointed out by the authors. The solution temperature falls to a steady value, T_s, which is 5–6°C below the ambient temperature at the nebulization flow rate of 6.3–5.0 L/min, and 11–15°C at 8 L/min air flow rate.

Drug aerosol delivery efficiency and particle size distribution: Delivery efficiency of aerosolized drug product and particle size distribution are the two most important parameters in assessing the performance of a nebulizer for aerosol therapy. The aerosol output from the nebulizer depends mainly on the nebulizer type, drug formulation, solution volume placed in the nebulizer, and the applied air pressure (and hence the airflow through the nebulizer). The simplest method to calculate the output from a nebulizer is to weigh the nebulizer before and after the nebulization, often expressed as the solution volume output per unit time (i.e., mg/min). However, this method of calculation is subject to at least two possible error sources: 1) neglecting the change in solution density when it is used to transfer the mass output per unit time to

Table 2 Final drug concentration (mg/ml) in the nebulizer reservoirs

	Nebulization flow rate			
Nebulizer type	6 L/min	8 L/min	10 L/min	12 L/min
Solution fill volume: 2 ml				
Bird	54.4	62.0	57.2	58.4
DeVilbiss	55.6	60.4	56.0	65.6
Inspiron	58.4	65.2	68.0	68.0
Upmist	64.4	58.0	58.0	58.0
Solution fill volume: 4 ml				
Bird	59.2	65.6	58.0	64.0
DeVilbiss	78.4	77.2	71.6	75.2
Inspiron	71.2	69.2	74.0	74.8
Upmist	76.8	75.6	62.8	62.8

(Adapted from Ref. 24.)

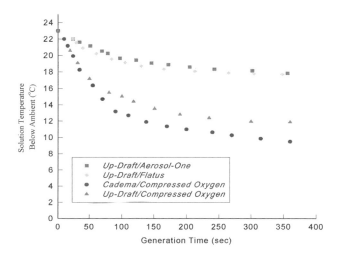

Fig. 4 Nebulizer solution temperature below ambient (23°C) vs. nebulization time. (Adapted from Ref. 20.)

volume output per unit time, and 2) neglecting the change in solution concentration as discussed previously. The delivery efficiency of the nebulizer can be expressed simply as

$$E = \frac{M_p - M_d}{M_p} \qquad (9)$$

where E represents the nebulizer delivery efficiency, M_p is the drug amount loaded into the nebulizer before nebulization, and M_d is the drug amount left in the nebulizer after the nebulization. Nebulizers are often operated until there is no visible aerosol or "sputtering," and a significant reduction in the nebulizer output occurs when the solution volume in the nebulizer reservoir becomes so low that it fails to maintain a continuous liquid supply to the nebulizer orifice. However, these are very crude measures and provide no indication of the amount of aerosolized drug a patient inhales.

The delivery efficiency, or the nebulizer output, can be expressed in many different ways, as widely documented in the literature. Sometimes it is represented as the volume output, or solution mass output. However, it is more practical to use the drug mass emitted from the nebulizer at or near the mouthpiece to estimate the nebulizer output, because the amount of aerosolized drug mass at this point in the system is the best measure of how much drug the patient has available to inhale.

Nebulizer output depends mainly on three variables: the type of the nebulizer, the operating conditions during nebulization, and the solution to be nebulized. Although solution density and viscosity play minor roles in nebulizer output for the majority of aqueous formulation, viscosity becomes an issue when aerosolizing highly viscous solutions. For any given solution and nebulizer, the operating pressure primarily determines the nebulizer output. Increasing the nebulization pressure usually increases nebulizer output. Increasing nebulizer output typically has a clinical benefit: it can reduce the time required to nebulize an effective dose, particularly for young patients who are less tolerant of the treatment procedure. As drug mass delivered per unit time is increased, treatment time is reduced leading to better acceptability and improved clinical outcome (27). Fig. 5 correlates drug mass output as a function of operating pressure (28).

A Pari LC Plus jet nebulizer (Fig. 6) was used in the study. The nebulizer was operated using a specially designed electronic unit to regulate the compressed air supplied to the nebulizer. The nebulizer was operated in a pulse mode, in which the time of nebulization was set at 3 s for each aerosol generation. The drug output was generally

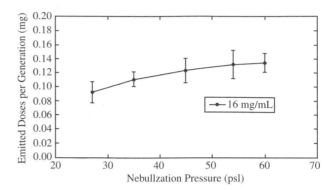

Fig. 5 Emitted dose per generation from the nebulizer vs. the nebulization pressure. (Adapted from Ref. 28.)

greater with each incremental increase in operating pressure. These increases were significant ($p < 0.05$) over a range of nebulization operating pressures of 27–45 psi. Additional increases in operating pressure of 45 to 60 psi did not significantly increase aerosol drug output.

Finlay et al. (29) recently tested 15 different jet nebulizers available commercially to investigate the performance of nebulizers. The drug compound used in the study was a 2.5 ml unit dose of Ventolin® (containing 1 mg/ml of salbutamol sulfate), which corresponds to a 2.5 mg in nominal dose per drug container. Table 3 shows the experimental results for the different nebulizers.

Nebulizers fitted with a T-mouthpiece have an unrestricted flow of ambient air passing through the nebulizer output, supplying inhaled air flow, which effectively increases drug output. In vented nebulizers,

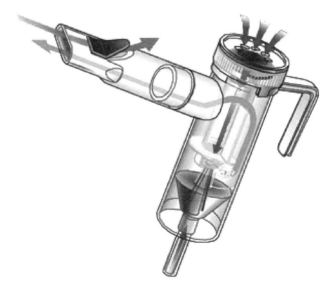

Fig. 6 The diagram of the Pari LC Plus jet nebulizer. (Courtesy of Pari GmbH.)

Table 3 Mass output of different nebulizers

Nebulizer name	Supplier	Flow rate (L/min)	In vitro inhaled dose		Methods[a]
			(mg)	% Nominal dose	
AirLife	Baxter, Valencia, CA	5.5	0.60 ± 0.02	24.1 ± 0.9	A
Disposible Sidestream	Medic-Aid, Pagham, U.K.	6.7	0.35 ± 0.01	13.8 ± 0.8	B
Sidestream	Medic-Aid, Pagham, U.K.	8.0	0.35 ± 0.02	24.1 ± 0.9	B
Ventstream	Medic-Aid, Pagham, U.K.	8.0	0.59 ± 0.01	23.6 ± 0.5	B
LCJet+ (ProNeb)	Pari, Richmond, VA	3.6	0.60 ± 0.02	23.9 ± 0.8	B
LCJet+ (Pulmo-Aid)	Pari, Richmond, VA	4.8	0.65 ± 0.02	26.0 ± 0.6	B
Pulmo-Neb	DeVilbiss, Somerset, PA	6.2	0.60 ± 0.02	24.0 ± 0.8	A
646	DeVilbiss, Somerset, PA	7.8	0.14 ± 0.02	5.5 ± 0.9	B
Raindrop	Puritan Bennett, Lenexa, KS	6.2	0.56 ± 0.02	22.3 ± 0.9	A
Salter	Salter Labs, Arvin, CA	6.1	0.65 ± 0.02	25.9 ± 0.6	B
T-Updraft	Hudson RCI, Temecula, CA	6.1	0.34 ± 0.02	13.8 ± 0.6	A
T-Updraft II	Hudson RCI, Temecula, CA	5.7	0.74 ± 0.02	29.7 ± 0.9	A
Up-Mist	Hospitak, Lindenhurst, NY	7.5	0.48 ± 0.02	19.1 ± 0.9	A
1405	Avion, Burlington, Ont.	6.2	0.47 ± 0.02	18.5 ± 0.9	A
1807	Avion, Burlington, Ont.	6.5	0.50 ± 0.02	19.8 ± 0.8	A

[a] A is a conventional T-mouthpiece, and B is a vented nebulizer.
(Adapted from Ref. 29.)

the inhaled air must flow through the droplet production region. Therefore, the breathing pattern of the patient has an effect on the aerosol characteristics produced by such devices. The delivery efficiency of the commercial nebulizers tested ranged from 6 to 30% of the nominal dose loaded into the nebulizers. For conventional nebulizers, the inhaled dose is approximated by the amount of drug leaving the nebulizer divided by 2, since inhalation is assumed to occupy half of the breathing cycle (29). However, this remains a very crude measure of delivered or inhaled dose.

The importance of particle size distribution in determining the site of the deposition of pharmaceutical compounds within the respiratory tract has been discussed extensively in the literature (1–7, 10, 12, 20, 24, 27, 30). For any given inhaled dose of aerosolized drug, the particle size distribution of drug aerosol, aerosol velocity, the breathing pattern (inspiratory flow and volume), and lung morphology, determine the location the aerosol is deposited in the respiratory airways. It is generally well accepted that the particle size of drug aerosols generated for inhalation should be within 1–5 μm in diameter. Because of polydispersity of the aerosol, the mass median aerodynamic diameter (MMAD) and geometrical standard deviation (GSD) are often used to describe the distribution of aerosol particles. The MMAD is defined as the mass median of the distribution of mass with respect to aerodynamic diameter (1). The mass median diameter

(MMD) and GSD of the salbutamol aerosol generated by 15 different nebulizers (29) are shown in Table 4, where $MMD = MMAD/(density)^{1/2}$.

Table 4 Particle size distribution of different nebulizers

Nebulizer name	Flow rate (L/min)	Particle size distribution	
		MMD (μm)	GSD
AirLife	5.5	5.8 ± 1.0	1.7
Disposible Sidestream	6.7	4.2 ± 0.2	1.5
Sidestream	8.0	4.3 ± 0.4	1.5
Ventstream	8.0	4.7 ± 0.4	1.5
LCJet + (ProNeb)	3.6	6.2 ± 0.4	1.7
LCJet + (Pulmo-Aid)	4.8	6.2 ± 0.3	1.7
Pulmo-Neb	6.2	5.6 ± 0.2	1.6
646	7.8	6.8 ± 0.6	1.7
Raindrop	6.2	5.0 ± 0.4	1.6
Salter	6.1	6.1 ± 0.9	1.7
T-Updraft	6.1	5.3 ± 0.5	1.7
T-Updraft II	5.7	5.9 ± 0.3	1.7
Up-Mist	7.5	4.5 ± 0.7	1.6
1405	6.2	5.0 ± 0.6	1.6
1807	6.5	6.1 ± 0.5	1.6

(Adapted from Ref. 29.)

The size distribution of aerosols generated using most commercial nebulizers is typically highly variable with somewhat large mean diameters. This not only results in poor transfer efficiency but poor and highly variable respiratory deposition patterns between and within patient populations.

Metered dose inhalers

Pressurized metered dose inhalers (pMDIs) have been widely used in the treatment of asthma and COPD. These devices are more popular than nebulizers and dry powder inhalers. The popularity of the pMDI has steadily increased since the 1950s due mainly to its compact and portable size, self-contained power source, and other rapid therapeutic effects in the use of bronchodilators. pMDIs appear to be simple to use, although this appearance is in fact deceptive. Many patients are not adequately trained to correctly use pMDIs or find it nearly impossible to effectively coordinate their breathing with the high velocity release of the aerosol. High ejection velocity of the aerosol at the mouthpiece (usually near 30 m/s) is the single largest deficit of pMDIs. At these high ballistic velocities, most of the drug aerosol impacts in the mouth or throat and can not be readily entrained within the respiratory flow (even when coordinated with aerosol release). Typically, about 60–90% of the emitted drug will be deposited in the oral-pharyngeal region. This not only reduces the amount of drug that reaches the intended action site, but often contributes to unwanted systemic side effects due to oral absorption. Spacers have been developed that help mitigate this problem. The spacers are placed in front of the pMDIs actuator to reduce the aerosol velocity, and reduce the number of large diameter droplets before entering into the airway. However, this occurs at the expense of delivery efficiency, further reducing the dose of drug inhaled.

A typical pMDI consists of a drug reservoir containing the drug compound suspended or solubilized in liquefied propellant, a metering valve, and an actuator that connects with the metering valve through a stem. The propellants historically have been chlorofluorocarbons (CFCs) which have high vapor pressures and are generally biologically inert. The pMDI delivers a metered dose of active drug compound using the propellants as a power source. In the rest position, the metering chamber is connected with the formulation reservoir. Depressing the drug canister activates the metering chamber and the formulation reservoir is then closed. Simultaneously, a connection is opened between the valve stem orifice and the metering chamber. The formulation contained in the metering chamber quickly escapes through the stem valve and spray orifice, atomizing the formulation. As the liquid CFCs vaporize, they generate sufficient energy to produce efficient two-phase atomization, without the need for an external power source (7).

The primary factors that will influence the performance of the pMDI are the propellant used, the physical properties of drug formulation, which partially governs droplet formation and drug uniformity, and the device itself.

Propellants: The propellants used in the pMDIs consist of CFCs with different molecular formulas. The propellants commonly used in inhalers to disperse the liquid into aerosols are CFC-11 (CCl_3F), CFC-12 (CCl_2F_2), and CFC-114 ($CClF_2$-$CClF_2$) (31, 32). These three propellants have been used for decades in pMDI products because of their unique properties, which include low toxicity, excellent physical and chemical stability, ideal vapor pressure, and generally good compatibility with drug compounds and surfactants. These propellants possess an appropriate degree of solvency that solubilizes the surfactants typically used in pMDI systems such as oleic acid, sorbitan trioleate, and soya lecithin, yet dissolve low quantities of most drugs. This combination of surfactant solubility and drug insolubility in the pMDI formulation is essential for maintaining uniform suspensions of appropriate particle size. The physical properties of these three propellants are shown in Table 5.

The vapor pressure of the formulation in a pMDI can be adjusted to a targeted value by mixing propellants with different vapor pressures. Propellants offer the additional advantage of having a narrow density range that may be adjusted to balance the density of the drug particle in suspension (33).

Table 5   Physical properties of CFCs propellants commonly used in pMDIs

Propellants	Molecular weight	Density (g/cm^3) at 21°C	Vapor pressure (psig) at 20°C	Boiling point (°C) at 1 atm	Atmospheric life (years)
CFC-11	137.4	1.49	−1.8	23.8	75
CFC-12	120.9	1.33	67.6	−29.8	111
CFC-114	170.9	1.47	11.9	3.6	200–300

Morén (32) investigated the influence of vapor pressure on the characteristics of aerosols generated using pMDIs. In these studies, nine healthy volunteers inhaled eight doses at one-minute intervals coordinated with the dose firing, and the amount of drug deposited in the actuator, extension tube, and mouth was determined spectrophotometrically. It was found that an increase in vapor pressure results in higher initial velocity of the aerosols, smaller initial aerosol particle size, and more rapid propellant evaporation. The amount of drug deposited in the actuator increased at the higher vapor pressure of 502 kPa, which was likely due to the high velocity of the aerosol exiting the spray nozzle and a wide spray angle.

Aerosol formation: Aerosol formation from pMDIs is a complex process influenced not only by the propellant as discussed above, but also by properties of the formulation and device design (e.g., valve volume and orifice size). After aerosol droplets form at the exit of the spray nozzle, an aerosol plume begins to expand, and large particles travel along the axis of the actuator. Fig. 7 shows photographs of aerosol formation using a commercially available pMDI.

Most large droplets fall out from the aerosol cloud, and those droplets are deposited in the mouthpiece or in the oral-pharyngeal region of the respiratory airways when the inhaler is used by a patient. When spaces are used, many large particles are collected within the spacers. The remaining aerosol cloud continues to evaporate, and the velocity of the aerosol reduces dramatically from about 35 m/s at 5 cm from the spray orifice to about 10 m/s at 20 cm (34). During aerosolization, surfactant molecules, used as dispersing agents and valve lubricants, will influence the evaporation rate of the propellants (33). The dimension and shape of the aerosol cloud significantly influence the transport efficiency of aerosol to the respiratory tract.

Physical stability of drug suspension: The physical stability of the nonpolar drug suspensions formulated in pMDIs again depends on many parameters, such as propellant type, chemical properties of the drug compounds, and the surfactants used in the formulation. A suspension is a liquid system in which insoluble solid particles are dispersed in a liquid medium. Suspensions can be divided into colloidal suspensions, in which the solid particles are less than 1 μm, and coarse suspensions, where particles are larger than 1 μm (35). The physical stability of a suspension can also be classified according to whether the formulation is flocculated or deflocculated. In a deflocculated system, the solid drug particles settle down slowly and form irreversible aggregates. As a result the particles form a distinct cake on the bottom of a container. The deflocculated system is impossible to redisperse by simple shaking, and the suspension is unlikely to be of use after caking. Therefore, it is necessary to develop the flocculated formulation systems for pMDIs. In flocculated systems, the particles form large aggregates, so that the

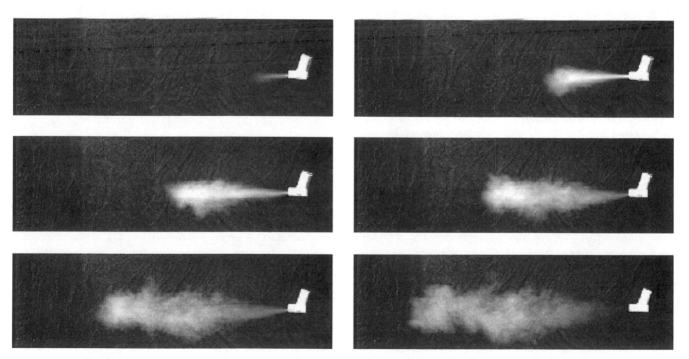

Fig. 7 Formation of the aerosol plume as a function of time. Each frame has a time interval of 30 mins.

solid particles can be resuspended upon shaking. The formulation of a flocculated system requires reducing or neutralizing the zeta potential around the drug compound. This means that repelling forces between the particles are neutralized and the particles can then interact with each other to form large aggregates which rapidly settle but, can be easily redispersed (36). In formulating a suspension for pMDI use, the drug particles are usually less dense compared with the suspension media. Therefore, in an unshaken inhaler the drug gradually separates as a layer, which floats on the propellant and surfactant mixture, and is resuspended immediately after shaking. The solubility of the drug compound in the propellant also plays an important role in the physical stability of the pMDI formulation. An extremely low solubility of drug compound is required in the nonpolar system. Therefore, pMDI formulations usually require a polar salt to be incorporated, because significant drug solubility in the propellant can lead to crystal growth, often associated with the caking of the suspension and a reduced amount of fine particles (37).

Sedimentation ratio is often used to assess suspension stability. Byron (37) reported the sedimentation ratios for a 1% sodium fluoresein suspension formulation with different amounts of surfactant (sorbitan trioleate) after standing for 20 days at room temperature. The suspension formulation with the lowest sedimentation ratio had the best-flocculated system. However, all formulations were easily redispersible: one complete revolution of the container was sufficient to produce a homogeneous dispersion. There was no clear difference in the times taken to reach apparent sedimentation equilibrium. Physical stability of the formulation was determined according to:

- Whether the drug material was adequately deaggregated during manufacture,
- Whether redispersibility was easy and allowed doses to be metered reproducibly,
- Surfactant concentration-drug combination gave the greatest respirable fraction of the aerosols (37).

Determination of dose and particle size distribution: The amount of drug reproducibly delivered from pMDIs per actuation is one of the most frequently reported performance parameters of these products. Several experimental configurations are used to characterize the pMDI's emitted dose. One of the most commonly used experimental protocols is described in the Official Compendia of Standards published by *U.S. Pharmacopeia* (38). The pMDI device is fitted with a sampling tube at one end, and a vacuum pump is connected with a filter holder at the other end. A continuous airflow is drawn through the sampling tube to avoid the loss of the drug material into the atmosphere. The active compound delivered from the pMDI is recovered from the filter and the sampling tube to determine the mass output from the device. There are no universal definitions for different terminologies used to express dosages provided by pMDIs, and the labeling requirements for pMDIs differ among nations (37). In the United States, the emitted dose (label claim) is defined as the amount of drug leaving the device, excluding the drug mass left in the actuator and valve stem of the device. However, in other nations, the metered dose is often used, which includes the amount left in the actuator but not that retained in the valve stem (37). Descriptions of the emitted dose often use different terms, which are often used for different purposes (39, 40). Because of the lack of consistency in the terminology used in the literatures and by regulatory agencies, it is often difficult to compare the experimental results between different research groups, devices, and experimental methods and procedures. Therefore, it would be beneficial to harmonize the terminology commonly used to describe drug doses from different parts of the pMDIs, and efforts are currently underway to standardize the way delivered dose and device performance are measured and reported. Table 6 shows the definitions for the various doses frequently used in the literatures.

However, even with a clear understanding of the dose delivered by a pMDI, there is no direct or consistent correlation to the amount of drug delivered to the patient's lungs. A typical drug distribution within patients and from devices is shown in Table 7 (41). The table is based on an experiment conducted on healthy volunteers with an average FEV_1 at 105% of predicted (range 92–119%). A terbutaline formulation was labeled with ^{99m}Tc and administered to patients using a pMDI. The average inspiratory flow rate was 33.8 L/min, (SD = 6.7), and the total inspired volume averaged 2.86 L (SD = 0.87), with an average of (SD = 0.7) 9.1s breath-hold. The intersubject variability in the patients' breathing patterns was relatively small, contributable to on-line monitoring of breathing patterns using a spirometer.

The amount of drug deposited in the lungs expressed as percentage of emitted dose (including drug left on actuator) was about 16.7% (SD = 9.6), and the percentage of emitted dose deposited in the oral-pharynx was 68.3% (SD = 10.2). The percentage of emitted dose deposited in the actuator was 13.4% (SD = 2.1). The intersubject variability for the percentage of emitted dose found in the actuator and oral-pharynx was 15.3 and 14.9%, and the variability for the total lung deposition was 57.7%. These

Table 6 Definition of various doses

Terminology	Description
Nominal dose (metered dose)	The dose represents the actual amount of the drug loaded into the pMDI device. It can be calculated using drug concentration times the metering valve volume.
Emitted dose (ex-valve dose)	The amount of drug emitted from the device, including the drug deposited on the actuator and inhaled dose.
Inhaled dose (label claim)	The amount of drug emitted from the device, not including the drug left on the actuator. This amount of drug is available for inhalation by patient.
Fine particle dose	The amount of drug with particle diameter less than 5.0 μm, which is a portion of the inhaled dose.
Deposited dose	The amount of drug deposited in the respiratory airways, which can further be divided into the drug amount in the oropharyngeal region and lungs.

large variations in the total lung deposition are typical of clinical results when inhaled drugs are given using pMDIs.

The particle size distribution of drug aerosol generated from the pMDI is another important performance parameter of the drug delivery device, which depends on the combination of the propellants and surfactants, the original size of the drug particle, and the design of the device (metering valve, orifice, actuator). The initial atomization process and subsequent spray evaporation govern the amount of drug aerosol deposited both in the oral-pharyngeal and pulmonary regions. Aerosol particles ejected from the pMDI experience constant changes in size due mainly to the drug formulation. Fig. 8 shows the change in particle size as a function of the distance from the actuator orifice. The experiment was conducted using a pMDI obtained commercially, and a laser diffraction instrument (Malvern, Mastersizer X) was used to determine the size of drug aerosol. The device was

mounted on a platform, and the distances between the actuator and the center of the laser beam were chosen to be about 5, 10, 15, 20, and 25 cm. The pMDI was operated according to the instructions given by the manufacturer, and five measurements were repeated for each chosen distance.

The size of the drug particle was about 8 μm at 5 cm between the actuator orifice, and gradually decreased to about 2.5 μm at 35 centimeters from the actuator orifice due to the evaporational shrinkage. The particle diameter was about 6.5 μm at a distance of 10 centimeters, which was about the distance to the oral-pharyngeal region from the actuator orifice. The amount of drug deposited in the oral-pharyngeal region is mainly due to the inertial impaction; therefore it depends more on particle size than on particle velocity. The inertial impaction is proportional to the square of the particle diameter, and is linearly proportional to the particle velocity. The decreases in particle diameter followed exponentially with the distance

Table 7 Deposition of radioactive drug after inhaling via pMDI

Subject	Actuator	Throat	Total lung	Regional lung			P/C ratio	Exhaled
				Central	Intermediate	Peripheral		
1	15.5	76.3	7.1	1.7	2.4	3.1	1.87	1.1
2	10.4	81.8	6.1	1.2	1.9	3.0	2.54	1.6
3	15.6	66.2	12.5	2.9	4.3	5.4	1.86	5.8
4	12.8	75.6	10.9	3.2	3.9	3.8	1.2	0.8
5	11.7	66.3	21.8	6.5	7.1	8.2	1.27	0.2
6	11.8	57.6	30.0	7.8	9.3	12.9	1.65	0.6
7	13.1	71.7	15.0	4.1	5.5	5.4	1.31	0.3
8	16.0	51.0	30.0	6.3	11.2	12.6	2.00	3.0
Mean	13.4	68.3	16.7	4.2	5.7	6.8	1.71	1.7
SD	2.1	10.2	9.6	2.4	3.3	4.0	0.45	1.9

(Adapted from Ref. 41.)

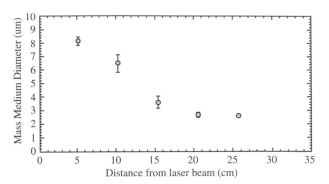

Fig. 8 The change in particle size vs. the distance from the actuator orifice.

from the actuator orifice. The exponential decrease rate of particle diameter differs with different drug formulations (vapor pressure, nonvolatile concentration, etc.).

High Frequency Oscillating Devices

Ultrasonic nebulizer

Ultrasonic nebulizers utilize high frequency sonic energy to convert liquid drug formulations into aerosol clouds. Although these devices have been used in clinical settings since the 1960s, they are not as widely used as the jet nebulizer and pMDIs. Ultrasonic nebulizers typically have higher drug mass output and significantly larger particle size distributions at the point of aerosolization compared with jet nebulizers (42). Advantages and disadvantages of the ultrasonic nebulizer for the delivery of pharmaceutical compounds to the human respiratory airways are listed in Table 8. The output of drug compound leaving the ultrasonic nebulizer is at a relatively slow velocity compared with the jet nebulizer. Therefore, less patient coordination is required during treatment.

The reservoir temperature in the ultrasonic nebulizer increases rapidly during operation. In the study by Phipps et al. (20), the solution in the nebulizer increased from room temperature (~23°C) to greater than 30°C after

about 5 min of operation, and exceeded 40°C after 30 min of nebulization. This significant temperature increase may cause some pharmaceutical compounds to be degraded during aerosolization (43). Changes in drug potency due to delivery by ultrasonic nebulizer have been reported in the literature, with degradation more profound for protein and peptide therapeutics compared to more stable small molecules.

Mechanism of aerosol generation: Ultrasonic nebulizers generate aerosols using a piezoelectric transducer that vibrates when subjected to high-frequency electric energy. When liquid is fed continuously through or over the vibrating surface, a wave pattern is formed as the liquid spreads over the liquid surface. Liquid droplets are formed when the amplitude of the vibrating surface increases to the point at which the capillary wave becomes unstable and collapses (44). An empirical equation to calculate the droplet diameter (D) produced from an ultrasonic nebulizer was described by Lang (44). The diameter is approximately proportional to the capillary wave length (λ), density (ρ) and surface tension (σ) of the liquid, and the excitation frequency (F).

$$D = 0.34\lambda = 0.996\frac{\sigma}{\rho F^2}. \tag{10}$$

As with jet nebulizers and pMDIs, the formulation characteristics include liquid density, surface tension, viscosity, and vapor pressure. Many of these that effect nebulizer performance of formulation properties are described in the above equation. The configuration of the device, such as the location of the baffles, mechanisms in the transport of the liquid formulation to the piezoelectric transducer, and the size of medication chamber, also affect the performance. The units frequency and amplitude of vibration, control the mass output and the particle size distribution permitting some adjustment in aerosol characteristics.

Performance characteristics: Greenspan (42) summarized the performance of commonly used ultrasonic nebulizers. The excitation frequency ranged from 1.3 to about 2.6 MHz, and the MMAD of the produced aerosols

Table 8 Characteristics of ultrasonic nebulizer

Advantages	Disadvantages
Little patient coordination	Large particle size and less efficient
Aerosol exited with low velocity	Microbiological contamination risk
Small dead volume and quite operation	Possibility of degrading drug compound
High dose output and fast drug delivery	Poor portability and is expensive
No propellants requirements	Requirement of electric power supplier

was approximately 1–7 μm. Several ultrasonic nebulizers generated relatively large aerosol particles, which were usually associated with low excitation frequency. Hager et al. (45) characterized the performance of two ultrasonic nebulizers using a pentamidine solution, which is used to treat *Pneumocystis carinii* pneumonia associated with acquired immunodeficiency syndrome (AIDs). The ultrasonic nebulizers used in the study were Fiso Neb (model FZV 40 BAMKI, Fisons) and Porta-Sonic (model 8500GB, Devilbiss). It was found that the mass output for FISO Neb at airflow rate of 6 L/min were 201.4 and 36.7 mg for drug concentrations of 50 and 10 mg/mL, respectively. Corresponding outputs decreased to 85.2 and 23.6 mg for Porta-Sonic nebulizer. However the MMD of aerosol generated from the Fiso Neb was 5.8–6.93 μm, and 1.96–3.04 μm for Porta-Sonic nebulizer. The higher mass output from the Fiso Neb compared to the Porta-Neb was due to the presence of larger aerosol particles produced by the Fiso Neb nebulizer. However, these larger droplets are typically nonrespirable, if they are transported at all to the patient inhalation port. Therefore, the overall dose efficiency of ultrasonic nebulizers tend to be poorer than jet nebulizers.

ADVANCED DRUG DELIVERY TECHNOLOGIES

Using the various drug delivery devices, such as pMDIs, nebulizers, and DPIs, discussed in the first half of this chapter, has had an enormous impact on patient quality of life, as inhaled drugs play an important role in the management of airway diseases. However, past successes in topical delivery of drugs to the lung owe more to the therapeutic properties of the drugs used than to the delivery device itself (30). Currently used delivery devices tend to be inefficient, with small amounts of drug delivered to the site of action, with a large portion of the drug compound lost in the device or deposited orally, often causing unwanted side effects.

The shortcomings described for the current devices limit their ability to meet the demands created by advancements in more potent small molecules and biotechnology therapies. More and more new drugs are potential inhalation candidate therapies to treat various diseases, including nonairway diseases such as diabetes. There is an urgent need for more advanced drug delivery technology, which can deliver the drug more precisely to the targeted area for action, with better efficiency and improved reproducibility. Over the last 10 years, many innovations have occurred in the field of inhalation drug delivery with advances in aerosol technology and electronics, spurred by the demand created by new drug

compounds. Most of the technologies have tried to tackle problems such as reducing the ballistic velocity of aerosol released from pMDIs by breath activated functions and developing new propellants with lower ejection pressures. Focus has shifted to defining and developing a more "ideal" inhaler to administering various pharmaceutical compounds for different diseases. The following describes many of the features these new pulmonary drug delivery devices are designed to include (30).

- Aerosol generation independent of the patient's inhalation.
- Duration of aerosol dose generation should occupy a substantial part of a slow inhalation cycle. A generation time of greater than 1 s will permit the patient to better coordinate aerosol delivery effectively during inhalation.
- The aerosol cloud should consist largely of particles of less than 5 μm in size. Fine aerosols are necessary for delivery to the lung periphery if this is the site of action or if systemic delivery is the objective. The ability to vary and then control the mean particle size distribution of the aerosol would be an added advantage for targeting deposition within different regions of the respiratory tract.
- The velocity of the aerosol should be minimal to reduce oral-pharyngeal deposition and provide maximum delivery to the lungs.
- The inhaler should be simple to use, require little patient coordination and preferably should be breath-actuate.
- The inhaler should have dimensions similar to those of the pMDIs, fitting the pocket or the handbag and permitting discrete use.
- The inhaler should contain a large number of doses (>50 doses).
- A dose counter should be included.
- The device should be easy to manufacture and reasonably priced.
- The device should generate uniform doses throughout its life, be resistant to microbial and other contamination, and have a suitable shelf life.
- Propellants should be avoided, or designed for low environmental impact.

Pressure Driven Devices

New generation pressurized metered dose inhaler

Asthma affects an estimated 100 million people worldwide, including over 15 million in the United States (45), and while the pMDI has many disadvantages, it still is the most prescribed drug product for the treatment of asthma. The long-term dominance of pMDIs in inhalation drug

Table 9 Physical properties of propellants (CFCs and HFAs)

Propellants	Density (g/cm³) at 21°C	Vapor pressure (psig) at 20°C	Boiling point (°C) at 1 atm
CFC-11	1.49	− 1.8	23.8
CFC-12	1.33	67.6	− 29.8
CFC-114	1.47	11.9	3.6
HFA-134a (replace CFC-12)	1.21	81	− 27
HFA-227 (replace CFC-12, CFC-114)	1.41	43	− 17

delivery is mainly due to its convenience. However, it is extremely difficult to use effectively. Everard (46) pointed out that the pharmaceutical industry elected to perpetuate the failings of the pMDI and develop replacements for CFCs, rather than develop novel devices to meet current demands. Extensive resources have been invested to preserve the pMDI when the industry was challenged with phasing out CFC propellants, and to reduce the oral-pharyngeal deposition by methods such as using attached spacers and breath-actuated devices.

pMDIs with new propellants: Since 1974, the CFCs have been believed to contribute to erosion of the earth's stratospheric ozone. Coyne (47) summarizes the history and progress of the Montreal Protocol negotiations and formation in great detail, and introduces the objectives and history of the Pharmaceutical Aerosol CFC Coalition (PACC) in the United States and the International Pharmaceutical Aerosol Consortium (IPAC) in Europe. The objectives of the organizations are to find replacements for CFC propellants that can be used in pMDIs.

Reformulation of drugs used in pMDIs to avoid CFC propellants presented numerous obstacles, because no approved alternative pharmaceutical propellants were available (48). Replacement of the propellants used in pMDIs requires changes in many fundamental aspects of formulation, device design, device components, and manufacturing. Several classes of propellants have been considered as alternatives for use in pMDIs, but each has its disadvantages, as shown below, in a listing based on Leach (49).

Alternative propellant	Disadvantage(s)
Dimethyl ether	Flammable
Hydrocarbons	Flammable, high volatile organic compound content
Hydrochloroflurocarbons	Some ozone depleting potential
Compressed gases (e.g., carbon dioxide and nitrogen)	Inconsistent pressure throughout the product life

So far, two alternative propellants, tetrafluoroethane (HFA-134a, CF_3CH_2F) and heptafluoropropane (HFA-227, CF_3CHFCF_3), have been successfully tested and developed as propellants in pMDIs. The physical properties of these two propellants are compared with those of CFCs in Table 9.

There are many similarities between pMDIs formulated with CFCs and HFAs, such as the operating principles and basic components. However, due to differences in the physical properties such as vapor pressure, density, and solvency characteristics, the pMDIs powered with HFA propellants encounter complex formulation challenges and the need for new hardware designs. The surfactants commonly used in the CFC-based pMDIs are oleic acid, sorbitan trioleate, and soya lecithin, which not only help to stabilize the formulation, but also help lubricate the metering valve system. These surfactants exhibit lower solubility when formulated with HFAs compared to CFCs. Therefore, sometimes a co-solvent will be added to the HFA formulation. New surfactants may need to be identified for drug formulations when using HFAs as propellants. However, with each change in product formulation, extensive testing is required before the product is approved for general clinical use.

Therefore, the phasing out of CFCs in pMDIs has provided an opportunity to improve the performance of the pMDIs and address the shortcomings of pMDI technology. Keller (50) compared the performance of three different active compounds, beclomethasone dipropionate (BDP), budesonide, and di-sodium-cromo-glycate (DSCG), formulated with both CFC and HFA propellants. The HFA formulations were compared with three types of commercial devices, Becotide 100®, Pulmicort®, and Intal®. The amount of drug deposited on the mouthpiece and USP throat was measured, and particle size distribution and fine particle dose were also determined accordingly. Table 10 compares the performance of the pMDIs using formulations with CFCs and HFAs propellants.

Table 10 Performance of pMDIs formulation with CFCs and HFAs

Product batch no. Formulation (label claim)	Becotide 100® 10072926 CFCs suspension (100 μg)	BDP 809/L86-04 Non-CFCs solution (100 μg)	Pulmicort® YK702 CFCs suspension (200 μg)
Mouthpiece (μg)	16.6	7.8	21.4
USP-throat (μg)	55.2	22.0	114.0
FPD (μg)	26.9	60.8	43.3
FPF (%)	26.9	60.8	21.7
MMAD (μm)	~3.1	~1.4	~4.5
GSD	1.63	1.87	1.63

Product batch no. Formulation (label claim)	Budesonide 821/372-05 Non-CFCs suspension (200 μg)	Intal® FEF2E CFCs suspension (1000 μg)	DSCG 802/352-01 Non-CFCs suspension (1000 μg)
Mouthpiece (μg)	33.4	419.3	116.8
USP-throat (μg)	46.7	385.7	488.4
FPD (μg)	86.2	147.8	300.0
FPF (%)	43.1	14.8	30.0
MMAD (μm)	~3.1	~4.0	~3.8
GSD	1.55	1.81	1.65

(Adapted from Ref. 51.)

For the BDP formulation, the fine particle dose increased from 27 to about 61 μg and the drug lost in the mouthpiece and USP throat was reduced from 17 μg and 55 μg to about 8 μg and 22 μg respectively, when using the non-CFC formulation. The increase in the fine particle dose resulted from the reduction in the MMAD, which changed from 3.1 to about 1.4 μm. The particle size distribution of a suspension formulation is expected to be controlled mainly by the drug powder particles used in the formulation. For a solution formulation, particle size distribution is dictated by other factors such as formulation and device configurations. The fine particle dose was also increased for the budesonide formulation associated with a decrease in the amount of drug deposited in the USP throat, and the particle size distribution of budesonide delivered from both pMDIs changed slightly since both formulations were suspensions. Similar results were achieved for the DSCG compared with the Intal pMDI, except that the increase in fine particle dose was likely due to the decrease in the drug amount deposited in the mouthpiece.

These performance changes typically reduce the drug deposition in the oral-pharyngeal region, providing an added advantage of producing fewer steroid side effects such as candida infection and hoarseness of the throat (49).

pMDIs with breath activated function: The firing of the pMDI and inhalation by the patient have to be coordinated or "synchronized," because the drug aerosol is produced by the pMDI for a very short time only, in the order of milliseconds. This presents a challenge for patients to inhale and capture the aerosol as it is generated. It has been estimated that more than half of the patients (47–89%) receive little benefit from their pMDIs because of failure to coordinate the firing of the pMDIs and inhalation (51,52). A breath-activated pMDI (Autohaler, 3M Riker) has been developed to minimize the need for the actuation-inhalation coordination. This device is intended to reduce the performance variability of the pMDIs caused by differences in use techniques. The Autohaler is triggered by the patient's inhalation flow rate. To use the Autohaler, the patient turns a level on the top of the device that engages a spring mechanism to load the canister against a vane mechanism that is used between the canister and the actuator. When the patient's inspiratory flow rate exceeds 30 L/min, the vane moves and allows the canister to be pressed into the actuator to deliver the drug.

Newman (53) conducted a clinical study to compare the performance of conventional pMDIs with the Autohaler using a scintigraphic technique to measure the drug deposition in the different sites of interest. The patients who participated in the study were divided into two groups classified as good coordinators and poor coordinators. Initially, patients used their own inhalers

Table 11 Percentage deposition at different sites

Deposition site	Own MDI	Taught MDI	Autohaler
Good coordinators			
Lungs	18.6 (2.9)	12.8 (1.8)	17.5 (2.8)
Oropharynx	64.4 (3.8)	71.1 (2.5)	61.2 (4.5)
Actuator	16.1 (2.0)	15.8 (1.2)	21.0 (2.8)
Exhaled	0.7 (0.4)	0.3 (0.1)	0.3 (0.1)
Poor coordinators			
Lungs	7.2 (3.4)	22.8 (2.5)	20.8 (1.7)
Oropharynx	67.7 (4.7)	59.3 (2.3)	60.7 (2.2)
Actuator	23.5 (3.8)	17.6 (0.9)	18.2 (1.3)
Exhaled	1.7 (0.9)	0.3 (0.1)	0.2 (0.1)

(Adapted from Ref. 53.)

as baseline deposition values. The depositions were then measured after those patients were instructed about the proper inhalation technique when using their own inhaler and after using the Autohaler. Table 11 shows the percentage of the aerosol dose located at various locations after inhalation by good coordinators ($n = 10$) and by poor coordinators ($n = 8$).

For the good coordinators, the deposition patterns were very similar for the patients using their own pMDIs and Autohaler, in which about 18% of the aerosol dose was deposited in the lungs and about 60% of the dose was deposited in the oral-pharyngeal region. There was a trend toward less deposition in the lungs after the patients had been taught the proper pMDI technique. It was possible that the patients had different abilities to familiarize themselves with the new technique as instructed during the study. There was a clear improvement in the lung deposition for the poor coordinators after they were given instruction or when they used the Autohaler, in which over 20% of the aerosol dose was deposited in the lungs. The increased lung deposition contributed to the improvement in the pulmonary function parameter, in which the FEV_1 increased significantly from the baseline.

New Pressure Driven Devices

Respimat™

The agreement to eliminate the use of CFCs in pMDIs for respiratory medication has stimulated interest in the development of propellant-free inhaled drug delivery technology. The Respimat developed by Boehringer Ingelheim (Ingelheim am Rhein, Germany) is one of the technologies under development (54–58). The device consists of a Uniblock, spring, drug cartridge with a capillary tube, and a nonreturn valve. The Uniblock is the major component of the device, which contains two nozzles positioned at opposing angles. The spring is the power source. Turning the lower part of the device, the rotation movement is transferred to a liner movement, which simultaneously tightens the spring and pushes the capillary tube with the nonreturn valve to the lower position. During this movement, about 13.5 μl of drug solution is drawn through the capillary to a pump chamber. When the patients press the release button, the mechanical force stored in the spring pushes the capillary tube and nonreturn valve to the upper position, driving the metered volume of drug solution through the two jet nozzles in the Uniblock, which generates two jets of liquid. The two jets are directed toward each other at a carefully controlled angle, and aerosol is generated by the impaction of the two jets.

Newman (55) examined the deposition profiles in patients of several developmental Respimat prototypes using gamma scintigraphic techniques. In these studies, the deposition of the bronchodilator fenoterol and the corticosteroid flunisolide were examined. Fenoterol in the Respimat was formulated in an aqueous medium, and flunisolide was formulated in 96% ethanol. The experimental data from these studies are shown in Table 12.

The performance of the Respimat was clearly improved for the final prototype compared with Prototype III. Drug deposition in the lungs increased from approximately 31 to 39% for the fenoterol, and from about 40 to 45% for the drug compound of flunisolide respectively. At the same time, the oral-pharyngeal deposition decreased from

Table 12 Average deposition data using the Respimat (% of the emitted dose)

Device	Formulation	Lung deposition	Oropharynx deposition	Reference
Prototype III	Fenoterol (100 μg, aqueous)	31.1	53.7	55
Prototype III	Flunisolide (250 μg, ethanolic)	39.7	39.9	56
Final Prototype	Fenoterol (100 μg, aqueous)	39.2	37.1	57
Final prototype	Flunisolide (250 μg, ethanolic)	44.6	26.2	57

(Adapted from Ref. 55.)

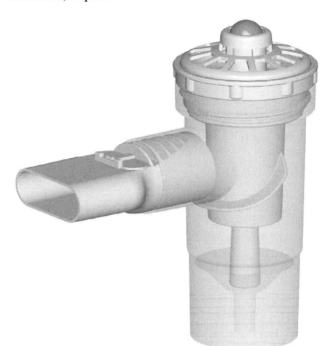

Fig. 9 The schematic diagram of the AeroEclipse nebulizer. (Courtesy of Monaghan/Trudell International.)

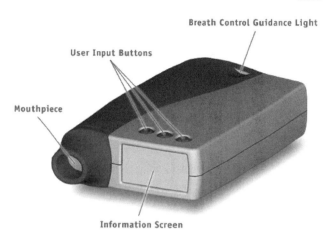

Fig. 10 The metered dose liquid inhaler as shown in Aradigm Corporation's website (www.aradigm.com).

approximately 54 to 37% for the fenoterol, and from 40 to about 16% for the flunisolide. Comparing the deposition data for the aqueous and ethanolic formulations, it can be seen that the ethanolic formulation had better performance, which may be due to the different particle size distribution for the formulations. The MMADs of the aerosols used in the Respimat were 2.0 ± 0.4 μm for the aqueous formulation and 1.0 ± 0.3 μm for the ethanolic formulation (53). The overall deposition efficiency of this device was apperently two to three times better than typically seen with pMDIs.

AeroEclipse™

The AeroEclipse (Monaghan/Trudell International) shown in Fig. 9, is a nebulizer powered by compressed air, which can be operated in both continuous nebulization and breath-actuated modes. The nebulizer was characterized,

in vitro, using different breathing patterns, with either continuous nebulization or breath-actuated nebulization (59). A piston pump was used to mimic a range of breathing patterns in pediatric patients.

Table 13 shows the experimental data. The average drug mass for the three breathing patterns were $11.1 \pm 0.74\%$ (P1), $22.9 \pm 2.74\%$ (P2), and $36.3 \pm 1.22\%$ (P3). The average mass median aerodynamic diameter was 3.55 ± 0.07 μm with the geometric standard deviation of 2.55. The test was also conducted to compare the device performance with other small-volume nebulizers (60), and found to be more efficient in the delivery rate (mass out per minute) than that of other SVNs.

AERx™

The AERx, developed by Aradigm (Hayward, CA), is a metered dose liquid inhaler designed to deliver various pharmaceutical compounds to the peripheral lungs. The system, as shown in Fig. 10, consists of a unit dose disposable container equipped with a nozzle array, a piston assembly, and electronics associated with breath actuation and compliance monitoring functions (61).

The unit dose package contains the unit dose reservoir and an array of laser drilled nozzles, and the reservoir and

Table 13 Breathing patterns

Pattern	Tidal volume (ml)	Breathing frequency (1/min)	Nebulization
P1	50	40	Continuous
P2	200	25	Continuous
P3	440	19	Breath-activated

(Adapted from Ref. 60.)

Table 14 Emitted dose (% of loaded dose) vs. inhalation flow rate ($n = 5$)

Flow rate (L/min)	Emitted dose (% loaded dose)
20	50.6 ± 2.0
30	68.6 ± 3.0
45	72.3 ± 2.5
60	70.9 ± 1.5
70	68.5 ± 1.3
85	66.1 ± 5.1
100	61.5 ± 1.9

(Adapted from Ref. 61.)

Table 15 In vitro performance of solution MDI and AERx system

	Solution MDI ($n = 4$)		AERx system ($n = 4$)	
	Mean	SD	Mean	SD
Emitted dose (%)[a]	63.2	8.2	60.8	7.1
FPF (%)[b]	71.0	5.6	90.6	1.6
MMAD (μm)	1.2	0.1	2.6	0.1
GSD	1.8	< 0.1	1.5	0.3

[a]Percentage of radioactivity contained in the AERx dosage form or ex-valve dose for the MDI.
[b]FPF = Amount of aerosolized radioactivity in droplets with less than 5.7 μm.
(Adapted from Ref. 63.)

nozzle array are connected with a heat seal that allows the formulation to flow from the reservoir to the nozzle after the seal is ruptured. The piston assembly consists of a motor, a piston, and a cam, which compresses the unit dose packet to extrude the drug under pressure through the nozzle array to produce aerosols suitable for inhalation. The AERx also has internal electronic monitoring, which measures the patient's inspiratory flow rate as a function of time of inspiration and triggers the dispensing of the dose at a predetermined inspiratory flow rate and time for optimal delivery. The dosage administered is also logged, thereby providing a record of treatments and an indication of patient compliance with therapy (62).

The performance of the AERx has been characterized both in vitro and in vivo (63–67). Schuster et al. (61) reported in vitro experimental data of emitted dose as a function of inhalation flow rates from 20 to 100 L/min, and Table 14 shows the emitted dose expressed as the percentage of loaded dose at different inhalation flow rates. The emitted dose was consistent at inhalation flow rates ranging from 30 to 70 L/min, which averaged approximately 60–70% of the loaded dose emitted from the device. The percentage of loaded dose emitted from the device was about 51% at the inhalation flow rate of 20 L/min. When the device was used at this low flow rate, the aerosol was not efficiently entrained into the air, which was confirmed by a large fraction of the drug compound recovered from the air channel opposite the nozzle (61). The emitted dose was also decreased with the increase in the inhalation flow rate, which may have been due to increase in turbulent deposition as explained by the authors.

A study was also conducted both in vitro and in vivo to compare the performance of the AERx with a pMDI device that was operated with a SmartMist™ system for in vivo study using the scintigraphic technique (64). Table 15 shows the in vitro experimental data for both the AERx and the pMDI devices.

The in vitro data showed that the fine particle fraction for the AERx was approximately 91% of emitted dose compared with 71% for the pMDI at the comparable emitted dose. The mass median aerodynamic diameter was 2.6 μm for the AERx and 1.2 μm for the pMDI, with a slightly larger GSD. An experiment was conducted to compare the in vivo performance of both devices using scintigraphy (64). The average depositions (expressed as the percentage of loaded dose for the AERx and percentage of ex-valve dose for the pMDI) in the oral-pharynx and stomach were 6.9% with a relative standard deviation (RSD) of 47% for the AERx and 42% with a RSD of 16% for the pMDI respectively. The average depositions in the lungs were 53.3% (RSD = 10.9%) and 21.7 (RSD = 30.9%) for the AERx and the pMDI, respectively. The experimental data also showed that uniform drug distribution in the lungs was achieved while using the AERx (c/p = 1.15) as compared with that of the pMDI (c/p = 1.66), where the c/p ratio is defined as the ratio of drug deposition in the central region to that of peripheral region.

HaloLite™

HaloLite, shown in Fig. 11, is a hand-held drug delivery system developed by Medic-Aid (Bognor Regis, United Kingdom). The device, which uses compressed air, consists of a medication chamber, a control unit, and an aerosol generation assembly that is operated by a portable, dedicated compressor. The aerosol is generated based upon conventional nebulization principles. The control unit allows the patient to select a budenoside nebulizing suspension, salbutamol, or terbutaline, since the device is calibrated to deliver preset doses of 50 μg of budenoside, 200 μg of salbutamol, or 500 μg of terbutaline from commercially available pre-mixed solution formulations

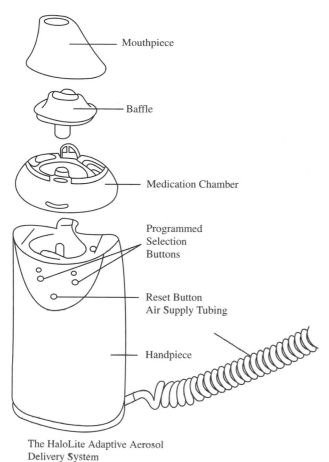

The HaloLite Adaptive Aerosol Delivery System

Fig. 11 The schematic diagram of the Halolite. (Courtesy of Medic-Aid.)

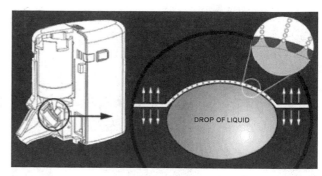

Fig. 12 The schematic diagram of AeroDose™ as shown in AeroGen, Inc.'s website (www.aerogen.com).

of each drug (68). The device has the capability to analyze the patient's breathing pattern (flow rate, frequency, etc.) to determine a) the aerosol pulse time for each inhalation, b) whether the patient is inhaling or exhaling, c) the start of inhalation, and d) trigger the aerosolization process.

In vitro experimental data show that the fine particle fraction (<5.0 μm) ranged from 70 to 80% of the device output, and the coefficient of variation for the dose output was 6% at a preset dose of 63 mg of 1% NaF solution (69). The device was also evaluated in vivo using healthy volunteers and asthmatics, and the coefficient of variations were 11% for the healthy volunteers and 21% for the asthmatics.

New High Frequency Oscillating Devices

AeroDose™

The AeroDose is a battery-operated drug delivery device under development by AeroGen, Inc. (Sunnyvale, CA),

which uses vibrating orifice technology to produce drug aerosols suitable for human inhalation. The schematic diagram of the device and its operation principle are illustrated in Fig. 12. The device consists of a drug canister, aerosol generator assembly, and electronic control unit. The aerosol generator contains a dome-shaped aperture plate with 600 tapered holes that vibrate due to the attachment to a piezoelectric crystal. The piezoelectric material will undergo small physical displacement at ultrasonic frequency to generate aerosols with low velocity. During each use, a droplet of formulation (~ 15 μL) is dispensed from a multidose canister to an aperture plate by a metering pump, as shown in Fig. 12, and an aerosol is then generated by breath activation.

Three AeroDose devices were characterized to determine the in vitro performance using albuterol sulfate with a nominal dose of 120 μg per actuation (70,71). The average liquid volume dispensed for three devices was 15.2 ml with a coefficient of variation (cv) of 2.7%. The emitted dose expressed as percentages of nominal doses were 80% (cv 5.9%), 81% (cv 3.7%), and 79% (cv 4.0%). The MMADs were 2.0 μm (cv 13%), 2.0 μm (cv 5.7%), and 1.9 μm (cv 21%), with GSDs of 2.1 (cv 7.2%), 2.2 (cv 4.5%), and 2.4 (cv 4.7%) for the three devices tested. A lung deposition study using ^{99m}Tc radiolabeled albuterol sulfate was also conducted to determine the amount of drug deposited in the lungs for both the AeroDose and the conventional pMDI. The average lung deposition was 18% (cv 32%) of the emitted dose for the pMDI and 70% (cv 28%) of the emitted dose or an overall delivery efficiency of approximately 56% for the AeroDose for the six volunteers who participated in the study.

Metered solution inhaler (MSI)

The metered solution inhaler (MSI), under development by Sheffield Pharmaceuticals, uses the same aerosolization principle as the AeroDose. The MSI is a portable, hand-held drug delivery device, as shown in Fig. 13. Using a

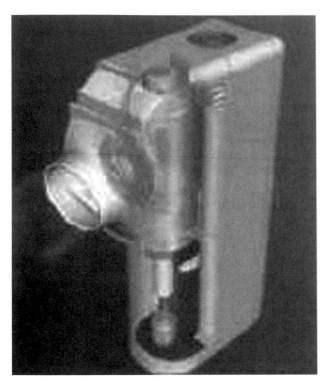

Fig. 13 The metered solution inhaler as shown in Sheffield Pharmaceutical's website (www.sheffieldpharm. com).

motorized pump, drug solution is delivered to the surface of a ultrasonic horn powered by a piezoelectric crystal upon actuation, and is then aerosolized in about 1 s (72, 73).

The performance of the MSI was characterized in vivo using morphine sulfate for systemic absorption (72). A total of 1.25 mg of morphine sulfate was delivered in five doses of 250 μg per actuation to the healthy volunteers. The average amount of drug deposited was approximately 800 μg in the lungs and less than about 500 μg in the oral-pharynx; therefore the average respiratory deposition efficiency was approximately 64% of the inhaled dose. The average amount of drug deposited in the peripheral respireto region was slightly over 300 μg, a little less than 300 μg was deposited in the intermediate lung, and about 200 μg was deposited in the central region. The ratio of deposition in the peripheral to central regions ranged from 1.1 to 2.2. The morphine sulfate concentration in the plasma reached a peak within 3 min after inhalation, compared with 15 min for the subcutaneous injection. The peak plasma concentration level for the inhalation route was more than double compared to the subcutaneous route.

Vibrating membrane nebulizer

The vibrating membrane nebulizer is currently under development by Pari GmbH, (Germany), which is based upon the TouchSpray technology developed by The Technology Partnership plc (United Kingdom). The main aerosol generation principle is similar to that of AeroDose, which uses piezoelectric material as a power source to vibrate a surface having on it a droplet of drug solution. The vibrating membrane nebulizer consists of two major components, a membrane and a piezoelectric ring, as shown in Fig. 14. The membrane is a circular, wafer-thin metal plate with small holes. A ring-shaped piezoelectric actuator excites the membrane to vibrate, thus ejecting the fluid through the holes as droplets and creating aerosols. Unlike the AeroDose, which is a single-dose device, the vibrating membrane nebulizer is a continuous generation device similar to the conventional nebulizer, which produces aerosols during both inhalation and exhalation (74, 75).

Experimental data obtained from in vitro testing using a functional model of the vibrating membrane nebulizer showed that the average percentage of emitted dose for a continuous aerosolization in approximately 8 min was about 79% of dose loaded in the device, and the output rate of the delivery device was found to be about 238 μg/min. The mass median diameter measured by the Malvern Diffraction Sizer was 4.6 μm. It was also found that the cumulative output from the device was linearly proportional to the time of aerosolization, which implied a constant output rate throughout the entire aerosolization process (75). Experimental data obtained from a prototype device developed based upon the functional model showed a reduction from 79 to about 50% in the emitted dose of the device. The amount of drug left in the device increased

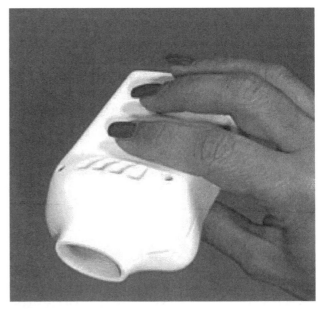

Fig. 14 Hand–held EHD device being developed by BPT.

from 477 to about 1060 mg, which changed from 19 to 43% in terms of percentage to the loaded dose. The increase in the drug amount left in the device reduced the delivery efficiency of the device. The delivery efficiency can be improved by redesigning the flow channel and incorporating a breath-activated function to eliminate the aerosolization process during exhalation, as suggested by the authors (74).

Novel Electrohydrodynamic (EHD) Devices

Electrohydrodynamic (EHD) aerosolization is a process of the disruption of a liquid surface into a spray of droplets when subjected to an electric field. The liquid meniscus at the outlet of a capillary tube takes a conical shape under the action of the electric field. The cone tip breaks up into a spray of fine, charged aerosol (76). The cone-jet mode offers the appealing feature of aerosol monodispersity. It can produce droplets/particles over a wide size range, from submicron to hundreds of microns in size, depending on liquid flow rate, applied voltages, and physical and chemical properties of the liquid. When considering the size range of interest to pulmonary drug delivery (1–5 μm), the production of monodispersed aerosols with relative ease by EHD aerosolization technology is unmatched by any other aerosol generation process. Additionally, the aerosols are generated from capillary nozzles having relatively large diameters (e.g., 100 μm), which are therefore, unlikely to clog at the atomization site or during the metering of each dose. When considering the particle size range of 1–5 μm, the capacity to produce monodispersed aerosols with relative ease by EHD is also unmatched by any other aerosol generation process (77). The particle size distribution of the aerosol can be controlled by adjusting a number of variables, such as physical and chemical properties of drug formulations, operating conditions, and electric field. Another key clinical and technical attribute of the EHD technology is that it delivers a soft (isokinetic) aerosol cloud of nearly monodispersed particles to the patient, because aerosol formation does not require any liquid propellants or other pressurized systems. The EHD process can aerosolize a broad range of drug formulations, requires low precision manufacturing (i.e., low-cost production), and is amenable to miniaturization. These fundamental features underpin the ability of EHD pulmonary drug delivery devices to aerosolize a wide array of drug formulations, and provide accurate, reproducible drug delivery with targeted dosing to the human respiratory tract. Battelle Pulmonary Therapeutics, Inc. (BPT) is currently developing an array of EHD pulmonary devices, ranging from small hand-held disposable units, home table-top aerosol delivery devices, to large benchtop clinical devices designed to operate continuously with high outputs (Fig. 15).

In vitro performance

Prior to clinical evaluations, comprehensive studies were conducted to characterize prototype EHD pulmonary drug delivery devices for emitted dose uniformity and reproducibility of particle size distribution (78). Table 16 shows the dose uniformity. The nominal dose is defined as the amount of active drug metered as a liquid solution from the device. The emitted dose is the amount of aerosolized drug obtained at the exit of the mouthpiece, and the device delivery efficiency is the ratio of the emitted to nominal dose. The mean delivery efficiency was approximately 94% (SD = 3.2) with a 3.4% coefficient of variation. The delivery efficiency for the two devices tested was 93% (SD = 3.60, $n = 5$) and 95% (SD = 2.8, $n = 5$), respectively. The intradevice variation was 1.7% (coefficient of variation, $n = 2$ prototypes). There were no significant differences ($p > 0.05$) in the drug mass output within the device throughout its life cycle, nor between devices tested in the study.

Fig. 15 shows the drug mass recovered from the various stages of the impactor and device at a nominal drug dose of 75 μg per actuation. The amount of drug deposited on each stage was used to calculate the MMAD and GSD. The calculated MMAD was 2.85 μm with a GSD of 1.6. The fine particle fraction (FPF) of the aerosol was 90% (<5.8 μm) of the emitted dose, and 95% (<5.8 μm) of the dose distal to the USP throat.

In vivo performance

A Phase I clinical study was conducted to evaluate the performance of the prototype EHD pulmonary drug delivery device in healthy volunteers (78). The EHD

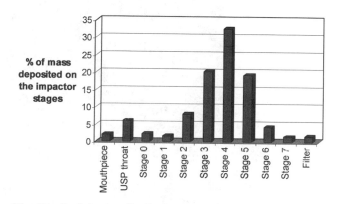

Fig. 15 Particle size distribution of a NCE from EHD device. (Adapted from Ref. 78.)

Table 16 Dose uniformity of a NCE delivered EHD pulmonary drug delivery device

Device ID	Actuation number	Nominal dose (μg)	Emitted dose (μg)	Device delivery efficiency (%)
Device 1	3	75	74.2	98.9
	15	75	68.5	91.3
	30	75	69.1	92.1
	45	75	67.8	90.4
	60	75	67.8	90.4
Device 2	3	75	71.3	95.0
	15	75	67.8	90.4
	30	75	73.4	97.9
	45	75	71.7	95.6
	60	75	71.7	95.6
Mean			70.3	93.7
SD			2.42	3.22
CV(%)			3.44	3.44

(Adapted from Ref. 78.)

device was compared with a commercially available capsule dry powder inhaler (DPI). The NCE was prepared in two formulations. The first was a powder formulation specific for the DPI, and the second was formulated in a liquid solution for the EHD device. Each formulation was radiolabelled with ^{99m}Tc, and the amount of drug deposited in the lungs from each device was quantified using gamma scintigraphy. Each volunteer was administered one dose of drug using the DPI and three different doses using the EHD device. The nominal doses were 1000 μg for the DPI and 150, 250, and 400 μg for the EHD device. Multiple blood samples were collected from each subject up to 8 h after dosing to measure plasma drug

concentration. An interval of 1 week was used between administration of the four doses.

The average whole lung deposition efficiency for the EHD device expressed as the percentage of the emitted dose was approximately 78% (cv 7.3%) for the 400-μg dose.

Fig. 16 shows representative scintigraphic images from both the DPI and the EHD pulmonary drug delivery device. It can be seen that the EHD pulmonary drug delivery device produced a uniform deposition distribution through the lung field with only ~16% deposition in the oral-pharyngeal region, and virtually no drug in the GI tract. However, the amount of drug

EHD Device (400 μg)   **DPI (1000 μg)**

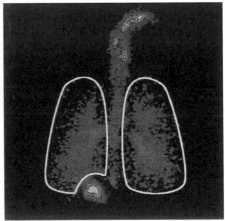

Fig. 16 Scintigraphic images of the EHD device and the DPI. (Adapted from Ref. 78.)

Table 17 Performance comparison of various devices

Delivery system for liquid	System features	Particle size	Device efficiency	In vivo deposition
Respimat	Mechanical spring	3.5–6.5 μm		30–45% of emitted dose
AeroEclipse™	Compressed air powered	~3.6 μm	11–36% of nominal dose	
AERx	Mechanical, battery powered	2–4 μm	50–72% of nominal dose	~53% of loaded dose
Halo*lite*	Compressed air powered	~3.0 μm		8–10% of nominal dose
AeroDose	Vibrating orifice	~2.0 μm	~80% of nominal dose	~70% of emitted dose
MSI™	Vibrating orifice	FPF >50% of emitted dose		~64% of emitted dose
Membrane nebulizer	Vibrating orifice, continuous mode	NA	50–80% of emitted dose	NA
EHD	Electrospray	2–4 μm, adjustable	~93% of nominal dose	~78% of emitted dose

deposited in the oral-pharyngeal region using the DPI averaged 67% of metered dose, which was nearly 6 times higher compared with that of the high dose delivered using the EHD device. The AUC for plasma drug concentration with the DPI was approximately 20% higher than that of the EHD device for a comparable deposited pulmonary dose. It appeared that the higher systemic exposure resulting from the DPI was likely due to absorption from the throat and GI tract.

Performance Comparisons

Comparison of the performance of various drug delivery devices based upon the data published in the literature is often difficult because of inconsistency in the experimental methods used in the characterization of those devices as well as differences in the devices. However it is also extremely important to understand the different features of the devices to help select the best device for a drug compound intended for delivery through the human respiratory tract. Table 17 summarizes the performance of devices currently under development.

The selection of a drug delivery system suitable for the administration of a particular drug compound to human respiratory airways depends not only on the device performance, but also on many other factors such as drug properties, formulation excipient, intended site of action, marketing preference, and regulatory requirements. It is important to fully understand the drug properties during the formulation development so that a proper excipient system can be identified. The

selection of an excipient for a particular drug also influences the particle size distribution of aerosol generated from a drug delivery device. For example, increasing the volatile components in the solution formulation can reduce the diameter of aerosol particles because of solvent evaporation, which is another variable available to optimize drug formulation and device performance for either local delivery or systemic absorption. The stability of drug product in the long term (usually ~2 years) has also to be considered in the device selection process. Some drug compounds can only be packaged in a unit dose because of instability of the drug product in the multidose reservoir; therefore, a device that can be fitted with a unit dose package is needed for such purpose. The drug delivery devices mentioned above have different features and different requirements for the drug formulation, and there is no single delivery device that can meet all the needs for such requirements. To ensure a successful launch of a new inhalation drug product, it is necessary to conduct a comprehensive evaluation of a potential drug candidate for administrating via inhalation.

REFERENCES

1. Hinds, W.C. *Aerosol Technology, Properties, Behavior, and Measurement of Airborne Particles*; 2nd Ed.; John Wiley & Sons, Inc.: New York, 1999.
2. Wood, R.E.; Knowles, M.R. Recent Advances in Aerosol Therapy. J. Aerosol Med. **1994**, 7 (1), 1–11.
3. Byron, P.R. Aerosol Formulation, Generation, and Delivery Using Nonmetered System. *Respiratory Drug Delivery*; Byron, P.R. Ed.; CRC Press, Inc.: Boca Raton, 1990, 143–165.

4. Patton, J.S.; Platz, R.M. (A) Routes of Delivery: Case Studies, (B) Pulmonary Delivery of Peptides and Proteins for Systemic Action. Adv. Drug Delivery Rev. **1992**, *8*, 179–196.

5. Gupta, P.K.; Adjei, A.L. Therapeutic Inhalation Aerosol. *Inhalation Delivery of Therapeutic Peptides and Proteins*; Adjie, A.L., Gupta, P.K. Eds.; Marcel Dekker, Inc.: New York, 1997, 185–234.

6. Newman, S.P.; Forward. *Inhalation Delivery of Therapeutic Peptides and Proteins*; Adjie, A.L., Gupta, P.K. Eds.; Marcel Dekker, Inc.: New York, 1997, xi–xii.

7. Clark, A.R. Medical Aerosol Inhalers: Past, Present, and Future. Aerosol Sci. Technol. **1995**, *22*, 374–391.

8. Thiel, C.G.; From Susie's Question to CFC Free: AN Inventor's Perspective on Forty Years of MDI Development and Regulation. *Respiratory Drug Delivery*; Byron, P.R., Dalby, R.N., Farr, S.J. Eds.; Interpharm Press, 1996, 349–351.

9. Lefebvre, Arthur H. Basic Processes in Atomization. *Atomization and Sprays*; Hemisphere Publishing Co.: Washington, DC, 1989, 27.

10. Newman, S.P.; Pellow, P.G.D. Valuation of Jet Nebulizer. *In Drug Delivery to the Respiratory Tract*; Ganderton, D., Jones, T. Eds.; Ellis Horwood Ltd.: Chichester, England, 1987, 124–132.

11. Klusener, O. The Injection Process in Compressorless Diesel Engines. VDIZ **1933**, *77* (7).

12. Niven, RalphW. Atomization and Nebulizers. *Inhalation Aerosols*; Hickey, A.J. Ed.; Marcel Dekker, Inc.: New York, 1996, 273–312.

13. Rizkalla, A.A.; Lefebvre, A.H.; Influence of Liquid Properties on Air-Blast Atomizer Spray Characteristics. ASME Gas Turbine Conference **1974**, 1–5, Paper No. 74-GT-1.

14. Searls, E.M.; Snyder, F.M. Relation of Viscosity to Drop Sizes. J. Econ. Entomol. **1936**, *29*, 1167–1170.

15. Hinds, W.C.; Macher, J.M.; First, M.W. Size Distribution of Aerosols Produced by the Laskin Aerosol Generator Using Substitute Materials for DOP. Am. Ind. Hyg. Ass. J. **1983**, *44*, 495–500.

16. McCallion, Orla, N.M.; Taylor, Kevin, M.G.; Thomas, Marian; Taylor, Anthony, J. Nebulization of Fluids of Different Physicochemical Properties with Air-Jet and Ultrasonic Nebulizers. Pharm. Res. **1995**, *12* (11), 1682–1688.

17. Clark, Andrew, R. The Use of Laser Diffraction for the Evaluation of the Aerosol Clouds Generated by Medical Nebulizers. Int. J. Pharm. **1995**, *115*, 69–78.

18. Davis, S.S. Physico-chemical Studies on Aerosol Solutions for Drug Delivery.] I. Water-Propylene Glycol Systems. Int. J. Pharm. **1978**, *1*, 71–83.

19. Newman, S.P.; Pellow, P.G.D.; Clarke, S.W. Dropsizes from Medical Atomisers (Nebulizer) for Drug Solution with Different Viscosities and Surface Tensions. Atomization Spray Technol. **1987**, *3*, 1–11.

20. Phipps, Paul, R.; Gonda, Igor; Droplets Produced by Medical Nebulizers Some Factors Affecting Their Size and Solute Concentration. Chest **1990**, *97* (6), 1327–1332.

21. Mercer, T.T.; Tillery, M.I.; Chow, H.Y. Operating Characteristics of Some Compressed-Air Nebulizers. Am. Ind. Hyg. Assoc. J. **1968**, *29*, 66–78.

22. Smye, S.W.; Jollie, M.I.; Cunliffe, H.; Littlewood, J.M. Measurement and Predication of Drug Solvent Losses by Evaporation from a Jet Nebuliser. Clin. Phys. Physiol. Meas. **1992**, *13*, 129–134.

23. Ferron, G.A.; Soderholm, S.C. Estimation of the Times for Evaporation of Pure Water Droplets and for Stabilization of Salt Solution Particles. J. Aerosol Sci. **1990**, *21*, 415–429.

24. Newman, S.P.; Pellow, P.G.D.; Clay, M.M.; Clarke, S.W. Evaluation of Jet Nebulizers for Use with Gentamicin Solution. Thorax **1985**, *40*, 671–676.

25. Wood, J.A.; Wilson, R.S.E.; Bary, C. Changes in Salbutamol Concentration in the Reservoir Solution of a Jet Nebulizer. Br. J. Dis. Chest **1986**, *80*, 164–169.

26. May, K.R. The Collison Nebulizer: Description, Performance and Application. Aerosol Sci. **1973**, *4*, 235–243.

27. Everard, M.L.; Clark, A.R.; Milner, A.D. Drug Delivery from the Nebulisers. Arch. Dis. Childhood **1992**, *67*, 586–591.

28. Ding, J.Y.; Brooker, M.J.; Andre, J.C.; Zimlich, W.C.; Imondi, A.R.; Placke, M.E. Performance Evaluation of the Pari LC Nebulizer Using Different Nebulization Pressures. *Respiratory Drug Delivery VII*; Dalby, R.N., Byron, P.R., Farr, S.J., Peart, J. Eds.; Serentec Press, Inc.: 2000, 349–351.

29. Finlay, W.H.; Stapleton, W.K.; Zuberbuhler, P. Variations in Predicted Regional Lung Deposition of Salbutamol Sulphate Between 19 Nebulizer Types. J. Aerosol Med. **1998**, *11* (2), 65–80.

30. Ganderton, D. Targeted Delivery of Inhaled Drugs: Current Challenges and Future Goals. J. Aerosol Med. **1999**, *12*, S3–S8.

31. Stapleton, K.W.; Finlay, W.H.; Zuberbuhler, P. An In Vitro Method for Determining Regional Dosages Delivered by Jet Nebulizers. J. Aerosol Med. **1994**, *7*, 325–344.

32. Morén, F.; Aerosol Dosage Forms and Formulation. *Aerosols in Medicine, Principle, Diagnosis and Therapy*; Morén, F., Dolovich, M.B., Newhouse, M.T., Newman, S.P. Eds.; Elsevier Science Publisher: Amsterdam, 1993, 321–350.

33. Hickey, A.J.; Evans, R.M. Aerosol Generation from Propellant-Driven Metered Dose Inhalers. In *Inhalation Aerosols*; Hickey, A.J. Ed.; Marcel Dekker, Inc.: New York, 1996, 417–439.

34. Clark, A.R. MDIs: Physics of Aerosol Formulation. J. Aerosol Med. **1996**, *9* (S1), s19–s26.

35. Edman, P. Pharmaceutical Formulations—Suspensions and Solutions. J. Aerosol Med. **1994**, *7* (S1), s3–s6.

36. Hallworth, G.W. The Formulation and Evaluation of Pressurized Metered-Dose Inhalers. *Drug Delivery to the Respiratory Tract*; Jones, D.G.T. Ed.; Ellis Horwood, Ltd.: Chichester England, 1987, 87–118.

37. Byron, PeterR.; Aerosol Formulation, Generation, and Delivery Using Metered System. *Respiratory Drug Delivery*; Byron, P.R. Ed.; CRC Press, Inc. Boca Raton, 1990, 167–205.

38. Physical Tests and Determinations: ⟨601⟩ Aerosols, The Official Compendia of Standards, USP 24 NF19; U.S. Pharmacopeia and National Formulary, 2000, 1895–1912.

39. Leach, C. Enhanced Drug Delivery through Reformulating MDIs with HFA Propellants—Drug Deposition and Its Effect on Preclinical and Clinical Programs. In *Respiratory*

Drug Delivery V; Byron, P.R., Dalby, R.N., Farr, S.J. Eds.; Interpharm Press, 1996, 133–144.

40. Fink, J.B. Metered-dose Inhalers, Dry Powder Inhalers, and Transitions. Respir. Care **2000**, *45* (6), 623–635.

41. Borgström, L.; Newman, S. Total and Regional Lung Deposition of Terbutaline Sulphate Inhaled via a Pressurised MDI or via Turbuhaler. Int. J. Pharm. **1993**, *97*, 47–53.

42. Sterk, P.J.; Plomp, A.; van de Vate, J.F.; Quanjer, P.H. Physical Properties of Aerosols Produced by Several Jet- and Ultrasonic Nebulizers. Bull. Eur. Physiopathol. Respir. **1984**, *20*, 65–72.

43. Greenspan, B.J. Ultrasonic and Electrohydrodynamic Methods for Aerosol Generation. In *Inhalation Aerosols*; Hickey, A.J. Ed.; Marcel Dekker, Inc.: New York, 1996, 313–335.

44. Lang, R.J. Ultrasonic Atomization of Liquids. J. Acoust. Soc. Am. **1962**, *34*, 6–8.

45. Hager, J.; Gober, K.-H.; Löhr, J.-P.; D ürr. Measurement of Particle and Mass Distribution of Pentamidine Aerosol by Ultrasonic and Air Jet Nebulizers. J. Aerosol Med. **1992**, *5* (2), 65–79.

46. Everard, M.L. Aerosol Therapy Past, Present, and Future: A Clinician's Perspective. Respir. Care **2000**, *45* (6), 769–776.

47. Coyne, T.C. Introduction to the CFC Problem. J. Aerosol Med. **1991**, *4* (3), 175–180.

48. Kontny, M.J.; Destefand, G.; Jager, P.D.; McNamara, D.P.; Turi, J.S.; Van Campen, L. Issues Surrounding MDI Formulation Development with Non-CFC Propellants. J. Aerosol Med. **1991**, *4* (3), 181–187.

49. Leach, C.L. Approaches and Challenges to Use Freon Propellant Replacements. Aerosol Sci. Technol. **1995**, *22*, 328–334.

50. Keller, M. Innovations and Perspectives of Metered Dose Inhalers in Pulmonary Drug Delivery. Int. J. Pharm. **1999**, *186*, 81–90.

51. Larsen, J.S.; Hahn, M.; Kochevar, J.W.; Morris, R.J.; Kasier, H.B.; Weisberg, S.C.; Halverson, P.C.; Quessey, S.N. Administration Errors with a Conventional Metered Dose Inhaler Versus a Novel Breath Actuated Device. Ann. All. **1993**, *71*, 103–106.

52. Epstein, S.E.; Manning, C.P.; Ashley, M.J. Corey, P.N.; Survey of the Clinical Use of Pressurized Aerosol Inhaler. Can. Med. Assoc. J. **1979**, *120* (7), 813–816.

53. Newman, S.P.; Weisz, A.W.B.; Talaee, N.; Clarke, S.W. Improvement of Drug Delivery with a Breath Actuated Pressurised Aerosol for Patients with Poor Inhaler Technique. Thorax **1991**, *46*, 712–716.

54. Zierenberg, B. Optimizing the In Vitro Performance of Respimat. J. Aerosol. Med. **1999**, *12*, s19–s24.

55. Newman, S.P. Use of Gamma Scintigraphy to Evaluate the Performance of New Inhalers. J. Aerosol. Med. **1999**, *12*, s25–s31.

56. Steed, K.P.; Towse, L.J.; Freund, B.; Newman, S.P. Lung and Oropharyngeal Depositions of Fenoterol Hydrobromide Delivered from the Prototype III Hand-held Multidose Respimat Nebuliser. Eur. J. Pharm. Sci. **1997**, *5*, 55–61.

57. Newman, S.P.; Steed, K.P.; Reader, S.J.; Hopper, G.; Zierenberg, B. Efficient Delivery to the Lungs of Flunisolide from a New Portable Hand-held Multidose Nebuliser. J. Pharm. Sci. **1996**, *85*, 960–964.

58. Newman, S.P.; Brown, J.; Steed, K.P.; Reader, S.J.; Kladders, H.; Lung Deposition of Fenoterol and Flunisolide Delivered Using a Novel Device for Inhaled Medications. Chest **1998**, *113*, 957–963.

59. Smaldone, G.C. *Enhanced In-Vitro Delivery of Budesonide via Continuous and Breath-Activated Nebulization*; European Respiratory Society, Florence Italy, Aug. 30–Sep. 3, 2000.

60. Blacker, R.; Morton, R.W.; Mitchell, J.P.; Nagel, M.W.; Hess, D.R. *The Effect of Small Volume Nebulizer (SVN) Design on Fine Particle Mass Delivery of a Bronchodilator* Present at Drug Delivery to the Lungs, London, UK, Dec., 1999.

61. Schuster, J.A.; Farr, S.J.; Cipolla, D.; Wilnbanks, T.; Rosell, J.; Lloyd, P.; Gonda, I. Design and Performance Validation of a Highly Efficient and Reproducible Compact Aerosol Delivery System: AERx™. In *Respiratory Drug Delivery VI*; Dalby, R.N., Byron, P.R., Farr, S.J. Eds.; Interpharm Press, 1998, 83–90.

62. Dolovich, M. New Propellant-Free Technologies under Investigation. J. Aerosol Med. **1999**, s9–s17.

63. Schuster, J.; Rubsamen, R.M.; Lloyd, P.; Lloyd, J. The AERx™ Aerosol Delivery System. Pharma. Res. **1997**, *14*, 354–357.

64. Farr, S.J.; Warren, S.J.; Lloyd, P.; Okikawa, J.K.; Schuster, J.A.; Rowe, A.M.; Rubsamen, R.M.; Taylor, G. Comparison of In Vitro and In Vivo Efficiencies of a Novel Unit-Dose Liquid Aerosol Generator and a Pressurized Metered Dose Inhaler. Int. J. Pharm. **2000**, *198*, 63–70.

65. Farr, S.J.; Schuster, J.A.; Lloyd, P.; Lloyd, L.J.; Okikawa, J.K.; Rubsamen, R.M. AERx™—Development of a Novel Liquid Aerosol Delivery System: Concept to Clinic. In *Respiratory Drug Delivery V*; Byron, P.R., Dalby, R.N., Farr, S.J. Eds.; Interpharm Press: , 1996, 175–185.

66. Cipolla, D.; Boyd, B.; Evans, R.; Warren, S.; Taylor, G.; Farr, S.J. Bolus Administration of INS365 Studying the Feasibility of Delivering High Dose Drugs Using the AERx™ Pulmonary Delivery System. In *Respiratory Drug Delivery VII*; Dalby, R.N., Byron, P.R., Farr, S.J., Peart, J. Eds.; Interpharm Press, 2000, 231–239.

67. Chan, H.K.; Daciskas, E.; Eberl, S.; Robinson, M.; Bautovich, G.; Young, I. Deposition of Aqueous Aerosol of Technetium-99m Diethylene Triamine Penta-Acetic Acid Generated and Delivered by a Novel System (AERx™) in Healthy Subjects. Eur. J. Nuclear Med. **1999**, *26*, 320–327.

68. Denyer, J. Adaptive Aerosol Delivery in Practice. Eur. Respir. Rev. **1997**, *7*, 388–389.

69. Denyer, J.; Nikander, K.; Halolite, T.M. A Novel Liquid Drug Aerosol Delivery System. *Respiratory Drug Delivery VI*; Dalby, R.N., Byron, P.R., Farr, S.J., Peart, J. Eds.; Interpharm Press, 1998, 311–314.

70. De Young, L.R.; Chamber, F.; Narayan, S.; Wu, C. The AeroDose Multidose Inhaler Device Design and Delivery Characteristics. In *Respiratory Drug Delivery VI*; Dalby, R.N., Byron, P.R., Farr, S.J., Peart, J. Eds.; Interpharm Press, 1998, 91–95.

71. De Young, L.R.; Chamber, F.; Narayan, S.; Wu, C. Albuterol Sulphate Delivery from the AeroDose Liquid Inhaler. In *Respiratory Drug Delivery VI*; Dalby, R.N., Byron, P.R., Farr, S.J., Peart, J. Eds.; Interpharm Press, 1998, 315–318.

72. Hirst, P.H.; Bacon, R.E.; Newman, S.P.; Armer, T.; Mohsen, N.; Pavkov, R.; Byron, D. Deposition, Absorption and Bioavailability of Aerosolized Morphine Sulfate Delivered by a Novel Hand-held Device, The Metered Solution Inhaler (MSI). In *Respiratory Drug Delivery VII*; Dalby, R.N., Byron, P.R., Farr, S.J., Peart, J. Eds.; Interpharm Press, 2000, 467–469.

73. van der Linden, K.; Haack, O.; Ruttel, M. US Patent, 5, 950, 619.

74. Stangl, R.; Luangkhot, N.; Liening-Ewert, R.; Jahn, D. Characterising the First Prototype of a Vibrating Membrane Nebuliser. In *Respiratory Drug Delivery VII*; Dalby, R.N., Byron, P.R., Farr, S.J., Peart, J. Eds.; Interpharm Press, 2000, 455–458.

75. Stangl, R.; Luangkhot, N.; Liening-Ewert, R.; Jahn, D. Characterising the Functional Model of a Vibrating Membrane Nebuliser. *Drug Delivery to the Lungs*; Aerosol Society: London, 1999.

76. Cloupeau, M.; Prunet-Foch, B. Electrostatic Spraying of Liquids in Cone-jet Mode. J. Electronics **1989**, *22*, 135–159.

77. Gomez, A.; Bingham, L.de Juan; Tang, K. Production of Protein Nanoparticles by Electrospray Drying. J. Aerosol Sci. **1998**, *29*, 561–574.

78. Zimlich, W.C.; Ding, J.Y.; Busick, D.R.; Moutvic, R.R.; Placke, M.E.; Hirst, P.H.; Pitcairn, G.R.; Malik, S.; Newman, S.P.; Macintyre, F.; Miller, P.R.; Shepherd, M.T.; Lukas, T.M. The Development of a Novel Electrohydrodynamic Pulmonary Drug Delivery Device. In *Respiratory Drug Delivery VII*; Dalby, R.N., Byron, P.R., Farr, S.J., Peart, J. Eds.; Interpharm Press, 2000, 241–246.

IONTOPHORESIS

J. Bradley Phipps
Erik R. Scott
J. Richard Gyory
Rama V. Padmanabhan
ALZA Corporation, Mountain View, California

INTRODUCTION

Iontophoresis is a method of transferring substances to and from the body for therapeutic or diagnostic purposes by applying an electric potential to enhance their movement across biological membranes. The most common applications of iontophoresis involve the delivery of therapeutic substances across the skin, though there are numerous examples of the use of iontophoresis to treat conditions of the eye, ear, nose, and mouth. Iontophoresis can also be used to remove substances (e.g., glucose) from the body. A technique known as microiontophoresis employs a small capillary probe to study cellular function by releasing precise quantities of active substances.

Banga (1) has stated that Veratti made the earliest references to the use of an electric potential to enhance the penetration of charged substances into tissues in the year 1747. Stephane Luduc (2) is generally recognized as the most important early researcher in the field because of his comprehensive studies of iontophoresis described in the 1907 publication "Les Ions et les Medications Ioniques."

Today, iontophoresis of drugs across skin or mucosal membranes is a noninvasive (needleless) method where the rate of delivery is primarily determined by the magnitude of the applied current, making patterned and on-demand delivery possible. Commercially available devices are typically bench-top systems with discrete patches connected to a power supply by electrical cables. However, due to recent innovations in electronic circuitry and battery technology, iontophoretic treatments can be administered with small, integrated patch-like systems.

The most common therapeutic applications of iontophoresis are topical administration of lidocaine as a local anesthetic and dexamethasone for treatment of local inflammation (Iomed, Inc., Salt Lake City, Utah and Empi Corp., Minneapolis, Monnesota). In addition to these therapeutic uses, iontophoretic systems are commercially available for the diagnosis of cystic fibrosis. For example, the CF Indicator® (Scandipharm, Birmingham, Alabam)

and the Webster Sweat Inducer (Wescor, Inc., Logan, Utah) deliver pilocarpine to cause local sweating: sweat is collected and analyzed for high levels of chloride. More recently, iontophoresis has been used to extract glucose from the skin as a means of detecting hypo- and hyperglycemia (Cygnus Corp., Redwood City, California).

Although these examples demonstrate the successful commercial use of iontophoretic technology for topical delivery of compounds, transdermal systems for systemic administration of medicinal agents have not been widely employed. There is, however, heightened interest in this field because of potential medical and economical benefits offered by iontophoretic technology, especially for meeting the delivery challenges posed by new biotechnology compounds.

A schematic diagram of a transdermal iontophoretic system on skin is shown in Fig. 1. A source of electrical energy, such as a battery, supplies electric current to the body through two electrodes. The first electrode, called the donor electrode, delivers the therapeutic agent into the body. The second electrode, called the counter or receptor electrode, closes the electrical circuit. Each electrode contacts an ionically conductive reservoir, normally present as a liquid or hydrogel. The reservoirs are placed on the patient's skin and contain either the drug (for the donor electrode assembly) or a biocompatible electrolyte (for the counter electrode assembly).

TRANSPORT MECHANISM

The term iontophoresis encompasses several processes for moving molecules across the skin: electromigration, electroosmosis, and electroporation. Electromigration is the movement of charged ionic species in response to an applied electric field. This process is usually of primary importance for delivering charged drug species. The movement of charged species within a solvent can induce solvent flow by a process known as electroosmosis. This process is useful for delivering both

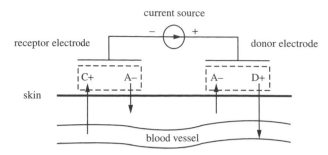

Fig. 1 Schematic diagram of an iontophoretic device on skin indicating the flow of ions in response to an applied voltage.

neutral and charged drug species. Electroporation is the temporary creation of aqueous pores through lipid bilayers by applying high-voltage pulses, typically 50–1000 V, across the bilayers of a biological membrane. This process is useful for delivering large hydrophilic drug species. For any given iontophoretic treatment, one or more of these processes may occur simultaneously and to a varying extent, depending on the magnitude and duration of the applied electric field, the composition of the donor reservoir, and the type of the tissue being treated.

The movement of charges due to electromigration is illustrated in Fig. 1. In this diagram, positively charged drug (D^+) and its counter ion (A^-) are formulated for delivery from the anodic donor reservoir. The cathodic counter reservoir contains biologically acceptable cations (C^+) and anions (A^-). When an electric field is applied, drug ions migrate into the skin and endogenous anions, mostly chloride, migrate from the body into the donor reservoir. Simultaneously, at the cathodic counter electrode, anions migrate from the counter reservoir into the skin, whereas endogenous cations, mostly sodium and potassium, migrate from the body into the counter reservoir. The movement of ions maintains local electroneutrality throughout this process.

For iontophoretic treatments involving placement of the system on the skin, the therapeutic agent in the donor reservoir must cross the outermost layer of the skin, known as the stratum corneum, which is the primary barrier to permeation of substances both into and out of the body. The stratum corneum's excellent barrier properties result from its unique structure: approximately 10–20 layers of flattened, keratin-rich cells cemented together by lipid bilayers composed primarily of ceramides. In general, lipophilic species are capable of traversing the stratum corneum because of their ability to partition into the intercellular lipid region. In contrast, most ionic and polar substances are largely excluded from this region.

At the typical voltages used in iontophoresis (e.g., 2–80 V), the nature and composition of the pathways in the skin remain matters of some debate. However, there is a growing body of evidence that the preferred path for ionic species across the stratum corneum is not spatially homogenous, but rather consists of a distribution of localized regions. These regions include endogenous shunt-like structures across the stratum corneum such as sweat ducts and hair follicles, but may also include pathways not associated with natural shunts. Direct physical measurements of the transport of model permeants through the skin of hairless and nude mice have shown that between 60 and 90% of the overall flux can be explained by such regions (3).

The rate of transport of a charged drug species across a biological membrane is generally modeled by the Nernst–Planck equation. This equation contains terms for diffusion, electromigration, and bulk convection. However, under optimized iontophoretic conditions the electromigration contribution is often much greater than that of the other two, therefore the expression for delivery of an ionic drug species is frequently simplified to include only the electromigration term. The molecular flow of drug is thus related to the electric current, according to Faraday's principle:

$$N = (t_d I M)/(z_d F) \qquad (1)$$

where N = total rate of delivery, t_d = transport number (the fraction of charge carried by the drug ion), I = current applied across the skin, M = drug molecular weight, z_d = charge of the drug molecule, and F = Faraday's constant (96,485 $coul$/Eq).

Many researchers have have used in vitro and in vivo studies to demonstrate that the rate of drug delivery is linearly proportional to the applied current over a wide range. Because studies are typically performed with a fixed skin contact area, this proportionality indicates that the transport number is a constant and not dependent on the current density. However, the transport number is unique for each drug, and is a function of the drug's mobility, charge, and concentration, as compared with those of other migrating species. These dependencies are summarized in the following expression:

$$t_d = \frac{\mu_d |z_d| C_d}{\Sigma_i \mu_i |z_i| C_i} \qquad (2)$$

where μ_d, z_d, and C_d are the mobility, charge and molar concentration, respectively, of the drug species, and μ_i, z_i, and C_i are the mobility, charge, and concentration for each mobile ion that competes with the drug for transport across the skin barrier. Competing ions are those in the formulation that have the same sign of charge as the drug (i.e., competing coions), as well as those ions in the body that have the opposite sign as the drug (competing counterions).

The transport number determines delivery efficiency; that is, the amount of drug delivered per unit charge passed across the skin. Because it is desirable to minimize current (for optimal biocompatibility and battery longevity), it is advantageous to develop a formulation that maximizes t_d. This can be accomplished by maximizing the mobility and concentration of drug species while minimizing, to the greatest extent possible, the mobility and concentration of the competing species. Simple measures to achieve this include incorporating the highest practical concentration of the drug in the formulation, as well as avoiding excipients or impurities that produce mobile coions in the formulation. Even if both of these measures are taken, a t_d value of unity (i.e., all current is carried by the drug ion) is still unattainable in practice, because of endogenous counterions in tissue (e.g., Na^+ and Cl^-). However, the efficiency-lowering effect of competing counterions can be reduced by exploiting the inherent permselectivity of skin. Permselectivity based on charge arises from the principle of Donnan exclusion. The skin has an isoelectric point of about pH 4. Therefore, for a formulation with a pH value below four the skin will have a net positive charge and favor transport of anions; and at a formulation pH > 4, skin will have a net negative charge and favor transport of cations. Thus, at the physiological pH 7.4, skin should be negatively charged and therefore be *cation selective*.

Efficient iontophoretic delivery depends on the materials and excipients used in the system. Selection of appropriate electrodes and formulations are critical to maximizing the efficiency of iontophoretic treatments. The following sections will summarize key criteria for selection of electrodes and formulations for transdermal applications, however, many of the same principles are applicable to iontophoretic systems used on mucosa or implanted within the body.

ELECTRODES

Electrodes apply the driving force for ion migration and are therefore critical components of the system. They serve as the bridge between the electric circuit and the two reservoirs, and perform both electrical and chemical functions. During iontophoretic therapy, electrodes undergo sustained electrochemical reactions and thus the migration of reactants is a critical functional consideration. In this aspect, electrodes used in iontophoretic devices are different from those of most other medical electrodes. For example, medical potentiometric electrodes (such as those used for electrocardiograms or electroencephalograms) undergo no net reaction because little or no electrode current is required by the measurement equipment. In other applications such as cardiac pacing or transcutaneous electrical nerve stimulation (TENS), the applied voltage pulses are extremely brief (milliseconds or less) or of alternating polarity so the net quantity of reaction products is not great. For these applications the management of electrochemical reactions is achieved merely by constructing the electrodes from inert materials, for example, gold, platinum, or stainless steel. In contrast, iontophoretic electrodes are usually inherently reactive materials and are chosen for their preferred electrochemical attributes, as is described below. Because of their reactivity, and also because electrodes contact the drug formulation directly and therefore the patient's body indirectly, it can be technically challenging to choose an electrode system that possesses adequate performance while avoiding adverse material and biological interactions during storage and use.

As indicated in Fig. 1, a transdermal iontophoretic system requires that two electrode assemblies contact the patient's skin. The donor electrode (also known as the delivery or active electrode) contacts the drug reservoir. The counter electrode (also known as the return or receptor electrode) contacts the counter reservoir and completes the electrical circuit by providing a path for the current. The two reservoirs are separated from each other and contact skin over a fixed area. The electrodes apply an electric field across the skin by converting electric current supplied by the battery into ionic current moving in the skin and body. In doing so, a Faradaic reaction takes place at the electrode/electrolyte interface. As described previously in this chapter, there is generally a linear dependence of the rate of drug delivery on this current.

The polarity of the donor and counter electrodes depends on the sign of the charge on the species to be delivered. To cause migration of positively charged species from the donor reservoir into the skin, the donor electrode must have a positive polarity (i.e., anode), and the counter electrode must have a negative polarity (i.e., cathode). For negatively charged species, the polarity is reversed, so that the donor electrode is the cathode, and the counter electrode is the anode.

A practical electrode system must meet a variety of performance, compatibility, and physical requirements. When possible, the electrode system should provide for maximum drug delivery efficiency (i.e., the rate of drug delivered per unit current), operate at low voltage (i.e., <1 V), have adequate longevity (e.g., 24 h), and distribute the current evenly over the entire area of skin surface (e.g., 10 cm^2). The electrode will provide maximum drug delivery efficiency if it does not contain or produce any competing ions (i.e., mobile ions of the same charge as the drug ion). For optimum compatibility, the electrodes should be made of materials that are nontoxic and compatible with other formulation components such as the drug, excipients, and matrix material. In addition, they must not generate reaction products that are toxic or that adversely affect drug and excipient stability.

Two classes of electrode are the nonconsumable or inert type and the consumable or sacrificial type. Nonconsumable electrodes are made from nonreactive materials, whereas consumable electrodes are electro-chemically active and are structurally altered by the passage of current during treatment.

Nonconsumable Electrodes

Early iontophoretic drug delivery systems (IDDS) used materials that were not consumed during use. Commonly used materials included metals such as stainless steel or platinum. Although these nominally inert materials may have long use and storage lives, they also have significant shortcomings.

In accordance with Faraday's Law, the operation of an IDDS requires redox reactions at the electrodes in proportion to the amount of charge passed. For non-consumable electrodes, contacting an essentially aqueous electrolyte solution, electrolysis of water is the likely redox reaction. Therefore, the reaction at the anode is:

$$2H_2O \rightarrow 4H^+ + O_2 \uparrow + 4e^- (E° = 1.229 \text{ V}) \quad (3)$$

and at the cathode, the most prevalent steady-state reaction is:

$$2H_2O + 2e^- \rightarrow 2OH^- + H_2 \uparrow (E° = -0.828 \text{ V}) \quad (4)$$

Both of these reactions have a number of undesired consequences. The generation of H$^+$ and OH$^-$ can shift the formulation pH, affecting both delivery efficiency (due to a shift in the skin permselectivity, formation of competitive ions, or alteration of the charge state of the drug) and skin tolerability. The gases that are produced can accumulate on the electrode or skin surface, interfering with the uniformity of current distribution. Furthermore, because these reactions take place at relatively high voltage, there is high power consumption and a risk of electrolytic decomposition of the drug or other excipients.

Some electrodes made from nonnoble metals, such as stainless steel, can release metal ions through direct oxidation at the anode, or indirectly by the creation of a caustic environment at the cathode. For example, nickel and chromium ions were released from a medical-grade steel anode following a few minutes of iontophoresis at 400 μA/cm^2. These ions can be toxic to the body (4).

Chemical methods that mitigate the deleterious effects of unwanted reaction products can be divided into three categories: blocking their migration, neutralizing (e.g., buffering) them, and preventing their formation by addition of sacrificial redox species to the reservoir electrolyte. Migration blocking is achieved by isolating the electrolyte adjacent to the electrode from the drug formulation or from the body by using ion-exchange or size-selective membranes or coatings. For example, an anion-selective coating at a non-consummable electrode composed of methacrylamido-propyltrimethyl ammonium chloride copolymerized with methyl methacrylate was found to prevent degradation of the drug oxymorphone at electrode potentials up to 800 mV by blocking migration of the drug to the anode surface (5).

Buffering agents can partially compensate for the generation of acid and base, but their duration of efficacy (buffering capacity) is limited by the quantity of buffer species present, and the addition of excess buffer salts can result in ionic competition. Ion-exchange polymers can effectively scavenge, neutralize, and immobilize generated reaction products (6); the advantage over simple buffer salts is that the polymer chains are immobile and therefore noncompeting.

Consumable Electrodes

As described above, approaches have been devised for resolving the disadvantages of nonconsumable electrodes. Although many of these schemes are simple in principle, their practical implementation can be difficult because of various physical, chemical, and biological requirements. A simpler alternative is to use consumable electrodes. Also known as sacrificial electrodes, they are altered by electrochemical reaction during operation. Appropriate consumable electrodes will have redox reactions that take place at low potentials, thus avoiding parasitic reactions (e.g., electrolysis of water, drug, or excipients) at the electrode surface. Also, the reactants and products of the redox reaction must meet formulation and biological compatibility requirements.

A sacrificial electrode has a finite operational lifetime, or capacity, defined as the amount of charge that can be passed before the reactants are effectively depleted. The capacity of an electrode can be empirically determined, or can be calculated from the following equation:

$$Q = \frac{umnF}{3.6\,M} \qquad (5)$$

where Q = capacity (mAh), u = utilization (fraction of reacting species available for reaction), m = mass of reactant (g), n = number of equivalents of charge per mole of reactant (eq/mol), F = Faraday's constant (96,485 C/eq), M = molecular weight of the reactant (g/mol), and the constant 3.6 is a conversion factor (C/mAh).

If depletion results in an open circuit, the electrode will cease to function. Otherwise if an electrically conductive pathway remains, the electrode will continue to function under suboptimal conditions (i.e., at a higher voltage where other redox reactions, such as water electrolysis, take place).

Use of materials and structures that maximize utilization of reactants are preferred, as this allows the electrodes to be thin while making the most economical use of the consumable electrode. Factors that limit utilization include a tendency for passivation of the active component (by formation of a uniform, insoluble, nonconductive product over the active surface), and formation of "islands" (electrical isolation of one or more active portions by nonuniform current distribution).

No single consumable electrode is ideal for all iontophoretic applications. Different materials meet different capacity needs, and because consumable electrodes consist of chemically reactive species, certain materials may be compatible with certain drugs or excipients but not all of them. The most popular electrodes are based on the silver/silver chloride redox couple. Silver and silver chloride have several advantageous characteristics: They are biocompatible, perform well, and have an established history of use in medical applications including sensing electrodes.

Silver as a Consumable Anode

The use of a silver anode in the presence of chloride or another halide ion in the electrolyte solution is the most commonly used consumable anode for delivery of positively charged drugs.

Metallic silver oxidizes according to the following reaction:

$$Ag^\circ \leftrightarrow Ag^+ + e^- \,(E^\circ = 0.800V) \qquad (6)$$

However, when chloride is present, it will immediately react with the silver ion, that is:

$$Ag^\circ + Cl^- \leftrightarrow AgCl^\circ \,(K_{sp} = 1.78 \times 10^{-10} mol^2/kg^2) \qquad (7)$$

The complete reaction is therefore:

$$Ag^\circ + Cl^- \leftrightarrow AgCl^\circ + e^- (E^\circ = 0.222V) \qquad (8)$$

The final product, silver chloride forms on the surface of the silver anode and is electrically neutral and practically insoluble. Therefore, this reaction couple does not generate species that compete with cationic drugs for delivery. Because the equilibrium potential is low and the reaction is kinetically fast, the silver anode operates at low voltage, avoiding undesirable side reactions such as water splitting or electrochemical degradation of the drug or excipients. The rapid reaction kinetics and immobility of silver chloride make the system highly reversible. A reversible electrode system is especially attractive in an alternating polarity IDDS (i.e., one in which the drug is present in both electrode reservoirs and is delivered alternately from each as the current is reversed). The electrode is effectively discharged on one phase of the cycle and recharged on the other phase, leading to extended capacity.

There is one significant limitation to the use of silver as an anode to form silver chloride. The silver surface of the electrode gradually passivates as the silver chloride layer builds up, causing an increase in discharge voltage with use. This passivation process can limit both the maximum allowable current density and the utilization of silver.

Chloride Ion Management with Silver Anodes

For optimal silver anode function, there must be sufficient chloride ion to react with the silver ion. When the anode is the donor electrode (i.e., delivers positively charged drugs), the addition of chloride salts can lead to ion competition and reduced delivery efficiency. To minimize cation competition the preferred method of adding chloride is by using the drug chloride salt (7). Not all drug substances are readily available as chloride salts, but many can be converted to the chloride form by ion exchange or to the hydrochloride salt form by protonation of amine groups through addition of HCl.

Because chloride ion is consumed as it reacts with silver ions to form insoluble AgCl, its concentration decreases during treatment. Chloride must be present in the electrolyte in sufficient quantity to ensure proper operation of the electrode throughout the therapy. If the concentration of chloride drops to the point where it can no longer scavenge free silver ions, there is the potential for silver to be delivered to the skin. The amount of bulk chloride in the electrolyte required to avoid silver migration depends on many factors, including the volume of the electrolyte, current density, duration of treatment, the rate at which chloride is replenished from the body (i.e., the chloride transport number), and the configuration of the electrode and reservoir. Because interaction among these factors is often complex, it is difficult to construct a generalized model purely from first principles. Rather, for a given electrode/reservoir combination, it is often simpler to experimentally determine the threshold chloride concentration at which silver migration begins to occur, and then use a mass balance calculation to compute the required starting composition. A helpful indicator of silver migration is the potential of the polarized silver electrode. As chloride becomes less abundant, the silver anode voltage increases in a Nernstian fashion. Empirically, it has been found that operation of the anode above approximately 400 mV (vs. Ag/AgCl standard reference electrode) can lead to free migration of silver ions (5).

If it is impossible to use the chloride salt of a drug or impractical to include it in the amount required to prevent silver migration, two alternative methods can prevent the onset of silver migration without introducing mobile cations into the delivery reservoir. One is to immobilize the silver by using anion-selective membranes or coatings, or by using chelating agents. Another is to precipitate the silver using chloride ion-containing resins (e.g., those with quaternary ammonium chloride functionality) in the donor reservoir (8).

Silver Chloride as a Consumable Cathode

The silver chloride cathode reaction is given by Eq. 8 in reverse; that is, silver chloride is reduced to form metallic silver and chloride ion. The silver chloride cathode shares many of the qualities of the silver anode, with some additional desirable traits: No electrolyte is depleted by its reaction; it is hydrophilic and therefore wetted by the reservoir electrolyte; and the insoluble reaction product, metallic silver, is electrically conductive, eliminating problems of polarization or isolation of the redox species. Because of this combination of properties, the operating voltage of silver chloride decreases with use, and the utilization of a silver chloride cathode is nearly 100%.

Operation of the silver chloride cathode can lead to an accumulation of chloride ions in the electrolyte. When the electrode is a counter electrode, chloride buildup is not a concern. However, when used as a donor electrode for delivery of anionic drugs, the accumulation of chloride ion can lead to decreased drug flux because of ionic competition. For short duration applications, this

effect may be negligible. However, if the molar concentration of chloride approaches some appreciable fraction of that of the drug, substantial competition will occur. A simple, yet not always practical, way to remain below this threshold fraction is to increase drug content. The amount of additional drug required can be computed from a mass balance calculation. The chloride accumulation rate is determined by the current, according to Faraday's law, and this can be compared with the drug content, which decreases over time as drug is delivered into the body.

FORMULATION COMPOSITION

The formulations of an IDDS are the ingredients in the drug and counter reservoirs, which typically consist of a solvent, a drug salt or a biocompatible salt, and a matrix-forming material. A formulation may also include additives such as buffers, antimicrobial agents, antioxidants and additional electrolyte salts or permeation enhancers. All of these can interact in a complex fashion to affect rate of delivery, biocompatibility, and product shelf life.

Solvent

Drug solubility and stability, in addition to solvent biocompatibility, are obvious considerations when selecting a solvent for a pharmaceutical formulation. For an IDDS, the effect of a solvent on the drug charge state is also an important consideration. Although a neutral drug molecule can be transported into the skin by electroosmosis (9), maximal drug-delivery efficiency is usually achieved if the drug has a net electric charge. For this reason, polar solvents with large dielectric constants are preferred. For example, the dielectric constants of water, glycerol, and ethanol are 80, 42, and 24, respectively. Use of solvents with large dielectric constants results in greater dissociation of the drug salt (i.e., less ion-pairing), enhancing drug mobility during application of an electric field.

Because of its large dielectric constant and inherent biocompatibility, water is the most commonly used solvent. Other cosolvents such as ethanol, glycerol, polyethylene glycol, or polypropylene glycol may be added to enhance drug solubility and drug stability, or to reduce the rate of water evaporation. Sanderson and colleagues (10) used a 40:60 mixture of water and ethanol to enhance the solubility of dobutamine hydrochloride and demonstrated a twofold enhancement in dobutamine flux. However, addition of a cosolvent to enhance drug solubility may, in some cases, decrease the rate of delivery by electromigration if excessive ion-pairing results.

Jadoul and coworkers (11) studied the effect of adding ethanol and propylene glycol (PG) to aqueous solutions of fentanyl and metoprolol. They reported that drug flux was diminished by up to 80% for solutions containing 60 vol% ethanol or PG. A fourfold drop in formulation conductance was also measured, indicating that more ion association was occurring in the cosolvents. In addition, the solvent may have a direct effect on the skin, thus altering its permeability to drug ions (12). In summary, the effect of a solvent or cosolvent on the drug solubility, ion interactions, and skin permeability are important considerations when choosing the formulations for IDDS.

Drug Salt

In addition to the usual solubility, stability, and biocompatibility considerations, several unique aspects should be considered when selecting the drug salt for an IDDS formulation. First, the counterion must be compatible with the electrochemical reactions occurring at the electrode. As noted previously, halide drug salts are preferred when using a silver anode. For example, fentanyl citrate is used in intravenous formulations, but citrate does not form an insoluble salt with electrochemically generated silver cation. For this reason, a formulation containing fentanyl hydrochloride was specifically developed for use in a patient-activated IDDS for treatment of pain (13). Clinical results using this formulation strategy are summarized latter in this chapter.

As mentioned previously, the extent of drug salt dissociation is an important consideration when selecting a solvent. Therefore, for a particular solvent (e.g., water), selection of a drug salt that more fully dissociates will likely result in more efficient drug delivery. Using aqueous solutions of the acetate, sulfate, and hydrochloride salts of morphine, a correlation between drug salt dissociation and transdermal delivery has been observed (14). From conductance measurements, it was determined that morphine hydrochloride was more fully dissociated in water than were the sulfate and acetate salts. The rate of morphine delivery, at currents ranging from 0.1 to 1 mA, was about 60% greater for the hydrochloride salt than for the sulfate and acetate salts.

Ion mobility (the velocity achieved by an ion per unit electric field) is largely determined by its ionic charge and by the extent of its physical interaction with the formulation or skin. The mobilities of a drug ion and its counterion in a formulation are likely to be different than their mobilities in the skin. In addition, the mobilities of ions that are endogenous to the skin

(e.g., Na^+, K^+, Cl^-, HCO_3^-) are likely to be different in the two environments. Therefore, during electromigration the ionic composition of the formulation in the vicinity of the skin can be substantially different than the bulk composition. As a result, it has been suggested that the drug counterion can alter the pH of the interface between the formulation and the skin, and thus alter transport efficiency (10). A twofold enhancement in transport efficiency for the succinate salts of verapamil, gallopamil, and nalbuphine relative to the hydrochloride salts was reported. This result was attributed to the ability of the weakly acidic succinate anion to buffer the boundary layer near the skin surface at about pH 4.8, thus avoiding significant hydronium ion competition.

Matrix

Use of drug dissolved in a liquid solvent is generally adequate for in vitro experimentation, but is not optimal for use in a commercial product. Not only must the formulation be biocompatible, but it must also be readily incorporated into the IDDS during commercial-scale manufacturing, be easily applied by the user, and leave little or no residue on the skin. To achieve these goals, two fundamentally different matrix-based formulation strategies have been adopted for use in IDDS.

In one approach, the drug solution is placed on an absorbent porous material. Such materials include hydrophilic fabrics composed of polyester or nylon, and hydrophilic porous films composed of polyurethane, polyvinyl alcohol (PVOH), or cellulose. To improve hydration kinetics and solvent retention, hydrophilic polymers and/or surfactants have been incorporated into the fabric or foam matrices (15). Examples of hydrophilic polymers are polyethylene oxide, PVOH, poly-N-vinyl pyrrolidone, polyacrylamide, polyhydroxyethyl methacrylate, and polysaccharides such as hydroxyethyl cellulose, modified starches, or natural gums. Nonionic surfactants such as Tween 20®, Neodol 91-6®, or Tergitol 15-S-7® can also be added to enhance the rate of hydration. The water-retentive properties of the polymers, combined with the structural integrity of a fabric or porous film, provide a composite matrix material that will readily absorb the drug solution during the manufacturing process or just prior to use by the patient. The addition of solvent just prior to use can enhance drug stability, particularly for polypeptides and proteins.

The second strategy utilizes drug-containing hydrogels and provides an alternative to the absorption of drug solution by porous composite matrices. With the hydrogel approach, drug salt is mixed with a solvent and a network-forming polymer to create a viscous solution. The solution is then dispensed into a cavity containing an electrode of the appropriate polarity, and the polymer is crosslinked. To minimize degradation of the drug during the crosslinking process, physical crosslinking is preferred over chemical or radiation-induced crosslinking reactions. For example, polyvinyl alcohol can be dissolved in water, mixed with drug salt, and then frozen at about −20°C. When thawed, a soft, cohesive, water-rich hydrogel results (16). Other hydrophilic polymers such as polyvinyl pyrolidone or polysaccharides (e.g., hydroxypropylmethyl cellulose) can be added to modify the rheological, adhesive, or water-retentive properties of polyvinyl alcohol hydrogels (17).

In general, polar nonionic polymers have been used as the matrix material in formulations for IDDS. Nonionic polymers are preferred because they typically do not have mobile ionic species and do not interact strongly with drug ions. However, results from studies of drug delivery from matrices composed of ionic polymers have been reported. For example, Gupta and coworkers reported a substantial reduction in cromolyn flux when a hydrogel composed of polyglycerylmethacrylate and water was employed, suggesting a strong interaction between the cromolyn anion and polymer (12).

In contrast, the transdermal iontophoretic delivery of the drug cation, hydromorphone, was enhanced by using a hydrogel formulation composed of water and poly-acrylamido-methylpropane-sulfonate (poly-AMPS) (8). A hydrogel composed of water and the acid form of poly-AMPS was imbibed with a stoichiometric amount of hydromorphone base to form the hydromorphone salt of poly-AMPS. Hydromorphone hydrochloride was also added, and the hydrogel was placed in contact with a silver anode. Hydromorphone was delivered at a current density of 0.05 mA cm^{-2} through dermatomed pig skin into a 0.1 M sodium chloride solution. The flux of hydromorphone from the poly-AMPS hydrogel was found to be about twice that of a nonionic PVOH hydrogel. This result suggests that migration of mobile chloride ions from the skin into the hydrogel was hindered by the presence of immobilized sulfonate anions (i.e., ionic repulsion or Donnan exclusion).

Excipients

Excipients such as buffers, antimicrobials, antioxidants and chelating agents may be required for optimal drug stability in IDDS formulations. Several unique criteria when selecting excipients must be considered.

As described earlier, excipients can contact the electrodes of the system. Therefore, excipients must be screened for their compatibility with the electrodes. Sacrificial electrodes (e.g., Ag and AgCl) are particularly reactive. If inherently nonreactive electrodes are used (e.g., platinum or carbon), then the excipient can be exposed to a relatively large electric potential at the electrode/reservoir interface during system use. In such cases, excipients that are inherently stable should be selected. Excipients are typically evaluated for their electrochemical stability using standard potentiometric techniques (e.g., cyclic voltammetry) before being selected for use in an IDDS formulation.

The effect of an excipient on drug transport must also be considered, especially if it is ionic. If the excipient has the same charge as the drug ion, then it will be delivered into the skin with the drug. In addition to the direct competitive effect on drug transport, the excipient may alter the permselectivity of the skin, causing a change in the drug transport efficiency. If an excipient of opposite charge to the drug ion is chosen, then the effect of the excipient counterion on drug transport must be determined.

Because IDDS formulations usually contain water, the use of lipophilic excipients may not be possible. Instead, salt forms of excipients are often employed. However, excipient salts often contain inorganic cations that are usually much more mobile than most drug cations. The detrimental effects of inorganic cations on the flux of drug cations have been well documented (18). In particular, since inorganic cations are depleted from the formulation more rapidly than the drug cations, the flux of the drug will not be constant but rather will increase with time during system use. The competitive effect of buffer anions on transport of anionic drugs has also been reported (19).

Standard phosphate and citrate buffers have been successfully used in formulations for transdermal ionto-phoresis of drug ions. However, because small inorganic and organic ions frequently have a negative effect on drug flux due to competition, selecting a buffer can be challenging. Several unique buffering strategies have been developed specifically for use in IDDS. In one strategy, zwitterionic buffering agents are used at their isoelectric pH (20). The net zero charge of the zwitterion largely avoids the ion competition effect. Two preferred zwitterionic buffers are N-2-hydroxyethylpiperazine-N-2-ethane sulfonic acid (HEPES) and 2-N-morpholino-propane sulfonic acid (MES).

Alternatively, the delivery of the buffer ion can be largely eliminated by using cationic buffers in the cathode reservoir and anionic buffers in the anode reservoir, so that the buffer ion moves away from the skin when an electric field is applied. In addition to common weak acids such as citric and phosphoric, the use of amino acids in the anode formulation has been suggested. Amino acids such as cysteine and histidine would be incorporated at neutral or basic pH, where they are predominately anionic (20).

In another buffering strategy, polymeric materials with pendant acid or base groups (e.g., carboxylic, phosphoric, amines) are dispersed in the formulation (10, 20). Examples of such polymeric buffers are polyacrylic acid and methacrylate/divinyl benzene copolymers (e.g., Amberlite IRP-64®). The exceedingly high molecular weight of these polymers renders them essentially immobile in an electrical field. The counterion to the ionic resin must still be considered; preferably it should have the opposite charge of the drug to avoid ionic competition. Alternatively, the counterion to the drug ion can be specifically selected for its inherent buffering capability (10).

In all of these strategies, the goal is to minimize the mobility of the buffering agent, or its counterion, relative to that of the drug ion. This is accomplished by choosing buffers with no net ionic charge, choosing buffers whose mobile species have a charge opposite that of the drug ion, or by increasing the molecular weight of the buffering agent.

Excipients may also be included in the formulation to enhance drug delivery efficiency. For example, Sanderson and colleagues (10) reported a threefold enhancement in delivery of dobutamine after the skin site was pretreated with an anionic surfactant, sodium lauryl sulfate (SLS). They attributed the enhancement in flux to an increase in the negative charge on the skin because of neutralization of fixed positive charges in the skin and to hydrophobic binding of the surfactant to the skin. More specifically, Sanderson and coworkers proposed that an increase in negative charge within the transport pathway enhanced the migration of drug cations by hindering the migration of chloride ions from the body. They noted that while SLS is not biocompatible, the charge-alteration strategy may be useful if other more biocompatible surfactants were identified.

Alternatively, Huntington and Cormier (21) used nonionic surfactants, including dodecanol and 1,2-dodecanediol, to enhance the delivery of the anionic drug, ketoprofen. Because nonionic surfactants are not directly affected by the applied electric field, their use may be preferred over ionic surfactants.

Some drugs and excipients may cause excessive skin irritation (22). Researchers have reduced skin irritation in humans by including an antiinflammatory agent in the formulation (23). Using the moderately irritating antiemetic drug, metoclopramide, they demonstrated improved biocompatibility by adding hydrocortisone to the formulation. As little as 0.05% hydrocortisone in the formulation significantly reduced erythema at the skin site following treatment. They also reported that hydrocortisone had no effect on the transport of the metoclopramide cation.

Formulation pH

Many drugs have a broad pH range in which drug solubility and stability are adequate for transdermal delivery by iontophoresis. However, optimal drug delivery and biocompatibility are usually restricted to a more narrow range of formulation pH. As discussed previously, skin is a permselective membrane with an isoelectric point of about pH 4. For this reason, formulation pH can affect the selectivity of the skin to cations and anions. As formulation pH increases, skin becomes more negatively charged, thus favoring cation transport. Therefore, to maximize the transdermal flux of a cationic drug, the formulation pH should be as basic as is practical, limited by drug solubility, charge state, stability, and biocompatibility. By analogy, for anionic drugs, acidic formulations are generally preferred.

The effect of formulation pH on skin permselectively has been clearly demonstrated (24): As the pH of a solution containing salicylate anion was increased from pH 4 to 6, and then to 8, the transdermal flux of salicylate anion at 200 $\mu A/cm^2$ decreased from 480 to 192, and then to 174 $\mu g\ h^{-1}\ cm^{-2}$, respectively. In contrast, with an identical increase in pH, the flux of triethylamine cation increased from 117 to 170, and then to 303 $\mu g\ h^{-1}\ cm^{-2}$, respectively.

A formulation must provide adequate drug transport, while ensuring good biocompatibility. Several investigators have found that formulation pH can have a substantial effect on skin irritation (10, 20, 25). By measuring the redness at treated sites on hairless guinea pigs, Cormier and Johnson (23) found that skin irritation was reduced by choosing different pH ranges for the anode and cathode formulations. For anode formulations, pH values between 4 and 10 produced the lowest skin responses. For cathode formulations, pH values between 2 and 4 were least irritating.

Electrolytes for Counter Reservoir

An appropriate electrolyte for the formulation in contact with the counter electrode must provide sufficient conductivity to minimize the voltage required during system use. The minimum conductivity, σ, needed to limit the voltage drop, ΔV, across a hydrogel formulation with a thickness of L and a cross-sectional area of A at a current of I is given by the expression:

$$\sigma = (IL)/(\delta VA) \qquad (9)$$

For example, a voltage drop of less than 1 V will occur across a hydrogel formulation with a thickness of 0.5 cm and a cross-sectional area of 5 cm^2 at a current of 0.5 mA, if the formulation has a conductivity of at least 50 μS/cm.

Because formulation conductivity is sensitive to solubility and ion-pairing effects, it can be used to characterize alternative formulations during formulation development. Gangarosa and colleagues (26) and Yoshida and Roberts (19) provide examples of the effect of drug and electrolyte conductivity on formulation performance in IDDS.

In addition to rendering the formulation sufficiently conductive, the ion delivered from the nondrug formulation must be biocompatible. Irritation resulting from use of four inorganic electrolytes has been reported by Anigbogu and coworkers (27). They reported that use of 0.9% NaCl or KCl in the anode reservoir at current densities of 0.5 mA/cm^2 and 1 mA/cm^2 for 1 h elicited no skin irritation in rabbits. In contrast, the use of 0.9% CaCl$_2$ or MgCl$_2$ caused moderate erythema.

Using weak acids and bases as electrolytes for the counter reservoir formulation at the proper pH (i.e., pH < 4 for cathode formulations and pH > 4 for anode formulations) provides adequate biocompatibility and low skin resistance (20). Low skin resistance is advantageous since less voltage output is required from the control circuit, and therefore a smaller battery may be required, potentially reducing the size and cost of the IDDS.

For current densities at or above 0.2 mA/cm^2, the sensation associated with transdermal iontophoresis is determined by the type of ion being delivered into the skin. When human subjects compared the sensation experienced during iontophoresis of different salt solutions applied to the right and left forearms, delivery of calcium caused less sensation than delivery of phosphate, magnesium, and zinc, which caused less sensation than delivery of chloride, acetate, citrate, and sulfate, which in turn caused less sensation than delivery of lithium, potassium, and sodium. In general, multivalent ions were found to cause less sensation than monovalent ions (28).

ELECTRONIC COMPONENTS

The unique electrical nature of an IDDS provides an enhanced level of control over drug delivery. In addition, the ability to provide information feedback is not often available in other modes of drug delivery.

There are two general electrical approaches used in iontophoretic treatments: One is to control the applied voltage; the other is to control the applied current. A simple example of a controlled-voltage circuit is a battery that applies a constant voltage to the electrodes. However, as will be pointed out later, the skin resistance is neither constant between individuals nor is it static from the start to finish of a single application. Thus, a constant voltage approach will result in variable current. Since the rate of drug delivered is directly proportional to the current passed, a controlled-current approach is generally preferred.

The electrical control components of an IDDS may be divided into two elements: the power source and the control circuitry.

Power Source

The electrical power source for portable IDDS is a battery. Commercially available primary batteries have cell voltages that range from about 1.2 to 3.0 V. To overcome the resistance of the skin and achieve the desired current, it may be necessary to use higher voltages. Voltage can be increased by combining cells in series, or by using circuitry to "step-up" the voltage at the cost of drawing a larger current from the battery. This additional current drain adds to the total battery capacity needed to provide the required therapy. Thus, the total battery capacity required is the sum of that needed to support the therapy plus any "overhead" associated with the electrical circuitry.

The first objective of the circuitry is to control the amount of drug delivered. For a zero-order (constant-delivery) system, for example, a specified current should be maintained regardless of the resistance of the application site. Computing the power requirement in this case is difficult because the resistive load of the skin

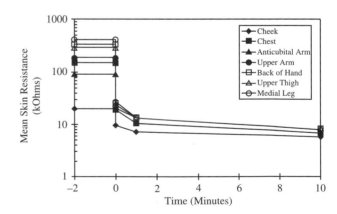

Fig. 2 Skin resistance of various body sites as a function of time of current application. (From Ref. 29.)

depends on both the application site and the time elapsed since current has been initiated (29). Fig. 2 shows the skin resistance at different application sites in response to the application of 1 mA to a 4 cm^2 area. Two minutes before applying 1 mA, a small current of 10 μA was applied to determine the skin resistance, which was highly variable and had a mean value of about 200 kΩ. Just 1 s after applying a current of 1 mA, the resistance decreased substantially to 16 ± 4 kΩ. As time progressed, the resistance continued to fall and all sites appeared to approach a quasi-steady-state value of 7.4 ± 1.3 kΩ. The small relative standard deviation (RSD) of the quasi-steady-state resistance of 18% compared with an initial RSD of 92% indicates that all body sites tested tend toward a common resistance, despite the large differences that are present prior to application of current. This fact has been attributed to an increase in ionic conductivity of the skin due to an increase in ion concentration within the stratum corneum and to "activation" of shunt pathways (3).

For a typical initial skin resistance of 200 kΩ, 200 V would be required to achieve a current of 1 mA. Therefore, a typical system having a modest output voltage of 10–20 V will operate below the desired current (i.e., will be noncompliant) during the initial moments of current application. However, because the resistance drops quickly, a voltage capability of about 10–20 V is generally sufficient to achieve compliance within an acceptably short time of about 1 min or less.

Control Circuitry

A controlled current circuit does not necessarily require a high level of electronic sophistication. A simple field-effect transistor with a feedback resistor can maintain the current delivered from a battery at a constant value over a wide range of skin resistances. Other types of delivery requirements such as pulsed current, patient-controlled on-demand dosing, dose titration, ramp-up or ramp-down dosing, and other special waveforms can be addressed with control circuitry. In these cases integrated circuits are usually employed to minimize system size.

Visual and audio feedback information is provided to the user by light-emitting diodes (LED), liquid crystal displays (LCD), and piezoelectric transducers. This information can indicate that the system is working, show errors or warnings, signal system maintenance needs (such as battery replacement), or display the amount of drug that has been delivered.

The ability of an IDDS to electronicallly control drug delivery gives rise to another potential advantage; the opportunity to create sensor-based or "closed-loop" therapy. If an appropriate sensor is available to measure

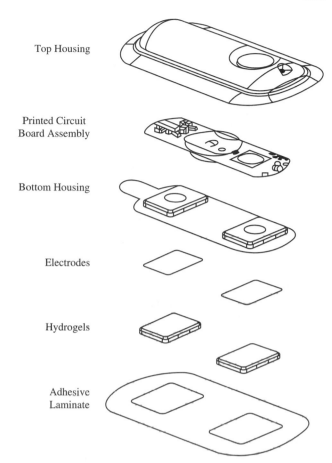

Fig. 3 Exploded view of an iontophoretic drug delivery system showing major components: top housing, printed circuit board assembly, a bottom housing containing reservoirs for placement of electrodes and hydrogels, and an adhesive laminate. (Diagram from International Patent Publication Number WO 96/39222.)

a biological response (e.g., to measure blood glucose levels in response to the delivery of insulin), then circuitry can be used to modulate the output current, and therefore drug delivery. In so doing, an automated, closed-loop system is created that ensures the proper amount of drug is delivered and avoids both over- and under-dosing the patient. As shown in Fig. 3, the electronic components are typically mounted on a printed circuit board and mounted within a protective housing containing the electrodes and formulation hydrogels.

CLINICAL ASSESSMENT OF SYSTEMIC DELIVERY

In the following clinical case studies, a number of delivery attributes discussed in earlier sections are exemplified. In addition, in vitro methodologies are briefly discussed to highlight the good correlation possible with observed in vivo results.

Fentanyl Clinical Study

Fentanyl has a molecular weight of 336 Da in the base form, an aqueous solubility of about 24 mg/ml as the HCl salt, and a charge of +1 over a wide pH range. Fentanyl is a synthetic opioid widely used in anesthesia and analgesia. A passive transdermal system is available for the treatment of chronic pain (Duragesic®, Janssen Pharmaceutica). This patch delivers fentanyl through the skin continuously over 72 h. For the management of acute pain, such as post-operative pain, the slow onset of action of fentanyl obtained with passive transdermal delivery is not appropriate. However, fentanyl delivery from an IDDS to quickly attain therapeutic blood levels and a quick onset of analgesia has been demonstrated clinically (30, 31). In addition, the electrical nature of iontophoresis allows the patient to initiate a dose of fentanyl when in pain, which is not possible with passive delivery (32).

The IDDS used in the clinical study consisted of a reusable, battery-operated controller capable of delivering user-actuated doses when connected to a disposable patch-like drug unit. The drug unit had a silver anode and silver chloride cathode in intimate contact with hydrogel reservoirs within a flexible foam housing. The drug unit contained 5 mg (base equivalent) of the hydrochloride salt of fentanyl and the donor hydrogel reservoir had a skin

contact area of 2 cm². The disposable drug units were applied to the upper outer arms of healthy volunteers. The opioid effects of fentanyl were blocked in the volunteers by oral administration of naltrexone every 12 h.

The study was a four-treatment crossover (three with IDDS plus an IV treatment), conducted in 12 subjects. All treatments delivered fentanyl for the first 20 min of every hour for 24 h. The three IDDS treatments employed currents of 150, 200, and 250 μA, while the IV treatment infused 50 μg of fentanyl. Blood samples were collected, and serum fentanyl concentrations were measured using a specific radioimmunoassay. Plasma data collected during and immediately following the 1st, 13th, and 25th treatments are shown in Fig. 4. The gradual upward shifts in concentration over time indicate a baseline increase due to incomplete fentanyl clearance between the hourly doses. For all treatment types, serum fentanyl concentrations rapidly increased within a few minutes after the start of each dose.

The average drug input fluxes during the 20-min dosing periods between hours 24 and 25 were calculated to be 81, 108, and 138 μg/h/cm² for currents of 150, 200, and 250 μA, respectively. These values, the mean maximum plasma concentration values, and the total AUC values (over the same time period) for the three IDDS treatments all increased proportionally with current. These results agree with theoretical expectations expressed by Equation (1). In addition, the variabilities in the fentanyl pharmacokinetic parameters were similar for the IDDS and IV treatments, indicating that the IDDS doses were delivered with an accuracy similar to the IV infusions.

The in vivo flux values for fentanyl agree closely with in vitro flux values obtained with human cadaver skin. In vitro transdermal experiments with fentanyl were conducted using two-compartment permeation cells.

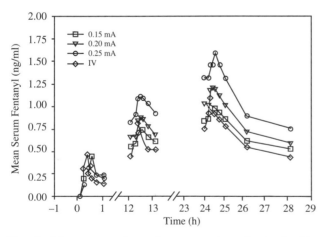

Fig. 4 Mean serum fentanyl concentrations for 12 healthy volunteers receiving fentanyl intermittently (20 min each hour over a 24-h administration period) from an iontophoretic system at three currents, and from IV fentanyl infusion (50 μg for 20 min hourly). Serum fentanyl concentrations were measured during and immediately after the 1st, 13th, and 25th doses. (From Ref. 31.)

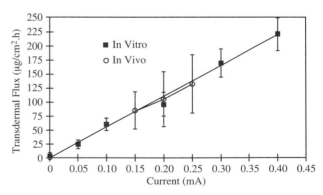

Fig. 5 Comparison of in vitro (n = 5) and in vivo (n = 13) fentanyl flux as a function of applied current. (From Ref. 13.).

Heat-stripped human epidermis was oriented so that the stratum corneum surface contacted the fentanyl hydrochloride solution in the donor compartment. The donor solution pH and fentanyl concentration were very similar to the pH and concentration of the donor formulation used in the clinical study.

To establish a good in vitro/in vivo correlation, the composition and ionic strength of the receptor solution must be adjusted (18). For fentanyl, the best correlation was obtained with a receptor solution comprised of a 10-fold dilution of modified Dulbecco' phosphate-buffered saline (without calcium or magnesium) at pH 7.4. The currents tested in vitro ranged from 0 to 400 μA and were applied to a silver anode and a silver chloride cathode using a constant current power supply. The in vitro data presented in Fig. 5 clearly demonstrate the expected linear dependence of fentanyl delivery on current and the excellent correlation to the in vivo data.

Lutelnizing Hormone-Releasing Hormone Clinical Study

Systemic delivery of polypeptides, proteins and oligonucleotides pose many significant delivery challenges to pharmaceutical scientists. Because of their extensive metabolism in the gastrointestinal tract, they are generally not good candidates for oral administration. These compounds typically have large molecular weights, are hydrophilic, and have a pH-dependent electrical charge. These qualities also make them poor candidates for passive transdermal delivery but excellent candidates for iontophoretic delivery (33).

Luteinizing hormone-releasing hormone (LHRH) is a native reproductive hormone containing 10 amino acids with a molecular weight of approximately 1200 Da and a charge of +1 near neutral pH. Pulsatile delivery of LHRH by the hypothalamus stimulates the production of gonadotropins, such as luteinizing hormone (LH), by the pituitary gland for the maintenance of normal female reproductive function. In contrast, continuous secretion of LHRH shuts down the reproductive axis.

It is possible to achieve continuous or pulsed LHRH delivery profiles using transdermal iontophoresis. Heit and colleagues have demonstrated that continuous transdermal iontophoresis of LHRH is possible (34). Continuous transdermal iontophoresis of leuprolide, a nine-amino acid analog of LHRH, has also proved clinically successful (35).

The iontophoretic delivery of discrete pulses of LHRH using an IDDS was investigated in a clinical study with healthy male volunteers (36). The clinical system comprised an 8 cm² hydrogel formulation containing 15 mM LHRH as the hydrochloride salt in contact with a

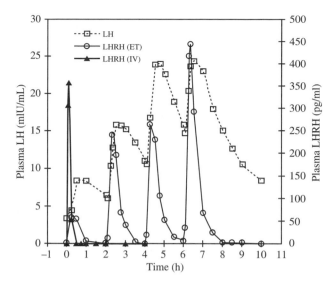

Fig. 6 Mean plasma LHRH concentrations of eight healthy male volunteers receiving four 15-min doses of LHRH at 0.1 mA/cm² every two h, and an IV LHRH bolus dose of 5 μg. Mean plasma LH levels resulting from the iontophoretic LHRH doses are also plotted. (From Ref. 36.)

silver anode. Plasma LHRH and LH concentrations obtained in eight subjects receiving one 15-min pulse at a current of 0.8 mA (0.1 mA/cm² current density) every 2 h for 8 h are shown in Fig. 6. The plasma LHRH concentration obtained following the administration of a single 5 μg IV bolus is also shown as a reference. These results demonstrate that pulsatile delivery of LHRH is possible using reasonable iontophoretic conditions. Significantly, the plasma LHRH profiles obtained with an IDDS are comparable with those obtained following IV bolus administration. The four consecutive 15-min doses resulted in plasma LHRH profiles with sharp peaks (C_{max} up to 450 pg/ml). Plasma LHRH levels rapidly declined to negligible baseline values between doses, consistent with IV administration. The plasma LHRH levels rose and fell much more rapidly than profiles obtained with subcutaneous injections (37).

Following each dose of LHRH, the pharmacodynamic plasma LH response also followed a pulsatile pattern with a mean maximum concentration of about 26 mIU/ml. As was discussed earlier for fentanyl, the variability in the iontophoretic LHRH plasma data was comparable to that obtained with IV administration.

While iontophoresis has not been widely employed, the field is rapidly evolving. The development of small patch-like devices for glucose extraction and for systemic delivery of therapeutic agents is occurring at several companies, including Cygnus, Becton Dickinson, and ALZA. If commercially successful, these efforts would greatly expand the applications of iontophoresis for systemic therapy.

REFERENCES

1. Banga, A.K. *Electrically Assisted Transdermal and Topical Drug Delivery*; Taylor and Francis: Bristol, PA, 1998.
2. Leduc, S. Electric Ions and Their Use in Medicine. Rebman Ltd.: Liverpool, UK, 1908.
3. Scott, E.R.; Phipps, J.B.; White, H.S. Direct Imaging of Molecular Transport Through Skin. J. Invest. Dematol. **1995**, *104*, 142–145.
4. Lindblad, L.E.; Ekenvall, L. Electrode Material in Iontophoresis. Pharm. Res. **1987**, *4*, 438.
5. Phipps, J.B. Electrode and Reservoir Design for Optimal Transdermal Delivery by Iontophoresis. *Transdermal Administration, A Case Study, Iontophoresis*; APGI/CRS European Symposium, Couvreur, P., Duchene, D., Green, P., Junginger, H.E., Eds.; 3–4 March 1997, Paris, France Editions de Sante: Paris, 1997; 30–39.
6. Sanderson, J.E.; Deriel, S.R. Method and Apparatus for Iontophoretic Drug Delivery. US Patent 4,722,726, 1988.
7. Philips, J.B., Untereker; D.F. Iontophoresis Apparatus and Methods of Producing Same. US Patent 4,744,787, 1988.
8. Philips, J.B.; Howland, W.W.; Jevne, A.H.; Holmblad, C. Device and Method for Iontophoretic Drug Delivery. US Patent 5,558,633, 1996.
9. Pikal, M.J. The Role of Electroosmotic Flow in Transdermal Iontophoresis. Adv. Drug Del. Rev. **1992**, *9*, 201–237.
10. Sanderson, J.E.; Reil, S.D.; Dixon, R. Iontophoretic Delivery of Nonpeptide Drugs: Formulation Optimization from Maximum Skin Permeability. J. Pharm. Sci. **1989**, *78*, 361–364.
11. Jadoul, A.; Regnier, V.; Preat, V. Influence of Ethanol and Propylene Glycol Addition on the Transdermal Delivery by Iontophoresis and Electroporation. Pharm. Res. **1997**, *14*, S308–S309.
12. Gupta, S.K.; Kumar, S.; Bolton, S.; Behl, C.R.; Malick, A.W. Effect of Chemical Enhancers and Conducting Gels on Iontophoretic Transdermal Delivery of Cromolyn Sodium. J. Controlled Release **1994**, *35*, 229–236.
13. Lattin, G.L.; Phipps, J.B.; Southam, M.A.; Klausner, M. Evaluation of Fentanyl Delivery in Humans Using E-TRANS Technology. *Transdermal Administration, A Case Study, Iontophoresis*; APGI/CRS European Symposium, Couvreur, P., Duchene, D., Green, P., Junginger, H.E., Eds.; 3–4 March 1997, Paris, France Editions de Sante: Paris, 1997; 365–368.
14. Corish, J.; Corrigan, O.I.; Foley, D. The Iontophoretic Transdermal Delivery of Morphine Hydrochloride and other Salts Across Excised Human Stratum Corneum, Proceedings of the Conference on Prediction of Percutaneous Penetration: Methods, Measurements, Modeling, April 1989 International Conference; Scott, R.C, Guy, R.H., Hagraft, J., Eds.; IBC Technical Services Ltd.: London, 1990; 302–307.
15. Beck, J.E.; Lloyd, L.B.; Petelenz, T.J. Iontophoretic Delivery Device with Integral Hydrating Means. US Patent 5,730,716, 1998.
16. Hyon, S.H.; Yoshito, I. Transdermal Therapeutic Composition. US Patent 4,781,926, 1988.
17. Jevene, A.H., Vegoe, B.R.; Holmblad, C.M. Hydrophilic Pressure Sensitive Biomedical Adhesive Composition. US Patent 4,593,053, 1986.
18. Phipps, J.B.; Gyory, J.R. Transdermal Ion Migration. Adv. Drug. Del. Rev. **1992**, *9*, 137–176.
19. Yoshida, N.H.; Roberts, M.S. Prediction of Cathodal Iontophoretic Transport of Anions Across Excised Skin from Different Vehicles Using Conductivity Measurements. J. Pharm. Pharmacol. **1995**, *47*, 883–890.
20. Cormier, M.J.; Ledger, P.W.; Johnson, J.; Philips, J.B.; Chao, S. Reduction of Skin Irritation and Resistance During Electrotransport. US Patent 5,624,415, 1997.
21. Huntington, J.A.; Cormier, M. Composition, Device and Method for Electrotransport Agent Delivery. US Patent 5,811,465, 1998.
22. Ledger, P.W. Skin Biological Issues in Electrically Enhanced Transdermal Delivery. Adv. Drug Del. Rev. **1992**, *9*, 289–307.
23. Cormier, M.; Johnson, B. Skin Reactions Associated with Electrotransport. *Transdermal Administration, A Case Study, Iontophoresis*; APGI/CRS European Symposium, Couvreur, P., Duchene, D., Green, P., Junginger, H.E., Eds.; 3–4 March 1997; Paris, France Editions de Sante: Paris, 1997; 50–57.
24. Nightingale, J.; Sclafani, J.; Kurihara-Bergstrom, T. Effect of pH on the Iontophoretic Delivery of Ionic Compounds, Proceedings of the 17th International Symposium on Controlled Release of Bioactive Materials, Reno, Nevada, July 22–25, 1990; Lee, H.E., Ed.; Controlled Release Society: Lincolnshire, IL, 1990; 17, 431–432.
25. Phipps, J.B.; Cormier, M.; Padmanabhan, R. *In Vivo* Ion Efflux from Humans and the Relationship to Skin Irritation. *Transdermal Administration, A Case Study, Iontophoresis*; APGI/CRS European Symposium, Couvreur, P., Duchene, D., Green, P., Junginger, H.E., Eds.; 3–4 March 1997; Paris, France Editions de Sante: Paris, 1997; 289–291.
26. Gangarosa, L.P.; Park, N.H.; Fong, B.C.; Scott, D.F.; Hill, J.M. Conductivity of Drugs Used for Iontophoresis. J. Pharm. Sci **1978**, *67*, 1439–1443.
27. Anigbogu, A.; Singh, P.; Liu, P.; Dinh, S.; Maibach, H. Effects of Iontophoresis on Rabbit Skin *In Vivo*. Pharm. Res. **1997**, *14*, S-308.
28. Philips, J.B. Method for Reducing Sensation in Iontophoretic Drug Delivery. US Patent 5,221,254, 1993.
29. Gyory, J.R.; Phipps, J.B. Effect of Current Density and Current Duration on the Membrane Resistance of Skin. *Transdermal Administration, A Case Study, Iontophoresis*; APGI/CRS European Synposium, Couvreur, P., Duchene, D., Green, P., Junginger, H.E., Eds.; 3–4 March 1997; Paris, France Editions de Sante: Paris, 1997; 262–265.
30. Gupta, S.K.; Bernstein, K.J.; Noorduin, H.; Van Peer, A.; Sathyan, G.; Haak, R. Fentanyl Delivery from an Electrotransport System: Delivery is a Function of Total Current, not Duration of Current. J. Clin. Pharmacol. **1988**, *38*, 951–958.
31. Gupta, S.K.; Southam, M.; Sathyan, G.; Klausner, M. Effect of Current Density on Pharmacokinetics Following Continuous or Intermittent Input from a Fentanyl Electrotransport System. J. Pharm. Sci. **1998**, *87*, 976–981.

32. Thysman, S.; Tasset, C.; Preat, V. Transdermal Iontophoresis of Fentanyl: Delivery and Mechanistic Analysis. Int. J. Pharm. **1994**, *101*, 105–113.

33. Delgado-Charro, M.B.; Guy, R.H. Iontophoretic Delivery of Nafarelin Across the Skin. Int. J. Pharmaceut. **1995**, *117*, 165–172.

34. Heit, M.C.; Williams, P.L.; Jayes, F.L.; Chang, S.K.; Riviere, J.E. Transdermal Iontophoretic Peptide Delivery: *In Vitro* and *In Vivo* Studies with Luteinizing Hormone Releasing Hormone. J. Pharm. Sci. **1993**, *82*, 240–243.

35. Meyer, R.B.; Kreis, W.; Eschbach, J.; O'Mara, V.; Rosen, S.; Sibalis, D. Transdermal versus Subcutaneous Leuprolide: A Comparison of Acute Pharmacodynamic Effect. Clin. Pharmacol. Ther. **1990**, *48*, 340–345.

36. Scott, E.R.; Phipps, J.B.; Gyory, J.R.; Padmanabhan, R.V. Electrotransport Systems for Transdermal Delivery: A Practical Implementation of Iontophoresis. *Handbook of Pharmaceutical Controlled Release Technology*; Wise, D., Ed.; Marcel Dekker, Inc.: New York, 2000.

37. Handelsman, D.J.; Jansen, R.P.S.; Boylan, L.M.; Spaliviero, J.A.; Turtle, J.R. Pharmacokinetics of Gonadotropin-Releasing Hormone: Comparison of Subcutaneous and Intravenous Routes. J. Clin. Endocrinol. Metab. **1984**, *59*, 739–746.

38. Banga, A.K.; Chien, Y.W. Iontophoretic Delivery of Drugs: Fundamentals, Developments and Biomedical Applications. J. Contr. Rel. **1998**, *7*, 1–24.

39. Burnette, R.R. Iontophoresis. *Transdermal Drug Delivery: Developmental Issues and Research Initiatives*; Hadgraft, J., Guy, R.H., Eds.; Marcel Dekker, Inc.: New York, 1989; 247–292.

40. Singh, P.; Maibach, H.I. Iontophoresis in Drug Delivery: Basic Principles and Applications. Crit. Rev. Ther. Drug. Carr. Syst. **1994**, *11*, 161–213.

41. Tyle, P. Iontophoretic Devices for Drug Delivery. Pharm. Res. **1986**, *3*, 318–326.

FURTHER READING

For additional examples of In Vitro and In Vivo Iontophoretic Drug Delivery Studies and Techniques, the Reader is Directed to the Comprehensive Reviews by Banga (1), Banga and Chien (38), Burnette (39), Singh and Maibach (40), and Tyle (41).

ISOLATORS FOR PHARMACEUTICAL APPLICATIONS

Gordon J. Farquharson

Bovis Lend Lease Pharmaceutical, United Kingdom

INTRODUCTION

The use of isolators in research and manufacturing in the health care and life science industries continues to develop rapidly. An overview shows many new applications being conceived, designed, constructed, and set into operation to satisfy many different processing needs. These applications frequently fall outside the accepted concepts and practice found in human scale rooms. It is only in the last 2 or 3 years that the technology has been recognized within cGMP guidelines and regulations. This article attempts to describe the practical experience gained from consultancy and design of isolators from the early 1970s up to and including state of the art applications developed today. For clarity, an isolator can be defined as:

> A device creating a small enclosed controlled or clean classified environment in which a process or activity can be placed with a high degree of assurance that effective segregation will be maintained between the enclosed environment, its surroundings, and any personnel involved with the process or manipulation. Isolators can be closed or open designs, and may be maintained at positive or negative pressure to their surroundings.

The following list summarises some essential features that help to expand on the definition as it is applied in the life science and pharmaceutical industry context:

- An isolator is an enclosed controlled environment of minimum volume.
- Isolators segregate people from processes.
- Isolators can contain processes hazardous to the surroundings, processes that are at risk from the surroundings, or in some cases activities where both types of risk coexist.
- Isolator walls or envelopes may be rigid or flexible; typical primary materials are stainless steel and glass, and polyvinyl chloride (PVC) flexible sheet welded to form an enclosure.
- Isolators are internally pressurized with air or inert gas to help achieve the required segregation between inside and outside. Pressurization can be positive or negative.

- Air filtration through High Efficiency Particulate Air (HEPA) or Ultra Low Particulate Air (ULPA) filters (9) is used to control the quality of air entering, leaving, and recirculating. For some applications in which very small inert gas quantities are used, nitrogen, for example, can be delivered through sterilizing-grade membrane filters.
- Isolators are frequently connected intimately to items of process equipment to provide an effective locally controlled environment.

The principal industry drivers generating the interest in isolators in the last few years have been focused on improvements in process integrity. This includes operator protection from potent and hazardous materials and, in the case of sterile products manufacturing, to reduce the potential of contaminated nonsterile units from being produced by a specific process. There are some circumstances in which reductions in occupied space and operational cost savings have been essential objectives.

TECHNICAL GUIDELINES AND STANDARDS

Although guidelines, such as the UK Pharmaceutical Isolator Guideline (1), and standards for microbiological safety cabinets (2, 3) and those for flexible-film isolators (4), satisfy part of the need for effective standards, further support is needed. During 2001, the ISO Technical Committee 209 should publish EN/ISO (DIS) 14644-7 (5). This standard will be entitled "Enhanced Clean Devices." Although it is not pharmaceutical industry specific, it will contain much excellent basic good practice guidance. 2001 should also see publication of PDA's Monograph "Design and Validation of Isolator Systems for the Manufacturing and Testing of Health Care products." Useful sources of reference can also be obtained from the nuclear industry. ISO 10648 "Containment enclosures" contains some valuable sections (6, 7).

For isolators, the barrier between the critical controlled environment and its surroundings is created by a single element, rather than the multilayer protection approach used in cleanroom technology. It is essential, therefore, to realize that the engineering solution, integrity, and reliability of the final operational isolator will have a direct impact not only on the enclosed process, but also on the quality required of the surrounding environment. This is particularly so when an isolator is used to contain a vulnerable aseptic process. This is usually be the most critical task for isolators, and the one that is most difficult to prove.

The design and construction of isolators should be carried out in an appropriate quality-assured way because the devices are frequently complex and require a high level of documentation to comply with both safety and good quality requirements. ISO 9000 compliant or similar quality assurance systems provide an appropriate management environment in which to design and build systems destined for quality or safety critical applications.

HEALTH CARE INDUSTRY REGULATORY DEMANDS AND EXPECTATIONS

Many operational applications are now in place, particularly in Europe. They can be found in manufacturing, R&D, and QC sectors. Experience continues to develop, and the users are at the forefront of the knowledge. Regulatory guidance can now be found in the European Union Guide to Good Manufacturing Practice (EU GMP) and will shortly appear in "Pharmaceutical Inspection Co-operation Scheme" (PICS) inspection guidelines. It is the responsibility of the isolator user, together with the designer or supplier, to effectively demonstrate an appropriate level of system integrity and performance. Regulators primarily hope to see that the use of isolators has been targeted at improvements in sterility or other attributes of quality assurance, as well as operator health and safety, and environmental protection. Such regulators may be less impressed by issues relating to reduction of unit manufacturing cost or amount of capital employed.

At present, the pharmaceutical industry regulatory requirements refer to isolators specifically in the context of the manufacture of sterile products. There is no reference to their role in broader areas of crosscontamination and operator safety control. Within Europe, the current EU GMP clearly states that isolators might produce improvements in sterility assurance of sterile products, and that aseptic processing manufacturing isolators should be placed in at least a Grade D surrounding environment. The Food and Drug Administration (FDA) requirements are less well defined, but it is likely that in equivalent circumstances, they would like to see an isolator located in a class 100,000 or M6.5 environment "In Operation."

As far as the configuration and performance of isolators is concerned, the pharmaceutical regulators have not made specific demands in their documentation. However, some of the main issues that have been identified by U.S. and European investigators or inspectors include:

- Concern that the use of isolators engenders a false sense of security, and that cGMP standards might be abandoned
- Concern over the effects of vibration caused by the process and the critical environment being physically connected
- Integrity of glove and half-suit systems
- Effective leak testing regimes that should be established
- Effectiveness of the physical cleaning of isolators applied in conjunction with gaseous or aerosol disinfection systems
- Evidence of good ergonomic design
- A well-defined and implemented personnel intervention policy, including intervention recording
- Tailored process simulation programs for aseptic processing
- Inappropriate sterility assurance level claims

APPLICATIONS

Isolator systems can be used for quality-critical, safety-critical, or combined applications. The examples given here are not exhaustive but focus on some of the most important applications, and clearly illustrate the broad range of devices that are created to satisfy particular needs.

Sterility Testing

For many years, isolators have provided a valuable tool for providing very clean conditions in the microbiological laboratory for testing the sterility of the end product. Both flexible-film and rigid-wall devices have been successfully utilized. These isolators are used to carry out manipulations with a growth-promotion medium. Any failures in the security of the isolator are likely to manifest themselves as growth in the culture medium. Such growths would be deemed false positives, and would result in a requirement to investigate the source of contamination. The security and effectiveness of isolators, operating in conjunction with sanitization techniques and transfer systems such as interlocking transfer ports, have been demonstrated to provide a more secure system than the traditional cleanrooms for this type of analytical work.

Sterility testing requires a strict control of microbial contamination challenge from outside the controlled environment, but not of the particulate contamination liberated by the process itself. Hence, a positive-pressure isolator in a controlled environment, using nonunidirectional airflow, is satisfactory. Flexible-film devices using half-suit manipulation techniques are frequently used in these applications. These isolators are usually configured as "closed" isolators because they don't have continuous-process discharges from the contained

volume. Fig. 1 shows an example of an isolator used in sterility testing.

Subdivision and Dispensing of Potent Compounds

As pharmaceutical products contain increasingly potent active constituents and as health, safety, and environmental protection issues increase in importance, isolators have been developed in many shapes and forms to permit

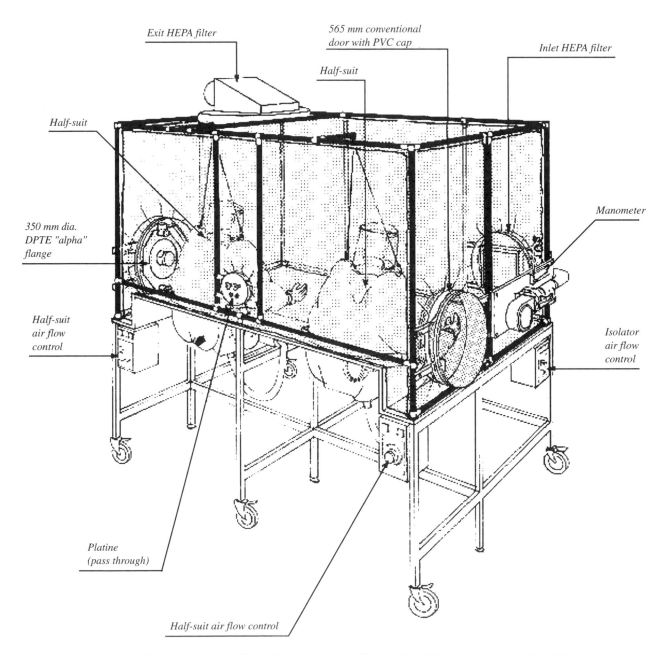

Fig. 1 Flexible-film isolator with half-suit used for sterility testing. (Diagram courtesy of La Calhene.)

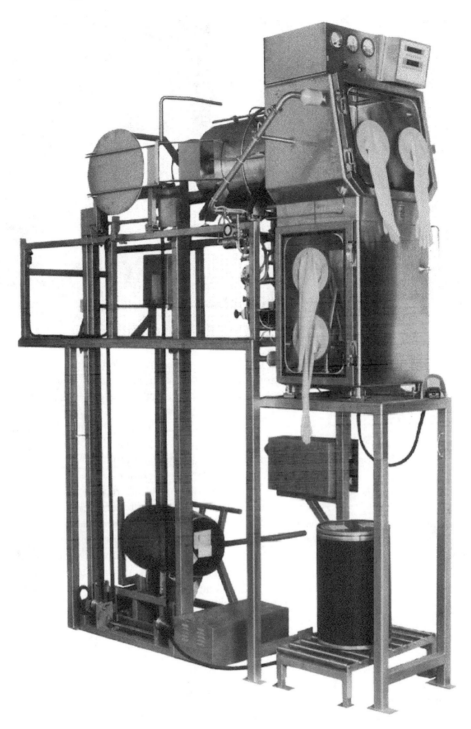

Fig. 2 Potent drug-dispensing isolator. (Photograph courtesy of TPC Microflow Ltd.)

the safe weighing and subdivision of highly active compounds. The most sophisticated applications, such as the subdivision of bulk sterile active compounds, require that the isolator maintain aseptic processing conditions internally at the same time as satisfying the

safety requirements. Fig. 2 shows an isolator device designed to allow a keg of potent raw material to be introduced into an isolator environment, and be securely subdivided into lots suitable for a subsequent formulation batch process. The device includes systems for mechanical

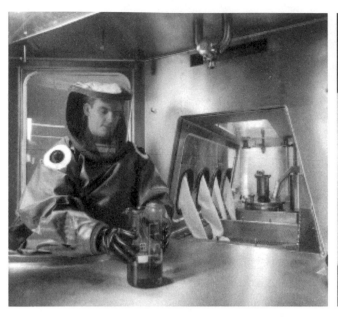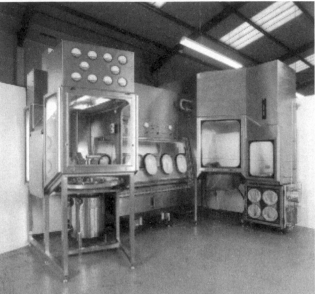

Fig. 3 Specialized isolator for potent drug processing and handling. (Photograph courtesy of TPC Microflow Ltd.)

handling of the kegs, and for washing their exterior to decontaminate them after completion of the manipulation.

Powder Processing Systems

A natural extension from the simple handling of potent compounds is to use barrier technology to provide highly secure mechanisms for processing and more complex manipulation of powders. Isolators of this type and configuration have the objectives of operator and environmental protection as well as the provision of a secure clean and aseptic environment around the process.

The example shown in Fig. 3 is a system used for the drying and handling of bulk powder. It provides a clean classified environment for handling bulk powder, a containment of the potent compound, and a nitrogen environment to allow the safe use of flammable solvents. It is a rigid positive-pressure device located in a EU GMP Grade D cleanroom. The cleanliness of the internal nitrogen environment is maintained using nonunidirectional airflow. Manipulations are achieved using a combination of glove and half-suit systems.

Small-Scale Manipulations

Many isolator applications at the clinical trial scale of manufacturing are based on the same scale of technology used for sterility testing. The aseptic dispensing of pharmaceutical products in hospital pharmacies is also carried out on this scale. Such manufacturing is not carried out on a continuous basis, but in relatively small batches

that can be transferred from the isolator with the help of one of the more secure transfer systems. In this type of application, one isolator is being used to dispense a variety of products or several isolators are used for separate tasks.

In the application shown in Fig. 4, a group of isolators are placed in an EC Grade C working environment (approximately equivalent to ISO 7 or Class 10,000 "At Rest"). The isolators are configured to provide an aseptic environment interfacing with a depyrogenating oven for handling and holding dry-heat-sterilized components. Additional individual isolators are provided in which separate formulation and/or filling operations can be undertaken. Materials are moved from one isolator to another using closed containers that dock with alpha/beta docking ports mounted in the sidewall and floor of the isolators. Internal cleanliness is maintained through positive pressurization and the supply of double HEPA-filtered unidirectional airflow to the critical process zones within the isolators.

LARGE-SCALE ASEPTIC PRODUCTION

Isolators are now used in industrial scale aseptic processing for both formulation and filling. Fig. 5 shows an example of a rigid interconnected network of isolators providing a complete component handling and aseptic filling capability in an integrated line. The internal control of the environment is achieved by a combination of nonunidirectional and unidirectional airflow within positively pressurized cells. The individual cells are

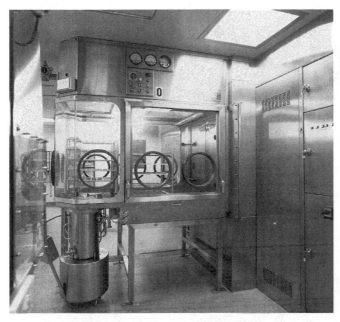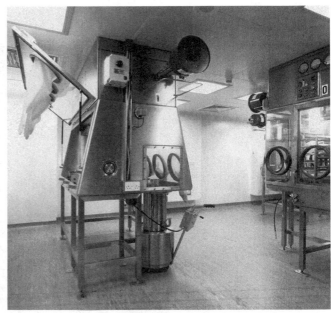

Fig. 4 Isolators used in clinical trials and specials manufacturing (the gloves have been removed for photographic clarity). (Photograph courtesy of Boots Contract Manufacturing and Bovis Tanvec Ltd.)

separated by "airlock" flap valves. The product flow through to aseptic filling operations is largely automatic, with gloves provided for specific manual interventions. The complete line is placed in a room in which the environment is controlled but unclassified in terms of cleanroom standards. Hydrogen peroxide vapor is used for the surface sterilization of the isolator network, and for the continuous surface disinfection of containers of product components that enter the system.

Technical Considerations for the Design, Manufacture, and Testing of Isolators

The susceptibility of the process to contamination is critical in terms of risk assessment. In aseptic processing, for example, open processes are at far greater risk than closed processes. Furthermore, systems requiring complex aseptic assembly prior to use are more difficult to manage in a small isolator environment than if cleaning and sterilization-in-place techniques were employed (referred to as *CIP* and *SIP*). It is essential, therefore, to evaluate all the process steps, including equipment transfers, assembly manipulations, and the processing activity itself. Effective documentation of such analysis is good practice in a validated operational scenario.

Barrier-integrity characteristics

Complex isolators are unlikely to be leak free. It is obvious that the better the barrier integrity is, the less will be the opportunity for contamination to be transferred across the isolator wall. The integrity is influenced by the basic materials of construction, design effectiveness, damage caused by cleaning, resistance to process chemicals, and robustness. The first fundamental option to consider is a rigid or a soft-wall construction. The former normally utilizes a combination of stainless steel and glass or Perspex windows; the latter uses a welded transparent PVC envelope connected to a stainless steel floor tray or machine bedplate. After choosing either a rigid or soft-wall solution, it is most important to ensure that an effective mechanism is selected to measure the leakage-air tightness of the isolator. Such tests should form part of the construction acceptance testing of a device, and should become part of routine operational leak testing. A pressure-hold test is the simplest method of determining that the complete assembly satisfies a set of acceptance criteria. Provided that the isolator, including its internal and external air systems, is configured in an appropriate way, simple isolating valves can be used to isolate the isolator, thus allowing convenient leakage-rate tests to be carried out. Such tests could ultimately be carried out on a batch basis if required. The most commonly used test methods are:

- Evaluation of pressure decay rate
- Leakage-rate measurement at constant pressure
- Tracer gas leak-rate detection
- Tracer particle transfer measurement (sometimes called a leak-induction test)

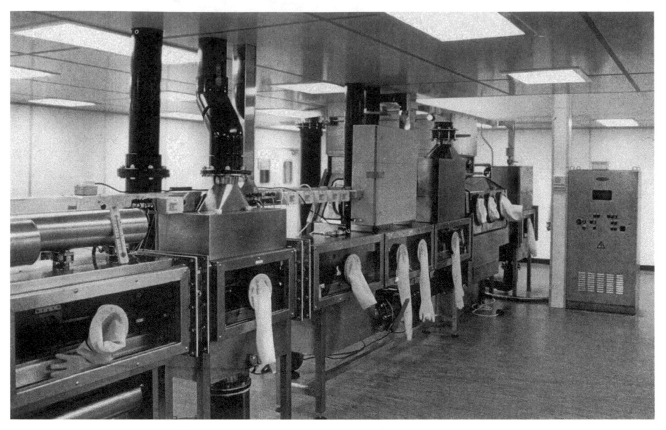

Fig. 5 A specialized network of isolators used for large-scale industrial syringe filling; process flow is from left to right. (Photograph courtesy of Medeva Ltd.)

Table 1 illustrates a range of four "Leakage Classes" that will be included in the "Enhanced clean devices" standard, EN ISO (CD) 14644-7. These classes are based on levels of leakage defined in the ISO 10648 (6,7) nuclear containment standards.

Manipulation technique

The manipulation technique influences the overall integrity of an isolator system, as in virtually all cases, the manipulation device presents a potential breach to the barrier of the isolator. Additionally, where the manipulation involves placing part of the human body within a specialised system component, such as gloves or a half-suit, a greater potential exists for process or product contamination than would occur with tong manipulators, remote manipulators, or robotics devices. Utilizing a simple pressure-hold or leakage test on a glove port and glove before and after a process work session can achieve a high level of glove integrity assurance. Such a technique is virtually impossible with half-suit applications due to their size and construction. Strategic inspections and pressure tests for integrity at

Table 1 Isolator leak rates (tentative levels)

Leakage class reference	Leak rate enclosure air change/hour	Leak rate: percentage enclosure volume/hour %
1	$<5 \times 10^{-4}$ (<0.0005)	<0.05
2	$<2.5 \times 10^{-3}$ (<0.0025)	<0.25
3	$<10^{-2}$ (<0.1)	<10
4	$<10^{-1}$ (<1.0)	<100

less frequent intervals are required for such devices. Alternative manipulation methods using tongs and remote manipulators (mainly for handling radioactive substances) can be of advantage in isolators, but currently are rarely found in pharmaceutical applications. However, it should be noted that tong manipulators, for example, have their own special problems and use a gaiter system to ensure air pressure integrity around the rotation and sliding gimbals. This gaiter is akin to the glove gauntlet, and its integrity and risk of failure are just as important.

Manipulations should always be minimised. An event report should be made, and a preprepared action plan must be implemented should damage occur to a glove. The selection of glove and gauntlet materials is most important. Half-suit and sleeve/glove systems use a technique where the glove can be detached from the sleeve by way of a specialized fitting in the wrist region. Some of these devices have the capability of allowing glove change while the system is in use. Gauntlet or one-piece systems are generally more durable, but do not have the same change in use capability. A balance has to be maintained between durability and "feel." Typical available materials are:

- Latex (natural rubber) allows great dexterity; if thick enough, these can be wear and abrasion resistant. It is chemically resistant to many mild chemicals, detergents, and disinfectants.
- Neoprene (synthetic) has high flexibility and allows good dexterity. It has low tensile strength, and is chemically resistant to materials with the exception of oxidizing agents such as hydrogen peroxide.
- Nitrile (synthetic copolymer) has poor flexibility, but is strong and highly chemical resistant.
- PVC (synthetic polymer) is strong and chemically resistant to materials except ketones and aromatic hydrocarbons; it is inflexible and subject to tearing.
- Urethanes have good abrasion, chemical resistance, and good tensile strength, but are not suitable for high temperatures.
- Laminated polymers exhibit high strength and selective resistance to chemicals; they are subject to failure when used with sharp objects.

A variation of the pressure-hold test can be used to test the integrity of manipulation gloves in situ. This provides a convenient way of determining the integrity of the glove without entering the controlled environment or unnecessarily changing an expensive commodity. An alternative, provided by a particular vendor, involves inert gas purging of a glove volume, followed by measurement of the build-up of oxygen that diffuses through glove pinhole leaks.

Transfer techniques

The transfer of materials into and out of an isolator represents the most likely and most common source of loss of internal environmental integrity. The more secure the transfer system, the less demanding is the surrounding environment. The simplest devices, such as single doors, present very little ability to separate the external from the internal environment. In fact, in these applications, the only facet of the device's performance that provides any protection is outward airflow when the door or cover is open. Security can be improved by a double-door pass-through hatch. The performance and effectiveness of such a device can be improved by introducing mechanical or electromechanical interlocking of the opposing doors. Furthermore, adding positive ventilation of the airlock space to dilute and remove contamination that may enter when the external door is open adds security to this form of transfer. The most secure techniques include a direct process connection to the isolator, interlocked docking port systems (often called alpha/beta systems), and airflow protected tunnels for continuous component discharge. Although no specific tests or standards exist to define the performance of such devices, tests can be adopted from other applications. Containment tests such as those used for open-fronted microbiological safety cabinets can be effectively used to determine a protection factor for airflow-protected product-discharge tunnels. In the case of alpha/beta interlocked docking port systems, certain manufacturers have developed and applied particulate and microbiological challenge tests to determine the effectiveness or a protection factor of these devices. This quantifies the segregation achieved by such a device in operation. Such tests may become the basis of type or performance testing and subsequent selection of specialized transfer devices. A typical alpha/beta port is illustrated in Fig. 6.

Internal pressurization

Internal pressure within an isolator clearly has a major influence on the ability of the isolator to exclude the external environment. The level of the pressurization should also be considered in relation to its ability to withstand the piston effect of rapid glove movement, and whether or not the internal isolator air system should achieve a specific outflow of air in the event of partial or total glove loss. The integrity and performance of pressurisation equally apply to negative-pressure systems. However, negative-pressure systems, used for clean and aseptic processing, are more likely to require a higher class of surrounding environment than that required for equivalent positive pressure systems. The glove piston

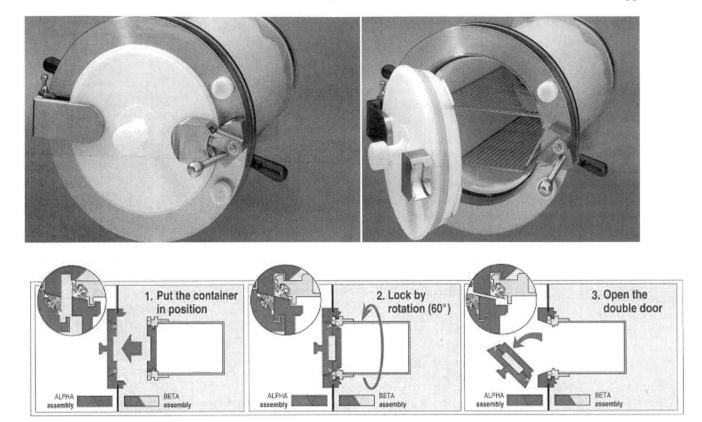

Fig. 6   A typical alpha/beta port. (Illustration of DPTE courtesy of La Calhene.)

effect is relative volume related (i.e., the volume displaced by the glove compared to the volume of the isolator). As a rule of thumb, devices with a pressure of 15–25 Pa compared to the surrounding atmosphere, are likely to be less secure (due to the piston effect) than devices with a pressure of 50–80 Pa compared to the surrounding area. When lost glove airflow protection is required, air velocities of 0.5–0.7 m/s should be considered. If extremely high velocities above these figures occur, reentrainment of external contamination due to high turbulence is a distinct possibility. In testing the effectiveness of the pressurisation, it is necessary to challenge not only the steady state conditions but also the transient conditions. It is therefore expected that a series of tests be carried out to investigate start and stop modes of the isolator control system, the influence of glove or other device manipulation, and of course, the interaction of the process itself. The most demanding processes in aseptic pharmaceutical applications are usually continuous depyrogenation tunnels, where the air leakage into the tunnel due to isolator overpressure, varies with time, and may well vary with different machine settings for various sizes. In this type of application, it is absolutely critical that the qualification of the isolator environment

is carried out in conjunction with all states of operation. Similarly, it is essential that the depyrogenation process in the tunnel is fully qualified with all states of the isolator.

Airflow configuration

As with cleanroom applications, isolators can use unidirectional or non-unidirectional airflow regimes, or in larger systems a combination of both. Isolators are very different from cleanrooms in that generally a physical barrier separates critical from noncritical zones rather than the use of managed airflow. It is possible therefore in isolators to obtain the necessary levels of environmental cleanliness with very low air velocities. Unidirectional airflow systems designed to achieve class 100/M3.5/ISO 5 cleanliness can be achieved with velocities as low as 0.10 m/s. When the velocity is set at such low levels, it is necessary to carefully evaluate the influence of heat sources and process disturbance. Having defined the airflow characteristics required for the isolator, it is necessary to determine both the airflow rate using flow anemometers and the uniformity of the airflow in the case of unidirectional airflow systems. The latter is best achieved using flow visualization smoke-tracing techniques. This is particularly important if an isolator environment itself contains a mixture of unidirectional and turbulent and/or conventional flow zones.

Filtered-air exchange rate in nonunidirectional flow systems should be based on the rate required to dilute internally generated contamination. The contamination decay rate of an enclosed volume can be used as a measure of effectiveness of the air-movement system in an isolator. This can be helpful for assessing the degassing rate at the conclusion of a gaseous sanitisation or sterilizing procedure. The decay rate can be measured using artificial aerosol generation combined with measuring the decay profile broadly in accordance with the method set out in IES recommended practice 006.2. Alternative gas-decay methods can be adapted from tracer-gas methods used to prove the effectiveness of ventilation systems.

HEPA filtration

The provision and location of air filters and the filtration integrity in isolators are as important as in clean or containment room technology. The filter and its installation must be designed with the utmost care, and special consideration should be given to the effect of vibration transferred from the isolator mechanical systems or the process. Final filters should be placed as close as possible to the critical zone. However, this sometimes makes the task of fitting the filters difficult due to restricted space and access. Maintenance convenience can be improved by locating filters close to, but away from the critical zone, in carefully engineered housings. When this technique is used, the duct between the filter and the isolator should be constructed of non shedding materials. Natural or artificial aerosol challenge tests are the appropriate way to test in situ final HEPA or ULPA filters and existing cleanroom oriented standards, and requirements are directly relevant to isolator applications.

Airborne cleanliness classification

Classification of the working environment by measuring the particulate concentration is normally carried out in accordance with the requirements stated within the accepted airborne-particle classification standards. If the isolator working volume is extremely small, it may be necessary to increase the number of test locations from the single point determined by using the formula within the standards. Two, three, or more locations focused on the critical points of process or product exposure. When continuous or cyclic automatic particle monitoring is being considered, care should be taken to ensure that the volume of air taken as a sample does not adversely influence the isolator pressurization.

Open aperture integrity

Open aperture protection is an important feature of some isolators. In addition to designing and testing for isolator pressurisation, some isolators need to be engineered to maintain segregation in case of partial or total glove loss. This is particularly the case when biological or chemical hazards are present internally, and need to be contained for safety reasons. Furthermore, in many production-scale isolator networks, particularly those filling parenteral containers, it is an advantage to pass the filled closed containers out of the isolator continuously via an airflow protected tunnel. In such cases, there is a protecting air velocity, entering or leaving the isolator, to contain a hazard or minimize the opportunity of internal contamination, respectively. The effectiveness of this inrush or outrush of air (protection factor) can be quantified by a biological or aerosol challenge test derived from adaptation of the method defined in British Standard 5726 (2) or the U.S. Standard NSF 49 (3). Both these standards relate to microbiological safety cabinets where the test is specified for the purposes of quantifying a containment factor. The containment test challenges the aperture with a test aerosol, and measures the quantity that escapes through the opening. The ratio of escape to generated quantity is used to calculate a containment factor. This test method can also be effectively deployed for testing and demonstrating the effectiveness of any other aperture inward or outward and is used to protect and segregate the internal from the external environment. In the classic case, there is a continuous discharge of filled containers across a dead plate, leaving an aseptic processing environment. Here it is important to determine that there is no turbulence causing induction of external contamination into the critical aseptic zone.

CLEANING AND SANITIZATION OF ISOLATORS

Effective cleaning and biodecontamination of the internal surfaces of isolators and their intimate product contact parts is of greatest importance, particularly for aseptic processing. The effectiveness and repeatability of the sanitisation method also has an impact on the quality of the surrounding environment required. This is particularly the case if it is anticipated that batch and machine format changes are carried out with the isolator open. If this procedure is adopted, it is necessary first to minimize the introduction of room contamination into the open isolator, and then to apply an effective cleaning procedure. If some contamination has entered the device, it is essential to use a repeatable and effective sanitization or surface sterilization method. The requirement to clean and disinfect would be lessened if changeover were achieved with a closed isolator. The least effective processes, such as surface swabbing and aerosol spraying with disinfectant, are unlikely to satisfy the requirements of a repeatable process of high efficacy. However, the use of highly controlled gaseous-phase processes, using materials such as formaldehyde, hydrogen peroxide, peracetic acid, and chlorine dioxide, can be very effective. These gaseous-phase processes are generally intolerant of soiling deposits on the surface. Therefore, the methods must be deployed in conjunction with effective physical cleaning.

DESIGN CONSIDERATIONS FOR THE SURROUNDING ENVIRONMENT

Finally, having taken all the above issues into account, and determined the type and nature of the isolator to be used and the quality of the surrounding environment, it is important to consider some of the broader issues relating to the design of the surrounding environment. It is essential to thoroughly consider all the attributes of the facility in which the isolator is placed, as this can have a major influence on the product. The facility in which the isolator is placed must provide a clear departmental separation from less critical adjacent activities. By layout and configuration, it must achieve the following:

- Provide appropriate physical security for the operation
- Control and manage access of personnel and materials
- Ensure the required background environment is maintained
- Provide the utilities required by the isolator

REFERENCES

1. Isolators for Pharmaceutical Applications. In *The UK Isolator Group*; ISBN 0 11 701829 5 Her Majesty's Stationery Office: London, 1994.
2. Microbiological Safety Cabinets. BS5926: 1992 & BS EN 12469: 2000.
3. NSF 49 Microbiological Safety Cabinets.
4. ACDP UK, Guidance on the Use, Testing, and Maintenance of Laboratory and Animal Flexible Film Isolators, Dec. 1995.
5. Clean Rooms and Associated Controlled Environments. A family of new standards produced by ISO and CEN. EN/ISO, 14644-1–14644-8, (Progressive Publication from May 1999).
6. Refer to ISO 10648 *Containment Enclosures—Part 1: Design Principles*; 1997.
7. Refer to ISO 10648 *Containment Enclosures—Part 2: Classification According to Leak Tightness and Associated Checking Methods*; 1994.
8. U.S. Fed. Standard 209E, Airborne Particulate Cleanliness Classes in Clean Rooms and Clean Zones.
9. Refer to *Air Filtration*, EN 1822 parts 1–5.
10. Air Cleanliness in Clean Rooms. JIS 9920 **1989**.

ISOMERISM

Thomas N. Riley
Jack DeRuiter
William R. Ravis
C. Randall Clark
Auburn University, Auburn, Alabama

BASIC PRINCIPLES

Isomers are defined as molecules of identical atomic compositions (molecular formulas), but with different bonding arrangements of atoms or orientation of their atoms in space. Based on this definition, several types of isomerism are possible including constitutional, configurational, and conformational isomerism. Constitutional isomers (also called structural or positional isomers) are molecules with the same atomic composition but different bonding arrangements between atoms, as illustrated by the examples of catechol, resorcinol, and hydroquinone (Fig. 1). All of these compounds have the same atomic composition ($C_6H_6O_2$), but different bonding arrangements of atoms and are thus distinct chemical entities with different chemical and physical properties.

Configurational isomers are defined as molecules of identical atomic composition and bonding arrangements of atoms, but different orientations of atoms in space, and these different orientations cannot interconvert freely by bond rotation. Since these types of isomers differ only in relative spatial orientations of atoms, they are commonly referred to as stereoisomers. Configurational stereoisomers are subcategorized as optical isomers (enantiomers) or geometric isomers (Fig. 2), depending upon the hybridization state and geometry of the atoms that impart the properties of stereoisomerism and the overall structure of the molecule. Stereoisomers of this type are distinct chemical entities that may have different chemical and physical properties.

Conformational isomers (conformers) are stereoisomeric forms characterized by different relative spatial arrangements of atoms that result from rotation about sigma bonds. Thus, unlike configurational isomers, conformers are interconverting stereochemical forms of a single compound. The nature of conformational and configurational stereoisomerism, as well as the role of stereoisomerism in drug activity is the subject of this article.

Optical Activity and Molecular Structure

Modern stereochemistry originated with the research of Malus in 1808 who discovered that plane-polarized light is generated when a beam of light is passed through calcium carbonate. In 1813, the mineralogist Biot reported that asymmetrically cut quartz crystals rotate the plane of a beam of polarized light. It also was noted that certain organic liquids, as well as solutions of certain organic compounds, can rotate the plane of polarized light. Biot attributed this effect on plane-polarized light to a property of the individual organic molecules through which the light is passed, a property now referred to as optical activity. The concept of optical activity was extended by Herschel in 1812, who observed that hemihedral quartz crystals, having odd faces inclined in one direction, rotated the plane of polarized light in one direction, whereas crystals whose odd faces were inclined in the opposite direction rotated plane-polarized light to the same extent but in the opposite direction.

Pasteur refined the observations of the mineralogists by proposing a link between optical activity and molecular structure. His landmark work of 1847 was based on earlier observations by Biot that chemically identical salts of tartaric acid rotated plane-polarized light differently. Pasteur discovered that two distinct crystalline forms of tartaric acid salt could be obtained from solutions of the optically inactive salt of "paratartaric acid" (also known as racemic acid), and that one crystal form has hemihedral faces that inclined to the right, whereas the other has faces that inclined to the left. He separated the distinct crystalline salts forms and observed that they, unlike paratartaric acid, are optically active; solutions of the left-handed crystals rotate the plane of polarized light to the right, and solutions of the right-handed crystals rotate the light to the same degree, but in the opposite direction. Pasteur further demonstrated that the left- and right-handed crystals were mirror images of each other and concluded that this property must reflect the handedness of the molecules that constitute the crystals.

Encyclopedia of Pharmaceutical Technology

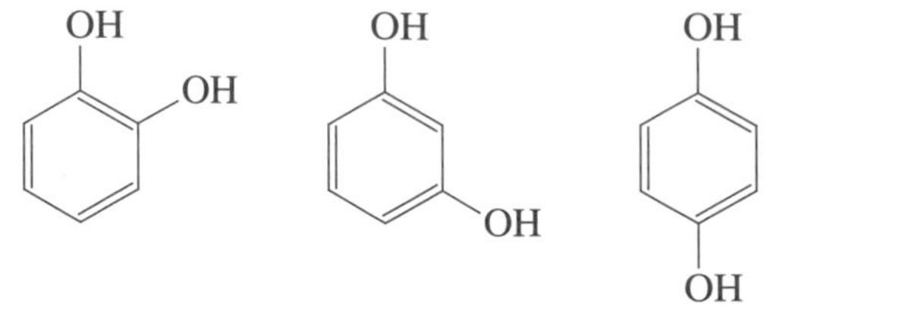

CATECHOL   RESORCINOL   HYDROQUINONE

Fig. 1   Constitutional isomers.

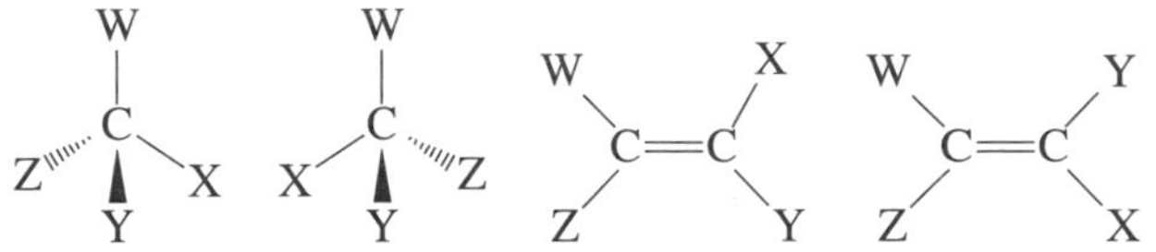

Optical Isomers
(Enantiomers)   Geometric Isomers

Fig. 2   Stereoisomers.

The molecular basis for the left- and right-handedness of distinct crystals of the same chemical substance and the associated differences in optical rotation was developed from the hypothesis of Paterno (1869) and Kekulé that the geometry about a carbon atom bound to four ligands is tetrahedral. Based on the concept of tetrahedral geometry, Van't Hoff and LeBel concluded that when four different groups or atoms are bound to a carbon atom, two distinct tetrahedral molecular forms are possible, and these bear a nonsuperimposable mirror-image relationship to one another (Fig. 3). This hypothesis provided the link between three-dimensional molecular structure and optical activity, and as such represents the foundation of stereoisomerism and stereochemistry.

Chirality and Optical Isomers (Enantiomers)

The property of nonsuperimposability became known as chirality, and molecules containing asymmetrically substituted carbons are referred to as chiral molecules. The term chiral was derived from the Greek word meaning "hand" and was applied as a description of the left- and right-handedness of crystal structure resulting from molecular asymmetry. The individual mirror image forms

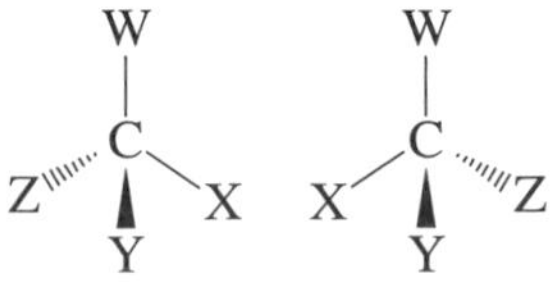

Fig. 3   Tetrahedral geometry and optical isomerism.

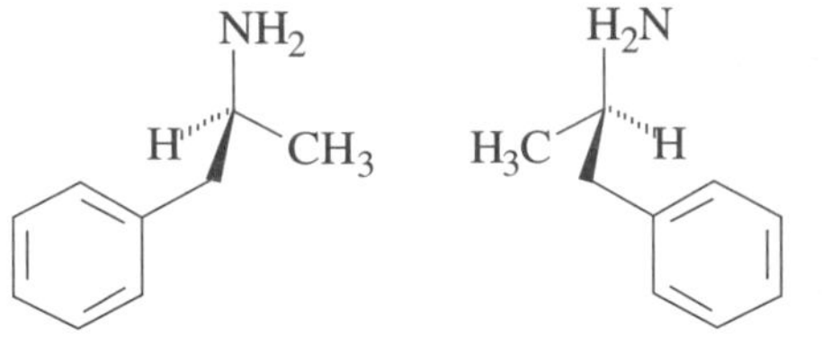

(+) - Amphetamine   (−) - Amphetamine
$[\alpha] = + 21.8°$ $[\alpha] = - 21.8°$

Fig. 4   Amphetamine enantiomers.

of a chiral molecule are called optical isomers because they rotate the plane of polarized light (are optically active) and differ in structure only in the orientation of atoms or groups about the asymmetric carbon (are isomers). Today, optical isomers are more commonly referred to as enantiomers or an enantiomeric pair.

Generally, optical isomers or enantiomers have identical physical and chemical properties, for example, the enantiomeric forms of amphetamine (Fig. 4) have identical melting points, pK_a, solubilities, etc. There are, however, two important differences in properties between the members of an enantiomeric pair. First, each member rotates the plane of polarized light to the same degree, but in opposite directions. The enantiomer rotating the plane to right (clockwise) is designated as the dextrorotatory (d) or (+)-enantiomer. The other enantiomer rotates the plane to the left (counterclockwise) and is designated as the levorotatory (l) or (−)-enantiomer. This is illustrated in Fig. 4 for the enantiomers of amphetamine, where the enantiomer with the specific optical rotation of (+)-21.8° is designated as dextrorotatory, whereas the mirror enantiomer with a specific rotation of (−)-21.8° is called levorotatory. A second difference between enantiomers is their interactions with other chiral substances. For example, enantiomers may have different solubilities in chiral solvents, they may react at different rates in the presence of an optically active reagent or enzyme, and many have different affinities for chiral surfaces and receptors.

Most optically active drugs are chiral as a result of the presence of an asymmetrically substituted tetrahedral carbon atom. However, chirality can result from the

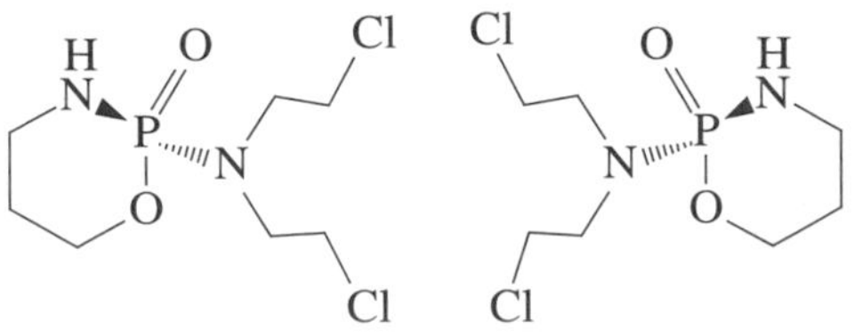

Fig. 5   Optical isomers of cyclophosphamide.

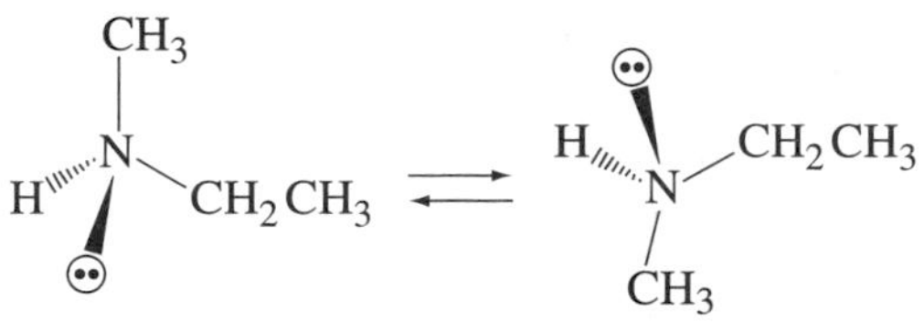

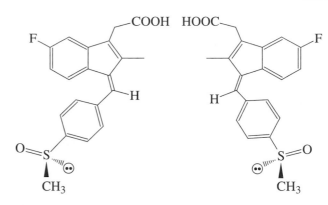

Fig. 6   Pyramidal inversion of chiral nitrogen.

Fig. 7   The chiral sulfoxide sulindac.

Definitions and Nomenclature

presence of other asymmetrically substituted atoms within molecules as illustrated below including phosphorous (Fig. 5), nitrogen (Fig. 6), and sulfur (Fig. 7).

As discussed in the preceding section, each member of an enantiomeric pair rotates the plane of polarized light to the same degree, but in opposite directions (dextrorotatory and levorotatory). However, the amount of optical rotation is not constant for an individual enantiomer but rather is dependent on the solvent, concentration, temperature, the wavelength of light used, and the path length of the sample cell employed to determine the rotation. Thus, meaningful optical rotation comparisons for chiral compounds are only possible when optical activities are determined under specified conditions. Such conditions are defined as specific rotations $[\alpha]$ and are expressed for solutions and neat liquids in Eq. 1 and 2, respectively.

$$[\alpha]_\lambda^t = \frac{100\alpha}{l \cdot c} \tag{1}$$

$$[\alpha]_\lambda^t = \frac{\alpha}{l \cdot d} \tag{2}$$

where α is the measured rotation; t, the temperature; λ the wavelength; c, the concentration; d, the density; and l, the length.

Specific rotation data may assist in the identification of a specific enantiomer, or may be used to determine the optical purity (enantiomeric purity) of a mixture of enantiomers. Optical purity is defined as the percent excess of one enantiomer over another in a mixture and is expressed in Eq. 3:

$$Optical purity = \frac{[d] - [l]}{[d] + [l]} \cdot \frac{\alpha_{obs}}{\alpha_o} \tag{3}$$

Based on Eq. 3, a mixture consisting of equal amounts of each enantiomer would have no net optical rotation; the optical rotation of one enantiomer is cancelled by the rotation of the other enantiomer. Such a mixture is referred to as a racemic mixture or racemate.

Other terms commonly applied in discussions of optically active compounds include resolution and racemization. Resolution describes the processes whereby a racemic mixture is separated (resolved) into its component enantiomers. Racemization refers to the conversion of either enantiomer into equal parts (racemic mixture) of both enantiomers.

Over the years, several nomenclature systems have been developed to characterize the relationship between enantiomers. The system based on optical activity and the classification of enantiomers as dextrorotatory [d or (+)] or levorotatory [1 or (−)] already has been described. However, this system of nomenclature is of limited applicability because the sign of rotation, (+) or (−), does not predict the absolute configuration or the relative spatial arrangement of atoms in the enantiomers. In an attempt to designate the precise configurations about carbon centers of asymmetry, the Cahn–Ingold–Prelog R/S system have been developed and adopted as the most commonly used nomenclature system for isomers.

In applying the Cahn, Ingold, and Prelog R/S system the compound is oriented in a Fischer projection and the four groups or atoms bound to an asymmetric carbon are ranked by the following set of sequence rules (Fig. 8):

1. Substituents are ranked (1–4) by the atomic number of the atom directly joined to the chiral carbon.
2. When two or more of the atoms connected to the chiral carbon are the same, the atomic number of the next adjacent atom determines the priority. If two or more atoms connected to the second atom are the same, the third atom determines the priority, etc.
3. All atoms except hydrogen are formally given a valence of 4. When the actual valence is less than 4 (N, O), phantom atoms are assigned an atomic number of zero and therefore rank the lowest.
4. A tritium atom has a higher priority than deuterium, which has a higher priority than hydrogen. Similarly, any higher isotope has a higher priority than any lower one.

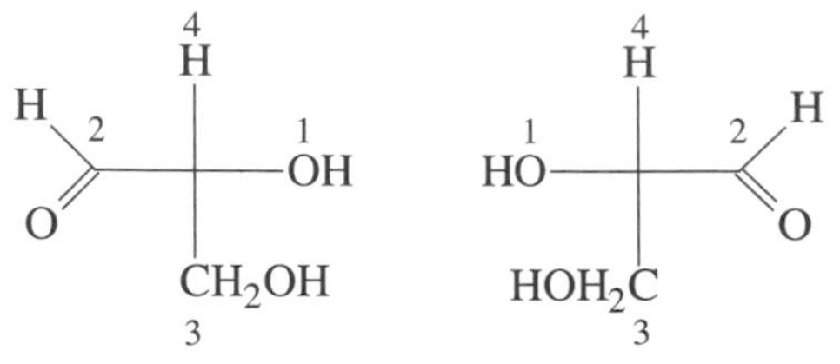

S-Glyceraldehyde   R-Glyceraldehyde

Fig. 8   Cahn–Ingold–Prelog sequence rule.

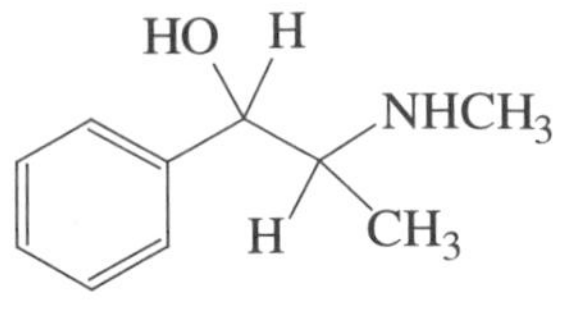

Ephedrine

Fig. 9   Ephedrine having multiple chiral centers.

5. Atoms with double and triple bonds are counted as if they were connected by two or three single bonds. Hence a CC is regarded as a carbon bound to two carbons; and a CO is regarded as a carbon bound to two oxygens.

Once the four groups bound to the chiral carbon are ranked, the compound is oriented in such a way that the lowest priority group (4) is projected away from the observer. Then, if the other groups (1–3) are oriented by priority in a clockwise fashion, the molecule is designated as R (rectus), and if counterclockwise, as S (sinister). These sequence rules are applied in the assignment of the absolute configurations for the enantiomers of glyceraldehyde in Fig. 8. According to the first rule, the highest priority substituent (1) is the hydroxy group (OH) and the lowest priority group (4) is the hydrogen atom; since the atomic number of carbon is higher than that of hydrogen but lower than that of oxygen, the two carbon substituents (CHO and CH_2OH) are assigned intermediate priorities. To determine the priority relative to the two carbon substituents, both the 2nd and 5th rules must be applied. The aldehyde carbon is part of a carbonyl (C=O) moiety which, by rule 5, is equivalent to a carbon bound to two oxygen atoms. The alcohol carbon (CH_2OH) is bound to one oxygen and two hydrogens. The "two oxygens" of the aldehyde take priority over the single oxygen of the alcohol moiety; the aldehyde is assigned priority 2, and the alcohol priority 3. With all substituents ranked and the enantiomers oriented in such a way that the lowest priority group (4) is projected away from the observer, the configurations can be assigned. The enantiomer in which the substituents are oriented by priority in a clockwise fashion, is designated as R, and the enantiomer in which the substituents are oriented by priority in a counterclockwise direction is designated as S.

Compounds with Multiple Centers of Asymmetry

Many stereoisomeric drugs contain more than one asymmetrically substituted atom. For example, ephedrine has two chiral centers (Fig. 9). In this case, a greater

number of configurational isomers is possible; the maximum number possible is 2^n, where n is the number of chiral atoms. Hence, the maximum number of possible configurational isomers for ephedrine is four, which are designated RR, SS, RS, and SR (Fig. 10). The RS and SR isomers are nonsuperimposable mirror images and hence are enantiomers. The same relationship exists for the RR and SS isomers. The relationship between each member of an enantiomeric pair and each member of the other enantiomeric pair is diastereomeric; they are nonsuperimposable nonmirror images. Thus, the RS isomer is a diastereomer of the RR and SS isomers, and the SS isomer is a diastereomer of the RS and SR isomers. In this case, the SR and RS enantiomers are referred to as ephedrines, whereas the RR and SS enantiomers are called pseudo-

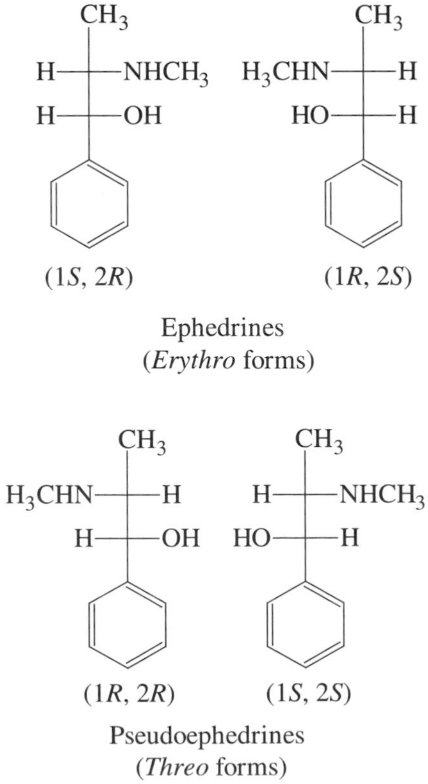

(1S, 2R)   (1R, 2S)

Ephedrines
(*Erythro* forms)

(1R, 2R)   (1S, 2S)

Pseudoephedrines
(*Threo* forms)

Fig. 10   Ephedrine and pseudoephedrine stereoisomers.

ephedrines. Diastereomers, unlike enantiomers, differ in their physicochemical properties including solubilities, acid-base strengths, melting points, etc.

In addition to the *R* and *S* designations, compounds with two chiral centers may also be identified by stereochemical nomenclature that describes the entire system. For example, the *erythro* and *threo* nomenclature derived from carbohydrate chemistry may be employed to describe the relative positions of similar groups on each chiral carbon. Thus, the ephedrines are designated as *erythro* forms since the similar groups (OH and $NHCH_3$) are on the same side of the vertical axis of the Fischer projection, and the pseudoephedrines are designated as *threo* forms since like groups are on opposite sites of the vertical axis of the projection (Fig. 10).

It is important to note that the 2^n rule predicts only the maximum number of stereoisomers possible in compounds with more than one center of chirality. For example, some compounds with two asymmetrically substituted carbon atoms may have only three stereoisomeric forms. This

occurs when three of the substituents on one asymmetric carbon are the same as those on the other asymmetric carbon, as shown for the antitubercular ethambutol (Fig. 11). In this case, one stereoisomer has a plane of symmetry even though two asymmetric atoms are present. Such an isomer is referred to as a *meso* compound and is optically inactive. Therefore, when a plane of symmetry is present in a compound with two centers of asymmetry, only three stereoisomeric forms are possible.

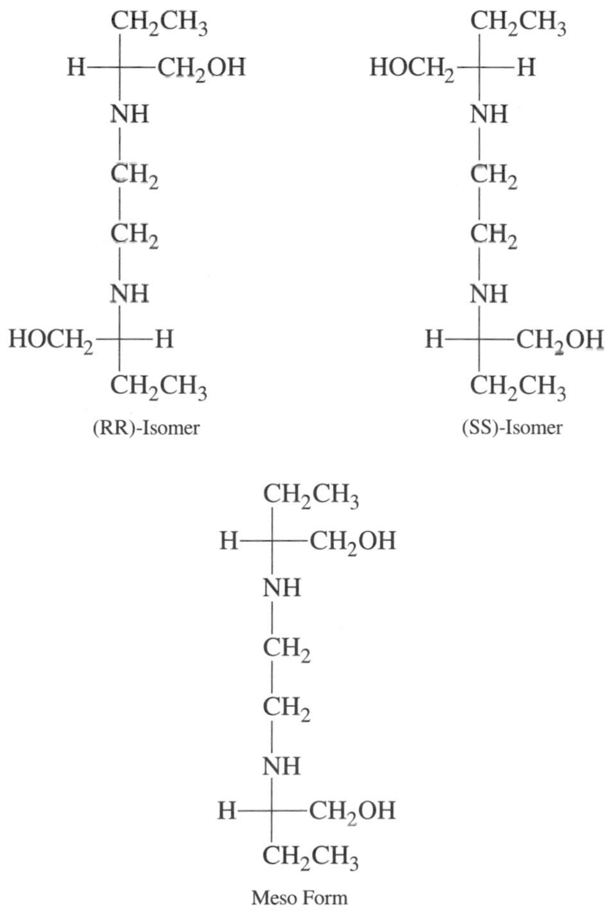

Geometric Isomerism

Geometric isomerism was first defined by Wislicenus in 1887 as isomerism occurring in compounds where rotation is restricted by double bonds or ring systems. Geometric isomers do not rotate the plane of polarized light (unless they also contain a chiral center), and hence are not optically active.

Geometric isomerism resulting from restricted rotation about double bonds

The sp^2 hybridized carbon atoms of alkenes (olefins) and the atoms or groups attached to these carbons all lie in the same plane, and rotation around the double bond is restricted. As a result, stereoisomerism is possible when each carbon atom of the double bond is asymmetrically substituted. Because geometric isomers are nonsuperimposable, nonmirror images they are classified as diastereomers and therefore possess different physical and chemical properties. A number of drugs contain dissymmetrically substituted carbon–carbon double bonds and therefore can exist as two distinct geometric isomers (Fig. 12).

Several systems of nomenclature have been developed to designate the configuration of geometric isomers. Historically, the *cis–trans* system of nomenclature has been applied most frequently. It was developed to assign the configuration of geometric isomers when each isomer contains a like group or atom on each carbon atom of the double bond. However, in more complex structures this

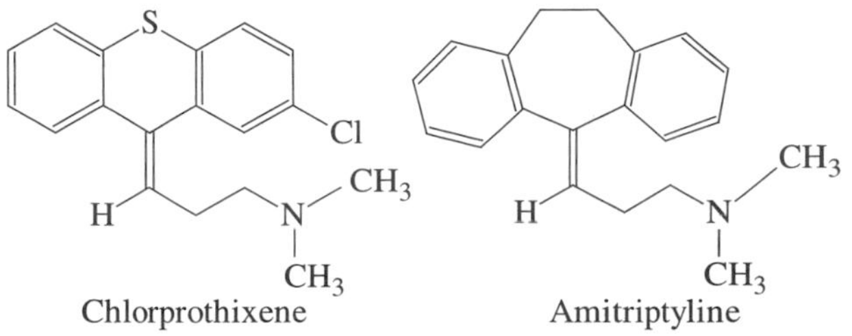

Fig. 11 Ethambutol stereoismoers.

Fig. 12 Pharmacologically active dissymmetrically substituted alkenes.

system cannot be used unambiguously to assign configurations for all geometric isomers. For example, the sp^2 atoms of the antipsychotic agent thiothixene do not contain a like atom or group (Fig. 13). Thus, the *E/Z* notation system was developed to unambiguously assign configurations in all cases of geometric isomerism.

1. Priorities are assigned on the basis of atomic number for the two atoms or groups attached to each carbon of the carbon–carbon double bond. The same priorities apply as in the Cahn–Ingold–Prelog sequence rules.
2. Configuration is assigned based on the relative positions of the highest priority atoms or groups on each carbon of the carbon–carbon double bond. If these groups are on the same side, the *Z* (zusammen) designation is used. If they are on the opposite side, the *E* (entgegen) designation is assigned.

Geometric isomerism is also possible in double-bonded carbon-heteroatom systems such as imines and oximes (CN), and in azo (NN) systems. For example, several cephalosporin derivatives contain an alkoxyimino side chain that may exist in *E* or *Z* isomeric forms; the azo compound prontosil may display similar isomerism (Fig. 14). A *syn–anti* system can also be applied to CN geometric isomers. In these cases, the priority assignments are made as described previously, and the isomer with highest priorities on the same face of the double bond are called *syn*, whereas those with these groups on opposite sides are named *anti*.

In a number of amides, thioamides, and related systems, rotation about the single bond is hindered, and distinct geometric isomers can be observed and even isolated. This type of geometric isomerism is referred to as atropisomerism and results from resonance contributions by the nitrogen atom that imparts significant double bond character to the system, thus slowing rotation. Such is the case for the thioamide aldose reductase inhibitor

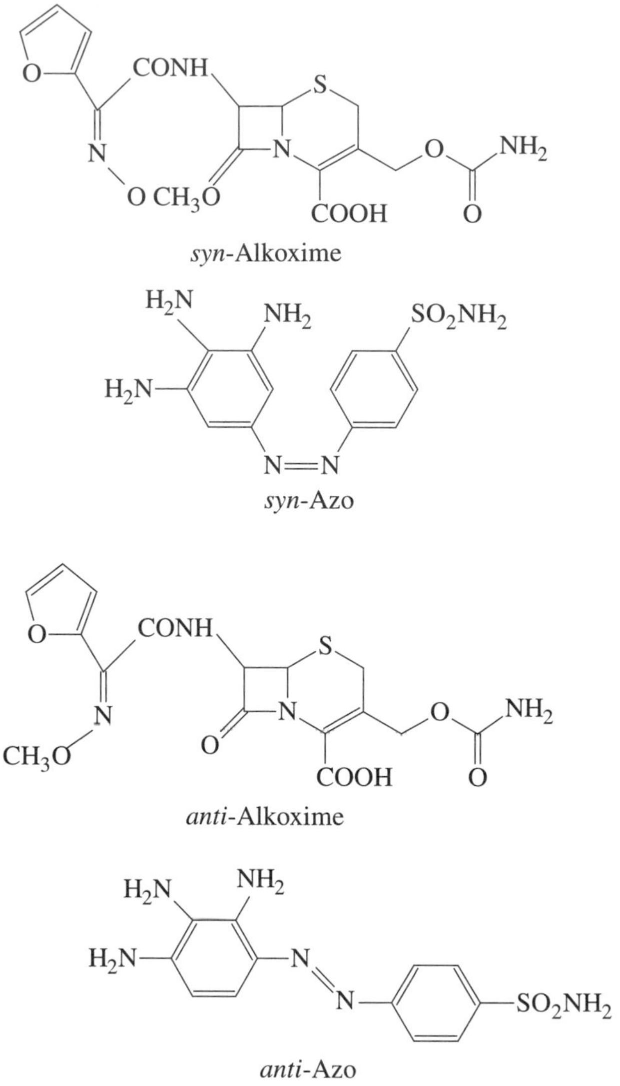

syn-Alkoxime

syn-Azo

anti-Alkoxime

anti-Azo

Fig. 14 Geometric isomerism about C-heteroatom double bonds.

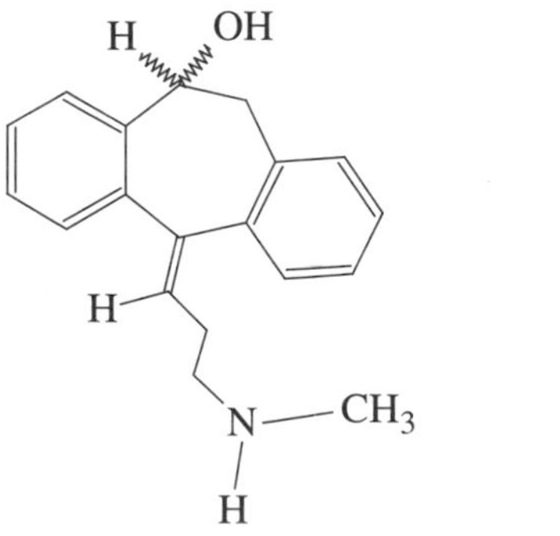

10-HYDROXYNORTRIPTYLINE

Fig. 13 Geometric isomer nomenclature—thiothixene.

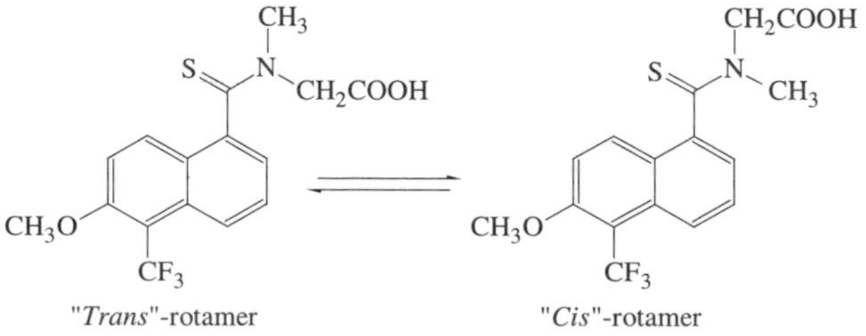

"*Trans*"-rotamer   "*Cis*"-rotamer

Fig. 15 Atropisomerism, tolrestat.

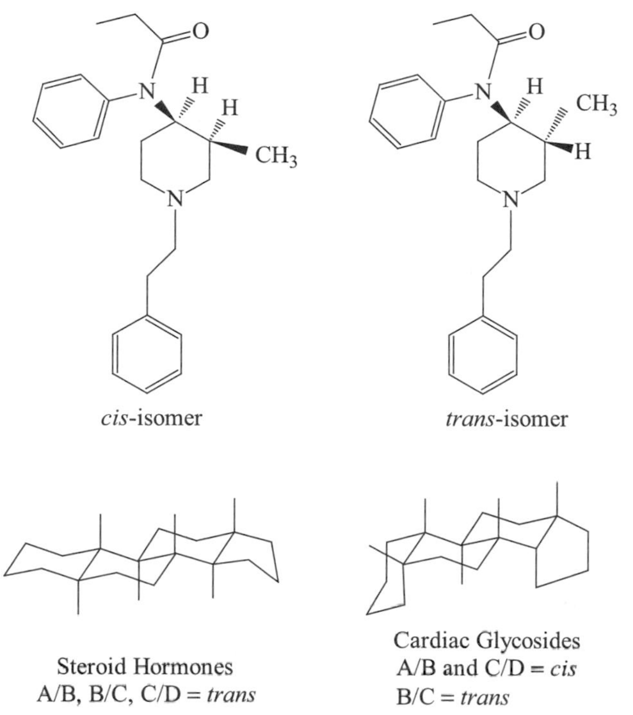

cis-isomer   *trans*-isomer

Steroid Hormones
A/B, B/C, C/D = *trans*

Cardiac Glycosides
A/B and C/D = *cis*
B/C = *trans*

Fig. 16 Geometric isomerism in cyclic drug structures.

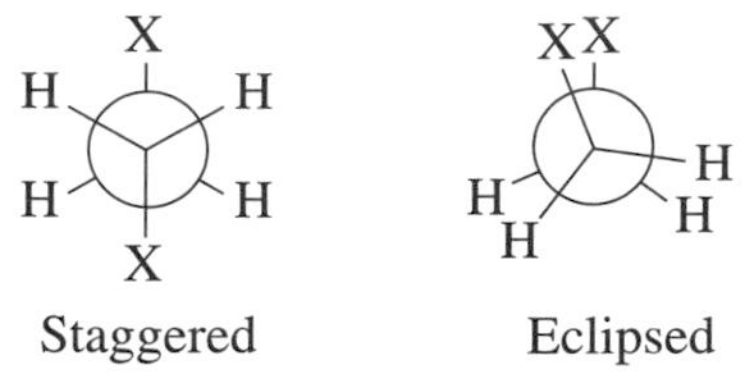

Staggered   Eclipsed

Fig. 17 Newman projection formulas for staggered and eclipsed rotamers.

tolrestat shown in Fig. 15. Isomers of this type are also called rotamers and are considered to be conformational isomers since they result from rotation about a single bond.

Geometric isomerism in cyclic compounds

The presence of a ring system, either cycloaliphatic or heteroaliphatic, like that of a double bond, prevents rotation, therefore giving rise to geometric isomers when two carbon atoms of the ring are each substituted by different groups. Structures of pharmacologically-important structures that display geometric isomerism are shown in Fig. 16.

When rings are fused through adjacent atoms, the fusion may be *cis* or *trans*, as illustrated by the steroid structure (Fig. 16). In the naturally occurring steroids the ring junctions are all *trans*, except in the case of the cardiac glycosides where both A/B and C/D junctions are cis. Rings fused through nonadjacent atoms, or bridged systems, may also display stereoisomerism.

Conformational Isomerism

In the preceding sections the nature and properties of configurational (optical and geometric isomers) were discussed. It is important to remember that configurational isomers are distinct, separable compounds.

Conformational isomers are different three-dimensional arrangements in space of the atoms of a single compound or configurational isomer. Such isomers are termed conformers and are interconvertible by free rotation about single bonds.

In alkanes or alkyl systems, an infinite number of conformations is possible as a result of rotation about CC single bonds, and each conformation has a certain potential energy. Two conformational extremes, one of low (minimal steric interaction between bond substituents) and one of high (maximal steric interaction) potential energy, have been described for these systems. These are depicted as Newman projections in Fig. 17. A more recent nomenclature system for conformational isomers arising from energy barriers associated with rotation about a C–C single bond is shown in Fig. 18. In this case, the most stable conformer is the antiperiplanar isomer, where the distance between the two bulky groups (X and Y) is maximized, thus minimizing steric interactions. The least stable conformer is the fully eclipsed or synperiplanar conformer where the two groups are closest together. The other conformers, the anticlinal and gauche or synclinal are of intermediate stability.

Conformational isomerism is believed to be of great significance for drug-receptor and drug-enzyme

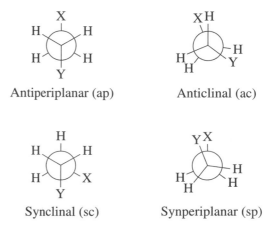

Antiperiplanar (ap)   Anticlinal (ac)

Synclinal (sc)   Synperiplanar (sp)

Fig. 18 Conformational isomers.

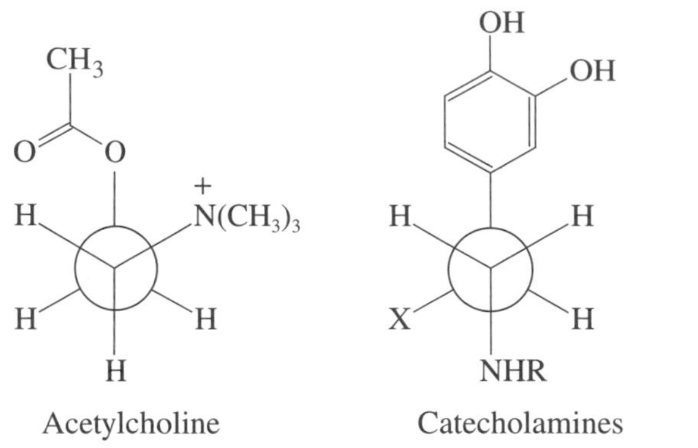

Acetylcholine   Catecholamines

Fig. 19 Pharmacophoric conformations of acetylcholine and norepinephrine.

interactions. For example, experimental data suggest that catecholamines such as norepinephrine and dopamine interact with their receptors in the antiperiplanar conformation. Furthermore, the preferred (pharmacophoric) conformation of acetylcholine at its muscarinic receptor sites is the synclinal conformer (Fig. 19).

Conformational isomerism in cycloalkyl and cycloheteroalkyl structures is characterized by several different conformational extremes. For example, cyclohexane systems can exist in three distinct conformations: boat, twist boat, and chair. Of these, the chair form is the most stable conformation because steric interactions are minimized (Fig. 20). The substituents present on a ring conformer are designated as axial or equatorial, depending on the direction of projection from the average plane of the carbon skeleton. Substituents that project directly up or down from the ring are axial, and those in the plane of the ring are equatorial. Because of the conformational flexibility of cycloalkanes such as cyclohexane, the ring conformation can invert. During inversion, all axial substituents become equatorial and all equatorial substituents become axial.

Ring conformations are believed to be important in drug activity. For example, experimental evidence suggests that the analgesic fentanyl binds to opiate receptors preferentially in the conformation shown in Fig. 21, where the

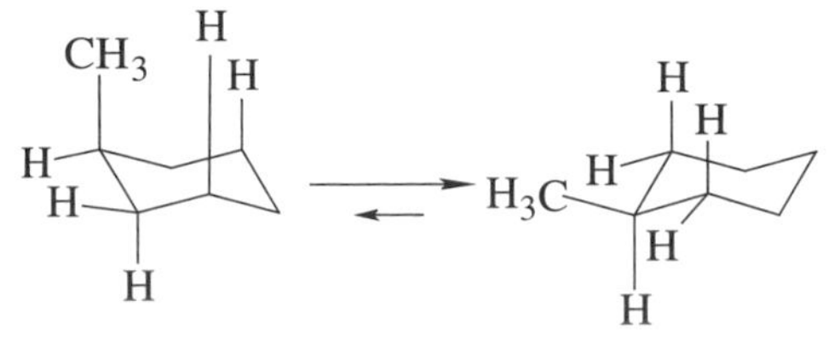

Fig. 20 Conformational isomerism of cycloalkanes.

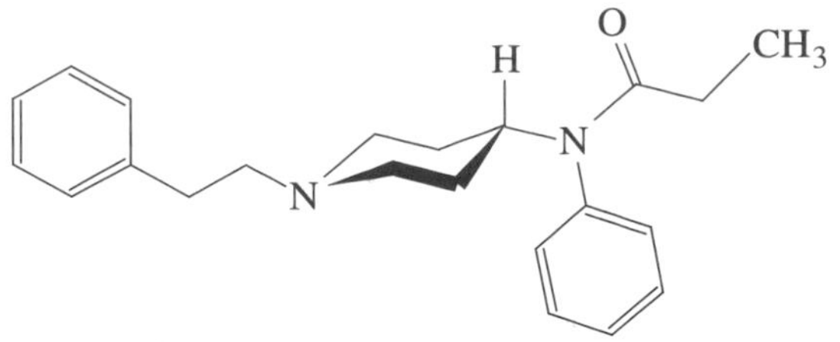

Fig. 21 Conformational isomerism, 3-methylfentanyl.

bulky substituents are positioned equatorially to minimize conformational instability.

PHARMACOLOGICAL ASPECTS OF ISOMERISM

Background and Definitions (1, 2)

Structural and steric complementarities of drug molecules with their target sites of action are essential criteria for the production of a pharmacological effect. The requirement of stereocomplementarity for organic medicinal agents reflects the inherent dissymmetry of the biological system comprised of stereoisomeric proteins, amino acids, lipids, carbohydrates, nucleic acids, etc. Molecular dissymmetry of biological systems was initially demonstrated in the 1880s by Pasteur. Then in 1908 Cushney explained differences in pharmacological actions of epinephrine enantiomers on the basis of dissymmetric drug receptors. Easson and Stedman in 1933 proposed a model for the molecular basis of sympathomimetic amines stereoselectivity at adrenergic receptors based on optimization of the number of interactions for each stereoisomer. Hence, the more efficacious (R)-$(-)$epinephrine isomer can achieve a three-point receptor interaction while the less active (S)-$(+)$-enantiomer and its achiral desoxy analogue, dopamine, can only achieve a 2-point interaction (Fig. 22). While Easson–Stedman's description of stereoisomeric drug action is a rather simplistic approximation of the steric aspects of drug action, it served to stimulate concerted chemical and pharmacological study of the phenomenon of stereoselectivity of drug action. Pfeiffer's rule, an attempt to quantifying drug stereoselectivity, states that, in the case of enantiomeric drugs, the greater the activity of the racemate the higher the ratio of the enantiomer's activity. A quantitative treatment of stereoisomeric drug action is the technique of eudismic analysis, which is most commonly applied to studies of enantiomeric drug action. In an eudismic analysis, the more active enantiomer (e.g., higher receptor

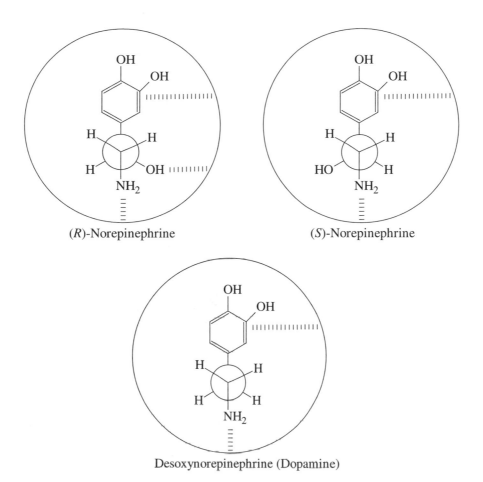

(R)-Norepinephrine   (S)-Norepinephrine

Desoxynorepinephrine (Dopamine)

Fig. 22 The Easson-Stedman hypothesis of stereoisomeric drug action.

affinity—aff) is termed the eutomer and its less active mirror image form (e.g., relatively lower receptor affinity) is referred to as the distomer. Stereoselective pharmacological profiles of an enantiomer can be quantitated as a ratio of specific pharmacological actions termed the eudismic ratios (Eq. 4). The logarithm of the eudismic ratio is termed the eudismic index (Eq. 5).

$$\text{Eudismic ratio (ER)} = \text{Aff}_{eu} + \text{Aff}_{dis} \qquad (4)$$

$$\text{Eudismic index (EI)} = \log \text{Aff}_{eu} + \text{Aff}_{dis} \qquad (5)$$

Steric Aspects of Drug Action (3–7)

It is estimated that approximately one-half of all drugs worldwide exist as stereoisomers. However, only one-half of stereoisomeric drugs are marketed as the individual stereoisomer and most of the latter are of natural or semi-synthetic origin. There is increasing awareness of the clinical importance of drug stereoselectivity because differences in the behavior of isomers in the chiral living system can result in significant differences in clinical outcomes. Table 1 presents a number of examples of these difference.

The previous examples have described the varying influences of chirality on pharmacological activity. Table 1 also illustrates the influence of other types of stereoisomerism on the pharmacological profiles of medicinal agents including that of geometric isomerism on the antipsychotic activity of thioxanthene derivatives. The eutomeric relationship of the Z-thioxanthene has been ascribed to its greater conformational complementarity with the pharmacophoric extended conformation of that natural receptor ligand dopamine. Both conformational and configurational isomerism are important in the pharmacological actions of the calcium-channel-blocking 1,4-dihydropyridines. Unsymmetrical ester substitutions at C3 and C5 result in chirality at C4 with the enantiomers of selected derivatives possessing opposite effects on calcium-channel function. Further, the availability of a "boat-like" conformation of the dihydropyridines has been

Table 1 Steric aspects of drug action

Stereoisomeric drug	Structure	Comments
R- and S-α-Methyldopa	R- and S-α-Methyldopa	Only the S isomer possess pharmacologic activity (stereo specificity of action) because only the S isomer can be stereoselectively bioactivated to (1R,2S)-α-methylnor-epinephrine, a presynaptic α1-sympatho-mimetic antihypertensive.
R- and S-Flecainide	Flecainide	An example of a lack of stereoselectivity of pharmacological action. The enantiomers of flecainide demonstrates an eudismic ratio of ∼1.0 on excitable tissue of the canine myocardium.
R- and S-Warfarin	Warfarin	The anticoagulant activity of warfarin is a classic example of stereoselective drug action. S-warfarin in vivo is from two- to five-fold more anticoagulant than its R-enantiomer. This potency difference is coincidentally offset by the two-or five-fold greater plasma clearance of the distomer.
R- and S-Albuterol	Albuterol	The S-isomer of albuterol has been shown to oppose the bronchodilatory effects of the eutomer, R-albuterol and may therefore contribute to paradoxic bronchospasm and the occurrence of severe reagenic-like reactions seen with racemic albuterol.
R- and S-Bupivacaine		Bupivacaine exhibits stereoselectivity of local anesthetic activity, CNS and cardiac toxicity and pharmacokinetics. R-Bupivacaine is more potent, more toxic and more rapidly cleared than its S-isomer.

(Continued)

Table 1 Steric aspects of drug action (*Continued*)

Stereoisomeric drug	Structure	Comments
Labetalol stereoisomers	 Labetalol stereoisomers	These stereoisomers provide an example of different but complementary pharmacological of stereoisomers contributing to overall therapeutic utility. *R,R*-labetalol is a selective β-sympatholytic whiole the *S,R*-isomer is an α₁-adrenolytic eutomer.
Antipsychotic thioxanthenes		*Z*-orientation of the propylamine side chain enhances dopamine receptor site recognition of these agents.
Dihydropyridine derivatives	 (*S*) : Ca⁺⁺-channel activator (*R*) : Ca⁺⁺-channel blocker	Unsymmetrical ester substitutions at C3 and C5 result in chirality at C4 of the dihydropyridines. Separation of pharmacological actions is seen in appropriately structures optical isomers of chiral dihydropyridines. Further, the availability of a "boat-like" conformation of the dihydropyridines has been proposed to facilitate the calcium channel blocking activity of this class of agents.

proposed to facilitate the calcium channel blocking activity of this class of agents.

Hence it is obvious that stereoisomeric influences as well as structural effects, play a major role in the production of the pharmacological profiles of medicinal agents. Variations noted in vitro that are related to the three-dimensional shape of a drug molecule originate primarily in stereoselective processes involved in the target site. In vivo variations related to stereochemical influences reflect selective interactions of the drug both at its site of action and in the various phases of biodisposition.

STERIC ASPECTS OF PHARMACOKINETICS

The macromolecules of the body can distinguish between drug isomers leading to stereoselective differences in tissue and protein binding, biotransformation, and renal excretion. Slight spatial differences in stereoisomers can have marked effects on the degree of association and interaction with proteins and enzyme systems. Stereoisomeric drugs often display stereoselectivity in pharmacokinetic processes and pathways that require interaction and association with macromolecules and enzymes systems. Furthermore, diastereomers display a higher degree of stereoselective than enantiomers due to their differences in solubility and partitioning. Since enantiomers have identical solubility and partitioning characteristics, their stereo selective pharmacokinetics are expected to reside in more structurally specific processes such as membrane transport, biotransformation, and binding to proteins and tissues.

Drug Absorption

The passive gastrointestinal absorption of enantiomeric drugs would be expected to be similar since the physical properties of partitioning and solubility of enantiomers are the same. Transdermal absorption of drugs such as ketoprofen also appears to be nonstereo specific (8).

Stereoisomers with structural similarities to endogenous entities and nutrients display differences in permeability rates across the gastrointestinal membrane and hence in bioavailability. L-DOPA, which is absorbed by an amino acid transport system, passes the gastrointestinal wall at a rate four to five times that of the D-enantiomer (9). L-methotrexate is absorbed by active processes in the gastrointestinal tract, and the D-isomer is reportedly absorbed by passive absorption. Another example of enantiomeric effects on gastrointestinal absorption is the

reported stereoselective absorption and intestinal biotransformation of cephalexin in rats (10).

In addition to stereospecific membrane permeability, there is a potential for stereoselective drug and dosage form effects. The crystalline forms of racemates may not be the same as the crystal structures of the individual stereoisomers and may be a source of differences in rates of dissolution between racemic and single enantiomer dosage forms. With respect to formulation, stereoselective interactions between solid dosage form excipients that are chiral, such as cellulose derivatives, may have the potential of altering the dissolution rates of stereoisomers. Further investigations of excipients and dosage form influences on the dissolution of chiral drugs are needed.

Drug Distribution

The extent and degree of interactions between chiral macromolecules of the body and stereoisomers is a source of observable differences in isomeric drug distribution. Stereoselectivity in drug distribution may occur when tissue or protein binding or uptake is associated with structurally specific receptor, protein, or enzyme binding. Since only unbound or free drug is susceptible to elimination and distribution to receptors and other tissues and fluids, differences in the protein and tissue binding of stereoisomers are reflected in their overall pharmacokinetic profiles.

Stereoselective interactions with both isolated human albumin and α_1-acid glycoprotein have been observed with a variety of protein-binding techniques. The interaction of an enantiomer with a plasma protein yields a diastereomeric association. The S isomer of warfarin is bound to a greater extent to albumin than the R isomer (11). α_1-Acid glycoprotein binds S-propranolol (87.3%) to a slightly higher degree than R-propranolol (83.8%), whereas human albumin binds R-propranolol more strongly than the S form (12).

The extent of binding differences between isomers is most readily noted from ratios of fractions free in the plasma; this ratio can be as high as three (Table 2). Recognizing that plasma protein binding impacts on drug distribution and elimination, differences in plasma protein binding between stereoisomers may lead to misinterpretation of pharmacokinetic comparisons between isomers, unless protein binding of the isomers is considered.

For enantiomeric drugs with low organ clearance, differences in renal or hepatic clearance between stereoisomers may reflect their free fraction in the plasma and not real stereoselectivity of the ability of the organ to remove the free enantiomers (intrinsic clearance) from the plasma. Clearance differences between stereoisomers of

Table 2 Stereoselective biodisposition

Parameter	Isomer	Warfarin	Ibuprofen[a]	Disopyramide[b]	Propranol[c]	Verapamil[d]
Total clearance	R	3.5 ml/h/kg	68 ml/min	111 ml/min	1210 ml/min	10.24 ml/min/kg
	S	4.9 ml/h/kg	74 ml/min	111 ml/min	1030 ml/min	18.1 ml/min/kg
	R/S	0.71	0.92	1.0	1.17	0.57
Volume of distribution	R	0.154 L/kg	9.9 L	48 L	4.8 L/kg	2.74 L/kg
	S	0.16 L/kg	10.5 L	50 L	4.1 L/kg	6.42 L/kg
	R/S	0.96	0.94	0.96	1.17	0.43
$t_{\frac{1}{2}}$, h	R	35	2	5.2	3.6	4.08
	S	24	1.7	5.5	3.5	4.81
	R/S	1.46	1.18	0.95	1.03	0.85
Unbound, %	R	1.2	—	34	20.3	11.0
	S	0.9	—	22.2	17.6	6.4
	R/S	3.3	—	1.53	1.15	1.72

[a](Ref. 26.)
[b](Ref. 14.)
[c](Ref. 12.)
[d](Ref. 59.)

verapamil and disopyramide may be a function of plasma protein binding differences. In addition, volumes of distribution as well as concentration ratios of stereoisomers in body fluids to total plasma and blood are influenced by plasma protein binding. For example, the larger volume of distribution and greater total body clearance of R-disopyramide compared to the S isomer may be explained by the lower plasma protein binding of the R isomer (13, 14). Also, the higher synovial fluid concentrations of S-ibuprofen following administration of the racemate appears to be related to the lower plasma protein binding of this isomer compared to that of the R isomer (15).

An unique example of stereoisomer selective tissue uptake of stereoisomers is noted with NSAIDs. The R enantiomer of ibuprofen shows preferential uptake into fat following the administration of the racemate and individual isomers (16). However, this apparent difference in fat distribution is probably a consequence of the selective metabolic uptake and formation of the coenzyme A thioester of the R isomer, which does not occur with the S isomer.

Drug Biotransformation

Numerous metabolic pathways involving mixed-function oxidases, esterases, transferases, and hydroxylases exhibit selectivity toward stereoisomeric substrates. Of all disposition differences that stereoisomers may display, the greatest stereoselectivity is expected in biotransformation, because of the specificity of metabolic enzymes and isoenzymes. The overall differences in hepatic clearance of stereoisomers reflect not only differences in intrinsic clearance (activity of drug metabolizing enzymes) for the isomers but also the steric effects of plasma protein binding and hepatic blood flow.

When stereoisomers are biotransformed by a variety of pathways, differences in the susceptibility of the separate isomers to these pathways result in stereoselectivity for their metabolite patterns. For example, S-warfarin is oxidized to form primarily 7-hydroxy-S-warfarin, whereas the R enantiomer predominantly undergoes hydroxylation in the 6-position (17, 18). Oxazepam glucuronidation is 3–3.4 times higher for the S isomer compared to the R isomer in man and dogs (19). Biotransformation may generate an additional chiral center in the drug structure and result in diastereomeric metabolites with markedly different disposition characteristics.

Some of the greatest differences in the pharmacokinetics of stereoisomers can be attributed to stereoselective hepatic biotransformation. The oral clearance of S-mephenytoin is 170 times that of the R enantiomer in extensive metabolizers of the drug (20). This large difference in clearance is reflected in a 2-h half-life for the S-mephenytoin compared to a 76-h half-life for the R enantiomer in the same patient group. Interestingly, the half-life of the S isomer (63 h) and the R isomer (77 h) are similar in poor metabolizers of mephenytoin. Numerous other examples of stereoselectivity in hepatic clearance can be found in the literature (21–23).

Metabolic processes in humans and animals may invert the configuration of several NSAIDs. For many

2-arylpropionic acid NSAIDs in humans, the S enantiomer is the pharmacologically active form. Following administration of the racemate or R enantiomer, a slow inversion of the R to the S enantiomer occurs. All the 2-arylpropionic acid NSA1Ds are administered as the racemate with the exception of naproxen. Based on investigations of ibuprofen, the R enantiomer is inverted to the S enantiomer via coenzyme A thioester formation (24, 25). It has been estimated, from pharmacokinetic studies of racemic ibuprofen that approximately 63% of the R isomer is inverted to the pharmacologically active S form (26). Stereoisomeric inversion is not universal for all 2-arylpropionic acids in humans with reports of inversion for ibuprofen, fenoprofen, and benoxaprofen and little or no evidence of inversion for tiaprofenic acid, ketoprofen, indoprofen, and carprofen (27–33).

Racemic drugs that experience hepatic "first-pass" metabolism of one or both isomers may experience stereoselectivity in biotransformation prior to the drug entering the systemic circulation, resulting in a route of administration effect on plasma concentration ratios and therapeutic response. Following IV doses of propranolol, plasma concentrations of both enantiomers appear to be similar, with only slight differences in total body clearance between the isomers (34). When propranolol is given orally, the higher rate of biotransformation and lower plasma binding of the less active R isomer results in lower plasma concentration of this isomer compared to the active S isomer. Other drugs administered as racemate such as verapamil, metoprolol, and prilocaine are reported to display stereoselective hepatic first-pass effects on the oral bioavailability of their isomers (35–38).

Renal and Biliary Excretion

The tubular secretory contribution to drug renal clearance has the potential of producing stereoselective renal elimination in the handling of stereoisomers. Enantiomers of terbutaline, disopyramide, and pindolol exhibit stereoselective renal clearance, probably due to differences in tubular secretion of individual stereoisomers (39–41). When examining the renal clearance of unbound disopyramide, the L-enantiomer has a renal clearance 29–86% higher than that of the D-isomer. The overall clinical significance of renal clearance differences for stereoisomers depends on the importance of renal elimination in the drug's total elimination. Biliary clearance of stereoisomers is difficult to evaluate in light of the techniques required and the many stereoselective factors influencing rate of biliary excretion. For these reasons, uncomplicated examples of stereoselective biliary excretion are not common.

Pharmacodynamics and Stereoselective Pharmacokinetics

The potency ratio (euduismic ratio) for stereoisomeric drugs reflects not only pharmacokinetic but also pharmacodynamic variations for the individual stereoisomers. In many respects, pharmacodynamic differences contribute more to large potency and activity differences of stereoisomers. Stereoselectivity at the level of drug-receptor interactions appears to be more pronounced than that noted for biotransformation or protein-binding interactions. A wide range of drug classes have been identified in which stereoselective pharmacodynamics are seen (4). Evidence for pharmacodynamic differences between stereoisomers is found in studies of isolated tissue and organ preparations and the relationships of drug response to plasma concentrations (42–44).

Analysis of pharmacological effects versus plasma concentrations of stereoisomers have been interpreted in terms of pharmacodynamic stereoselectivity. Pharmacological and toxicologic effects should be related to free plasma concentrations of stereoisomers in order to be able to appropriately compare activity or potency. Comparison of the free warfarin plasma concentration required to produce a 50% inhibition in synthesis of the prothrombin-activity complex reveals that S-warfarin has five times the inhibitory activity of the R isomer (45). The impact of the higher pharmacodynamic activity of S-warfarin on the dose-effect relationships of warfarin stereoisomers is partially offset by the fact that the S isomer is metabolically cleared more rapidly.

Pharmacokinetic Implications and Considerations

Recognizing that stereoisomers may vary markedly in their pharmacokinetic and pharmacodynamic profiles raises questions as to the usefulness of drug disposition, bioavailability, and pharmacodynamic modeling studies in which racemic forms are administered and nonstereospecific assays are utilized. Total body clearances, volumes of distribution, and bioavailability parameters become complex when the plasma concentrations of both stereoisomers are added. Clearance and bioavailability values observed after dosing of a racemic agent reflect a value falling between that of the two isomers (46–49). The observed half-life of the racemate is that of the stereoisomer with the longest half-life. The necessity of providing pharmacokinetic and pharmacodynamic data for both stereoisomers as well as their possible interaction could discourage the development of individual stereoisomers of drugs.

Since the administration of a racemate involves two separate drug entities, there can be intersubject variability in pharmacokinetic and pharmacodynamic profiles for both stereoisomers. Intersubject variability in the pharmacokinetics of both isomers leads to a large range of plasma concentration ratios across populations of patients. Factors such as disease, age, genetics, and concurrent drug therapy have been shown to lead to differing effects on stereoisomers of a drug. For example, the ratio of S- to R-tocainide plasma concentrations may vary over a 1.5- to threefold range (50, 51). R-Tocainide is believed to be several times more active than the S isomer (52). Factors such as disease, age, genetics, and concurrent drug therapy have been shown to lead to differing effects on stereoisomers of a drug. Liver disease patients have lower S/R ratios of plasma concentrations for ibuprofen stereoisomers than healthy subjects and this may be related to decrease conversion of the S- to R-isomer (53).

A major source of intersubject variability for stereoisomers is polymorphism in drug biotransformation (54). Extensive metabolizers of metoprolol display higher clearances of both stereoisomers than poor metabolizers, but the magnitude of the differences between stereoisomers is not the same within each population (38). Extensive metabolizers of metoprolol require lower total (R and S) plasma concentration of metoprolol for the same degree of beta blockade (51). In addition, R-mephenytoin shows similar oral metabolic clearance in extensive and poor metabolizers, whereas S-mephenytoin, which undergoes 4-hydroxylation, has markedly higher clearances in extensive metabolizers (55).

The area of clinical pharmacology that first directed attention to the consequences of stereoisomerism on therapeutic and pharmacokinetics was that of drug interactions, particularly those of the anticoagulant warfarin. Not only may drug interactions be stereoselective, but there is a potential for one stereoisomer to alter the pharmacokinetics and pharmacodynamics of the other. A classical example is the interaction with achiral phenylbutazone, which inhibits the metabolism of active S-warfarin but stimulates the metabolism of the less active R isomer (56). Other stereoselective drug interactions include the induced elimination of misonidazole by phenytoin (57). Phenytoin enhances the clearance of (4−)-misonidazole by 56%, which is higher than the increase in clearance of 33% noted for (−)-misonidazole.

Identical chemical and physical properties of enantiomers represent a potential source for enantiomer−enantiomer interactions at both pharmacokinetic and pharmacodynamic levels. Whether by competition for plasma- or tissue-binding sites or for drug-metabolizing enzymes, enantiomers may exhibit changes in pharmacokinetics when administered as a racemate compared to individual stereoisomers. The enantiomers of disopyramide exhibit similar clearance and volumes of distribution when given separately (14). However, when administered as the racemate, the S isomer has higher clearance and volume of distribution. Ibuprofen enantiomers have also been shown to undergo enantiomer-enantiomer interactions (58).

In the past, pharmacokinetic and pharmacodynamic investigations of chiral drugs have neglected the influences of stereoisomerism. This is primarily a result of the lack of stereospecific analysis procedures. Nonstereospecific assays give pharmacokinetic and pharmacodynamic information which represents a complex combination of the characteristics of the separate stereoisomers. With the advent of stereospecific analysis procedures a better understanding of drug kinetics and action as possible.

ANALYTICAL METHODOLOGY AND ISOMERISM

A diastereoisomeric interaction is always required for the resolution of enantiomeric substances. This interaction occurs between the enantiomers of interest and a second enantiomeric species often referred to as the chiral selector. The diastereoisomeric interaction between the enantiomers and the chiral selector may involve a covalent bond or other less stable noncovalent associations. In the example below, a mixture of R and S isomers associates with the R isomer of the chiral selector to yield two diastereoisomeric products:

$$R + R, S \longrightarrow R \cdots R + R \cdots S$$

In this process, enantiomers (R and S) of the heterochiral substance of interest interact with the homochiral selector (R) to yield two products having a diastereoisomeric relationship. The formation of diastereoisomeric complexes is the basis for enantiomeric separations. The ability to use smaller differences in the rates of formation, stability, and properties of these complexes has been responsible for the major advances in stereochemical separations.

Chromatographic Techniques

The chromatographic separation of enantiomers, often referred to as enantioseparation, has received a great deal of attention in recent years. Both liquid (LC) and gas (GC) chromatographic procedures are used. The former is extremely useful for enantioseparations because of the available variations in scale, mechanism, and technique. It has been used in enantioseparations from analytical to preparative in scale, taking advantage of various modes of diastereoisomeric interactions and using elution and displacement techniques. All the chromatographic methods involve diastereoisomeric interactions between the enantiomers of interest and a second chiral substance, the chiral selector. The difference in the interaction of the two enantiomers with the chiral selector is the enantio selectivity, $\alpha = k'_R/k'_s$; it can be thermodynamic or kinetic in nature. The choice of k'_R or k'_s as the numerator of the enantioselectivity expression is made for a ≥ 1.0. The k' (capacity factor) is defined in the customary manner in Equation (6).

$$k' = (V_R - V_o)/V_o \qquad (6)$$

It represents the number of column volumes required to elute the enantiomer. The volume of mobile phase required to elute the component V_R (the elution volume, retention volume) and the void volume, V_o, are the chromatographic measurements needed to calculate the capacity factor. The void volume is defined as the volume of mobile phase required to elute an unretained solute.

Chromatographic enantioseparations can be achieved when the diastereoisomeric interaction is established via a precolumn covalent derivatization, or a noncovalent association formed within the chromatographic system through the use of chiral mobile phase additives (primarily an LC technique) or chiral stationary phases.

PRECOLUMN DERIVATIZATION

The reaction of a homochiral derivatizing agent with a heterochiral sample to yield covalently linked diastereo-isomeric products is a precolumn technique used for the analysis of the individual enantiomers. The diastereo-isomeric products are separable under a variety of chromatographic conditions (GC and LC), including both normal and reversed-phase procedures (59–61). Fig. 23 shows the LC separation of two diastereoisomeric products formed by the reaction of a heterochiral amine and a homochiral derivatization reagent. The derivatization reaction involves the formation of an amide by treating an N-substituted S-prolyl chloride with racemic amphetamine (Fig. 24).

The configuration of the asymmetric center in the prolyl moiety is homochiral S and the racemic amphetamine (R and S) yields diastereoisomeric amides S,R and S,S. Thus, these amides have the same configurations (S) at the center

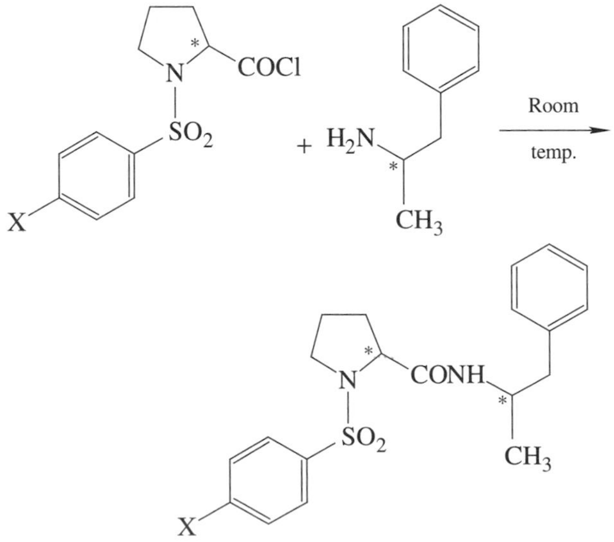

Detector Response (254 nm)

Time (minutes)

Fig. 23 Normal-phase liquid chromatographic separation of 4-nitrophenylsulfonyl-S-prolylam-phetamine. $1 = R$-amphetamine, $2 = S$-amphetamine. (Ref. 60.)

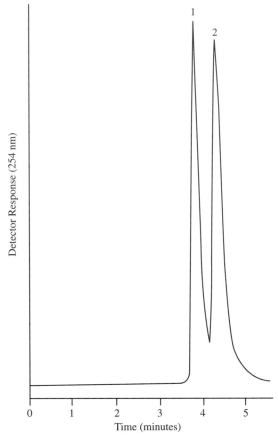

Fig. 24 Precolumn diastereomeric derivatization.

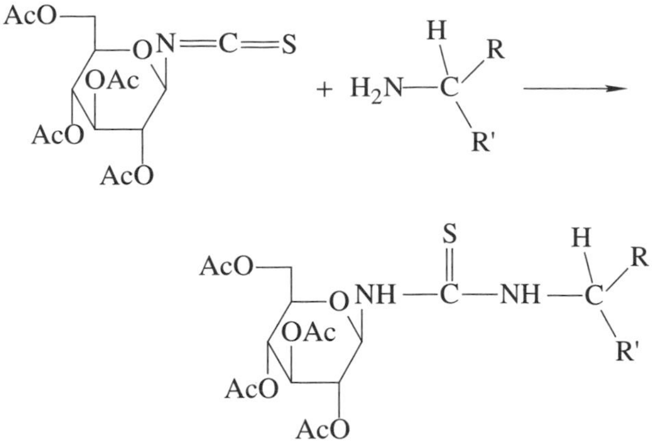

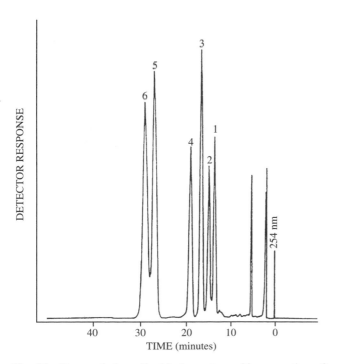

Fig. 25 GITC derivatization of a primary amine.

originating from the prolyl moiety, and differing configuration at the chiral center originating from heterochiral amphetamine. A similar derivatization procedure with *N*-trifluoroacetyl-*S*-prolyl chloride is used in GC to form diastereoisomeric amides. The *N*-TFA moiety imparts volatility and electron capture detectability to the derivatives for GC analysis (62).

The homochiral derivatization reagents are usually modified compounds that are available in high enantiomeric purity. Cost and availability make naturally occurring substances such as amino acids excellent sources of enantiomeric purity. A reagent widely used in the diastereoisomeric derivatization of amines is 2,3,4,6-tetra-*O*-acetyl-13-D-glucosyl isothiocyanate (GITC) (Fig. 25). The isothiocyanate moiety reacts with primary and secondary amines yielding thiourea products, thus covalently linking the homochiral acetylated glucose and the amine (63). If the amine is racemic, the products are a diastereoisomeric pair. The configurations of all the chiral centers in glucose remain the same and the two configurations in the amine yield diastereoisomeric products (60). Fig. 26 shows the reversed-phase LC separation of diastereoisomeric ureas following derivatization of a racemic amine sample with GITC.

Mobile-Phase Additives

The direct separation of enantiomers by chromatography can be achieved by two fundamentally different processes: The diastereoisomeric interaction can occur between the sample molecules and the stationary phase or between the sample and chiral mobile-phase additives. Consequently, two different results can be obtained: A chiral stationary phase with an achiral mobile phase or an achiral stationary phase with a chiral mobile phase. The use of chiral mobile-phase additives is limited to LC procedures. The most widely applied examples include ligand exchange, ion-pair and inclusion complexation.

The exact sequence of events in the case of chiral mobile-phase additives varies, depending on the affinity of the additive for the achiral stationary phase. The chiral additive may associate with the stationary phase to become a dynamic chiral stationary phase, or the additive and sample molecules may form a diastereoisomeric complex in the mobile phase which associates that the achiral stationary phase.

Cyclodextrins

The cyclodextrins are perhaps the most widely used mobile-phase additives which form diastereoisomeric inclusion complexes. The cyclodextrins (α, β, and γ-cyclodextrins) are made up of α-D-glucose units (6, 7, or 8 α-D-glucose molecules) cyclized to form a truncated cone-like molecule (Fig. 27). The interior cavity of this molecule contains hydrogens and glycoside oxygens and is relatively lipophilic, whereas the exterior of the cyclodextrin molecule is composed primarily of hydroxyl groups and therefore is relatively hydrophilic. The wider end of the cone is composed of secondary hydroxyl groups and the narrow (truncated) end is composed of the primary

Fig. 26 Reversed-phase liquid chromatographic separation of GITC-derivatized amines. 1 = *R,R*-pseudoephedrine, 2 = *S,S*-pseudoephedrine, 3-*R,S*-ephedrine, 4 = *S*, *R*-ephedrine, 5 = *S*-methamphetamine, 6 = *R*-methamphetamine. (From Ref. 61.)

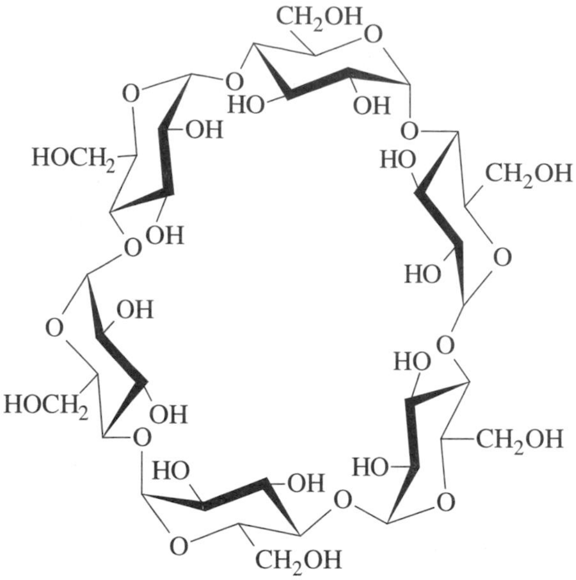

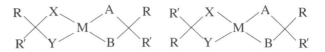

Fig. 28 Diastereoisomeric chelates.

It involves the formation of a dissociable diastereoisomeric complex between a homochiral additive and a heterochiral solute about a central metal ion (Fig. 28). The mobile phase contains both the homochiral ligand and the metal ion as additive components. These species probably exist as the fully complexed species with at least two molecules of the homochiral additive complexed to the metal ion. The ligand exchange with the components of the heterochiral sample enantiomers yields diastereoisomeric products. Obviously the concentration of the homochiral additive ligand is relatively high compared to the heterochiral sample molecule. Thus, the probability of displacing two molecules of homochiral ligands from the metal ion is extremely small, limiting the number of possible products to just two, as seen in Equation (6).

$$(HoL)_n \cdots M + HeL \longrightarrow (HoL)_{n-1} \cdots M \cdots HeL + HoL \quad (7)$$

where HoL, is the homochiral ligand,; HeL, is the heterochiral ligand, and; M, is the metal.

Ligand exchange has found extensive use in the resolution of amino acids, amino acid derivatives, and other bidentate ligands (68, 69). These separations are done using an aqueous or organic modified aqueous mobile phase in which the metal ion, such as copper(II) from copper sulfate, is soluble. The stationary phase is usually a hydrocarbon such as C_8. Some of the widely used homochiral ligands such as L-proline and L-hydroxyproline (70) are N-alkylated with large hydrocarbon moieties such as C_8 to enhance the dynamic chiral stationary-phase process. The hydrocarbon moieties of the ligand and the stationary phase associate in the usual solvophobic process, leaving the chelating functional groups exposed to the mobile phase and its components.

The mobile-phase-additive ligand-exchange chromatography has been applied to the resolution of some chiral amino alcohols. The enantiomers of norephedrine, norpseudo−ephedrine, metaraminol, and phenylephrine were resolved (70) in a reversed-phase procedure using a $0.05\,M$ acetate buffer mobile phase containing N-octylhydroxyproline and $5-8\,\mathrm{m}M$ copper(II). All these enantioseparations show base-line resolution

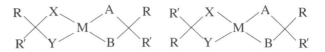

Fig. 27 Structure of α-cyclodextrin.

hydroxyl groups from the individual D-glucose units. Thus, complexation reactions occur only from the secondary OH side. The dimensions of the cavity in the cyclodextrin depend upon the number of glucose units in the compound.

The cyclodextrin-solute inclusion complexation is a reversible reaction with an equilibrium constant similar to that for diffusion-controlled processes. Thus, the effect of underivatized cyclodextrins as mobile-phase additives is often a reduction in column efficiencies. The increase in peak width in cyclodextrin systems compared to that of conventional reversed-phase systems requires a decrease in flow rates for best resolution. Some enantioseparations using this technique report flow rates between 20 and 40 µl/min (64). Considerable column efficiency changes occur over a flow range of 0.02–2.0 ml/min. In addition to flow rate, the concentration of cyclodextrin in the mobile phase can be adjusted to optimize enantioseparations.

The pH, temperature, and ionic strength of the mobile phase also affect the cyclodextrin-solute complexation and retention properties. Many enantio-separations using cyclodextrin-modified systems involve solutes with an aromatic ring substituent or similar cyclic structure at the chiral center. A variety of chiral barbiturates, hydantoins, and related compounds (65–67) have been resolved by using β-cyclodextrin and alkylated B-cyclodextrin-modified systems.

Ligand Exchange

The ligand-exchange process has been applied as a mobile-phase-additive technique for enantioseparations.

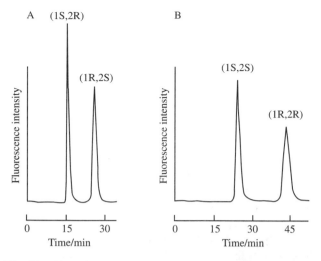

Fig. 29 Ligand-exchange liquid chromatographic separation of norephedrine (A) and norpseudoephedrine (B), using a C_{18} stationary phase coated with N-n-dodecyl-L -hydroxyproline and a mobile phase containing 5 mM copper(II). (From Ref. 72.)

with norpseudoephedrine (Fig. 29), yielding an enantioselectivity in the 2.0 range ($\alpha = 2.0$) and the $1S$, $2S$-isomer eluting before the $1R$, $2R$-enantiomer.

Diastereoisomeric Ion Pairs

The addition of a homochiral counterion to the mobile phase for the LC resolution of enantiomers can yield enantioseparations with only slight differences in the properties of the resulting diastereoisomeric ion pairs. Derivatives of L-proline and 10-camphorsulfonic acid have been used to resolve enantiomeric amines through the formation of diastereoisomeric ion pairs (71). The concept of reciprocity in these separations (72) has been shown to occur in such a way that if the R enantiomer of acid HA resolves base B into its R- and S-enantiomers, an enantiomer of B (for example, R-B) can be used to resolve R-HA and S-HA.

Chiral Stationary Phases

The use of chiral stationary phases (CSP) in liquid chromatography continues to grow at an impressive rate. These CSPs contain natural materials such as cellulose and starch as well as totally synthetic materials, utilizing enantioselective and retentive mechanisms ranging from inclusion complexation to π-electron interactions. The major structural features found in chiral stationary phases include cellulose, starch, cyclodextrins, synthetic polymers, proteins, crown ethers, metal complexes, and aromatic w-electron systems.

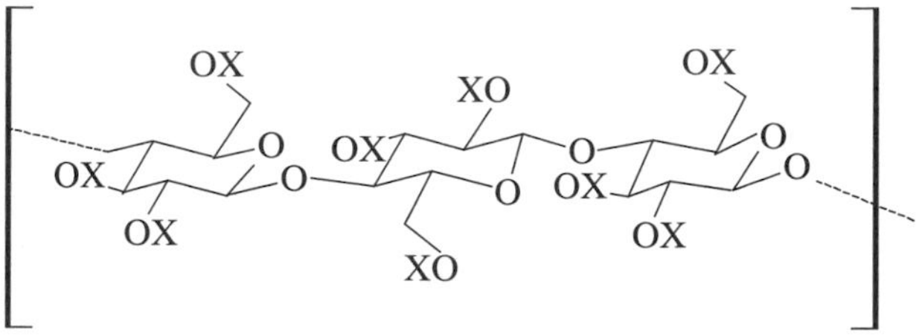

Fig. 30 Cellulose (XH) and derivatives.

Cellulose and Starch

Cellulose and starch are naturally occurring polysaccharides exhibiting enantioselective properties. Cellulose is a linear polymer of D-glucose units with individual fibers arranged in parallel bundles through hydrogen bonding between the fibers (Fig. 30). Starch is a similar material, containing a higher degree of branching with enantioselectivities similar to those of cellulose. The mechanism of retention and enantioselectivity for cellulose involves hydrogen bonding and possibly the formation of inclusion complexes within the cellulose structure. The chromatographic procedures used for these materials involve normal-phase conditions (nonpolar solvents), which allow for strong hydrogen-bond formation between the solute and CSP. A variety of stationary phases of varying enantioselective and retention properties have been prepared by chemical modification of the hydroxyl groups by esters, nitrates, carbamates, and ethers. Because of their excellent chiral recognition properties, these materials have been used to resolve a large number of pharmaceutically significant compounds (73).

Synthetic Polymers

Synthetic polymers can be prepared to contain chirality as is the case for cellulose and other natural polymers. Chirality can be introduced into the monomer before polymerization to yield the chiral polymer. Alternatively polymerization of an achiral monomer in the presence of some chiral catalyst yields the chiral polymer. Polymethacrylates exhibiting chirality due to single-handed helicity have been prepared via polymerization in the

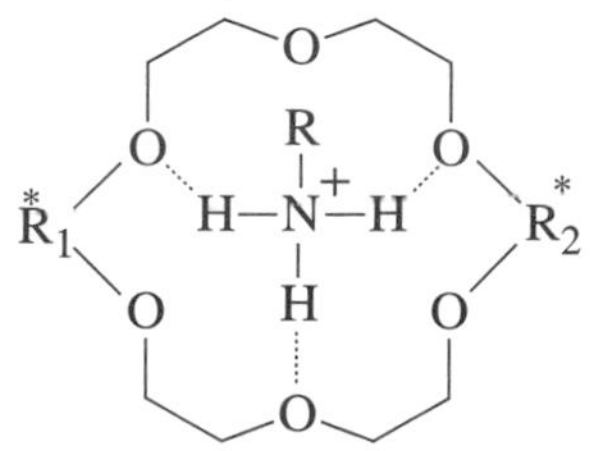

Fig. 31 Crown ether complexes.

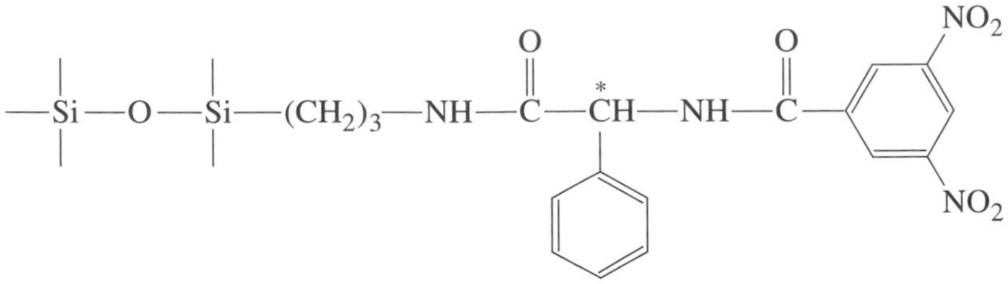

Fig. 32   3,5-Dinitrobenzoylphenylglycine (DNBPE) stationary phase.

presence of a chiral catalyst. These materials are used in liquid chromatography primarily under low-pressure conditions and have shown good resolution for compounds capable of hydrogen-bond formation.

Proteins

Proteins are naturally occurring chiral polymers that interact selectively with chiral solutes. The proteins most widely used as chiral selectors in liquid chromatography are albumin and α_1-acid glycoprotein. These proteins are covalently linked to silica particles and are used primarily in the reversed-phase mode of separation.

Bovine serum albumin has a molecular weight of about 6.6×10^4 and consists of 581 amino acids. The tertiary structure of the protein is controlled by the 17 disulfide linkages, and at pH 7.0 the net charge on the protein is -18. The human plasma protein, α_1-acid glycoprotein, contains five carbohydrate units and has a molecular weight of 4.1×10^4. The 14 sialic acid residues in the sugar units are involved in binding various cationic species and are believed to play a role in the chiral selectivity of this protein.

The mechanism of solute retention and chiral recognition is similar for both albumin and α_1-acid glycoprotein and involves charge and dipolar interactions in addition to hydrophobic associations. The mobile-phase variables that can be adjusted to affect retention and chiral recognition include pH, ionic strength, and organic modifier (74). Such changes affect the properties of the solute as well as the stationary-phase protein. Thus, pH changes can alter the retention of a neutral solute by changing the properties of the binding site on the CSP.

Crown Ethers

These macrocyclic ethers assume a crown-like shape in solution with a central cavity capable of containing a small solute. They bind to small cationic species through association with the electron-rich oxygens of the ether linkage. Chiral crown ethers (Fig. 31) serve as selectors for enantiomeric amines in the protonated state (75). They have been used as mobile-phase additives and been covalently linked to the surface of silica particles. The chromatographic procedure for these materials is primarily the reversed-phase mode, and many separations are done in a purely aqueous mobile phase modified to pH $1-2.0$ with perchloric acid.

Chiral recognition in these phases is achieved when a chiral center is introduced into the crown ether to serve as a barrier to one enantiomer of the guest amine. The chiral barrier is usually a large bulky group that selectively affects the association of one enantiomer of the amine.

Aromatic π-electron Systems

These CSPs have in common a strong aromatic $\pi-\pi$ interaction, dipolar stacking process as a central component of the retention process. They are often referred to as Pirkle columns based on the pioneering work by Pirkle and coworkers (76, 77). These π-donor and π-acceptor interactions occur though the tendency of some electron-rich aromatic systems to donate π-electrons (π-base) to an electron-deficient acceptor aromatic system (π-acid). These CSPs offer the clear advantage of complete structural characterization of the stationary phase. Since these are totally synthetic phases prepared by linking small chiral substances to silica particles, all the solute-stationary phase interactions can be readily predicted. The solute-CSP interactions include hydrogen bonds, steric, dipole–dipole, and conformational as well as $\pi-\pi$ interactions. These phases generally consist of an acylated amino acid covalently linked to aminopropyl silica (Fig. 32). The acyl group is usually an aromatic acid, with the π acceptor 3,5-dinitrobenzoyl group among the most common. Phenylglycine and leucine provide chirality of general utility for the resolution of many chiral substances.

The major advantage of these phases is the ability to manipulate structure and the reciprocity of chiral recognition. The reciprocity approach is not readily available for the naturally occurring polymeric CSPs such as cellulose, proteins, and others. Those solutes not containing the complementary π-acid or π-base functionality can often be derivatized to incorporate these features into the molecules of interest.

REFERENCES

1. Williams, K.M. Molecular Asymmetry and its Pharmacological Consequences. Adv. Pharmacol. **1991**, *22*, 57–135.
2. Lehmann, P.A. Stereoisomerism and Drug Action. Trends Pharmacol. Sci. **1986**, *7* (7), 281–285.
3. Ariens, E.J. Implications of the Neglect of Stereochemistry in Pharmacokinetics and Clinical Pharmacology. Drug lntell. Clin. Phar. **1987**, *21*, 827–829.
4. Jamali, F.; Mehvar, R.; Pasutto, F.M. Enantioselective Aspects of Drug Action and Disposition: Therapeutic Pitfalls. J. Pharm. Sci. **1989**, *78* (9), 695–715.
5. Smith, D.F. *Handbook of Stereoisomers: Therapeutic Drugs*; CRC Press, Inc.: Boca Raton, FL, 1989; 405.
6. Wainer, I.W.; Drayer, D.E. *Drug Stereochemistry: Analytical Methods and Pharmacology*; Marcel Dekker, Inc.: New York, 1988; 276.
7. Hyneck, M.; Dent, J.; Hook, J. Chirality: Pharmacological Action and Drug Development. *Chirality in Drug Design and Synthesis*; Brown, C., Ed.; Academic Press: San Diego, 1990; 1–28.
8. Panus, P.C.; Campbell, J.; Kulkarni, S.B.; Herrick, R.T.; Ravis, W.R.; Banga, A.K. Transdermal Iontophoretic Delivery of Ketoprofen Through Human Cadaver Skin and in Humans. J. Control. Rel. **1997**, *44* (2), 113–121.
9. Wade, D.N.; Mearrick, P.T.; Morris, J.L. Active Transport of L-DOPA in the Intestine. Nature (London) **1973**, *242* (5398), 463–465.
10. Tamai, I.; Ling, H.Y.; Timbul, S.M.; Nishikido, J.; Tsuji, A. Stereospecific Absorption and Degradation of Cephalexin. J Pharm. Pharmacol. **1988**, *40* (5), 320–324.
11. Brown, N.A.; Jahnshen, E.; Muller, W.E.; Wollert, U. Optical Studies on the Mechanism of the Interaction of the Enantiomers of the Antiocagulant Drugs Phenprocoumon and Warfarin with Human Serum Albumin. Mol. Pharmacol. **1977**, *13* (1), 70–79.
12. Walle, U.K.; Walle, T.; Bai, S.A.; Olanoff, L.S. Stereoselective Binding of Propranolol to Human Plasma, Alpha 1-acid Glycoprotein and Albumin. Clin. Pharmacol Ther. **1983**, *34* (6), 718–723.
13. Takahashi, H.; Ogata, H.; Shimizu, M.; Hashimoto, K.; Mashuhara, K.; Kashiwada, K.; Someya, K. Comparative Pharmacokinetics of Unbound Disopyramide Enantiomers Following Oral Administration of Racemic Disopyramide in Humans. J. Pharm. Sci. **1991**, *80* (7), 709–711.
14. Giacomini, K.M.; Nelson, W.L.; Pershe, R.A.; Valdevieso, L.; Turner-Tamayasu, K.; Blaschke, T.F. In Vivo Interaction of the Enantiomers of Disopyramide in Human Subjects. J. Pharmacokinet. Biopharm. **1986**, *14* (4), 335–355.
15. Day, R.O.; Williams, K.M.; Graham, G.G.; Lee, E.J.; Knihinicki, R.D.; Champion, G.D. Stereoselective Disposition of Ibuprofen Enantiomers in Synovial Fluid. Clin. Pharmacol. Ther. **1988**, *43* (5), 480–487.
16. Williams, K.; Day, R.; Knihinicki, R.; Duffield, A. The Stereoselective Uptake of Ibuprofen Enantiomers into Adipose Tissue. Biochem. Pharmacol. **1986**, *35* (19), 3403–3405.
17. Lewis, R.J.; Trager, W.F. Warfarin Metabolism in Man, Identification of Metabolites in Urine. J. Clin. Invest. **1970**, *49* (5), 907–913.
18. Toon, S.; Low, L.K.; Gibaldi, M.; Trager, W.F.; O'Reilly, R.A.; Motley, C.H.; Goulart, D.A. The Warfarin–Sulfinpyrazone Interaction, Stereochemical Considerations. Clin. Pharmacol. Ther. **1986**, *39* (1), 15–24.
19. Sisenwine, S.F.; Tio, C.O.; Hadley, F.V.; Liu, A.L.; Kimmel, H.B.; Ruelius, H.W. Species-Related Differences in the Stereoselective Glucuronidation of Oxazepam. Drug Metab. Disp. **1982**, *10* (6), 605–608.
20. Wedlund, P.J.; Aslanian, W.S.; Jacqz, E.; McAllister, C.B.; Branch, R.A.; Wilkinson, G.R. Phenotypic Differences in Mephenytoin Pharmacokinetics in Normal Subjects. J. Pharmacol. Exptl. Ther. **1985**, *234* (3), 662–669.
21. Godbillon, J.; Richard, J.; Gerardin, A.; Meinertz, T.; Kasper, W.; Jahnchen, E. Pharmacokinetics of the Enantiomers of Acenocoumarol in Man. Br. J. Clin. Pharmacol. **1981**, *12* (5), 621–629.
22. Gill, T.S.; Hopkins, K.J.; Bottomley, J.; Gupta, S.K.; Rowland, M. Cimetidine –Nicoumalone Interaction in Man, Stereochemical Considerations. Br. J. Clin. Pharmacol. **1989**, *27* (4), 469–474.
23. Chandler, M.H.; Scott, S.R.; Blouin, R.A. Age-Associated Stereoselective Alterations in Hexobarbital Metabolism. Clin. Pharmacol. Ther. **1988**, *43* (4), 436–441.
24. Hutt, A.J.; Caldwell, J. The Metabolic Chiral Inversion of 2-arylpropionic Acids–A Novel Route Wlth Pharmacological Consequences. J Pharm Pharmacol **1983**, *35* (11), 693–704.
25. Caldwell, J.; Winter, S.M.; Hutt, A.J. The Pharmacological and Toxicological Significance of the Stereochemistry of Drug Disposition. Xenobiotica **1988**, *18* (Suppl 1), 59–70.
26. Lee, E.J.; Williams, K.; Day, R.; Graham, G.; Champion, D. Stereoselective Disposition of Ibuprofen Enantiomers in Man. Br. J. Clin. Pharmacol. **1985**, *19* (5), 669–674.
27. Rubin, A.; Knadler, M.P.; Ho, P.P.; Bechtol, L.D.; Wolen, R.L. Stereoselective Inversion of (*R*)-fenoprofen to (*S*)-fenoprofen in Humans. J. Pharm. Sci. **1985**, *74* (1), 82–84.
28. Bopp, R.J.; Nash, J.F.; Ridolfo, A.S.; Shepard, E.R. Stereoselective Inversion of (*R*)-(−)-benoxaprofen to the (*S*)-(+)-enantiomer in Humans. Drug Metab. Disp. **1979**, *7* (6), 356–359.
29. Simmonds, R.G.; Woodage, T.J.; Duff, S.M.; Green, J.N. Stereospecific Inversion of (*R*)-(−)-benoxaprofen in Rat and Man. Eur. J. Drug Metab. Pharmacokinetics **1980**, *5* (3), 169–172.
30. Singh, N.N.; Jamali, F.; Pasutto, F.M.; Russell, A.S.; Coutts, R.T.; Drader, K.S. Pharmacokinetics of the Enantiomers of Tiaprofenic Acid in Humans. J. Pharm. Sci. **1986**, *75* (5), 439–442.
31. Foster, R.T.; Jamali, F.; Russell, A.S.; Alballa, S.R. Pharmacokinetics of Ketoprofen Enantiomers in Young and Elderly Arthritic Patients Following Single and Multiple Doses. J. Pharm. Sci. **1988**, *77* (3), 191–195.
32. Tamassia, V.; Jannuzzo, M.G.; Moro, E.; Stegnjaich, S.; Groppi, W.; Nicolis, F.B. Pharmacokinetics of the

Enantiomers of Indoprofen in Man. Int. J. Clin. Pharmacol. Res. **1984**, *4* (3), 223–230.

33. Stoltenborg, J.K.; Puglisi, C.V.; Rubio, F.; Vane, F.M. High-Performance Liquid Chromatographic Determination of Stereoselective Disposition of Carprofen in Humans. J. Pharm. Sci. **1981**, *70* (11), 1207–1212.

34. Von Bahr, C.; Hermansson, J.; Tawara, K. Plasma Levels of (+) and (−)-propranolol and 4-hydroxypropranolol after Administration of Racemic (+/−)-propranolol in Man. Br. J. of Cli. Pharmacol. **1982**, *14* (1), 79–82.

35. Tucker, G.T.; Mather, L.E.; Lennard, M.S.; Gregory, A. Plasma Concentrations of the Stereoisomers of Prilocaine after Administration of the Racemate, Implications for Toxicity? Br. J. Anaesthesia. **1990**, *65* (3), 333–336.

36. Echizen, H.; Brecht, T.; Niedergesass, S.; Vogelgesang, B.; Eichelbaum, M. The Effect of Dextro-, Levo-, and Racemic Verapamil on Atrioventricular Conduction in Humans. Amer. Heart J. **1985**, *109* (2), 210–217.

37. Echizen, H.; Vogelgesang, B.; Eichelbaum, M. Effects of D,L-verapamil on Atrioventricular Conduction in Relation to its Stereoselective First-Pass Metabolism. Clin. Pharmacol. Ther. **1985**, *38* (1), 71–76.

38. Lennard, M.S.; Tucker, G.T.; Silas, J.H.; Freestone, S.; Ramsay, L.E.; Woods, H.F. Differential Stereoselective Metabolism of Metoprolol in Extensive and Poor Debrisoquin Metabolizers. Clin. Pharmacol. Ther. **1983**, *34* (6), 732–777.

39. Borgstrom, L.; Nyberg, L.; Jonsson, S.; Lindberg, C.; Paulson, J. Pharmacokinetic Evaluation in Man of Terbutaline given as Separate Enantiomers and as the Racemate. Br. J. Clin. Pharmacol. **1989**, *27* (1), 49–56.

40. Lima, J.J.; Boudoulas, H.; Shields, B.J. Stereoselective Pharmacokinetics of Disopyramide Enantiomers in Man. Drug Metab. Disp. **1985**, *13* (5), 572–577.

41. Hsyu, P.H.; Giacomini, K.M. Stereoselective Renal Clearance of Pindolol in Humans. J. Clin. Invest. **1985**, *76* (5), 1720–1726.

42. Raschack, M. Relationship of Antiarrhythmic to Inotropic Activity and Antiarrhythmic Qualities of the Optical Isomers of Verapamil. Arch. Pharmacol. **1976**, *294* (3), 285–291.

43. Giacomini, K.M.; Cox, B.M.; Blaschke, T.F. Comparative Anticholinergic Potencies of *R*- and *S*- Disopyramide in Longitudinal Muscle Strips from Guinea Pig Ileum. Life Sci. **1980**, *27* (13), 1191–1197.

44. Wise, R.; Wills, P.J.; Bedford, K.A. Epimers of Moxalactam, In Vitro Comparison of Activity and Stability. Antimicrob. Agts. Chemother. **1981**, *20* (1), 30–32.

45. Levy, G.; O'Reilly, R.A.; Wingard, L.B., Jr. Comparative Pharmacokinetics of Coumarin Anticoagulants. XXXV. Examination of Possible Pharmacokinetic Interaction between (*R*)-(+)- and (*S*)-(−)-Warfarin in Humans. J. Pharm. Sci. **1978**, *67* (6), 867–868.

46. Tucker, G.T.; Lennard, M.S. Enantiomer Specific Pharmacokinetics. Pharmacol. Ther. **1990**, *45* (3), 309–329.

47. Ravis, W.R. Pharmacokinetics and Pharmacodynamics. *Stereoisomerism in Pharmaceuticals*; Riley, T.N., Ed.; Technomics Publishing Company: Lancaster, PA, 1991.

48. Ravis, W.R.; Owen, J.S. Stereochemical Considerations in Bioavailability Studies. *Generics and Bioequivalence*; Jackson, A.J., Ed.; CRC Press: Ann Arbor, MI, 1994; 113–137.

49. Mehvar, R.; Jamali, F. Bioequivalence of Chiral Drugs. Stereospecific Versus Non-Stereospecific Methods. Clin. Pharmacokin. **1997**, *33* (2), 122–141.

50. Thomson, A.H.; Murdoch, G.; Pottage, A.; Kelman, A.W.; Whiting, B.; Hillis, W.S. The Pharmacokinetics of *R*- and *S*-tocainide in Patients with Acute Ventricular Arrhythmias. Br. J. Clin. Pharmacol. **1986**, *21* (2), 149–154.

51. Sedman, A.J.; Gal, J.; Mastropaolo, W.; Johnson, P.; Maloney, J.D.; Moyer, T.P. Serum Tocainide Enantiomer Concentrations in Human Subjects. Br. J. Clin. Pharmacol. **1984**, *17* (1), 113–115.

52. Block, A.J.; Merrill, D.; Smith, E.R. Stereoselectivity of Tocainide Pharmacodynamics In Vivo and In Vitro. J. Cardiovasc. Pharmacol **1988**, *11* (2), 216–221.

53. Li, G.; Treiber, G.; Maier, K.; Walker, S.; Klotz, U. Disposition of Ibuprofen in Patients with Liver Cirrhosis. Stereochemical Considerations. Clin. Pharmacokin. **1993**, *25* (2), 154–163.

54. Testa, B.; Mayer, J.M. Stereoselective Drug Metabolism and its Significance in Drug Research. Prog. Drug Res. **1988**, *32*, 249–303.

55. Wedlund, P.J.; Aslanian, W.S.; Jacqz, E.; McAllister, C.B.; Branch, R.A.; Wilkinson, G.R. Phenotypic Differences in Mephenytoin Pharmacokinetics in Normal Subjects. J. Pharmacol. Exptl. Ther. **1985**, *234* (3), 662–669.

56. O'Reilly, R.A.; Trager, W.F.; Motley, C.H.; Howald, W. Stereoselective Interaction of Phenylbutazone with [12c/13c]Warfarin Pseudoracemates in Man. J. Clin. Invest. **1980**, *65* (3), 746–753.

57. Williams, K.M. Kinetics of Misonidazole Enantiomers. Clin. Pharmacol. Ther. **1984**, *36* (6), 817–823.

58. Lee, E.J.; Williams, K.; Day, R.; Graham, G.; Champion, D. Stereoselective Disposition of Ibuprofen Enantiomers in Man. Br. J. Clin. Pharmacol. **1985**, *19* (5), 669–674.

59. Barksdale, J.M.; Clark, C.R. Liquid Chromatographic Determination of the Enantiomeric Composition of Amphetamine and Related Drugs by Diastereomeric Derivatization. J. Chromatogr. Sci. **1985**, *23* (4), 176–180.

60. Noggle, F.T., Jr.; DeRuiter, J.; Clark, C.R. Liquid Chromatographic Determination of the Enantiomeric Composition of Methamphetamine Prepared from Ephedrine and Pseudoephedrine. Anal. Chem. **1986**, *58* (8), 1643–1648.

61. Barksdale, J.M.; Clark, C.R. Synthesis and Liquid Chromatographic Evaluation of Some Chiral Derivatizing Agents for Resolution of Amine Enantiomers. Anal. Chem. **1984**, *56* (6), 958–961.

62. Hengstmann, J.H.; Falkner, F.C.; Watson, J.T.; Oates, J. Quantitative Determination of Guanethidine and Other Guanido-Containing Drugs in Biological Fluids by Gas Chromatography with Flame Ionization Detection and Multiple Ion Detection. Anal. Chem. **1974**, *46* (1), 34–39.

63. Debowski, J.; Sybilska, D.; Jurcyak, J. β-Cyclodextrin as a Chiral Component of the Mobile Phase for Separation of Mandelic Acid Enantiomers in Reversed Phase Systems of High Performance Liquid Chromatography. J. Chromatogr. **1982**, *237* (3), 303–306.

64. Zukowski, J.; Sybilska, D.; Bojarski, J.; Szejtli, J. Resolution of Chiral Barbiturates into Enantiomers by Reversed-Phase High-Performance Liquid Chromatography Using Methylated Beta-Cyclodextrins. J. Chromatogr. **1988**, *463* (3), 381–390.

65. Magurie, J.H. Some Structural Requirements of Resolution of Hydantoin Enantiomers with a β-cyclodextrin Liquid Chromatographt Column. J. Chromatogr. **1987**, *387* (5), 453–457.

66. Sybilska, D.; Zukowski, J.; Bojarski, J. Resolution of Mephenytoin and Some Chiral Barbiturates into Enantiomers by Reversed Phase High Performance Liquid Chromatography via β-cyclodextrin Inclusion Complexes. J. Liq. Chromatogr. **1986**, *9* (6), 591–606.

67. Debowski, J.; Sybilska, D.; Jurcyak, J. The Resolution of Some Chiral Compounds in Reversed Phase High Performance Liquid Chromatography by Means of β-cyclodextrin Inclusion Complexes. Chromatographia **1982**, *16* (2), 198–200.

68. LePage, J.N.; Lindner, W.; Davies, G.; Seity, D.E.; Karger, B.L. Resolution of the Optical Isomers of Dansyl Amino Acids by Reversed Phase Liquid Chromatography with Optically Active Metal Chelate Additives. Anal. Chem. **1979**, *51* (3), 433–435.

69. Horikawa, R.; Sakamoto, H.; Tanimura, T. Separation of α-Hydroxy Acid Enantiomers by High Performance Liquid Chromatography Using Copper (II)-L-Amino Acid Eluent. J. Liq. Chromatogr. **1986**, *9* (4), 537–549.

70. Yainazaki, S.; Takeuchi, T.; Tanimura, T. Direct Enantiomeric Separation of Norepinephrine and its Analogues by High Performance Liquid Chromatography. J. Liq. Chromatogr. **1989**, *12* (7), 2239–2248.

71. Pettersson, C.; Schill, G. Separation of Enantiomeric Amines by Ion-Pair Chromatography. J. Chromatogr. **1981**, *204* (1), 179–183.

72. Pettersson, C.; Schill, G. Chiral Resolution of Amino-alcohols by Ion-Pair Chromatography. Chromatographia **1982**, *16* (2), 192–197.

73. Shibata, T.; Mori, K.; Okamota, Y. Polysaccharide Phases. In *Chiral Separations by HPLC*; Krstulovic, A.M., Ed.; Ellis Horwood, Ltd.: Chichester, U.K., 1989; 336–398.

74. Allenmark, S.; Bomgren, B.; Boren, H. Direct Liquid Chromatographic Separation of Enantiomers on Immobilized Protein Stationary Phases. IV. Molecular Interaction Forces and Retention Behaviour in Chromatography on Bovine Serum Albumin as a Stationary Phase. J. Chromatogr. **1984**, *316* (12), 617–624.

75. Shinbo, T.; Yamaguchi, T.; Nishimura, K.; Sugiura, M. Chromatographic Separation of Racemic Amino Acids by Use of Chiral Crown Ether-Coated Reversed-Phase Packings. J. Chromatogr. **1987**, *405* (9), 145–153.

76. Pirkle, W.H.; Sikkenga, D.L. Resolution of Optical Isomers by Liquid Chromatography. J. Chromatogr. **1976**, *123* (3), 400–406.

77. Pirkle, W.H.; Dazzsen, R. Reciprocity in Chiral Recognition: Comparison of Several Chiral Stationary Phases. J. Chromatogr. **1987**, *404* (1), 107–111.

78. March, J. *Advanced Organic Chemistry: Reactions, Mechanisms, and Structure*; Wiley-Interscience: New York, 1985; 82–140.

79. Brown, C. *Chirality in Drug Design and Synthesis*; Academic Press: San Diego, 1990; 243.

80. Wainer, I.W.; Drayer, D.E. *Drug Stereochemistry Analytical Methods and Pharmacology*; Marcel Dekker, Inc.: New York, 1988; 276.

LAMINAR AIRFLOW EQUIPMENT: APPLICATIONS AND OPERATION

Gregory F. Peters

Lab Safety Corporation, Des Plaines, Illinois

INTRODUCTION

The number and complexity of pharmaceutical manufacturing and compounding processes requiring protection from airborne contaminants has increased substantially in recent years. Because pathogenic viable and nonviable contamination may be readily introduced into a patient along with a therapeutic parenteral drug, the sterility and purity of parenterals must be controlled in the manufacture and assured in the compounding of these products. Laminar airflow (LAF) equipment is widely used as an engineering control in aseptic processing to provide a production environment free of airborne and resulting surface contamination by microorganisms, pyrogenic and drug residues, and other materials that present a risk of intravascular infection, pyrogenic response, or occlusion of the peripheral vasculature. With the growth of the small- and intermediate-size generic drug manufacturing, drug repackaging, and diverse hospital pharmacy and home health care IV admixtures, compounding industries, clean space design and management has become the direct responsibility of an increasing number of middle- and line-management personnel. As such, a working knowledge of LAF theory, aseptic processing, and clean space management is integral to the conceptualization, construction, and operation of a safe and effective clean space, and an important consideration in the selection or retention of the clean space manager and operative personnel.

CONTAMINATION CONTROL

All manufactured products are vulnerable to contamination by a myriad of aerosolized contaminants, including microorganisms, pyrogenic dust, ash, pollen, smoke, hydrocarbons, and other chemicals that are omnipresent in the environment (Fig. 1). Because of the potential dangers to the patient resulting from a parenteral product containing even minute quantities of these contaminants, exceptional measures are required to exclude them from the finished product. Careful planning is essential in preventing contamination of the environment leading to occupational exposure of personnel to hazardous substances, which are routinely manipulated in pharmacy operations. The primary objective of the aseptic process is control and elimination of viable contaminants. These contaminants are numerous and varied, normally consisting of bacteria, fungi, and viruses. Viruses are usually short-lived upon exposure to air, and require host systems to remain viable and reproduce; they are generally not of direct concern, except in excluding their vector, or transport mechanism. Aseptic processes are designed to exclude bacteria and fungi as well as their spore forms and breakdown products. Many of these contaminants are naturally airborne and occur commonly in the atmosphere. However, the contamination of greatest concern in aseptic processing is the endogenous microbiologic material generated by the operative personnel and others involved in the manipulation of parenteral products. This type of contamination is easily aerosolized and introduced into air currents by normal "shedding" of endogenous microbiota, and by mechanical means as microscopic droplets of sputum, produced by talking, laughing, or sneezing. Endogenous contamination is generated in enormous quantities on the skin[a] (1) and may be deposited on the surfaces of containers, equipment, gowns, and materials introduced into the aseptic work field during the course of manipulations.

Waterborne contaminants may also be introduced by contaminated cleaning agents or poor cleaning and sanitizing techniques. All types of gross microbiologic contamination are found on work surfaces, gloves, and compounding materials following contact with contaminated objects. Pyrogenic and nonpyrogenic dust must also be excluded from parenteral products. Even minute quantities of this material may cause acute inflammation or abscess at the injection site, and induce a life-threatening pyrogenic response. In addition, evidence of long term dangers of fiber emboli in producing pulmonary and

---

[a]The average adult human sheds 25,000–50,000 *Staphylococcus epidermidis* particles per minute; one person in five is a carrier and active producer of *Staphylococcus aureus*, the organism responsible for toxic shock syndrome, a bacteremia fatal in 50–90% of reported cases.

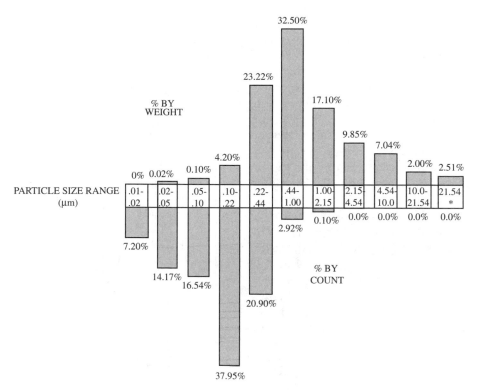

Fig. 1 Distribution by size and weight percent of particulates in normal atmospheric air. (Courtesy of American Air Filter Research, Louisville, Kentucky.)

cerebral granulomas, stenosis, and occlusion of microcirculation, as well as clouded vision, and neurological sequelae in patients receiving particulate-contaminated intravenous admixtures has emerged (2, 3). Additionally, drug product residues remaining in the aseptic processing field as a result of improper line-clearance are a threat to the patient for whom they are not intended.

History

LAF is an "offshoot technology" stemming from development of the high efficiency particulate air (HEPA) filter, spearheaded by the U.S. Army Chemical Corps, Naval Research Laboratories, and the Atomic Energy Commission in the 1940s and 1950s. Known as an absolute filter, the HEPA filter was further developed by the nuclear industry to provide fail-safe removal of extremely hazardous microscopic airborne particulates[b] at nuclear facilities. In the late 1950s, a proliferation of laminar flow clean benches (LFCBs), incorporating a HEPA filter, made it possible for the hospital pharmacy to achieve a small, but exclusive compounding environment of sterile air and sanitized, bacteriostatic worksurfaces in

[b]99.97% of particulates smaller and larger than 0.3 microns.

which to prepare small numbers of individual, patient-specific sterile products.

On a broader scale, pharmaceutical manufacturers were beginning to utilize absolute filtration as a primary engineering control in the maintenance of large, carefully controlled clean spaces in the batch production of quality-controlled parenteral products. In this application, LAF was supplied directly to production lines and extended critical worksurfaces within defined, nonturbulent entrance and exit planes as parallel or "columnated" airflow (misnamed "laminar flow").[c] This highly controlled laminar airstream was supplied to the critical worksurface, in addition to conventionally supplied turbulent airflow to the general space, provided through terminal diffusers for filtration of the balance of room air. In this manner, the "stepped" control of all critical, as well as support areas was achieved.

In the mid-1970s, increased control of manufacturing process air quality became possible with the refinement of LAF clean space design, the growing body of

[c]Laminar flow is defined as a fluid stream having discernible differentiations (laminations or layers) of velocity, pressure, temperature, or other characteristic, whereas parallel flow is uniform throughout its vertical, horizontal and longitudinal extent.

historical process quality data, the refinement of statistical process controls (SPCs), and the emergence of industry operating standards (4). In 1979, concern for the safety of pharmacy personnel compounding anti-neoplastic drugs in LFCBs was expressed, following studies that clearly identified the potential health risks to these personnel (5). The introduction and widespread use of the Class II laminar flow biological safety cabinet (BSC) by oncology/hematology pharmacy occurred in the late 1970s, and was almost universal by the end of the 1980s. Additional studies conducted in the late 1990s clearly indicated that, in spite of pharmacy-wide implementation of Class II BSC containment technology, the same potential health risks identified in 1979 continued to exist in the workplace (6). The swift, anecdotal response in some segments of the pharmacy industry was to strongly recommend immediate retrofit of the Class II design with the Class III BSC, or Barrier Isolator (sometimes referred to as a "barrier hood") in the glovebox or half-suit configuration, as an alternative to "open" Class II units used by pharmacy in a manner that had ostensibly failed to protect workers and the environment. This recommendation, however, was not based upon adequate and careful engineering failure analysis (FA) of the Class II design as implemented in pharmacy operations, by which the Practice might rationally evaluate and address the reasons for such failure. Neither, as of this writing, have any systematic, scientifically based feasibility studies, validation and monitoring protocols, or operating specifications leading to proper, corrective retrofit with the Class III or barrier isolator designs been developed as a corollary to such FA. (It should be noted that not all "barrier isolators" or "gloveboxes" are Class III BSCs.) These steps are absolutely essential in preventing a repeat failure of any type of BSC in the engineering control of hazardous substances manipulated by pharmacy personnel, and the resulting characterization of the IV pharmacy as a serious occupational risk environment.

THE HEPA FILTER

The essential element common to all LAF equipment is the HEPA filter.

Construction

The HEPA filter is normally constructed of borosilicate microfibers, formed into a flat sheet by a process similar to papermaking (Fig. 2). This sheet is pleated to increase the

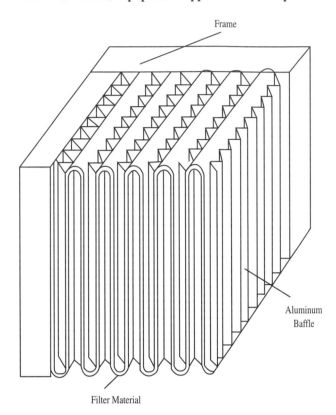

Fig. 2 HEPA filter cross-section showing pleated construction. (Courtesy of the Baker Company, Sanford, Maine.)

overall filtration surface area, in order to minimize the static pressure drop across the filter to a predetermined value[d] at a given airflow specification. The pleats are separated by serrated aluminum baffles or stitched fabric ribbons, which direct airflow through the filter. This combination of pleated sheets and baffles facilitates maximum exposure of the upstream filtration area to the airstream and is referred to as the filtration medium. It is constructed in a predetermined size, and installed into an outer frame made of fire-rated particle board, aluminum, or stainless steel. The frame-media junctions are permanently glued or "pot-sealed" to ensure a leakproof bond. The frame is fitted with a continuous, closed-cell neoprene gasket or other suitable occlusive seal to provide a gas-tight installation of the filter into the air handling system.

Filtration Efficiency

Refinement of HEPA filter manufacturing and testing technology and development of the ultra low particulate air (ULPA) filter, have led to an increase of absolute

---

[d]Normally 0.50–1.2 inches. water column (WC) or water gauge (WG).

filtration retention efficiency of greater than two orders of magnitude above 99.97%. HEPA filtration efficiencies range from a minimum of 99.97 to 99.99%, with ULPA efficiencies above 99.9999% for particulates larger and smaller than 0.3 μm in diameter (Fig. 3). (HEPA filters used in pharmaceutical and pharmacy-compounding applications rarely exceed 99.99%.) Expressed another way, the HEPA filter is capable of trapping and retaining 999,700–999,900 of every 1,000,000 particles smaller and larger than 0.3 μm in diameter.

Filtration Mechanisms

The three principal filtration mechanisms (Fig. 4) by which aerosols are collected on the HEPA filtration medium are:

- Inertial impaction, where particle inertia causes it to leave the flow streamlines and impact on the fiber;
- Interception, a screening effect dependent upon particle fiber-size relationships; and
- Diffusion, a Brownian motion diffusion of very small particles due to molecular bombardment (7).

Other filtration mechanisms, such as sedimentation and electrostatic attraction, provide some degree of aerosol collection, however most particulates are removed from the airstream by the above methods.

Shipment, Storage, and Handling

The HEPA filter is extremely fragile and should be shipped, stored, and handled in the same manner as delicate instrumentation. Personnel responsible for receiving and handling HEPA filters should receive training in proper handling technique. All incoming HEPA filters should be visually inspected for apparent damage due to

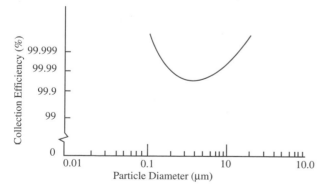

Fig. 3 Theoretical HEPA filter-collection efficiency. (Courtesy of the Baker Company, Sanford, Maine.)

mishandling, and all damage described in detail on the shipping documentation prior to acceptance.

Filtration Performance Certification

Individual HEPA filter efficiencies are established by an exacting challenge of the filter frame and medium, usually incorporating a "cold-boil," polydisperse aerosol of dioctylpthalate (DOP) or equivalent (8), which is introduced into the upstream plenum-side of the filter in a manner that ensures even distribution of the test aerosol behind the filter, at its rated airflow.

Following verification of acceptable airflow velocities, expressed by the manufacturer in linear feet per minute (LFPM) or meters per second (m/s), leakage is determined by measuring the penetration of the test aerosol through the filter as a percentage of the upstream plenum aerosol concentration, using an aerosol photometer (4) or optical particle counter (9) to carefully scan the entire filter media face and frame. Penetration of the test aerosol at or above 0.01% of the upstream concentration is considered a leak requiring repair. Leakage should be repaired only with room temperature-vulcanizing (RTV) silicone caulk, which is easily applied, and exhibits long term stability and resistance to deformation. Repairs to the filtration medium should be made in the manner specified in the literature (10). Individual repair "patches" should not exceed 1.5 in. in length or width, nor should the sum total of all repairs exceed 3% of the total area of the filter face. During operation and at all times no object, drug residue, or debris should be permitted to come into contact with the HEPA filter.

LAF AS A BARRIER TECHNIQUE

LAF has long been the primary method of controlling airborne contamination in the aseptic processing of pharmaceutical and pharmacy products. Also known as nonturbulent, or unidirectional airflow, LAF is generally defined as "HEPA-filtered air having parallel streamlines, flowing in a single pass and direction through a clean zone" (4). LAF is technically defined as fluid flow without macroscopic fluctuations, which generally occur when the Reynolds number[e] is less than 2000. Industry standards require that 80% or more of the total airflow exhibit this characteristic, in order to meet the

[e]The "Reynolds number" is the ratio of inertial to viscous forces in a pipe or duct.

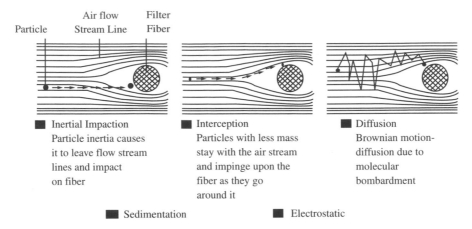

Fig. 4 Air filtration theory particle-collection mechanisms. (Courtesy of the Baker Company, Sanford, Maine.)

definition of LAF (11). LAF is necessary to maintain the most stringent air cleanliness classes[f] (4) in the production of "first air"[g] at the critical worksurface of the LFCB and BSC, and in operational cleanrooms (4,11). It is important to note that the terms "laminar airflow" and "Class 100" are not interchangeable; LAF first air incorporating properly validated HEPA filtration produces air cleanliness of approximately Class 1, nearly two orders of magnitude cleaner than Class 100. Class 100 nonlaminar airflow does not constitute first air within a critical work zone, and should not be substituted in applications requiring or designating LAF.

Conventional Airflow

Conventional airflow (also known as turbulent, or non-unidirectional airflow) incorporates HEPA filters, located in-duct, or as room terminal filtration modules (TFMs; Fig. 5). Often confused with LAF, conventional airflow does not meet that definition because it allows multiple-pass circulating characteristics or a nonparallel airflow direction, or both. This type of airflow is incapable of producing first air, and is normally used as secondary or "buffer" filtration in treating a processing or compounding space that contains laminar airflow devices (LAFDs) to maintain primary critical work surface conditions, or in treating other processing or

support areas about which a definitive air cleanliness statement must be made. Properly designed, a conventional airflow system is effective in maintaining the less-stringent air cleanliness classes[f] in operational cleanrooms (4, 11).

Advantages

When used properly by trained personnel, employing adequate process controls, the LAF environment provides a reliable barrier to measurable airborne viable and nonviable, solid particulate contamination, which may defeat the aseptic process. LFCBs, BSCs, and heating, ventilation, and air conditioning (HVAC) installations are easily validated. These systems normally continue in operation with little or no variation in output quality for long periods of time, and are easily maintained and tested.

Limitations

Any discussion of LAF equipment must include consideration of aseptic technique and the aseptic process as a whole. Often relied upon as an infallible process support, LAF is in fact a fragile, protective envelope of slow-moving, aerosol-free air[h] (4) the effect of which is easily disrupted and defeated by improper placement of processing materials, poor manufacturing and personnel practices, inadequate aseptic technique, or failure to maintain the HVAC components. Although the laminar slip stream itself is free of particulates, it does not eliminate particulates or other surface contaminants present in the aseptic field, or contamination introduced into the aseptic field on the surfaces of improperly prepared

---

[f]"... Most stringent air cleanliness classes ..." are defined as class 10–100, (F.S. 209e); Classes C, D, and E (British Standard 5295); Classes 4–5 (EN ISO); Grades A-B (EC). "...less stringent air cleanliness classes..." are defined as Class 1,000–100,000 (F.S. 209e); Classes F through K (B.S. 5295); Classes 6–8 (EN ISO); Grades C-D (EC).

[g]"First air" is uninterrupted air issuing directly from a HEPA filter in a laminar-airflow environment.

[h]Airflow velocity exiting an unobstructed workstation should be maintained at *90 LFPM average with a uniformity within ± 20%* across the entire area of the exit.

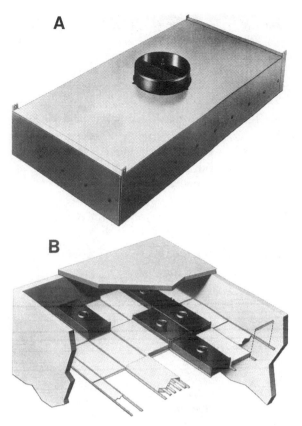

Fig. 5 (A) The self-contained terminal HEPA filtration module (TFM). (B) Arrangement of TFMs in the T-Bar ceiling in a conventional-flow application. (Courtesy of American Air Filter, Inc., Louisville, Kentucky.)

processing materials, and their manipulation and storage within the aseptic environment. Neither is LAF a substitute for proper manipulative and aseptic technique. Excessive confidence in any LAF system should not lead to the neglect of proper precleaning and staging of processing materials, personnel selection, training, and validation[i] (12); effective routine housekeeping and maintenance procedures (13); and aseptic process monitoring and auditing methods.[j] This may result in a breakdown of the process and a compromise of product integrity. In addition,

[i]1) Personnel selection and screening criteria; 2) a formalized training program to include a period of supervised manufacturing or clinical experience culminating in a recommendation for validation by the supervisor; 3) a personnel validation method, including a written exam with a required passing grade, and a practical assessment of aseptic technique, utilizing sterile microbiologic growth media in a process simulation incorporating all processing steps encountered by the candidate during the actual processing operation.

[j]Quality assurance (QA) testing and recertification of LAF systems and other engineering controls, which support the aseptic process (process auditing), irrespective of quality control, or procedures to demonstrate conformance with product specifications of identity, purity, sterility, and apyrogenicity (product auditing).

the use of improper manipulative technique in BSCs and containment systems may result in a compromise of the waste-stream, resulting in cumulative contamination of operative personnel and the environment.

Operating procedures

Although the design of each type of LAFD dictates certain specific operating procedures, several general principles apply to all LAFDs (9).

Cleaning and preparation: *LFCB*: The LFCB should be allowed to run for at least 30 min before the commencement of aseptic operations. All work-zone accessible surfaces, with the exception of the filter-protective screen, should be cleaned and sanitized by application and recovery of a low-residuing, water-base disinfectant cleanser (household bleach or other hypochlorite solutions should not be used at any time on stainless steel surfaces), followed by application of 70% ethyl or isopropyl alcohol sprayed evenly length-wise across the work surface from the back of the cabinet to the front, and allowed to dry (14). (The combination of a water-base disinfectant cleanser with alcohol provides both the broadest antimicrobial action and widest range of surfactant and solubility factors for recovery of surface residues during the cleaning process.)

BSC: The BSC should operate continuously to ensure containment of hazardous substances. All work-zone interior surfaces with the exception of the HEPA filter-protective screen should be cleaned and sanitized in the manner of the LFCB in the proper order to ensure protection of operator's garb from contaminants and cleaning residues during the cleaning process. This will also prevent transfer of drug residues to the general environment (14).

Staging

After drying of the work surface, operations in the LAFD should begin with staging of all working materials for introduction into the aseptic work area (14). This should include:

- assembly of required working materials: drug components, syringes and sterile fluid pathways, diluents, dispensing and venting devices, wipes, final containers, etc.
- preparation, in a Class 100,000 environment (4), of all working materials to go into the aseptic field by sanitizing with 70% ethyl or isopropyl alcohol spray, wiping all containers, careful removal of gross contamination and filth from any container that does not have an outer wrapper, removal of inner containers from their outer wrappers, and placement of all materials on a sanitized, stainless steel surface. This is preferably a cart or tray at a close proximity to the LAFD for direct loading of materials into the aseptic work zone.

Materials such as paper, labels, writing implements, etc., should not be placed into the work zone.

Aseptic manipulation

Prior to introduction of the working materials into the LAFD, the gloved hands of the operator should be thoroughly washed and rinsed to remove dry lubricants, sanitized by spraying with 70% alcohol, and allowed to dry in the laminar airstream. The working materials may then be transferred to the work zone, and aseptic manipulations begun. The operator's hands should be slowly inserted into, and removed from the laminar airstream, in order to minimize backwash and cross-stream contamination of the work zone. Working materials should be arranged in such a way that work progresses laterally, from right to left or left to right, so that non-interrupted first air is continuously supplied to the critical surfaces of all working materials at all times. If the operator must leave the work zone area, his or her gloved hands should be resanitized with 70% ethyl or isopropyl alcohol prior to reentering the work zone. This practice takes little time and minimizes contamination of the work zone by endogenous and residual environmental flora. An alcohol-spray bottle or other suitable dispenser should be provided close to the work zone entrance for this purpose, with the alcohol filtered and the dispenser sanitized each time the dispenser is refilled. Good aseptic technique is essential to retain the sterility of compounded products, and properly fitting surgeon's gloves, mask, laboratory coat (or arm barrier), and hair cover are recommended for all pharmacy operators working in the LAFD[a] (1, 14).

LFCB

The oldest and most basic LAFD is the LFCB, universally referred to as a "hood"—an enclosed work area with its own HEPA-filtered air supply (Fig. 6). It provides only product protection by capturing room air, passing it through a HEPA filter, and directing the filtered air horizontally or vertically uniformly across the work surface toward the operator at a constant speed.

Limitations

The LFCB should not be used in operations requiring manipulation of cytotoxic, radioactive, microbiologic, or other hazardous materials, which may become aerosolized and aspirated by the operator. Reconstitution and manipulation of antineoplastics and vesicants, mass reconstitution of antibiotics, antivirals, vaccine formulation, and similar manipulations should be done in a laminar flow BSC.

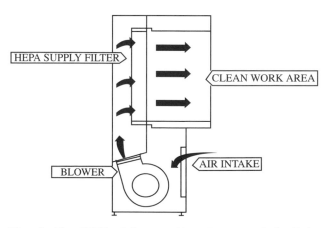

Fig. 6 The LFCB airflow profile. (Courtesy of the Baker Company, Sanford, Maine.)

Placement of materials in the work zone

Working materials placed into the LFCB should be positioned a minimum of three object-diameters in from the open end of the unit when the object is exposed to the laminar airstream on all sides, and a minimum of six diameters in from the open end when working at either end of the unit or when the object is exposed to the laminar airstream on only one side (14). This general method counteracts backwash contamination, which may compromise the aseptic field. The introduction of any large object (automated, high speed compounding devices, water baths, carboys, etc.), obstruction, or complicated process into the laminar airstream may likewise induce backwash contamination, and should be validated to maintain cohesion of the airstream and exclude both backwash and cross-stream contamination during the process. This may be accomplished by the use of visual tracers, such as smoke sticks or other smoke-producing devices, to introduce quantities of smoke both upstream of the critical worksurface and at the open end of the unit during a process validation or qualification run for visual observation of airstream behavior. Work should take place not less than 6 in. in from the open end of the work surface. Although engineering improvements in the laminar airstream recovery have been made, the laminar airstream is slow-moving,[k] and care should be exercised in the location, operation, and maintenance of this unit.

Location and performance testing

The LFCB should be located in an area free of ventilation or other air currents, steady or intermittent, which might hamper the laminar airstream by backwash effect.[l] Performance testing of the LFCB by a qualified inspector is recommended at least every 6 months, and servicing or replacement of the unit prefilters every 60 days or less.

Applications

The LFCB is used in hospital, clinical, and home health care pharmacies to provide a sterile field in which to conduct aseptic manipulations in the compounding of large-volume parenterals (LVPs) in the form of IV admixtures, hyperalimentation, and small-volume parenterals (SVPs) in the form of piggybacks, syringes, or other parenteral products of less than 250 ml, and for general sterile manipulation of nonhazardous materials.

---

[k]Normally *90 LFPM* ±20% or as specified by the user.
[l]"Backwash contamination" is the general term given to the reflux entry of unfiltered room air into the LAFD work zone.

In industry, the LFCB is used to conduct small batch sterile filling operations, in the general manipulation and isolation of nonhazardous materials, and in quality assurance/quality control (QA/QC) sterility testing.

Laminar Flow BSC

Pharmaceutical and clinical research in the past four decades has led to the development of drug products and other hazardous substances, the manufacture, handling, and compounding of which are considered hazardous to operative personnel in both the short and the long term (15). In addition to protection of the purity and sterility of the product, it is necessary to consider protection of personnel and the environment. The need to protect both the product and personnel has resulted in the adaptation and use of a variety of laminar flow BSCs in the manufacture and compounding of numerous biological, radioactive, cytotoxic, allergenic, and antibiotic drug products. It is necessary that proper containment and barrier techniques be followed in the preparation, operation, and cleanup of any BSC. Although both are considered to be LAFDs, a clear distinction between the LFCB and BSC should be made in the training of operative personnel. There should be no generalized "grouping" of BSCs and LFCBs as "hoods" requiring similar use and maintenance patterns; each type of LAFD has airflow patterns, containment characteristics, and operating requirements unique to its design (Fig. 7). Operative personnel must understand that the containment and barrier techniques used in the operation of the BSC are significant not only as protection against sudden, overt contamination, but more importantly, as barriers to traces of residual contamination to which constant exposure may present long term health risks (15,16). Current pharmacy practices and contamination control manipulative techniques have been shown to be inadequate to contain hazardous substances in all phases of compounding and administration, and a pharmacy-wide study and standardized, remedial training programs must by quickly developed and carried out to protect operative personnel (6, 17).

Classification

BSCs are divided into three classes. Class I and Class II are used for low to moderate risk agents, and Class III for high risk agents. The risk level serves as a guide for pharmaceutical manufacturing and pharmacy compounding operations based on a reasonable extrapolation from the personnel risk levels, containment models, and product/personnel protection factors encountered in operations using the biological agents for which this type of equipment was originally designed.

The BSC in pharmacy operations

Although the BSC was not specifically designed for pharmaceutical manufacturing or pharmacy compounding operations, reasonable analogies in the management of hazardous aerosols may be made, justifying use of the BSC in such operations. Such was the case in 1979, following a comprehensive study (5) that determined that pharmacy and nursing personnel were experiencing occupational exposures to antineoplastic agents following their compounding in LFCBs and routine administration. As a prudent response to these findings, recommendations based upon such analogies by segments of the pharmacy community facilitated pharmacy-wide use of Class II BSCs. The Class II design was quickly implemented without attendant feasibility studies, validation and monitoring protocols, or standardized operating, cleaning, and line-clearance procedures, resulting in the installation and operation of this equipment with wide variation in its effectiveness from institution to institution.

Recent studies have indicated the unabated occupational exposure of pharmacy personnel to these substances, causing an inference of the inadequacy of the Class II system in controlling environmental contamination (6). These findings have again prompted vendors and segments of the pharmacy community to aggressively promote use of the Class III BSC, or barrier isolator, postulating that a so-called "closed system" would unfailingly prevent the transfer of hazardous agents to the environment, thus preventing personnel exposures. Pharmacy-wide promotion of a containment technology is

thus being repeated without the benefit of comprehensive engineering studies to both identify the reasons for any "failure" of the Class II system, and to provide standardized procedures to properly implement and operate the Class III system. It must be noted that Class II systems are completely effective in the management of particulate and aerosol contaminants in the microbiologic and toxicologic procedures for which they were originally designed. These contaminants include numerous dangerous agents, for which exacting, albeit decades-old manipulative and management techniques remain effective. No applications' failure of the Class II system has yet been reported by these industries, implying that it is improper use of this equipment and/or poor manipulative, product transfer, and cleaning techniques by pharmacy and nursing personnel, rather than any inherent design or applications' flaw in the Class II system, which would account for unabated occupational exposures (17). At this writing, insufficient evidence appears to exist supporting the remedial, pharmacy-wide retrofit of the Class II system with the Class III BSC, or barrier isolator. The pharmacy community should, rather than prematurely dispose of an effective and functional containment system for a more complex and expensive design, seek to identify and correct the cause(s) of such personnel exposures. A controlled study measuring the nature and magnitude of personnel exposures prior to, and following implementation of carefully designed and executed training exercises, containment procedures, and waste-streaming techniques should be carried out prior to any measures to retrofit these engineering controls.

Following any scientific determination of the inadequacy of the Class II technology in providing the necessary

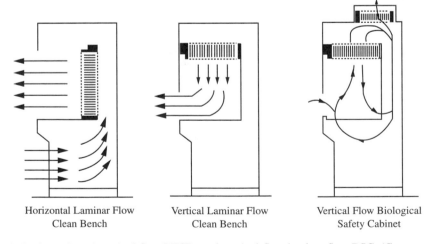

Horizontal Laminar Flow	Vertical Laminar Flow	Vertical Flow Biological
Clean Bench	Clean Bench	Safety Cabinet

Fig. 7   Airflow patterns in horizontal- and vertical-flow LFCBs and vertical-flow laminar flow BSC. (Courtesy of the Baker Company, Sanford, Maine.)

levels of operator and environmental protection, the Class III and barrier isolator systems should, without presumptions, be carefully evaluated for use in this application. Such evaluation should systematically encompass the full range of performance, operational, and maintenance factors, which bear upon gloveboxes or other closed systems, such as lowered productivity because of the cumbersome nature of gloves, half-suits, and reduction of dexterity; difficulty in effective cleaning, resulting in increased residual and cross-contamination of products; inferior product protection characteristics of turbulent Class 100 supply airflow; lowered throughput; increased compounding time and errors; and the manner in which these factors may inhibit the product protection capabilities of the Class III design.

Suitability

Prior to choosing a BSC for any pharmaceutical manufacturing or pharmacy compounding operation, all risks should be assessed by a qualified process engineer, safety officer, or industrial hygienist, ensuring that the equipment meets occupational safety as well as process requirements.

Class I BSC: The Class I BSC is an open containment unit suitable for work involving agents of low to moderate risk to the user and environment, where there is a need for containment but none for product protection or isolation. The Class I BSC provides protection to personnel using the cabinet by means of constant, controlled airflow into the work area and away from the operator, preventing the escape of aerosols through the front opening. It is of limited use in manufacturing and has no reported use in the current practice of pharmacy.

Class II BSC: The Class II BSC (Fig. 9) provides product, personnel, and environmental protection, and is the most common BSC employed in pharmaceutical manufacturing and pharmacy-compounding operations. The Class II BSC has several subclassifications, based upon cabinet ventilation design (18) (Table 1). The Class II BSC (Fig. 8), the most widely used by hospital and home-care pharmacies, features a front access opening

with carefully maintained inward airflow for replacement of air exhausted from the cabinet, a HEPA-filtered vertical laminar flow airstream within the entire work area, and HEPA-filtered exhaust air. The vertical laminar flow airstream and front access opening are common to all Class II cabinets, although LAF velocities and patterns, HEPA filter sizes and position, ventilation rates, and cabinet exhaust methods vary considerably in different designs (Fig. 7).

Class III BSC: The Class III BSC (Fig. 9) provides the highest level of personnel, product, and environmental protection from high-risk microbiologic and toxicologic agents. It is usually employed in pharmaceutical manufacturing operations involving weighing, diluting, and high volume aerosol generation of high-risk agents, as well as for handling contaminants that are slowly or rapidly vaporized. This type of laminar flow device affords the maximum containment and product protection barrier, and is used only in cases of extreme exposure hazard or product sensitivity.

The Class III BSC is a gas-tight enclosure, utilizing total air displacement ventilation that protects personnel from exposure to the products contained within the enclosure, the product from contaminants found in the ambient environment, and the environment from release of potentially hazardous substances. The Class III BSC is used where absolute containment of hazardous agents is required, and is normally configured with glove ports housing gas-tight, full length latex, neoprene, PVC, urethane, or laminated polymer gloves (19).

Operating procedure

In addition to cleaning all accessible work zone surfaces, the Class II BSC worksurface tray should be lifted up and back, and the area under the tray should be thoroughly cleaned with the same frequency as the other user-accessible worksurfaces; this is of particular importance in preventing the buildup of potentially harmful product residues. All materials used in cleaning and sanitizing should be treated as toxic waste, and disposed of in accordance with state and local

Table 1 BSC cabinet ventilation

(Type) Class II	Cabinet air characteristics	Air recirculated (%)
Type A	30% Vented back into room	70
Type B3	30% Ducted to outdoors	70
Type B1	70% Ducted to outdoors	30
Type B2	100% Ducted to outdoors	0

*

ordinances. Following complete drying of the worksurface, operations may begin by staging all working materials for introduction into the aseptic work area. The working materials may then be transferred to the work zone, and aseptic manipulations begun. Work should be performed only on the worksurface, taking care not to handle or store materials on or near the ventilation grilles. First air should be maintained at the critical surfaces of all working materials in the aseptic field; interference with the vertical flow of first air by passing anything over critical orifices or septa in the aseptic field must be prevented. Good aseptic technique is essential to retain the sterility of compounded products[m] (14) and surgeon's gloves, mask, laboratory coat (or arm barrier), and hair cover are recommended for all pharmacy operators working in the BSC.[n]

Location

The location, operation, and maintenance of the BSC should be carefully planned. Similar to LFCB, the BSC should be located in an area free of steady or intermittent air currents, which might defeat the laminar airstream by a backwash effect[l]. The BSC should be connected to an adequate power source, having the minimum possible current fluctuation. The effects of voltage variation on cabinet performance can be pronounced (Fig. 10A), causing a variation in intake and supply velocities sufficient to result in an unacceptable unit performance (Fig. 10B), thereby compromising personnel and product protection design features (Table 2). Performance testing of the BSC by a qualified inspector is recommended at least every 6 months and always after relocation of the unit. Appropriate surface decontamination is recommended prior to moving or refiltering the unit.[o]

---

[m]The importance of good aseptic technique is occasionally deemphasized by personnel compounding cytotoxic and antibiotic agents in the BSC, based on the belief that these substances are themselves toxic or germicidal to any microbiologic contaminants. It should be noted that numerous microbiologic organisms remain viable and replicate in cytotoxic compounds, and that no antibiotic has a universal antimicrobial action. Proper aseptic technique is therefore mandated in all operations carried out in the LAF environment.

[n]These are basic barriers, proven to aid in the retention of gross endogenous contamination at close working proximity to the critical field, but as importantly, these barriers protect the operator from direct contact with potentially hazardous substances, and should be used in accordance with established guidelines (see "Regulatory Issues").

[o]Although microbiologic decontamination of the BSC is not required, except as used in the manipulation of microbiologic agents, proper containment technique should be employed when refiltering or servicing these units.

Table 2 Protection provided by various BSC designs

Design	Personnel	Product	Environmental
Clean benches		●	
Class I	●		●
Class II			
Type A	●	●	●
Type B1	●	●	●
Type B2	●	●	●
Type B3	●	●	●
Class III	●	f(design)[a]	●

[a]Characteristic a function of design

Applications

The BSC is used in hospital, clinical, and home health care pharmacies to provide a sterile field in which to conduct aseptic manipulations in the compounding of LVPs, SVPs, antineoplastics, antibiotics, antivirals, and vaccines, the direct exposure to which may be hazardous to the operator and the environment. Most hospital and clinical pharmacy operations are currently carried out in a Class II(B3) BSC, which is vented to the outside by a dedicated, nonrecirculating HVAC exhaust, directly connected to the BSC.[p] Although direct connection to an HVAC exhaust is not required for proper Operation of the Class II(a) BSC in the containment of biological aerosols, such direct connection is recommended in all pharmaceutical manufacturing or pharmacy-compounding applications. The Class I BSC is almost never used in pharmacy compounding operations, and the Class III BSC technology is currently being evaluated for use in pharmacy compounding following comprehensive evaluation of any Class II FA, and outcomes of feasibility studies of the Class III system in such operations.

In industry, the BSC is used to conduct small batch sterile-fill operations, manipulation (weighing and

---

[p]Current guidelines may recommend use of the Class 11 Type B2 (total exhaust) BSC in certain manufacturing and compounding applications, but proper operation of this unit is difficult to maintain because of non-interlocked operation of separate BSC supply and in-house exhaust air-handling systems. B2s in the configurations currently available frequently develop a supply–exhaust flow imbalance, which may readily compromise product or personnel protection. Until a reliable system for direct interlock of the supply and exhaust air handlers is available that synchronizes the operation of the components, facilitating changes in operation by either air handler being proportionately matched by the other, use of the Class-11 Type B2 BSC is not recommended for pharmaceutical manufacturing and pharmacy compounding applications as a containment LAFD.

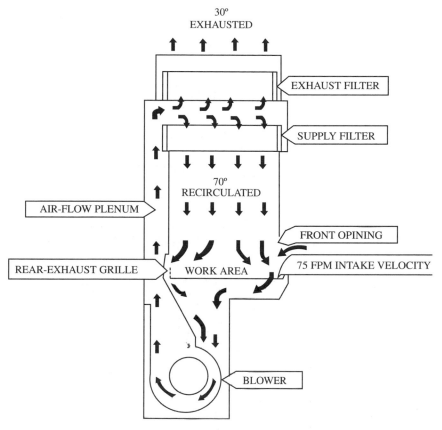

Fig. 8 Airflow patterns of the Class II(a) laminar flow BSC. (Courtesy of the Baker Company, Sanford, Maine.)

pouring), isolation of hazardous materials, and in QA/QC testing applications. All classes of BSC are encountered in pharmaceutical manufacturing operations for a wide variety of processing applications.

Terminal HEPA Filtration Module

The terminal HEPA filtration module (TFM) is a self-contained HEPA filter and plenum unit (Fig. 11), which may be used to provide laminar or conventional airflow[q] to a clean space, or may be dedicated as a LAF workstation (20). The TFM is available with a 10 in. (optional 12 inch) collar for connection by a circular supply duct to a central air handling system (Fig. 5A) or as a free-standing, fully powered unit containing a motor

[q]Laminar-airflow room is defined as a cleanroom in which filtered air entering the room makes a single pass through the work area in a parallel-flow pattern, with a minimum of turbulent flow areas. Laminar-flow rooms must have HEPA filter coverage of at least 80% of the ceiling (as vertical flow), or one wall (as horizontal flow), producing a uniform and parallel airflow (net filter medium face area versus gross area = 0.80).

and blower. It is normally installed in a "T-bar" grid ceiling system, suspended by seismic restraints from the architectural ceiling or building supports (Fig. 5B), which constitutes the inner clean space ceiling. Permanently installed or modular air handling systems are available that provide treatment (heating, air conditioning, dehumidification, etc.) of recirculated and make-up air to the clean space. Self-powered TFMs do not provide supply air treatment, and care should be taken in installing this type of unit because of high noise level and heat output factors, which may fatigue operative personnel or adversely affect temperature-sensitive stored drug products.

The TFM may also be used to provide a Class 1–100 work surface of almost any size, and may be installed in the ceiling (vertical downflow), or in a wall (horizontal flow). Using this design, shrouded laminar flow Class 1–100 "first air" is provided directly to the critical worksurface in the same quantity and quality as by a LFCB. Outflow from the critical worksurface is used to treat the general space, in combination with additional room "buffer" HEPA filtration, thus

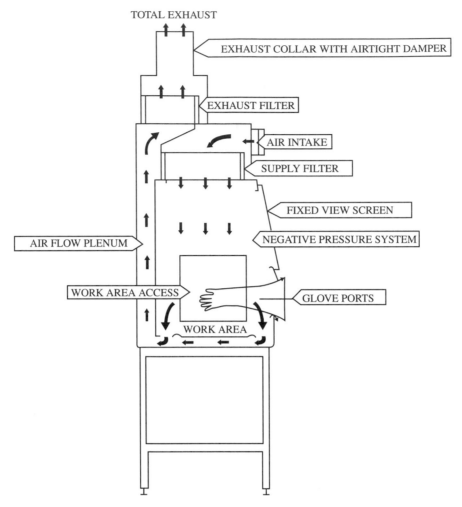

Fig. 9   Airflow patterns of the Class III laminar flow BSC. (Courtesy of the Baker Company, Sanford, Maine.)

providing both the highly-controlled critical worksurface, and the less-controlled general room area. Several inexpensive concept designs are available to develop reliable worksurfaces and buffer areas, which support both pharmacy and pharmaceutical manufacturing operations (20).

In-duct HEPA filtration

In this type of filtration the HEPA filter is placed within the supply duct system, providing Class 100 air from the point immediately downstream of the filter to the supply diffusers within the general clean space. This arrangement is used where a comparatively small volume of supply air is required for the clean space operation, when filter handling and disposal is critical (requiring remote "bag in/out" containment isolation or other special handling considerations), or where space

limitations prevent the installation of TFMs. Induct HEPA filtration provides conventional airflow and is recommended as secondary or "buffer" filtration in clean spaces where critical work zones are treated using an LAFD. In-duct HEPA filtration is not recommended for LAF applications to provide required Class 1–100 conditions at critical worksurfaces, where uninterrupted "first air" is necessary to achieve the highest levels of contamination control.

The plenum ceiling

The plenum ceiling is an arrangement of ductless terminal HEPA filter modules which, in a manner similar to TFMs, are installed in a "T-bar" grid system. These filter modules are not connected directly to an air handling system by means of ducts. The uniform flow of air through all modules results rather from a

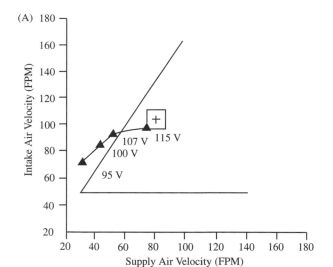

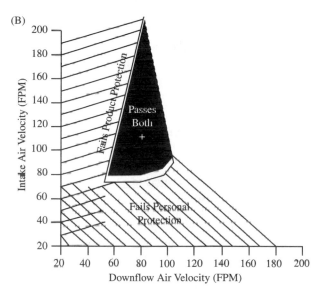

Fig. 10 (A) Effects of voltage variation on cabinet performance; National Sanitary Foundation (NSF) range, +: Normal setpoint; ——: Performance envelope; ▲—▲ Airflow balance. (B) Performance envelopes for Class II BSCs determined by conducting a series of microbiological aerosol tests at a variety of airflow settings. (Courtesy of the Baker Company, Sanford, Maine.)

pressurized common space or "plenum" immediately above the entire T-bar ceiling assembly. This plenum is supplied directly by an air handler, eliminating the need for extensive ductwork. The plenum ceiling is normally used in overhead space-limited LAF applications.

The cleanroom

The cleanroom is a dedicated clean space with exacting as-built, at-rest, and operational specifications of airborne and surface cleanliness, temperature, relative humidity, and lighting and noise levels, in which specific critical operations are carried out (11). The cleanroom may be designed to provide vertical or horizontal LAF throughout the entire room for large-scale operations requiring extended critical work zones (sterile conveyors, sterile fill operations, etc.), or may be designed as a conventionally-supplied, controlled secondary or "buffer" area, housing one or more smaller LAFD for aseptic processing steps requiring comparatively limited critical work zones.

The cleanroom is normally constructed in an existing building or structure as a core unit, surrounded by supporting access and staging anterooms, service chases, and machine rooms necessary to support the aseptic operation, supply working materials, and remove finished products and waste materials without cross-contamination or interference with the critical work stream.

TESTING AND CERTIFICATION OF LAF SYSTEMS

Thorough, periodic testing of LAF equipment is necessary to optimize performance and demonstrate compliance with established operating procedures and industry standards.

Certification

The term "certification" is widely used in connection with this type of testing. Certification may, however, only be provided by a registered testing or metrology laboratory, or other organization that derives its certification authority directly from a legitimate regulatory agency (FDA, EPA, AIHA, etc.) and which is subject to review. For a test procedure to qualify as a performance certification, the procedure must be performed and documented in accordance with the current good laboratory practices (21). All on-site testing of this nature constitutes a laboratory field certification of performance, with each test report accession-numbered in the laboratory test notebook as an actual laboratory test procedure. If the vendor of this service does not have such regulatory oversight, the buyer must qualify the vendors adequacy of experience, equipment, and efficacy of all test procedures to be performed (22), regardless of the vendor's professional affiliations or memberships.

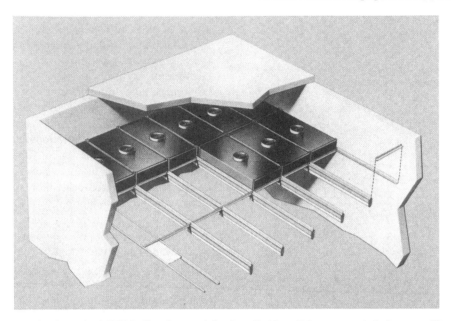

Fig. 11 Self-contained terminal HEPA filtration modules installed in a T-bar suspended plenum ceiling in a laminar-flow application. (Courtesy of American Air Filter, Inc., Louisville, Kentucky.)

Vendor Qualification

Although large manufacturers often have in-house personnel and facilities available to carry out LAF equipment testing, this task is frequently performed by an outside testing contractor, whose procedures and findings are relied upon without question by the buyer. Because the pharmaceutical manufacturer and pharmacy practitioner bear the ultimate responsibility to regulatory groups for ensuring compliance with all testing standards and requirements, it is essential that they select a qualified testing contractor. The buyer should interview the prospective contractor and review all aspects of the tester's training and experience, the test procedures and equipment to be used, equipment calibration and traceability, and the proposed documentation (22). The prospective contractor should be prepared to provide both company and individual resumes of qualifications, including at least three references of clients for whom the contractor has recently provided similar services (20).

Test Equipment Calibration and Traceability

The LAF equipment tester should have the equipment necessary to carry out the required challenge of the LAF system (20). This equipment should be in good working order and calibrated to a National Institute of Standards and Testing (NIST)-traceable[r] standard at least annually, or more often as indicated by the manufacturer's specifications or equipment performance (23). NIST-traceable calibration ensures the uniformity, accuracy, and serviceability of all test equipment as well as proper maintenance and care by the user. The NIST-traceability of equipment calibration is substantiated by a detailed calibration certification letter, issued by the calibrating authority for each piece of equipment.

Certification Standards

The primary standard for testing LAF equipment is a standard operating procedure (SOP), unique to the equipment or system. This SOP is normally established by the using organization to define the calibration and testing requirements of a specific LAF system, and should include the scope, intent, and frequency of testing; the equipment to be used in conducting the test; test equipment calibration; test methods and performance criteria; documentation of results; and corrective actions and acceptance. The SOP should cite the applicable references and industry standards from which it has been derived. In the absence of an organizational SOP, LAF equipment should be tested in accordance with industry standards applicable to the specific LAF

[r]Formerly the National Bureau of Standards (NBS), Washington, DC.

application or area of operation (Table 3). In this case, regulatory groups will defer to these standards for proof of proper LAF system function and serviceability.

Test Reports

A comprehensive report should be issued upon completion of the test procedures, which should include all values measured for compliance, a listing of all test equipment, calculations, conversions, and all appropriate statistical justification along with comments pertaining to system function and operation. A dated test-completion or certification sticker should be affixed to the LAF unit referring any examining authority to the completed test report. All reports should include floor plans or maps of the clean space, which identify sample locations, probe heights, unusual performance characteristics, system adjustments, and repairs.

Test Procedures

Air velocity

Measurement of air velocity and laminar profile quality is the first step in LAF system testing. Using the appropriate instrument and measurement technique (4, 11, 18), the velocity of the laminar airstream for all LAFDs, and conventional buffer supply airflow volume for all controlled areas should be measured and adjusted to conform with pertinent SOPs or industry standards, consistent with the system manufacturers specifications and limitations (20).

HEPA filter performance

Following verification of the proper velocities, the HEPA filter should be aerosol-challenged in accordance with industry standards (4, 11, 18). Because this challenge is based upon the effectiveness of the filter in retaining aerosols, the upstream concentration of test aerosol should be verified before commencing this test and should not be assumed to be adequate, regardless of the circumstances.

Particle counting

Only through discrete particle counting can air cleanliness be verified, and the cleanliness class of the sampled environment established (4). Periodic in-process monitoring of workstations, buffer rooms, anterooms, production areas, and any other area about which a definitive air cleanliness statement is made or reasonably assumed, should be carried out in accordance with

SOPs or industry standards (4, 11). A discrete particle counter (DPC) with an adequate sampling rate, calibration features, and dynamic range should be used for sample acquisition, based on the specified air cleanliness level (4, 17).

Noise levels

Noise in excess of recommended levels within the LAF environment or clean space may cause operator discomfort and premature fatigue, and may indicate HEPA filter failure, or a malfunction of the LAFD or clean space air handling unit (20, 24). Cabinet pressure integrity and vibration analysis are recommended for all biological safety cabinets.

Visible and ultraviolet light levels

Visible light levels should be monitored for operator comfort and total visibility of the worksurface (20, 22). Ultraviolet germicidal light should be measured for effectiveness in all LAFDs having this feature (18).

LAMINAR FLOW CLEAN SPACE PROJECT DEVELOPMENT

As an engineering control, the demands normally placed upon an LAF system should not exceed the system's ability to provide a sterile, aerosol-free work area in which to conduct the desired aseptic operations with a high degree of confidence. Neither should a facility be overbuilt; unnecessary complication of clean space operation to achieve control levels that provide no demonstrable improvement in the process or finished product is counterproductive and an expensive waste of resources. To develop a system that is adequate for the aseptic processing task at minimum expense, a definitive, phased approach to design and implementation of the LAF system should be taken, regardless of the size or complexity of the system. The method described below ensures that any project, from a simple hood installation to a complex process cleanroom, will have the most comprehensive development and planning, thus maximizing the probability of a successful outcome.

Conceptualization

As the initial step, a thorough and complete conceptualization of the process, and the steps that will be taken to achieve the desired results should be defined in a protocol.

Table 3 Regulations and guidelines pertaining to LAF systems[a,b]

	Guidelines										Regulations					
	ASHP (Proposed)	EN ISO 14644-1 TO 6	IES-RP-CC-001-86 (Testing HEPA Filters)	IES-RP-CC-006-84-T (Testing cleanrooms)	IES-RP-CC-018.2 (Cleanroom Housekeeping operating and monitoring)	NSF 49	USP 1074 (Proposed)	FED. STD. 209c	CGMP-CFR	CGLP-CFR	JCAHO	Regional Pharmacy Practice Acts	Regional Department of Public Health Acts	OSHA 8.1.1	NRC: FEDERAL	NRC: STATE Municipal Codes
Pharmacy (IV/TPN)	●						●				●	●			●	
Pharmacy (CYTA)	●										●	●			●	
Home health care (IV/TPN)		●	●	●	●	●					●	●	●		●	
Home health care (CYTA)		●	●	●	●	●					●	●	●		●	
Nursing home (IV/TPN)											●	●			●	
Nuclear pharmacy	●						●				●	●		●	●	
Pharmaceutical manufacturing		●		●			●	●	●	●		●				
Nuclear pharmaceutical manufacturing		●	●	●	●		●	●		●		●		●	●	
Pharmaceuticals repackaging		●	●	●	●		●	●	●			●			●	

[a] Courtesy Lab Safety Corp., Chicago.

[b] Reactor products on site: nonagreement states.

TPN: Total parenteral nutrition; CYTA: Cytotoxic agent; CGMP: Current Good Manufacturing Practices; CGLP: Current Good Laboratory Practices; CFR: Code of Federal Regulations; NRC: Nuclear Regulatory Commission.

This document is to be used as the basis of communication with design and mechanical engineers in developing specifications for an effective and workable design, to be constructed, validated, and operated within existing cost constraints.

Protocol and Project Management

The protocol should be developed under the supervision of a project manager, selected on the basis of experience and understanding of the product, existing and intended markets, regulatory issues, the intended aseptic process, the engineering controls normally required for such a process, and the design, construction, validation, operational, and maintenance methods to be employed (25). The manager represents the owners' interests, and acts as liaison in all dealings with outside vendors and contractors. He or she should seek direct input from key personnel and representatives of all groups having direct involvement with the planned clean space (26) in meetings and discussions, as the concept evolves, with appropriate sign-off by the participants on the finished protocol. This method prevents after-the-fact, unforseen demands upon system operation, or dissatisfaction with system performance by essential personnel. Conceptualization is based upon the following considerations:

- Space constraints vs. process requirements.
- Product or process quality statements.
- Output capacity and growth expectations.
- Industry standards and regulatory issues (Table 3).
- Cleanliness class(es) required. Identification of critical work zones and areas requiring LAF, rather than mere characterization of these areas as Class 100.
- Work streaming. Inclusion of the necessary QA/QC steps in the overall process.
- Necessary process equipment (Table 4).
- Identification of all process steps requiring an LAF environment to facilitate the desired cleanliness class. What facility and equipment performance alert and action limits are necessary, and how are these to be monitored?
- Process equipment portability and flexibility requirements. Will the process(es) be expanded or modified at some time in the future? What equipment must be permanently installed and "hard wired" within the clean space?
- Process equipment service and maintenance requirements.
- Number of personnel required.

- Personnel disciplines. What type and arrangement of anterooms are required for scrubbing, gowning, and storage of barrier materials?
- Process materials staging and waste management.
- Health and safety requirements.
- Facility housekeeping and maintenance procedures.
- Facility validation, testing, and recertification.
- Documentation, i.e., the necessary process records, logs, labels, etc., and how, when, and where these documents are produced and used.

Regulatory Issues

Operation of LAF systems in the course of pharmaceutical manufacturing and pharmacy compounding operations is ultimately scrutinized by several regulatory and quasi-regulatory groups responsible for the control and oversight of these industries. Because these regulatory groups require, almost without exception, operation of manufacturing or compounding systems in accordance with "current industry standards," the distinction between regulations and guidelines has become unclear. Guidelines, as a reflection of the most current application of any technology, often take on the weight of regulations as determinants of industry standards. As such, operation in accordance with specific industry guidelines is often required to demonstrate compliance with nonspecific or generalized regulations—i.e., current good manufacturing practices (cGMPs) or Joint Commission on Accreditation of Health Care Organizations (JCAHO) Standards. Table 3, although not intended to be all inclusive, provides a list of regulations and guidelines that are pertinent to the operation of LAF systems in several different pharmaceutical manufacturing and pharmacy-compounding applications.

Design

Based upon the protocol, the facility and process design is the next step. Whether a simple hood installation to an existing space, an upgrade retrofit of an existing space, or construction of a totally new space, the design responsibility has to be assigned and a designer chosen. The designer's obligations are considerable and should be thoroughly understood by the individual or firm retained to provide the clean space design (20).

Construction

Following completion of the design, the building contractor is chosen. The construction phase is normally

Table 4 Equipment Features and Performance[a,b,c]

	Cleanliness Class-Fed Std 209°C					Applications									Airflow and Equipment Configuration							
	Class 10	Class 100	Class 1,000	Class 100,000	Pharmacy IV corresponding	TPN (HA) compounding	CYTA compounding	Product protection	Personnel protection	Technology, screening	Microbiology	Sterility testing	Work station	Cleanroom	Laminar flow	Conventional flow	First air work station	Terminal filtration	In-duct filtration	Ventable to room	Direct connection	Thimble unit
LFCB	2	1			3	1	1	1			1	1	1		1		1	1		1		
LFBSC Class I	2		1		1	1	1	1	1	3	1	1	1			1	1			1	1	
LFBSC Class IIA	1	1			1	1	2	1	1	1	1	1	1		1	1	1	1	1	1	1	
LFBSC Class IIB		1[d]			2	1	2	1	1	1	1	1	1		1	2	2		2		1	1
LFBSC 3 glovebox	2	1			1	1		1		1		1	1		2	1	1		1		1	
In-duct HEPA filter		2	2	4	4	4	4	4			4	4		4	1					1		
Terminal HEPA filter module (TFM)	2	2	1	4	4	4	4	4		4	4	4	2	1	2	1	2	2	1	1		
Filter plenum ceiling	2	1			2	2	2	2		2			1	1	1	2	2	1				

[a] See also Appendix B.
[b] 1: Primary engineering control; 2: With optimization or modification; 3: Obsolete application; 4: Secondary or "buffer" control.
[c] Courtesy Lab Safety Corp., Chicago.
[d] Early designs.

carried out with the input and assistance of the designer in conducting vendor audits for the selection of contractors with sufficient experience and facilities to complete the building tasks efficiently. Materials and workmanship audits should be carried out periodically by the project manager and the designer.

Validation and certification

Validation is described as proof that the system performs as stated. As an engineering control, the LAF system must demonstrably support the intended aseptic or controlled process. Validation of the aseptic manufacturing process and the LAF systems that support terminal sterilization in pharmaceutical manufacturing applications should be carried out in accordance with industry standards (1, 27–31). Such validation should be accomplished in three phases, consisting of installation qualification (IQ), operational qualification (OQ), and process qualification (PQ), with full and detailed documentation of all activities and outcomes (20).

Cleanroom Construction and Validation: A Low-Cost Approach

The following is a consolidation of steps leading to the construction and operation of a low-cost clean space of the type required for small- and intermediate-size drug repackagers, home health care pharmacies, and small pharmaceutical manufacturers.

Cleanroom design

The cleanroom should be conceptualized, designed, constructed, validated, operated, and maintained in a manner that supports the aseptic process. A construction plan, including reasonable time frames for the acquisition of labor and materials should be developed, followed, and updated. All work and materials should comply with local building codes and safety ordinances.

HEPA Filtration

Computation of the air change rate (AC) necessary for the desired cleanliness class is the initial step in determining the ceiling module filter density required for the clean space, and should be calculated accurately, with sufficient redundancy to assure the required airflow and resulting cleanliness levels (20, 32,33).

Air Handling

Air handling requirements should be calculated, and air handler type and capacity should be matched to the AC rate, heating, cooling, and dehumidification requirements of the facility (34), as calculated from the reflected ceiling plan. At almost any intended level of processing, low cost, "turn-key" air handling systems are available with a minimum of lead time. They are easily installed, operated, and maintained. The installation of a modular air handler of this type provides conditioned air, allowing operation of the core and anteroom areas as an independent facility, without dependence upon a central building air handling apparatus for process control. This type of low-cost, modular air handler, in a single-or multiple-unit installation, facilitates complete treatment and conditioning of the supply air to be provided in quantities adequate to maintain the most stringent air cleanliness classes for workstations and general room air, as well as temperature and relative humidity at recommended core and anteroom internal operating pressures. In addition, several manufacturers of this type of unit have experienced, on-staff mechanical engineers qualified to assist the buyer in determining the exact air treatment and handling requirements for a specific application at no additional charge. Qualification of the knowledge and experience of all individuals involved in the conceptualization and design phases is necessary, and references should be obtained and checked by the buyer.

Differential Pressurization

The cleanroom facility should be carefully designed to control the ingress of contaminants, and be positively pressurized to the surrounding area in accordance with industry standards. The core and anterooms are positively pressurized by varying the amount of incoming "make-up" air (20). In the case of "soft wall" clean space facilities, such pressurization (potential outflow) is not possible, and a sufficient amount of constant, active outflow (kinetic outflow) should occur to prevent ingress of contaminants.

Lighting and Electrical

Electrical service should be provided in the normal fashion in accordance with local building and electrical codes. Clean space service requires no special treatment, and should provide a 25–50 A surplus over worst-case processing demands, to allow for additional electrical equipment and source power fluctuations. Fixture types, sealable outlets, and hard-wiring of processing equipment should be selected and carried out in accordance with industry standards and electrical codes (20).

Walls and Windows

Walls should be typical 5/8-in. drywall over metal studs at 16-in. centers, and may be insulated or not as deemed appropriate. The inner clean space wall should be finished with enameled panels (available at most building supply outlets) that are butted and sealed with RTV silicone, to provide gas-tight seams between the wall panel, ceiling T-bar, and floor base junctions. (Clear RTV silicone is recommended, neatly and sparingly "mopped in," with all residues cleared away while still wet; this method creates an invisible, water-tight seal facilitating long term serviceability and ease of cleaning.) The outer walls should be painted with cleanable epoxy enamel or suitably covered, and a long, narrow observation window (recommended aspect 1:8–10, without ledge), or a series of double-pane, ledgeless windows should be installed and finished to provide complete observation of the operational process by prospective clients, supervisory personnel, and others.

Floor

The anteroom and core flooring should be an attractive, highly durable, one-piece vinyl or other suitable floor material, providing a minimum of seams. This flooring should ideally radius in a cove at the wall base and continue upward to a height of 8 inches. to 1 ft above the floor. At that point it should be capped with a suitable beading, sealed by RTV silicone, neatly "mopped in," and allowed to dry. No drain or other floor opening should be permitted in the core; a small, single drain may be permitted in the anteroom in the event carts or other materials are to be cleaned and staged in that area. The floor should be routinely cleaned by a wet-vac recovery of a spread floor cleaning solution (with hose and head located within the clean space, with pass-through connection to a vacuum source located and vented outside the clean space).

Ceiling

The anteroom and core ceilings should be of typical 1.5 in. T-Bar construction, with seismic restraints adequate

to support the HEPA terminals, lighting fixtures, and ceiling panels. The panels may be obtained from clean space suppliers in the form of finished "cleanroom" ceiling panels, or by reduction of additional enameled wall panels to 2 × 4 ft (nominal) panels, affixed by permanent adhesive to standard, plain face (nontextured), fire-rated, 0.5 inches. commercial ceiling panels, which are easily installed and RTV silicone-sealed in place. This allows installation of a permanent, gastight ceiling, washable like the walls and floor, and attractive in that it provides visual continuity of the wall material.

Doors and Pass-Throughs

Doors and pass-throughs should facilitate easy, integral entry and exit of personnel and working materials (20).

Construction

Construction of the facility should be based upon the completed design and incorporate normal construction methods, tools, and techniques. Special preparation of components is necessary, including a general cleaning and protection of components and equipment from potential sources of contamination during the construction phase. The working materials should be protected from atmospheric dust, sawdust, grease, aerosols of oil, and other residues, which may be encountered during construction, using "clean construction" methods (20).

Validation

Following completion of all testing and certification of the facility, documentation should be developed and retained, which may be used as proof of performance in accordance with the protocol in the as-built configuration (4, 11). Periodic retesting and monitoring at specified intervals in the at-rest and operational modes (4, 11) should be carried out to maintain operation of the facility in accordance with SOPs or industry standards.

Operation

Operation of the facility in accordance with validation conditions, through the use of appropriate SOPs and industry standard quality management parameters (28) should be commenced following validation, incorporating the necessary alert and action limits, monitoring procedures and maintenance steps to be carried out and included in the production cycle documentation. All microbiologic monitoring of the clean space anterooms, core, worksurfaces and personnel barriers should be carried out in a systematic manner by experienced personnel (35).

Personnel Selection and Validation

Because the effectiveness of operative personnel is potentially the greatest variable in any controlled process, a selection, training, examination, and grading system should assure the suitability of candidates, the adequacy of training, and the ultimate uniformity and consistency of clean space operating procedures (12, 14, 15, 36).

Maintenance

Clean space maintenance SOPs and documentation should be developed and followed in strict accordance with industry standards (13) to ensure the consistency of operation in accordance with validation conditions.

REFERENCES

1. Frieben, W.R. Validation of Aseptic Processing Operations. Encyclopedia of Pharmaceutical Technology; Swarbrick, J., Boylan, J.C., Eds.; Marcel Dekker, Inc.: New York, 1988; 1, 355–359.
2. Kleinberg, M.; Shatsky, F.; Lumkin, B. Particulate Matter in In-Line Burettes. Particulate and Microb. Control 1983, 2 (5), 77–150.
3. Wilson, J. Infection Control in Intravenous Therapy. Heart Lung 1976, 5 (3), 430–436.
4. Commissioner, Federal Supply Service, General Services Admin. Clean Room and Workstation Requirements, Controlled Environment; U.S. Government Printing Office: Washington, 1976.
5. Falck, K.; Grohn, P.; Sorsa, M. Mutagenicity in Urine of Nurses Handling Cytostatic Drugs. Lancet 1979, 1, 1250–1251.
6. Connor, T.H.; Anderson, R.W.; Sessink, P.J.; Broadfield, L.; Power, L.A. Surface Contamination with Antineoplastic Agents in Six Cancer Treatment Centers in Canada and the United States. AJHP 1999, 56 (14), 1427–1432.
7. Laminar Flow Biological Safety Cabinets, A Training Manual for Biomedical Investigators; National Cancer Institute: Washington, 1972.
8. Hinds, W.C.; Macher, J.M.; First, M.W. Size Distribution of Aerosols Produced by the Laskin Aerosol Generator Using Substitute Materials for DOP. J. Am. Ind. Hyg. Assoc. 1983, 44 (7), 495–500.
9. Recommended Practice for Laminar Flow Clean Air Devices; Institute of Environmental Sciences: Mt. Prospect, IL, 1986.
10. Recommended Practice for HEPA Filters; Institute of Environmental Sciences: Mt. Prospect IL, 1989.
11. Recommended Practice for Testing Cleanrooms; Institute of Environmental Sciences: Mt. Prospect IL, 1984.
12. Dirks, I.; Smith, F.M.; Furtado, D. Methods for Testing Aseptic Technique of Pharmacy Personnel. Am. J. Hosp. Pharm. 1982, 39, 457–459.
13. Cleanroom Housekeeping-Operating and Monitoring Procedures; Institute of Environmental Sciences: Mt. Prospect IL, 1989.
14. McKeon, M.R.; Peters, G.F. VALITEQ Aseptic Technique Validation System Compounding Manual; Boylan, J.C., Ed.; Lab Safety Corp. Des Plaines IL, 1999; 35–37.
15. OSHA. Work Practice Guidelines for Personnel Dealing with Cytotoxic [Antineoplastic] Drugs; U.S. Dept. of Labor: Washington, 1986.
16. American Society of Hospital Pharmacists. ASHP Technical Assistance Bulletin on Handling Cytotoxic and Hazardous Drugs. Am. J. Hosp. Pharm 1990, 47, 1033–1049.
17. Galatowitsch, S. Technique May Be Culprit Behind Class II BSC Contamination. Cleanrooms 1999, 13(11), 1, 4–45.
18. National Sanitation Foundation. NSF Standard 49; Advisory Committee for Biohazard Cabinetry: Ann Arbor, MI, 1995.
19. Farquharson, G.J. Isolators for Pharmaceutical Applications. Encyclopedia of Pharmaceutical Technology; Swarbrick, J., Boylan, J.C., Eds.; Marcel Dekker, Inc.: New York, 1999; 18, 121–136.
20. Peters, G.F. Laminar Airflow Equipment: Engineering Control of Aseptic Processing. Encyclopedia of Pharmaceutical Technology; Swarbrick, J., Boylan, J.C., Eds.; Marcel Dekker, Inc.: New York, 1993; 8, 317–359.
21. Food and Drug Administration. Current Good Laboratory Practices; Washington, 1992.
22. Bryan, D.; Marback, R. Laminar-Airflow Equipment Certification: What the Pharmacist Needs to Know. Am. J. Hosp. Pharm. 1984, 41, 1343–1349.
23. Recommended Practices for Equipment Calibration or Validation Procedures; Institute of Environmental Sciences: Mt. Prospect IL, 1986.
24. OSHA. Standard 1910.95; U.S. Dept. of Labor: Washington, 1971.
25. Facility Design Considering Safety, Monitoring and Detection: A Team Approach (Verbal Communication) Microcontamination Conference, Santa Clara, CA, 1988.
26. Whyte, W. Cleanroom Design; Wiley: New York, 1991.
27. Food and Drug Administration. Current Good Manufacturing Practice for Finished Pharmaceuticals; Washington, 1992.

28. Kozicki, M.; Hognie, S.; Robinson, P. *Cleanrooms*; Van Nostrand, Reinhold, Eds.; New York, 1991.

29. Parenteral Drug Association. *Validation of Aseptic Filling for Solution Drug Products*; Philadelphia, 1980.

30. American Society of Hospital Pharmacists. Technical Assistance Bulletin on Quality Assurance for Pharmacy-Prepared Sterile Products. Am. J. Hosp. Pharm. **1993**, *50*, 2386–2398.

31. *Sterile Drug Products for Home Use*; The United States Pharmacopoeial Convention, Inc.: 1998.

32. Dixon, A. *Cleanroom Management Manual*; Cleanroom Management Association: Tempe, AZ, 1991.

33. *Guideline on Sterile Drug Products Produced by Aseptic Processing*; Food and Drug Administration: Washington, 1987; 20–27.

34. High Performance-Low Energy-Cost Cleanroom: A Case Study Microcontamination Conference, Santa Clara, CA 1990.

35. Peters, G.F.; McKeon, M.R. Microbiologic Monitoring of Aseptic and Controlled Processes. *Encyclopedia of Pharmaceutical Technology*; Swarbrick, J., Boylan, J.C., Eds.; Marcel Dekker, Inc.: New York, 2000; 19, 239–278.

36. Dixon, A. Training Cleanroom Personnel. J. Parent. Sci. Technol. **1991**, *45* (6), 276–278.

LENS CARE PRODUCTS

Masood Chowhan
Ralph Stone
Alcon Laboratories, Fort Worth, Texas

INTRODUCTION

Contact lenses are made of polymeric materials designed and fabricated to correct vision. Because these lenses are removed from the eye after a prescribed wear time, lens care products are required to clean, disinfect and rinse them prior to reinsertion to avoid ocular infections and other complications. Lens care products are also required to enhance the comfort of lens wear.

HISTORICAL OVERVIEW

Lens care products are relatively new compared to many other pharmaceutical products. Leonardo da Vinci was the first to conceive the concept of the contact lens. In 1508 he illustrated the concept of vision involving "upside down" images with a water-filled sphere covering the eye. However, the actual development of contact lenses did not occur until about 100 years ago (1887–1888) when scleral contact lenses were fabricated. The three innovators credited for this are Dr. A.E. Fick, a physician in Zurich, F.A. Mueller, a maker of prosthetic eyes in Germany, and Dr. Eugene Kalt, a French physician. The earlier lenses were made of glass. In the late 1930s (1937–1939), Mullen, Obrig and Gyorrfy are credited with fabricating plastic contact lenses made from methyl methacrylate (PMMA). However, Kevin Tuohy, who filed a patent for contact lens design in 1948, is recognized as the "father" of modern day corneal contact lenses. These early lenses were rigid and uncomfortable with very low oxygen transmission. Advances in rigid lens technology have provided materials capable of oxygen transmission required to maintain corneal health. In the 1960s Otto Victerle developed the hydrophilic soft contact lens from polyhydroxyethyl methacrylate (HEMA). Hydrophilic soft contact lenses are the primary lenses available today. Since then, significant technological advances have been made in contact lens material, designs, and manufacturing processes. In 1990, the estimate of contact lens wearers in the United States alone was around 30 million.

The commercialization of the first pharmaceutical quality lens care products occurred in the 1950s. Harry Hind, a pharmacist and founder of the Barnes-Hind Company, has been credited as one of the first to develop and commercialize a wetting and storage solution for the rigid PMMA plastic lenses. Prior to his efforts, the literature mentions formulation of a saline solution containing sodium bicarbonate to be used with scleral lenses made from glass.

CURRENT CONTACT LENS MATERIALS AND FUTURE DIRECTIONS

Most of the materials currently used in fabricating contact lenses have been available since the mid-1960s with the exception of polymethyl methacrylate. Lens materials can be broadly classified as follows:

Rigid Gas-Permeable Lenses:

- Cellulose acetate butyrate
- Silicone
- Silicone acrylate
- Fluoro silicone acrylate
- *t*-Butylstyrene
- *t*-Butylstyrene-*co*-silicone acrylate

Soft Hydrophilic Lenses:

- Polyhydroxyethyl methacrylate
- Polyhdroxyethyl methacrylate-*co*-methacrylic acid
- Polyglyceryl methacrylate
- Polyhydroxyethyl methacrylate-*co*-polyvinylpyrrolidone
- Polyvinylpyrrolidone-*co*-methyl methacrylate
- Polyhydroxyethyl methacrylate-*co*-silicone (silicone hydrogel)

In addition to these materials, several others, such as polyurethanes, polysulfones, polyvinyl alcohol, and various copolymers, have been tried or are under development. Recently, silicon hydrogel lenses with high oxygen permeability were marketed. The future trends in material development will continue to include polymers which have a high degree of oxygen permeability, resist accumulation of metabolic products of the cornea, and materials that resist lens deposits and bacterial attachment on lens surfaces to minimize the potential for ocular infection.

Classification of Contact Lenses Currently Marketed

During a period beginning from mid-1970, numerous hydrophilic and rigid gas-permeable lenses were introduced into the market. Although many had similar basic chemical compositions, they contained different additives designed to achieve desirable properties or to avoid infringement of existing patents. Such a proliferation of contact lens materials created confusion regarding Food and Drug Administration (FDA) criteria for approval of contact lenses and their care products. In the mid-1980s, the FDA worked with the contact lens manufacturers and evolved a classification for soft contact lenses based on the ionic or nonionic nature of polymers constituting the lens material and the water content. A classification was also worked out for rigid gas-permeable (RGP) lenses based on the chemical nature of the polymers. It is interesting to note that contact lenses and their care products were originally considered as drugs. However, upon passage of the U.S. Medical Device Act in 1996, contact lenses were reclassified as devices. Contact lenses and their care products were considered Class-III devices, which mandate the filing of a premarket approval application and obtaining FDA approval prior to marketing. Recently these products were reclassified as Class II devices and are currently cleared for marketing under the 510(k) premarket notification section of the regulations.

LENS CARE PRODUCTS BY FUNCTIONAL PURPOSE

Marketed lens care products fall mainly into the following categories: cleaners, disinfectants, lubricants, and multipurpose products. Cleaners are subdivided into daily or weekly cleaners. Disinfectants comprise solutions containing chemical antimicrobial agents, which do not require heating the lenses, and preserved or unpreserved saline solutions, which are used with an electrical thermal device for lens disinfection. These products are also used to rinse contact lenses. Lens lubricants are intended to enhance the comfort of lens wear and are used prior to insertion and during wear. Multipurpose solutions are intended to

accomplish two or more of the functions described earlier (cleaning, rinsing, and disinfection).

Rigid lens care also includes conditioning solutions to make the basic hydrophobic polymers wettable when placed on the eye.

PRODUCTS FOR CLEANING SOFT CONTACT LENSES

Lens Deposits

Composition

Basically there are two types of deposits: those resulting from tear components and those derived from other sources. Tear components especially proteins can accumulate on the lens surface. These proteins can denature or change conformations during absorptions on over tissue. Most deposits, with the exception of those that are tenaciously bound to the lens, can be cleaned easily with a surfactant-type of daily cleaner. Deposits resulting from tear components include proteinacieous deposits such as lysozyme, lactoferrin, albumin, globulins, etc. Proteinaceous deposits are present on all types of lenses. However, the amounts differ, depending on the number of ionic charges on and in the lens, the pore size, and the relative hydrophobicity of the polymers. For example, conventional nonporous and uncharged hard PMMA lenses with a hydrophobic surface attract very little proteinaceous deposits. Among the soft contact lenses with hydrophilic surfaces, the extent of deposits differs among various groups. For example, Group-4 lenses, which exhibit considerable negative charges due to methacrylic acid content, interact readily and heavily with a positively charged protein (lysozyme). Group-2 hydrogel lenses have no ionic charges, but can acquire substantial amounts of protein because of their large pore size. Besides protein deposits, lipid deposits are also found on contact lenses. These deposits are more common with rigid gas-permeable lenses because of their lipophilic nature. Such deposits may include cholesterol esters, wax esters, triglycerides, sterols, fatty acids, etc. Calcium present in tears results in calcium carbonate or phosphate-type of deposits as well as so-called mixed deposits (calcium bonded to organic compounds). Such deposits are common mainly in high water content soft contact lenses and are difficult to remove without damaging the contact lenses. Other deposits result from the patient environment. These include deposits resulting from cosmetics, make-up, and hair-spray, as well as materials from the wearing environment such as pollen dust and debris.

Table 1 Daily cleaners with shearing particles

Trade name	Manufacturer	Type of particle	Used with
OPTI-CLEAN	Alcon	Nylon	Soft, PMMA, RGP
OPTI-CLEAN II	Alcon	Nylon	Soft, PMMA, RGP
OPTI-FREE daily cleaner	Alcon	Nylon	Soft, PMMA, RGP
Boston cleaner	Polymer technology	Silica	PMMA, RGP
Boston advance cleaner	Polymer technology	Silica	PMMA, RGP

Problems associated with lens deposits

Cleaning is one of the most important steps in contact lens care. It helps in the removal of surface debris and contaminating microorganisms, thus facilitating the disinfection process. Improperly cleaned lenses can cause discomfort, red eye, decrease in visual acuity, and giant papillary conjunctivitis (GPC). The last often requires discontinuance of lens wear, at least until the symptoms clear. The change from heat to cold disinfection technology and the introduction of disposable lenses may have reduced the incidence of GPC. However, since these lenses can be worn on an extended basis for up to seven days without cleaning, GPC can still occur, as has been noted in the literature.

Classification of Lens Cleaners

Daily cleaners versus weekly cleaners

Daily cleaners generally contain surfactants and are used every day. They may also contain abrasive (deposit-shearing) particles, which enhance product performance. Commonly used daily cleaners with deposit shearing particles are listed in Table 1.

There are two types of weekly cleaners: those containing enzymes and those containing concentrated surfactants. Products containing enzymes for daily use are usually accepted by the patients and recommended by practitioners. Commonly used enzymatic products are listed in Table 2.

In-the-eye versus out-of-the-eye cleaners

Most of the cleaners marketed are out-of-the-eye cleaners; however, in recent years there has been a trend to try to develop cleaners for use while the lenses are inserted. A specific instance where such products could be beneficial is the case of the extended-wear lenses, which are not removed daily but are worn up to a week at a time. Generally, these cleaners are less effective in removing deposits already formed on the lens surface. However, they may play a role in retarding deposit formation.

Consumer versus professional use cleaners

Cleaners for lens wearers are used either on a daily or weekly basis and are fairly innocuous. Even upon gross misuse, they are not likely to be sight-threatening. Professional cleaners, however, are potent as well as toxic if not used properly. They are also more likely to damage the lens if used too frequently.

Active Components of Lens Cleaners

Surfactants

Surfactants are broadly classified into nonionic, anionic, cationic, and amphoteric types. Nonionic and amphoteric surfactants are most commonly used in contact lens cleaners, because strong anionic surfactants are generally toxic to the cornea. The recommended procedure by the manufacturer removes several types of deposits, except the most tenaciously bound and denatured proteins, lipids, and mucins. Surfactant-type cleaners are also effective in removing greater than 99.9% of microorganisms contaminating the lens. There are several mechanisms for their effectiveness, which include displacement of contaminants from the surface by mechanical force after the surface debris has been loosened as a result of a reduction in the interfacial tension. In addition, surfactants act by emulsification and micellar solubilization. They may also play a role in preventing or retarding deposition of contaminants.

Enzymes

Enzymes are biochemical molecules responsible for catalyzing reactions in which certain chemical bonds are broken. Their mechanism of action in cleaning involves attacking substrate protein, lipid, and mucin deposits, and fragmenting them into smaller molecules which are readily removed by the mechanical action of rubbing with the fingers and rinsing. Marketed products contain different enzymes, such as papain, pancreatin, and subtilisin. Papain and subtilisin are only proteolytic in nature, whereas pancreatin is a broad-spectrum enzyme

Table 2 Enzymatic products for contact lenses

Trade name	Manufacturers	Enzyme	Source	Dosage form
OPTI-FREE enzymatic cleaner	Alcon	Pancreatin	Mammals	Tablet
OPTI-ZYME enzymatic cleaner	Alcon	Pancreatin	Mammals	Tablet
SupraClens daily protein remover	Alcon	Pancreatin	Mammals	Liquid
Allergan enzymatic contact lens cleaner	Allergan	Papain	Plant	Tablet
ProFree/GP weekly enzymatic cleaner	Allergan	Papain	Plant	Tablet
Ultrazyme enzymatic cleaner	Allergan	Subtilisin-A	Microrganisms	Tablet
ReNu effervescent enzymatic cleaner	Bausch & Lomb	Subtilisin	Microrganisms	Tablet
ReNu thermal enzymatic cleaner	Bausch & Lomb	Subtilisin	Microgranisms	Tablet
Sensitive eyes enzymatic cleaner	Bausch & Lomb	Subtilisin	Microrganisms	Tablet

containing protease, lipase, and amylase enzymes that digest proteins, lipids, and mucins. Enzyme cleaners are effective in attacking all lens proteins, including the removal of tenaciously bound and denatured deposits, that cannot be removed by surfactant cleaners. Traditional enzymatic cleaning of contact lenses is recommended usually once a week. The soaking time varies from 15 min to overnight, followed by a disinfection process. However, more recently products have been introduced that can be used simultaneously during disinfection on a daily process. Certain enzyme products are recommended for this single-step cleaning and disinfection, using a heat or chemical regimen that enhances convenience and increases user compliance.

Oxidizing agents

Oxidizing agents such as sodium perborate and sodium percarbonate have also been used in cleaning contact lenses. None of these products are currently marketed for that purpose in the United States. Products marketed earlier were withdrawn because of their deleterious effects on lens polymers.

Deposit-shearing particles

Deposit-shearing particles are incorporated in suspension form in some daily cleaners. These formulations are more effective than daily surfactant cleaners as they are capable of removing tenaciously bound and denatured deposits. Some of the marketed products contain polymeric beads or silica. When used as recommended, these products are very effective and do not scratch the lens surface.

Chelating agents

Chelating agents such as disodium edetate (EDTA) are commonly used in lens care products to enhance the antimicrobial activity of preservatives and remove calcium and magnesium from the lens. EDTA is the most effective chelating agent known for calcium and magnesium. Other chelating agents have been used such as phosphonates, which are most effective against iron.

Solvents

Solvents such as isopropyl alcohol have been incorporated in daily cleaners to aid in removing lipid type of deposits. Such solvents have been reported to affect certain lens materials, especially silicone acrylate rigid gas-permeable lenses.

Accessory Cleaning Products

Hand soaps

In the daily care of contact lenses, wearers are instructed to clean their hands with soap and to dry hands their hands with lint-free towels prior to handling their lenses. Selection of the specific soap product is important. In addition, to cleaning the hands thoroughly, it should be rinsing and should not cause ocular irritation even if residual amounts are transferred to the lens. With these considerations in mind, some hand soaps have, therefore, been designed specifically for contact lens users.

Cleaning devices

The general method of daily lens cleaning involves rubbing lenses between the index finger and thumb or placing the lens in the palm of the hand and rubbing with the index finger after applying cleaning solution to the surface. However, there are also special devices available in the market for cleaning lenses. They are said to clean lenses more effectively and avoid potential scratching by the fingers. These devices involve mechanical agitation and are manually or electrically operated. Ultrasound devices have been used mainly by lens practitioners in their office. None of those devices per se are effective in removing tenaciously bound, denatured deposits.

PRODUCTS FOR DISINFECTING CONTACT LENSES

Disinfection of contact lenses is an important step in preventing ocular irritation, red eye, and potential loss of eyesight due to corneal ulcers resulting especially from *Pseudomonas aeruginosa* infections. The pore openings of hydrophilic soft contact lenses are estimated to be between 3.0 and 7.0 nm, and are considerably smaller than the average bacterial particle size of 0.2–1.0 μm or fungus particle size of 2–6 μm. Even viruses ranging in particle size from 25 to 200 nm are large in size compared to the pore openings of soft lenses. None of the microorganisms can penetrate an intact lens matrix. However, when lenses are not properly cared for, some fungus growth facilitates the penetration of fungal hyphae into the matrix.

Contact lenses and their cases are frequently contaminated by microbes. Although studies have indicated that as many at 30% of lens cases are contaminated, the incidence of permanent ocular damage due to this is very low. Nevertheless, it is critical to properly instruct lens wearers and emphasize the importance of disinfection in order to avoid the potential risk of ocular infection or damage to the eyesight.

Thermal Versus Chemical Disinfection

Both thermal and chemical methods are commonly used for the disinfection of soft contact lenses. With the former, a case containing the lenses immersed in saline solution is heated by an electrical unit with a predesigned heating cycle. The current FDA requirement for thermal disinfection by saline solution requires a minimum temperature of 80°C for 10 min within the contact lens case. This ensures elimination of vegetative forms of ocular pathogens but not the spores.

The chemical method involves antimicrobial compounds with an adequate antimicrobial spectrum and biocidal action. The FDA guidelines include the methods for determination of efficacy for all disinfecting solutions. The initial testing process is defined as the elimination or reduction of microorganisms achieved over the disinfection period. The FDA guidelines also provide a method for manufacturers to conduct use tests on purposely contaminated contact lenses, following a complete disinfection regimen, which includes cleaning and rinsing. This test is generally known as the FDA regimen test. The FDA guidelines specify the types and levels of organisms as well as the details of the test. Other methods using ultraviolet light, microwave, and ultrasonics, have been tried for lens disinfection but are not widely applied because of ineffectiveness or deleterious effects on lens materials.

The advantage of the thermal method is that it ensures complete elimination of vegetative forms of microorganisms, whereas chemical disinfectants may encounter some resistant organisms. Although the thermal method is preferable from the microbiological viewpoint, it has several disadvantages: It is a complex method involving the use of electrical devices. The failure of an electrical heating unit to perform properly presents a potential risk of ocular infection. Malfunctioning units and improper use may result in electrical shock to users and fires have been reported. If the saline solution in the lens container evaporates during the heating cycle as a result of carelessness in not properly tightening the lens case cap, the lens might be damaged. Thermal disinfection has been cited in shortening lens life and enhancing the formation of deposits on the surface. This occurs especially if the lens has not been properly cleaned prior to thermal disinfection. The method is not practical for campers who are frequently without an electrical outlet.

Chemical disinfection, on the other hand, is not as effective in killing organisms as thermal disinfection, but has several advantages: It is simple to use, thereby ensuring greater user compliance. Lens life is longer with chemical disinfection as lenses are not subjected to daily heat treatment. The method results in fewer deposit problems as surface debris left on the lens surface due to improper cleaning is not baked by heat.

The choice between thermal and chemical disinfection depends, to a large extent, on the recommendation of the lens practitioners. Factors involved include the wearer's sensitivity to preservatives, needs, personal hygiene habits, and product cost. Today fewer heat disinfection units are available.

Thermal Disinfection

Soft contact lenses were introduced in the United States in 1972. At that time, the thermal disinfection method was the only method available. It uses either preserved or unpreserved saline solution.

Unpreserved versus preserved saline solutions

Prior to the commercial availability of pharmaceutically prepared saline solutions, they were prepared by the lens wearer using salt tablets and distilled water. This method was undesirable and created many problems as the pH and osmolarity of such solutions were not controlled, which often resulted in parameter changes in some soft lenses. The major problem stemmed from noncompliance.

In order to reduce cost, tap water was often used instead of distilled water for preparing saline solutions, which resulted in mineral deposits on the lens surface. Microorganisms proliferated in nonsterile saline solution prepared with distilled water stored for a number of days and instilled in eyes directly to hydrate contact lenses while they were worn. Such gross misuses resulted in ocular infection affecting vision. By the mid-1980s products label and package inserts warned against the use of tap water for contact lens care. In the mid-1970s, pharmaceutically prepared sterile saline solution preserved with thimerosal was introduced to eliminate the disadvantages of home-made saline. However, thimerosal often caused a brownish and grayish lens discoloration and also led to red-eye and sensitization reactions in some patients. Soon after the introduction of pharmaceutically prepared preserved saline solutions, most salt tablets were withdrawn from the market. They were, however, reintroduced because of the red-eye and sensitization problems associated with thimerosal-preserved salines. In 1987, the FDA asked companies marketing salt tables for their voluntary withdrawal because of several incidences of keratitis caused by *Acanthamoeba* species, resulting in significant loss of vision or eyesight of several lens wearers. Most of these cases were associated with the use of salt tablets to prepare home-made saline solution.

In the United States today saline solutions are marketed in preserved and unpreserved forms; both are sterile and pharmaceutically prepared. The unpreserved solutions are available in unit dose or multidose plastic containers and multidose aerosols. In the latter instance, the pressurized container and the construction of the valve prevents innoculation of microorganisms into the container during its use, thus maintaining sterility more effectively in comparison to multidose nonpreserved saline solution in plastic containers. Nonpreserved saline solution in an aerosol container is, therefore, preferred over nonpreserved saline solution because it eliminates the potential of irritation and sensitization reactions caused by thimerosal and sorbic acid preserved salines. Such reactions may result in considerable patient discomfort and require temporary discontinuance of lens wear. However, the newer preservatives Polyquad and Dymed do not cause significant levels of such reactions. The disadvantage of unpreserved saline solution in unit dose is higher cost. There is also a potential risk of ocular infection as it is a common practice among lens wearers to leave their lenses in a lens case containing an unpreserved saline for several weeks, often without appropriate disinfection. Unpreserved saline does not protect against proliferation of microorganisms.

In contrast, preserved saline helps to prevent microbial growth when lenses are not worn and stored in lens cases. They are also less costly in comparison to unit dose or multidose pressurized nonpreserved saline solution containers. As already noted, the principal disadvantage of preserved saline solution is that some of the preservatives, such as thimerosal and sorbic acid, have the potential of causing irritation and sensitization in some patients. However, these reactions are not sight-threatening. In most instances these symptoms clear on discontinuance of the product without requiring any drug therapy. Again, this problem now appears to have been eliminated or greatly minimized with the introduction of newer preservatives such as Polyquad and Dymed.

Both preserved and unpreserved saline solutions are multifunctional solutions. In addition to thermal disinfection, they are also used to dissolve enzyme tablets in cleaning contact lenses, as a rinsing solution following cleaning and chemical disinfection, and as a lens storage solution.

Thermal disinfecting units

The FDA guidelines require that thermal disinfecting units must attain a minimum temperature of 80°C for 10 min in the saline solution, which is placed in the lens cases. There are several units on the market, which meet these requirements; they vary in their time–temperature profiles. Certain lenses such as those belonging to the FDA Group-4 classification (ionic, high-water-content lenses) do not withstand repeated heat treatment and tend to discolor. In general, FDA Group-4 lenses are not heat disinfected. Units on the market today have a thermostat, which cuts off the electrical current when a certain temperature is reached, eliminating the need for patients to switch it off. However, malfunctioning of units occasionally does occur.

Units on the market today are much different from those available earlier. The first unit was analogous to a "baby bottle warmer." Lenses were placed in a lens case, which was placed in a reservoir of water in an electrical heating unit. The temperature in the reservoir reached almost the boiling point of water and the time for disinfection was 30 min. To ensure not only disinfection but also sterilization of lenses, a unit was introduced capable of achieving 120°C for 20 min to ensure complete elimination of vegetative organisms as well as spores. This unit, however, was not successful since the high temperature was detrimental to many lens polymers. The current trend is toward developing a heating unit, which reaches temperatures below 80°C but ensures elimination of vegetative forms of ocular pathogens.

Chemical Disinfecting Agents (Oxidizing and Nonoxidizing)

There are two categories of chemical disinfecting solutions: The first category comprises those containing nonoxidizing chemical antimicrobial agents, which are nontoxic at the concentration level used in the products. The second category constitutes those containing oxidizing agents, which are toxic at the level used for disinfection but are degraded to a nontoxic level during the disinfection process over a course of time or by use of a second step that involves a neutralizing ingredient. Disinfecting solutions containing oxidizing agents (specifically hydrogen peroxide) gained popularity among lens practitioners in the mid- to late-1980s because of the absence of traditional preservatives, which often caused red eye and delayed hypersensitivity. However, the neutralizing solution used with hydrogen peroxide often contains preservatives that can cause ocular reactions. Lens practitioners liked the concept of hydrogen peroxide decomposing to innocuous water and oxygen. Fewer reactions have been observed with such products, but the long term toxic effects on the eye of the free radicals which are generated by low concentrations of undergraded oxidizing agents are not well known. Hydrogen peroxide products can cause severe toxic reactions if the products are not used properly and the patient inserts a lens without neutralizing the hydrogen peroxide.

The ideal chemical disinfecting agent should possess the following properties: It should have excellent wearer's acceptance in terms of being nonirritating, nonsensitizing, and easy to use. It should be relatively nontoxic compared to the earlier preservatives in terms of cytotoxicity, including its effects on epithelial and endothelial cells as well as its ability to maintain mitotic activity of corneal epithelial cells. It must have an adequate antimicrobial spectrum and be able to eliminate ocular pathogens in short lens-soaking regimens. It should not bind or bind minimally to the lens surface. It should be compatible with the lens and not cause discoloration or alter the tint of colored contact lenses.

A hydrogen peroxide disinfection system for soft lenses was tried initially in the early 1970s. The system failed to gain FDA approval because of the potential toxic nature of the chemical, the complexity of several steps, and the cost. The system was approved by the FDA in the early 1980s after having undergone significant refinements compared to the original system.

All products currently marketed in the United States under the oxidizing agent category contain hydrogen peroxide. In the international market, products containing chlorine-releasing agents are also available. These products are generally indicated for the disinfection of hydrophilic soft contact lenses and are contraindicated for rigid gas-permeable lenses. Most of the hydrogen peroxide is decomposed by catalytic degradation (platinum ring); chemical neutralization using pyruvate, sodium bisulfite, or sodium thiosulfate; dilution and rinsing; and enzymatic neutralization (catalase).

Hydrogen peroxide, on degradation, forms water and oxygen and, hence, it is perceived by practitioners as a superior product. However, most of the neutralizers used in the second step contain preservatives such as thimerosal and sorbic acid, and stabilizers such as stannates or phosphonates. Consequently, they have the associated disadvantages of those ingredients. On the other hand, not having a preservative in a neutralizer makes these products vulnerable to microbial growth on accidental contamination. A single-step product containing hydrogen peroxide is also available on the market, which is convenient, but has the same disadvantage of not having any preservative effect at the end of the disinfection cycle. The disinfecting time recommended by various companies ranges from 10 min to an overnight soak. This category of disinfecting agents has a better antimicrobial spectrum and a faster kill rate. However, their shortcomings included toxicity if the regimen was not followed properly, complexity of use, and zero to minimal protection against microbial recontamination once the disinfection cycle was complete.

The first generation nonoxidizing chemical disinfection solution contained a combination of antimicrobial agents incorporating thimerosal with chlorhexidine or alkyltriethanol ammonium chloride. These solutions are now not commonly used because of the thimerosal problems as discussed previously. The newer antimicrobial agents, Polyquad and Dymed, because of their molecular structure and large molecule size have a better profile. These antimicrobial agents were introduced in the late 1980s and their long-term use has not caused reactions similar to those observed for older antimicrobial agents. Products with these agents currently dominate the lens care market.

PRODUCTS FOR ENHANCING SOFT CONTACT LENS WEAR COMFORT

Factors Contributing to Wear Comfort

It has already been noted that hydrogel contact lenses are inherently more comfortable that rigid (RGP or PMMA) lenses. This is related to the former's superior flexibility and hydrophilic character which permits incorporation of substantial amounts of water (38–74%) into the lens material. However, after periods of wear time, some lenses may experience changes in hydration, that may be related to deposits, environmental (e.g., temperature and humidity) changes and improper care. In particular, "dry spots" may become evident on the lens with attendant reduction in comfort and visual acuity. When this happens, the wearer may benefit from periodic administration of rewetting (or soothing or comfort) solutions onto the lens while being worn. These solutions are usually low-viscosity aqueous compositions containing polymers or surfactants, which enhance the wettability of the surface, facilitating the spreading tears, and enhancing the stability of the tear film. They may also provide cushioning and lubricating actions, lessening impact, and reducing the frictional forces of the eyelids as they move across the lens on the corneal surface. The frictional forces would be especially important in instances where deposits or debris on the lens are present in sufficient amounts to cause physical irritation to the ocular tissue. In addition to wetting, cushioning, and lubricating, the ability of the solutions to facilitate removal of contaminants and retard further soilage are also desirable attributes. It is also desirable, in terms of convenience to the lens wearer, that the frequency of administration of drops of the above-mentioned types be minimal. Therefore, the use of polymers and surfactants that associate with the (deposited) lens and resist removal by the rinsing action of the tears is called for (i.e., polymers and surfactants with good substantivity).

Although rewetting efficacy is usually the primary requirement for hydrogel lens wearers, all three actions (rewetting, cushioning, and lubrication) may be of considerable significance for RGP or PMMA lens wearers. The practitioner should seek to help the wearer find the product best suited for his or her specific comfort needs. Solutions designed for hydrogel lenses generally have lower viscosities, whereas solutions for rigid hard lenses usually have higher viscosities. Although high viscosities can be of distinct benefit in enhancing cushioning action, a solution that is too viscous can cause blurred vision and hinder normal lid movement to an undesirable extent.

Components of Lens Comfort Solutions

Among the polymers used in lens comfort solutions are polyvinyl alcohol, polyvinylpyrrolidone, dextran, and various cellulose derivatives such as hydroxyethyl cellulose, hydroxypropyl cellulose, and hydroxypropyl methylcellulose. Surfactants include certain poloxamer and poloxamine compounds. Other normal components comprise appropriate preservative(s) as well as buffering and tonicity-adjusting agents.

LENS CARE PRODUCTS FOR RIGID GAS-PERMEABLE LENSES

Several types of RGP lenses are marketed (Table 2) and others are under development. Because of their rigid nature, they have certain characteristics in common with conventional hard PMMA lenses. In many cases, care products available for use with the latter have been found to be also suitable for the care of the RGP lenses. Although they may not have optimal characteristics, they are still preferred by many practitioners in comparison to products that were originally designed for use with soft lenses and were subsequently approved by the FDA also for use with RGP materials.

Most categories of products indicated for the care of soft contact lenses are applicable to rigid gas-permeable lenses. These include daily cleaners, wetting and cushioning drops, and weekly enzymatic cleaners. While disinfecting solutions are necessary for RGP lens care, they are often positioned as conditioning solutions. Conditioning is important in providing a hydrophilic lens surface during wear. Because RGP lenses do not withstand heat, saline solutions (both preserved and unpreserved) are not needed for these lenses, except for dissolving enzymatic cleaners for weekly cleaning or rinsing.

Because RGP lenses are not as porous or water absorbing as soft lenses, wearers do not experience the problems that are specific to soft lenses, resulting from preservatives penetrating and concentrating within the lens polymer matrix, which often cause toxic and hypersensitivity-type reactions. However, certain preservatives bind with RGP surfaces and can create clinical problems. Binding may involve ionic and/or hydrophobic interactions.

In addition to accumulation of proteinaceous deposits, such as those occurring on soft hydrophilic lenses, the molecular make-up of many RGP lenses also tends to attract lipid deposits, such as cholesterol esters, wax esters, triglycerides, etc. This is especially true of the more hydrophobic materials such as silicone acrylates with high Dk (oxygen permeability) values. Accordingly, more recent developments in material science related to contact lenses have resulted in materials such as fluorosilicone acrylates and fluorocarbons with purportedly less propensity for deposits.

Wearing rigid lenses is much less comfortable than wearing soft contact lenses. In fact, this is generally perceived to be the major factor limiting the growth of the RGP lens market segment. Consequently, the need for superior wetting, cushioning, and lubricating products is clearly recognized. Superior combination products are also required for RGP lenses, which provide convenience and enhance product performance.

MULTIPURPOSE SOLUTIONS

Multipurpose solutions are designed to increase wearer compliance and the convenience of product use. Such solutions are not commonly used for the conventional PMMA hard lenses and rigid gas-permeable lenses. They combine two or more basic functions of lens care, including cleaning, disinfection, soaking, wetting, and lubricating. Combination of these functions in a single product may compromise certain aspects of product efficacy. For instance, a solution designed to clean and disinfect may not clean as well the cleaner would alone. However, a combination cleaning and disinfection solution provides the convenience of a single step and would be particularly useful for wearers whose lenses do not attract deposits as readily because of their tear chemistry.

Multipurpose solutions for soft lenses are primarily limited to cleaning and disinfecting. Wetting and lubricating combinations are not a major need because of the inherent hydrophilic nature of soft lenses that makes them comfortable to wear. The technology advances made in identifying preservatives with broader spectrum and capacity along with the ability of chemicals to clean while disinfecting has further simplified care of lenses. Recently, a new product has been developed in a multipurpose solution format that has allowed removal of the rubbing step.

PACKAGING OF CONTACT LENS PRODUCTS

All lens care products are packaged in plastic containers or pressurized metal containers with the exception of enzymatic or disinfecting tablets. The tablets are generally effervescent and packaged in laminated foil or blister packs to ensure adequate shelf life. The packaging materials normally used by the pharmaceutical industry for effervescent tablets are adequate for this purpose. The plastic containers are usually fabricated from low-density polyethylene, high-density polyethylene, or polypropylene materials. Many of the containers are opaque for protection against light. Several types of colorant mixtures, which usually contain titanium, are used in squeeze bottles, and the composition and thickness of the container wall should be designed to allow easy delivery. Another important

consideration is the orifice at the tip, which allows the desired product to flow. For instance, a disinfecting or saline solution needs to be delivered in a large volume of 3 to 5 ml to fill the lens case. A steady stream is desirable and acceptable here, but not for products like wetting, lubricating, and cushioning drops, which are directly instilled in the eye. For these products, the tip has to be designed to allow drop-by-drop instillation. Formulation characteristics such as viscosity and surface tension determine the tip design. The tip must be smooth and rounded as it can come into contact with the eye. The caps for the bottle are normally constructed of polystyrene or polypropylene material.

Because all lens care products, with the exception of the tablet dosage form, have to be sterile, the containers must be sterilized prior to filling unless the process involves form, fill, and seal technology. Containers are usually sterilized by ethylene oxide or gamma irradiation. The latter method is preferred because of stringent government regulations and requirements regarding ethylene oxide residues and its degradation products. Recent years have also seen strict controls regarding the exposure of workers to ethylene oxide and its by-products. Terminal sterilization of the final product is normally not done for lens care products, with the exception of nonpreserved saline solutions in aerosol containers, which are sterilized by gamma irradiation.

ACCESSORY CONTACT LENS PRODUCTS

Accessory contact lens products include cases and devices for cleaning contact lenses and facilitating insertion.

Lens Cases

Lens cases are utilized for disinfection and storage while the lenses are not being worn. Lens cases may have a single compartment with a barrel shape, generally holding 7 to 10 ml of solution, or they may have two compartments in a flat case design, each compartment holding 3 to 5 ml of solution. Lens cases are also used by lens manufacturers as mailers to ship RGP and PMMA lenses in the dry state. Recently, shipping the lenses in conditioning solution has been approved. On the other hand, hydrophilic soft contact lenses are generally shipped in sealed sterile glass vials containing buffered isotonic saline solution. Plastic lens cases are fabricated from polymeric materials such as polyethylene, polypropylene, polysulfone, or polycarbonate.

Devices Facilitating Cleaning

Cleaning devices are useful for lens wearers who lack the manual dexterity to clean lenses with their fingers. They are also used for cleaning lenses that could be scratched easily by fingertips. The consumer versions provide mechanical action by manual swirling or by agitation with the help of an electrical motor or sonication The professional versions are usually ultrasonic-type devices. None of these devices are capable of removing tenaciously bound protein. The reservoir of the cleaning device is filled with special cleaning fluid or a saline with a few drops of a surfactant-type daily lens cleaner. The device should allow easy lens placement and retrieval and minimize the potential of damage. Lens baskets that allow for rinsing after the cleaning regimen without additional handling are a desirable feature.

Devices Facilitating Lens Insertion

These devices are generally helpful to elderly patients, especially those wearing aphakic lenses. They consist usually of a rubber bulb with a suction cup. They can cause severe corneal damage if used improperly as well as ocular infection if they are not properly cleaned and disinfected.

Future Directions in Lens Care Products

Of the persons fitted with contact lenses (both soft and hard), 40% discontinue wearing them within the first three years. One of the reasons cited is the time and effort required in taking care of them. Therefore, lens care systems will be developed that are simple and more convenient to use, requiring fewer products, and less time. The new products will minimize patient problems through safer preservatives, which are nontoxic even on misuse and do not produce hypersensitization. More effective cleaners as well as products which minimize protein and microbial attachment to lens surfaces will also be forthcoming as well as cleaners that can be instilled in the eye during lens wear to retard deposit formation on extended-wear lenses or to clean lenses while they are being worn. Other future product types may include special artificial tears and comfort drops for older patients who are prone to dry eye. There is also a need for diagnostic products that can detect potential problems before they are manifested clinically. Universal products that could be used with all contact lenses (i.e., hard PMMA, RGP, and soft lenses) may be desirable; however, it is unlikely that such products will be available as different contact lenses vary significantly in their chemical and surface characteristics. The main emphasis in the future will be on the development of convenient, easy-to-use products that can increase patient compliance and reduce the dropout rate, while ensuring desirable efficacy without compromising product safety. Products specifically designed for the care of disposable and frequent replacement lenses will also be forthcoming.

COMPONENTS OF LENS CARE PRODUCTS

Active Components

Active components play a primary role in the intended use of a product. The active components in lens care products are usually limited to either one or two chemical entities. However, a product may contain several active components if it is designed for multiple functions or indications.

Chemicals with disinfecting capability

Active chemical entities must have bactericidal and fungistatic properties. However, cidal properties for fungal organisms is preferable. The product performance criteria encompassing the types of organisms to be tested, levels of inoculum, and method of testing are defined by guidelines developed by the FDA. Current chemical systems have disinfection times of 4–6 h. This fits with most wearing schedules, because more than 90% of patients remove their lenses overnight between wear periods. Overnight removal seems to help the eye recover from the stress of lens wear. Recently, some efforts to move to shorter disinfection time are under way to increase convenience. The products will require dramatically enhanced disinfection efficacy than currently available or strict compliance to a regimen to achieve the required level of disinfection.

Surface-active and other agents with cleaning capability

Surfactants of various types have been traditionally used for cleaning conventional PMMA hard lenses. They are considered effective in removing surface deposits on these lenses, such as cosmetics, hair spray, mascara, etc. However, they are not effective in removing tenaciously bound deposits (e.g., proteins, lipids, lipoproteins, mucoproteins) that are commonly encountered with soft hydrophilic contact lenses and rigid gas-permeable lenses. Such deposits are more effectively removed by products containing enzymes, strong oxidizing agents, or suspended abrasive (deposit-shearing) particles. The types of surfactants used and representative products on the market are discussed later under Products for

Cleaning Soft Contact Lenses. A few other agents such as citrate and some phosphates have been used as cleaning agents.

Components with wetting, lubricating, and cushioning capabilities

Polymers and surfactants are the two main classes of compounds used as wetting, lubricating, and cushioning agents. Contingent on the nature of the specified polymers, they are used in various combinations to achieve desired product characteristics.

Both synthetic and natural polymers are commonly used in lens care products. These agents can provide a cushioning effect as a result of increased viscosity. The need for products with such action is greater for the wearers of conventional hard PMMA lenses and rigid gas-permeable lenses, for these are inherently not as comfortable as soft contact lenses because of the lens design and the physiochemical nature of the polymers. Viscosity-building agents provide the necessary initial coatings on the lens surface before it is coated by natural tear components. Besides contributing to viscosity, the ability of polymers to adsorb on lens surfaces and to elicit surface-active (wetting) properties are important considerations.

Surface-active agents are adsorbed on the lens surface and allow ready spreading of tears when the lenses are inserted, thus making them more comfortable to wear. The use of surface-active agents to impart wettability to the lens surface is of lesser value for products used for hydrophilic soft contact lenses, which have built-in wetting characteristics because of their water content. Addition of surfactants may be of value, however, in retarding deposit formation or for cleaning while the lenses are worn. The methodology for measuring both advancing and receding contact angles, as an indication of wetting efficacy, has been standardized for contact lenses. Various polymers have different degrees of wettability as measured by contact angle using a goniometer. However, the in vitro contact-angle measurement of contact lenses made from various polymers is of little clinical value. No discernible differences in in vivo contact angle can be detected on insertion of a contact lens in the eye following a few blinks that result in coating the lens surface with tear components. Surfactants are usually combined with polymers to impart substantivity and cushioning characteristics. The types of polymers and surfactants used in representative products in the market are discussed later under Products for Enhancing Soft Contact Lens Wear Comfort. Again, the need for surface-active agents which can facilitate wetting of lenses and spreading of tears is greater for

PMMA and rigid gas-permeable lenses because of their hydrophobic surface characteristics.

Ancillary Components

Preservatives

Preservatives are used in almost all multidose contact lens products. Because the potential for misuse of products by lens wearers is significant, preservatives prevent the potential proliferation of microorganisms. A contaminated product could ultimately lead to an ocular infection and possible loss of eyesight. Preservatives are considered active components when incorporated in products for the purpose of disinfecting contact lenses. The preservative must possess the antimicrobial activity described in the FDA guidelines for contact lens care.

The FDA has issued guidelines for preservative efficacy, which include an additional safety factor to compensate for potential misuse of products. These requirements are more stringent than the requirements of the *United States Pharmacopeia* (USP) for preservative efficacy. The FDA requires rechallenging the preserved products on day 14 with a defined inoculum of microorganisms; this is not required by the USP. The preservatives generally used are mainly the same as those used for thermal or chemical disinfection of contact lenses. The concentrations could be different than in the chemical disinfection of contact lenses. The concentration is generally higher in cleaners and comfort-enhancing solutions because of possible binding with polymer and surfactant components, which result in a decrease in preservative efficacy.

Different countries have different standards for preserving contact lens solutions; the requirements of the *British Pharmacopoeia* are the most stringent. Many marketed products do not meet these requirements. The three major preservative efficacy tests, which must be considered in developing products, are delineated in the United States Pharmacopoeia (modified test to meet FDA guidelines), the *British Pharmacopoeia* and the *German Pharmacopoeia* (DAB). In terms of difficulty to comply, the *British Pharmacopoeia* test is the most stringent and the modified USP test the least stringent. The main differences among the test requirements are the exposure times and use of *Escherichia coli* as a challenge organism. The *British Pharmacopoeia* utilizes a 6-h criterion for antimicrobial activity, whereas the USP uses a 14-day criterion. Recently, an International Standard has been approved which is comparable to the US FDA procedure. The types of preservatives used are described in the tables related to various product categories.

Buffers for adjusting pH

The use of buffers and pH adjustment is an important consideration in lens care products. It is a general practice that all products which are likely to come in direct contact with ocular tissues should be buffered for ocular comfort around physiologic pH and preferably in the range 6–8.0. The most commonly used buffers in contact lens care products are phosphates and borates. Buffers used occasionally are acetate, citrate, and others. Besides buffers, sodium hydroxide and hydrochloric acid are generally used to achieve a desirable pH in the final product. They are also used to adjust the final pH in products, which do not have any buffering system. The selection of an appropriate buffering system should consider the pH necessary for optimal performance of the product, as well as products stability and potential incompatibility with other components of the product.

Although it is desirable to have a product as close to physiologic pH as possible, it is often essential to formulate a product outside the physiologic pH range in order to achieve the desired stability of the product, optimal efficacy, or appropriate solubility of active and ancillary components. Products formulated outside the physiologic pH range should have low buffer capacity to allow quick equilibration to tear pH by the bicarbonate buffer system present in the tears. The maintenance of pH close to physiologic pH is essential for products intended for soaking and disinfection of hydrophilic soft contact lenses in order to maintain the parameters of some lenses, especially those belonging to FDA Group 4. Such changes in parameters can cause not only discomfort but can also produce blurred vision.

Tonicity-adjusting agents

Contact lens products should be formulated as closely as possible to the tonicity of tears. This is important for optimal comfort. Prolonged exposure to hypotonic solutions can induce edema in corneal epithelial cells, which can cause blurred vision and discomfort, whereas prolonged exposure to hypertonic solutions can cause corneal epithelial cells to shrivel and cause discomfort by exposing nerve endings. None of the currently available contact lens solutions have been responsible for such symptoms as most of them are formulated close to isotonicity and many contact lens products have minimal contact with the cornea. Nevertheless, maintaining the tonicity of products close to the isotonic value of 280 ($\pm$50) mOsm/kg is important for optimal comfort as well as for maintaining the integrity of certain hydrophilic soft

contact lenses (especially those belonging to FDA Group 4). The type of compounds commonly used for imparting isotonicity include buffering agents, sodium chloride, potassium chloride, propylene glycol, mannitol, dextrose, etc.

Viscosity-building agents

Viscosity-building agents such as synthetic and natural polymers are used as active ingredients in solutions providing comfort and rewetting products. However, they are also used as ancillary agents in contact lens cleaning products. These agents allow better cleaning of contact lenses by enhancing the contact of the cleansing agent with the soiled lens and by facilitating the process of rubbing the lens between fingers or between the palm of the hand and an index finger. Highly viscous or gel-type cleaners are also available. However, they are not very popular as they are difficult to rinse and may cause ocular irritation. The types of polymers used as ancillary agents are the same as those used for solutions providing comfort or rewetting solutions.

PHARMACEUTICAL TECHNOLOGY CONSIDERATIONS IN PRODUCT DESIGN

With few exceptions, contact lens products are sterile solutions. The sterility requirements are important because of the potential of sight-threatening ocular infections. The sterility test procedures and pass–fail criteria as described in the *United States Pharmacopeia* must be met for FDA approval of contact lens products. The technology practiced in the development of pharmaceutical products, such as injectable and large volume intravenous fluids, is generally acceptable, with somewhat less stringent requirements for contact lens care products because most of these products do not come into direct contact with the eye (i.e., its interior cells and fluids). Products that are packaged in unit dose containers or multidose pressurized aerosol containers do not have to be preserved. However, multidose products other than aerosol containers should be preserved and should pass the FDA preservative efficacy test. Manufacturers intending to develop lens care products should consult with the FDA for the latest guidelines.

Apart from solutions, there are other pharmaceutical dosage forms for contact lens products that are less commonly used. They include gel- and suspension-type cleaners, powders, and tablet dosage forms for enzymatic cleaners or disinfectants. All of these products are formulated as sterile products with the exception of powders and tablets. These, however, must comply with

USP requirements for bioburden with added specifications for absence of colony-forming units of *Staphylococcus aureus* and *Pseudomonas aeruginosa* among other organisms. The choice of components in formulating these products is much more restrictive in comparison to pharmaceutical products intended for systemic or topical use because of the potential of causing irritation to the sensitive ocular tissues.

Chemical components must be nonirritating and compatible with ocular tissue as well as with lenses. The choice of components for tablets, such as binding and lubricating agents, is much more restrictive, as these ingredients must be soluble and form a clear solution when dissolved in saline solutions. Formulation components generally used and acceptable for ophthalmic products may be unacceptable for contact lens products, as many contact lens materials can concentrate components used in contact lens products as much as several hundredfold. On insertion of the lenses, these ingredients are released in toxic levels to the cornea, causing minor to severe ocular reactions. The binding and release of ingredients can be further complicated by the condition of the lens. For instance, thimerosal and chlorhexidine, commonly used ingredients in contact lens products, concentrate differently in new, deposit-free lenses as compared to used lenses with protein deposits on the surfaces. Appropriate studies must be designed to address these issues to minimize the potential of ocular irritation. Certain ingredients such as thimerosal, when used initially are well tolerated. However, on prolonged exposure, some lens wearers develop hypersensitivity, resulting in intolerance of thimerosal products. Such intolerance is difficult to predict and currently no satisfactory method is available to predict delayed hypersensitivity-type reactions, which are modulated immunologically. The commonly used guinea pig maximization test is not predictive of delayed hypersensitivity reactions.

As noted previously, formulating products close to physiological pH is desirable. However, for optimal product performance or meeting regulatory requirements, it is sometimes necessary to formulate products outside the physiologic pH range. Sorbic acid, a commonly used preservative for lens care products, is a marginally effective antimicrobial agent with a pKa value of 4.8. A product fails the FDA preservative efficacy test if it is formulated around a physiologic pH of 7–7.4 at a concentration of 0.1 sorbic acid normally used in marketed products. To maximize its antimicrobial activity without compromising ocular comfort to a significant extent, it is necessary to formulate such products around pH 6.5–6.8. Thus, a consideration of the dissociation constants of preservatives is essential as the antimicrobial activity of many preservatives depends on the undissociated species, which should be present in an adequate amount at physiological pH without causing ocular irritation.

The product design should also consider the nature of the lens polymer and its surface charges. For example, FDA Group-4 lenses, which carry negative surface charges, can react with positively charged product components, resulting in severe ocular toxic reactions. Such toxic reactions can be prevented by incorporating nonionic surfactants to form micelles with the cationic components, thus minimizing surface interactions and toxicity. If a cationic agent in the product is a primary disinfecting agent, efforts to minimize toxicity or surface interactions often result in reduced antimicrobial performance. It is, therefore, essential to minimize surface interactions and yet have a product, which meets the requirements for disinfection or preservation.

The hydrophilic–lipophilic balance (HLB) and molecular dimensions of a preservative should also be considered in the design of contact lens products. For example, chlorobutanol (a nonionic preservative used in ophthalmic products) penetrates into the matrix of rigid gas-permeable (RGP) lens materials because of the molecule's substantial lipophilic characteristics. The preservative present in the lens matrix may change the parameters or may be gradually released during wear, causing irritation and toxicity to the corneal cells. On the other hand, the molecular dimensions of a preservative are very important in designing a product for hydrophilic, soft contact lenses. Generally, preservatives with a high molecular weight and appropriate molecular configuration are less likely to penetrate the porous matrix of hydrogel lenses. Products containing preservatives like Dymed and Polyquad, with molecular weights above 1000, are currently available.

ACKNOWLEDGMENT

The authors wish to acknowledge the unstinting assistance of Cathy Hughes in the preparation of this article.

BIBLIOGRAPHY

Bailey, N.J. Contact Lens Spectrum **1987**, *2* (7), 6–31.
Bennett, E.S.; Grohe, R.M. *Rigid Gas-Permeable Contact Lenses*; Professional Press Books/Fairchild Publications: New York, 1986.
British Pharmacopoeia 1988; [Appendix SVIC (Efficacy of Antimicrobial Preservatives in Pharmaceutical Products)] Her Majesty's Stationery Office: London, 1988; 2, A200–A203.

Chowhan, M.; Bilbault, T.; Quintana, R.P.; Rosenthal, R.A. Contactologia **1993**, *15*, 190–195.

US Patent, 5,370,744, Alcon Laboratories, Inc.

CLMA Standards Subcommittee, Technical Affairs Committee (Q.A. Cappelli, chair). Industry Accepted Reference Procedure for Determining Wetting Angle **1979**, *4* (4), 35–39, Contact Lens Manufacturers Association (CLMA), Chicago [cf. *Contact Lens Forum*].

Dabezie, O.H., Jr. Ed. *Contact Lenses: The CLAO Guide to Basic Science and Clinical Practice*; Little, Brown and Company: Boston, 1989; 1 and 2.

Deutsches Arzneibuch; [Anhang VIII.N1 (Prufung auf ausreichende Konservierung)] 9. Ausgabe, Deutscher Apotheker Verlag: Stuttgart, 1986; 369–370.

Food and Drug Administration, Draft Testing Guidelines for Class III Soft (Hydrophilic) Contact Lens Solutions United States Food and Drug Administration, Silver Spring, MD, 1985.

Food and Drug Administration, Guidance Document for Class III Contact Lenses United States Food and Drug Adminstration, Silver Spring, MD, 1989.

Gossel, T.A.; Wuest, J.R. Contact Lenses and Lens Care Products. In *Handbook of Nonprescription Drugs*; Feldmann, E.G., Ed.; American Pharmaceutical Association: Washington, 1990, 601–631.

Harris, J.K. Solutions for Cleaning, Disinfection, and Storage. In *Contact Lenses*; Aquavella, J.V., Rao, G.N., Eds.; J.B. Lippincott Company: Philadelphia, 1987; 226–263.

Hartstein, J., Ed. *Extended Wear Lenses for Aphakia and Myopia*; The C.V. Mosby Company: St. Louis, 1982.

Hartstein, J.; Swanson, K.V.; Harris, C.R. *Contemporary Contact Lens Practice*; Mosby-Year Book, Inc.: St. Louis, 1991.

Holly, F.J., Ed. *The Preocular Tear Film in Health, Disease, and Contact Lens Wear*; Dry Eye Institute, Inc.: Lubbock Texas, 1986.

Houlsby, R.D.; Ghajar, M.; Chavez, G. J. Am. Optom. Assoc. **1988**, *59*, 184–188.

Kreiner, C.F. *Kontaktlinsen-Chemie*; Median-Verlag: Heidelberg, 1980.

Lippman, J.I. CLAO J. **1990**, *16*, 287–291.

Lowther, G.E. Preparations Used with Contact Lenses. In *Clinical Ocular Pharmacology*; Bartlett, J.D., Jaanus, S.D., Eds.; Butterworth's: Boston, 1989; 337–353.

MacKeen, D.L. Am. Pharm. **1986**, *NS26* (10), 27–31.

Mandell, R. *Contact Lens Practice*; Charles C. Thomas: Springfield, IL, 1981.

Philips, A.J., Stone, J., Eds. *Contact Lenses: A Textbook for Practitioner and Student*; Butterworth's: Boston, 1989.

Randeri, K.J.; Quintana, R.P.; Chowhan, M.A. Contact Lenses Cleaning. In *Contact Lenses: The CLAO Guide to Basic Science and Clinical Practice*; Kastl, P.R., Ed.; Kendall/Hunt Publishing Company: 1995; 215–236.

Ruben, M. *Color Atlas of Contact Lenses & Prosthetics*; The C.V. Mosby Company: St. Louis, 1989.

Tripathi, R.C.; Tripathi, B.J.; Silverman, R.A.; Rao, G.N. Int. Ophthalmol. Clin. **1991**, *31*, 91–120.

The United States Pharmacopoeia, 24, NF19; United States Pharmacopeial Convention, Inc.: Rockville, MD, 2000; 1809–1823.

White, P.; Scott, C. Contact Lenses & Solutions Summary. In *Supplement to Contact Lens Spectrum*; Viscom Publications, Inc.: Norwalk, CT, Feb. 1991.

Yeager, M.D.; Benjamin, W.J. Int. Contact Lens Clin. **1987**, *14* (8), 61.

LIPID EXCIPIENTS IN PHARMACEUTICAL DOSAGE FORMS

Alan L. Weiner

Alcon Research, Ltd., Fort Worth, Texas

L

THE ROLE OF LIPIDS

Biologically, lipids function as structural elements in plants and animals, transport vehicles, mediators of chemical reactions, energy sources, and as messenger molecules. It is from an understanding of these functions that lipids have been applied to pharmaceutical applications. Lipids can be appropriately manipulated to conform to various physical states such as solutions, suspensions, emulsions, creams, gels, or solids. Because a combined lipid–drug formulation will present a very different conformation and/or molecular size than the drug alone when introduced into a biological environment, changes in both the distribution and the recognition of the drug by the host defense system will occur. These changes may be either intended or undesired.

Overall, the uses of lipids in pharmaceutical dosage forms can be grouped into four categories: 1) improvement in the processing or stability of the formulation in the preferred physical state; 2) enhancement or reduction in cellular or systemic absorption of the drug from the formulation; 3) more effective drug targeting; and 4) sustained or more controlled delivery of the drug. In this article, the problems and opportunities in utilizing lipids for these applications will be explored from various aspects of pharmaceutical formulation, analysis methods, and other commercial issues.

CATEGORIES OF LIPIDS IN PHARMACEUTICAL PREPARATIONS

The principal material categories discussed in this article are illustrated in Fig. 1. Categories shown are: fatty chain acids, salts, alcohols or amines, oils and waxes, phospholipids, glycolipids, neutral lipids, and nonlinear chain compounds, such as sterols.

Fatty Acids and Derivatives

Fatty acids, salts, alcohols, and amines have been utilized in pharmaceutical formulations. Fatty acids are present in cosmetics, ointments, and suppositories and are used in tablet coating applications and as carriers in inhalant products. Fully saturated fatty acids are solid materials at chain lengths above eight, whereas longer chain polyunsaturated forms may exist as liquids, unless the double bonds are conjugated. Fatty acid salts are used widely in tableting applications and often include magnesium, calcium, and aluminum stearates. The handling properties and physical interaction with other solids make them ideal as conditioning agents to effect even distribution of particles, improve compressibility, and control the eventual release of active agent. The fatty alcohols, including cetyl and palmityl alcohol, are well known and are used extensively in ointments or creams as an emollient or emulsion modifier. Fatty amines are generally utilized as precursor compounds in coupling reactions to produce lipophilic drug derivatives. Fatty amines, like the acids, are solid at higher chain lengths and insoluble in aqueous solution. Finally, aldehydes of fatty chain compounds have application in fragrances and flavorings. The unsaturated liquid forms of fatty aldehydes are most often employed.

Oils, Waxes, and Neutral Lipids

Fatty acids, when esterified to glycerol, form mono-di-and triglycerides. Depending on the number of substituted fatty acids, the carbon chain lengths and the unsaturation level, the resultant product may exist in either liquid state (oil) or solid state (wax). Products in this category may either be naturally derived or synthetically produced and, thus, a wide diversity of products is commercially available. Oils have drug-carrying and solubilization functions in oral, topical, or injectable products. Waxes are presently used in topical and oral preparations to improve desired physical properties and control dissolution of the final product. Common materials in this group that are present in commercialized pharmaceutical preparations include castor oil, hydrogenated vegetable oil wax, paraffin, carnauba wax, white wax, olive oil and olive oil ethyl ester, mineral oil, petrolatum, cetyl ester wax, and beeswax. Neutral lipids, such as steroids, are also of value in pharmaceutical practices. For example, cholesterol and cholesterol esters can be exploited to broaden liposome phase transitions and to allow easier manipulation and or emulsification.

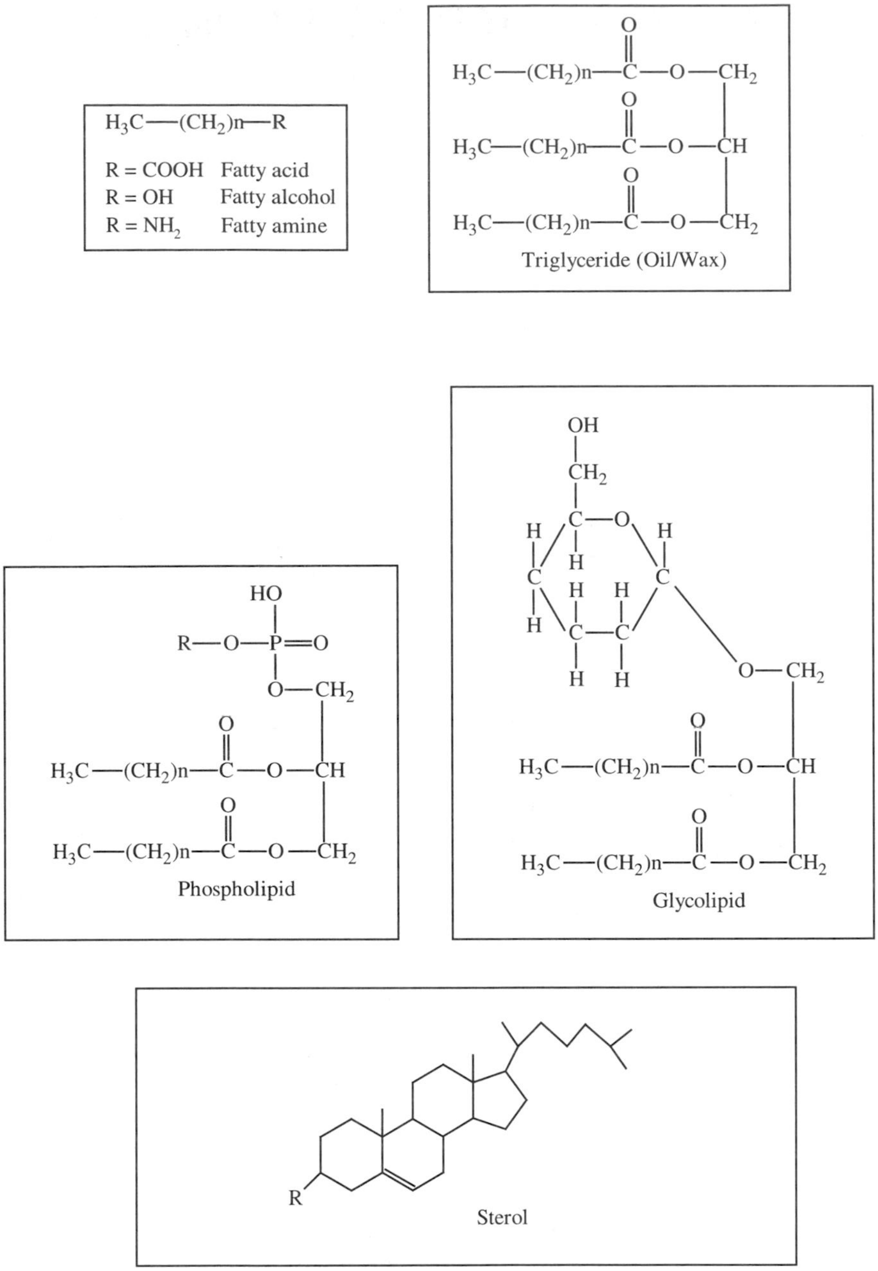

Fig. 1 Lipid structures.

Phospholipid Compounds

The complexity of glycerides advances by modification of the terminal hydroxyl with phosphate linked head groups to form phospholipids. Common phospholipid head groups include choline, ethanolamine, serine, inositol and inositol phosphates, glycerol, and glycerol esters. As with the triglycerides, numerous species are possible by various combinations of different headgroups and fatty acyl substitution at the 1st and 2nd positions of the glycerol backbone. Fluidity differences are evident as a function of the gel to liquid crystalline transition temperatures (Table 1). Solubility of phospholipids is intimately linked to the conformation of the aggregate material rather than strictly a chemical function of the molecule. Monoacyl phospholipids, which tend to form micelles, are usually more readily

Table 1 Transition temperatures of common phospholipids

Head group	Fatty acid component	Transition temperature (°C)
Hydrogen (phosphatidic acid)	Dimyristoyl	51
	Dipalmitoyl	67
Choline	Dioleoyl	−22
	Natural (mixed unsaturated)	−15
	Dilauryloyl	−1.8
	Dimyristoyl	23
	Dipalmitoyl	41
	Distearoyl	55
Ethanolamine	Dimyristoyl	50
	Dipalmitoyl	66
Glycerol	Dioleoyl	−18
	Dilauryloyl	4
	Dimyristoyl	23
	Dipalmitoyl	41
	Distearoyl	55
Serine	Natural (mixed unsaturated)	7
	Dimyristoyl	38
	Dipalmitoyl	51
Sphingomyelin	Natural	32
	Dipalmitoyl	41
	Distearoyl	57

soluble in aqueous solution. Diacyl phospholipids generally form liquid crystalline suspensions as long as the temperature is held at or above the phase transition. Overall, because phospholipids are amphipathic, they function well as emulsifying or dispersing agents. Although most often found in topical products, phospholipids have been employed in oral capsule formulations as well as in liposomal parenteral formulations.

Glycolipid Compounds

Glycolipids include compounds formed by the linkage of a sugar moiety to a glyceride backbone. Classical glycolipids such as glycosyl glycerides or ceramides are not common in pharmaceutical preparations primarily due to low abundance and high cost; however, glycosyl modifications can be used to impart targeting mechanisms to aggregate lipid formulations.

LIPID CONFORMATION

The colligative and solubilizing properties of lipids have been known since the early part of the 20th century. What had been perceived as clusters of amphipathic molecules (soaps) in aqueous solution are now better understood as micelles (1–3). Micellar solubilization of pharmaceuticals is now a familiar classical technique, which has been reviewed in detail (4, 5). Additional understanding of drug dissolution and impact of lipid conformations can be gained from studies that utilized macro and microemulsions to solubilize drugs (5–9).

Beyond the concept of micelles and emulsions, the combination of lipid and aqueous components can result in formulations that exhibit a variety of physical states. These result from lipid orientations, which may be either random, in thermotropic crystalline lattices, or in aggregate structures with long-range order (lyotropic liquid crystals) (10). Figure 2 illustrates possible lipid conformations with micellar and emulsion/surface monolayer orientations being the earliest of recognized microstructures. Lipid molecules are also capable of packing tightly together to give more ordered states, such as a bilayer. In fact, depending on the components in the formulation, lipids may contribute to distinct phase diagrams containing up to at least six different regions (11). The "neat" or lamellar (liposomal) phase (12) physically can appear as a suspension to a highly viscous cream (13), depending on the final volume. Lamellar organizations further include liquid crystalline,

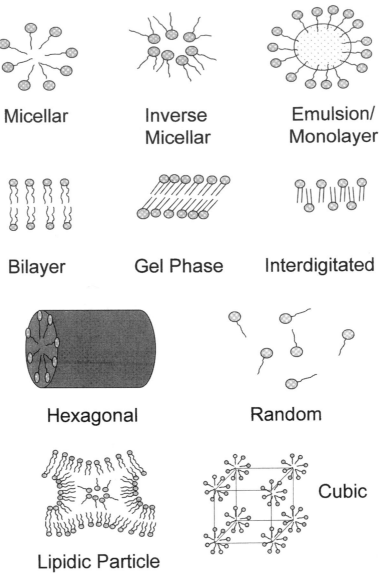

Fig. 2 Conformational states and spatial organizations of lipids. Small circles indicate the polar head group region of the molecules, whereas hydrophobic chains are represented as single lines.

gel state, and interdigitated phases. The middle phase (hexagonal) is a cylindrical arrangement with a hydrocarbon core, surrounded by an interfacial layer of hydrated polar groups. This orientation can be reversed to yield the hexagonal II structure, which appears stiff, and suspends as hard particles in water and will not dilute in additional aqueous solution. Lipids can also organize into cubic structures that appear clear, brittle, and viscous in character (14). Mixed conformations of lipids have also been observed, as is the case for lipidic particles, with inverse micelles distributed between a lamellar matrix.

These different aggregated states are sometimes reached by transitions through other phases simply by changes in temperature or by nature of the external environment (such as solvent concentration). Phase transitions of lipids can be regulated by changes in pH, temperature, cation concentrations, and presence of amphipathic additives. A comprehensive database on lipid phase transitions has been recently compiled by Caffrey (15). Polymorphic transitions are common in the preparation of lipid-containing formulations and can account for the differences in physical handling properties of the material during manufacture in which varying amounts of solvents, or energy input, are encountered at the different process steps. Geometric preferences of lipids can be better understood by considering the relative volume occupied by each portion of the molecule. Cullis et al. (16) and Gruner et al. (17) have described such molecular shape analysis of lipids in detail (Fig. 3).

The various macromolecular aggregates of lipids also make it possible to associate with drugs through physical entrapment. In these cases, the concentration of lipid associated drug is dictated by the size or conformation of the drug and the spaces created in the lipid aggregate. Entrapment levels of drug can vary from less than 1% to as high as complete encapsulation. Excluding chemical interactions or solubilization phenomena, drug encapsulation efficiency is linked to both the lipid conformation and the manufacturing method, which juxtaposes the two components. This is particularly true of liposome formulations in which factors of temperature, pressure, solute concentration, solvent volumes, or energy application all contribute to the final amount of drug incorporated within the lipid matrix (18).

MANUFACTURING OF LIPID-CONTAINING PRODUCTS

Manufacturing issues should be evaluated as part of overall lipid formulation development. Although lipid addition may be desirable for pharmacological purposes there are often commercial issues which present hurdles to eventual marketing. Among those factors are the availability and cost of raw materials, handling of intermediate mixed-phase systems, particulate control, stability of the lipid ingredients, sterilization, packaging interactions, qualification of noncompendial ingredients, and development of validated methods for analysis of either raw material or product.

Availability and Cost of Lipid Raw Materials

For commercial formulations, raw material sources should be of high purity and quality consistently meeting defined specifications, preferably compendial when available. Fortunately, high-purity lipids have

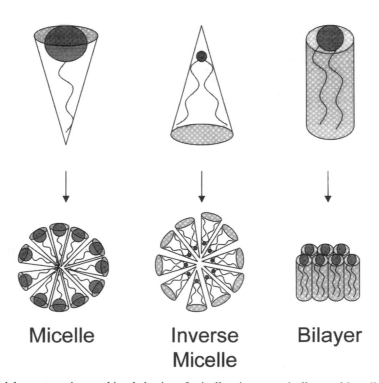

Fig. 3 Geometric models representing packing behavior of micelles, inverse micelles, and lamellar structures. Lipid molecules with domains that occupy a large lateral distance compared to adjacent domains of the molecule will conform to corresponding shapes and packing behavior. Micelles and inverse micelles approximate cone shape, whereas lamellar systems resemble cylinders. (Adapted from Refs. 16 and 17.)

become increasingly available in large supply, and in particular, phospholipid supply has advanced in recent years due to the approval and marketing of parenteral liposome formulations.

Large supply of naturally derived lipids can be obtained from plants in which many oils and fatty acids can be readily extracted and purified. Animal sources (e.g., eggs or milkfats) are used to derive complex lipids such as phospholipids and cholesterol. Yield from natural sources is dependent on the weight-percent composition and the efficiency of the extraction procedure. The constitution of fatty acids in vegetable oils varies widely from different sources (19). For example, oleic acid is present at 64.6% by weight in olive oil but is present at only 0.7% in palm kernel oil. Similarly, castor oil triglyceride is comprised of almost entirely ricinoleic chains. There are numerous raw material suppliers of oils and oil fractions worldwide. As such, the relative cost of bulk purified fractions and their derivatives such as salt forms and alcohols is quite low ($\approx$\$50–150/kg). Costs for high purity synthetic phospholipids (>97%) continue to drop when compared to prices 8 to 10 years earlier (18, 20, 21). This is primarily due to the advent of marketed liposome products. Phospholipids are available worldwide from companies such as Genzyme (U.S./U.K.), Avanti Polar Lipids (U.S.), Matreya Inc. (U.S.), American Lecithin Co. (U.S.), Lipoid GmBH (Germany)/Vernon Walden (U.S.), Lucas Meyer (Germany), Nichiyu Liposome/Nippon Oil and Fat (Japan) and Northern Lipids (Canada). Also now available in larger supply are PEGylated phospholipids, lysopholipids, and various cationic lipids used in gene therapeutic applications.

Compounding of Lipids into Formulations

Lipids may be supplied either as lyophilized or dried powders, as liquids, or dissolved or suspended in an appropriate solvent. Dried powders are typically waxy or sticky in character, making aliquoting of the product troublesome. Lipid lyophilates can also be hygroscopic, thus presenting some difficulty for fluidized bed operations. Fluid bed applications however, may be successful if the concentration of lipid is held fairly low (22).

Handling of lipid products in a liquid state allows for more accurate compounding. Solubilization vehicles may involve dissolution into either polar or nonpolar solvents or surfactant solutions. Aside from safe handling, a primary concern when introducing lipids

from solvent environments is the compatibility of the solvent with processing equipment, in particular the gaskets and seals found in the pumps, transfer lines, mixers, and extractors. Elevated temperatures, which are used to dissolve or maintain the phase transition of the lipid or to initiate solvent evaporation, can further induce problems for gaskets and seals. In systems with nonvolatile solvents and detergents, removal of the dissolution vehicle can be achieved with flow centrifugal separation, chromatography or diafiltration.

Introducing a lipid-containing solvent to an aqueous solution of drug will require some means for energy input to mix the components, whether by simple rotating blade stirring, more vigorous homogenization, or milling, by sonication and filtration, or by high-pressure extrusion (23). Unless cosolvation is achieved a suspension of nonmiscible aqueous and nonpolar phases will offer more resistance to flow and may present problems for extrusion through filters, which tender a surface that is of opposite character to one of the phases. Binding of active agent, such as proteins, must also be considered (24). The conformational state of the lipid and the concentration also will govern the workability of the formulation. Lamellar orientations will flow fairly readily at concentrations below about 400 mg/ml whereas cubic or hexagonal phases will present difficulty even at very low concentrations.

Particulate and Particle Size Control

For lipids dissolved in solution, particulate control may be necessary, depending on administration route. For parenterals the large- or small-volume parenteral particulate tests of the USP are applicable, as would be the Ph. Eur. clarity test and JP foreign matter insoluble test. For suspended or opaque lipid formulations, compendial particle size tests and specifications for suspensions will apply (i.e., light obscuration or microscopy). Size reduction of lipid formulations can be achieved with a variety of processing equipment including paddle stirrers, homogenization and high shear mixers, Microfluidizer, colloid mills, ultrasonic and piezoelectric emulsifiers, and pressurized filtration or membrane extrusion.

Lipid Stability

A characteristic of lipid products, particularly those with unsaturated lipids is peroxide formation with oxidation (25). Free radicals such as ROO$^\bullet$, RO$^\bullet$, and OH$^\bullet$ can damage the drug and induce toxicity. Lipid peroxides may also form due to autoxidation, which increases with unsaturation level. Hydrolysis of the lipid may be accelerated due to the pH of the solution (26) or from processing energy such as ultrasonic radiation (27). Antioxidants (i.e., α-tocopherol, propyl gallate, ascorbate, or BHT) may be required.

Sterilization Methods

Because of possible oxidation, steam or heat sterilization of lipids may not be an attractive option. Validations at nonstandard autoclave cycles or F_o values may prove valuable. In some instances, as in ophthalmic ointments made with white petrolatum or oleagenous components, the base can be sterilized by dry heat (160–180°C for 1–3 h) and combined aseptically with the sterile drug and additives (28). Ointments with lipids such as lanolin, petrolatum, and mineral oil have been terminally sterilized by cobalt-60 gamma irradiation with success (28–30). In less viscous solutions, end terminal filtration with aseptic fill is often necessary, requiring justification to regulatory authorities for lower sterility assurance levels. High pressures may be required to force lipid through membranes, thus adequate filter integrity checks are critical. High-pressure extrusion through straight channel membranes (polycarbonates/ceramics) may reduce the pressures and improve flow rates (23).

Packaging and Processing Surface Considerations

Lipids will be attracted to hydrophobic surfaces where losses might be expected. Overall binding will be affected if the molecule also contains ionic regions. Generally, lipids are chemically compatible with most plastics or glass used in packaging. Residual solvents that partition into the lipid phase may interact with plastic resins such as polystyrene or polycarbonate or with rubberized seals. Extractables from plastic packaging may be accelerated by the presence of lipid. Extraction of silicone polymer into lipid phases also occurs from silanized surfaces or coated gaskets. Compendial tests and regulations on extractables and impurities will apply here. Presence of metals coming from process or package surfaces are a potential source of catalysis leading to degradation of lipid components. In addition, reducing oxygen headspace should be considered to minimize potential degradation. Inert gas purging can improve lipid stabilities.

ANALYSIS OF LIPID PHARMACEUTICAL PRODUCTS

Because lipids exhibit primary through quaternary conformations, the analysis of lipid-containing pharmaceutical products must therefore involve both chemical and physical determinations to define the product on the molecular level as well as the aggregate state of the product. Stability-indicating assays can be developed from both approaches.

Chemical Determinations

Lipids can be measured by standard analytical methods such as wet chemistry, HPLC, thin-layer chromatography, and gas chromatography (31). Because lipid formulations may have several components and because the formulation may have an overall aggregate structure, it is usually necessary to develop further strategies for isolation and detection of the lipid ingredients (32). Dissociation of the individual components using temperature, solvents, detergents, reducing or oxidizing agents, or mechanical disruption prior to analysis may be necessary. Further separation or extraction of the components before analysis is required if interference is encountered. With lipid solvent extraction, there is a greater likelihood for losses of material. More often than not, a combination of techniques will be required for validation of the product. There are worldwide compendial procedures for analysis of various lipids by wet chemistry procedures to determine concentration, end group analysis, acid value, hydroxyl value, iodine value, and saponification value. A listing of the USP/NF methods for lipids is shown in Table 2.

HPLC Methods

Analysis of nonpolar lipids by HPLC is best carried out using normal phase columns. However, for mixed phases with polar drug or drug within an aqueous phase some compromise may be necessary. Good separation of polar and neutral lipids with a C8 column and a four-solvent mobile phase has been reported (33). Elution of neutral lipids like triglycerides from C18 columns is slow, however, good resolution can been achieved. Mobile-phase development is usually necessary to effect a high degree of separation and resolution of similarly eluting components (34). Heated columns are beneficial for increasing temperature above the phase-transition temperature of the lipid and thus minimize clogging. Lipids with predominantly saturated chain lengths will

Table 2   USP 24/NF 19 methods for lipids

Lipid category	Method
Steroids and steroid esters	Cholesterol, betamethasone, calcifediol, cholcalciferol, clocortolone pivate, cortisone acetate, dehydrocholic acid, desoximetasone, desoxycortisone (acetate and pivalate), dexamethasone, difluorosone diacetate, dihydrotachysterol, dydrogesterone, ergocalciferol, estradiol, estriol, conjugated estrogens, estrone, estropipate, ethynodiol diacetate, fludrocortisone acetate, flumethasone pivalate, flunisolide, fluocinolone acetonide, fluocinonide, fluoromethalone, fluoxymesterone, flurandrenolide, halcinonide, hydrocortisone, levonorgetstrel, medroxyprogesterone, meprednisone, mestranol, methylprednisone, methyltestosterone, mibolerone, mometasone furoate, nandrolone (decanoate and phenproprionate), norethynodrel, norgestrel, oxymethalone, prednisone, progesterone, rimexolone, spironolactone, stanozolol, testolactone, testosterone, trenbolone acetate, and triamcinolone
Fatty-acids, salts and esters	Aluminum monostearate, calcium stearate, ethyl oleate, isopropyl myristate, isopropyl palmitate, magnesium stearate, oleic acid, polyoxyl 40 stearate, proprionic acid, sodium stearate, stearic acid, purified stearic acid, and zinc stearate
Fatty alcohols	Benzyl alcohol, butyl alcohol, cetostearyl alcohol, cetyl alcohol, cetyl esters wax, lanolin alcohols, octyldodecanol, oleyl alcohol, and stearyl alcohol
Oils and oil esters	Almond oil, castor oil, cod liver oil, corn oil, cottonseed oil, diacetylated monoglycerides, ethiodized oil injection, glyceryl behenate, glyceryl monostearate, hydrogenated castor oil, hydrogenated vegetable oil, light mineral oil, mineral oil, mono- and diglycerides, mono- and diacetylated monoglycerides, oil-soluble vitamines, oliver oil, orange flower oil, peanut oil, peppermint oil, perflubron, persic oil, polyoxyl 35 castor oil, polyoxyl 40 hydrogenated castor oil, rose oil, safflower oil, sesame oil, soybean oil, squalane, tocopherols excipient, vitamin E, and vitamin E PEG succinate
Phospholipids	Lecithin
Waxes	Caranuba wax, emulsifying wax, hard fat, hydrophilic ointment, hydrophilic petrolatum, microcrystalline wax, paraffin, petrolatum, rose water ointment, synthetic paraffin, white wax, yellow ointment, and yellow wax

have poor ultraviolet (UV) absorption even at the lower wavelengths (190 nm). Alternative detectors should then be considered.

Thin Layer Chromatography

One- and two-dimensional thin-layer silica gel chromatography remains a cornerstone of lipid analysis (31, 35). Sensitivity by this method is typically as low as 2 μg/spot. Lipid visualization can be achieved by many methods, including iodine vapor or charring of plates following exposure to sulfur-dichromic acid, cupric reagents, Phospray, or α-naphthol. Other useful reagents include stains and dyes such as fluorescamine, rhodamine 6G, bromothymol blue, molybdenum blue, phosphomolybdic acid, and silver nitrate, which may be impregnated into the silica. Validation of lipid

purity and quantitation is performed using gel or plate scanners.

Gas Chromatography (GC)

Capillary and packed (GC) columns are of value in the analysis of complex mixtures of lipids. The best capillary column length will depend on the complexity of the material injected, however, 30-m columns are often employed. In packed columns, many types of stationary phases are available for lipid separation, and these include silicone and alkylated or cyanogenated derivatives, polyesters, polyglycol, and carboranes. It is also common to derivatize the fatty-acid side chains to the corresponding methyl esters by reaction in BF_3/methanol prior to chromatographic analysis to achieve more distinct and uniform separations.

Physical Determinations

The aggregate states of lipids are discernable from measurements provided by a host of analytical devices, which yield information on physical properties. These techniques may also be used to give clues as to the interaction of the lipid carrier and the drug.

Particle sizing

Lipid particulate analysis can be achieved with most commercial laser particle counters. Compendial requirements for suspensions also allow for sizing via electron microscopy determinations, which can provide for qualitative assessments in addition to quantitation. Lipid suspension particles can be detected by negative-stain, freeze-fracture, critical-point drying and scanning techniques.

Nuclear magnetic resonance (NMR)

NMR is a valuable technique in the analysis of lipid phases (36). More specifically, proton, deuterium, carbon-13, fluorine-19, and phosphorus-31 NMR have been utilized for analysis of the dynamic and motional properties of lipids, lipid diffusion, ordering properties, head-group hydration, lipid asymmetry, quantitation of lipid composition, and head-group conformation and dynamics. Cullis et al. (16) and Gruner et al. (17) have shown the importance of P-31 NMR as a tool in the determination of phase properties and lipid asymmetry and the identification of bilayer, hexagonal, and isotropic phases.

Electron spin resonance (ESR)

ESR is used to give information on the local environment of a lipid molecule (37). In normal state these molecules inherently do not exhibit ESR spectrums. However the necessary signal can be generated from reporter labels such as nitroxide or doxyl probes, which can either be linked directly to the lipid molecule or prelinked to a lipid chain and then partitioned into the lipid aggregate formulation. Data from ESR spectrums are valuable for determining molecular properties of the formulation, such as phase transitions and separations, order parameters (anisotropy), polarity, lateral diffusion, segregation and clustering, surface and transbilayer potentials, permeability and internal volumes, surface determinants (antigens), pH gradients, lipid asymmetry, flip flopping, and fusion.

Differential scanning calorimetry

Differential scanning calorimetry is a well known technique in the study of the thermal behavior of lipids and can be used to assess purity and stability of lipids, perturbation of aggregate structures, phase transition temperatures, lipid mixing behavior, and influence of other molecules and ions on structure (38).

X-ray and neutron diffraction

Diffraction patterns of lipid solutions can yield strong evidence for the presence of specific repeating conformational structures as well as the spacing between lipid molecules in organized films or layers (12, 39–41).

Spectroscopic analysis

Appraisals of the optical properties of lipid solutions and dispersions will provide information on concentrations, aggregation and stability, phase transitions, densities, and repeating structures (42–44). Measurements of refractive index, scattered light intensity (polarized and depolarized), and birefringence are relatively easy laboratory methods on which certain product specifications may be based. Also, fluorescent techniques can readily provide information on lipid movements and transfer of lipid between particles (45, 46).

COMMERCIAL AND EXPERIMENTAL LIPID DOSAGE FORMS

The key purposes of lipid materials in dose forms include: 1) improving the solubility or physical workability of the drug for ease of administration or to enhance stability; 2) augmentation or reduction in absorption of the drug from the formulation; 3) specific drug targeting to maximize response and minimize side effects; and 4) controlled or slow delivery of the drug from the formulation. Currently, the largest use of lipids in pharmaceuticals is in products for oral or topical dosage administration, although there is growing use in parenteral, pulmonary and nasal products.

The mechanics of drug delivery from lipid systems is governed by five structural features: primary structure, that is, chemical or molecular interactions, secondary organization into aggregate structures such as inverse micelles, tertiary organization of the aggregate projected into three dimensions such as three dimensional inverse micelles or hexagonal phase tubules; quaternary associations, agglomeration or interaction of the three dimensional structures such as lateral stacking of hexagonal tubules, and final packing of the molecules in solution (concentration effects) to produce liquids, creams, solids, etc. Mammalian systems have natural degradative pathways for the rapid metabolism of most lipid raw materials. However, the release of drug to a biological system will be controlled at least as much by these structural features as by simple natural degradative mechanisms.

Lipophilic Derivatives and Prodrugs

Lipophilic derivatives and prodrugs are a prudent tactic to alter the normal interaction of drug compounds with cells and cellular barriers. The type of modification desired may be a permanent one if the drug compound maintains its activity following conjugation, or a reversible type subject to biological cleavage. A variety of strategies for chemical coupling of lipids to drugs can be developed to produce the desired modified product (20). Briefly, nonreversible reaction approaches include conjugation to drugs with amine residues either via glutaraldehyde, lipid anhydrides or halides, or succinimidyl derivatives of the fatty acyl chain via carbodiimide activation. Nonreversible conjugations have also been accomplished via carbodiimide-activated carboxyl moieties of drugs reacted with amine containing lipids. Permanent conjugation to phenolic residues of drugs can be accomplished with diazo derivative of lipids bearing available amines. This approach has been successfully employed to prepare lipophilic derivatives of peptides containing tyrosine residues. Lipid conjugation reactions have also taken advantage of available sulfhydryl groups on drugs, particularly for modification of antibodies. On the other hand, bioreversible conjugates have been made via use of the Schiff base reaction to couple an aldehyde-bearing lipid to amines present on the drug. It is possible to convert the hydroxyl groups of more abundant glycolipids to the corresponding aldehydes using periodate. An extension beyond the Schiff base reaction is the Mannich base condensation, which introduces a nucleophilic reactant such as an enolate anion or amide to the reaction between the aldehyde and amine. In these reactions the amine component is generally a lipophilic primary or secondary amine. Extensive literature is available on the production and biological activities of lipophilic N-Mannich base derivatives and stabilized α-acyclo-alkyl forms. The effect of lipophilic derivatized drugs given by various administration routes has been discussed in detail in several reviews (47–50).

Permeation Enhancers

There are a number of excellent reviews on the requirements for enhancing drug permeability across lipophilic biological barriers, with particular reference to the importance of the lipophilic properties of formulations (51–55). A listing of some penetration enhancing lipids can be found in Table 3. Administration sites include buccal, oral, nasal, ocular, transdermal, rectal, and pulmonary.

Vehicles for Dispersion

There is fairly extensive use of lipid materials in oral liquid dose forms strictly as vehicles. Primary applications have been as surfactants to promote drug suspension or dissolution (fatty glycols and fatty acids), as flavoring agents (natural or synthetic oils), and as thickening agents (hydrogenated oils). Aspects of

Table 3 Lipid permeation enhancers

Category	Compounds
Ionic lipids	Lauryl sulfate, dodecyl-2-pyrrolidone, N-dodecyl azacycloheptan-2-one (Azone), N-dodecyl-N,N-dimethyl betaine, calcium dodecylbenzene sulfonate, dioctyl sodium sulfosuccinate, dodecyl N,N-dimethylamino (acetate or proprionate), and cetyltrimethylammonium bromide
Steroid and steroid esters	Cholate, deoxycholate, taurocholate, glycocholate, taurodeoxycholate, sodium taurodihydrofusidate, and cholesterol esters
Fatty-acids/fatty-acid esters/fatty alcohols	Oleic acid, lauric acid, capric acid, heptanoic acid, stearic acid, palmitoleic acid, palmitelaidic acid, octadecanoic acid, sucrose laurate, and isopropyl myristate
Phospholipids	Phosphatidylcholines, lysophosphatidylcholine, monooleoyl phosphatidylethanolamine
Oils	Monoolein, cocoa butter, cardamom oil, tricaprylin, mineral oil, terpenes, and terpenoids

pharmaceutical oral suspensions have been discussed in greater depth (56). Solution based-lipid vehicles have been applied in softgel applications, the primary category being oils that are compatible with gelatins and that that have had applications as both lubricants for processing of the gelatin sheets and as drug vehicles for liquid fill operations into the softgel. High lipid concentrations may allow for higher ethanol content in softgel fills (57).

Lipids may also be used to create solutions for injectable products, particularly intravenous preparations. Fatty acids, fatty glycols, and fatty alcohols may be used to enhance the dissolution of certain insoluble drugs, act as preservatives, or function as active agents as demonstrated by Scleromate injection (Glenwood, Tenafly, NJ), a mixture of fatty acid salts derived from cod liver oil. As another example, benzyl alcohol preservative has been useful in formulations for water insoluble drugs such as etoposide (VePesid®, Bristol-Meyers Squibb, Princeton, NJ) and is a primary active agent in Zilactin gel (Zila, Phoenix AZ). Polyoxyethylated fatty-acid derivative has been used in the dissolution of phytonadione, a lipid-soluble vitamin (AquaMEPHYTON, Merck, Sharp & Dohme, Rahway, NJ) for subcutaneous or intramuscular injection. Injectable amphotericin B is solubilized with sodium desoxycholate in Fungizone (Bristol-Meyers-Squibb, Princeton, NJ). Polyoxyethylated or PEGylated castor oils are also used in dissolution of injectable drugs such as cyclosporine (Sandimmune, Novartis/Sandoz, East Hanover, NJ), paclitaxel, and teniposide (Taxol, and Vumon, Bristol-Myers Squibb) and miconazole (Monistat, Janssen Pharmaceutica, Piscataway, NJ). Clear colloidal dispersions are also possible using a wide varity of phospholipids, cholesterol esters, and tocopherol esters (13, 18).

Solid- and Liquid-Crystalline Suspensions, Creams, and Gels

Suspensions and creams are most often developed for aqueous insoluble drugs, as typified by ophthalmic and otic preparations of corticosteroids. In suspensions such as Cortisporin or Pediotic (Glaxo Wellcome, Research Triangle, NC), components such as cetyl alchol, glyceryl monostearate, mineral oil, and propylene glycol are commonly used to effect a homogeneous suspension of drug particles.

The creation of fine suspensions may also be necessary to administer a highly insoluble product by parenteral injection. In these instances lipids may be used as either wetting agents or suspension vehicles (58). Lecithin (phosphatidylcholine) is a suitable agent for wetting or

suspending of drug particles in either aqueous or nonaqueous solutions. This common formulation additive is used for injectable long-acting IM suspensions of penicillin (e.g., Bicillin L-A®, Wyeth-Ayerst, Philadelphia, PA) for the bronchodilator inhalation aerosol, Atrovent® (Boehringer Ingelheim, Ridgefield, CT), and for the otic suspension Cipro HC (Bayer, Germany). Naturally derived and synthetic lecithins, in mixtures with neutral lipids, also serve as the active ingredient in lung surfactants products such as Exosurf (Glaxo Wellcome), Survanta (Ross, Columbus OH), and Infasurf (Forest Labs, St. Louis, MO).

Lipid materials are used extensively as vehicles in topical creams, ointments, gels, and lotions, and usually serve as the base material for many such preparations. These formulations are principally presented as emulsions and may contain fatty acids, fatty-acid salts, fatty alcohols, petroleum based and natural oils, waxes, fatty glycols, lanolin, and other hydrophobic surfactants. Such emulsions are common in dermal topicals, for which the list of products is too numerous to elaborate. Some of these ingredients also are present as vehicles in suppositories such as semisynthetic glycerides existing in Nembutal (Abbott Laboratories, North Chicago, IL), hydrogenated vegetable oil as found in Dulcolax (Novartis Consumer Health), and glycerides of fatty acids or oils that can be found in vaginal suppositories such as Prostin E2 (Pharmacia and Upjohn, Kalamazoo, MI) and Crinone Gel (Wyeth-Ayerst). Mineral oil is frequently present in transdermal products such as Catapres-TTS (Boehringer Ingelheim) and Estraderm (Novartis Pharmaceuticals Corp). In addition, numerous ocular or topical ointments, such as TobraDex (Alcon Labs, Fort Worth, TX) and Nitro-Bid (Hoechst Marion Roussel, Kansas City, MO), use white petrolatum and mineral oil as a base. Short-chain triglycerides such as triacetin can be found in products such as Prepidil Gel (Pharmacia-Upjohn, Kalamazoo MI), a cervically administered prostaglandin.

Oil-in-water emulsions have also been applied for intravenous use. Commercial parenteral emulsions include Dizac (Schein, Florham Park, NJ) and Diprivan (Zeneca Pharmaceuticals, Wilmington, DE). Many commercial or experimental parenteral products have been based on vegetable oil (most often soybean, safflower, or cottonseed) stabilized with phosphatides and monoglycerides, which nicely match the hydrophile–lipophile balance (HLB) requirements of those oils ($\approx$6–7). Further prospects for expanded nontoxic parenteral emulsions may come with use of other phosphatide-based surfactants with high HLB values (24, 59, 60). A number of excellent reviews and articles on the application of parenteral emulsions for drug delivery have been written (61–65). Drug delivery from oil/phosphatide emulsions stems from earlier development and marketing of intravenous nutrient emulsion products such as Intralipid (KabiVitrum, Clayton, NC) and Aminosyn II, (Abbott Laboratories), which are sterile and nontoxic. The development of these emulsions as well as distribution profiles of these and similar emulsion compositions have been studied (63, 64, 66–68). A cursory scan of the literature on parenteral oil emulsion formulations will obtain studies on amphotericin B, prostaglandin E1, halothane, pregnanolone, paclitaxel, perilla ketone, penclomedine, F-octylbromide, flurbiprofen axetil (Lipfen), lasalocid, lignin, podophyllotoxin, tacrolimus, doxorubicin, epirubicin, menatetrenone, chlorpheniramine maleate, naproxin, cyclosporin A, propranolol, testotsterone, benzocaine, phenylazoaniline, palmitoylrhizoxin, pilocarpine, diazepam, and various peptide and proteins for vaccine delivery.

Liposomal Dosage Forms

Extensive studies on liposomes date back to the 1960s. Many good comprehensive review references exist on compositions and manufacturing of liposomes (18, 23, 24, 69–73) including the article "Liposomes as Pharmaceutical Dosage Forms" in this volume. The earliest commercial liposomal formulations were developed for veterinary application (Novasome, IGI, Vineland, NJ) or over-the-counter cosmetic creams promoted for improved hydration (L'Oreal, Paris and Dior, Paris). More recently, parenteral liposome formulations of amphotericin B, doxorubicin, and daunorubicin have been approved and marketed (ABELCET, Elan, the Liposome Co., Inc, Princeton, NJ; AmBisome and DaunoXome, Nexstar/Fujisawa, Deerfield Park, IL; Amphotec and Doxil, Sequus/Alza, Menlo Park, CA), with others on the horizon for applications in photodynamic therapy (74). Although the vast majority of liposome preparations are constructed from phospholipids, other nonphospholipid materials can be used either alone or in mixtures to form bilayer arrays. One such example is Amphotec, which utilizes sodium cholesteryl sulfate as the primary lipid. Other liposome forming materials may include but are not limited to fatty-acid compositions, ionized fatty acids, or fatty acyl amino acids, longchain fatty alcohols plus surfactants, ionized lysophospholipids or combinations, nonionic or ionic surfactants and amphiphiles, alkyl maltosides, α-tocopherol esters, cholesterol esters, polyoxyethylene alkyl ethers, sorbitan alkyl esters, and polymerized phospholipid compositions (20).

Low Density Lipoprotein Carriers

Lipoproteins are naturally occurring particulate emulsion carriers for the transport of cholesterol and other lipids such as triglycerides in the blood. Because low-density lipoprotein (LDL) particle clearance is receptor mediated, they have been proposed as drug carriers for targeting applications, specifically for targeting of cytotoxic agents to tumor cells, delivery of antiviral agents to parenchymal liver cells, targeting of immunomodulators, antiviral and antiparasitic drugs to Kupffer and endothelial cells, and as gene vectors (75–78).

Solid Dosage Forms

The main use of lipids in solid form has been for oral tableting applications. Fatty-acid salts such as magnesium and calcium stearates, and various waxes and glycerides are most often used as conditioners and binders during compaction and provide more even, controlled, or slower disintegration of the tablet once administered. Extensive literature is available in which these materials are discussed in context of the preparation of oral tablets or capsules (79–81). The use of lipids for solid-implant formulations has also been investigated. Materials such as cholesterol, and high-melting-point fatty-acids, fatty anhydrides, and glycerides have been utilized in compressed implants to prolong systemic delivery of drugs (82, 83). Lipids are also well suited for suppository and vaginal insert formulations.

Safety of Lipid Products

The safety of a lipid product will in part be a reflection of 1) the purity of the compounds administered; 2) biological toxicity of the basic chemical ingredients; and 3) reactions to structural presentations of the lipid. Noncompendial lipid materials will necessitate significant toxicology testing.

Contaminants and impurities

Sensitive analytical procedures will be required to distinguish contaminants from lipid peaks within the preparation. By-products may be present from the synthetic processes used to produce the lipids or if copurified from the natural source. For example, common impurities in synthetic diacyl chain lipids are the monoacyl forms, which are generally more toxic to biological systems. Endotoxins and pyrogens either may be detectable in a lipid preparation (23, 84) or difficult to detect due to the lipids shielding against the analytical reagents (85).

Immune reactivity

Consideration should be given to immune reactivities when administering lipids to mammalian systems. Oils are well known for their adjuvancy; different oils will produce varying levels of reactivity (86). Biological responses such as leukocyte attraction, encysting of the oil, and edema reactions vary in severity simply as a function of the chemical nature or purity of the oil itself. Importantly, most lipids, including normal endogenous compounds possess antigenic potential to varying degrees (87). These possible reactivities should be monitored as part of the overall clinical design.

Conformational considerations

There may be biological sensitivities to the conformational presentation and sizing of the lipid formulation. For example the ability of antibodies to distinguish between lamellar organizing lipids and hexagonal-phase lipids are known and may form the basis for certain types of autoimmune dysfunction (88). Biological factors such as reticuloendothelial cell recognition of particles provide further impetus for control of the particle size and stability.

REFERENCES

1. Harkins, W.D.; Mattoon, R.W.; Corrin, M.L. Structure of Soap Micelles Indicated by X-rays and the Theory of Molecular Orientation. I. Aqueous Solutions. J. Am. Chem. Soc. **1946**, *68*, 220–228.
2. Jones, M.N., Chapman, D., Jones, M., III Eds.; *Micelles, Monolayers and Biomembranes*; John Wiley & Sons: New York, 1994; 264.
3. Mittal, K.L., Shah, D.O. Eds., *Surfactants in Solution*; Plenum Publishing Corp.: New York, 1992; 720.
4. Florence, A.T. Drug Solubilization in Surfactant Systems. *Techniques of Solubilization of Drugs*; Yalkowsky, S.H., Ed.; Marcel Dekker, Inc.: New York, 1981; 15–89.
5. Mittal, K.L. *Micellization, Solubilization and Microemulsions*; Plenum Publishing Corp.: New York, 1977; vol. 1 and 2, 945.
6. Gelbart, W.M., Ben-Shaul, A., Roux, D., Eds. *Micelles, Membranes, Microemulsions, and Monolayers (Partially Ordered Systems)*; Springer Verlag: New York, 1994; 608.
7. Shah, D.O., Ed. *Micelles, Microemulsions and Monolayers: Science and Technology*; Marcel Dekker, Inc.: New York, 1998; 610.
8. Sjoblom, J., Ed. *Emulsions and Emulsion Stability*; Marcel Dekker, Inc.: New York, 1996; 474.
9. Shinoda, K.; Friberg, S. *Emulsions and Solubilization*; John Wiley & Sons: New York, 1986; 174.
10. Tyle, P. Liquid Crystals and Their Applications in Drug Delivery. In *Controlled Release of Drugs: Polymers and Aggregate Systems*; Rosoff, M., Ed.; VCH Publishers: New York, 1989; 125–162.
11. Lo, I.; Florence, A.T.; Treguier, J.P.; Seiller, M.; Puisieux, F. The Influence of Surfactant HLB and the Nature of the Oil Phase on the Phase Diagrams of Nonionic Surfactant-Oil-Water Systems. J. Colloid Interface Sci. **1977**, *59*, 319–327.
12. Gruner, S.M. Material Properties of Liposomal Bilayers. *Liposomes: From Biophysics to Therapeutics*; Ostro, M.J., Ed.; Marcel Dekker, Inc.: New York, 1987; 1–38.
13. Weiner, A.L. Lamellar Systems for Drug Solubilization. *Liposomes: From Biophysics to Therapeutics*; Ostro, M.J., Ed.; Marcel Dekker, Inc.: New York, 1987; 339–369.
14. Brown, G.H.; Wolken, J.J. *Liquid Crystals and Biological Structures*; Brown, G.H., Wolken, J.J., Eds.; Ch. 2 and 3 Academic Press: New York, 1979.
15. Caffrey, M. *Lipidat a Database of Thermodynamic Data and Associated Information on Lipid Mesomorphic and Polymorphic Transitions*; CRC Press Inc.: Boca Raton, FL, 1993; 305.
16. Cullis, P.R.; de Kruijff, B.; Hope, M.J.; Verkleij, A.J.; Nayar, R.; Farren, S.B.; Tilcock, C.; Madden, T.D.; Bally, M.B. Structural Properties of Lipids and their Functional Roles in Biological Membranes. *Membrane Fluidity in Biology. Concepts of Membrane Structure*; Academic Press: New York, 1983; 1, 39–81.
17. Gruner, S.M.; Cullis, P.R.; Hope, M.J.; Tilcock, C.P.S. Lipid Polymorphism: The Molecular basis of Nonbilayer Phases. Ann. Rev. Biophys. Biophys. Chem. **1985**, *14*, 211–238.
18. Weiner, A.L.; Cannon, J.B.; Tyle, P. Commercial Approaches to the Delivery of Macromolecular Drugs with Liposomes. *Controlled Release of Drugs: Polymers and Aggregate Systems*; Rosoff, M., Ed.; VCH Publishers: New York, 1989; 217–253.
19. Bailey, A.E. Composition and Characteristics of the Individual Fats and Oils. *Industrial Oils and Fat Products*; Interscience Publishers, Inc.: New York, 1951; 967.
20. Weiner, A.L. Lipids in Pharmaceutical Dosage Forms. *Encyclopedia of Pharmaceutical Technology*; Swarbrick, Boylan, Eds.; Marcel Dekker, Inc.: New York, 1993; Vol. 8, 417–476.
21. Weiner, A.L. Developing Lipid-Based Vehicles for Peptide and Protein Drugs. Part I: Selection and Analysis Issues. Biopharm. **1990**, *3* (3), 27–32.
22. Chen, C-M.; Alli, D. Use of Fluidized Bed in Proliposome Manufacturing. J. Pharm. Sci. **1987**, *76*, 419.
23. Martin, F.J. Pharmaceutical Manufacturing of Liposomes. *Specialized Drug Delivery Systems. Manufacturing and Production Technology*; Tyle, P., Ed.; Marcel Dekker, Inc.: New York, 1990; 267–316.
24. Weiner, A.L. Liposomes for Protein Delivery. Immunomethods **1994**, *4*, 201–209.
25. Bressler, R. Fatty-Acid Oxidation. *Lipid Metabolism*; Florkin, M., Stotz, E.H., Eds.; Comprehensive Biochemistry Ch. 8 Elsevier Publishing Co. Amsterdam, 1970; 18.
26. Ho, R.J.Y.; Schmetz, M.; Deamer, D.W. Non-enzymatic Hydrolysis of Phosphatidylcholine Prepared as Liposomes and Mixed Micelles. Lipids **1987**, *22*, 156–158.
27. Jana, A.K.; Agarwal, S.; Chatterjee, S.N. Ultrasonic Radiation Induced Lipid Peroxidation in Liposomal Membrane. Radiat. Environ. Biophys. **1986**, *25*, 309–314.

28. Turco, S.J.; King, R.E. *Sterile Dosage Forms. Their Preparation and Clinical Application*; Lea & Febiger: Philadelphia, 1974; 326–328.
29. Tsuji, K.; Goetz, J.F.; Vanmeter, W. Effect of 60 Co-Irradiation on Penicillin G Procaine in Veterinary Mastitis Products. J. Pharm. Sci. **1979**, *68*, 1075–1080.
30. Nash, R.A. Radiosterilized Tetracycline Ophthalmic Ointment. Bull. Par. Drug Assoc. **1974**, *28*, 181–187.
31. Kates, M. *Techniques in Lipidology. Isolation, Analysis and Identification of Lipids*, 2nd Revised Ed.; Elsevier: Amsterdam, 1986; 464.
32. Kuksis, A.; Myher, J.J. General Strategies For Practical Chromatographic Analysis of Lipids. *Journal of Chromatography Library Monographs*; Kuksis, A., Ed.; (Chromatography of Lipids in Biomedical Research and Clinical Diagnosis) Elsevier: Amsterdam, 1987; Vol. 37, 1–47.
33. McCracken, M.S.; Holt, N.J. High-Performance Liquid Chromatographic Determination of Lipids in Vesicles. J. Chromatog. **1985**, *348*, 221–227.
34. Jungalwala, F.B. High-Performance Liquid Chromatography of Phosphatidylcholine and Sphingomyelin with Detection in the Region of 200 nm. Biochem. J. **1976**, *155*, 55–60.
35. Fried, B.; Sherma, J. *Thin Layer Chromatography*; Marcel Dekker, Inc.: New York, 1986; 394.
36. Browning, J.L. NMR Studies of the Structural and Motional Properties of Phospholipids in Membranes. *Liposomes: From Physical Structure to Therapeutic Applications*; Knight, C.G., Ed.; Elsevier/North-Holland Biomedical Press: Amsterdam, 1981; 189–242.
37. Marsh, D.; Watts, A. ESR Spin Label Studies of Liposomes. *Liposomes: From Physical Structure to Therapeutic Applications*; Knight, C.G., Ed.; Elsevier/North-Holland Biomedical Press: Amsterdam, 1981; 139–188.
38. Mabrey-Gaud, S. Differential Scanning Calorimetry of Liposomes. *Liposomes: From Physical Structure to Therapeutic Applications*; Knight, C.G., Ed.; Elsevier/North-Holland Biomedical Press: Amsterdam, 1981; 106–138.
39. Luzzati, V.; Tardieu, A. Lipid Phases-Structure and Structural Transitions. Ann. Rev. Phys. Chem. **1974**, *25*, 79–94.
40. Mitsui, T. X-Ray Diffraction Studies of Membranes. Adv. Biophys. **1978**, *10*, 97–135.
41. Franks, N.P.; Lieb, W.R. X-ray and Neutron Diffraction Studies of Lipid Bilayers. *Liposomes: From Physical Structure to Therapeutic Applications*; Knight, C.G., Ed.; Elsevier/North-Holland Biomedical Press: Amsterdam, 1981; 243–272.
42. Mishima, K.; Satoh, K.; Ogihara, T. Optical Birefringence of Phosphatidylcholine Liposomes in Gel Phases. Biochim. Biophys. Acta **1977**, *898*, 231–238.
43. Yi, P.N.; MacDonald, R.C. Temperature Dependence of Optical Properties of Aqueous Dispersions of Phosphatidylcholine. Chem. Phys. Lipids **1973**, *11*, 114–134.
44. Powers, L.; Pershan, P.S. Monodomain Samples of Dipalmitoyl Phosphatidylcholine with Varying Concentrations of Water and Other Ingredients. Biophys. J. **1977**, *20*, 137–152.
45. Tanaka, Y.; Schroit, A.J. Calcium/Phophate-Induced Immobilization of Fluorescent Phophatidylserine in Synthetic Bilayer Membranes: Inhibition of Lipid Transfer Between Vesicles. Biochemistry **1986**, *25*, 2141–2148.
46. Nichols, J.W.; Pagano, R.E. Resonance Energy Transfer Assay of Protein-Mediated Lipid Transfer Between Vesicles. J. Biol. Chem. **1983**, *258*, 5368–5371.
47. Bundgaard, H. Prodrugs as a Means to Improve the Delivery of Peptide Drugs. Adv. Drug Del. Rev. **1992**, *8* (1), 1–38.
48. Lee, V.H.L.; Li, V.H.K. Prodrugs for Improved Ocular Drug Delivery. Adv. Drug Del. Rev. **1989**, *3* (1), 1–38.
49. Sloan, K.B., Ed. *Prodrugs. Topical and Ocular Drug Delivery*; Marcel Dekker, Inc.: New York, 1992; 313.
50. Roche, E.B. *Bioreversible Carriers in Drug Design: Theory and Application*; Pergamon Press: New York, 1987; 292.
51. Lee, V.H.L.; Yamamoto, A.; Kompella, U.B. Mucosal Penetration Enhancers for Facilitation of Peptide and Protein Drug Absorption. CRC Critical Reviews in Therapeut. Drug Carriers **1991**, *8* (2), 91–192.
52. Lee, V.H.L. Enzymatic Barriers to Peptide and Protein Absorption and the Use of Penetration Enhancers to Modify Absorption. *Delivery Systems for Peptide Drugs*; Davis, S.S., Illum, L., Tomlinson, E., Eds.; Plenum: New York, 1986; 87–104.
53. Wearley, L.L. Recent Progress in Protein and Peptide Delivery by Noninvasive Routes. CRC Critical Reviews in Therapeut. Drug Carriers **1991**, *8* (4), 331–394.
54. Bodde, H.E.; Verhoeven, J.; van Driel, L.M.J. The Skin Compliance of Transdermal Drug Delivery Systems. CRC Critical Reviews in Therapeut. Drug Carriers **1989**, *6* (1), 87–115.
55. Knepp, V.M.; Hadgraft, J.; Guy, R.H. Transdermal Drug Delivery: Problems and Possiblities. CRC Critical Reviews in Therapeut. Drug Carriers **1987**, *4*, 13.
56. Carstensen, J.T. *Theory of Pharmaceutical Systems*; (General Principles) and 2 (Heterogeneous Systems) Academic Press: New York, 1972 and 1973; Vol. 1.
57. Weiner, A.L. Integrity Protected Gelatin. US Patent 5,376,381, 1994.
58. Wang, Y.-C.J.; Kowal, R.R. Review of Excipients and pH's for Parenteral Products Used in the United States. J. Parent. Drug Assoc. **1980**, *34*, 452–462.
59. Weiner, A.L. Emulsions. US Patent 5,626,873, 1997.
60. Weiner, A.L. Emulsions. US Patent 5,171,737, 1992
61. Collins-Gold, L.C.; Lyons, R.T.; Bartholow, L.C. Parenteral Emulsions for Drug Delivery. Adv. Drug Del. Rev. **1990**, *5* (3), 189–208.
62. Benita, S., Ed. *Submicron Emulsions in Drug Targeting and Delivery (Drug Targeting and Delivery)*; Harwood Academic Publishers/Gordon and Breach Publishing Group: Newark, NJ, 1999; Vol. 9, 352.
63. Davis, S.S.; Washington, P.W.; Illum, L.; Liversidge, G.; Sternson, L.; Kirsh, R. Lipid Emulsions as Drug Delivery Systems. Ann. N.Y. Acad. Sci. **1987**, *507*, 75–88.
64. Davis, S.S.; Hadgraft, J.; Palin, K. Medical and Pharmaceutical Applications of Emulsions. In *Encyclopedia of Emulsion Technology*; Beecher, P., Ed.; Marcel Dekker, Inc. New York, 1985; Vol. 2, 159–238.
65. Singh, M.; Ravin, L. Parenteral Emulsions as Drug Carrier Systems. J. Parenter. Sci. Technol. **1986**, *40*, 34–41.

L

66. Hansrani, P.K.; Davis, S.S.; Groves, M.J. The Preparation and Properties of Sterile Intravenous Emulsions. J. Parent. Sci. and Technol. **1983**, *37*, 145–150.

67. Davis, S.S.; Hansrani, P.K. The Evaluation of Parenterally Administered Emulsion Formulations. *Radionuclide Imaging in Drug Research*; Wilson, C.G., Hardy, J.G., Frier, M., Davis, S.S., Eds.; Croom Helm, 1982; 217–241.

68. Davis, S.S.; Illum, L. Colloidal Delivery System. *Site Specific Drug Delivery*; Tomlinson, E., Davis, S.S., Eds.; John Wiley & Sons: Chichester, 1986; 93–110.

69. Shek, P.N., Ed. *Liposomes in Biomedical Applications (Drug Targeting and Delivery)*; Harwood Academic Publishers/Gordon and Breach Publishing Group: Newark, NJ, 1995; 6, 304.

70. Ostro, M.J., Ed. *Liposomes: From Biophysics to Therapeutics*; Marcel Dekker, Inc.: New York, 1987; 393.

71. Janoff, A.S., Ed. *Liposomes: Rational Design*; Marcel Dekker, Inc.: New York, 1998; 451.

72. Lasic, D.D., Papahadjopoulos, D., Eds. *Medical Applications of Liposomes*; Elsevier Science Ltd.: Amsterdam, 1998; 779.

73. Barenholtz, Y.; Crommelin, D.J.A. Liposomes as Pharmaceutical Dosage Forms. *Encyclopedia of Pharmaceutical Technology*; Swarbrick, J., Boylan, J., Eds.; Marcel Dekker, Inc.: New York, 1993; 9, 1–39.

74. Husain, D.; Miller, J.W.; Michaud, N.; Connolly, E.; Flotte, T.J.; Gragoudas, E.S. Intravenous Infusion of Liposomal BPD for Photodynamic Therapy of Experimental Choroidal Neovascularization. Arch. Ophthalmol. **1996**, *114*, 978–985.

75. de Smidt, P.C.; van Berkel, Th.J.C. LDL-mediated Drug Targeting. CRC Critical Reviews in Therapeut. Drug Carriers **1990**, 7 (2), 99–120.

76. Bijsterbosch, M.K.; van Berkel, Th.J.C. Native and Modified Lipoproteins as Drug Delivery Systems. Adv. Drug Del. Res. **1990**, 5 (3), 231–252.

77. Hara, T.; Tan, Y.; Huang, L. In Vivo Gene Delivery to the Liver Using Reconstituted Chylomicron Remnants as a Novel Nonviral Vector. Proc. Nat. Acad. Sci. **1997**, *94* (26), 14547–14552.

78. de Smidt, P.C.; Bijsterbosch, M.K.; van Berkel, T.J.C. LDL as a Carrier in Site Specific Delivery. *Targeted Therapeutic Systems*; Tyle, P., Ram, B.P., Eds.; Marcel Dekker, Inc.: New York, 1990; 355–383.

79. *Tableting Specification Manual*, 4th Edn.; American Pharmaceutical Association, Tableting Specification Steering Committee: Washington, D.C., 1995; 114.

80. Banker, G.S.; Rhodes, C.T. *Modern Pharmaceutics*, 3rd Ed.; Marcel Dekker, Inc.: New York, 1996; 943.

81. Lieberman, H.A.; Lachman, L.; Schwartz, J.B. *Pharmaceutical Dosage Forms:Tablets*; Marcel Dekker, Inc.: New York, 1990; 1–3.

82. Wang, P.Y. Lipids as Excipient in Sustained Release Insulin Implants. Int. J. Pharmaceut. **1989**, *54*, 223–230.

83. Joseph, A.A.; Hill, J.L.; Patel, J.; Patel, S.; Kincel, F.A. Sustained Release Hormonal Prparations XV: Release of Progesterone from Cholesterol Pellets In Vivo. J. Pharm. Sci. **1977**, *66*, 490–493.

84. Kuo, H.S.; Muthua, S.C.; Thompson, C.R. Fat Emulsion Pyrogenicity Test. US Patent 4,245,044, 1981.

85. Dijkstra, J.; Mellors, J.W.; Ryan, J.L.; Szoka, F.C. Modulation of the Biological Activity of Bacterial Endotoxin by Incorporation into Liposomes. J. Immunol. **1987**, *138*, 2663–2670.

86. Leenaars, M.; Koedam, M.A.; Hendriksen, C.F.; Claassen, E. Immune Responses and Side Effects of Five Different Oil-Based Adjuvants in Mice. Vet. Immunol. Immunopathol. **1998**, *61* (2–4), 291–304.

87. Alving, C.R.; Richards, R.L. Immunologic Aspects of Liposomes. *Liposomes*; Ostro, M.J., Ed.; Marcel Dekker, Inc.: New York, 1983; 209–287.

88. Rauch, J.; Janoff, A.S. Antibodies against Phospholipids other than Cardiolipin: Potential Roles for Both Phospholipid and Protein. Lupus **1996**, *5* (5), 498–502.

LIQUID ORAL PREPARATIONS

Jagdish Parasrampuria
Galderma R&D, Cranbury, New Jersey

INTRODUCTION

Liquid oral preparations are composed of many types of formulations, both aqueous and nonaqueous, including solutions, suspensions, and emulsions. Oral solutions are homogeneous mixtures of one or more solutes dissolved in a suitable solvent or mixture of mutually miscible solvents. In pharmaceutical terms, solutions are defined as "liquid preparations that contain one or more soluble chemical substances, usually dissolved in water and they do not, by reasons of their ingredients, method of preparation, or use, fall into another group of products" (1). Solutions are classified on the basis of physical properties, method of preparation, use, and type of ingredients (Table 1) (2). The distinction among different types of solutions is not always clear because of overlap in definitions. Therefore, in some instances, definitions are not important for commercial products.

APPLICATIONS

Liquid oral preparations are useful for a number of reasons. Patient compliance is often a problem with oral solid dosage forms, especially with young children and the elderly. This refusal to accept medication stems from the difficulties experienced by these age groups in swallowing tablets or capsules. Such difficulties can be overcome by administering the active compound in a palatable liquid form. An oral liquid can be readily administered to children and the elderly who are unable to swallow. Because solutions are homogenous mixtures, the medication is uniformly distributed throughout the preparation. The dose can be easily adjusted as fractional doses by dilution to meet the needs of the patients. Extracts eliminate the need to isolate the drug in pure form, allowing several ingredients to be administered from a single source (e.g., pancreatic extract) and permit the preliminary study of drugs from natural sources. Some deliquescent and hygroscopic powders are more easily dispensed as liquids. Some drugs that are not tolerated in a concentrated form may be less irritating if dissolved in soothing liquid (3). Occasionally, solutions of drugs such as potassium chloride are used to minimize adverse effects in the gastrointestinal tract. Because drugs are absorbed in their dissolved state, the rate of absorption of oral dosage forms usually decreases in the following order: aqueous solution > aqueous suspension > tablets or capsules. A drug administered in solution is immediately available for absorption from the gastrointestinal tract and is more rapidly and efficiently absorbed than the same amount of drug administered in a tablet or capsule.

LIMITATIONS

Drug substances in general are less stable in liquid media than in the solid dosage form. Special techniques are required to solubilize poorly soluble drugs. Masking the taste of inherently very bitter drugs is sometimes difficult. Extremely potent drugs with a low therapeutic index cannot be given in an oral liquid dosage form because dosage measurement errors could be made by the patients. As with other oral dosage forms, liquid oral preparations cannot be administered to the unconscious patient.

DESIGN AND FORMULATION

The design of liquid oral solutions involves the combination of ingredients with medicinal agents to enhance the acceptability or effectiveness of the product. The formulation of pharmaceutical liquids requires several considerations: concentration of the drug; solubility of the drug; selection of the liquid vehicle; physical and chemical stability; preservation of the preparation; and appropriate excipients such as buffers, solubilizers, sweetening agents, viscosity-controlling agents, colors, and flavors.

Pharmacists can handle liquid preparations in three ways (4): They may dispense the product in its original container; they may buy the product in bulk and repackage it at the time of dispensation; or they may compound a solution. Compounding may involve nothing more than mixing two marketed products in the manner indicated on the prescription or may require the incorporation of an active ingredient in a logical and pharmaceutically

Table 1 Classification of oral solutions

Type	Description
Syrup	Solutions containing high concentrations of sucrose or other sugars
Elixir	Sweetened solutions containing alcohol as a cosolvent
Spirit	Hydroalcoholic solutions of aromatic or volatile substances
Aromatic Water	Aqueous solutions of aromatic or volatile substances
Tincture	Hydroalcoholic solutions prepared from vegetable materials or chemical substances by dissolution or extraction
Fluid extract	Concentrated alcoholic solutions of animal or vegetable drugs obtained by removal of active constituent by extraction (maceration, percolation)

(From Ref. 2.)

acceptable manner into the aqueous or nonaqueous solvents forming the bulk of the product. Most prescriptions today are dispensed in their original containers. In these cases, the pharmacist depends on the manufacturer to provide a product that is effective, pharmaceutically acceptable, and stable when stored under recommended conditions. Most drug manufacturers attempt to guarantee efficacy by evaluating their products in a scientifically acceptable manner. However, in some instances, such efficacy is relative. For example, cough mixtures marketed by two different manufacturers may contain active ingredients of the same therapeutic class and concentration. It therefore becomes difficult to assess the relative merit of the two products. In such cases, the commercial advantages gained by one over another may be based on other product characteristics. Thus, color, odor, taste, pourability, and homogeneity are important pharmaceutical properties, Hence, the successful design and formulation of liquids, as well as other dosage forms, require both scientific and pharmaceutical acuity (5).

Solubility

Solubility is of prime importance in developing liquid oral solutions. The drug and other dissolved substances should remain solubilized throughout the shelf life of the product. Therefore, the drugs are present in solution at unsaturated concentrations; otherwise, the drug may crystallize as a result of changes in temperature or by "seeding" from other ingredients or particulate matter present. The taste of organic drugs has been shown to be a direct function of aqueous solubility (6). For example, increasing the chain length of clindamycin esters (thus reducing aqueous solubility) dramatically improves the taste (7).

It is also important to determine solubility at refrigeration temperature (2–8°C) to establish the usable concentration in the range of 2–25°C without the risk of

saturation and crystal growth. This procedure is necessary to cover the wide range of temperature conditions to which the product may be exposed during the normal distribution process. If the exact solubility has not been determined, general expressions of relative solubility may be used. These terms are defined in the *United States Pharmacopeia* (USP) and are listed in Table 2 (8).

The solubility of the drug substance is attributable in large part to the polarity of the solvent, often expressed in terms of dipole moment, which is related to the dielectric constant. Solvents with high dielectric constants dissolve ionic compounds (polar drugs) readily by virtue of ion–dipole interactions, whereas solvents with low dielectric constants dissolve hydrophobic substances (nonpolar drugs) as a result of dipole or induced dipole interactions (Van der Waals, London, or Debye forces). This principle is illustrated in Fig. 1 (9). The former is classified as polar solvents, with examples such as water and glycerin; the latter are nonpolar solvents, with example such as oils. Solvents with intermediate dielectric constants are classified as semipolar. The dielectric constants of some solvents are shown in Table 3 (8).

Table 2 USP terms of solubility

Terms	Part of solvent required to dissolve 1 part of solute
Very soluble	<1
Freely soluble	1–10
Soluble	10–30
Sparingly soluble	30–100
Slightly soluble	100–1000
Very slightly soluble	1000–10,000
Practically insoluble, or insoluble	>10,000

(From Ref. 2.)

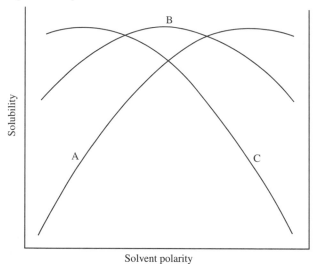

Fig. 1 Influence of solvent polarity on the solubility of drugs: A) Polar drug: B) semipolar drug; C) nonpolar drug. (From Ref. 9.)

A substance often exists in more than one crystalline form, such as chloramphenicol, dehydroepiandrosterone (DHEA), progestrone, sulfathiazole, cortisone or prednisolone, to name a few. Polymorphic transformations are structural differences resulting from different arrangements of molecules in the solid state.

Solubilization Techniques

Sometimes the desired drug concentration in a liquid dosage form cannot be reached because of the drug's low water solubility. Solubilization is the process by which the apparent solubility of a poorly water-soluble substance is increased. Solubilization techniques include addition of a cosolvent, salt formation, prodrug design, complexation,

Table 3 Dielectric constants of solvents at 25°C

Solvent	Dielectric constant
Water	78.5
Glycerin	40.1
Ethanol	24.3
n-Propanol	20.1
Benzyl alcohol	13.1
Polyethylene glycol 400	12.5
Cottonseed oil	3.0

(Modified from Ref. 8.)

Table 4 Comparison of drug solubilization techniques

Method	Approximate range of solubility increase	Reference
Cosolvency	1–1000×	(10)
Salt formation	1–1000×	(11)
Prodrug formation	1–1000×	(12)
Complexation	1–100×	(13)
Micellization	1–50×	(14)

(From Ref. 9.)

particle size reduction, and the use of surface-active agents (micellization). Table 4 shows a comparison of the magnitude of increase in solubility obtained in general with various solubilization techniques (9).

Cosolvency

Cosolvents are defined as water-miscible organic solvents that are used in liquid drug formulations to increase the solubility of poorly water-soluble substances. Cosolvency, then, refers to the technique of using cosolvents. The need to use cosolvents in the formulation of new drugs as solutions remains high, especially with the increasing structural complexity of new therapeutic agents. The importance of using cosolvents in the formulation of a peptide drug has been reported (14).

Cosolvency is highly effective in increasing drug solubility. Advantages include not only the large increases in drug solubility but also simplicity. In the past, ethanol was the most commonly used solvent in oral preparations because of its excellent solvent properties for many nonpolar drugs as well as its favorable taste. Its use is often undesirable, however, in preparations intended for pediatric patients. Ethanol may also accentuate the saline taste of ionic salutes (15). Sorbitol, glycerin, propylene glycol, and several polyethylene glycol polymers are cosolvents that are both useful and acceptable in the formulation of oral liquids. For example, Fig. 2 shows solubilization curves of alprazolm in cosolvent–water systems (16). Cosolvents are used not only to effect solubility of the drug but also to improve the solubility of volatile constituents used to impart a desirable flavor and odor to the product. The primary limitation of consolvency is the toxicity of most water-miscible solvents that have a high potential for increasing drug solubility. The toxicological a properties of a solvent that may limit or eliminate its use in drug formulations include its general toxicity, target organ toxicity, or tissue irritation. Even if found to be relatively nontoxic, a cosolvent can rarely be administered as a neat or 100%

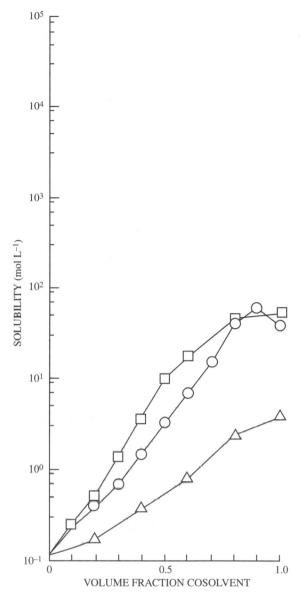

Fig. 2 Solubilization of alprazolam by ethanol (□), propylene glycol (○), and glycerin (△). (From Ref. 16.)

data. Moore (17) reported a method using approximate dielectric constants of the pure and mixed solvents. The basic assumption is that all vehicles with the same dielectric constant solubilize a given drug to the same extent. However, the dielectric constant alone is a poor predictor of the degree of drug solubility. Rubino (9) has described various mechanisms and equations that were derived with the objective of establishing a basic understanding of and developing a mathematical approach to interpreting and predicting drug solubility behavior.

Salt formation

Many poorly soluble drugs can be solubilized in salt form (18). The compound (α-(2-Piperidyl)β-3,6-bis (trifluoromethyl)-9-Phenanthrenemethanol, an antimalarial agent, and its hydrochloride salt are both only slightly soluble in water. However, its lactate salt is approximately 200 times more soluble than the hydrochloride. This enhanced aqueous solubility is attributed in part to the decrease in crystal lattice energy, as indicated by a reduction in the melting point. If a particular salt form cannot be isolated because of its very highly solubility, the same end result (i.e., desired aqueous solubility) can be achieved by in situ salt formation. This is accomplished by using an appropriate acid or base to adjust the pH level while formulating the drug product solution.

Prodrug method

The solubility characteristics of a drug can be altered by chemical modification; this is referred to as the "prodrug" approach. The term was first used by Albert (19) for a compound that undergoes biotransformation before eliciting a pharmacological response. This method has been successful in the case of corticosteroids. The solubility of betamethasone in water, for example, is 5.8 mg/100 ml at 25°C. The solubility of its disodium phosphate ester is more than 10 g/100 ml, an increase in solubility greater than 1500-fold. Although methods such as salt and prodrug formation can result in high increases in solubility, they require synthesis of essentially new drug entities as well as additional animal studies to confirm their efficacy and safety. Thus, an undertaking of this magnitude can be justified only if no other reasonable approach is available.

Complexation

Complexation is another means of improving the aqueous solubility of insoluble compounds; it is described by Eq. 1:

$$n[D] + m[L]_s \rightarrow [D_{rmn} : L_{rmm}]_{rms} \qquad (1)$$

where $[D]_s$ = concentration of drug in solution; $[L]_s$ = concentration of ligand in solution; and

solvent because of its poor taste or objectionable odor. Although a cosolvent may increase the solubility of the drug, it may also affect the solubility of other polar or ionic components of the formulation such as buffer materials.

Early formulation work using cosolvency involved an empirical approach for choosing the type and amount of cosolvent for a liquid vehicle. An improvement in the purely empirical approach was the introduction of alligation methods that could be used to reformulate vehicles based on experimental formulation or solubility

$[D_n:L_m]_s$ = concentration of the drug-ligand complex solution.

A complex is an entity formed when two molecules, such as a drug and a solubilizing agent (ligand), are bound by weak forces (e.g., dipole–dipole interaction or hydrogen bonding). For complex formation to occur, drug and ligand molecules must be able to donate or accept a pair of electrons.

Complexation has several advantages, such as the reversibility of the interactions. Dissociation of the complex to the individual reactants occurs rapidly and spontaneously on dilution. Consequently, the biological effects of complexes can be predicted on the basis of knowledge of the pharmacological properties of each of the reactants. Another advantage is the predictability and physical stability of the systems. Because complex formation involves equilibrium attainment, once the necessary data defining the system parameters such as stability constants and solubility properties of the complexes have been gathered, the behavior of the system is totally reproducible and predictable. This is in contrast to the polymorphs and other crystal modifications, which can be thermodynamically unstable; they may undergo time-dependent changes, that may lead to changes in solubility behavior.

The disadvantage of complexation is the presence of the ligand in molar ratios equivalent to and often higher than those of the drug. However, its sensory or pharmacological effects may be unacceptable. The formulator must also take into account detrimental interactions of the ligand with the exicipients. Furthermore, the apparent solubility increase realized by complexation compared with other techniques is usually less by an order of magnitude.

Micellization

Micellization has been defined by McBain as the spontaneous passage of poorly water-soluble solute molecules into an aqueous solution of a soap or a detergent in which a thermodynamically stable solution is formed (20). The mechanism for this phenomenon has been studied extensively and involves the property of surface-active agents forming colloidal aggregates known as micelles. When surfactants are added to a liquid at low concentrations, they tend to orient at the air–liquid interface. As additional surfactants are added, the interface becomes fully occupied, and the excess molecules are forced into the bulk of the liquid. At still higher concentrations, the molecules of surfactant in the bulk of the liquid begin to form oriented aggregates or micelles; this change in orientation occurs rather abruptly, and the concentration of surfactant in which it occurs is known as

the critical micelle concentration (CMC). Solubilization is thought to take place by virtue of the solute entrapped in or absorbed onto the micelle. Thus, the ability of surfactant solutions to dissolve or solubilize water-insoluble materials starts at the critical micelle concentration and increases with the concentration of the micelles.

It has been observed that lyophilic surface–active agents with hydrophilic–lipophilic balance (HLB) values above 15 are the best solubilizing agents. The commonly used solubilizing agents in pharmaceutical systems include polyoxyethylene sorbiton fatty acid esters (Tween series), polyoxyethylene monoalkyl ethers (BRIJ and MYRJ series), and sorbiton fatty acid esters (Span series). The choice of solubilizing agents is based on phase-solubility studies in which the solubility of the drug is determined as a function of surfactant concentration; several surfactants are included in these studies. The appropriate surfactant can then be selected on the basis of its efficacy as a solubilizer and its effect on other product characteristics and formulation adjuvants.

STABILITY

Drug substances in general are less stable in liquid media than in the solid dosage form. As a class of formulations, oral liquids are more complex in their composition than are parenterals, and more interactions can occur that might affect the stability of the product. Not only is it necessary to consider the solution stability of the drug, but also the effects on stability caused by excipients such as colorants, flavors, preservatives, solubilizers, thickening agents, and sweetening agents.

Chemical Stability

The techniques for predicting the chemical stability of homogeneous drug systems are well-defined (21, 22). The formulation chemist should consider both the pH-solubility profile and pH-stability profile to select the optimum pH for formulating the liquid oral dosage form. For example, Figs. 3 and 4 show that pH-stability and pH-solubility profiles (23, 24), respectively, for acetazolamide are approximately 4, which is the pH of optimum stability. However, the solubility above pH 7 is much higher because of sodium salt formation.

Physical Stability

Physical instability of liquid formulations involves the formation of precipitates, less soluble polymorphs,

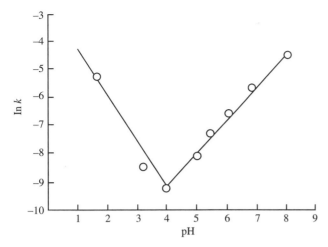

Fig. 3 pH-Stability profile of acetazolamide. (From Ref. 23.)

adsorption of the drug substances onto container surfaces, microbial growth, and product appearance (25). The acceptability of the product is a subjective evaluation and includes properties such as color, odor, taste, and clarity. Dye stability depends on the excipients used in the formulation. For example, FD&C Blue No. 2 has been

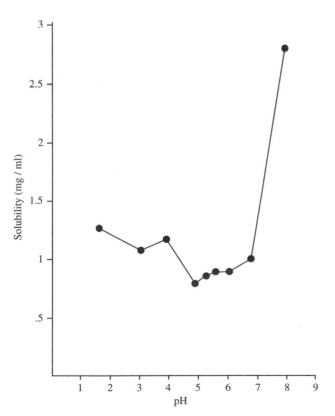

Fig. 4 pH-Solubility profile of acetazolamide. (From Ref. 24.)

found to fade more rapidly in the presence of several sugars (sorbitol, mannitol, dextrose, sucrose, lactose). In addition, trace amounts of impurities and nonionic surfactants such as pluronic F-68 contribute to the fading (26, 27).

Preservatives have been shown to bind to macro-molecules (28); for example, the binding of methyl *p*-Hydroxybenzoate to nylon was found to be dependent on the size of the nylon membrane and the concentration of free methylparaben. The complexation of methyl *p*-Hydroxybenzoate with Tween 80 depends on the amount of free methylparaben and the concentration of Tween 80. Similar results have been reported for propyl *p*-Hydroxybenzoate.

COMPONENTS AND ADDITIVES

Sweetening Agents

Sweeteners are indispensable for liquid oral dosage forms. They are used to mask bitter or unacceptable tastes of constituents. Sweetening agents constitute a major portion of the solid content in most liquid oral dosage forms. The most commonly used sweeteners include sucrose, sorbitol, mannitol, liquid glucose, honey molasses, sacchrin, and aspartame (Table 5). The types and concentrations of sweeteners for common prescription liquid medications are reported by Hill et al. (29).

Sucrose is the most widely used sweetener with a long history of use. It is a white crystalline powder, soluble in water and alcohol. It inhibits the growth of micro-organisms in solution at a sucrose concentration above 65 wt% by reducing the water-activity coefficient. Official Simple Syrup is an 85% w/v solution of sucrose in water. During the preparation of sucrose solution, care should be taken to avoid charring and caramalization caused by heat. Sucrose is chemically and physically stable in the pH range of 4.0–8.0. It is frequently used in conjunction with sorbitol, glycerin, and other polyols, which reduce its tendency to crystallize. One of the manifestations of the sucrose crystallization is "cap-locking" which occurs when sucrose crystallizes on the threads of the bottle cap and interferes with opening.

Liquid glucose is an extremely viscid substance that imparts both body and sweetness to liquid formulations. It is obtained by the incomplete hydrolysis of starch and consists chiefly of dextrose, dextrins, maltose, and water. It imparts a characteristic odor and flavor to the formulation in a manner similar to that of honey and molasses but to a lesser degree. Although liquid glucose is

Table 5 Sweetening agents

Sweetener	Sweetening power	Chemical structure	Comment
Sucrose	≈ 1		Most commonly used
Saccharin	≈ 500		Unpleasant aftertaste
Sodium cyclamate	≈ 30		Banned
Aspartame	≈ 200		Not very stable in solution

not a pure chemical entity, its method of manufacture can be well-controlled, and batch-to-batch variability is usually not a significant problem. The same is not true of honey and molasses, in which the quality depends on the sources, the time of the year they are produced, and natural factors that cannot be controlled.

Saccharin is a synthetic sweetening agent. It has approximately 500 times the sweetening power of sucrose, depending to some extent on the strength of the solution. The relative sweetening power of sucrose, depending to some extent on the strength of the solution. The relative sweetening power is greatest in dilute solution. Saccharin is a sucrose substitute for diabetics, the obese, and others who do not wish to ingest sucrose. It has no food value and is commonly used in the form of its sodium salt, which is more palatable than saccharin and comparatively free of unpleasant aftertaste. Sodium cyclamate is another synthetic sweetening agent that is approximately 30 times as sweet as sugar. However, its use as an artificial sweetener is no longer permitted in most countries because of the possible toxicity of its metabolite cyclohexylamine.

Aspartame, N-L-α-Aspartyl-L-Phenylalanine methyl ester, is 200 times sweeter than sucrose and, unlike saccharin, has no aftertaste. Its aqueous solubility is adequate for formulation purposes. It is stable in the sold form, but its stability in solution depends on temperature and pH. It hydrolyzes to aspartylphenylalanine and diketopiperazine, with a loss in sweetness by aspartame synergistic with saccharin, sucrose, glucose, and cyclamate. In addition, its taste can be improved by adding sodium bicarbonate, gluconate salts, and lactose (30).

Flavoring Agents

The flavoring of pharmaceuticals is of great importance to liquid dosage forms intended for oral use in that it can mask the disagreeable taste of drugs (31).

Coloring Agents

Although the use of colorants in medicinal products affords no direct therapeutic benefit, the psychological effects have long been recognized. The appearance of clear liquid products depends primarily on the color and clarity of the solution. Many patients rely on color to recognize the prescribed drug and proper dosage. Unattractive medication can be made acceptable to the patient by careful selection of color. Color is usually chosen according to the flavor of the product (for example, yellow for lemon or red for cherry).

The current list of Food, Drug, and Cosmetics (FD&C)-certified colorants contains both dyes and lakes. The latter are pigments that are insoluble in water and that impart color by dispersing and reflecting light; they are not used for aqueous solutions. In contrast, FD&C dyes are water-soluble and exhibit color by transmitting light. Dyes should be used at the lowest possible concentration required to produce the desired color; higher concentrations can result in a dull color. Most liquid drug products have dye concentrations of less than 0.001%. Because dyes are usually present in trace amounts, they should be dissolved before mixing with the bulk of the formulation. This ensures complete dissolution before further processing. If dye is added directly to the bulk mixing tank, the presence of small amounts of undissolved materials is difficult to determine and can cause problems later during the compounding. Factors influencing the shade and stability of dyes in liquid systems must be carefully considered. Among these are pH level, microbiological activity, exposure to light in the final package, and compatibility of the dye with other ingredients. Because color shades vary greatly at different pH levels, pH control is extremely important. All soluble dyes contain reactive sites, and some dyes may be incompatible with compounds containing polyvalent cations (such as

calcium, magnesium, or aluminum) and precipitate. Certain dyes, such as FD&C Blue No. 2 and FD&C Red No. 3, exhibit poor stability in aqueous solutions and should never be used for coloring aqueous liquid pharmaceutical products (32).

Preservatives

Liquid oral preparations are the most likely of all nonsterile pharmaceutical products to be contaminated by micro-organisms. Most of these preparations are marketed in a multidose form, enhancing the risk of exposure to microbes. The inclusion of sugars and other excipients enriches the preparation with growth-supporting substrates. The manufacturing process also contributes to possible microbiological contamination. In addition to the risks associated with even purified (USP) water, many raw materials of natural origin are used that may contain a large number of viable spores. Many over-the-counter pharmaceutical products have been prepared traditionally at low costs without sufficient care to prevent microbiological contamination. Therefore, it is essential that these preparations are protected against microbiological deterioration by adequate preservation.

Preservatives must fulfill certain criteria for acceptability. The major factors are those of safety and lack of toxicity after oral intake, particularly because liquid

Table 6 Preservatives used in pharmaceutical systems

Preservative	Usual concentration (%)
Acidic	
Phenol	0.2–0.5
Chlorocresol	0.05–0.1
α-Phenylphenol	0.005–0.01
Alkyl esters of *p*-Hydroxybenzoic acid	0.001–0.2
Benzoic acid and its salt	0.1–0.3
Boric acid and its salts	0.5–1.0
Sorbic acid and its salts	0.05–0.2
Neutral	
Chlorobutanol	0.5
Benzyl alcohol	1.0
β-Phenylethyl alcohol	0.2–1.0
Mercurial	
Thiomersal	0.001–0.1
Phenylmercuric acetate and nitrate	0.002–0.005
Nitromersol	0.001–0.1
Quaternary ammonium compounds	
Benzalkonium chloride	0.004–0.02
Cetylpyridinium chloride	0.01–0.02

(From Ref. 5.)

Table 7 Buffers commonly used in liquid pharmaceutical products

Buffer	pH	Usual concentration (%)
Acetic acid and a salt	3.5–5.7	1–2
Citric acid and a salt	2.5–6	1–3
Glutamic acid	8.2–10.2	1–2
Phosphoric acid salts	6–8.2	0.8–2

(From Ref. 5.)

medications are often administered to children and the elderly. Preservatives must be soluble, stable, microbiologically active, and compatible with the active ingredient as well as with other components of the formulation.

An ideal preservative that meets all the requirements does not exist. The choice must be made on an individual basis, balancing antimicrobial efficacy against safety. Frequently, a combination of two or more preservatives is needed to achieve the desired efficacy. The antimicrobial preservatives are classified into four major types: acidic, neutral, mercurial, and quaternary ammonium compounds (Table 6) (5).

Acidic preservatives are the most widely used for oral preparations, such as the *p*-Hydroxybenzoic acid esters and the salts of benzoic acid. These are adequately soluble in aqueous systems and possess both antifungal and antibacterial properties. Methyl and propyl *p*-hydroxybenzoic acid are often used together in a ratio of 10:1. The use of more than one ester makes possible a higher total preservative concentration owing to the independent solubilities of each and, according to some researchers, maximizes the antimicrobial effect.

The other three classes of preservatives have been widely used in ophthalmic, nasal, and parenteral products, but not frequently in oral liquid preparations. The neutral preservatives are volatile alcohols; their volatility introduces problems of odor and loss of preservative on aging in multidose preparations. The mercurials and quaternary ammonium compounds are excellent preservatives but are subject to incompatibilities (33). Mercurials are readily reduced to free mercury, and the quaternary compounds are inactivated by anionic substances.

Buffers

Changes in the pH level of a preparation may occur during storage because of degradation reactions within the product, interactions with container components, or dissolution of gases and vapors. To avoid these problems,

buffers are added to stabilize pH levels. A suitable buffer system should have adequate capacity to maintain the pH level of the product during storage. It can be based on the pH profile of the drug in solution. Commonly used buffer systems are acetates, citrates, phosphates, and glutamates (Table 7). Although buffers ensure pH stability, the buffer system can affect other properties such as solubility and kinetics. Buffers can act as general-acid or general-base catalysts and cause degradation of the drug substance. The ionic-strength contributions of the buffer systems can also affect stability. Therefore, the effect of buffer species should be studied before selecting any buffer system.

Antioxidants

Many drugs in solution are subject to oxidative degradation. Such reactions are mediated by free radicals or molecular oxygen and often involve the addition of oxygen or the removal of hydrogen. Drugs possessing favorable oxidation potential are especially vulnerable to degradation. Agents with an oxidation potential lower than that of the drug in question is called antioxidants. They are added to solutions alone or in combination with a chelating agent or other antioxidants and function by being preferentially oxidized and gradually consumed or by blocking an oxidative chain reaction where they are not consumed. Sulfites are the most common antioxidants in aqueous solutions. Irrespective of which sulfite salt is added, the antioxidant moiety depends on its final concentration and the final pH level of the formulation; metabisulfite is used at low pH. A single antioxidant may not provide complete protection. Certain compounds (e.g., ascorbic and citric acids) have been found to act as synergists, increasing the effectiveness of antioxidants, particularly those that block oxidative reactions. Frequently, chelating agents such as ethylenediaminetetraacetic acid derivatives (EDTA) are used in formulations containing trace amounts of heavy metals that would otherwise catalyze oxidative reactions.

Viscosity-Controlling Agents

It is sometimes desirable to increase the viscosity of a liquid to provide or to improve palatability or pourability. This can be achieved by viscosity-controlling agents such as polyvinylpyrrolidone or carboxymethylcelluloses. These compounds give aqueous solutions that are stable over a wide pH range. Methylcellulose and carboxymethylcellulose are available in a number of different viscosity grades. The latter may be used in solutions containing up to 50% alcohol without precipitating. However, care should be taken to avoid precipitation, which occurs with the insoluble salts to a number of multivalent metal ions such as Al^{3+}, Fe^{3+}, and Ca^{2+}. Methylcellulose polymers do not form insoluble salts with metal ions but can be salted out when the concentration of electrolytes or other dissolved materials exceeds certain limits. These limits may vary from 2 to 40%, depending on the electrolyte and the type of methylcellulose involved. Viscosity-inducing polymers should be used with caution. They are known to form molecular complexes with a variety of organic and inorganic compounds. It is conceivable that highly viscid systems that resist dilution by gastrointestinal fluid may impede drug release and absorption.

MANUFACTURE

The preparation of liquid drug preparations involves choosing the ingredients (using principles already addressed) and the manufacturing equipment. The basic principles involved are the same, regardless of the materials and the quantities involved. Carstensen and Mehta report the scaling-up of solution dosage forms (34), including heating, agitation, and clarification along with basic equations and calculations.

Liquid processing lends itself to computer-controlled automation. A few pharmaceutical firms have already instituted automated or semiautomated processes for several large-selling liquid products (35).

Raw Materials

Although purified water (USP) is required in all operations, it is particularly important in liquid manufacturing. If de-ionized and other water-treatment equipment is used, special attention must be given to routine microbiological and chemical testing. Storage tanks for glycerin and propylene glycol should be constructed to facilitate examination as well as cleaning.

Equipment

Simple solutions are most straightforward to scaleup but require tanks of adequate size and suitable mixing capacity (35). Most equipment should have heating and cooling capabilities for rapid dissolution of formulation components. Adequate transfer systems and filtration equipment are required, but they must be monitored to ensure that they can clarify the product without removing active or adjuvant ingredients. All equipment must be made of suitable, nonreactive sanitary materials and be designed and constructed to facilitate easy cleaning. Liquid pharmaceutical processing tanks, kettles, pipes, mills, filter housings, and so forth are most frequently fabricated from stainless steel. Of the three types commonly used in the industry (304, 308, and 316), type 316 is most often used because it is the least reactive. Stainless steel is virtually nonreactive but may react with some acidic pharmaceutical liquids (36). This problem can be minimized by treating the stainless steel with acetic acid or nitric acid solution to remove surface alkalinity. This process, known as passivation, may be needed periodically. For example, if an alkaline cleaning agent is used between batches of a reactive product, passivation may be required before the subsequent batch can be prepared.

Interaction with metallic surfaces can be minimized by using polytetrafluoroethlylene (Teflon) liners. Although Teflon is inert, these liners have the potential disadvantages of cracking, breaking, flaking, and peeling, with resulting product contamination.

A valuable and practical discussion on the design of piping, valves, mixers, pumps, and controls to produce high-quality liquid products is given by FitzSimon (37).

Methods of Preparation

Dilute solutions of rapidly dissolving materials are prepared by adding the solute to the solvent and agitating until the solution in homogeneous. Heat may be required for more concentrated solutions or when the solute is slow to dissolve. Excipients are usually added in a specified order to increase the rate of dissolution and to facilitate a rapid approach to equilibrium. For this reason, menthol and flavors are charged as alcoholic solutions to the batch. Solutes present in small concentrations, particularly dyes and other intensely colored materials, should be dissolved before mixing with the main portion of the batch to ensure complete dissolution. If the solutes were charged directly to the bulk mixing tank, it would be difficult to detect small amounts of undissolved material at the bottom of the tank. As a rule, complete solution should be confirmed at every stage in the manufacture of a homogeneous liquid. In the laboratory, liquids are usually measured by volume. However, in large-scale production, gravimetric means of measurement are used. For this reason, all liquids components of the formulation are expressed in units of both volume and weight.

Solutions must be filtered and clarified; this stage of the process is called "polishing." A highly polished solution requires the removal of particulate matter down to at least 3 μm. Filters used in the manufacturing, processing, or packing of liquid drug products intended for human use should not release fibers. If a fiber-releasing filter needs to be used, it must be followed by a nonfiber-releasing filter of optimum porosity. Filter aids are commonly used to improve clarity and increase the flow rate, thus decreasing filtration time. The amount and type of filter aid must be determined during the development of the product; the amount usually does not exceed 0.5 g/L. Examples of filter aids are diatomaceous earth, carbon, expanded perlite, and cellulose.

Filling and Sealing

A liquid may be removed from a bulk container in portions to individual-dose containers more easily and uniformly than a solid. Certain fundamental features are found on all machines used for filling containers with liquid. A means is used for repeatedly forcing a measured volume of the liquid through the orifice of a delivery tube designed to enter the constricted opening of a container. The size of the delivery tube is governed by the opening in the container, the viscosity and density of the liquid, and the desired speed of delivery. The tube must freely enter the neck of the container and deliver the liquid deep enough to permit air to escape without sweeping the entering liquid onto the neck or out of the container; the tube should have the maximum possible diameter. Excessive delivery force causes splashing and troublesome foaming if the liquid has a low surface tension.

Small volumes of liquids (usually for pediatric use) are delivered by the stroke of the plunger of a syringe, which forces the liquid through a two-way valve that provides for an alternative filling of the syringe from a reservoir and delivery to a container. For heavy, viscous liquids, a sliding piston valve provides more positive action. A drop of liquid normally hangs at the tip of the tube after a delivery, which is removed by a retraction device. Filling machines should be designed so that the parts through which the liquid flows can be easily dismantled for cleaning. These parts should be constructed of nonreactive materials such as stainless steel. Small-volume filling machines are designed to deliver volume precisely. Syringes are typically also made of stainless steel. The stroke of the syringe can be repeated precisely; therefore, once a particular setting has been calibrated for a delivery, high precision is possible. The precision can be affected by certain operating factors such as the speed of delivery, the

uniformity of speed, the expansion of rubber tubing connecting the valve to the delivery tube, and the rapidity of the action of the valves.

Large-volume filling does not normally require the precision required for small volumes. Therefore, bottles of solution are usually filled by gravity, pressure, or vacuum devices. Gravity filling is relatively slow but simple. The liquid reservoir to a shut-off device at the filling line, which is usually hand-operated; the bottles are filled to a graduation mark. The pressure-pump filler is often operated semiautomatically and differs from the gravity filler principally in that the liquid is under pressure. It is usually equipped with an overflow tube connected to a receiver to prevent excess filling.

Vacuum filling is commonly used for large liquid volumes because it is easily adapted to automation. A vacuum is produced in a bottle when the nozzle gasket makes a seal against the lip of the bottle to be filled. The vacuum draws the liquid from a reservoir through the delivery tube into the bottle. When the liquid level reaches the level of an adjustable overflow tube, the seal is mechanically loosened, and the vacuum is released. Any liquid that has been drawn into the vacuum line is collected in a receiver and returned to the reservoir.

Accuracy and precision of filling with liquids vary with the method. Therefore, a method is selected to provide the degree of accuracy and precision required. A slight excess is required in each container to provide for the loss that occurs at the time of administration resulting from adherence to the wall of the container. The danger of overdose as well as economic factors limits the amount of excess desirable in a given container.

Highly viscous solutions require specially designed equipment. To obtain a reasonable flow rate, high pressure must be applied, or containers with large openings must be used to permit the entry of large delivery tubes. Sometimes jacketed reservoir tanks can be used to raise the temperature of the product and thereby lower its viscosity.

A problem common to all types of machines that fill containers with liquid but that is particularly bothersome in high-speed automatic equipment is excessive foaming. Foaming during the filling operation can be reduced by using filling equipment that minimizes product turbulence, closed-system filling to limit the introduction of air or other gases that cause foaming, mechanical defoaming devices, or reduction in the speed of the filling line. All these methods introduce considerable engineering and production difficulties. It would be preferable to formulate the product with careful consideration of the problems that might eventually be encountered in large-scale production and high-speed filling operations.

A microbial survey should be performed on all packaging materials that come in contact with the product to ensure the absence of microbial contamination. Attention must also be given to details during packaging operations. For example, on small-volume orders, bottle closures or tips for plastic squeeze-spray containers are often placed on the product by hand. This procedure can be a source of microbial contamination unless operators use gloves that are sterilized and disinfected periodically during use.

REFERENCES

1. Ansel, H.C. Popvich, N.G. *Pharmaceutical Dosage Forms and Delivery Systems*; Lea & Febiger: Philadelphia, 1990; 196–224.
2. *United States Pharmacopoeia XXIV-National Formulary XIX*; United States Pharmacopeial Convention, Inc.: Rockville, MD, 2000; 2107–2118.
3. Ecanow, B. Liquid Medications. *Dispensing of Medication*; King, R.E., Ed.; Mack Publishing Co.: Easton PA, 1984; 100–139.
4. Nairn, J.G. Solutions, Emulsions, Suspensions, and Extractives. *Remington's Pharmaceutical Sciences*; Gennaro, A., Ed.; Mack Publishing Co.: Easton, PA, 1990; 1492–1517.
5. Boylan, J.C. Liquids. *The Theory and Practice of Industrial Pharmacy*; Lachman, L., Lieberman, H.A., Kanig, J.L., Eds.; Lea & Febiger: Philadelphia, 1996; 457–458.
6. Valvani, S.C. Yalkowsy, S.H. Solubility and Partitioning in Drug Design. *Physical Chemical Properties of Drugs*; Yalkowsky, S.H., Sinkula, A.A., Valvani, S.C., Eds.; Marcel Dekker, Inc.: New York, 1980; 201–229.
7. Sinkula, A.A. Morozwich, W. Rowe, E.L. J. Pharm. Sci. **1973**, *62*, 1106–1111.
8. DeLuca, P.P. Boylan, J.C. Formulation of Small Volume Parenterals. *Pharmaceutical Dosage Forms: Parenteral Medications*; Avis, K.E., Lachman, L., Lieberman, H.A., Eds.; Marcel Dekker, Inc.: New York, 1986; 1, 139–201.
9. Rubino, J.T. Cosolvents and Cosolvency. *Encyclopedia of Pharmaceutical Technology*; Swarbrick, J., Boylan, J.C., Eds.; Marcel Dekker, Inc.: New York, 1990; 3, 375–398.
10. Martin, A.; Swarbrick, J. Cammarata, A. *Physical Pharmacy*; Lea & Febiger: Philadelphia, 1983; 577–579.
11. Melby, J.C. Cyr, M., St. Metabolism **1961**, *10*, 75–82.
12. Repta, A.J. Alternation of Apparent Solubility Through Complexation. *Techniques of Solubilization of Drugs*; Yalkowsky, S.H., Ed.; Marcel Dekker, Inc.: New York, 1981; 135–158.
13. Florence, A.T. Drug Solubilization in Surfactant Systems. *Techniques of Solubilization of Drugs*; Yalkowsy, S.H., Ed.; Marcel Dekker, Inc.: New York, 1981 15–90.
14. Sanders, L.M. Abstracts of American Pharmaceutical Associations 133rd Annual Meeting **1986**, *16*, 14–16.
15. Pernarowski, M. Solutions, Emulsions, Suspensions and Extractives. *Remington's Pharmaceutical Sciences*; Osol, A., Hoover, J.E., Eds.; Mack Publishing Co.: Easton PA, 1970; 1488–1489.
16. Yalkowsky, S.H. Roseman, T.J. Solubilization of Drugs by Cosolvents. *Techniques of Solubilization of Drugs*; Yalkowsky, S.H., Ed.; Marcel Dekker, Inc.: New York, 1981; 91–134.
17. Moore, W.E. J. Am. Pharm. Assoc. Sci. Ed. **1958**, *47*, 855–857.
18. Agharkar, S. Lindenbaum, S. Higuchi, T. Am. Pharm. Sci. **1976**, *65*, 747–749.
19. Albert, A. Nature **1958**, *182*, 421–423.
20. McBain, J.W. *Advances in Colloid Science*; Interscience: New York, 1942; 1.
21. Streng, W.H. Drug Develop. Indus. Pharm. **1985**, *11*, 1869–1888.
22. Cartensen, J.T. *Drug Stability: Principles and Practices*; Marcel Dekker, Inc.: New York, 1990; 15–108.
23. Parasrampuria, J. Gupta, V.D. J. Pharm, Sci. **1989**, *78*, 855–857.
24. Parasrampuria, J. University of Houston: Houston, 1989, 94.
25. Shami, E.G. Bernardo, P.D. Rattie, E.S. Ravin, L.J. J. Pharm. Sci. **1972**, *61*, 1318–1321.
26. Kuramoto, R. Lachman, L. Cooper, J. J. Am. Pharm. Assoc. Sci. Ed. **1958**, *47*, 175–180.
27. Scott, N.W. Goudie, A.J. Huettman J. Am. Pharm. Assoc. Sci, Ed. **1960**, *49*, 467–472.
28. Patel, N.K. Kostenbauder, H.D. J. Am. Pharm. Assoc. Sci. Ed. **1958**, *47*, 289–293.
29. Hill, E.M. Flaitz, C.M. Frost, G.R. Am. J. Hosp. Pharm. **1998**, *45*, 135–142.
30. Beck, C.I. Application Potential for Aspartame in Low Calorie and Dietetic Food. *Low Calorie and Dietary Food*; Dwivedi, B.K., Ed.; CRC Press, Inc.: Boca Raton, FL, 1978; 68.
31. Adjei, A. Doyle, R. Reiland, T. Flavors and Flavor Modifiers. *Encyclopedia of Pharmaceutical Technology*; Swarbrick, J., Boylan, J.C., Eds.; Marcel Dekker, Inc.: New York, 1992; 6, 101–139.
32. Woznicki, E.J. Schoneker, D.R. Coloring Agents for Use in Pharmaceuticals. *Encyclopedia of Pharmaceutical Technology*; Swarbrick, J., Boylan, J.C., Eds.; Marcel Dekker, Inc.: New York, 1990; 3, 65–100.
33. Lachman, L. Bull. Parent. Drug Assoc. **1968**, *22*, 127–144.
34. Carstensen, J.T. Mehta, A. Pharm. Technol. **1982**, *6*, 64–77.
35. Yelvigi, M. Pharm. Technol. **1984**, *8*, 47–56.
36. Narurhar, A.N. Sheen, P.C. Corrosion in Pharmaceutical Processing. *Encyclopedia of Pharmaceutical Technology*; Swarbrick, J., Boylan, J.C., Eds.; Marcel Dekker, Inc.: New York, 1990; 3, 353–360.
37. FitzSimon, R. Drug Dev. Commun. **1976**, *2*, 1–31.

LOZENGES

Robert W. Mendes
Massachusetts College of Pharmacy and Health Sciences (Retired), Dedham, Massachusetts

Hridaya Bhargava
Massachusetts College of Pharmacy and Health Sciences, Boston, Massachusetts

INTRODUCTION

Lozenges are solid preparations that contain one or more medicaments, usually in a flavored, sweetened base, and that are intended to dissolve or disintegrate slowly in the mouth. They can be prepared by molding (gelatin and/or fused sucrose and sorbitol base) or by compression of sugar-based tablets. Molded lozenges are sometimes referred to as pastilles, whereas compressed lozenges may be referred to as troches. They are intended to be allowed to dissolve on the back surface of the tongue to provide drug delivery locally to the mouth, tongue, throat, etc., to minimize systemic and maximize local drug activity.

The USP (1) currently recognizes Cetylpyridinium Chloride Lozenges and Nystatin Lozenges. However, more than five dozen over-the-counter (OTC) lozenge products are currently marketed (2). These contain a variety of active ingredients including antimicrobials and local anesthetics for throat pain; aromatics, herbals, zinc salts, decongestants, and cough suppressants for colds, allergy, cough, and congestion; and nicotine-like substances for smoking cessation.

HARD CANDY LOZENGES

Raw Materials

The types of raw materials used in medicated lozenges may vary according to a number of factors. Most medicated lozenges contain sugar, corn syrup, acidulant, colorant, flavor, and the medicament.

Sucrose, a disaccharide of glucose and fructose, is obtained from sugarcane or beet. The choice of beet or cane sugar is based on availability and geographical considerations. Sucrose and sucrose products are used in medicated lozenges because of their value as neutral sweeteners, their ready solubility, and their function as a "drier" to reduce the weight of the confection through crystallization. Invert sugar, derived from sucrose, possesses the very desirable physical property of controlling the crystallization of concentrated sugar solutions and maintaining freshness of the finished product through its humectant properties.

Corn syrup is used in almost every type of confection to control sucrose and dextrose crystallization, which may lead to crumbling. Corn syrup in appropriate proportion with sucrose and dextrose allows the formation of an amorphous glass and produces a candy with the desirable appearance. The following physical properties of corn syrup are extremely important in the preparation of medicated candies: density, dextrose equivalent (DE), hygroscopicity, sugar crystallization, viscosity, freezing-point depression, and osmotic pressure.

Colorants are incorporated into medicated lozenges for appearance, product identification, and masking of physical degradation. Dyes and other organic colorants may degrade by heat or light via oxidation, hydrolysis, photooxidation, etc., and their compatibility with drug, excipients, and process conditions should be studied before selection. Suppliers of colors are excellent sources of information on current regulatory status of colorants.

Acidulants are generally added to medicated lozenges to fortify and strengthen their flavor profile. Organic acids such as citric, malic, fumaric, and tartaric acids are most commonly used. Citric acid alone or in combination with tartaric acid is the most common. Another use of acids in medicated lozenges is to alter the pH to maintain the integrity of the drug. Regular conversion corn syrup has a pH of 5.0–6.0. Addition of a weak organic acid to improve flavor lowers it to 2.5–3.0, a pH at which some medicaments exhibit maximum stability (3). If necessary, some drugs can be stabilized by adjusting the pH to 7.0–8.0 with a suitable weak base such as calcium carbonate. Some research has shown that excessive use of acidic lozenges could have the potential to enhance existing dental erosion (4), and that low pH (2.6–3.7) leads to dissolution of calcium and phosphorous from hydroxyapatite (5). Others have shown that excessive use of citric and tartaric acids may effect bioavailability of zinc in zinc lozenges (6, 7). Another report indicated that the activity of cetylpyridinium chloride in candy-base lozenges is influenced by pH, with >5.5 being most desirable (8).

Acceptable taste is necessary to ensure patient acceptability, and this can be the determining factor between commercial success and failure of an OTC product. Flavors used in medicated lozenges must be compatible with the drug and excipients and capable of withstanding the rigors of the manufacturing conditions. Flavors consist of numerous chemicals that may interact with excipients or medicaments and that degrade by heat and light. Aldehydes, ketones, and esters may react with drugs. A classic example of flavor–drug interaction is that of a primary amine drug (benzocaine, phenylpropanola-mine) with aldehyde-containing flavor components like cherry, banana, etc., resulting in the formation of a Schiff base, drug decomposition, and loss of efficacy. Adjustment of lozenge base pH to accentuate certain flavors (e.g., citrus) may also result in incompatibility with some medicaments (e.g., benzocaine).

The last major ingredient in lozenges is salvage obtained from lozenge batches rejected because of imperfect shape or size, presence of air bubbles, or unacceptable drug concentration. Salvage, if properly heated, can be reused in finished products without altering color, texture, lozenge base composition, or drug concentration (9). Before any salvage can be used as part of a medicated lozenge base, it should be adjusted to a pH of 4.5–7.5 to prevent excessive and uncontrolled formation of reducing sugars, and the stability of the drug at cooking cycles should be determined.

Processing Methods

There are three types of candy-base cookers: fire cookers, high-speed atmospheric cookers, and vacuum cookers. Vacuum cooking is the process of choice for manufacturing hard candy lozenges. It is based on the principle that water boils at a lower temperature under vacuum, and can thus be removed. Sugar solutions and corn syrup are boiled at 125–132°C, vacuum is applied, and, due to the heat of the batch, additional water is boiled off without further heating. The resulting vapor is condensed and removed by the cooling water of the vacuum pump (3).

The continuous batch process cooker installation consists of an automatic sugar dissolver, a sugar solution and corn syrup storage unit, metering pumps, precookers and a holding tank, a vacuum pump, and a collection kettle (10). Precookers are standard steam-jacketed kettles equipped with an additional heat exchanger to provide better circulation in addition to more exchange surfaces. Each component (water, sugar, corn syrup, and

salvage) is added by pumps and metering devices controlled by one gearing system, in order to bring the finished precooked syrup to the desired temperature (110–120°C) in 1 min or less (3). The short dwell time significantly reduces the Browning reaction and the amount (1–2%) of invert sugar developed (11). Cooking machines consist of a heating coil, intermediate chamber, vacuum chamber, flow metering valve, turning device that charges the receiving kettle, receiving kettle, kettle turning device, and rotary vacuum. In the standard procedure, a precooked sugar–corn syrup solution at 110–120°C is passed through a chrome–nickel steel cooking coil housed in a steam dome at a temperature of 135–150°C. The coil leads to an intermediate chamber that is vented to the atmosphere. From the intermediate chamber, the syrup is sprayed into the vacuum chamber, which is regulated by a vacuum-actuated metering valve. This affects reevaporation of the sugar mass (12), further increasing the content of dry substance. An adjustable timing device charges the receiving kettle by opening an air valve the moment the batch is cooked. The filled receiving kettle drops from the vacuum hood and is held in front of the cooker by a spring-activated timing device; it is replaced by an empty one (3). The kettle is charged by the syrup pump, resulting in uniform weight of all batches. By selecting an appropriate model, more than 3000 kg of candy can be produced per hour.

Replacement of the collection kettle by a continuously moving stainless steel belt to carry the candy base away from the cooker at a predetermined rate in an unbroken stream has resulted in the continuous process cooker, which has some advantages and some limitations. Its advantages are high-speed production, improved organo-leptic characteristics, extended shelf life for physical properties, and cost effectiveness. The disadvantages are reduced controls, the addition of flavor at very high temperature, and increased possibility of nonuniform candy-base production. Preparation of candy base from gear metering of sugar solution and corn syrup to vacuum drying is identical to the batch process described above. However, candy base is continuously drawn off in a thin ribbon. As it leaves the cooker the flavor, preheated to 50–60°C, is injected. The flavored candy mass is dropped onto a variable-speed rotary cone head where it is mixed. Medicament as a solution or dispersion, preheated to 110–120°C, can be metered into the candy mass through dosing pumps. The candy mass then slides down the delivery chute onto the stainless-steel belt where it is mixed and sized by plows and rollers. The temperature of the conveyor belt is controlled by a spray of heated water that can be adjusted as necessary. The acidulant may be deposited onto the candy mass via a vibratory dosing auger (9); the subsequent steps are identical to those of the batch process.

Candy-Base Manufacturing

The first step in the manufacture of medicated lozenges is the preparation of candy base, followed by the addition of medicament, flavor, acidulants, colors, etc., and finally by lozenge formation. Irrespective of process, the manufacture of medicated lozenges involves the cooking of candy base, mixing, batch forming, "rope" sizing, adjustment of weight, lozenge formation, cooling, and storage of lozenges.

Candy base is prepared from liquid sugar (67% sugar) and corn syrup (liquid glucose 43°Bé, 80% solids) in a ratio of about 60:40. Precooking is initiated under vacuum at controlled temperature. The precooked solution is transferred into the steam-heated coil, where it is boiled and from which it is moved to the intermediate chamber where final mixture is produced (3). The final moisture content of candy base should be about 1%, its temperature about 135°C, and its consistency plastic-like. The candy base is transferred into a kettle mounted on a suitable scale and, if necessary, batch weight is adjusted.

Heat-stable colors are added at this point as cubes or paste. The colored candy base is transferred to a cold stainless-steel cooling plate for the mixing operation. Mixing can be manual or mechanical, using a series of plows and rollers, or a mixer consisting of two arms, a plunger, and a slowly rotating table top.

The temperature of the mixing table is maintained at 40–50°C. Flavor, medicament, acidulant, and ground salvage are added to the colored candy mass when mixing is initiated. After completion, the medicated candy base is transferred to a warm slab and allowed to equilibrate to a uniform temperature.

The mass is cut into workable portions, properly tempered, and placed into batch-forming (holding) machines. For candy formers requiring a flat sheet, heated tables are used. For candies requiring cylindrical pieces to be fed into the batch formers, batch rollers are used. A plastic-like mass is formed into a sugar cone and transferred at a predetermined rate to the sizing roller. The operation of the batch former is synchronized with the rope sizer (12). In order to maintain a temperature at which the outer shell of the candy would not crack, the batch formers are kept at 80–90°C (3).

The height to which the batch formers are adjusted and the amount of material in them dictates the delivery rate of the candy flowing as a rope from the batch former to the sizing rollers. The sizers consist of sets of successively smaller forming rolls. The thickness of the rope is determined by the diameter of the sizing rollers and governs the weight and size of the candy. The sizers are generally heated to maintain temperatures of 50–60°C, preventing the candy from cracking by rapid cooling (12).

For the formation of the final lozenge, the candy rope is discharged into a forming machine. The formed lozenges are then fed onto the distribution belt, which provides intensive cooling and shaking to prevent deformation of the still plastic lozenge (12).

The formed candy must be cooled as quickly as possible to prevent loss of shape. The candy is usually cooled on a conveyor belt made of chain or canvas. Multibelt coolers are designed in such a way that the first narrow belt (15–20 cm wide) runs as rapidly as the candy-forming machine. At the end of the first belt, a breaker separates the candy and distributes the lozenges uniformly across a wider, slower-moving second belt. The third belt is still wider and travels even more slowly, allowing enough time to cool the lozenge to the desired temperature (below 35°C) (3).

In the sizing operation, the medicated lozenges are collected as they leave the cooling belt and transferred to a series of counterrotating rollers separated via caliper adjustment (12). The sizing operation removes all oversized and undersized lozenges, ensuring uniformity.

The properly sized lozenges are collected and stored in a climate-controlled room at 15–20°C and a relative humidity of 25–35% until the product is cleared by the quality control unit for packaging.

Recent technological advances in lozenge manufacture include a patent (13) that teaches a continuous process for producing dextromethorphan lozenges. A new lozenge cutter apparatus consisting of a drum with an array of cutter elements is described in a 1997 patent (14). A distributing device for feeding lozenges (or other flat products) via a feed conveyor to a "user" machine, such as a packager, is described in a 1993 patent (15).

COMPRESSED TABLET LOZENGES

Commercially, the preparation of lozenges by tablet compression is less important than hard-candy manufacturing techniques. Essentially, lozenge tablets differ from conventional tablets only in their organoleptic and nondisintegrating properties and slower dissolution rate. The associated attributes of pleasant taste with or without matching color, smoothness, and mouthfeel during prolonged dissolution on the tongue, and the physical consideration of holding the tablet in the mouth while swallowing its dissolved components, present unusual

L

formulation requirements compared to those of tablets intended for swallowing or chewing. The commonly used drugs mentioned previously tend to be bitter, unpleasant tasting compounds. The desire to release these agents slowly in the mouth, in constant contact with the tongue, demands a formulation approach unlike that found in any other dosage form.

Processing and Excipients

Any of the common tablet-processing methods, such as wet granulation, dry granulation, or direct compaction, may be utilized in the production of lozenge tablets. However, because the tablets should dissolve very slowly without disintegration, wet granulation is preferable because it generally provides better control. Through the judicious use of wet binders that retard dissolution, it should be possible to design a formulation having the appropriate dissolution rate.

Formulating for slow dissolution, plus smoothness and good mouthfeel, requires careful excipient selection and appropriate process development to ensure that the controlling variables are dealt with correctly. Several important aspects of lozenge tablet manufacture are critical to all of the desired performance attributes of the finished product. These include assurance of necessary particle size and distribution, maintenance of correct moisture content, and achievement of proper tablet hardness. Process development and scale-up considerations must be thoroughly explored to ensure the establishment of proper specifications for these parameters. As always when the process involves wet granulation, the extent of wetting and the rate and extent of drying must be defined. Overwetting almost certainly produces harder granules that may have poor compressional characteristics, resulting in softer and more friable tablets unacceptable for lozenge application. Because of the lesser degree of particle deformation, such granulations produce tablets having a gritty mouthfeel. Overwetting also leads to longer drying times in order to achieve the desired moisture level or, to a higher moisture level due to failure to compensate through adjustment of the drying cycle.

Lozenge tablets are generally formulated as relatively large-diameter (>12.5 mm), flat-faced (beveled edge), heavy (>700 mg) tablets with high hardness (>15 kp). These physical attributes lead to ease of use in the mouth and contribute to the desired slow dissolution. The formulation factors primarily responsible for controlling dissolution, hardness, and mouthfeel are the presence of a high strength, dissolution-retarding binder and the absence of a disintegrant. Several commonly employed binders (16–18) meet these criteria and provide the

added benefit of delivering a demulcent-like action in the throat.

Gelatin (in the form of a warm 10% aqueous solution) and acacia gum (in the form of an aqueous mucilage) in wet granulation form very hard tablets with slow dissolution. Guar gum, used as an aqueous thixotropic mucilage, exhibits behavior similar to that of acacia gum.

The sugar bases frequently associated with lozenge tablets are sucrose or compressible sugar, dextrose, mannitol, and sorbitol, which are available in special tableting grades from a variety of excipient manufacturers. Generally intended for direct compaction applications, they may also be utilized with the above binders in wet-granulation systems. Lactose, because of its extremely low sweetness (15% of sucrose), is limited for use in lozenges because it would require the addition of an artificial sweetener of sufficient potency to overcome its blandness. Xylitol is relatively sweet and has an advantage in lozenge formulation with respect to its lack of caries production.

Artificial sweeteners are of significant importance to lozenge tablet formulations. As noted above, some sugars may not be sweet enough to mask the bitterness or sourness of many drugs. Presently, there is considerable regulatory disagreement worldwide concerning these materials; some are approved for use in certain countries but not others. Aspartame, asulfame-K, cyclamate, saccharin, and sucralose appear to be technically usable, but their selection requires care from the regulatory perspective. All have potency (sweetness) levels orders of magnitude higher than that of sucrose, permitting the use of very low concentrations (less than 1%) to cover most bitter drugs. Semisynthetic sweeteners, derived from glycyrrhiza, have enjoyed some degree of popularity over the years. They are much sweeter than sucrose, but less sweet than saccharin. It is strongly recommended that the formulator validate the current regulatory acceptance of the intended sweetener prior to its use for a particular product and market country. In addition, a recent report suggests that the common lubricant, magnesium stearate, reduced the effectiveness of cetylpyridinium chloride in compressed tablet lozenges, and that the concentration of this ingredient in such a formulation should be maintained at not more than 0.3% (19).

QUALITY CONTROL

Lozenges require the same quality assurance and control measures as any pharmaceutical dosage form. Because of their unique composition, however, certain additional methods are necessary.

In-Process Testing

In addition to all of the common in-process tests used for all dosage forms, certain specialized procedures are necessary for hard candy lozenges. These include checking the corn syrup and sugar delivery gears, temperature, steam pressure, and the cooking speed of precooker and cooker; analysis of the candy base and its moisture content, and determination of the sugar-to-corn syrup ratio using the dextrose equivalent method, percent-reducing sugar (by reacting candy with copper sulfate and alkaline cupric tartrate and titrating with dextrose solution), pH, cooked candy batch weight, lozenge weight, and lozenge size. The usual in-process tests for compressed tablets apply to lozenge tablets, including particle-size distribution, moisture content, flow, blend uniformity, tablet weight and thickness control, hardness, etc.

Batch-Release Testing

In addition to the usual quality control procedures and the above in-process tests, batch-release testing includes dosage uniformity and a test for grittiness, performed by partially dissolving lozenges under running tap water until one-third to one-half has been removed. No grittiness must be felt when rubbed between thumb and forefinger.

Test procedures that are ordinarily applied to compressed tablets are also employed for lozenge tablets. However, because the lozenge is intended to dissolve slowly in the mouth, typical disintegration and dissolution testing is inappropriate. Lozenges should be nondisintegrating; therefore, there is no need for disintegration testing. Dissolution specifications should be developed on the basis of a minimum and maximum time to physically dissolve, rather than on the basis of minimum percent drug released in the maximum time interval. As with hard candy lozenges, microbial testing may be appropriate, especially when wet granulation has been used in processing the materials and high concentrations of carbohydrates are present.

Stability

For both hard candy lozenges and compressed tablet lozenges, stability considerations extend to areas not usually of concern with other types of tablets. These products should not only conform to chemical and physical specifications, but should also exhibit satisfactory stability of organoleptic attributes. Because lozenges are flavored, flavor stability is important. There is, however, no objective method for measuring flavor stability in a finished dosage form, although GC may be used for chemical analysis of flavor compounds. Even subjective methods such as tasting are difficult because formal taste

panels are needed to acquire reliable data. Subtle changes in flavor with time, although not affecting product performance, may have a significant impact on product market acceptability. This could also be true of minor changes (increase or decrease) in tablet hardness, which could affect dissolution time and therefore acceptability.

PACKAGING

Medicated lozenges, especially those of hard candy base composition, are hygroscopic because of their unique ingredients. In order to be competitive in the marketplace, they need a shelf life longer than 3 years. For these reasons, they are usually packaged individually wrapped in polymeric moisture-barrier material. The wrapped lozenges are placed in a tight or moisture-resistant glass, polyvinyl chloride, or metal container that is overwrapped with cellophane or aluminum foil. This complex, multiple packaging is intended to provide the maximum possible protection from moisture in order to ensure the longest possible shelf life for the product.

SUMMARY

Lozenges are medicated confections designed to locally deliver drug to the mouth and throat. Very widely sold as OTC products, there are also prescription products marketed in the lozenge dosage form. Lozenges are used to deliver local anesthetics, cold and allergy treatments, antimicrobial drugs, antismoking drugs, and anticariogenic drugs. They are usually produced in the form of cooked, hard candies based on sugar and corn syrup or sorbitol. They are totally different from any other pharmaceutical dosage form in terms of ingredients and method of manufacture and, therefore, require specialized facilities. Compressed tablet lozenges differ from conventional tablets by requiring materials and methods that provide slow dissolution and drug release.

For these and other reasons, lozenges are produced by few pharmaceutical manufacturers, and represent a very small percentage of total pharmaceutical sales. No significant growth can be currently anticipated in these areas.

REFERENCES

1. *United States Pharmacopeia 24/National Formulary 19*; United States Pharmacopeial Convention, Inc.: Rockville, 1999.

L

2. *Non-Prescription Drug Products: Formulations & Features*; Knodel, L.C., Ed.; American Pharmaceutical Association: Washington, 1998.

3. Peters, D. Medicated Lozenges. *Pharmaceutical Dosage Forms: Tablets, 2nd Ed.*; Lieberman, H.A., Lachman, L., Schwartz, J.B., Eds.; Marcel Dekker, Inc.: New York, 1989; I, 419–463.

4. Lussi, A.; Portmann, P.; Burhop, B. Erosion on Abraded Dental Hard Tissues by Acid Lozenges: An In Situ Study. Clin. Oral Investig. **1997**, *1* (4), 191–194.

5. Grenby, T.H. Dental Properties of Antiseptic Throat Lozenges Formulated with Sugars or Lycasin. J. Clin. Pharm. Ther. **1995**, *20* (4), 235–241.

6. Marshall, S. Zinc Gluconate and the Common Cold. Review of Randomized Controlled Trials. Can. Fam. Physician **1998**, *44*, 1037–1042.

7. Garland, M.L.; Hagmeyer, K.O. The Role of Zinc Lozenges in Treatment of the Common Cold. Ann. Pharmacother. **1998**, *32* (1), 63–69.

8. Richards, R.M.; Xing, J.Z.; Weir, L.F. The Effect of Formulation on the Antimicrobial Activity of Cetylpyridinium Chloride in Candy Based Lozenges. Pharm. Res. **1996**, *13* (4), 583–587.

9. Clarke, W.T. The Re-use of Chocolate and Confectionary Rejects. Manuf. Confec. **1975**, *55* (6), 37–40.

10. Meiners, A. Incorporating Flavor and Acid in Continuous Manufacturing Systems. Manuf. Confec. **1973**, *53* (10), 58–59.

11. Hartel, R.W. Sugar Crystallization in Confectionary Products. Manuf. Confec. **1987**, *67* (10), 59–65.

12. Technical Bulletin. *Machines, Production Lines and Process Technologies for the Confectionery Industry*; Robert Bosch Corp.: Bridgman MI, 1998.

13. Dextromethorphan Continuous Lozenge Manufacturing Process, US Patent 5,302,394, April 12, 1994.

14. Lozenge Cutter Apparatus US Patent 5,676,982, Oct 14, 1997.

15. Distributing Device for Feeding Flat Products to a User Machine, US Patent 5,199,546, April 6, 1993.

16. Peck, G.; Bailey, G.E.; McCurdy, V.E.; Banker, G.S. Tablet Formulation and Design. *Pharmaceutical Dosage Forms: Tablets,* 2nd Ed.; Lieberman, H.A., Lachman, L., Schwartz, J.B., Eds.; Marcel Dekker, Inc.: New York, 1989; I, 98–107.

17. Bandelin, F.J. Compressed Tablets by Wet Granulation. *Pharmaceutical Dosage Forms: Tablets,* 2nd Ed.; Lieberman, H.A., Lachman, L., Schwartz, J.B., Eds.; Marcel Dekker, Inc.: New York, 1989; I, 160–164.

18. Mendes, R.W.; Anaebonam, A.O.; Daruwala, J.B. Chewable Tablets. *Pharmaceutical Dosage Forms: Tablets,* 2nd Ed.; Lieberman, H.A., Lachman, L., Schwartz, J.B., Eds.; Marcel Dekker, Inc.: New York, 1989; I, 362–387.

19. Richards, R.M.; Xing, J.Z.; Mackay, K.M. Excipient Interaction with Cetylpyridinium Chloride Activity in Tablet Based Lozenges. Pharm. Res. **1996**, *13* (8), 1258–1264.

MANAGEMENT OF DRUG DEVELOPMENT

James E. Tingstad

Tingstad Associates, Green Valley, Arizona

The most successful new drug-development programs require competent, caring, people-oriented leaders at all levels. Overwhelming social science data show that this approach will optimize productivity, efficiency, and creativity, while fostering employee growth, enthusiasm, cooperation, and loyalty.

THE DRUG DEVELOPMENT PROCESS

Before addressing the components of good management, here is a review of the basic new drug (new chemical entity or NCE) development process.

Brief Overview

The NCE works its way through the following groups before it can be marketed:

Synthetic Chemistry → Pharmacology → Toxicology → Pathology →
Regulatory Affairs [Investigative New Drug (IND) application] →
Product R&D → Clinical Research → Regulatory Affairs [New Drug]
Application (NDA)] → Approval by government regulatory agency

Additional Important Contributors

Other involved departments/disciplines that are equally important as the above groups include Analytical Chemistry, Biochemistry, Biopharmaceutics/Pharmacokinetics/Drug Metabolism, Chemical Pilot Plant, Experimental Engineering, Packaging Development, and Statistics. Additional significant contributors include Purchasing and Quality Assurance/Documentation.

Post-NDA Departments

After NDA approval, non-R&D functions—after being partially involved at various stages of NCE development—take over, including Chemical Manufacturing, Engineering, Marketing, Packaging, Pharmaceutical Manufacturing, Quality Control, and Sales.

Departmental Responsibilities

Companies are organized differently; for example, the various engineering responsibilities may be in one or more departments. A brief description of typical functions follows:

- Synthetic chemistry synthesizes NCE candidates for pharmacological testing.
- Pharmacology examines the in vivo activity of the NCE in animals (1).

  1. For economic reasons, activity is determined in animals before safety, whereas in humans, preliminary safety studies need to come first.

     - Toxicology determines the "macro" negative effects of the NCE in animals.
     - Pathology examines the "micro" negative effects of the NCE in animals.
     - Product R&D designs a simple, preliminary dosage form for initial clinical trials (2).

  2. Additioxnal dosage-form development is deferred until safety/activity experiments in humans show promise. Eventually, scale-up experiments are conducted in cooperation with Pharmaceutical Manufacturing.

- Clinical research determines the safety and efficacy of the NCE in humans.

  - Phase I examines small-dose tolerance and safety in a limited number of young adult, usually male, volunteers.
  - Phase II, involving hundreds of patients, investigates efficacy, dosage, and prominent side effects.
  - Phase III, utilizing thousands of patients, broadens Phase II experiments and determines safety, efficacy, and marketability.
  - Phase IV, conducted after regulatory approval and marketing, investigates additional medical uses.

- Regulatory Affairs works closely with all relevant organizational units and is the primary contact with government regulatory agencies.
- Analytical Chemistry develops stability-indicating assays for NCEs and identifies/quantifies impurities; cooperates with Product R&D on product stability studies.
- Biochemistry determines, among other experiments, the cell-level effects of NCEs.
- Biopharmaceutics, Pharmacokinetics, and Drug Metabolism examines the absorption, distribution, metabolism, and elimination of NCEs.
- Chemical Pilot Plant produces NCEs for R&D groups.
- Experimental Engineering helps design new processes and equipment.
- Packaging Development develops containers for new products with stability and consumer issues in mind.
- Statistics is involved in planning and interpreting many R&D experiments.
- Purchasing works with R&D to ensure consistent, high-quality raw materials from vendors.
- Quality Assurance/Documentation monitors procedures and records to comply with government-regulated Good Laboratory and Manufacturing Practices.
- Chemical Manufacturing supplies the bulk NCE to Pharmaceutical Manufacturing.
- Engineering offers process/equipment services to post-NDA groups.
- Marketing, in cooperation with Sales and Advertising, determines the overall strategy for supplying NCE products to primary customers (physicians and other healthcare professionals).
- Packaging packages and labels manufactured drug products for sale.
- Pharmaceutical Manufacturing produces finished drug products for consumer use.
- Quality Control monitors the quality and stability of manufactured/marketed drug lots.
- Sales supplies products to customers.

Departmental Interactions

It's important for managers and laboratory workers to meet with colleagues from other departments to learn about interrelations and interdependencies and to use that knowledge to ensure mutual understanding, respect, support, and cooperation. Here are examples:

Sales ⟵⟶ All R&D groups

R&D managers and laboratory workers should be encouraged to spend a day or two (one-on-one) with a salesperson "on the road," for two primary reasons:

1. R&D individuals can observe first hand the results of their labors.
2. Salespersons can learn important, relevant scientific facts about what they are selling and can directly inform the R&D person about problems their customers experience.

Synthetic chemistry ⟵⟶ Biopharmaceutics

Oral absorption data can help lead synthetic chemists in the most promising directions for NCE variations.

Synthetic chemistry ⟵⟶ Product R&D

Formulators usually prefer the most water-soluble form of an NCE; this can conflict with Synthetic Chemistry and Chemical Manufacturing's interest in high yields.

Biopharmaceutics ⟵⟶ Pharmacology

Interactional benefits go both ways, but Biopharmaceutics can help pharmacologists determine whether lackluster potency is attributable to inherent inactivity or poor oral absorption.

Product R&D ⟵⟶ Toxicology

True event: Product R&D helped Toxicology determine that the apparent intestinal irritation of an orally administered NCE was caused not by the drug, but by the "innocuous" solvent (glycerin).

Analytical chemistry ⟵⟶ Quality control

Analytical Chemistry develops stability-indicating assays for R&D, then transfers them to Quality Control when the product is marketed. Too often these groups are at loggerheads concerning what is an adequate, efficient assay procedure for the NCE. Management's mutual respect and cooperation, plus voluntary temporary interdepartmental transfers, can usually minimize these difficulties.

Pharmaceutical manufacturing ⟵⟶ Product R&D

1. These two groups need to interact at the appropriate stages in new drug development (especially scale-up) to ensure that a dependable, high-quality product can be consistently and economically manufactured.
2. Hands-on Manufacturing employees may feel most comfortable interacting with R&D scientists at the B.S./Associate degree level rather than at the Ph.D. level.

3. Product R&D laboratory workers at all educational levels should spend their first month or two in Pharmaceutical Manufacturing—working hands-on rather than just observing.

Marketing ←→ All R&D groups

True event: A Marketing executive was touring R&D laboratories and asked a key synthetic chemist working on antibacterials what she thought was the most important quality in an antibiotic after therapeutic activity. She replied, "lack of bacterial resistance." When the executive emphasized that Marketing was most concerned about lack of side effects, the scientist said, "No one ever told me that."

Quality assurance and documentation ←→ All R&D groups

Quality Assurance and Documentation should be thought of—and think of itself and operate accordingly—as helpful and supportive, not punitive.

Experimental engineering/product R&D ←→ Pharmaceutical manufacturing

True events:
1. Experimental engineering and Product R&D developed a computer-controlled automatic lyophilization process that was then transferred to Pharmaceutical Manufacturing.
2. Air-suspension particle/tablet coating and electronic monitoring of Pharmaceutical Manufacturing's tablet presses improved product quality and manufacturing efficiency.

DEVELOPING LINE-EXTENSION PRODUCTS

Once the first NCE product has been approved by the government regulatory agency, additional products (Product Line Extensions, or PLEs) are often developed. Requests for PLEs usually come from Marketing and Sales, but ideas can come from any employee/department, particularly from Product R&D. Regulatory approval of most PLEs is less demanding than for NCEs, e.g., there are fewer safety and clinical experiments.

SUCCESSFUL MANAGEMENT OF DRUG DEVELOPMENT

Successful management consists of a series of thoughts, attitudes, feelings, and skilled practices, not simply (and

counterproductively) an "I-am-the-boss-so-do-what-I-say" culture.

Characteristics of a Fertile R&D Work Environment

Psychiatrist Abraham Maslow (1) emphasizes that managers should not be sculptors (molding/forcing/shaping workers) but farmers who create a fertile work environment wherein all employees can learn, grow, and do their best. R&D managers can optimize group spirit, cohesiveness, innovation, and performance by looking at the team as a circle (in which everyone has a significant contribution to make), and not as the usual organizational pyramid with the boss at the top.

Here are characteristics of a fertile R&D work environment, starting with six cornerstones.

- Ethics—This is noted first for obvious reasons.
- Empathy—Empathy is the key to proper treatment of hands-on workers, e.g., managers should ask themselves how they would want their boss to treat them.
- Respect—Feeling respected (valued) as a unique person and as a contributor to group success is as important as anything in the workplace.
- Trust—This is an identical twin to respect. Without mutual trust, two or more people cannot survive a joint effort. The manager's genuine trust of employees as well intentioned, responsible adults is crucial to an efficient, productive work atmosphere.
- Caring—Managers need to have a genuine concern for employees' personal and professional well-being.
- Communication—Keeping employees informed fosters feelings of importance and "being in on things." Managers who listen carefully and inform abundantly will soon be surrounded by good communicators.
- Sense of Purpose—The manager and group members need to know how their department fits into the R&D division.
- Commitment—Everyone has a strong commitment to the long-term health of the division and to harmonized company, R&D, group, and personal goals.
- Competence and Dedication—Group members are competent and confident in each other's ability and dedication.
- Urgent but Well-reasoned, Goal-Focused Activity— Activity is goal-focused, with the general work pace being a healthy blend of urgency and contemplative, well reasoned, deliberate progress.
- Involvement—Productivity, personal growth, and morale will be high if everyone feels involved in the

planning, decision-making, and movement of the department toward its goals.

- Individuality—Everyone wants to be treated as an important, unique individual.
- Acceptance—Related to individuality, each person is valued just as they are; idiosyncrasies are tolerated, even appreciated, because variety is the "spice of life," and no one is perfect.
- Civility—"Good management starts with good manners, society's means of ensuring consideration of others as people" ... Anonymous.
- Agreeableness, Amiability, Friendliness—These are potent antidotes for nervous tension and anxiety and create as much tranquility in a work environment as civility.
- Honesty, Candor, Openness—If trust is basic to all good things in human relationships, honesty, candor, and openness are basic to sustaining/strengthening those relationships.
- Stability, Security, Predictability—The manager needs to be ethical, fair, and consistent without being inflexible. This minimizes uncertainty and anxiety and makes employees feel safe and secure. More energy can then be focused on productive work.
- Cooperation—When co-workers respect and care for one another and when all people feel safe and secure about their "place in the sun," the stage is set for cooperation rather than for competition, for mutual esteem and pride rather than for envy.
- Recognition—Everyone is recognized for his or her accomplishments and value to the organization. Consequently, they feel good about themselves, their colleagues, their boss, and the corporation.
- Thoughtfulness (Consideration for Others)—It has been said that nothing is more contagious than nervous tension, but surely thoughtfulness must run a close second. This can take many forms, but it generally involves getting outside oneself, being significantly oriented toward others rather than solely toward oneself. It means giving rather than taking.
- Genuineness, Realness—A quality work environment helps workers feel safe, secure, and accepted, thus encouraging them to be themselves, "warts and all." This reduces facades, protectiveness, and defensiveness, and allows people to focus their energy on productive work.
- Independence and Interdependence—When employees are valued for their basic worth and respected for their individuality, they develop a strong sense of independence. Consequently, they will have little need to "throw their weight around" or assert their individuality at the expense of others. When people feel good about themselves and receive emotional support from colleagues, they develop a strong sense of both independence and interdependence.
- Cohesive Group Spirit—Under good management, a group develops a close, family-type working relationship in which individual members care for, trust, and respect, and have confidence in one another.
- Deference—If the aforementioned characteristics are operative and the manager seeks advice from and defers to hands-on workers, group members will defer to one another's expertise and judgment when appropriate.
- Pride (but not Arrogance)—Realistic pride in oneself and in the work group strengthens group cohesiveness and individual self-confidence and fosters a "can-do" attitude toward innovation and technical challenges.
- Loyalty and Enthusiasm—When colleagues work at being civil and respectful, loyalty and enthusiasm will arise spontaneously. As Napoleon said, "An army's effectiveness depends on its size, training, experience, and morale ... and morale is worth more than all the other factors combined."

Honorable and Successful Management Practices

The following are specific suggestions for managing drug development. Two quotes say it all:

Honor is the quality of personal integrity. It is won slowly by a lifetime of small decisions where one places the virtues of compassion and justice ahead of his own advancement. — *Anonymous*

The only way to be a successful manager is to learn to behave like one. — *Jay Hall*

Behaving Ethically

This is listed first because everything must be based on consistent ethical principles and behavior. R&D managers work in an especially complex environment: they hold great power and interact in complicated ways with hands-on workers, peers, upper management, customers, local and national government agencies, and citizen groups. R&D managers also face a unique situation because often results must be taken on faith. Most projects involve extensive experimentation and complex interpretation; some involve equivocal results. Managers must:

1. Trust the competence and honesty of laboratory workers, and
2. Make honest use of the group's experimental results.

The leader is primarily responsible for the ethical attitude, behavior, and performance of the department. Here are three ways to ensure success:

1. Set a good example—The manager sets the tone for any group, acting as a role model. When employees observe that the boss is consistently ethical, they will set similar high standards for themselves.
2. Minimize unethical conformity and group-think—Peer pressure dominates most teenagers ("All my friends do it ... "), but adults must resist the slightest unethical behavioral norms.
3. Create a safe, stable, predictable work environment— Unless they are pathological, people suffer ethical lapses out of confusion, fear, and insecurity, not out of evil. When workers are afraid of punishment or dismissal if schedules aren't met, work tends to become sloppy. When R&D vice-presidents fear their jobs are in jeopardy, they might manipulate the information going to corporate management so that their organization will look good.

In summary, leaders need to have the personal qualities of candor, genuineness, and integrity. If not, they are in danger of becoming manipulators of people and situations.

Empathizing (The Golden Rule of Management)

As one of the six cornerstones of successful management, the importance of empathy cannot be overemphasized. Before managers make decisions affecting workers (read "almost all decisions"), they need to remember the Golden Rule of Management: How would I like to be treated? This safeguard on managerial behavior is nearly infallible; here are two examples:

Promotions

Case A: An experienced laboratory scientist believes that he deserves a promotion to the next grade. He raises the issue with his supervisor; she tells him that he has potential, but she is not yet convinced that he has sufficiently proven himself. Nineteen months later he is promoted.

Case B: An experienced research scientist's manager comes into his laboratory and informs him that he has been promoted to the next grade. The scientist is delighted but surprised; he didn't expect promotion for another year. The manager says that it may be a little early, but based on his performance and obvious potential, she believes that he deserves to be promoted now.

Reading this example, managers need to play the role of the laboratory scientist and ask themselves how would they would like to be treated by their boss; and would A or B elevate their spirit and incentive to work hard?

Treating employees as well-intentioned, responsible adults

Case A: Laboratory workers discover that, inadvertently, they are not in compliance with several Good Laboratory Practices regulations. When they inform the manager, he calls a department meeting, scolds all of them, orders them to shape up or else, and demands a full report within 3 days.

Case B: When the manager is informed of the GLP violations, he calls a department meeting, thanks them for alerting him to the problem, and asks them if he can be of any help; who would like to take charge of correcting the situation; and what deadline should be set so that he can reassure his boss.

Again, managers should play the role of laboratory workers and ask themselves how they would like to be treated, A or B.

Communicating

Here are two quite different definitions of communication:

1. The goal of communication is to persuade the listener to agree with the speaker. In this case, one gives little thought to the other's position. Most time and energy are spent thinking about what to say next rather than listening.
2. The purpose of communication is to create understanding. Here the emphasis is on listening, accepting differences of opinion, and freely expressing feelings.

Many sounds (street noise, small talk at a party) are assimilated through a process of hearing. This is primarily a physical phenomenon, with only a small mental element and virtually no emotional component. But when someone tries to communicate something they consider important, hearing becomes inadequate; instead, the other person needs to listen to and understand what they have to say. Now the process requires three components—physical, mental, and emotional—and becomes much more complex.

Generalizations aside, managers need to look at how communication skills apply to their job. First, the leader needs to communicate to employees the kind of person he or she is. Good working relationships, the cornerstone of good performance, depend on people getting to know one another. It is the manager's responsibility to initiate and encourage the communication process that brings about understanding. For example, he should meet at least once a year with each employee to find out:

- How things are going, personally and on-the-job;
- What is good and what is bad about the work environment;
- Always refer to the department as "ours," never "mine";
- Always say, when introducing a group member to someone else, "she works with me," never, "she works for me";
- Encourage being called by his first name, because hierarchy tends to disappear when people are on a first-name basis;
- Try to be the first one at department meetings; too many managers, for various reasons, wait until everyone else is assembled and then walk into the room. Making people wait is an inherent sign of disrespect, intended or not;
- Keep employees informed by posting all nonconfidential memos and notices on a large bulletin board under the categories of "urgent," "new," and "old." These actions are not gimmicks as long as they represent a sincere effort by the manager to communicate clearly and emphatically that everyone in the group is important.

Another valuable communication tool is seldom used—anonymous employee opinion surveys conducted by the manager, in addition to those of the Human Resources department. Annually, workers are asked to submit to the secretary their answers for three questions. The secretary then combines all responses:

1. What I like about my job;
2. What I don't like about my job; and
3. What my boss can do to make things better. Then (and most important), the manager should call a department meeting and ask the group to decide the priorities for improving the work environment.

Organizing

Hands-on laboratory workers

Experts agree that the number-one problem in any corporation is the underutilization of employees. This stems from management's failure to appreciate their intelligence and potential. Douglas McGregor (2) says that most people enjoy working and, given the chance, prefer to exercise self-direction and self-control. They are highly motivated, seek responsibility, and can be a major positive force in company operations if management allows them.

For example, too often Ph.D.s (scientists) are informal project leaders when B.S.- level laboratory workers (associate scientists) can do that job very well, allowing the Ph.D. to act as theoretical science advisors for several project teams. Then Laboratory Assistants (Technicians or Assistant Scientists) with high school diplomas or 2-year degrees can do most of the daily laboratory work with relatively little supervision rather than being treated as a "pair of hands." When employees feel respected and are encouraged to grow and take as much responsibility as possible, they will consult with higher-level scientists when necessary to minimize mistakes and to ensure group success.

First-line supervisors

Group Leaders/Section Heads should be responsible for approximately 15 laboratory workers and should think of themselves as supervisors, not superscientists. The nonsupervisory Ph.D.s should make most of the broad scientific decisions; the Group Leader/Section Head should concentrate on becoming a successful manager of people.

Management

Most organizations have too much management; the number of supervisors at all levels should be minimized.

Supervising

Douglas McGregor says that the supervisor should act as a helper, teacher, consultant, and colleague. Rarely should she assume the role of authoritative boss. Tom Peters agrees, saying "Leaders are servants." Hands-on workers produce results; the manager's primary job is to support them and remove obstacles that prevent them from doing their best. The best supervisor will ask workers what she can do to help; rather than making sure the jobs get done, she assists the workers in doing so.

Many leaders feel this approach reduces their organizational power (using "power" in the good sense), but the exact opposite is true.

1. The manager "sees over" more clearly because discussions with employees will sharpen the view of the situation for everyone.
2. Control and communication are enhanced because employees will interact frequently with a manager who is viewed as a source of help rather than as a giver of orders.
3. Treating employees as competent, responsible adults will greatly increase her influence with them.

Controlling

Originally, controlling meant running a tight ship; the boss watched over everyone and everything, told employees what to do and when to do it, and made all the important decisions himself. But this made the leader and hands-on workers antagonists, resulting in the manager knowing relatively little about what really went on in the trenches. In contrast, appropriate (nonauthoritarian) control means emphasizing employees' self-control simply because most people are trustworthy. This is especially true in R&D organizations in which the emphasis is on high technology, creativity, and innovation.

Peter Drucker, Tom Peters, and Douglas McGregor agree:

1. Drucker says that to be productive, workers need to have control over their work; control is a tool of employees and must never be their master.
2. Peters calls this the control paradox: less is more. Less central control and more genuinely delegated self-control for those closest to the action translates into tighter overall control.
3. McGregor believes that successful supervision is largely dependent on the manager's ability to predict and control human behavior, and the essence of control is selective adaptation. People control the physical world around them, not by expecting nature to do their bidding, but by adjusting their actions to natural laws. For example, humankind does not control surface water by commanding it to flow uphill; rather, people dig channels, adjusting to the fact that water obeys the law of gravity.

Similarly, effective management control consists of channeling workers' energies, interests, and capabilities into activities that meet organizational objectives. Management controls the work force by adjusting its decisions and actions to the realities of human nature, and not by telling people what to do and expecting blind obedience.

Delegating

Managers should delegate because employees like, want, and need to do things their own way. The wise leader assigns research projects only after consulting with laboratory workers, preferably at a department meeting, because bench scientists tend to have a much better feel than the manager concerning who has the time; who is most qualified; and how best to divide up responsibilities.

Also, employees feel more respected and involved when they are part of the work-assignment process.

Delegation, not relegation

Since the biggest waste in any organization is under-utilization of employees, delegation makes sense. Unfortunately, too many leaders confuse delegation with relegation. Delegation means assigning responsibility and authority to a representative. Relegation, on the other hand, connotes consignment to an inferior position. When managers give employees narrow, menial tasks and expect them to do all "delegated" work exactly as they would, their action is relegation, not delegation.

Goals of delegation

Three primary goals of true delegation are to:

1. Relieve managers of some of their workload so that they have more time to think, meditate, plan, learn, and grow;
2. Move work and responsibility as far down the organizational ladder as possible, increasing efficiency; and
3. Offer all employees maximum challenge and opportunities for growth, even when formal promotions are not immediately available. This increases productivity and develops future leaders.

In harmony with these goals, proper delegation has two distinguishing characteristics:

1. Most of the delegated tasks are a meaningful part of the manager's job and not just drudgery to avoid;
2. Workers are allowed, even encouraged, to perform the delegated work in their own way, with the manager helping only when asked.

Case study: In the movie *Bullitt*, a police lieutenant is working on a case that is of intense interest to a powerful U.S. senator. The senator is not happy with the way the lieutenant is conducting the investigation, so he pressures the lieutenant's boss to force him to proceed differently. As it happens, the captain agrees with the senator but refuses to interfere, saying "It's his case, Senator."

Monitoring

Here managers can be either authoritarian (running a tight ship) or smart. They can foolishly spend much of their valuable time monitoring their operation or they can wisely delegate most of that function to employees, thus improving productivity and orderliness, fostering growth, and freeing up more time for broader, long-range tasks.

In a good work environment, the impetus for monitoring comes from below, not from above. This places a positive focus on the process. The manager trusts group members and does not feel a need to monitor the operation closely. At the same time, employees are eager to keep managers informed because they sense that they are interested in their work and in departmental progress. They also recognize the need for management to know the general situation, to be informed of major progress or problems.

On the other hand, authoritative monitoring will yield negative results.

- Workers can't help but feel that managers don't trust them—else why would two people do one person's job? Most employees feel, correctly, that it is part of their job to monitor progress and to address problems.
- The situation is inherently inane, and perceived management inanities contribute to employee disrespect and alienation.
- Workers tend to lose interest in doing a careful job of monitoring when they see the boss repeating what they do.
- Management seldom performs lower-level tasks well. Hands-on employees, to whom such tasks are often challenging, are much more motivated and equipped to do them properly.
- Efficiency and productivity suffer, not only because of the redundancy, but because employees are forced to spend time educating the manager about the details.
- If managers get too involved with minutia, they tend to meddle in workers' jobs, and soup is not the only brew spoiled by too many cooks.

Advocating

This management task never appears in a job description, yet it is vital to enhancing the culture, environment, and performance of an R&D operation.

The world is not a fair place, and the world of work is even less fair. Why? In a free society, adults make most of their own decisions, but not in the workplace, where management and corporate rules reign supreme. Employees feel vulnerable, and "results only" oriented management practices can adversely affect their performance and well-being.

In unionized organizations, the agent or steward serves as employees' advocate (although R&D scientists are seldom part of a labor union); in nonunion companies, the Human Relations department usually fills that role. Seldom is management viewed as an advocate for workers, and rarely does management perceive itself that way. In fact, employees often consider the boss a powerful adversary—the very reason they need an advocate! Surely productivity, not to mention loyalty and enthusiasm, suffers when workers and management consider themselves adversaries.

The manager as advocate

In a well managed, people-oriented organization, the primary advocate for each employee is the immediate supervisor. Not only is that individual in the best position to know and help workers, but she is the major beneficiary of the increased productivity, loyalty, and enthusiasm that follow. Experience has shown that if workers believe their manager is for them and wants them to succeed, and a helper and facilitator rather than an overseer; there is little they won't do for the manager. In fact, when she is under great stress or trouble, the roles become reversed and employees will rush to her aid.

Some managers believe that they should be neither advocates nor adversaries but impartial judges. However, social science professionals have shown that managers are no more rational or impartial than anyone else, that everyone labors under a cloud of personal bias. Furthermore, strict impartiality usually results in impersonal treatment, and no one likes being regarded as a "nonperson." How do managers go about becoming primary personal and organizational advocates for employeehs?

Personal advocacy guidelines

- Managers should get to know each person as an individual and develop a relationship based on mutual trust, respect, and caring. Then employees will feel comfortable bringing them their concerns, and the manager will be able to give employees optimum help.
- Managers need to be perceptive observers of employees, not to check up on them, but to pick up subtle signs of trouble. For example, if an ebullient person becomes very quiet on the job, and this persists for a week or two, the manager may want to say, "I don't want to be nosy, but is anything wrong? Anything I can do to help?" If the employee does not want to talk, the manager should not force the issue, but observe the situation. Showing genuine interest in individuals has a positive effect, even though they may not want to confide in their supervisor. When an employee's performance starts to decline and the manager is quite sure it is not because of any action or inaction on his part, it is best not to intrude on one's privacy; treat the employee as an adult and provide her every chance to work out the difficulties.

- If the employee's performance continues to deteriorate, there will come a time when the manager needs to meet with her and talk. But if he has built a good relationship with the employee she will most likely confide in him long before that point is reached. If the manager finds himself growing impatient with an employee during a difficulty, it's best that he wait a bit longer; it usually pays off. People appreciate a supervisor who shows patience and faith in them during times of trouble.
- When the worker does confide in the manager, he should refrain from giving advice unless asked. Any troubled individual coming to a supervisor needs, first of all, a sympathetic ear and then appropriate reassurance.
- Even when she presses him for advice, both individuals are best off if the manager simply outlines options and their advantages and disadvantages, leaving the ultimate decision to the employee.
- The manager should not try to do too much. If he senses that professional help may be appropriate, a suggestion to that effect or a referral to the company's employee assistance program may be in order.

Organizational advocacy guidelines

Not all problems are highly personal or greatly troubling. Then it is best for the manager to use his administrative ingenuity to deal directly with such problems as a temporarily stalled promotion, a continuing problem with another department, tension or a disagreement with a colleague, or resentment over an ill-defined or apparently unfair company policy. The no-advice rule softens considerably when the manager has some control over the situation. Employees do not expect management to solve all their problems, but they do expect their supervisor to try when it's important to them.

The advocating manager serves as a bridge between employees and the organization. A key girder in that bridge is "loyalty up and down." Workers need to feel that the manager is truly for them, whereas the manager's boss has to be confident that the subordinate is looking out for the company's interests as well. If the manager has a reputation as a strong advocate for employees, when irreconcilable conflicts arise (assuming no violations of ethics or the law are involved), he can come down on the side of the company without straining his relationship with workers.

One of managers' primary responsibilities is to remove impediments to employees productivity. This can be viewed as advocacy as well, because such assistance improves workers' well-being.

Sheltering

Here is another managerial task that is missing from job descriptions, but it is very important, especially in these days of high-pressure, 60-h workweeks. What is sheltering? No matter what the weather outside, the roof, siding, and windows of a house provide a hospitable, safe environment for occupants. So, too, do managers need to create an optimum work atmosphere by sheltering hands-on workers.

Shelter them from what? Swirling about any organization are tensions, antagonisms, organizational red tape, and inanities—unpleasant and distracting. For example, perhaps the R&D vice-president, a tense, caustic individual who is uncomfortable with the deliberate pace of research, is constantly berating department managers to speed things up and increase productivity. The strong tendency in such a situation is to translate at least some of that unpleasantness and pressure down to hands-on workers—the "kick-the-dog" syndrome. With this response, not only are managers relieving some of their own frustrations and resentments, but they are convincing themselves, and trying to convince their boss, that they are team players who are bottom-line oriented. Unfortunately, such a reaction seriously damages the group's work environment and will likely reduce, not enhance, performance, especially in R&D, in which innovation and creativity require a positive atmosphere.

To avoid such debilitating problems, managers need to prevent disruption of the group's productive, relatively tranquil work environment by absorbing as much of the pressure and unpleasantness as possible. By taking most of that burden on their own shoulders, the managers protect the department from contamination by poor management practices elsewhere in the organization. This does not mean that legitimate pressures and emergencies should not filter down; employees can and will respond with vigor and enthusiasm to them, especially when the crisis is viewed as a challenge to the entire group. But no one can do their best when they are constantly pressured to hurry! hurry! hurry! Remember, "if you don't have time to do it right, where will you find the time to do it over?"

Successful sheltering is highly dependent on the level of mutual trust, respect, and confidence within the work group. When there is a strong, caring sense of family, intense sheltering is unnecessary because intrusions from the outside have minimal effect. Quality sheltering requires that managers get out of their offices and see what's going on in the department. If they have no sense of the group's day-to-day moods, detecting rising patterns of tension or indifference becomes difficult. Also, employees are more apt to call problems to the manager's attention if they perceive her as interested, friendly, and accessible.

Five important personal qualities required for good sheltering are:

1. *Strength.* The manager needs to swim against a strong current (i.e., the system or an unreasonable, autocratic boss).
2. *Courage.* There is risk to the manager who stands up for her people against superiors or the system.
3. *Stamina.* Sheltering is a never-ending task.
4. *Ingenuity.* Deflecting a rushing stream (again, the system) usually works better than constructing a dam.
5. *Tact.* Diplomacy usually makes deflection acceptable to the system.

Managers who provide effective shelter for their employees will succeed, both with their workers and with their bosses.

Fostering Creativity

Managers contribute to creativity by:

1. Demonstrating enthusiasm and excitement for new ideas;
2. Managing with a light touch, allowing laboratory scientists the freedom to grow in their own way and at their own pace;
3. Encouraging employees to take risks and explore new territory—and being there with encouragement rather than criticism if they fail;
4. Being both flexible and secure and creating a work atmosphere with those same characteristics;
5. Being committed, not just to today's and this year's comfort and well-being, but to the long-term health of the organization and its employees; and
6. Hiring competent, innovative scientists.

Tips for encouraging creativity

1. "Two heads are better than one" is not a cliché. Ideas are often enriched through discussions with others.
2. Brain-storming sessions involving multidisciplinary groups often produce marketable ideas. The cardinal rule of brainstorming is that no expressed thought be evaluated during the session, because the threat of critique inhibits the free flow of ideas.
3. Managers should refrain from judging employees' ideas. It's best to ask workers to research their concepts with the help of their colleagues (e.g., R&D, Marketing, and Sales) and then evaluate it themselves.

4. When innovation involves replacement of old technology, management often entrusts development of the new technology to old-technology experts. At times this succeeds, but the effort often fails because these veterans have too much intellectual and emotional investment in the old way. It is usually best to assign development of new technology to competent but relevantly inexperienced scientists who will take a fresh, unencumbered approach to the problem.
5. Formal suggestion systems can be beneficial, but management must guard against calcification, by which the suggestions nourish the bureaucratic system instead of the other way around.

Motivating

When thousands of supervisors were asked to list, in descending order, what they thought motivated workers, they got it all wrong. They listed:

1. "Interesting work" as #5, but in the same questionnaire workers chose it as #1.
2. "Full appreciation for work done" as #8, whereas employees rated it #2.
3. "Feeling of being in on things" as #10 whereas workers assigned it #3.

It is clear that managers need to learn more about motivation.

Experts agree that human behavior is not random, but caused; internally motivated; and always directed toward some goal.

Strictly speaking, managers do not and cannot motivate employees. The best they can do is provide the stimuli to which workers react, driven by their own internal motivation.

Psychologist Abraham Maslow (3) hypothesized a hierarchy of needs that classifies human motivation, listed in descending priority:

1. Physiological (hunger, thirst);
2. Safety (security, stability, predictability);
3. Belongingness and social integration (companionship, being part of a group);
4. Esteem (self-respect and recognition/respect from others); and
5. Self-actualization or self-fulfillment (each person's drive to move toward being the very best of which he or she is inherently capable).

The basic needs (physiological) are most important, but once satisfied, they no longer motivate, and the next set becomes operative. Because most employees are not starving nor threatened by anarchy, unless job security is a factor managers should be concerned with:

1. belongingness or social needs.
2. esteem, and
3. self-fulfillment.

Fostering Employee Growth

Human beings have innate pleasure in a sense of growth and improvement. — *Psychiatrist Willard Gaylin*
   To foster workers' growth, managers must:

1. Understand people so that their efforts will harmonize with the realities of human nature;
2. Understand the learning process to ensure the optimal rate of growth; and
3. Apply that understanding on the job with diligence and patience.

Let's examine these three components.

Understanding people

The human characteristics most relevant to the learning/growing process are:

1. *Desire to grow.* Everyone has an inherent tendency to move toward psychological health and maturity.
2. *Personal freedom.* The more people have a say about what they do, how and when they do it, and the direction and pace of personal growth, the faster and surer they will progress.
3. *Uniqueness.* People are different from each other. Everyone is a unique individual, as varied as fingerprints. Each individual has different needs and distinct ways of satisfying those needs.

Understanding the learning process

What does an R&D manager need to know about the learning process?

- Learning can be cognitive, as in memorizing multiplication tables or reading books; or experiential, as when riding a bicycle or working effectively in groups. Most learning is a combination of the two, especially in technical organizations, in which cognitive scientific knowledge must be integrated with a wide variety of experiential skills.
- Personal growth is best achieved experientially. Carl Rogers (4) defines the elements involved:

1. Primarily self-initiated, involving the entire person, physically, intellectually, and emotionally. A person learns best when he is ready and wants to learn;
2. Pervasive, making a difference in the attitudes and behavior of the learner;
3. Self-evaluated, in that the learner is the one who decides whether the learning experience is meeting his needs; and
4. Comprehensive, so that total (intellectual and emotional) meaning is experienced.

Application

Here are some general guidelines (keeping in mind the characteristics of a fertile work environment mentioned earlier). Leaders should:

- Manage with a light touch;
- Set a good example;
- Get to know workers as individuals;
- Involve employees as much as possible;
- Encourage risk-taking and creative thinking;
- Not underestimate employees' potential; and
- Consider overall personal growth.

Recruiting

When competent workers are hired, a manager is almost guaranteed good results. However with inadequate employees even a brilliant leader is in serious trouble. Therefore, good recruiting practices are basic to a successful R&D operation.

Effective recruiting depends first on good management of the people already on hand; the motivation, enthusiasm, and loyalty of group members will be obvious to visiting prospects.

True event. Under autocratic management, a division had 18 consecutive rejections; after changing to people-centered supervision, nine of 10 candidates accepted.

Two major steps in recruiting scientific personnel are:

1. Identifying quality candidates, and
2. Bringing them to the organization for in-depth interviews (including a seminar).

The best way to succeed with the first step is to visit universities for interviews with students. The ethical way to succeed with the second step is to have the candidate talk to as many hands-on workers as possible and to encourage interviewers to be honest and candid in answering questions about the organization. The more welcome and respected candidates feel, the better the chances they will accept an offer.

Recruiters should gather information about the candidate by talking with major advisors, other faculty members, former classmates, and formal references. The following personal characteristics are especially important:

competence, productivity, genuineness, growth potential, flexibility, open-mindedness, cooperativeness, deference, communication, self-confidence, motivation, thoughtfulness, ethics, independence, and commitment.

Conducting Formal Performance Reviews

Moral or diagnostic evaluations are always threatening.
—*Carl Rogers.*

The typical formal performance review is similar to a trip to the dentist: There is apprehension before, pain during, and a sense of relief afterward, when the session is over.

Douglas McGregor (2) explains why:

1. Evaluating an employee's performance is highly dependent on the manager's psychological makeup.
2. For various reasons (including managerial malfeasance), the appraisal often has little relation to reality.

True event. Roger, a first-line R&D supervisor, had always received above-average performance reviews. He made no waves, followed orders, did the required paperwork, and sleep-walked his way through corporate life for 10 years, totally ignoring employees' concerns and frustrations. When a new, highly competent department manager arrived, she quickly recognized Roger's incompetence and pressed for his demotion, transfer, or termination. This caused a great uproar because the "record"—a decade of innocuous, relatively positive performance appraisals by a variety of managers—painted an entirely different picture.

1. Experts agree that to a great extent, a worker's performance is a function of how he is managed.
2. Concerning criticism, the effectiveness in communication is inversely proportional to the employee's need to hear it. The more harsh the criticism, the less likely the person can/will accept it.
3. The manager may be able to convey negative judgments, but this will seriously damage the relationship.
4. Performance reviews accentuate the worker's dependence on the manager.
5. It's an open question if a troubled individual really wants to hear about his deficiencies.
6. Concerning amateur counselors (which managers are) Carl Rogers (5) says that the most they can accomplish is a temporary change, which then disappears, leaving the person more than ever convinced of his inadequacy.

There's a better, well-proven, successful approach (which assumes that all employees are performing

adequately; if that's not the case, then the manager needs to transfer or terminate unacceptable performers—see the next section).

1. Well before the actual reviews, employees are reminded that the "system" demands a formal performance appraisal and that certain rituals must, as in the past, be followed.
2. Then the manager reminds them that she has been in close contact with each of them throughout the year, and that consequently, there will be no surprises during the formal interview.
3. The manager assures everyone that their performance review will be a pleasant experience.
4. Then the manager holds formal reviews only when in a relaxed, reassuring mood.
5. When the person first comes into her office, she reiterates the first 3 points.
6. The manager emphasizes—genuinely—what a good job the employee is doing and how glad she is to have him in the department.
7. Then the manager goes into specifics concerning what she likes about the employee and his performance over the past year; he is encouraged to add accomplishments the manager has failed to mention.
8. Next, the manager reminds the employee that the system requires that she record some negatives and asks for suggestions (e.g., he often puts things off until the last minute).
9. The manager then reassures him—genuinely—concerning any weaknesses he brings up, e.g., "If you were perfect, you'd make the rest of us look bad." "Your intentions are always good, and your strengths far outweigh your weaknesses." Any additional discussion in this area should consist exclusively of the manager asking the employee how he feels about the negatives and, most important, where she—or the work situation—is deficient in helping him do his best.
10. The manager then records—honestly—the weaknesses the employee mentions, but puts them in as positive a light as possible (e.g., "Employee tends to complete some assignments at the last minute, but has a good sense of priorities and is always on schedule").
11. Then—and this is especially important—the manager asks the employee what she can do to help him improve even more. She then sits back and listens in a non defensive manner, thanking the employee—genuinely—for the candid feedback (and follows up on the suggestions).

12. The manager sums up by re-emphasizing—again, genuinely—an appreciation for the contributions to the group's accomplishments and her delight in having him as a member of the department.

In summary, criticism should be avoided here and in all management behavior, simply because it's counterproductive, and employees who feel accepted and valued by their supervisor will engage in self-criticism. This is, by far, more productive over the long term.

Transferring or Terminating Unproductive Employees

If, in spite of good management practices, a hands-on worker cannot do the job adequately, the manager is obliged to transfer the employee to a more suitable position elsewhere in the corporation. If that is not an option, then the employee should be terminated if legally possible and ethically acceptable.

Here's a recommended procedure to follow:

1. The manager should consult the Human Resources department personnel for official guidance. In fact, it is wise to work with them unofficially at a much earlier stage.
2. After ensuring that his actions have been consistent with company policy, the manager should bring the employee into his office for a private, candid, uninterrupted, and caring conversation.
3. He should begin by saying, "I'm sorry, but things are not working out and you are facing termination. You don't have to leave tomorrow, but if you were still here 6 months from now it would be a problem. Sometime between tomorrow and 6 months from now you need to find a job with a different company. I'll help you all I can, but in the end, that's your responsibility."
4. The person will almost certainly be upset and antagonistic toward the manager. At that point, he needs to remember that the employee is going through an ultratraumatic process and needs all the sympathy and support he can muster. The last thing the manager should do is try to defend his decision unless pressured by the employee, which usually does not occur.

Managers who recruit and manage well will seldom have to perform this unpleasant task.

Promoting

Proper selection of new supervisors is crucial to organizational success.

Promoting the wrong people

The most common mistakes made when choosing people for R&D management positions are:

1. Assuming the best laboratory worker will make the best supervisor (management is an entirely different world than laboratory research);
2. Choosing autocratic, results-oriented people rather than person-centered individuals; and
3. Going outside the company instead of promoting from within, which lowers employee morale and motivation.

Promoting the right people

A key element in promoting the right people is having the right people to promote; thus, recruiting the best candidates and creating a growth-fostering environment are crucial. It is also important to recognize the personal qualities (especially interpersonal orientation) needed to make a good supervisor. Managers should avoid promoting people with little talent for or interest in management. The best way to prevent this is to provide potential supervisors with temporary responsibilities and then evaluate their performance.

Organizing Project Teams

There are two common ways to organize project teams:

1. Informal (in which team members belong to scientific discipline-oriented departments with the leader's role being coordinator, not boss).
2. Formal (in which the project leader has organizational authority over team members).

In pharmaceutical R&D, it seems best to have informal project teams because:

1. Everyone needs an organizational "home" for emotional stability and security reasons, and formal project teams tend to make scientists migrant workers, e.g., when the project is completed, they are often assigned to another project with a new boss.
2. Formal project teams tend to inhibit intergroup cooperation and create unhealthy competition among teams (we should have the highest priority regarding limited joint resources and we want to make sure that our project comes out first in upper management's rating).

International R&D

Domestic R&D managers face special challenges in a multinational corporation; in general, they need to do the following:

1. Know the organizational specifics of their company's international operations;
2. Learn as much as possible about the cultural, economic, technical, and governmental differences among the various countries;
3. Establish close ties with their international R&D colleagues.

A multilingual R&D manager is especially valuable.

R&D Management and Corporate Management

R&D management needs to:

1. Understand and appreciate the views and concerns of corporate management;
2. Develop a broad vision for R&D that is harmonious with long-range corporate plans; and
3. Decide, with workers' help, what is in the best interests of the corporation.

Corporate management must learn enough about the world of R&D to:

1. Appreciate R&D's point of view;
2. Understand the R&D process so that funding is steady, not sporadic; and
3. Recognize the danger signals (confusion, aimlessness, consistently poor decisions, laboratory worker malaise) of poor R&D management to distinguish them from bad-luck cycles inherent to all R&D.

Industry and Academia

Interactions between industry and academia have mutual benefits.

Advantages for academia

1. Educational benefits:

   - Encourages the cross-fertilization of ideas;
   - Offers temporary, education-focused work in industry for faculty, undergraduates, and graduate students; and
   - Develops joint projects for increased knowledge.

2. Financial and other benefits:

   - Support for research
   - Possible employment opportunities for students after graduation
   - Consultantships for faculty
   - Rapid commercialization of academic research

Advantages for industry

1. An increased knowledge base for:

   - Cross-fertilization of ideas
   - More options for new and better products
   - More flexibility in R&D spending (academic support can be enlisted for an urgent but speculative project without making long-term internal commitments)

2. Greater professional development of employees through:

   - Teaching and lecturing opportunities in academia
   - Research sabbaticals
   - Internal short courses given by academic consultants

3. Successful recruiting of new personnel owing to:

   - More thorough evaluation of potential job candidates via summer employment of students
   - Improved corporate image among students and faculty.

BIBLIOGRAPHY

Argyris, C. *Personality and Organization: The Conflict between the System and the Individual*; Harper & Row: New York, 1976.

Bennis, W.; Nanus, B. *Leaders' Strategies for Taking Charge*; Harper Collins: New York, 1997.

Drucker, P.F. *The Practice of Management*, 2nd Ed.; Harper Collins: New York, 1993.

Goleman, D. *Emotional Intelligence: Why it can matter more than IQ*; Bantam Books: New York, 1995.

Hall, J. *The Competence Process: Managing for Commitment and Creativity*; Teleometrics International: Woodlands, TX, 1980.

Leavitt, H.J.; Bahrami, H. *Managerial Psychology: Managing Behavior in Organizations*, 5th Ed. University of Chicago Press: Chicago, 1988.

Likert, R. *New Patterns of Management*; McGraw-Hill: New York, 1987.

Maslow, A.H. *Eupsychian Management: A Journal*; Irwin-Dorsey: Homewood, IL, 1965.

Maslow, A.H. *Motivation and Personality*, 2nd Ed.; Holtzman, W.G., Murphy, G., Eds.; Harper & Row: New York, 1970.

McGregor, D. *The Human Side of Enterprise*; McGregor, C., Bennis, W.G., Eds.; McGraw-Hill: New York, 1985.

Rogers, C.R. *Freedom to Learn for the 80s*; Charles, E.Merrill, Ed.; Columbus, OH, 1983.

Rogers, C.R. *Carl Rogers on Personal Power: Inner Strength and its Revolutionary Impact*; Delacorte Press: New York, 1977.

Sampson, R.C. *Managing the Managers*; McGraw-Hill: New York, 1965.

Tingstad, J.E. *Good Technical Management Practices: A Complete Menu*; Interpharm Press: Buffalo Grove, IL, 1999.

MATHEMATICAL MODELING OF PHARMACEUTICAL DATA

David W.A. Bourne
University of Oklahoma, Oklahoma City, Oklahoma

INTRODUCTION

The intent of this article is to give the reader an overview of mathematical modeling as it can be applied to pharmaceutical and especially pharmacokinetic data. The emphasis is on the application of nonlinear regression techniques for the determination of suitable models and best-fit parameter estimates. A number of topics are discussed, including simulation of models described as explicit, implicit, or differential equations; numerical integration methods; optimization algorithms; weighting schemes; evaluation of program output; and approaches for designing future experiments.

The discussion begins with a rationale for modeling and a general approach to the development of suitable models. A brief review of various pharmacokinetic and other pharmaceutical models are followed by a description of methods used to determine calculated values of the dependent variable. The next step in modeling the data involves parameter estimation using a suitable optimization procedure. Not all data points have the same error or uncertainty, thus a weighting scheme should be considered. A variety of schemes are commonly used and all have some advantages. An extremely important part of any modeling exercise is the evaluation of the computer output. Each computer program will provide various information such as plots of the data and residuals, tables of observed, calculated, and residual data, and a variety of statistical parameters. These all can be important in the overall evaluation of the results. The first experiment and the first model are usually not final. Determination of the best model to explain the available data may be required. More experiments may be necessary, thus optimal sampling times or sample sites may need to be explored.

REASONS FOR MODELS

Successful modeling of experimental data should result in a concise and, it is hoped, precise representation of the real world. Successful models allow the exploration of mechanisms, simplify the reporting of experimental results by the condensation of the data collected allowing useful prediction of future results.

Mechanisms Exploration

Modeling allows the investigator to explore the underlying mechanism controlling various processes. The investigator may develop a hypothesis theoretically or based on preliminary observations. When fully developed, this hypothesis may result in one or more mathematical descriptions. On the basis of this hypothesis, experiments are planned and conducted and the results are analyzed. The most successful hypothesis or mathematical model will best explain the collected data. Variations between the predicted and measured observations may lead to refinement of the hypothesis (or the experimental techniques). An extension of the original experiments may be used to support and confirm the hypothesis. For example, a pharmacokinetic model developed after single-dose administration of a drug may be tested by changing the route of administration or by using multiple-dose administrations.

Data Condensation

Mathematical models allow for considerable data compression. Data that fill many notebooks and/or tables may be summarized by means of the few parameters of a well chosen model. Plasma concentration versus time data collected during a pharmacokinetic study in many patients may be summarized using a volume of distribution term and an elimination half-life. Other models may include more parameters, but there is always a considerable compression in the information required to describe the overall results of the study. An extensive drug stability study involving many samples stored at various elevated temperatures may be summarized as a single time for 10% decomposition at room temperature. Determination of appropriate models can be a very useful method of summarizing an experimental study.

Prediction

A thoroughly tested model with numerically determined parameter values should have very good prediction potential. A successful drug regimen design relies on the development of suitable pharmacokinetic models. With a good pharmacokinetic model and parameter values determined in similar patients, it becomes possible to calculate successful dosage regimens for future patients, either directly or by using a Bayesian analysis with limited patient data.

GENERAL METHOD

The detailed design of an experimental study varies considerably depending on the area of research, the objectives of the study, the study material available, and available methods of data collection. As many variables as possible should be controlled or measured. Study material and assay methods should be well defined. The sample schedule should be optimized to collect the most informative data. (Optimal sampling strategies are discussed later.) Once the experiment is designed and the data collected, a mathematical model can be used to analyze the results. Typically, a number of models will be evaluated, as will the utility of the data and data schedule. The cycle may include revised analyses and/or revised experiments (Fig. 1). Methods for distinguishing between models and for selecting optimal sampling times are covered later in more detail.

This discussion of mathematical modeling is limited to methods based on the assumption of error in the y (dependent) term only. The objective or minimization function will generally be restricted to the sum of the weighted residuals between the observed and calculated data, weighted sum of squared residuals (WSS). The objective of the mathematical modeling approaches is to adjust the parameter values so that a minimum value of the WSS is achieved.

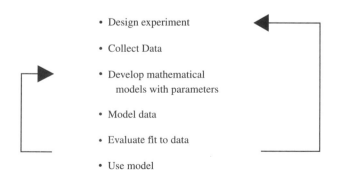

- Design experiment
- Collect Data
- Develop mathematical models with parameters
- Model data
- Evaluate fit to data
- Use model

Fig. 1 Mathematical modeling: A general approach.

Error in y Term Alone

With any experiment, measurement or random error may be found in the independent variables, the dependent variables, or both. However, most common modeling programs assume that the independent variable can be set or measured without significant error. Thus, all the error is assumed to be with the dependent variable. Therefore, it is important that the independent variables are carefully measured or controlled. For example, when time is the independent variable, actual times should be recorded and used in the data analyses rather than scheduled times. Although most modeling of pharmaceutical data has confined the error to the y term, there have been attempts to include error in the x value during the fitting process (1).

Least-Squares Criteria

The objective of any modeling exercise is to place a calculated line (based on some relevant mathematical model) as close to the data collected as possible. The difference between individual data points and the calculated line (in a vertical direction—no error in the x terms) is called the residual. The sum of residuals could be zero even with very large residuals for individual points if the negative residuals canceled the positive values. An absolute residual might solve this problem, but more usefully, the squared residual will also achieve the desired result. This is the least-squares criterion. An extension of this is to weight each data point by the inverse of the estimated variance. This term is the objective function, WSS, shown in Equation (1), calculated for "n" data points:

$$\text{WSS} = \sum_{i=1}^{i=n}(\text{Calculated Value}_i - \text{Observed Value}_i)^2$$
$$\times \text{ Weight}_i \qquad (1)$$

With normal weighted nonlinear regression, the objective is to minimize this objective function. As it is described later additional terms may be added to the objective function when performing extended least-squares (Eq. 23) or Bayesian analyses (Eq. 24).

Parameter Adjustment

The minimization of the WSS value is achieved by systematic modification of the values of the adjustable parameters of the model chosen. Changing the parameters moves the calculated line and thus the WSS.

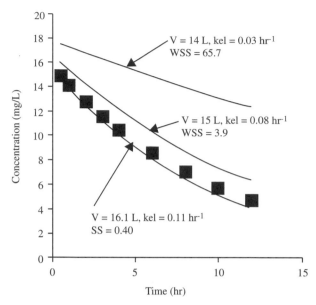

Fig. 2 Illustration of the effect of parameter values on WSS value. Calculated using a one-compartment IV bolus model with weighting by $1/\mathrm{Val}^2$.

Achieving the minimum WSS most efficiently is the objective of the minimization algorithms incorporated into the various nonlinear regression programs. Fig. 2 illustrates how the WSS value changes with different parameter values.

MATHEMATICAL MODELS

Most pharmaceutical results can be quantitated and represented by a mathematical model. The model thus developed consists of the dependent variables measured during the experiments (y), independent variables (x), parameters (p; adjustable or unknown), and constants (c). Thus, a mathematical model may have the general form shown in Eq. 2.

$$y = f(x, p, c) \qquad (2)$$

A number of equations will be presented as examples of mathematical models in use in pharmacokinetics and pharmaceutics.

Pharmacokinetics

Pharmacokinetics is the mathematical description of drug absorption and disposition. As such, it lends itself to mathematical modeling and the use of the models developed previously. Within the field of pharmacokinetics,

a different types of models are used. These include compartmental, physiologically-based, and pharmacodynamic models.

Compartmental models: With this type of model, the subject is represented as a number of well mixed compartments. When all the rate processes are first-order, equations in the form of sums of exponential terms are commonly used. Thus a two-compartment model is illustrated by Eq. 3:

$$Cp = A \bullet \exp(-\alpha \bullet t) + B \bullet \exp(-\beta \bullet t) \qquad (3)$$

where Cp is the dependent variable (concentration); t is the independent variable (time); and A, B, α, and β are parameters.

With more involved compartmental models, including, for example, Michaelis–Menten elimination kinetics, the model may be described more easily using differential equations. Thus, for a drug eliminated by a first-order excretion process and a Michaelis–Menten metabolic process, Eq. 4 holds:

$$\frac{dCp}{dt} = -\frac{Vm \bullet Cp}{Km + Cp} \qquad (4)$$

$$\text{Initial condition} = \frac{\text{Dose}}{V}$$

where dCp/dt is rate of change of drug concentration; Cp is the dependent variable; ke, Vm, Km, and V are parameters; and Dose is a constant. The differential equation is solved numerically to provide Cp values versus time. More information concerning the various equations associated with compartmental pharmacokinetic models can be found in the text by Gibaldi and Perrier (2), Bourne, Triggs, and Eadie (3), Wagner (4, 5).

Physiologically based pharmacokinetic models (PBPK): In contrast to compartmental models where most of the parameters are abstract and empirically based, PBPK models include many physiologically relevant parameters. These parameters include tissue or organ volumes, blood or plasma flow rates, and partition coefficients between blood and tissue. In some studies, protein binding or tissue binding parameters may be included. Drug elimination is commonly expressed as renal, hepatic, or other clearance. These models are expressed as mass balance-based differential equations. Thus, the rate of change of drug concentration in any organ or tissue of interest is given by Eq. 5:

$$V \bullet \frac{dC}{dt} = [\text{Mass of drug flowing in} -$$

$$\text{Mass of drug flowing out}] \qquad (5)$$

For a single noneliminating organ, this becomes Eq. 6:

$$V \bullet \frac{dCp_i}{dt} = \left[Q_i \bullet C_b - \frac{Q_i \bullet C_i}{R_i} \right] \qquad (6)$$

where C_i and C_b (drug concentration in tissue "i" and blood) are the dependent variables; t is the independent variable (time); and Q_i, R_i, and V_i are tissue blood flow rate, tissue to blood partition coefficient, and tissue volume, respectively. More detailed descriptions of these types of models can be found in the text by Gibaldi and Perrier (2) or in the papers of Bischoff and Dedrick (4, 6).

Pharmacodynamic models: These models are designed to relate drug effect (dependent variable) to drug concentration or time (independent variable). Included in these models may be disposition parameters, such as volumes and rate constants, as well as drug effect parameters such as E_{max} (maximum effect) and $EC_{50\%}$ (concentration eliciting 50% of maximum effect). The Hill equation has been used successfully to describe the relationship between effect and drug concentration. More information about these types of models may be found in the text by Gibaldi and Perrier (2) or the paper by Sheiner et al (7). Jusko proposed an alternative model involving equilibrium with the hypothetical receptor site (8). Recently, Jusko et al. have described four basic models to describe indirect drug effects that include tolerance or rebound, which should be useful (9, 10).

Stability

Drug stability studies may require the use of zero-, first-, or second-order reaction models. Reaction rates may be measured as a function of pH and buffer concentrations to determine the influence of various catalysis possibilities. For example, the hydrolysis of a compound may be pseudo first-order, as shown in Eq. 7:

$$\frac{dC}{dt} = -k' \bullet [C] \qquad (7)$$

where the first-order rate constant, k', can be expressed as in Eq. 8:

$$k' = k_0 + k_H \bullet [H^+] + k_{OH} \bullet [OH^-]$$
$$+ k_{HB} \bullet [HB] + k_B \bullet [B^-] \qquad (8)$$

Here the terms, k_0, k_H, k_{OH}, k_{HB}, and k_B, refer to noncatalyzed and specific acid, specific base, buffer (acid), and buffer (base) catalysis. Additional details regarding the models required to describe drug stability studies can be found in textbooks such as the one by Carstensen (11).

SIMULATION OF DATA

Mathematical models involve many different types of equations. These may be explicit, implicit, or differential equations. Dependent variables expressed as explicit equations are easily calculated. For example, plasma concentrations after a single oral dose can be calculated as in Eq. 9:

$$C_p = \frac{F \bullet \text{Dose} \bullet ka}{V \bullet (ka - kel)} \bullet \{\exp(-kel \bullet t) - exp(-ka \bullet t)\} \qquad (9)$$

Implicit equations include the dependent term in a form not readily separated from the other terms in the equation. One example in Equation (10) for drug concentrations after IV bolus administration, following Michaelis–Menten elimination kinetics as described by Wagner (12):

$$C_0 - C + K_m \bullet \ln\left(\frac{C_0}{C}\right) = V_m \bullet t \qquad (10)$$

Here the dependent variable C is found in two parts of the equation and cannot be solved directly. Thus, an iterative method (13) may be necessary to determine the value of C at each value of t, the independent variable.

Integration Methods

Many processes in the pharmaceutical sciences are dynamic. Thus, models of these processes may commonly involve differential equations, which must be numerically integrated at each step in the optimization procedure. A variety of numerical integration methods can be used, and some of these are discussed later.

When a model is expressed as differential equations, they usually must be integrated before the optimization can be performed. Thus, the differential terms must be converted into values for the dependent variable. For example, the differential Eq. 11:

$$\frac{dCp}{dt} = -kel \bullet Cp \qquad (11)$$

could be converted into the integrated Eq. 12:

$$Cp = \frac{\text{Dose}}{V} \bullet \exp(-kel \bullet t) \qquad (12)$$

Conversion from the differential equation form can be performed by analytical methods or numerically, using appropriate computer algorithms. Analytical integration may be mathematically intensive (or impossible), and numerical integration tends to be computationally intensive. Selection of the best approach depends on the equations involved.

Laplace transforms

Integration of differential equations can be quite involved and the subject of complete college courses (14). However, one useful technique is the method of Laplace transforms. An excellent tutorial is presented in the two papers by Mayersohn and Gibaldi (15, 16). Benet and Turi (17), and Benet (18) present more advanced techniques, such as the input and output disposition functions and the "fingerprint" technique for the solution of differential equations.

Another approach presented by Yamaoka et al. (19), uses a fast inverse Laplace transform to generate the integrated equation data. Thus the model is described in terms of the Laplace transform equations and solved numerically.

Numerical integration

Numerical integration also starts with a number of differential equations and initial conditions. However, now the computer program performs the integration. Using carefully defined algorithms, the computer program is able to start with the initial condition(s) and project forward with increasing values of the independent variable (often time) according to the slope given by the differential equation(s). With a careful selection of algorithm, accurate approximations to the required result can be calculated efficiently. The general approach can be understood more easily by looking at a simple point-slope method such as Euler's method. However, these methods are not

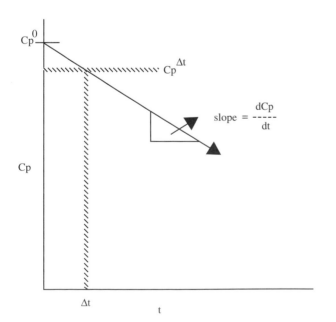

Fig. 3 Illustration of the point-slope method.

necessarily the most efficient. Runge–Kutta methods, including the Fehlberg modification, have advantages with the usual differential equations encountered in pharmacokinetics and pharmaceutics. For systems where the rate constants are widely disparate, so-called "stiff" systems, other methods become more useful.

Point-slope methods: Euler's method follows directly from the initial condition as a starting point and the differential equation as the slope (Fig. 3). Consider the simple model of a single differential Eq. 13 with one first-order rate process:

$$\frac{dCp}{dt} = -kel \bullet Cp \tag{13}$$

with an initial condition of Cp at time $= 0$ of Cp^0. Thus, the change in the value of Cp from time $= 0$ to time $= \Delta t$ is shown by Eq. 14:

$$\Delta Cp = \frac{dCp}{dt} \bullet \Delta t \tag{14}$$

and the value of Cp at time Δt by Eq. 15:

$$Cp^{\Delta t} = Cp^0 - kel \bullet Cp \bullet \Delta t \tag{15}$$

If Δt is sufficiently small, relatively accurate calculations can be performed. Unfortunately, very small step sizes are often required for reasonable accuracy and truncation errors then can be significant. Thus, this method is not generally used with nonlinear regression programs.

Euler's methods can be derived from a more general Taylor's algorithm approach to numerical integration. Assuming a first-order differential equation with an initial value such as $[dy/dx] = y' =$ function of x, and $y = f(x,y)$ with $y(x_0) = y_0$, if the $f(x,y)$ can be differentiated with respect to x and y, then the value of y at $x = (x_0 + h)$ can be found from the Taylor series expansion about the point $x = x_0$ with the help of Eq. 16:

$$y(x) = y_0 + hy'(x_0) + \frac{h^2}{2!} \bullet y''(x_0) + \dots \tag{16}$$

where h is an increment in x, that is Δt. It can be seen that including only the first two terms on the right side of Eq. 16 leads directly to Euler's method. This method gives increased accuracy with more terms on the right side of the equation. However, it is not readily applicable as a general-purpose procedure because of the requirement for higher-order derivatives. It has been useful theoretically in the development of more general-purpose methods such as the Runge–Kutta methods.

Runge–Kutta methods: The Runge–Kutta methods attempt to improve the accuracy of the calculation and avoid the evaluation of higher-order derivatives. The general approach is to determine values of the first-order differential equation at subintervals of the chosen step size. The way in which these subinterval results are combined can be derived from the Taylor series expansion. The most common of these Runge–Kutta methods is the classical fourth-order version. The values of the function are calculated four times for each step to improve the accuracy of the calculation. For complex functions, this may be a disadvantage. Another problem with this method is that it lacks any automatic step-size control. Additional details of these Runge–Kutta methods may be found in textbooks on numerical analysis (13).

The Runge–Kutta–Fehlberg is a further modification of the Runge–Kutta fourth-order method. It uses a fifth function evaluation to determine the appropriate step size. This method appears to be very efficient for nonstiff systems of differential equations. Additional details regarding this method and a computer listing can be found in a report by Fehlberg (20) and in the chapter by Watt and Shampine (21).

Multistep methods: Another class of methods, called multistep methods, involves the use of more than one previous value in the calculation of the "next" value. With the slope-point and Runge–Kutta methods, a single starting point (and the differential equation) is all that is required for the calculation of the next value at $(x + h)$. With a commonly used four-step method, values at $(x-3h)$, $(x-2h)$, $(x-h)$, and x are required in the calculation of y at $(x + h)$. One such method is that of Adams and Bashford (22).

The advantage of these techniques is that they require only one (additional) function evaluation for each step compared with four or five evaluations for the typical Runge–Kutta method. Thus, they should be faster. Their principle disadvantage is that they are not self-starting. Another method, Euler's or Runge–Kutta, is required to calculate the first (three) values at x, $(x + h)$, and $(x + 2h)$ before the Adams–Bashford multistep equation can be used to continue the calculation. Additional starting values are also required whenever the step size is changed.

An extension of the multistep methods is the predictor-corrector approach. Here, the Adams–Bashford equation may be used to calculate a "predicted" value for y at $(x + h)$. Then a second, corrector, equation is used to refine the value of y. If the difference between the predictor and corrector values is within specified error limits, the calculation is continued to the next step, otherwise the step size will be adjusted to maintain the error limits specified. With fewer function evaluations per step, these methods can be faster than the Runge–Kutta methods; however, they are not self-starting.

Methods for stiff equations: Stiff systems of differential equations occur commonly with physiologically based models. That is, very fast processes and very slow processes occur in the same model. The ratio between the fastest and the slowest rate constant can be used as an index of stiffness. With ratios greater than 500, a number of the "nonstiff" numerical integration methods become very inefficient. Gear's method for solving stiff systems has achieved wide acceptance (23, 24) and has been incorporated into a number of nonlinear regression programs such as SAAM II and Boomer. Adam and Gear's methods are both included in Gear's DIFSUB algorithm. The user has to specify which method they wish to use. The differential equation solver LSODA included in the ADAPT II program automatically switches between Adam and Gear's methods as required.

FITTING MODELS TO DATA

Fitting the model to the observed data is an important task. Each mathematical model studied consists of independent and dependent variables, constants (possibly), and parameters that have to be estimated. The objective is to reduce the overall difference between the observed data and the calculated points by adjusting the values of the parameters. As mentioned earlier, the methods to be discussed assume that there is no error in the independent variable. Also, in general, the criteria of "best" fit will be the weighted sum of squared residuals between the observed and calculated data, the WSS. The chosen model can be validated in part by accurately describing the observed data.

Graphical Methods

It is often possible to manipulate the mathematical model into the form of a straight-line equation. For example, the one compartment pharmacokinetic model after an IV bolus can be expressed as a differential equation or as an exponential equation as shown earlier. By taking the natural log of the exponential equation, Eq. 17 in the form of a straight line can be derived:

$$\ln(Cp) = \ln(Cp^0) - kel \bullet t \qquad (17)$$

Thus, by graphing the data on semilog graph paper and drawing a straight line through the data it is possible to read Cp^0 from the intercept and calculate kel from the natural log slope, as in Eq. 18:

$$kel = -\text{ slope} = \frac{\ln(Cp^1) - \ln(Cp^2)}{t_2 - t_1} \qquad (18)$$

Graphical methods have a number of advantages. They are usually fast and, when performed carefully, can give accurate results. A major plus for the method is the ability to "see" the data and visually determine whether there are systematic deviations from the chosen mathematical model. Graphical evaluation of the data may lead to consideration of alternative models. Graphical methods can be very useful in the estimation of initial parameter values. Unfortunately, these methods are not universally available, because it may not be possible to produce a straight-line equation. When manipulating the model to produce a straight line, the observed data is often "transformed," which may involve taking the logarithm or the reciprocal of the observed data. With other models, more involved transforms are required. This not only distorts the data but also the error or variance of the data. When using linear regression by the graphical approach, it is assumed that the error in each x-value is similar. Once the data are transformed, this may not be true. Another problem that is especially relevant with the use of log transforms and semilog graphical data representation involves the visual distortion that can occur. Typically, much of the graph is taken up by the least accurate data points; i. e., the last few data points at the lowest (and thus, the least well defined) concentrations may dominate the graph. Thus, although graphical techniques such as semilog data plots may be useful in the determination of initial estimates, they are not as suitable for complete data analysis or presentation of the final results.

Other approaches have been used for more complex models. These include curve stripping or the method of residuals (2), either manually or using a computer program

such as CSTRIP and ESTRIP (25, 26). These techniques can separate a multiexponential curve into its component parts for initial estimates. Other techniques include deconvolution methods specific to the one and two compartment pharmacokinetic models (27, 28). The objective of the deconvolution method is to mathematically "subtract" the results obtained after IV administration from the oral or extravascular data. This results in information about the input or absorption process alone. More general methods have been presented by various researchers that do not rely on a particular compartmental model (29–31).

Nonlinear Regression Analysis

For all mathematical models that are not "naturally" straight lines, nonlinear regression analysis is often the best approach. The observed data and the corresponding dependent variable can be analyzed without transformation. Thus, the data and the error or variance are not distorted during the analysis. If necessary, clearly defined weighting schemes can be applied. Furthermore, multiple observation sets can be readily accommodated.

Nonlinear regression analyses involve relatively complex calculations and thus are well suited to computer assistance. However, the program must have a well developed sequence of steps or algorithm to follow. Some methods are better than others. The program is asked to find the minimum point on a weighted sum of squares (objective or minimized function) surface. For two parameters, this can be represented as a three-dimensional surface (Fig. 4).

With more parameters, it is difficult to represent the shape of the WSS surface, but the program still moves to a minimum value of the WSS. Depending on the shape of this surface, there may be a number of local minima. That is, regions that are "lower" than the surrounding surface but *not* the "global" minimum. The objective of the nonlinear regression analysis is to reach the global minimum. Helpful strategies include: 1) careful calculation of initial estimates; 2) repeated analyses with different sets of initial estimates; and 3) careful evaluation of the program output, especially the plot of calculated and observed data versus time (x-value).

Many basic algorithms, each with a number of refinements, are useful in the search for a global minimum. Some of these methods are described briefly. These are the grid search, steepest descent, Gauss–Newton, Marquardt, and simplex methods.

Grid search

This method is more informative, but it can be quite slow. Its major objective is to produce a weighted sum

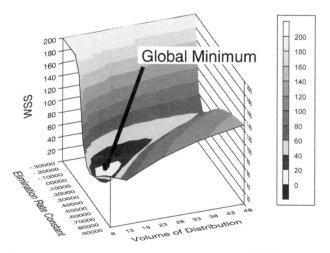

Fig. 4 A three-dimensional surface plot of WSS versus elimination rate constant and volume of distribution for a two-parameter model.

of squares surface diagram. In addition the minimum calculated WSS is estimated. The three-dimensional plot in Fig. 4 was calculated by this method. The calculation is set up by inputting the upper and lower limits of each parameter of interest. This range is split into a number of steps, and the program calculates the WSS at each point on the grid. The more steps, the smoother the surface but the longer the calculation. A three-parameter problem with only 10 steps per parameter (a relatively coarse grid) requires 1000 ($= 10 \times 10 \times 10$) calculations of the WSS. With many parameters and steps, these calculations can be very lengthy. This method is not usually used for nonlinear regression analyses, but its output may be educational.

Steepest descent

If the WSS surface is seen as similar to a geographical section with hills and valleys (at least for the two-parameter surface), the steepest-descent method would appear to follow the path of a round ball moving towards the minimum. When translated to a computer algorithm, some of the disadvantages become more apparent. The basic approach is to calculate the slope of the surface at the point of the initial (or current) parameter values. This can be calculated as $d\text{WSS}/dP$ over some small increment for each of the parameters P. By combining each of these partial derivatives over all the parameters, the direction of movement towards the minimum can be calculated. The second part of the problem is the distance h to move in the specified direction. This must be determined by finding the minimum WSS in the direction calculated from the slope. This means extra calculations of the WSS, which makes this process less efficient, especially as it approaches the minimum. The new parameter value is calculated with the help of Eq. 19:

$$P_{\text{new}} = P_{\text{old}} - h \bullet \frac{d\text{WSS}}{dP} \tag{19}$$

This new value is used as the P_{old} for the next iteration.

Gauss-Newton

If we can assume that the WSS surface between the initial estimate and the global minimum is convex, a Taylor series expansion leads to the Gauss–Newton approximation for a step closer to the minimum (32). Thus, the next point on the surface can be calculated as in Eq. 20:

$$P_{\text{new}} = P_{\text{old}} - \frac{d\text{WSS}}{dP} \left/ \frac{d^2\text{WSS}}{dP^2} \right. \tag{20}$$

This method gives both a direction and a distance. Close to the global minimum, where the surface is

typically more regular, the convergence can be dramatic. Farther from the minimum, the surface may not be convex or as smooth, and the method may become slow or even move away from the minimum. Thus, good initial estimates are very helpful.

The Gauss–Newton method can be improved by using two modifications. The first is a damping process. Thus, the new WSS is calculated with the help of P_{new} calculated using Eq. 20. If this WSS is worse than the original WSS, the step size is halved, and the WSS is calculated again. This is repeated until a preset number of halvings (dampings) occur or a better WSS is achieved. Excessive damping can occur close to the minimum if the WSS surface is very flat, owing to numerical instability. In this case, the uncertainty in the final parameter values (expressed as coefficients of variation or confidence intervals) may be large.

A second method of improving the Gauss–Newton method is the Marquardt modification (33). In this case, the equation for P_{new} is modified by the addition of another term, μI, as in Eq. 21:

$$P_{\text{new}} = P_{\text{old}} - \frac{d\text{WSS}}{dP} \left/ \left(\frac{d^2\text{WSS}}{dP^2} + \mu\text{I} \right) \right. \tag{21}$$

The analysis is started with a large value of μ, which has the effect of moving the equation in the direction of the steepest-descent method, which is better farther from the minimum. As the calculation approaches the minimum, μ is reduced progressively to automatically approach the Gauss–Newton method, which is better near the minimum.

Simplex

Another approach that is different from the previous methods is the simplex method of minimization (34). It involves the formation of a simplex, a geometric shape with $(m + 1)$ sides, where m is the number of parameters on the WSS surface. The WSS is calculated at each corner of the simplex and compared. The movement of the simplex across the WSS surface (toward the minimum) is controlled by a small number of rules. For example, the point with the highest WSS is reflected across the centroid (center of the simplex) to produce a new point. If this point has the lowest WSS, it is extended again. A point with a larger WSS causes the simplex to contract. By a series of such steps, the simplex moves across the WSS surface to approach the minimum value. Although the simplex method can be relatively slow, it has the advantage of computational simplicity that makes it useful for a variety of nonlinear regression problems.

Weighting Schemes

After selecting and describing an appropriate model, choosing a numerical integration method (if necessary) and a fitting algorithm, the mathematical modeler may need to select a weighting scheme for the data to be analyzed. Ideally, each data point is independent and has normally distributed error. Even when this is true, the magnitude of the variance or error in each data point may not be equal. Thus, a weight equal to the reciprocal of the variance may be applied to each data point in the calculation of the overall WSS. Information about the variance, standard deviation (SD), or coefficient of variation (CV) for each data point or how these values vary over the complete data set to be analyzed can be very useful in the selection of a "best" weighting scheme. The weighting scheme is best evaluated by looking at the weighted residual plots as described later.

If a single data set is to be analyzed (at one time) and the variance is similar for each data point, an unweighted regression may be appropriate; i.e., each data point may be given an equal weight. Unweighted regression may be appropriate when the variance is small. With physical systems, the weighting scheme may become less important. The weighting scheme becomes much more important when there is significant error or uncertainty in the data. With biological studies, such as pharmacokinetic determinations, the error in the measured data may be considerable, and the choice of weighting scheme becomes more important.

When the values of the dependent variable have considerable error and cover a relatively large range of values, a carefully selected weighting scheme may be useful or necessary. When the CV about a series of data points is constant, that is, there may be $\pm 5\%$ error in each data point, a weighting scheme can be estimated. Because the CV is equal to SD/Value:

$$SD = \text{Observed value} \times CV \text{ and Variance}$$
$$= \text{Observed value}^2 \times CV^2$$

With a single data set, the CV^2 can be ignored. However, when fitting more than one data set simultaneously, this value is important. Thus, the weight would be proportional to 1/observed value^2. Other weighting schemes include a more general expression, with a and b as constants (35):

$$\text{Variance} = a \times \text{Observed value}^b$$

Provision may be made for an assay sensitivity term:

$$\text{Variance} = a + b \times \text{Observed value}^c$$

Another possibility, especially useful in a clinical setting with older concentration-versus-time data, is to apply a smaller weight to older data (36):

$$\text{Variance} = a + b \times \text{Observed value}^c \times d^{(\text{tlast} - \text{time})}$$

with d typically equal to 1.01 to 1.05.

Careful consideration of the data may suggest a number of equations for the estimated variance of the error in the data. The analyst should consider the overall results produced by the chosen weighting scheme and especially confirm that the weighted residual plots are satisfactory.

Selection of appropriate weighting schemes is even more important if the analyst is modeling more than one data set simultaneously. For example, drug concentration in plasma and cumulative amounts of drug eliminated into urine may have been collected. Consequently, plasma concentrations may range from 0 to 25 μg/ml and will have quite different variance values to cumulative amount of drug in urine data ranging from 0 to 250 mg. If an unweighted analysis was undertaken, the plasma data (numerically lower values for concentrations) would tend to be ignored. Alternately, if the amount of drug excreted into urine was expressed in grams, not in milligrams, these data would be ignored during the fit because they are now much smaller numerically than the plasma concentration. Obviously, an appropriate weighting scheme must be developed. The same problem may occur if plasma concentrations after intravenous and oral administration is to be analyzed together. Again, consideration of the computer program output, especially the weighted residual plots, can help to confirm a chosen weighting scheme.

Iteratively Reweighted Least Squares

The variance formulas used in ordinary weighted least-squares analysis use the observed data values. This is easier to calculate because the observed values do not change during the fitting process. However, there can be advantages to using the calculated data values, instead of the observed values, in the variance formulas. For example, very low data points (which may have considerable error) are not given disproportionate weight. Thus, the technique of iteratively reweighted least squares may be useful (37).

Extended Least Squares

Another approach to weighting the data uses the data itself to develop the variance equation. This is the extended least squares (ELS) method (37, 38). Parameters for the variance equations are included in the fitting process as well as parameters for the chosen model. Thus, extra data points are necessary for a successful analysis. Futhermore, the analyst must decide the form of the variance equation. An example of a typical variance equation is:

$$\text{Variance} = a \times \text{Calculated value}^b$$

where a and b are parameters to be fitted to the data. The objective function must also be altered with the ELS method because driving the calculated variance to a very large value would automatically make the WSS very small, regardless of the fit to the data. Thus, a ln (variance) term is added to the WSS formula as a penalty, and the objective function to be minimized becomes Equation (22):

$$\text{Objective function} = \sum_{i=1}^{i=n} \frac{\left(C(\text{obs})_i - C(\text{calc})_i\right)^2}{\text{variance}(P, PV, t_i)}$$
$$+ \ln\left(\text{variance}(P, PV, t_i)\right) \quad (22)$$

where P values are the parameters of the model, PV values are the parameters of the variance equation, and n is the number of data points. This method is available in the nonlinear regression programs ADAPT II and NONMEM.

Bayesian Analysis

The analysis of clinical pharmacokinetic data offers additional challenges. Typically, the number of samples available from an individual patient can be limited. In some cases, only one or two samples may be available. If population-based pharmacokinetic values are available, it may still be possible to analyze this limited clinical information using a Bayesian approach (36). Using patient and population information, the objective function becomes a function of both the residual between the observed and calculated data (as in weighted least squares) and the residual between the population and the calculated values of the parameters, as shown in Eq. 23:

$$\text{Objective function} = \sum_{i=1}^{i=n} \frac{\left(C(\text{obs}) - C(\text{calc})_i\right)^2}{\text{Variance for data point}}$$
$$+ \sum_{j=1}^{j=m} \frac{\left(P(\text{pop})_j - P(\text{calc})\right)^2}{\text{Variance for parameter}_j} \quad (23)$$

Analysis of Population Data

A typical pharmacokinetic analysis of data from a single individual results in estimates for the values and variance (or SD) of each parameter. The calculated variance gives an estimate of the closeness of fit, the adequacy of the number of data points, and the error in the data values. If this analysis is repeated in a number of individuals, it is also possible to obtain some information about the average population value and intersubject variance. With sufficient data available from each subject, this two-step approach can be efficient using any number of nonlinear regression programs.

A few programs are now available that allow the efficient simultaneous data analysis from a population of subjects. This approach has the significant advantage that the number of data points per subject can be small. However, using data from many subjects, it is possible to complete the analyses and obtain both between- and within-subject variance information. These programs include NONMEM and WinNONMIX for parametric (model dependent) analyses and NPEM when nonparametric (model independent) analyses (39) are required. This approach nicely complements the Bayesian approach. Once the population values for the pharmacokinetic parameters are obtained, it is possible to use the Bayesian estimation approach to obtain estimates of the individual patient's pharmacokinetics and optimize their drug therapy.

Evaluation of computer program output

Once the computer program completes the calculations, it is time to evaluate the output, which should be scrutinized very carefully. Each line is there for a reason. Obvious errors of data entry can be found by looking at the data tables and plots. Model misspecification may be more difficult to access. Each computer program will present users with an array of information. During the evaluation of this output, the fit to the data, the weighting scheme used, and parameter values can be assessed. Each of the items that may be output by a nonlinear regression program should be considered.

Observed and calculated data

The table of observed and calculated data includes the observed x and y values. Some programs are sensitive about how the data should be entered, and data entry errors may be common. This table should be checked to ensure that the program is working with the correct numbers. The calculated data can be compared with the observed data. If the numbers are not similar, there may be problems with parameter value limits or model specification. A residual or weighted residual is often included. These values should be of similar magnitude and randomly positive and negative. The most important use of this table is to ensure correct entry of the observed data.

Most programs provide plots of observed and calculated data versus the independent variable x. On both linear or semilog axes, these should be similar, with the calculated line running close to the observed data. If the observed and calculated data appear to be going in different directions, incorrect model specification should be suspected. If the two lines have a similar shape but do not coincide, may be a parameter value limit is causing a problem. Alternately, the program may have fallen into a local minimum. Rerunning the analysis with better (different) initial estimates may help. This plot can be useful in the identification of incorrectly entered data or outliers.

Another plot often presented is a plot of calculated data versus observed data (with a line representing identity). This can be a sensitive plot for the assessment of the model chosen. Significant systematic deviations from the identity line may indicate the need for additional parameters in the model.

Final Parameter Values

Most programs present the final "best-fit" values of the parameters with some indication of the uncertainty in these values. Parameter values far from the expected results may indicate an incorrectly specified model. Possibly a model constraint has been incorrectly specified. Incorrect units may be causing a problem. The uncertainty in the values may be expressed as an SD or CV. Alternately a CI may be calculated. A high CV, higher than 20% and especially higher than 50%, generally indicates a parameter that is not well described by the data. Maybe the model has too many parameters. High CV values may be caused by small number of data points or data with larger error. Samples may need to be taken from additional parts of the model to fully specify the parameters of interest. This becomes a problem of identifiability, as described below. Many programs also provide a correlation matrix of the estimated parameters. A high correlation (>0.95) may suggest that the model has too many parameters and that a simpler model may be satisfactory.

Weighted Residual Plots

The weighted residual plots can be very useful in the evaluation of the chosen model and weighting scheme. The basic approach is to look for a pattern in the plot. Two types of patterns may be evidence of a problem in the analysis. Residuals larger on one side of the plot compared with the other may indicate a problem with the weighting scheme. A trend in the residuals either sloping up or down, or a "U" or inverted "U" shape, would suggest that one or two additional parameters should be added the model as seen in Fig. 5. The best result is a plot with no discernible pattern. This would support both the model and the weighting scheme selected for the analysis. A more complete discussion of residual plots can be found in the text by Draper and Smith (40).

Statistical Output

The WSS or other objective function is the major statistical parameter provided by any of the nonlinear regression programs. Typically, the analyst is looking for a minimum WSS value. However, this can be misleading if a variety of weighting schemes has been used throughout the analysis phase. For example, with observations greater than 1, the WSS when using an equal weight scheme will be much larger than with a reciprocal observed value or observed value-squared weighting scheme. Thus, comparisons of WSS (or WSS-related functions) must be made between analyses using identical weighting schemes. Some programs will normalize the sum of the weights to be equal to the number of data points. This may help in the comparison of results across the weighting scheme, but all

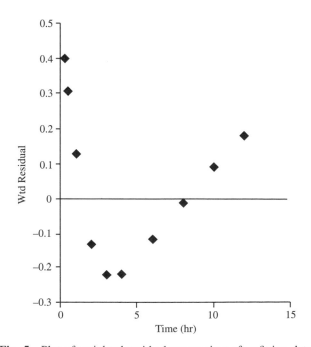

Fig. 5 Plot of weighted residual versus time after fitting data generated with a two-compartment model using a one-compartment model.

comparisons should be made with the same weighting scheme. Comparison of WSS values between similar data sets may help in the identification of sampling or analysis problems.

The correlation coefficient R and the coefficient of determination R^2 are often provided. Both terms are meant to indicate closeness of fit, with a value of 1 representing a perfect fit. With many data sets, a high value of R (greater than 0.9) seems relatively common even with a fit that visually looks poor. Thus, the analyst should not put too much emphasis on this parameter. Similarly, high values of R^2 are relatively easy to achieve. Although these parameters are widely used with unweighted linear least squares, they do not appear as useful in weighted nonlinear regression.

Comparison Between Different Models

A number of the output items already described are useful in the selection of a "best" model. Systematic deviations in the observed and calculated data plots may suggest the need for a model with additional parameters. Large values for the parameter CV values (or wide confidence intervals) may indicate a model with too many parameters. A number of patterns in the weighted residual plots may suggest the addition of parameters to the chosen model. The guiding rule is to start with the simplest model consistent with the data (and theory). As more parameters are added, it is expected that the WSS will decrease. The question becomes, has the inclusion of additional parameters produced a significant decrease in the WSS. Although developed for unweighted analyses, a number of approaches to this question have been used with weighted nonlinear regression. As suggested by Mandel (41) and Boxenbaum et al.(42), an F value can be calculated after the analysis using two different models (with different numbers of parameters), as shown by Eq. 24:

$$F\left(df_j - df_k, df_k\right) = \frac{\mathrm{WSS_j} - \mathrm{WSS_k}}{\mathrm{WSS_k}} \times \frac{df_k}{df_j - df_k} \qquad (24)$$

If the calculated F value is higher than the tabled F at the chosen level of significance (often 0.05), the use of the more detailed model is supported. Another commonly used parameter is the Akaike's Information Criterion (AIC) value (43, 44). It is calculated for each model, and the model producing the lowest value (most negative value) is considered the better model. The AIC value is calculated using the number of data (n), WSS, and the number of parameters (m), as in Eq. 25:

$$\mathrm{AIC} = n \ln(\mathrm{WSS}) + 2 \times m \qquad (25)$$

A variety of other criteria have been developed that may also be useful. It is hoped that each criterion (parameter variability, graphical output, AIC, F test, etc.) will complement each other, allowing the analyst to make an objective decision.

THE DESIGN OF FUTURE EXPERIMENTS

Once the first modeling phase is complete, the analyst may wish to consider revision of the experimental design to test the chosen model or to determine more reliable values for the parameters of the model. This leads to a number of approaches.

Extend the Range of the Current Model

Typically, a series of experiments is performed within a fixed framework. From these results, a "best" model may be selected and parameters determined. One test of this model is to make predictions beyond the range of the original experiments. These predictions can be tested by performing more experiments in the region of the new predictions and determine how well the model simulates the data. For example, a single-dose study may be conducted with data collected and analyzed to give a two-compartment pharmacokinetic model as most appropriate. This model could be tested by predicting and measuring drug concentrations after multiple-dose administration. Alternately a different route of administration may be used.

Identifiability and the Determination of Appropriate Sampling Sites

When working with complex models, it is easy to try to build a model more complicated than the data allow. For example, if a drug is metabolized and excreted unchanged, it is not possible to identify or determine a rate constant for excretion and for metabolism without measuring either drug or metabolite in urine. If the analyst attempted to model this overparameterized model with just drug-in-plasma data, the uncertainty (CV values, etc.) about the parameter values would be very high no matter how many data points were collected or how accurately they were measured. This is a problem in identifiability. The problem is to determine whether the minimum number of sampling sites for a particular model or a given number of sampling sites can adequately define a proposed model. There are a number of approaches to this problem. For linear, time-invariant systems, the Laplace transform method is convenient, whereas the Taylor series method is a more general analytical method (45–47). Numerical approaches have been presented by Jacquez et al.(48, 49) with the development of the IDENT computer program. Another method is to simulate error-free data for the sample sites and the model chosen and "refit" these data. If the uncertainties in the parameters estimated are large (using numerous, error-free data), then an identifiability problem should be expected. The identifiability of a sample and model set should be determined during the initial experimental design stage. This can avoid considerable time and expense.

Determine Optimal Sampling Times to Reduce Parameter Uncertainty

Once the sampling sites have been identified, the next question is, at what times should the samples be collected. Without any previous knowledge of the model or system, sampling times are typically determined from intuition or from similar studies. Because of the uncertainty in the expected result, more samples are typically collected over as wide a range in time as possible. Once these first (pilot study) results have been analyzed, it is possible to make a more rational decision regarding the best sampling times. Some methods use the model selected and the parameter values first determined to obtain the best sampling times. The program SAMPLE, part of the ADAPT II package, uses the C- or D-optimality method. The result typically is one optimal sample time for each parameter to be estimated. Many investigators are uneasy about such a small sample number, thus additional samples may be included. By repeating the SAMPLE calculation with a range of parameter values, it would be possible to determine additional sample times. These times should give the "best" information about the parameters of interest.

Computer Programs

A large number of computer programs are available to perform the functions of mathematical modeling. Some of these are listed below. See http://www.boomer.org/pkin/soft.html for a more complete and up-to-date list.

1. ADAPT II is supplied as FORTRAN code for VAX VMS, MS DOS, and SUN UNIX systems. It performs simulations, fitting, and optimal sampling and includes extended least-squares and Bayesian optimization. Models can be expressed as integrated or differential equations using FORTRAN statements.

2. BOOMER is supplied as a compiled program for Macintosh and MS DOS systems. It performs simulation and fitting and includes Bayesian optimization. Models, integrated or differential equations, are expressed as a sequence of parameters.

3. IDENT2 and IDENT3 are provided as FORTRAN source code (IDENT2C is provided in C) for VAX VMS and other systems. It performs identifiability analysis.

4. MULTI programs by K. Yamaoka and colleagues (44) are provided as BASIC source code within the manuscripts. Different versions include fitting to integrated or differential equations, Bayesian analysis, and extended least squares.

5. NONMEM is provided as FORTRAN source code for UNIX, IBM, and other computers. The program performs nonlinear regression of individual or population data.

6. NPEM is a program for performing nonparametric expectation maximization.

7. SAAM II is provided as a compiled program for Windows or Macintosh systems and performs nonlinear regression analysis. It has a graphical user interface for model specification.

8. WinNonlin is provided as a compiled program for Windows systems and performs nonlinear regression analysis.

REFERENCES

1. Ko, H.C.; Jusko, W.J.; Ebling, W.F. Nonlinear Perpendicular Least-Squares Regression in Pharmacodynamics. Biopharm. Drug Dis. **1997**, *18*, 711–716.
2. Gibaldi, M.; Perrier, D. *Pharmacokinetics* 2nd Ed.; Marcel Dekker, Inc.: New York, 1982.
3. Bourne, D.W.A.; Triggs, E.J.; Eadie, M.J. *Pharmacokinetics for the Non-Mathematical*; MTP Press Ltd: Lancaster, UK, 1986.
4. Wagner, J.G. *Biopharmaceutics and Relevant Pharmacokinetics*; Drug Intelligence Publications: Hamilton, IL, 1971.
5. Wagner, J.G. *Pharmacokinetics for the Pharmaceutical Scientist*; Technomic Publishing: Lancaster, PA, 1993.
6. Bischoff, K.B. Physiological Pharmacokinetics. Bull. Math. Biol. **1986**, *48*, 309–322.
7. Sheiner, L.B.; Stanski, D.R.; Vozeh, S.; Miller, R.D.; Ham, J. Simultaneous Modeling of Pharmacokinetics and Pharmacodynamics: Application to *d*-tubocurarine. Clin. Pharmacol. Ther. **1979**, *2*, 358–371.
8. Jusko, W.J. Conceptualization of Drug Distribution to a Hypothetical Pharmacodynamic Effect Compartment. Clin. Pharmacol. Ther. **1993**, *54*, 112–113.
9. Sharma, A.; Jusko, W.J. Characterization of Four Basic Models of Indirect Pharmacodynamic Responses. J. Pharmacokin. Biopharm. **1996**, *24*, 611–635.

10. Sharma, A.; Ebling, W.F.; Jusko, W.J. Precursor-Dependent Indirect Pharmacodynamic Response Model for Tolerance and Rebound Phenomena. J. Pharm. Sci. **1998**, *87*, 1577–1584.
11. Carstensen, J.T. *Drug Stability: Principles and Practice*; Marcel Dekker, Inc.: New York, 1990.
12. Wagner, J.G. *Fundamentals of Clinical Pharmacokinetics*; Drug Intelligence Publications: Hamilton, IL, 1975; 35.
13. Gerald, C.P.; Wheatley, P.O. *Applied Numerical Analysis,* 4th Eds.; Addison-Wesley: Reading, MA, 1990.
14. Boas, M.L. *Mathematical Methods in the Physical Sciences*, 2nd Ed.; Wiley: New York, 1983.
15. Mayersohn, M.; Gibaldi, M. Mathematical Methods in Pharmacokinetics. I. Use of the Laplace Transform for Solving Differential Rate Equations. Am. J. Pharm. Ed. **1970**, *34*, 608–614.
16. Mayersohn, M.; Gibaldi, M. Mathematical Methods in Pharmacokinetics. II. Solution of the Two Compartment Open Model. Am. J. Pharm. Ed. **1971**, *35*, 19–28.
17. Benet, L.Z.; Turi, J.S. Use of General Partial Fraction Theorem for Obtaining Inverse Laplace Transforms in Pharmacokinetic Analysis. J. Pharm. Sci. **1971**, *60*, 1593–1594.
18. Benet, L.Z. General Treatment of Linear Mammillary Models with Elimination from Any Compartment as Used in Pharmacokinetics. J. Pharm. Sci. **1972**, *61*, 536–541.
19. Yano, Y.; Yamaoka, K.; Tanaka, H. A Nonlinear Least Squares Program, MULTI(FILT), Based on Fast Inverse Laplace Transform for Microcomputers. Chem. Pharm. Bull. **1989**, *37*, 1035–1038.
20. Fehlberg, E. *Low-Order Classical Runge-Kutta Formulas with Stepsize Control and Their Application to Some Heat Transfer Problems*; NASA TR R-315; NASA Tech. Report: 1969.
21. Watt, H.A.; Shampine, L.F. Subroutine RKF45. *Computer Methods for Mathematical Computation*; Forsythe, G.E., Malcolm, M.A., Moler, C.B., Eds.; Prentice-Hall: Englewood, NJ, 1977, 133–147.
22. Press, W.H.; Teukolsky, S.A.; Vetterling, W.T.; Flannery, B.P. *Numerical Recipes in FORTRAN*; 2nd Ed. Cambridge University Press: Cambridge, UK, 1992; 741.
23. Gear, C.W. DIFSUB for Solution of Ordinary Differential Equations. Algorithm 407. Collected Algorithms. Communications of the Association for Computer Machinery (CACM): New York, 1971.
24. Gear, C.W. The Automatic Integration of Ordinary Differential Equations, Communications of the Association for Computer Machinery (CACM): New York, 1971; 14, 176–179.
25. Sedman, A.J.; Wagner, J.G. CSTRIP, A FORTRAN IV Computer Program for Obtaining Initial Polyexponential Parameter Estimates. J. Pharm. Sci. **1976**, *65*, 1006–1010.
26. Brown, R.D.; Manno, J.E. ESTRIP, A BASIC Computer Program for Obtaining Initial Polyexponential Parameter Estimates. J. Pharm. Sci. **1978**, *67*, 1687–1691.
27. Wagner, J.G.; Nelson, E. Kinetic Analysis of Blood Levels and Urinary Excretion in the Absorptive Phase after Single Doses of Drug. J. Pharm. Sci. **1964**, *53*, 1392–1403.
28. Loo, J.C.K.; Riegelman, S. New Method for Calculating the Intrinsic Absorption Rate of Drugs. J. Pharm. Sci. **1968**, *57*, 918–928.
29. Kiwada, H.; Morita, K.; Hayashi, M.; Awazu, S.; Hanano, M. A New Numerical Calculation Method for Deconvolution in Linear Compartmental Analysis of Pharmacokinetics. Chem. Pharm. Bull. **1977**, *25*, 1312–1318.
30. Vaughan, D.P.; Dennis, M. Mathematical Basis of Point-Area Deconvolution Method for Determining In Vivo Input Functions. J. Pharm. Sci. **1978**, *67*, 663–665.
31. Cutler, D.J. Numerical Deconvolution by Least Squares: Use of Prescribed Input Functions. J. Pharmacokinet. Biopharm. **1978**, *6*, 227–241.
32. Hartley, H.O. The Modified Gauss-Newton Method for the Fitting of Non-Linear Regression Functions by Least Squares. Technometrics **1961**, *3*, 269–280.
33. Marquardt, D.W. An Algorithm for Least-Squares Estimation of Non-Linear Parameters. J. Soc. Indust. Appl. Math. **1963**, *11*, 431–441.
34. Nelder, J.A.; Mead, R. A Simplex Method for Function Optimization. Comput. J. **1965**, *7*, 308–313.
35. Wagner, J.G. *Fundamentals of Clinical Pharmacokinetics*; Drug Intelligence Publications: Hamilton IL, 1975, 289.
36. Peck, C.C. Computer-Assisted Clinical Pharmacokinetics. *Pharmacokinetic Basis for Drug Treatment*; Benet, L.Z., Massoud, N., Gambertoglio, J.G. Eds.; Raven Press: New York, 1984, 353–354.
37. Peck, C.C.; Sheiner, L.B.; Nichols, A.I. The Problem of Choosing Weights in Nonlinear Regression Analysis of Pharmacokinetic Data. Drug Metab. Rev. **1984**, *15*, 133–148.
38. Peck, C.C.; Beal, S.L.; Sheiner, L.B.; Nichols, A.I. Extended Least Squares Nonlinear Regression: A Possible Solution to the Choice of Weights Problem in Analysis of Individual Pharmacokinetic Data. J. Pharmacokinet. Biopharm. **1984**, *12*, 545–558.
39. Schumitzky, A. Nonparametric EM Algorithms for Estimating Prior Distributions. App. Math. Comput. **1991**, *45*, 143–157.
40. Draper, N.R.; Smith, H. *Applied Regression*; Wiley: New York, 1966.
41. Mandel, J. *The Statistical Analysis of Experimental Data*; Interscience: New York, 1964; 164.
42. Boxenbaum, H.G.; Riegelman, S.; Elashoff, R.M. Statistical Estimation in Pharmacokinetics. J. Pharmacokin. Biopharm. **1974**, *2*, 123–148.
43. Akaike, H. A New Look at the Statistical Model Identification. IEEE Trans. Automat. Control. **1973**, *19*, 716–723.
44. Yamaoka, K.; Nakagawa, T.; Uno, T. Application of Akaike's Information Criterion (AIC) in the Evaluation of Linear Pharmacokinetic Equations. J. Pharmacokin. Biopharm. **1978**, *6*, 165–175.
45. Brown, R.F.; Godfrey, K.R. Problems of Determinacy in Compartmental Modeling with Application to Bilirubin Kinetics. Math. Biosci. **1978**, *40*, 205–224.
46. Godfrey, K.R.; Fitch, W.R. The Deterministic Identifiability of Nonlinear Pharmacokinetic Models. J. Pharmacokin. Biopharm. **1984**, *12*, 177–191.
47. Wang, Y.-M.C.; Reuning, R.H. An Experimental Design Strategy for Quantitating Complex Experimental Models: Enterohepatic Circulation with Time-Varying Gallbladder Emptying as an Example. Pharm. Res. **1992**, *9*, 169–177.
48. Jacquez, J.A. Identifiability: The First Step in Parameter Estimation. Fed. Proc. **1987**, *46*, 2477–2480.

49. Jacquez, J.A.; Perry, T. Parameter Estimation: Local Identifiability of Parameters. Am. J. Physiol. **1990**, *258*, E727–E736.

50. See http://www.boomer.org/pkin/book.html for a more complete and up-to-date list.

51. Bourne, D.W.A. *Mathematical Modeling of Pharmacokinetic Data*; Technomic Publishing: Lancaster, PA, 1995.

52. Carstensen, J.T. *Modeling and Data Treatment in the Pharmaceutical Sciences*; Technomic Publishing: Lancaster, PA, 1996.

53. Draper, N.R.; Smith, H. *Applied Regression Analysis*; Wiley: New York, 1966.

54. Gerald, C.F.; Wheatley, P.O. *Applied Numerical Analysis*, 4th Ed.; Addison-Wesley: Reading, MA, 1990.

55. Gibaldi, M.; Perrier, D. *Pharmacokinetics*, 2nd Ed.; Marcel Dekker, Inc.: New York, 1982.

56. Mandell, J. *The Statistical Analysis of Experimental Data*; Interscience: New York, 1964.

57. Sadler, D.R. *Numerical Methods for Nonlinear Regression*; Queensland Press: St. Lucia, Australia, 1975.

58. Wagner, J.G. *Biopharmaceutics and Relevant Pharmacokinetics*; Drug Intelligence Publications: Hamilton, IL, 1971.

59. Wagner, J.G. *Pharmacokinetics for the Pharmaceutical Scientist*; Technomic Publishing: Lancaster, PA, 1993.

MEDICATION ERRORS

Diane D. Cousins
United States Pharmacopeia, Rockville, Maryland

INTRODUCTION

A report issued by the Institute of Medicine (1) in November 1999 has drawn unprecedented national attention to the prevalence of medical error, including medication error. The issues and complexities surrounding this problem are compounded by the array of players and solutions that must address it for the public health and safety of the U.S. population. Medical products and their manufacturers are reported not only as part of the problem but also as part of the solution. Ongoing national efforts in medication error reporting and prevention place the pharmaceutical industry far ahead of other medical product manufacturers. These efforts, headed by the *United States Pharmacopeia* (USP), have involved the industry since 1991 by sharing reports received from healthcare practitioners and documenting industry actions to the reported problems. The Institute of Medicine fosters a systems approach to error analysis that focuses on identifying the root cause of error within the system and not on blame of the individual. The report postulates that individuals who commit errors are often well trained, experienced, well intentioned individuals whose misfortune is a result of the unsafe systems in which they operate. With the advent of new technologies and the healthcare-delivery processes surrounding them, new problems are likely to surface, particularly as health systems are redesigned in response to this national call to action. The challenge to the pharmaceutical industry is to learn from its own experiences and the USP national database of errors. The industry will be expected to be knowledgeable of the medication use process for the health setting in which its products are used and to anticipate misuse by designing error out of products.

SCOPE OF THE PROBLEM

Incidence of Medication Errors and Related Morbidity and Mortality

That medication errors occur frequently in U.S. hospitals has been well documented (2–4). In observation studies carried out between 1962 and 1995 on the rate of administration errors in a variety of inpatient settings, rates ranged from 0 to 59% (5). Estimates that medication errors occur in almost 7% of hospitalized patients have been reported (6). One study found that the frequency of medication errors was 1.4 per admission (4). When approximately 290,000 medication orders were analyzed, Lesar et al. estimated that there were almost two serious errors for every 1000 orders written. Based on a review of death certificates, it was estimated that nearly 8000 people died from medication errors in 1993 compared with almost 3000 people in 1983 (3). Researchers found an error rate at two children's hospitals of 4.7 per 1000 orders (7). Several excellent and comprehensive reviews of the literature on medication errors have recently been published (1, 5).

A variety of error rates for different aspects of the medication use process have been reported. Researchers use different methodologies and definitions of "medication error" and study different aspects of the medication use process (i.e., prescribing, dispensing, and administering). Because there is no national standardization for the denominator used to report medication error rates, the denominator can vary among several: doses dispensed, doses administered, doses ordered, patient days. Therefore, the rates reported in the literature are limited in their use for comparative purposes (5).

Research supports a systems approach to error prevention as well as to investigation of errors (8–11). This means that all aspects of the medication use process, including characteristics of the products themselves, should be explored for ways to improve safety in use.

Cost of Medication Errors

Medication errors are costly to both the patient (direct costs such as additional treatment and increased hospital stay) and to society (indirect costs such as decreased employment, costs of litigation) (1, 5). The cost of medication errors in a 700-bed teaching hospital, based on a study in 11 medical and surgical units in two hospitals over a 6-month period, was estimated at $2.8 million annually (2). The increased length of stay associated with a medication error was estimated at 4.6 days (2). In a 4-year study of the costs of adverse drug events (ADEs) in a tertiary care center, 1% of these events were classified as medication errors. The excess hospital costs for ADEs over the study period were almost $4,500,000, with nearly 4000 days of increased hospital stay (12).

Harm attributable to drugs is a major reason for malpractice claims associated with medical procedures (8). The average compensation for medication errors between 1985 and 1992 was almost $100,000. Most compensation for medication errors is for larger amounts that are agreed on in out-of-court settlements (5). None of the costs cited above include the cost of patient harm or subsequent hospital admissions (1, 3).

USP's EFFORTS TO STANDARDIZE MEDICATION ERRORS

History of USP and Its Involvement in Medication Errors

The USP is a private, not-for-profit organization whose mission is to promote public health through the creation of standards and authoritative information for the use of medicines and related technologies. The USP's authority to set standards is established by the Pure Food and Drug Act and by the Federal Food, Drug and Cosmetic Act. These standards include those for quality, strength, purity, packaging, labeling, and storage of drug products. The USP also creates the official name for drug products and is a member of the United States Adopted Names (USAN) Council that sets the nonproprietary name for drugs in the United States. The USP has been involved in reporting programs for health professionals for nearly 30 years through its USP Practitioners' Reporting Network (USP PRN). These programs support the standards-setting activity by providing practitioner-based experiences about the quality and safe use of medicines in the marketplace.

Nearly a decade ago, the USP agreed to coordinate the medication errors reporting program for the Institute for Safe Medication Practices. The Institute was seeking a home for its grass-roots program and believed the program could have greater impact on the national level. Through the program, the USP hoped to learn of those circumstances in which the product labeling, packaging, or name of product caused or contributed to an error. Then, the USP envisioned setting standards to address the issues and thereby to prevent future errors. In 1994, the USP signed an agreement to purchase the program from the Institute, established the USP Medication Errors Reporting (MER) Program, and began its long-term commitment to

the program as an important part of the USP's standards-setting process. As a condition of the agreement, the ISMP continues to receive copies of reports submitted to this program for its education and advocacy work.

Healthcare professionals report errors in which they are involved as well as errors that they observe or are party to. Reported information forms a database used by the USP to identify problematic situations, to heighten practitioners' awareness of these situations, and to make appropriate interventions regarding issues with drug products.

USP Medication Errors Reporting Program

The prevention of medication errors is the primary objective of the USP MER Program. It collects and analyzes potential and actual medication errors submitted by healthcare practitioners. The program affords health-care professionals the opportunity to report medication errors and thereby to contribute to improving patient safety by sharing their experiences.

To report an error, practitioners may phone USP toll-free at 1-800-23ERROR. A voice-mail system allows a report to be left 24 hr a day, 7 days a week. Reporters may submit reports anonymously or speak directly to one of USP's health professional staff. Alternatively, a report may be submitted to USP in writing. Report forms (Figs. 1 and 2) may be obtained by calling the USP directly or via an on-demand fax-back system. Practitioners may also access the form online on the USP's website.

Medication error information submitted to the USP is entered into a nationally recognized repository for medication error reporting. This database serves to track, monitor, and analyze medication errors from a systems-based perspective. The USP develops educational resources and materials to disseminate best-practice solutions and error-avoidance strategies to students and practitioners.

The MER Program is presented in cooperation with the Institute for Safe Medication Practices and is a partner in MED WATCH, the FDA's medical products reporting program. Although the FDA does not usually assert jurisdiction over practice issues, which are often involved in medication errors, it is concerned with issues relevant to product quality such as labeling and packaging, and product names, both trade and generic. When medication errors concerning product labeling and packaging are reported through the MER Program, pharmaceutical manufacturers are notified. They respond frequently and voluntarily make changes in labeling and packaging. Depending on the nature of the medication error, the MER Program reports provide material for ongoing discussions between the FDA and manufacturers and, if warranted, for

MEDICATION ERRORS REPORTING PROGRAM

Medication Errors Do Occur

Medication errors can occur anywhere, any time along the drug therapy course, from prescribing through transcribing, dispensing, administering, and monitoring. An error can cause confusion, alarm, and frustration for the health care provider and for the patient. And YES, an error can even cause a death or injury to your patient. The causes of errors are many; for example, lack of product knowledge or training; poor communication; ambiguities in product names, directions for use, medical abbreviations, handwriting, or labeling; job stress; poor procedures or techniques; or patient misuse. Along this continuum, any health care professional may be the cause of or contribute to an actual or potential error.

A Safer Environment for Your Patients

It is important to recognize that health care providers learn from medication errors. By sharing your experience through the nationwide USP Medication Errors Reporting (MER) Program you help your colleagues to gain an understanding of why errors occur and how to prevent them. You can also have a positive impact on the quality of patient care and influence drug standards and information. When others are informed about an error, the chance of recurrence may be lessened. Education regarding medication errors assists health care professionals to avoid errors by recognizing the circumstances and causes of actual and potential errors.

Easy Access

Just call 800-233-7767 to reach a USP health care professional, who will take your report and respond to your concerns. Reports may also be submitted in writing or faxed. All reported information is reviewed by USP for possible impact on USP standards and information development. Reports are forwarded to the Food and Drug Administration, the ISMP, and when appropriate, the product manufacturer/labeler. If you wish to remain anonymous to any of these sources, the USP will act as your intermediary in all correspondence. While including your identity is optional, it does allow for appropriate follow-up with you to discuss your observations or provide feedback.

USP: A Partner in MEDWATCH

The USP Practitioners' Reporting Network is a partner in MEDWATCH, the FDA's medical products reporting program. As a partner, USP PRN contributes to the FDA's efforts to protect the public health by helping to identify serious adverse events for the agency. This means that your reported information is shared with the FDA on a daily basis, or immediately if necessary.

 The USP PRN® is designed to collect experiences and observations from health care providers through three separate reporting programs:

- The USP Drug Product Problem Reporting Program
- The USP Medication Errors Reporting Program
- The USP Veterinary Practitioners' Reporting Program

The Institute for Safe Medication Practices, and the American Veterinary Medical Association cooperate in presenting the USP PRN.

Your Input Could Make the Difference!
USP PRN...CALL US WHEN YOU NEED US.

 U.S. Pharmacopeia
12601 Twinbrook Parkway
Rockville, MD 20852-1790

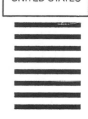 NO POSTAGE
NECESSARY
IF MAILED
IN THE
UNITED STATES

BUSINESS REPLY MAIL
FIRST-CLASS MAIL PERMIT NO 39 ROCKVILLE MD

POSTAGE WILL BE PAID BY ADDRESSEE:
DIANE D COUSINS RPh
THE USP PRACTITIONERS' REPORTING NETWORK
12601 TWINBROOK PARKWAY
ROCKVILLE MD 20897-5211

Fig. 1 USP medication errors reporting program form.

USP MEDICATION ERRORS REPORTING PROGRAM
Presented in cooperation with the Institute for Safe Medication Practices
The USP Practitioners' Reporting Network℠ is an FDA MEDWATCH partner

❑ ACTUAL ERROR   ❑ POTENTIAL ERROR

Please describe the error. Include sequence of events, personnel involved, and work environment (e.g., code situation, change of shift, short staffing, no 24-hr. pharmacy, floor stock). If more space is needed, please attach separate page.

Was the medication administered to or used by the patient? ❑ No ❑ Yes   Date and time of event: _____

What type of staff or health care practitioner made the initial error? _____

Describe outcome (e.g., death, type of injury, adverse reaction). _____

If the medication did not reach the patient, describe the intervention. _____

Who discovered the error? _____

When and how was error discovered? _____

Where did the error occur (e.g., hospital, outpatient or retail pharmacy, nursing home, patient's home)? _____

Was another practitioner involved in the error ? ❑ No ❑ Yes If yes, what type of practitioner? _____

Was patient counseling provided? ❑ No ❑ Yes If yes, before or after error was discovered? _____

If a product was involved, please complete the following:

	Product #1	Product #2
Brand name of product involved		
Generic name		
Manufacturer		
Labeler (if different from mfr.)		
Dosage form		
Strength/concentration		
Type and size of container		
NDC number		

If available, please provide relevant patient information (age, gender, diagnosis, etc.). Patient identification not required.

Reports are most useful when relevant materials such as product label, copy of prescription/order, etc. can be reviewed.
Can these materials be provided? ❑ No ❑ Yes If yes, please specify. _____

Suggest any recommendations you have to prevent recurrence of this error or describe policies or procedures you have instituted to prevent future similar errors.

A copy of this report is routinely sent to the Institute for Safe Medication Practices (ISMP), to the manufacturer/labeler, and to the Food and Drug Administration (FDA). **USP may release my identity to: (check boxes that apply)**
❑ ISMP ❑ The manufacturer and/or labeler as listed above ❑ FDA ❑ Other persons requesting a copy of this report ❑ Anonymous to all

Your name and title

Your facility name, address, and ZIP

Telephone number (include area code)

Signature   Date

Return to the attention of:
Diane D. Cousins, R.Ph.
USP PRN
12601 Twinbrook Parkway
Rockville, MD 20852-1790

Call Toll Free: 800-23-ERROR (800-233-7767)
or FAX 301-816-8532
USP home page: http://www.usp.org
Electronic reporting forms are available. Please call for additional information and/or your free diskette.

Date Received by USP: File Access Number:

699
M1305DM

Additional forms can be found in the USP DI Vol. I and Vol. III.

Fig. 2 USP medication errors reporting program form.

regulatory action. Furthermore, reported information identifies broader issues that may become the basis for instituting industry-wide changes. The reported concerns of practitioners have prompted the USP, FDA, and various drug manufacturers to institute numerous changes and improvements to drug products and have contributed to safer medication prescribing and use.

Facility-Based Reporting May Help Define Denominator of Errors

Because of its leadership and experience in the prevention of medication errors, the USP began to receive inquiries from hospitals seeking a nationally standardized database that would help them meet its accreditation requirements and also to compare rates of medication errors among hospitals. Hospitals were willing to share their adverse experiences with other participating hospitals but only if the report could be shared on an anonymous basis. In 1998, the USP developed MedMARx^{SM}, an Internet-accessible database of medication errors for hospitals. Reports submitted to the system are anonymous so that participating hospitals will share information openly. The database is structured to become part of the hospital's internal quality-improvement program and captures not only errors but prevention strategies taken by each hospital in response to errors. This valuable aspect of the national database enables hospitals to practice risk prevention, not just risk management, by learning from the unfortunate experiences of others. It is expected that this database will become a rich repository of information not only for hospitals but for the pharmaceutical industry as well.

USP's First Advisory Panel on Medication Errors

In 1996, the USP created an ad hoc Advisory Panel on Medication Errors. The mission of the Panel was to provide practitioner review of reports received through the USP MER Program and to make recommendations

relative to USP's standards-setting, information, and reporting programs. The Panel chairperson also has a unique opportunity to make broader recommendations through its seat on the National Coordinating Council for Medication Error Reporting and Prevention (NCC MERP). The chairperson of the Advisory Panel on Medication Errors is an ex-officio nonvoting member of the NCC MERP.

The USP Advisory Panel on Medication Errors is a unique and unprecedented opportunity for healthcare professionals to provide peer review of medication errors occurring nationally and to recommend far-reaching strategies for medication error prevention.

The Panel consists of 12 actively practicing volunteers representing medicine, nursing, and pharmacy. This year a Safe Medication Use Expert Committee will be elected to replace the Panel. For the first time, with the formation of this committee, a formal mechanism will be in place in the standards-development process for the purpose of providing direct practitioner input to standards development for the safer use of pharmaceuticals.

A National Coordinating Council Is Initiated

After a few years operating the MER Program, the USP realized that the solutions addressing the myriad issues identified through the program were beyond the mission of its standards-setting capacity. Indeed, errors proved to be multidisciplinary in origin and multifactorial in cause. These other practice-related and process-related aspects surrounding medication errors needed to be addressed. In 1995, the USP spearheaded the formation of the NCC MERP. The NCC MERP promotes the reporting, understanding, and prevention of medication errors relative to professional practice, healthcare products, procedures, and systems (Table 1). The Council is composed of 20 national organizations and agencies, representative of health professions, licensing boards, healthcare facilities, pharmaceutical manufacturers, regulators, standards-setters,

Table 1 The goals of the NCC MERP are far-reaching and encompass the full spectrum of healthcare goals

Goals of NCC MERP
Examine and evaluate the causes of medication errors
Increase awareness of medication errors and methods of prevention throughout the healthcare system
Recommend strategies relative to system modifications, practice standards and guidelines
Stimulate development and use of medication-error reporting and evaluation systems and stimulate reporting to a national system for review, analysis, and development of recommendations to reduce and prevent medication errors

Table 2 The membership of the NCC MERP is interdisciplinary and represents cross-functional groups in the delivery of healthcare products and services

National Coordinating Council for Medication Error: Reporting and Prevention Organizations Represented

American Association of Retired Persons
American Health Care Association
American Hospital Association
American Medical Association
American Nurses Association
American Pharmaceutical Association
American Society of Consultant Pharmacists
American Society of Health-System Pharmacists
American Society for Healthcare Risk Management
Department of Veterans Affairs
Food and Drug Administration
Generic Pharmaceutical Association
Healthcare Distribution Management Association
Institute for Safe Medication Practices
Joint Commission on Accreditation of Healthcare
     Organizations
National Association of Boards of Pharmacy
National Council of State Boards of Nursing, Inc.
Pharmaceutical Research and Manufacturers of America
United States Pharmacopeia

and others (Table 2). The USP is a founding member of and Secretariat to the Council.

Since the Council's formation, it has produced several important work products. Among them are the standardization definition of the "medication error," the development of a series of recommendations designed to reduce errors in the medication use process, and the adoption of a severity index for categorizing the outcome of medication errors. The "Recommendations to Correct Error-Prone Aspects of Prescription Writing," the first set of suggestions issued by the Council, included a list of "Dangerous Abbreviations," abbreviations that are frequently misunderstood or have often been implicated in medication errors and should never be used (Table 3). In addition to being used in prescription writing, these abbreviations can be found in proprietary product names, on manufacturers' product labels, and in advertising by pharmaceutical manufacturers. The pharmaceutical industry can support this effort by avoiding the use of these abbreviations. The Council also produced an extensive set of recommendations to reduce errors attributable to labeling and packaging. The recommendations are targeted to regulators and standards-setters, healthcare organizations and professionals, and the industry (Tables 4–7). The practical importance of the Council's

recommendations lies in a joint endorsement by a diverse group of organizations ranging from experts in safety issues to manufacturers of drug products to regulators. The importance of achieving consensus through a collaborative effort by these national leading healthcare and consumer organizations furthers the adoption of nonpunitive, systems-based approaches to reduce medication errors.

ERROR AVOIDANCE STRATEGIES FOR THE INDUSTRY—DESIGNING ERROR OUT OF PRODUCTS

The USP's medication error-reporting programs have uncovered a number of reported error-prone situations that could help industry consider the problems that should be addressed in advance, starting with the selection of a drug name and including the development of labeling, packaging, and dosing devices. Some of these cases are presented here. In many, the manufacturer corrected design flaws immediately and successfully. These should be considered showcase examples of industry responsiveness. The cases should also serve to teach certain designs in labels or packaging that should be avoided. And finally, the cases demonstrate how products can be misused because of the systems with which they interface.

Characteristics of Product Errors

Keep in mind that the medication use process is a complex continuum that requires the successful interaction of multiple allied health professionals, technology, and the patient. It can be described as a succession of joined, but distinct processes, known as nodes (Table 8). Each node in the medication use process is, in actuality, a discrete system and presents an opportunity for the occurrence and prevention of medication errors.

Medication errors have been defined in many ways depending on research methodologies, incident reporting systems, risk management, or total quality-improvement systems. The USP uses the broad definition of medication error from the NCC MERP.

A medication error is any preventable event that may cause or lead to inappropriate medication use or patient harm, while the medication is in the control of the healthcare professional, patient, or consumer. Such events may be related to professional practice, healthcare products, procedures, and systems including: prescribing; order communication; product labeling, packaging, and nomenclature; compounding; dispensing; distribution; administration; education; monitoring; and use.

Table 3 Dangerous abbreviations to never use owing to misunderstanding or misinterpretation

Abbreviation	Intended meaning	Common error
U	Unit	Mistaken as a zero or a four (4) resulting in overdose. Also mistaken for "cc" (cubic centimeters) when poorly written
μg	Microgram	Mistaken for "mg" (milligrams) resulting in overdose
Q.D.	Latin abbreviation for every day	The period after the "Q" has sometimes been mistaken for an "I", and the drug has been given "QID" (four times daily) rather than daily
Q.O.D.	Latin abbreviation for every other day	Misinterpreted as "QD" (daily) or "QID" (four times daily). If the "O" is poorly written, it looks like a period or a "I"
SC or SQ	Subcutaneous	Mistaken as "SL" (sublingual) when poorly written
T I W	Three times a week	Misinterpreted as "three times a day" or "twice a week"
D/C	Discharge; also discontinue	Patient's medications have been prematurely discontinued when D/C (intended to mean "discharge") was misinterpreted as "discontinue," because it was followed by a list of drugs
HS	Half-strength	Misinterpreted as the Latin abbreviation "HS" (hour of sleep)
Cc	Cubic centimeters	Mistaken as "U" (unit) when poorly written
AU, AS, AD	Latin abbreviations for both ears; left ear; right ear	Misinterpreted as the Latin abbreviation "OU" (both eyes); "OS" (left eye); "OD" (right eye)

Table 4 Recommendations on labeling and packaging to industry manufacturers of pharmaceuticals and devices (adopted May 12, 1997)

The Council recommends that industry not use any printing on the cap and ferrule of injectables except to convey warnings.

The Council encourages industry to employ failure mode and effects analysis in its design of devices, and the packaging and labeling of medications and related devices.

The Council encourages industry to employ machine-readable coding (e.g., bar coding) in its labeling of drug products. The Council recognizes the importance of standardization of these codes for this use.

The Council encourages printing the drug name (brand and generic) and the strength on both sides of injectables, and IV bags, containers, and overwraps. For large volume parenterals and IV piggybacks (minibags), the name of the drug should be readable in both the upright and inverted positions.

The Council encourages industry to support the development of continuing education programs focusing on proper preparation and administration of its products.

The Council encourages industry to use innovative labeling to aid practitioners in distinguishing between products with very similar names, for example, the use of tall letters such as VinBLAStine and VinCRIStine.

The Council encourages industry to avoid printing company logos and company names that are larger than the type size of the drug name.

The Council encourages collaboration among industry, regulators, standards-setters, healthcare professionals, and patients to facilitate design of packaging and labeling to help minimize errors.

Table 5 Recommendations on labeling and packaging to regulators and standards-setters (adopted May 12, 1997)

The Council recommends that FDA restrict the use of any printing on the cap and ferrule of injectables except to convey warnings.

The Council recommends the use of innovative labeling to aid practitioners in distinguishing between products with very similar names, for example, the use of tall letters such as VinBLAStine and VinCRIStine.

The Council recommends that FDA discourage industry from printing company logos and company names that are larger than the type size of the drug name.

The Council supports the recommendations of the USP-FDA Advisory Panel on Simplification of Injection Labeling. Furthermore, the Council encourages USP/FDA to consider expansion of the concepts of simplification to apply to: package inserts; and labeling of other pharmaceutical dosage forms.

The Council encourages further development of FDA's error prevention analysis efforts to provide consistent regulatory review of product labeling and packaging relative to the error-prone aspects of their design.

The Council encourages collaboration among regulators, standards-setters, industry, healthcare professionals, and patients to facilitate design of packaging and labeling to help minimize errors.

The Council encourages USP/FDA to examine feasibility and advisability of use of tactile cues in container design and on critical drugs. Such cues may be in the design of the container or embedded in the label.

The Council encourages the printing of the drug name (brand and generic) and the strength on both sides of injectables and IV bags, containers, and overwraps. For large volume parenterals and IV piggybacks (minibags), the name of the drug should be readable in both the upright and inverted positions.

Table 6   Recommendations to health care professionals to reduce errors due to labeling and packaging of drug products and related devices (adopted March 30, 1998)

The Council encourages healthcare professionals to routinely educate patients and caregivers to enhance understanding and proper use of their medications and related devices. Furthermore, the Council encourages healthcare professionals to regularly participate in error prevention training programs and, when medication errors do occur, to actively participate in the investigation.

In addition, the Council makes the following recommendations to healthcare professionals to reduce errors due to labeling and packaging of drug products and related devices:

1.   The Council encourages healthcare professionals to use only properly labeled and stored drug products and to read labels carefully (at least three times—before, during, and after use).
2.   The Council encourages collaboration among healthcare professionals, healthcare organizations, patients, industry, standard-setters, and regulators to facilitate design of packaging and labeling to help minimize errors.
3.   The Council encourages healthcare professionals to take an active role in reviewing and commenting on proposed regulations and standards that relate to labeling and packaging (i.e., Federal Register and Pharmacopeial Forum).
4.   The Council encourages healthcare professionals to report actual and potential medication errors to national (e.g., FDA MedWatch Program and/or the USP Practitioners' Reporting Network), internal, and local reporting programs.
5.   The Council encourages healthcare professionals to share error-related experiences, case studies, etc., with their colleagues through newsletters, journals, bulletin boards, and the Internet.

Table 7   Recommendations to healthcare organizations to reduce errors due to labeling and packaging of drug products and related devices (adopted March 30, 1998)

The Council recommends the establishment of a systems approach to reporting, understanding, and prevention of medication errors in health care organizations. The organization's leaders should foster a culture and systems that include the following key elements:

1.   an environment that is conducive to medication error reporting through the FDA MedWatch Program and/or the USP Practitioners' Reporting Network;
2.   an environment which focuses on improvement of the medication use process;
3.   mechanisms for internal reporting of actual and potential errors including strategies that encourage reporting;
4.   systematic approaches within the healthcare organization to identify and evaluate actual and potential causes of errors including Failure Mode and Effects Analysis (FMEA) and root cause analysis;
5.   processes for taking appropriate action to prevent future errors through improving both systems and individual performance.

In addition, the Council makes the following recommendations to healthcare organizations to reduce errors due to labeling and packaging of drug products and related devices:

1.   The Council recommends that healthcare organizations employ machine readable coding (e.g., bar coding) in the management of the medication use process.
2.   The Council recommends reevaluation of existing storage systems for pharmaceuticals by healthcare organizations and establishment of mechanisms to insure appropriate storage and location throughout the organization from bulk delivery to point of use. The following issues should be considered when applicable: storage and location that will help distinguish similar products from one another; storage and location of certain drugs, (e.g., concentrates, paralyzing agents) that have a high risk potential; scope, access, and accountability for floor stock medications; safety and accountability of access to pharmaceuticals in the absence of a pharmacist (e.g., floor stock, eliminate access to pharmacy after hours); labeling and packaging of patient-supplied medications.
3.   The Council recommends the development of policies and procedures for repackaging of medications that will clarify labeling to help avoid errors.
4.   The Council encourages collaboration among healthcare organizations, healthcare professionals, patients, industry, standard-setters, and regulators to facilitate design of packaging and labeling to help minimize errors.
5.   The Council recommends that healthcare organizations develop and implement (or provide access to) education and training programs for healthcare professionals, technical support personnel, patients, and caregivers that address methods for reducing and preventing medication errors.

Table 8 Nodes in the medication-use continuum

Medication use process nodes
Prescribing
Documenting
Dispensing
Administering
Monitoring

Thorough documentation of medication errors provides information about the severity of the error as it relates to the outcome of the patient, the product(s) involved, the level of staff handling the product or processing the order, any contributing factors that may predispose a product to misuse, and the suspected root cause of the error. The USP adds certain codes to MER Program data to characterize the error as it was reported. These codes include the type of error and the possible cause(s) of error. Table 9 lists product characteristics that have been recorded over 9 years to have caused or contributed to a medication error.

The pharmaceutical industry should pay close attention to these items in the earliest stages of product development, including clinical stages. Several years ago the drug zidovudine (an antiviral) was referred to as "AZT" in clinical trials. The abbreviation was brought along as the product was marketed. However, "AZT" had been a common abbreviation for azathioprine (an immunosuppressant), and several errors were made. The Institute of Medicine report (1) suggests that the FDA develop and enforce standards for the design of drug packaging and labeling that will maximize safe product use. Table 9 should serve as a starting gate of areas to examine.

Case 051133: Poor label design; confusing or incomplete label information; packaging

A pediatric patient was presented to the emergency room (ER) experiencing seizures for which 150 mg of I.V. Cerebyx® (fosphenytoin, an anticonvulsant) was ordered. The pharmacy technician took the call for Cerebyx® and delivered three 10-ml vials of Cerebyx 50-mg PE (phenytoin sodium equivalents) per milliliter to the ER as a "floor stock" transaction. A nurse then misread the 50 mg PE/ml on the 10-ml container label, making the assumption that the entire vial contained 50 mg PE. The contents of all three vials were prepared for administration. Instead of 150 mg PE, the patient was administered 10 times the intended dose, or 1500 mg of PE. The patient later died. ER staff only discovered the error after the patient's blood phenytoin levels were returned from the laboratory.

Discussion: Serious medication errors, including some leading to death, have resulted from the interpretation of the Cerebyx® product labeling. The terminology

Table 9 Product characteristics from medication errors as reported to USP

Abbreviations—Includes symbols and acronyms used in drug names as well as directions for use.

Dosage form confusion—Confusion due to similarity in color, markings, shape and/or size to another product, or to a different strength of the same product.

Equipment design confusing/inadequate for proper use—Example: administration pump makes it difficult to set precise fluid rate or is confusing to use.

Label (manufacturer's) design—Physical label design, e.g., contrast of label information and background, letter font, symbol(s), or logo causes information to be overlooked or difficult to read.

Measuring device inaccurate/inappropriate—Scale of graduation markings on medical device (e.g., syringe, dropper) is inaccurate or inappropriate for administering the correct dose.

Names, a brand name/generic name of different products look alike—self-explanatory

Names, a brand name/generic name of different products sound alike—self explanatory

Names, brand names look alike—brand names of different products look alike.

Names, brand names sound alike—brand names of different products sound alike.

Names, generic names look alike—generic names of different products look alike.

Names, generic names sound alike—generic names of different products sound alike.

Nonmetric units of measurement (apothecary)—use of apothecary units of measurement results in misinterpretation (e.g., "cc" (cubic centimeter) written and misinterpreted as "u" (units).

Packaging/container design—the design of the package, bag, syringe, etc., caused or contributed to the error.

Similar packaging/labeling—example: packaging/labeling of two or more different products look similar, causing one product to be mistaken for the other.

on the label, which previously indicated the concentration as being 50 mg of PE per milliliter, was misinterpreted as the total number of PEs per vial. Also, health professionals were reportedly confused by the use of "phenytoin equivalents," a prodrug concept introduced for this product. As a result, massive fosphenytoin overdoses were mistakenly administered.

Fosphenytoin is a prodrug, a compound that undergoes chemical conversion in the body to become the therapeutically active compound phenytoin. Cerebyx dosage will continue to be expressed in PEs. This terminology was adopted in an effort to simplify therapeutic conversions between phenytoin sodium and fosphenytoin sodium (i.e., 500 mg of phenytoin sodium injection is equal to 500 mg PE of fosphenytoin sodium injection). The manufacturer pointed out that by using PEs, prescribers will not have to make dosing adjustments when converting from phenytoin sodium to Cerebyx or vice versa. To reduce the risk of incorrect dosing, all healthcare providers should prescribe and dispense Cerebyx in PEs.

Parke-Davis has taken action to prevent future errors. The labeling for Cerebyx vials and packaging has been changed to further reinforce the total amount of drug in each vial. This is effective for both the 2- and 10-ml vials of the product. Although the new labeling further clarifies the total quantity of drug contained in the vial, the concentration of Cerebyx will remain 50 mg PE/ml.

Case 51832, 51845: Line extension creates confusion

Muro Pharmaceutical, Inc., introduced a new line extension, Prelone® Syrup 5 mg/5 ml (prednisolone, a steroid), to the existing product, Prelone 15 mg/5 ml. Because only one strength of Prelone had been available for many years, it was a general practice for prescribers to write for "Prelone Syrup" without indicating the strength.

Discussion: Manufacturers need to consider the transition time needed by practitioners to become familiar with the existence of a new strength. Confusion of this type is also seen when "long-acting" versions of a product are added to a product line, thereby changing the dosing regime to less frequent intervals. The product name is prescribed without the "long-acting" designation, and a medication error results. In similar cases, suffixes also cause errors when the product line extension adds a second strength and places a suffix such as "XL" after the product name to indicate long-acting release. Prescribers omit the suffix out of habit (for the initial formulation), and the patient receives the shorter-acting medication at the long-acting interval.

Muro Pharmaceutical, Inc., anticipated that a new concentration of an established product could indeed cause confusion and developed new packaging for both concentrations. Muro also sent mailers that announced the availability of two concentrations of Prelone to 32,000 pediatricians and 65,000 pharmacies, wholesalers, HMOs, and PPOs.

Cases 50446, 50499, 50519, 50534, 50736, 50820, 50918: Poor contrast compromises readability

The unit-dose packaging of the quinolone Levaquin (levofloxacin, an antibacterial) is silver foil with black letters. The dose is reverse shaded. A reporter noted that the packages have to be held at just the right angle to be able to read the label. It was reported to be especially difficult to differentiate between the 250- and 500-mg strengths because the numbers were so difficult to read.

Discussion: Ortho-McNeil is redesigning the packaging for Levaquin to improve readability. Manufacturers should be aware that practitioners often operate in areas that have poor lighting. This makes double-checking the label to prevent errors even more difficult. For some products, there may not be adequate time to read the label carefully the first time without having to look again because of poor contrast. The use of embossed printing on plastic containers has also been reported to be difficult to read because there is no contrast and no paper label to aid in distinguishing the products visually or identifying them properly.

Total volume is the key

Eight reports received from pharmacists expressed concern about the labeling on the Bentyl® (dicyclomine hydrochloride, an antispasmodic) 2-ml ampul. Practitioners reported that the label indicates only the drug concentration, 10 mg/ml, and not the total volume. Some practitioners believe the label information is incomplete. In one report, a 20-mg dose was ordered, but two ampuls were administered (4 ml total instead of 2 ml), leading to an overdose. This happened because the reporter mistook 10 mg as the total contents of one vial.

Discussion: Reports received by Hoechst Marion Roussel have prompted the company to return to the old-style labeling that includes the product's total volume data. According to the firm, this change will be implemented as quickly as possible.

Reports to the USP have identified the need for three items of information to appear on the vial or ampule: 1) the total volume, 2) the strength per milligram and 3) the total strength per total volume.

Although some manufacturers feel it would be unreasonable to include this amount of information on the container (especially containers of 1- and 2-ml sizes), this information would assure little chance of misinterpreting the contents or strength.

Cases 040925, 050419, 041485: Wholesaler errs due to label similarity

A pharmacist reported that vials of Marsam's cefazolin sodium 1 g and 10 g appear identical in shape and have the same color flip-top closures. The pharmacy ordered the 1-g product from the wholesaler. Instead, the wholesaler sent 10-g bulk vials of cefazolin sodium along with stickers for the 1-g vial The pharmacy, which does not normally stock the 10-g vials, interspersed the 10-g vials with the 1-g vials in their stock. Several vials were reconstituted in error. Fortunately, no patients received the wrong dose of cefazolin sodium.

In another reported incident, a pharmacist ordered the 10-g vials of cefazolin sodium but received the 1-g vials in error. Intending to reconstitute and then divide the 10-g vials into 1-g doses, a pharmacy technician inadvertently reconstituted the 1-g vials and proceeded to divide the total solution of each vial into ten 100-mg doses. Some of the prepared 100-mg doses of cefazolin sodium were administered to patients instead of their scheduled 1-g doses. No adverse effects to the patients were reported. The pharmacist felt the error occurred, in part, because the vials are identical in size and have similar labels.

Discussion: The pharmacist suggested that the color of the flip-top of the 10-g vial be changed. The company replied that although it is common practice to use color-coded labels and flip-tops to differentiate product lines or strengths, it tries to indicate the individual products in other ways, e.g., by varying the style and format of the label. Marsam revised the labeling of the cefazolin sodium 10-g bulk vial to help distinguish it from the 1-g, single-dose vial. The newly revised labeling included the following:

● the word "BULK" added in two places on the side panel
● screened color added to the box surrounding the product name
● "10 grams" printed in color
● the product name and strength on the back of the label printed in color

The use of color-differentiation is favored, whereas the use of color-coding is controversial because of the limited number of colors, color-blindness in our population, and inappropriate reliance on color in lieu of reading the label.

Case 042031: Packaged measuring devices

An order was written for 30 mg of Cyclosporine (an immunosuppressant) oral solution to be administered to a pediatric patient. However, for several days, the nurse administered 300 mg, believing that the syringe was calibrated in milligrams, not in milliliters. The oral solution is available as 100 mg/ml. As the pharmacist reviewed the error, he noted that the syringes accompanying the medication were never designed with pediatric patients in mind. It is not possible to calculate any dose less than 50 mg. It is understandable how the nurse assumed that the "3" mark was for 30 mg—it is positioned between "2,5" and "3,5" (which are European expressions for the decimals 2.5 and 3.5). To harmonize products in the global market, the manufacturer chose to follow European convention for expressing numbers, which uses commas and decimals in the reverse manner as that as in the United States.

Discussion: This error is unusual because it involves a global trade issue. Manufacturers would prefer to harmonize products used in the United States with those available in other markets. If dose preparation was centralized in the pharmacy, this error might have been avoided.

Other medication errors involving medication-dispensing devices reported to the USP have included the interchange of devices supplied with specific products. Each device packaged with a medication is calibrated for that medication based on the viscosity and concentration of the specific liquid it delivers. These devices are not calibrated in any standardized way; some are measured in milligrams (mg), others in milliliters (ml), and others in cubic centimeters (cc). Still others have calibrations for the strength per drop or per teaspoonful. Policies should be in place so that the dispensing or use of droppers or calibrated cups provided with specific medications is restricted to those medications. Manufacturers that supply droppers with a stock bottle should supply enough droppers to enable breakdown of the liquid to usable volumes. For example, one company supplied only one dropper with its 8-oz bottle of morphine sulfate, even though the more common quantities dispensed are 2- and 4- oz. Alternatively, manufacturers should package medication in the volume expected to be dispensed per medication order.

Case 52348: Abbreviations

The USP received a medication error report involving the products Neumega® (oprelvekin) and Proleukin® (aldesleukin). Oprelvekin, a recombinant human interleukin-eleven product used to stimulate platelet production in selected patients undergoing chemotherapy, is sometimes abbreviated as IL-11. Aldesleukin, a recombinant human interleukin-two derivative indicated in designated patient populations for the treatment of metastatic renal cell carcinoma, is sometimes abbreviated as IL-2.

In the reported error, a physician used the abbreviation "IL-11" when ordering oprelvekin for a patient. Unfortunately, the order was misinterpreted to be interleukin-two (i.e., the number eleven was perceived to be the Roman numeral two). Five or more healthcare professionals, including pharmacists and nurses, mistook the order to be aldesleukin. The error went undetected for 4 days, until it was noted that the inventory of aldesleukin was nearly depleted.

Discussion: Practitioners should be especially vigilant when orders for these interleukin products are received. If abbreviations have been used in an order, the order should be clarified to ensure that patients receive the intended medication. This medication error exemplifies the value of implementing prescribing guidelines, such as the recommendations adopted by the NCC MERP. Specifically, when writing an order, prescribers should avoid the use of abbreviations, including those for drug names. Drugs names should not have accepted abbreviations. Reference materials sometimes refer to these abbreviations as synomyns for the approved drug names. Manufacturers should discourage the use of abbreviations because of the potential to cause medication errors.

The following cases demonstrate how products can be misused because of the systems with which they interface.

Case 052718: Electronic drug reference products

A pharmacist asked one of the clinical pharmacists for information about Cartia®. Because an electronic drug reference listed the active ingredient as aspirin, the pharmacist was prepared to substitute an aspirin product for Cartia. The clinical pharmacist recognized the new product as Cartia XT® (diltiazem, a calcium channel blocker) and prevented the error.

Discussion: The manufacturer of Cartia XT shared the reporter's concern and contacted the electronic reference source to investigate the matter. The publisher of the electronic reference stated that a salicylate product called "Cartia" is manufactured by Lusofarmaco in Portugal and Smithkline Beecham in Australia. Both Cartia products were verified as active current products by the publisher. The publisher said it has no way of excluding the foreign marketed Cartia because it is an active product imported from a master database that contains many foreign drug products. The electronic reference is published quarterly. "Cartia XT" was entered into the database that is currently being shipped to customers, who will now be able to choose between "Cartia" and "Cartia XT". This should reduce confusion between the products.

As with many hard copy drug reference books, electronic drug references have lag time between production and the customer's receipt of the reference databases. Unfortunately, this may result in inaccurate/outdated information and omission of current drug information, causing confusion and misinterpretation of drug information by the users. Healthcare providers should realize that reference sources, including electronic reference databases, are not infallible, and that they are only good as their contents of updated information. As a safeguard, the healthcare providers should make it a practice to check at least two different drug information sources to confirm information.

Case 52125: Computers and processing software

A pharmacist entered an order for Diflucan (an antifungal) for a patient who had been receiving Propulsid (a gastrointestinal emptying adjunct), which is a documented drug interaction. The pharmacy computer system had multiple drug interaction screens. The pharmacist passed these screens by pressing "next screen" without any resistance by the system for this dangerous drug interaction. The patient received two doses of Diflucan. On the second day, the patient coded and later died.

Case 51088

A patient died after 12 mg of I.V. Colchicine (an antigout medication) was given instead of 2 mg I.V. "until diarrhea," as ordered. The physician was contacted by the pharmacist but the physician insisted on the dose. The computer program did not warn about the dangerous dose, and nurses had no idea they were giving an overdose.

Case 50908

Amoxicillin was prescribed and dispensed to a patient with a penicillin allergy. The front of the patient's chart was not marked for an allergy, and the problem list indicating the allergy was covered with a misfiled document. The pharmacy software program does not screen for allergies, and the pharmacy profile was not marked with any allergies.

Digoxin pediatric elixir

Because the computer in one facility was limited to entering doses in milligrams, a neonate patient's 20 microgram dose of digoxin first had to be converted to the equivalent milligram dose before it could be entered into the computer. A pharmacist incorrectly converted the 20 mcg dose and then entered it into the computer as 0.2 mg (instead of 0.02 mg). Consequently, the patient received four 200 microgram doses of digoxin instead of the 20 microgram dose as ordered. The patient experienced digoxin toxicity before the error was discovered.

Teaspoonful versus mL

By default, a certain software program printed "teaspoonful" for any syrup preparation when a numerical figure was not followed by a specific measure, such as ml, for the dose. A prescription for $\frac{1}{2}$ ml albuterol syrup every 6 h for a 9-week-old infant was presented to the pharmacy, and the pharmacist entered "$\frac{1}{2}$" into the computer but did not enter ml. Therefore, by default, the label printed $\frac{1}{2}$ teaspoonful every 6 h if needed for wheezing. The child was administered the overdose and was consequently admitted to the hospital emergency room for observation. Fortunately, the child was released with no permanent damage.

One versus one-half

New computer software was used to enter the directions for a cough medicine with a dose of "1–2 teaspoonsful." Instead, the new software printed the label as $\frac{1}{2}$ teaspoonful. The pharmacist did not check the label against the prescription and dispensed the product with the incorrect directions on the label.

Discussion: Computerized systems have become important tools in today's pharmacy settings. Computers have made prescription processing faster, easier, and more efficient. Computers have also provided for patient information to be readily available. However, as reliance on computers systems grows, care should be taken not to become totally dependent on these systems as the sole check in preventing medication errors.

Similar drug names

Confusion over similarity of drug names, either written or spoken, accounts for approximately one-quarter of all reports to the USP MER Program. Such confusion is compounded by illegible handwriting, incomplete knowledge of drug names, newly available products, similar packaging or labeling, and incorrect selection of a similar name from a computerized product list. The USP has produced a list of more than 1000 drug name pairs that have been reported as confusing. Manufacturers should refer to this list when selecting drug names. Recently, the USP voted to change Amrinone to Inamrinone when it was being confused with Amiodarone and caused fatal errors. This type of change is expensive to the industry and can be avoided by considering the potential for similarity in advance. Technologies and testing protocols, including voice and handwriting recognition, are available to help determine whether a drug name looks or sounds like another.

SUMMARY

The ability to predict error and thus avoid it is the focus of the science of human factors engineering. The adaptation of this science to the medication use process can help to predict the chances that a medication error will occur. Pharmaceutical manufacturers should design products including their names, labeling, and packaging so that errors can be avoided and safer systems and healthcare delivery result.

REFERENCES

1. Institute of Medicine. *To Err is Human: Building a Safer Healthcare System*; www.nas.org (accessed Dec 1999), November 1999.
2. Bates, D.W.; Spell, N.; Cullen, D.J.; Burdick, E.; Laird, N.; Peterson, L.A.; et al. The Costs of Adverse Drug Events in Hospitalized Patients. J. Am. Med. Assoc. **1997**, *277* (4), 307–311.
3. Phillips, D.P.; Christenfeld, N.; Glynn, L.M. Increase in U.S. Medication-Error Deaths between 1983 and 1993 [Research Letter]. Lancet **1998**, *351*, 643–644.
4. Bates, D.W. Frequency, Consequences and Prevention of Adverse Drug Events. J. Qual. Clin. Pract. **1999**, *19*, 13–17.
5. Flynn, E.A.; Barker, K.N. Medication Errors Research. *Medication Errors*; Cohen, M.R., Ed.; American Pharmaceutical Association: Washington, DC, 1999; 6.4–6.5.
6. Bates, D.W.; Cullen, D.J.; Laird, N.; Peterson, L.A.; Small, S.D.; Servi, D.S. et al. Incidence of Adverse Drug Events and Potential Adverse Drug Events. J. Am. Med. Assoc. **1995**, *274* (1), 29–34.
7. Bates, D.W. Preventing Medication Errors. *Medication Use: A Systems Approach to Reducing Errors*; Cousins, D.D., Ed.; Joint Commission on Accreditation of Health Care Organizations: 1999; 57–73.
8. Leape, L.L.; Bates, D.W.; Cullen, D.; Cooper, J.; Demonaco, H.J.; Gallivan, T. et al. Systems Analysis of Adverse Drug Events. J. Am. Med. Assoc. **1995**, *274* (1), 35–43.
9. Leape, L.L.; Woods, D.; Hatlie, M.; Kizer, K.; Schroeder, S.A.; Lundberg, G.D. Promoting Patient Safety by Preventing Medical Error [Editorial]. J. Am. Med. Assoc. **1998**, *280* (16), 1444–1445.
10. Phillips, D.L. "New Look" Reflects Changing Style of Patient Safety Enhancement [Medical News and Perspectives]. J. Am. Med. Assoc. **1999**, *281* (3), www.jama.ama-assn.org/issues/v281n3/full/jmn0120-1.html (accessed Jan 2000).
11. Bates, D.W.; Miller, E.B.; Cullen, D.J.; Burdick, L.; Williams, L.; Laird, N. Patient Risk Factors for Adverse Drug Events in Hospitalized Patients. Arch. Intern. Med. **1999**, *159*, 2553–2560.
12. Classen, D.C.; Pestotnik, S.L.; Evans, S. et al. Adverse Drug Events in Hospitalized Patients. J. Am. Med. Assoc. *277*, 301–306.

METERED DOSE INHALERS

Sandy J.M. Munro
Alan L. Cripps
GlaxoSmithKline, Ware, Hertfordshire, United Kingdom

INTRODUCTION

Metered dose inhalers (MDIs) are pharmaceutical delivery systems designed for oral or nasal use, which deliver discrete doses of aerosolized medicament to the respiratory tract. The MDI contains the active substance, dissolved or suspended in a liquefied propellant system held in a pressurized container that is sealed with a metering valve. Actuation of the valve discharges a metered dose of medicament as an aerosol spray through an actuator during oral or nasal inhalation.

The MDI may provide up to several hundred actuations, each containing typically from about 10 to 500 μg of drug dispersed in a 25 to 100 μl metered volume of liquid. The discharged liquid undergoes flash evaporation of the propellant to produce a finely dispersed aerosol spray. The deposition, and hence the clinical efficacy, are critically dependent on the mass of inhaled particles, which must have an appropriate aerodynamic size, typically less than 5 μm, to be deposited in the lungs (the respirable fraction) (1).

The first MDI products were developed by Riker Laboratories and marketed in 1956, using a newly patented design of metering valve. In most countries the MDI is now established as the principal dosage form of inhalation drug therapy for bronchial asthma and chronic obstructive pulmonary disease (COPD). Since its introduction, MDI technology has evolved steadily. However, with the phase-out in the commercial use of chlorofluorocarbon (CFC) propellants, which have been the mainstay of pharmaceutical MDIs, the pace of MDI technology development has accelerated with the transition to hydrofluorocarbon (HFC) propellants (2).

Despite their apparent simplicity in use, MDIs are complex devices involving the integration of formulation, container, metering valve and actuator (Fig. 1). Changes to any one of these components will affect the overall performance of the MDI, which is designed to ensure that the delivered dose and the particle size distribution of the drug in the aerosol spray are consistent over both the labelled number of actuations in the MDI and for the duration of the shelf-life (3).

The design and evaluation of MDIs are reviewed in references (4–7).

PROPELLANTS

The propellant or propellant mixture used in the MDI provides the energy necessary to generate a fine aerosol of drug particles suitable for delivery to the lungs or nasal cavity. Liquefied compressed gases are preferred over nonliquefied compressed gases such as nitrogen or carbon dioxide because they offer the following critical advantages for inhalation therapy:

- The discharge of defined aliquots of propellant from the MDI will undergo flash evaporation to give an aerosol of very small particles.
- The pressure inside the MDI remains consistent throughout the use of the entire contents, thus ensuring that the aerosol characteristics remain uniform during repeated discharges. At constant temperature, the vapor pressure remains constant while liquefied propellant remains. In contrast, aerosols generated using nonliquefied compressed gas coarsen during emptying of the MDI due to the decrease in gas pressure.

However, unlike nonliquefied compressed gases, the vapor pressure of liquefied propellants decreases significantly with decreases in temperature, such that below a certain temperature, the flash evaporation process is sufficiently retarded to give poor aerosol formation. For the propellants commonly used in MDIs, unacceptable aerosol formation is likely to occur below 0°C.

The ideal propellant for use in an MDI will exhibit the following properties (8):

- Nontoxic
- Inert and unreactive in the formulation
- Chemically stable under a range of conditions
- High purity
- Acceptable taste and odor
- Compatible with the packaging components (can, valve, actuator)

- Suitable vapor pressure
- Suitable density to facilitate suspension stability
- Suitable solvency properties
- Preferably nonflammable
- Acceptable cost

Until recently, only three chlorofluorocarbon (CFC) propellants, namely CFCs 11, 12 and 114 (Table 1), had been approved worldwide for use in medical MDIs. Their widespread acceptance was due to their ability to substantially meet the ideal propellant properties. All the CFC MDIs that are currently marketed employ CFC 12 as the major constituent mixed with either CFC 11 or with a mixture of CFC 11 and CFC 114. These mixtures of propellants closely obey Raoult's law and therefore the blend selected can be used to give a defined vapor pressure (Table 1). The inclusion of CFC 11 in the formulation also offered advantages in that it increased the solvency of most propellant systems, thereby facilitating the dissolution of surfactants in suspension formulations. By virtue of it being a liquid below 24°C, it was used as the primary dispersion medium for either suspending or dissolving the drug.

In 1974, Rowland and Molina (9) published their hypothesis that CFCs could lead to the depletion of stratospheric ozone. With confirmation of this theory through subsequent studies, an international agreement, The Montreal Protocol on Substances that Deplete the Ozone Layer (10), was drawn up and set in motion a timetable for the phase-out of both the manufacture and use of CFCs. Although the consumption of CFCs in inhalation products is probably insignificant in ozone depletion, representing approximately 0.4% of the world-wide CFC consumption in 1986 (11), the pharmaceutical industry has been working since 1987 to find alternative propellants with which to replace the CFCs used in MDIs. The establishment of the safety and suitability of such alternatives for use in medical aerosols is a lengthy and complex process. As a consequence, MDIs have been identified as an essential use of CFCs and have remained exempt from the provisions of the Montreal Protocol during the transition process.

The search for propellants of low or zero ozone depletion potential (ODP) has led to the identification of a number of potential compounds. A number of chemical industry consortia were established to investigate the acute toxicity of the most promising candidates under The Programme for Alternative Fluorocarbon Toxicity Testing (PAFTT) (8).

The use of HCFCs has been considered, although they still have an appreciable ODP. For instance, HCFC 22 could provide a technically satisfactory replacement for CFC 12. However, revisions to the Montreal Protocol in 1990 require the phase-out of HCFCs by 2020.

The use of hydrocarbons such as isobutane is common in general consumer aerosols. However, their odor and flammability have deterred their use in medical aerosols although purer grades, which are odorless are now available. Dimethylether (DME) is used similarly because it combines zero ODP with superior solvency for various active components and appreciable miscibility with water, which may be important in the formulation. However, the high flammability of both the hydrocarbons and DME would require expensive modification of facilities for the manufacture, storage, and transportation of MDIs. Flame extension studies have shown that the flammability of these propellants is unlikely to present a significant risk during inhalation use due to the small metered volumes (12). Another challenge in the use of both hydrocarbons and DME as propellants in suspension MDI formulations may be their low density, compared with most drug substances, which would give rise to poor suspension stability leading to the potential for inconsistent dose delivery.

Of the alternatives identified, the hydrofluoroalkanes (HFAs) or HFCs were targeted for development as replacements for the CFCs in MDIs. Within this class, 134a and 227ea were adopted for inhalation toxicity testing by two consortia of pharmaceutical companies: IPACT 1 for 134a and IPACT 2 for 227ea (IPACT: International Pharmaceutical Aerosol Consortium for Toxicity Testing). These programs established the safety profile of both propellants, which has led to the recommendation by the Committee of Proprietary Medicinal Products (CPMP) of their suitability for use in MDIs (13).

The vapor pressure of 134a is higher than that of 227ea, but both are seen as alternatives for CFC 12. To date, no suitable replacement for CFC 11 has been identified. In some HFA MDI formulations, ethanol has been used as a

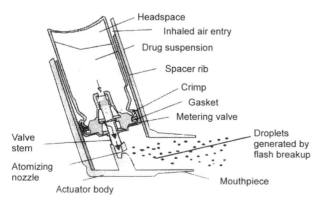

Fig. 1 Sectional view of a metered dose inhaler.

Table 1 Properties of fluorocarbon propellants and dimethyl ether[a]

Propellant	Molecular formula	Molecular weight	Boiling point at 101.3 kPa (1 atm.) (°C)	Gauge vapor pressure (barr at 21 °C)	Liquid density (g/cm³) at 21°C	Flammabil.b limits (vol. % in air)
CFC-11[b]	CCl₃F	137.4	23.8	−0.1	1.49	NF[c]
CFC-12[b]	CCl₂F₂	120.9	−29.8	4.84	1.33	NF
CFC-114[b]	CF₂ClCF₂Cl	170.9	3.6	0.89	1.47	NF
CFC-115[b]	CClF₂CF₃	154.5	−38.7	7.10	1.31	NF
HCFC-22	CHClF₂	86.5	−40.8	8.37	1.21	NF
HCFC-123	CF₃CHCl₂	152.9	27.1	0.79	1.47	NF
HCFC-124	CF₃CHClF	136.5	−0.11.1	2.28	—	NF
HCFC-141[b]	CCl₂FCH₃	117.0	32.1	0.69	1.24	7.6–17.7
HCFC-142[b]	CH₃CClF₂	100.5	−9.8	2.00	1.12	6.0–15.0
FC-C-318	C₄F₃(cyc.)	200.0	−5.8	1.75	1.51	NF
HFA-125[d]	CF₃CHF₂	120.0	−72.8	11.4	—	NF
HFA-134a[c]	CF₃CH₂F	102.0	−26.7	5.59 (20°C)	1.22	NF
HFA-152a[c]	CH₃CHF₂	66.1	−23.9	4.35	0.91	3.71–18.0
HFA-227[c]	CF₄CHFCF₄	132.0	−17.0	3.99 (20°C)	1.41	NF
DME[d]	CH₃OCH₃	46.1	−23.7	4.35	0.66	3.4–18.2

[a]Based on data of E.I. du Pont de Nemours & Co Ltd., except for propellants HFA-134a and HFA-227.
[b]Permitted used in most countries for specified MDI product.
[c]NF = nonflammable Ozone depletion potential (ODP), relative to CFC-11 with ODP of 1.
[d]HFA hydrofluoroalkane DME = dimethylether.

cosolvent to enhance the solubility of surfactants in place of CFC 11. The HFA propellants meet many of the criteria of the ideal propellant for use in an MDI, although the solvency properties of both 134a and 227ea are markedly different from those of the CFCs. Hence the conventional surfactants used in CFC MDIs were found to be incompatible. As a consequence, the development of HFA MDIs has required the resolution of a significant number of technical problems (3).

FORMULATION

In general, MDI formulations can take the form of either suspensions or solutions. Traditionally the preferred route has been to formulate a suspension of the micronized drug substance in the liquid propellant (CFC or HFA). In some cases, additional excipients (e.g., surfactants and/or cosolvents) have been added to improve the quality of the dispersion. The various MDI formulation options are described in detail later together with a description of some of the alternative options for the input drug substance.

Historical Overview of CFC-Based MDI Formulations

These typically comprised a suspension of the micronized drug substance in various ratios of propellants 12 and 11 and/or 114. A surfactant was usually added to improve the suspension behavior by decreasing the rate of flocculation and sedimentation or creaming and also by reducing the amount of drug deposition on the internal surfaces of the valve and container (4). The addition of a surfactant to moderate the suspension behavior and reduce internal drug deposition, can make the valve sampling and hence the dose delivery more reliable. Some CFC MDI products have also been formulated as solutions (14). Typically, the drug substance is solubilized by adding a small quantity of ethanol. The potential strengths and weaknesses of both suspension and solution formulations are discussed in detail in the following section, which covers formulation options for HFA-based MDIs (15).

HFA MDI Formulations

Input drug substance

The microfine drug powder used in suspension-based MDIs has typically been prepared using an air-driven fluid energy mill and this is still the method predominantly used for the currently marketed suspension-based MDIs.

In recent years, there has been a recognition that although the micronization process is a cost-effective method of producing a material with the correct particle size distribution for inhalation, the process, which relies on particle–particle collisions and attrition to gradually reduce the particle size, may also impart some undesirable characteristics to the particles produced.

As a consequence of the limitations of the micronization process, various particle engineering (16, 17) techniques are under investigation with a view to providing superior input microfine drug for MDI manufacture. Some of these techniques, for example, SEDS (Solution Enhanced Dispersion by Supercritical Fluids) (18) rely on alternative crystallization technologies to go straight from a solution of the required drug substance to crystals with exactly the required surface characteristics and particle size distribution without going through the high-energy micronization process. Other techniques extend spray drying technologies to produce particles with controlled density, porosity, particle size distribution, and shape as well as allow for coformulation with other solid excipients to produce particles with controlled drug release characteristics as well as potentially controlled regional deposition within the lung (19, 20). Particle engineering techniques may also offer enhanced performance to meet increasingly stringent regulatory requirements (21, 22).

HFA MDI solution formulations

In an HFA MDI solution formulation, the drug is completely dissolved using an HFA propellant (e.g., 134a) plus an appropriate cosolvent to produce a pure solution product. The cosolvent most commonly used is ethanol. This approach has been used successfully to produce a solution aerosol product for BDP (23). There are a number of advantages to a formulation of this type:

1. Potentially fewer issues around homogeneous valve sampling from the bulk.
2. As in the case of the BDP solution aerosol, enhanced efficiency of aerosolization, leading to high lung deposition compared with an equivalent suspension product.
3. Overcomes issues with suspension systems where the drug has measurable solubility in the propellant, i.e., formulation does not suffer from particle growth issues.
4. Provided there is always sufficient cosolvent present to preserve the true solution status of the product, no issues with drug deposition on the valve components and container.
5. May be a simpler filling process than for a suspension-based HF MDI.

There are also a number of disadvantages to true solution MDI products:

1. Solution products can be more susceptible to drug losses into the elastomeric components of the valve than for an equivalent suspension product. Drug losses of this kind can be an issue particularly for low dose products.
2. There are currently few options beyond ethanol in terms of cosolvents that would be Generally Regarded As Safe (GRAS). Thus, to develop a solution formulation using a cosolvent other than ethanol could necessitate an extensive toxicology testing program. Of the currently available respiratory drugs, there are few that are sufficiently soluble in ethanol or sufficiently low in strength to easily yield a solution product.
3. If too much ethanol is used to dissolve the drug, the vapor pressure may drop below that required to achieve efficient atomization.
4. If the product under development is transitioning from an existing CFC suspension-based product, it may be difficult to replicate the fine particle mass, the particle size distribution and/or the absorption characteristics. This can lead to problems in providing a seamless transition from the CFC product because of the potential to have to change the dose and because the product can smell and feel different to the original suspension formulation.

More recently, other (less volatile) organic modifiers, e.g., glycerol, have been added to solution-based HFA MDIs to modify the particle size distribution so that it more closely resembles that of the originator suspension product (24).

HFA MDI suspension formulations

There are a number of possible approaches to a suspension-based formulation. A micronized drug can simply be suspended in an HFA propellant or a mixture of HFA propellants. The principal advantage to a formulation of this type is that it is simple and contains no additional excipients with their inherent toxicological implications. The performance of a formulation of this simplicity will be dependent on the inherent properties of the drug substance and the propellants used. For example, if the drug substance is significantly more dense than the propellant(s) is, then rapid sedimentation of the suspension is likely to occur following agitation. This could create issues in terms of the valve sampling homogeneously from the bulk container contents. Further differences between the drug and propellant in terms of relative hydrophobicities and hydrophilicities can also result in rapid flocculation immediately postshaking or a tendency for the drug to deposit on the MDI container walls and valve components. For the approach of creating a dispersion of drug in propellant to be successful, the drug should essentially be insoluble in the propellant(s) to provide good product stability. The formulation should also possess reasonable characteristics such that the suspension is easy to redisperse so that the valve still samples homogeneously from the bulk suspension contents in a time-scale consistent with the gaps a patient would typically leave between shaking and firing the inhaler. The tendency for drug to deposit on the inner surfaces of the container and valve can be controlled via sophisticated packaging technologies, e.g., can coating, making this kind of MDI formulation successful for a number of drug substances.

For CFC-based suspension formulations, a surfactant was typically included. A variety of surfactants were used in these systems, e.g., lecithin, oleic acid, sorbitan trioleate (14). All these surfactants were freely soluble in the CFC propellants and allowed for a degree of control over the suspension characteristics. Rates of flocculation, sedimentation, and creaming could be controlled and deposition on the internal container components was minimized. The transition to HFA-based MDIs has created significant issues in that none of the surfactants, previously used with the CFC products are soluble in HFA propellants alone. Some formulations have still used these surfactants, but the addition of a cosolvent (ethanol) has been required to solubilize the surfactant.

In addition to HFA formulations using the traditional surfactants plus cosolvents, there has also been some research work to identify novel surfactant molecules for use with HFA propellants. As yet none of these research programs have successfully yielded molecules with suitable properties to control the suspension characteristics whilst also retaining a suitable toxicology profile.

An interesting alternative approach to suspension formulations in HFA propellants is via engineered drug substance particles. Porous drug substance/excipient particles can be produced via spray drying techniques. It is theoretically possible to match the density of the particles with that of the liquid propellant to produce a formulation with desirable suspension characteristics (19).

CONTAINERS

The essential requirements of containers used for MDIs are that they are compatible with the formulation, have an ability to withstand internal pressures up to 1500 kPa, and can be manufactured with reproducible quality. The most widely used containers for MDIs are made from an

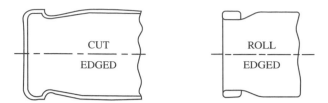

Fig. 2 Types of aluminum cans used with MDIs.

aluminum alloy, although glass bottles have also been used. Aluminum containers (cans) are preferred due to their light weight, strength, break resistance, compactness, and ability to provide light protection. There are two main types of aluminum cans—the cut-edge can and the rolled-edge can (Fig. 2). The cut-edge can, which is most commonly used in the manufacture of MDIs, is manufactured by a deep-drawing process to leave a sharp edge to the can rim (Fig. 3). After formation, the cans are washed with solvent and aqueous detergent to remove residues of oil, which is used as a lubricant in the drawing process. Rolled-edge cans are formed by impact extrusion (slugging) of a slug of high purity aluminum. The excess material is trimmed off and the can neck is externally rolled. The deep-drawing process is preferred because the cans have a more uniform weight and wall thickness, which facilitates fill weight control during the MDI manufacturing process.

Although aluminum cans generally show good compatibility with the propellant systems used in MDIs, drug degradation or drug deposition on the internal walls of the can may require the use of internal coatings. A suitable epoxy resin or phenolic vinyl type coating may be used (25). More recently, low-surface-energy coatings based upon perfluoropolymers have been proposed for use with HFA propellant systems (26).

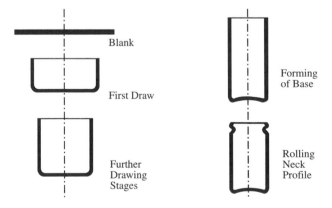

Fig. 3 Stages in the manufacture of aluminum cans by a deep-drawing process.

Glass bottles are not widely used because of their greater weight and potential fragility. Glass containers used with pressurized liquefied propellants are externally coated with a plasticized polyvinyl chloride (PVC) layer to retain glass fragments in the event of breakage. In the past, glass bottles may have been preferred for MDI formulations containing ethanol and CFC 11. Hydrogen chloride, formed via a free radical reaction, can result in corrosion of aluminum cans (27).

METERING VALVES: DESIGN AND FUNCTION

The primary function of the metering valve is to meter accurately and repeatably small volumes of the propellant-based formulation containing the drug. Secondly, it helps seal the pack to ensure minimal leakage of propellant. Most of the commercially available MDI products are fitted with metering valves designed to operate in the valve-down orientation, which eliminates the need for a dip tube. The typical MDI metering valve consists of two coupled valves placed on either side of a volumetric metering chamber (28). It is essential that during depression of the valve stem, the inner "valve" closes to isolate the container contents before the outer "valve" opens to allow discharge of the contents of the metering chamber. Reversal of this sequence would give rise to "continuous spraying," placing the patient at risk of overdosage. The metering performance of the valve is a critical aspect of quality control. A diagrammatic representation of the sequence of operation of a metering valve is shown in Fig. 4.

A metering valve comprises a number of essential components (Fig. 5) having specific functions (Table 2). The most significant feature of the valve are the two seals or seats. These are separated by the metering chamber, which is created by the space between the stem, the body, and the seals. The cylindrical stem passes through the flat elastomeric seals to create a dynamic seal during movement of the stem along its axis. With the exception of the aluminum ferrule, all other components are either press-formed in stainless steel or injected-moulded in suitable plastics such as nylon, polyacetal, or polyester, which are dimensionally stable when in contact with the propellant. The stem return spring is invariably made in stainless steel. Good surface finish and careful dimensional control of all the components and their correct assembly are critical in ensuring satisfactory valve performance.

The valve is sealed against the container by a rubber flat cut or "O" ring gasket that is compressed by crimping the aluminum valve ferrule to the container neck.

1. At rest

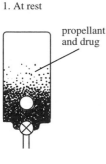

propellant
and drug

2. During actuation

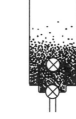

3. Discharging

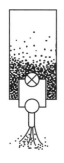

4. During release

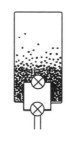

5. Chamber refilling

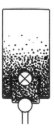

Fig. 4   Operation of an aerosol valve.

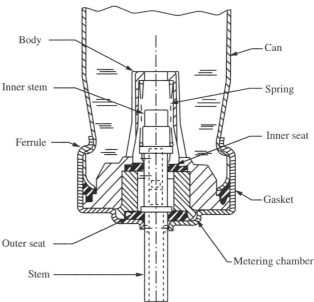

Fig. 5   Components of a metering valve.

Crimping during the filling operation is controlled by monitoring the crimp height and diameter to ensure adequate compression of the gasket. The optimum crimp parameters will permit correct valve function and minimize propellant leakage.

ELASTOMER COMPONENTS

The elastomeric sealing components of the metering valve are particularly critical. In those valves used with CFC propellants, the elastomeric seals have typically been formed from an acrylonitrile/butadiene rubber, which has been cured with sulfur. These rubber seals may not be fully compatible with HFA propellants; hence, alternative elastomeric materials have been used. These materials include peroxide-cured acrylonitrile/butadiene, ethylene–propylene diene monomer (EPDM), and chloroprene and thermoplastic elastomers (TPE). The elastomeric materials used to form the dynamic seals around the stem and the static gasket seal between the can and valve may differ based on the required properties of the rubber for the specific function of the seal (29). The most important characteristics of the elastomeric seals include their composition and degree of curing, which control the physical properties and swelling characteristics in situ, compatibility with the propellant and drug, their affinity for drug absorption, their dimensions and surface finish, and their potential to release foreign particulate matter and extractable material. The solvency properties of both CFC and HFA propellants is such that low levels of extractives from the elastomers can appear in the MDI formulation during storage. These may not present any safety concerns and their levels can be further minimized by using solvent-extracted elastomeric seals. The elastomeric seal material may also be selected, in part, to influence other changes that can occur during storage of an MDI. Under normal storage conditions, moisture will diffuse through the elastomeric seals into the MDI contents. The rate and quantity is dependent on the environmental conditions and the nature of the elastomeric material, the water vapor transmission properties of which can differ significantly (30).

Propellant leakage from an MDI is characteristic of this product and occurs by diffusion through both stem seals

Table 2 Function of the valve components

Valve component	Function
Gasket	Seal between the valve and can; usually made of rubber.
Ferrule	An aluminum cup that holds the valve components together and attaches them to the can in the crimping process.
Stem	Moving part of the valve that provides the metering action and connects the valve to the actuator. Its design provides entry and exit ports to the metering chamber to permit filling and discharge of the metered dose respectively.
Seat	Provides the main seal around the valve stem and is usually made from rubber. Most valves have two seats to provide the metering action.
Spring	Returns and holds the stem of the valve in the rest position after actuation. May be located inside or outside of the metering chamber.
Metering chamber	Defines the volumes of liquid discharged. Valves with 25-, 50-, 63-, and 100-μl nominal metering volumes are available.

and gasket of the valve. The leakage rate increases with increase in environmental temperature, and tends to parallel the rubber swell for a particular propellant–rubber combination. Propellant leakage from an MDI may shorten the product shelf-life by raising the drug concentration of the liquid contents, thereby increasing the metered dose of medicament. Additionally, excessive leakage may prevent the labelled number of actuations being delivered by the MDI.

ACTUATORS AND SPACERS

Overview of the Components for the Basic MDI Actuator

For a simple MDI, the actuator is a one-piece plastic molding that performs a number of critical functions as a key packaging component in the overall system. The main plastic body of the actuator surrounds and protects the aerosol canister, and veins within the actuator help to locate the canister so that when it is depressed by the patient to release the dose, the canister moves straight down without flexing the valve stem. A high degree of flex could result in

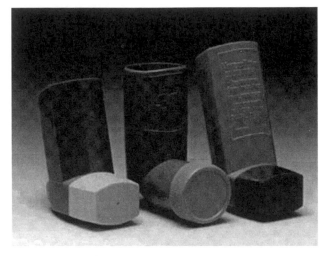

Fig. 6 Typical MDI actuators.

poor performance, e.g., as a result of continuous spraying of the valve. The veins also serve to centrally locate the canister within the actuator body to create airflow paths with minimum resistance so that air can be easily drawn through the device as the patient inhales (67). Some typical MDI actuators are shown in Fig. 6.

The actuator also incorporates the stem block containing the spray nozzle. The stem block contains a socket that the valve stem pushes into when the canister is placed inside the actuator. The socket is designed to provide a tight interference fit with the valve stem such that there is no tendency for the canister to fall out of the actuator on transportation and also so that the complete dose is pushed out of the spray orifice and does not leak back up the side of the valve stem to deposit on the valve ferrule. The final critical component of the actuator is the mouthpiece. The design of this component needs to be such that the patient is easily able to form a seal around it to draw air through the device and inhale the dose. The mouthpiece should also be designed to minimize the extent of drug deposition on the actuator during dose delivery. Typically, 10% to 20% of the dose delivered from the valve is deposited on the actuator and is therefore not available for delivery to the patient. Mouthpiece designs are usually a compromise of what is cheap and easy to mold, what is easy for the patient to use and form a seal around, and what will result in a small and portable device with acceptable drug delivery characteristics. A huge advantage to the MDI is that it is small, light, easy to carry, and discrete to use. A large and complicated design optimizing the delivery characteristics would probably be expensive for the manufacturer and unattractive to patients. A further component of most MDI actuator designs is a dust cap. This is most usually a separate plastic molding that

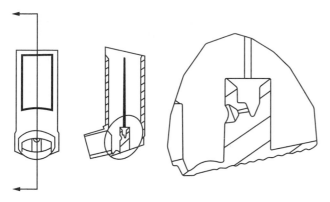

Fig. 7 Detailed diagram of MDI actuator stem block.

snap-fits onto the main actuator body. The main purpose of the dust cap is to prevent foreign matter from entering the mouthpiece and valve stem area while the device is being transported. Foreign matter in this area could either be inhaled by the patient during use or could potentially block the spray nozzle. A detailed cut-away drawing of a typical actuator stem block is shown in Fig. 7.

For a simple MDI actuator, the spray nozzle and valve stem socket are formed by metal pins that enter the stem block as part of the actuator molding process. It is essential to retain accurate dimensional control for these critical areas, to ensure absence of leakage and correct and consistent spray performance during discharge. Various combinations of nozzle diameter and length and expansion chamber volume (volume between the metering chamber and the actual spray nozzle, principally the internal volume of the valve stem), have been investigated. In practice, nozzle diameters range between 0.2 and 0.5 mm. Small nozzle diameters tend to give higher fine particle masses but also increase the length of time it takes to deliver the dose and can be more prone to blocking (31). The actuator parameters cannot be optimized in isolation but must be designed to work in harmony with a specific metering valve, container, and formulation combination (32).

Spacers

As mentioned earlier, the simplest MDI actuators are a compromise between portability, cost, and performance. When a simple MDI is used, a significant portion of the dose is deposited in the oropharyngeal cavity. This is because when the canister is pushed down for the dose to be delivered, the spray emerges from the actuator orifice at such a rate that there is insufficient space for the cloud to decelerate before it strikes the back of the throat or other parts of the oropharyngeal cavity. Simple low-volume spacer devices (70–150 ml) provide an extension to the mouthpiece to allow space for the deceleration of the aerosol cloud to occur. These can either push-fit onto the simple classical type of actuator or can unfold as part of an integral actuator/spacer design (33–37). They significantly reduce the amount drug deposition in the oropharyngeal cavity (35) by allowing more time for the aerosol to decelerate. As a consequence, slightly more drug may be deposited in the lungs but the majority of the reduced throat deposition is accounted for by higher device/spacer deposition. The principal benefit in using this type of simple spacer is in reducing oropharyngeal irritation and hoarseness caused by the deposition of inhaled steroids (34, 38).

Spacer/Holding Chambers

In addition to the simple spacer devices that have been described, there are also much larger volume spacer devices (500–750 ml). These devices provide all the benefits of the simple devices but are capable of capturing and holding the dose prior to the patient inhaling. A one-way valve (or paired valves) may also be incorporated into the mouthpiece region to allow natural breathing cycles so that the patient breathes out into the atmosphere but breathes in through the spacer to inhale the dose held within the spacer. These larger spacers may be beneficial for asthmatic patients who show poor coordination of inhalation with inhaler actuation (33, 34) because actuating the canister to deliver the dose does not have to be coordinated with breathing in (39, 40). Drug deposition in a spacer increases with decreasing chamber size (as a function of width and length) (35, 36). Spacer deposition may be influenced by the size of the metering valve and the propellant composition (37). The delivery of a respirable drug from MDIs is generally similar with or without a larger spacer but with the advantages of lower oropharyangeal deposition and lower need for accurate coordination.

The materials used to manufacture spacers are also key to their performance. A build-up of static electricity on a spacer device can significantly affect the amount of drug deposited on it and, consequently, the dose the patient could receive (41). Similarly, the way in which spacer devices are washed or dried can also result in a build-up of static electricity (42).

BREATH OPERATED INHALERS AND OTHER DEVICE ENHANCEMENTS

The MDI has proved itself over many years of successful use as a highly effective method for delivering drug to the lungs for the treatment of respiratory disease. The MDI is simple to use for most people, but there are difficulties that certain sectors of the patient population may have with the use of this device type.

Very young children and older people have significant difficulty coordinating their actuation of the device with breathing in (43). Patients who have this coordination difficulty can either be supplied with a dry powder inhaler (where the inspiration through the device is also responsible for the release and aerosolization of the powdered drug so that coordination is no longer an issue), or they may be be prescribed a Breath Operated Inhaler (BOI).

Several of these device types are marketed; they are still MDIs but the device takes over the responsibility for actuating the can as the patient breathes in. Typically, the device is primed immediately before the patients takes their dose. This priming can be achieved either via the opening of the dust cap to reveal the mouthpiece or by operating a special priming lever. For the currently marketed devices, this results in a spring being compressed above the aerosol canister that has enough strength to actuate the can on release. The device contains a triggering mechanism that is released when the patients breathe in through the device to take their medicine. The release of the triggering mechanism allows the coiled spring to push the MDI canister down and deliver the medicine, negating the need for the patients to coordinate the activities (44). Although there is significant merit to devices of this type, they need to be carefully developed to ensure that the altered pattern of use in terms of priming, shaking, and taking the medicine works in harmony with the other device components to ensure that consistent doses of medicine are always delivered from the device.

More BOI devices are likely to reach the market. They could be either mechanical or electronic in operation. The incorporation of electronics into a device of this type opens up the possibility of including other patient features, e.g., counters and other data logging.

MDI COUNTERS

One significant issue with MDIs is that because of the aluminum canister used for most device types, it is impossible for the patient to know exactly how much medicine is left in the inhaler. Shaking the canister prior to taking the medicine can give the patient some confidence that formulation is still there within the device, but this is a very crude measure. MDIs are always filled with more medicine (termed the overfill) than the number of actuations mentioned on the label. Thus a 200 actuation

product might actually be filled with 240 actuations. There are a number of reasons for this:

1. There is always some leakage from devices of this type throughout their life. Including an overfill guarantees that the device is still capable of delivering the claimed number of actuations at the end of the shelf life.
2. There can be some variability in the dosing performance of an MDI as the formulation level becomes very low. Including an overfill guarantees that the MDI will perform consistently throughout the number of actuations claimed on the label.
3. There is a portion of the formulation that is not removable from the canister because of the positioning of the metering valve sampling port.

Using a glass container is one method of overcoming the difficulty by knowing how much medicine is left, but because of the overfill factor there will always appear to be medicine left even after the patient has exceeded the number of actuations claimed on the label. Also, glass containers may be more bulky than their aluminum counterparts and are certainly more expensive to produce.

The alternative to a transparent container is to fit the MDI with some kind of actuation counter or level indicator. The level indicator, much like the fuel gauge within a car, will give some idea of the amount of medicine that remains, but will not be an exact measure. A numerical counter is probably the preferred solution as it leaves the patient in absolutely no doubt about the amount of medicine remaining in the device. When the number of actuations claimed in the label have been taken from the device, the patient will know that a replacement is needed, thereby completely avoiding the uncertainty that would arise from continuing to use the device during the overfill phase between label claim and final device exhaustion. The counting mechanism could be either applied to the top of the aerosol canister or the valve area or be an integral part of the actuator and be mechanical or electronic in operation.

OTHER DEVICE ENHANCEMENTS

The incorporation of breath activation and/or counting mechanisms into the MDI opens the possibility of including other device features, particularly if the above-mentioned two features are achieved via electronic means. MDIs that feature data gathering technology allow the patient or physician to monitor how and when the medicine is being taken (compliance) or to monitor lung function and control the amount of medicine that the patient is taking are distinct possibilities.

Spray Atomization and Evaporation

The respirable fraction or Fine Particle Mass (FPM) of a finely aerosolized drug delivered from an MDI is highly dependent on the atomization of the formulation and the subsequent spray dynamics. The aerosol characteristics depend heavily on interactions between the propellant(s), the (typically) micronized drug particles, the formulation excipients, and the design and dimensions of the metering valve and the key actuator variables (stem block, atomization orifice, actuator airflow paths, and mouthpiece design). The importance of these inhaler variables has been demonstrated previously (45–47). MDIs give a much slower metered delivery and a much finer spray droplet size distribution than what would be expected for simple hydraulic atomization because a mixture of gas and liquid is discharged from the metering chamber.

Partial flash evaporation of the propellant occurs in the metering chamber and in the expansion spaces of the valve stem and actuator stem block (47). Further evaporation also occurs within the discharge nozzle, and alternating segments of liquid and gas pass through the nozzle in a process of effervescent atomization.

The spray droplets are ejected at a high velocity of about 25–30 m/s (48), and although the aerosol decelerates rapidly the velocity is still much higher than the inhaled air velocity, resulting in significant drug impaction in the oropharyngeal region. This effect has been mimicked crudely in simple throat models (49) and more accurately in throat models having carefully matched human dimensions (50).

The probability of oropharyngeal deposition is determined more by droplet size than by velocity and density because the particle inertia is proportional to the density, velocity, and the square of the diameter. It, therefore, follows that oropharyngeal drug deposition is reduced and the respirable drug delivery is increased when MDI sprays are finely atomized and evaporate rapidly. Such MDI sprays are generally promoted by increasing the propellant vapor pressure (45, 47, 51) and reducing the actuator spray nozzle diameter (45, 46, 52).

Spray evaporation is impeded by the inclusion of appreciable concentrations of nonvolatile miscible excipients in the formulation. These include ethanol as a cosolvent (53), and CFC 11, both having low volatility in the spray, which is also chilled by propellant evaporation, thereby further reducing the rate of evaporation. The particle size distribution of the resulting aerosol depends not only on the spray dynamics but also on the number and primary size distribution of the drug particles in liquid suspension and their degree of deagglomeration during spray atomization. The evaporated aerosol particle size increases with the concentration of drug (45, 54) and nonvolatile excipients (45, 55) in suspension formulations and also in solution products.

MANUFACTURING

In the manufacture of MDIs, liquid filling procedures have been developed based on either a cold-filling method or a pressure-filling method. Both methods are suitable for either solution or suspension formulations and regardless of the process, it is important to maintain a low atmospheric relative humidity in the filling area to minimize condensation and possible absorption of water by the product.

The cold-filling process involves chilling the propellant and drug formulation to approximately −60°C in tanks to maintain the liquid state and metering it into the open cans in a single step. The cans are then sealed immediately by crimping on the valves.

The potential advantages of this procedure are that it is simple and can accommodate any valve, with minimal changes to the production line. The potential disadvantages include high energy consumption (refrigeration), inconsistent fill weights due to propellant evaporation, contamination from moisture condensation, and possible irreversible physical changes in the formulation at low temperature.

The pressure-filling process is now more commonly used and relies on the injection of at least part of the fill through the valve, which is crimped to the container. Pressure filling with CFC propellants generally involves preparing a concentrated suspension (or solution) of the drug in the high-boiling CFC 11, together with any excipients. This concentrate is metered into the open container in a cool area to minimize evaporative losses of propellant before crimping on the valve. The low-boiling propellant, CFC 12 or a CFC 12/CFC 114 blend, is then filled through the valve by high-pressure injection, a process commonly known as gassing. For this process, the potential advantages are that accurate fill weights are achievable and that filling can be undertaken at or near room temperature. The potential disadvantages are that the filling equipment is complex and expensive to install and that the valves must be suitable for pressure filling.

With the transition to HFA/HFC propellants, the lack of a direct replacement for CFC 11 has resulted in the development of a single-stage pressure-filling process. For the HFA/HFC propellants, a concentrated suspension (or solution) of drug is prepared in the propellant

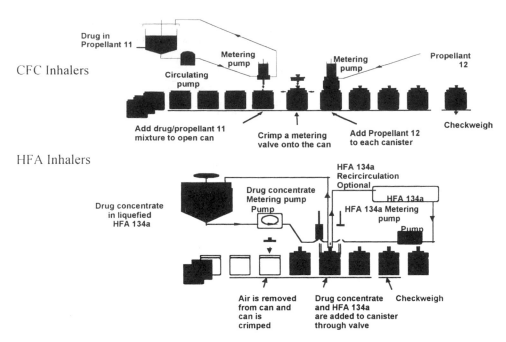

Fig. 8   Production pressure-filling sequence for MDI cans.

(134a or 227ea) contained in a pressurized system. A valve is crimped to a container and the concentrate is pressure-filled through the valve, followed by an aliquot of pure propellant (56). Such a process requires the development of a total pressurized filling system with compatible elastomeric seals and the use of pumps capable of recirculating, without cavitation, high-pressure liquids.

During the filling process, it is normal to displace the air from the container before valve crimping to avoid internal pressure changes in the MDI at the time of progressive discharge of the contents during use. For the cold filling and two-stage pressure-filling processes, air displacement occurs after filling the initial propellant liquid into the container. However, in the single-stage pressure-filling process, air is purged from the container in a separate operation prior to crimping the valve, using either a small injection of propellant or vacuum (Fig. 8).

High-speed rotary filling machines are widely used to provide concentrate filling, valve placement, and crimping and gassing in a continuous sequence. Similar set-ups are used for HFA/HFC MDIs with appropriate modifications to permit container purging. Intermittent indexing machines are often employed for small-scale filling. Filling lines may also be equipped with a checkweighing station to reject any over- or under-filled canisters. In addition, a heat-stressing facility may be employed after filling to raise the temperature of the MDIs to a predetermined value (e.g., 50–55°C) to increase the

internal pressure and thereby challenge the integrity of the crimp seal. After a defined quarantine period, further checkweighing, normally as part of the final packaging operation, can be used to reject canisters that have leaked.

QUALITY CONTROL

Quality control testing of MDI batches is applied to the individual inhaler components prior to manufacture, as in-process controls during the manufacturing, and to the finished product (Table 1). A number of publications describe quality control procedures for MDIs (21, 57, 58).

Component and In-Process Quality Control

Typical QC procedures for the aluminum canisters would include careful assessments of their dimensions, weight, strength, surface finish, and cleanliness. Important canister characteristics are neck finish and dimensions, regional can wall thickness, and external size of the canister, which influence valve sealing, canister strength and volume, and the fit into the actuator. Canister strength is typically monitored by the manufacturer, using a hydraulic pressure test. Glass bottles may be subjected to impact fracture drop tests.

The metering valve is generally the most critical inhaler component in terms of its effect on product performance;

Table 3 Quality control and analytical tests for the characterization of metered dose inhalers

Name of test/test area	Type of data/comments
Individual component testing prior to manufacture of active product:	
Containers	Dimensional accuracy and surface quality; strength testing by canister manufacturer
Metering valves	Dimensional accuracy and surface quality of individual components from dismantled valves
Mean weight per actuation and leakage rate	Samples filled on the production line and shot weight through use data generated to guarantee correct valve function; samples tested after a period of equilibration to ensure leak rates within specification
Input micronized drug	Chemical, physical, and particle size specifications
Propellant	Chemical and physical specifications
Surfactant	Chemical specification
Actuators	Dimensional accuracy and finish; accuracy and centralization of the atomization orifice
In-process control testing that occurs during manufacture:	
Atmospheric conditions	Monitoring of atmospheric temperature and humidity in manufacturing areas
Drug suspension concentration	Rapid analysis initially and during filling
Drug suspension	Periodic fill weight checks (if separate suspension followed by gassing)
Filled canisters	Automatically checkweigh all canisters
Gross leakage and safety	Containers heated to raise internal pressure; visable leakage and pack distortion examination
Control of leakage rate	Checkweigh all containers after a suitable quarantine period to meet specified limits
Metering-valve function	Each filled container is spray-tested after quarantine, following a number of priming actuations
Analytical testing applied to completed product:	
Appearance	Description of the suspension; absence of corrosion of canister; completeness of inhaler components
Identity	HPLC or infrared confirmation of identity and absence of polymorph or incorrect solvate
Microbial limit testing	e.g., to USP requirements
Spray pattern	Consistent, concentric pattern fired straight with respect to mouthpiece geometry
Water content	Karl Fischer or similar method
Foreign particulate matter	BP 1993
Leachables	Consistent profile between batches, careful consideration of levels versus specifications based on individual components
Pressure test	USP
Leak test	USP
Drug related impurities	Comparison with specifications based on preclinical/clinical batches
Characterization of particle size distribution:	
Multistage impactor	Careful consideration of particle size distribution profile data and a multipoint specification; individual stage data may be combined for comparison with the specification for QC purposes
Laser particle sizing	Tends to be used to characterize products more in development
Microscopy	Tends to be used to characterize products more in development
Characterization of drug delivered from the MDI	
Mean dose delivered and content uniformity	Careful consideration against various specifications covering mean and individual actuations through use assessing inter- and intracan variability; regulatory guidance varies from region to region (see Refs. 22, 58, 59)
Number of primes	Test to demonstrate the number of priming actuations the patient must fire to waste before performance is nominal
Number of actuations	To demonstrate that the product delivers nominal dose at the end of label claim (can be derived from CU data)
Actuator deposition	Generated during development to determine how much drug deposits on the actuator with each dose and thus what the ex-actuator dose is

therefore, it also requires detailed testing prior to use. The disassembled valve components are examined for dimensional accuracy and surface quality. Assembled valves are tested for correct metering function and formulation delivery. Test packs are stored until equilibration and the units are tested for propellant leakage (weight loss) and weight of metered delivery. The reproducibility of delivery has been reported for various valve propellant combinations (59). Where propellant mixtures are used in the product, there is some progressive fractionation during discharge of the pack contents because of greater loss of the more volatile component (59). The associated change in liquid propellant density can cause a small progressive change in metered delivery weights, but this does not influence the drug delivery, which is determined by the metered volume.

Common in-process control procedures for MDIs are provided in Table 3. In addition, stringent environmental controls are required for air cleanliness, humidity, and temperature during the manufacturing run. Rapid verification of the drug content of the fresh bulk suspension or solution may be important prior to commencing the filling run because reworking of aerosol products for recovery is not practical. It may be necessary to monitor the dispersion quality and drug concentration of suspension during filling. Various online monitoring methodologies are under development but still the principal method is via measuring the total drug per can for a sample taken from the manufacturing run. Inline checkweighing of the crimped units provides an indirect record of the suspension fill weight per canister.

MDI BATCH ACCEPTANCE

MDI products are subject to batch control and acceptance tests similar to those for other pharmaceutical dosage forms, that is, active drug identification, dose delivery, and dose uniformity. Additional special tests unique to inhalers, e.g., characterizing the particle size distribution of the delivered aerosol, are also applied. Typical tests are shown in Table 3.

It is now rare to specify determination of the metered drug delivery by discharging directly from the metering valve (without the actuator) into a solvent (60). Via this route, correction is subsequently made for the amount of drug that typically deposits on the actuator to leave the ex-device dose available to the patient. The preferred method now is to discharge the inhaler with the actuator fitted, into a trapping system with an airflow being drawn through it (e.g., the USP/NF method) (61). This method of

characterizing the ex-actuator dose is much more representative of the real patient case. Typically, the mean specified delivery ex-actuator is controlled to within 85–115% of the label claim, with additional limits also applied to the spread of individual doses.

PARTICLE SIZE ANALYSIS OF SPRAYS AND AEROSOLS

The characterization and quality control of the particle size distribution of the discharged aerosol has become one of the key tests applied to MDI and other inhaler products, and a wide variety of methods have been developed to make this possible. The available methods can be broadly split into two categories: optical (typically laser) methods or methods based on inertial impaction.

Optical methods typically have the advantage of producing detailed results very quickly on a small number of actuations, but the disadvantage is that they do not characterize the whole spray emerging from the device. They are also not able to distinguish drug particles from drug-free excipient particles or propellant alone droplets or even between two different drug substances as in the case of a combination product. The sizing results obtained via optical methods may give an incorrect or biased impression of the true particle size distribution for the pharmaceutically active substance. Nevertheless, these methods can prove to be extremely useful from a qualitative perspective.

SPRAY DROPLET SIZE ANALYSIS

The spray droplet size distribution has a major influence on the amount of oropharyngeal deposition and the amount of drug delivered to the lungs and the regions of lung deposition. Methods for spray droplet particle sizing from MDIs (4, 6) have been reviewed.

For the quality control of actuators, spray flume appearance and profile are often used (62). These methods potentially highlight any gross issues with the moulding of the actuator atomization orifice and stem block (e.g., firing off-centre or poor spray homogeneity). Flume profiles can also obtained by timed flash photography (4, 63), but an even better picture of dynamic flume changes can be provided by high-speed video recording (62, 64).

Spray droplets have also been analyzed microscopically after impacting the spray on to specially coated slides. Microscopic laser holography has been used to measure droplet size distributions and concentrations for MDIs

(65). Laser video imaging has also been applied to MDI sprays (66).

Laser diffraction (LD) size analysis is a rapid and convenient noninvasive method used extensively for measuring the droplet size distribution of industrial sprays. LD analysis has been used for nonmetered dispenser sprays to study the effects of varying the propellants (67, 68) and valve orifices (69).

Oropharyngeal spray impaction depends on the droplet velocity and size. Both these parameters can be measured simultaneously and recorded for each droplet. With Phase Doppler Anemometer (PDA) instruments, useful results have been obtained on MDI sprays (70).

MDI AEROSOL PARTICLE SIZE DISTRIBUTION ANALYSIS

Methods for the size analysis of MDI aerosols have been reviewed (6, 71–73). Various sizing methods are available. Microscopic examination of particles based on discharging the spray against a slide (72, 73) can provide a limit test for unduly large single particles resulting from poor micronization or poor physical stability of the drug in liquid suspension, but this is only a very gross measure.

INERTIAL IMPACTORS

Inertial impactors fractionate aerosol particles aerodynamically according to their inertia, which increases with size. Inertial impaction is the most widely used method for sizing MDI aerosols, partly because a large sample is measured, consisting of the total aerosol generated from a number of actuations. Methods of this type have the advantage that the aerodynamic measurement accounts for the effects of particle shape and density and that the aerodynamic size distribution is measured specifically in terms of the drug mass independently of any other aerosolized constituents that may be present, giving a specific measure of the aerodynamic size distribution of the drug.

The most commonly used tool for the aerodynamic classification of particle size distributions is the Andersen cascade impactor. The Andersen impactor was originally developed for the environmental monitoring of air samples but is now commonly applied to characterizing medical aerosol size distibutions. Particle size distribution profile data can be generated or an overall figure can be derived to loosely determine the mass of drug that falls into the respirable range. This is achieved by combining several impactor stages with particle size cut-offs roughly

corresponding to respirable particles (74). To gather the particle size distribution data, the MDI is actuated a number of times into the cascade impaction apparatus via a connecting elbow (termed the throat or induction port). On entering the impactor, the aerosol is passed through successive impaction plates with decreasing jet diameters. Velocities increase as the particles go down through the impactor to the point where they impact on the collection plate below. Cascade impactors (particularly the Andersen) have been used extensively to assess MDI aerosols (72). A schematic diagram of the Andersen impactor is given in Fig. 9.

To collect and deliver the MDI discharge to the impactor, two main types of collector system have been used: a large chamber to permit extensive or complete spray droplet evaporation before impaction (72, 75, 76), and a restrictive induction port (51, 73, 78) in which considerable droplet impaction occurs in a very crude analogy to the behavior for the human oropharynx. The extent of droplet evaporation before impaction, and therefore the size distribution measured, is a function of the lag time between spray discharge and impaction. The lag time depends on the size and shape of the particular inlet duct and upper impactor stages and also the volumetric airflow rate. The droplet evaporation rate depends on the volatility of the particular propellant/excipient system (75) and the effect of the airflow rate and air vapor mixing on vapor diffusion from the droplets. Clearly, it is essential in comparing inhaler systems to standardize the induction port, cascade impactor, and airflow rate (72, 77).

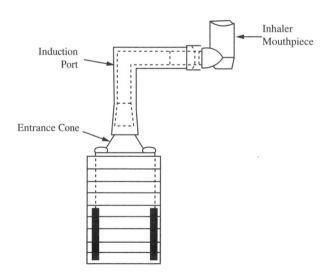

Fig. 9 Schematic representation of the Andersen cascade impactor.

The impacted drug fractions are normally measured via a specific chemical assay, although mircoweighing the plates has also been investigated (75, 78). A number of actuations are normally accumulated for each cascade impaction determination to collect sufficient drug for accurate assay. The United States Pharmacopoeia includes a test for MDIs, using a cascade impactor coupled to a throat of specified dimensions (74).

Simple two-stage impactors (or impingers) with a defined throat geometry have also been used to generate simple data more rapidly than for the multi-stage cascade impactors (or impingers) or for QC purposes (74, 79–81). The Twin Impinger (TI) has gradually become a much less widely used technique as it cannot provide the more detailed distribution data required for in-house product development or by the regulatory authorities, but it can be sensitive enough to reveal formulations that are unstable due to crystal growth or particle aggregation.

SINGLE PARTICLE OPTICAL SIZERS (SPOS)

Single particle optical sizers measure each aerosol particle passing through a small optical sensing zone to give rapid "real time" measurement of particle number diameter distribution and concentration. Low particle concentrations are necessary to avoid coincidence errors arising from multiple particle occupancy in the sensing zone. SPOS methods are rapid, but they have the following disadvantages for MDI aerosol evaluation:

- Drug containing particles are not distinguished from excipient or foreign particles.
- Aerosol sampling may not be representative due to inadequate measurement of the large particles and their possible partial loss in the sampling probe (82).
- Equivalent mass distribution is derived based on the assumption that the particles are spherical and of equal density.

Optical single-particle counters offer much more rapid aerosol size analysis than do impaction methods. They need to be applied with caution to MDIs for the reasons stated previously.

REFERENCES

1. Bisgaard, H. Respir. Med. **1997**, *91* (Suppl A), 20–21.
2. Tansey, I.P. Pharm. J. **1997**, *259*, 896–898.
3. Vervaet, C.; Byron, P.R. Int. J. Pharm. **1999**, *186*, 13–30.
4. Hallworth, G.W. The Formulation and Evaluation of Pressurised Metered Dose Inhalers. *Drug Delivery to the Respiratory Tract*; Ganderton, D., Jones, T., Eds.; Ellis Horwood: Chichester, UK, 1987; 87–118.
5. Atkins, P.J.; Barker, N.P.; Mathisen, D. The Design and Development of Inhalation Drug Delivery Systems. *Pharmaceutical Inhalation Pressurised Metered-Dose Inhaler Technology*; Hickey, A.J., Ed.; Marcel Dekker, Inc.: New York, 1992.
6. Moren, F. Aerosol Dosage Forms and Formulation. *Aerosols in Medicine—Principles Diagnosis and Therapy*; Moren, F., Newhouse, M.T., Dolvich, M.B., Newman, S.P., Eds.; Elsevier: Amsterdam, 1993; 2.
7. Purewal, T.S.; Grant, D.J.W. *Metered Dose Inhaler Technology*; Interpharm, Press Inc.: Illinois, 1998.
8. IPAC (International Pharmaceutical Aerosol Consortium). *Ensuring Patient Care—The Role of the HFC MDI*, 2nd Ed.; 1999.
9. Molina, M.J.; Rowland, F.S. Nature **1974**, *249*, 810.
10. Montreal Protocol on Substances that Deplete the Ozone Layer, Liaison Office of the United Nations Environmental Programme, New York, 1989.
11. Dalby, R.N.; Byron, P.R.; Sherpherd, H.R.; Papadopoulos, E. Pharm. Technol. **1990**, 26–33.
12. Dalby, R.N.; Byron, P.R. Pharm. Technol. Int. **1992**, *4* (1/2), 42–45.
13. CPMP (Committee for Proprietary Medicinal Products) Result of the Coordinated Review of 1, 1, 1, 2 - Tetrafluoroethane HFC-134a **13 July 1994.**
14. Harnor, K.J.; Perkins, A.C.; Wastie, M.; Wilson, C.G.; Sims, E.E.; Feely, L.C.; Farr, S.J. Effect of Vapor Pressure on the Deposition Pattern from Solution Phase Metered Dose Inhalers. Int. J. Pharm. **1993**, *95* (1–3), 111–116.
15. Byron, P.R. Towards the Rational Formulation of Metered Dose Inhalers. J. Biopharm. Sci. **1992**, 1–9.
16. Vanbever, R.; Mintzes, J.D.; Wang, J.; Nice, J.; Chen, D.; Batycky, R.; Langer, R.; Edwards, D.A. Formulation and Physical Characterization of Large Porous Particles for Inhalation. Pharm. Res. **1999**, *16* (11), 1735–1742.
17. Edwards, D.A.; Hanes, J.; Caponetti, G.; Hrkach, J.; Ben, J.A.; Eskew, M.L.; Mintzes, J.; Deaver, D.; Lotan, N.; Langer, R.S. Large Porous Particles for Pulmonary Drug Delivery. Science **1997**, *276* (5320), 1868–1871.
18. Shekunov, B.Yu. Crystallization Processes in Pharmaceutical Technology and Drug Delivery Design. J. Cryst. Growth **2000**, *211*, 122–136.
19. Dellamary, L.A.; Tarara, T.E.; Smith, D.J.; Woelk, C.H.; Adractas, A.; Costello, M.L.; Weers, J.G. Hollow Porous Particles in Metered Dose Inhalers. Pharm. Res. **2000**, *17*, 168–174.
20. BenJebria, A.; Eskew, M.L.; Edwards, D.A. Inhalation System for Pulmonary Aerosol Drug Delivery in Rodents Using Large Porous Particles. Aerosol Sci. Technol. **2000**, *32*, 421–433.
21. FDA Centre for Drug Evaluation and Research (CDER), DRAFT Guidance for Industry, Metered Dose Inhaler (MDI) and Dry Powder Inhaler (DPI) Products. http://www.fda.gov/cder/guidance/index.htm.

22. Adams, W.P.; Poochikian, G.; Taylor, A.S.; Patel, R.M.; Burke, G.P.; Williams, R.L. Regulatory Aspects of Modifications to Innovator Bronchodilator Metered Dose Inhalers and Development of Generic Substitutes. J. Aerosol Med. Deposition, Clearance, and Effects in the Lung **1994**, *7* (2), 119–134.

23. Ruffin, R.E.; Southcott, A.M. Chlorofluorocarbon-Free Inhalation Devices in Asthma: Are there Clinical Implications?. Biodrugs **1998**, *10* (2), 91–96.

24. Brambilla, G.; Ganderton, D.; Garzia, R.; Meakin, B.; Ventura, P. Proceedings of Drug Delivery to the Lungs IX. *Modulation of Aerosol Clouds Produced by HFA Solution Inhalers*; 1998, 155–159.

25. Williams, R.O.; Hu, C. European J. Pharm. Biopharm. **1997**, *44*, 195–203.

26. Novartis A.G. European Patent Application No. 94810478.1.

27. Downing R.C.; Parmalee H.M. Proc CSMA 37th Annual Meeting Freon Aerosol Report A19, E.I. Du Pont de Nemours and Co. Ltd. New York 1950.

28. Howlett, D. Spray Technol. Market. **1994**, 18–22.

29. Pischtiak, A.H. *Proceedings of Drug Delivery to the Lungs X*; 1999, 171–174.

30. Williams, G.; Tcherevatchenkoff, A. *Proceedings of Drug Delivery to the Lungs VIII*; 1997, 91–94.

31. Dunbar, C.A. CA129 –153066/12 Journal 19981231. Part. Sci. Technol. **1997**, *15*, 253–271.

32. Tansey, I.P. The Challenges in the Development of Metered Dose Inhalation Aerosols using Ozone-Friendly Propellants. Spray Technol. Mark. **1994**, *7*, 26–29.

33. Weeke, E.R. Eur. J. Dis. **1982**, *63* (Suppl. 119), 105–109.

34. Konig, P. Chest **1985**, *82*, 276–284.

35. Moren, F. Int. J. Pharmacol. **1978**, *1*, 205–212.

36. Corr, D.; Dolovich, M.; McCormack, D.; Ruffin, R.; Obminski, G.; Newhouse, M.J. Aerosol Sci. **1982**, *13*, 1–7.

37. Moren, F. Int. J. Pharmacol. **1978**, *1*, 213–218.

38. Newman, S.P.; Newhouse, M.T. Effect of Add-On Devices for Aerosol Drug Delivery: Deposition Studies and Clinical Aspects. J. Aerosol Med: Depositions, Clearance, and Effects in the Lung **1996**, *9*, 55–70.

39. Zanen, P. Inhalation Anti-asthma Therapy with Spacers: Technical Aspects. Monaldi Arch. Chest Dis. **1994**, *49*, 258–264.

40. Barry, P.W.; O'Callaghan, C. Inhalational Drug Delivery from Seven Different Spacer Devices. Thorax **1996**, *51*, 835–840.

41. Wildhaber, J.H.; Devadason, S.G.; Eber, E.; Hayden, M.J.; Everard, M.L.; Summers, Q.A.; LeSouef, P.N. Effect of Electrostatic Charge, Flow, Delay and Multiple Actuations on the in Vitro Delivery of Salbutamol from Different Small Volume Spacers for Infants. Thorax **1996**, *51*, 985–988.

42. Dewsbury, N.J.; Kenyon, C.J.; Newman, S.P. The Effect of Handling Techniques on Electrostatic Charge on Spacer Devices: A Correlation with in Vitro Particle Size Analysis. Int. J. Pharm. **1996**, *137*, 261–264.

43. Crompton, G.K. Problems Patients have using Pressurised Aerosol Inhalers. Eur. J. Respir. Dis. **1982**, *63*, 101–104.

44. Newman, S.P.; Weisz, A.W.B.; Talee, N.; Clarke, S.W. Improvement of Drug Delivery with a Breath Actuated Pressurised Aerosol for Patients with Poor Inhaler Technique. Thorax **1991**, *46*, 712–716.

45. Polli, G.P.; Grim, W.M.; Bacher, F.A.; Yunker, M.H. J. Pharm. Sci. **1969**, *58*, 484–486.

46. Clark, A.R. *Metered Atomisation for Respiratory Drug Delivery*; Ph.D. Thesis Loughborough University of Technology: 1991.

47. Hickey, A.J. *Inhalation Aerosols—Physical and Biological Basis for Therapy, Lung Biology in Health and Disease*; Marcel Dekker, Inc.: 1996; 94.

48. Newman, S. *Deposition and Effects of Inhalation Aerosols*; AB Draco: Lund Sweden, 1983; 13–22.

49. Kim, C.S.; Eldridge, M.A.; Sackner, M.A. Am. Rev. Respir. Dis. **1987**, *135*, 157–164.

50. Swift, D.L. J. Aerosol Sci. **1992**, *23*, 495–498.

51. Backstrom, K.; Nilsson, P.G. J. Aerosol Sci. **1988**, *19*, 1097–1100.

52. Ranucci, J.A.; Cooper, D.; Sethachutkul, K. Pharmacol. Technol. **1992**, *4*, 84–92.

53. Miller, J.F.; Schatzel, J.F.; Vincent, B.J. Colloid Int. Sci. **1991**, *143*, 532–554.

54. Najafabadi, A.R.; Ganderton, D. J. Pharm. Pharmacol. **1991**, *43*(67P).

55. Najafabadi, A.R.; Ganderton, D. J. Pharm. Pharmacol. **1990**, *42* (Suppl. 12P).

56. Patent UK GB2236146B

57. Committee for Proprietary Medicinal Products. Replacement of Chlorofluorocarbons (CFCs) in Metered Dose Inhalation Products. 1993, MCA Eurodirect Publication No. 5378/93.

58. Inhalanda, Preparations for Inhalation, European Pharmacopoeia. Supplement: 1999, 671.

59. Contractor, A.M.; Richman, M.D.; Shangraw, R.F. J. Pharm. Sci. **1970**, *59*, 1488–1489.

60. British Pharmacopeia. Her Majesty's Stationery Office: London, 1988; II, 875–876.

61. USP. United States Pharmacopeia. 23rd Revision U.S. Pharmacopeial Convention, Inc.: Rockville, MD, 1994; 1839.

62. Miszuk, S.; Gupta, B.M.; Chen, B.C.; Clawans, C.; Knapp, J.Z. J. Pharm. Sci. **1980**, *69*, 713–717.

63. Hallworth, G.W.; Kedgley, D. J. Pharm. Pharmacol. **1986**, *38* (Suppl), 27.

64. Dhand, R.; Malik, S.K.; Balakrishnan, M.; Verma, S.R. J. Pharm. Pharmacol. **1988**, *10*, 429–430.

65. Moren, F.; Hathaway, D. Proc. 3rd International Conference on Liquid Atomization and Spray Systems 1985. 1,111B.1 ICLASS–85: London, 1985; 1–6.

66. Hotham, G.A. Particle Size Analysis of Aerosols in Medicine. *Respiratory Aerosols*; Gale, A.E. Ed.; Gordon Harris: St. Agnes, South Australia, 1981; 47–71.

67. Johnsen, M.A. *The Aerosol Handbook*, 2nd Ed.; Dorland: Wayne NJ, 1982; 271, 273–354.

68. Hind, G. Manf. Chem. **1990**, *61*, 23–30.

69. Tsuda, S.; Dohara, K.; Shinjo, G. Chem. Pharm. Bull. **1988**, *37*, 2777–2781.

70. Burton G.R. Negus C.R. Proceedings of the Fourth Annual Conference of the Aerosol Society University of Surrey 1909; 211–216

71. Byron, P.R. Respiratory Drug Delivery. CRC Press, Inc.: Boca Raton, FL, 1973.

72. Hallworth, G.W.; Andrews, U.G. J. Pharm. Pharmacol. **1976**, *28*, 898–907.

73. Hallworth, G.W.; Hamilton, R.R. J. Pharm. Pharmacol. **1976**, *28*, 890–897.

74. The Pharmacopeial Convention. 7th Suppl.: Rockville, MD, 1992; 3122–3129, United States Pharmacopeia (USP/NF).

75. Kim, C.S.; Trujillo, D.; Sackner, M.A. Am. Rev. Respir. Dis. **1985**, *132*, 137–142.

76. Nilsson, G.; Nrunzell, A.; Helberg, H. Acta Pharmac. Suec. **1977**, *14*, 95–104.

77. Phillips, E.M.; Byron, P.B.; Fults, K.; Hickey, A.J. Pharmacol. Res. **1990**, *7*, 1228–1233.

78. Malton, C.A.; Hallworth, G.W.; Padfield, J.M. J. Pharm. Pharmacol. **1982**, *34* (Suppl), 65.

79. Hallworth, G.W.; Westmoreland, D.G. J. Pharm. Pharmacol. **1987**, *39*, 966–972.

80. Atkins, P.J. Pharmacol. Technol. **1992**, *4*, 26–32.

81. British Pharmacopoeia. Appendix XV11C Her Majesty's Stationery Office: London, 1988.

82. Bouchikhi, A.; Becquemin, M.H.; Bignon, J.; Roy, M.; Teillac, A. Eur. Respir. J. **1988**, *1*, 547–552.

83. CPMP (Committee for Proprietary Medicinal Products) Result of the Coordinated Review of 1, 1, 1, 2, 3, 3, 3 - Heptafluoropropane (HFC-227)   **13 Sept 1995.**

MICROBIAL CONTROL OF PHARMACEUTICALS

Nigel A. Halls

GlaxoSmithKline Global Manufacturing and Supply, Uxbridge, United Kingdom

INTRODUCTION

Pharmaceutically active products (drug products) are expected to be efficacious, however; the presence of microorganisms in these products may have adverse effects on their efficacy. The severity of the effects that microorganisms may have on any particular drug product is a function of the nature of the product, its intended use, and the nature of the microorganism concerned. At one end of the spectrum, microbial contamination of a sterile parenteral product may, on injection into a debilitated patient, result in fatality; at the other, patients may refuse to begin or continue a course of medication because of aromas, off-flavors, or discolorations of microbial origin. In either situation, or in any related situation, the presence of microorganisms ought to be avoided in drug products.

Microbiological standards for drug products are published in the pharmacopoeias and/or are required by regulatory agencies for their registration. Generally, these standards are concerned with the protection of the public from infection by limiting the numbers and types of microorganisms to levels that are unlikely to be harmful. In addition to standards applying to the products themselves, there are also microbiological standards applying to the conditions under which drug products are allowed to be manufactured. These manufacturing standards (Good Manufacturing Practices, or GMPs) are intended to ensure that finished product standards are being attained consistently.

Microbial control of pharmaceuticals is primarily concerned with minimizing the opportunities for drug products to be contaminated by microorganisms. It is secondarily concerned with minimizing the potential for any microorganisms that may have contaminated drug products to increase to levels that may risk the efficacy of the product. The testing of product samples for compliance with microbiological standards is only one small part of this. By and large, microbiological test methods are product-destructive and, as a consequence, it is unusual to find valid statistical sampling and testing being done at batch release. Finished product testing is at best confirmatory and in some cases may be dispensed with when manufacturing controls ensure that products are highly unlikely to become microbiologically contaminated (parametric release in its broadest sense).

Minimizing the risk of microbiological contamination of drug products is assured by the application of microbiological and physical standards and controls to starting materials, product-contact packaging components, manufacturing facilities, manufacturing processes, and equipment. By and large, these assurances are obtained by applying controls that protect materials, equipment, and processes from sources of microbiological contamination. In recognition of the fraility of protective measures in all but the most extreme circumstances, microbiological contaminants are also routinely controlled by removal, inactivation, or destruction.

The microbiological standards applying to drug products are expected to be maintained until time of use by the patient (or healthcare professional) and throughout their shelf-lives. This presents two areas of concern relevant to microbiological control: first, that the product should be protected (usually by its packaging) from additional contamination after release to market, and second, that the product should be formulated to prevent proliferation of any microorganisms that may have been present at tolerable levels at the time of release.

Different types and levels of microbial control are applicable to different types of products. The single major division is between sterile and nonsterile products.

MICROBIAL CONTROL OF STERILE PRODUCTS

Sterility is defined as the total absence of all viable life forms. Parenteral products and ophthalmic products are expected to be sterile. Parenteral products must be sterile because their route of administration overrides the body's external physical barriers to infection. Ophthalmic products must be sterile because eye damage is often irreparable. No distinction can be made between microorganisms that are known to be specific causative agents of disease and those that are not. Any microorganism may be opportunistically pathogenic if administered parenterally or if applied to susceptible tissues (the transparent parts of the eye have a particularly poor blood supply and, therefore, a less sensitive immunological response than do other parts of the body) or to debilitated or immunocompromised patients.

Sterility, the Sterility Test, and Sterility Assurance

Sterility has an absolute definition (absence of ALL viable life forms). As with all absolutes, it is difficult, if not impossible, to prove.

Sterility tests

The pharmacopoeial standard applying to sterile products is that they must be capable of passing a Test for Sterility. A Test for Sterility is described in *U.S. Pharmacopeia* (USP) under Section 71 and in the *European Pharmacopoeia* (PhEur) under Section 2.6.1. These were "harmonized" along with the *Japanese Pharmacopoeia* and the requirements of the Australian Therapeutic Goods Administration in 1999, but they still have some minor differences in detail.

The Test for Sterility relies on the detection of viable microorganisms within a sample that is directly or indirectly inoculated into broad-spectrum microbiological recovery media. Detectable microbial growth is confirmation of nonsterility, whereas sterility can be assumed from the absence of growth. In other words, the Test assumes sterility unless nonsterility can be demonstrated. The Test for Sterility is really a test for nonsterility, and even within that redefinition of its terms of reference, its indication is limited to those microorganisms capable of producing discernible growth under the specified test conditions. Many microorganisms are not recoverable under these conditions.

When the Test for Sterility first appeared in the USP and in the *British Pharmacopoeia* (BP) in the 1930s, it was described in the same terms as any other pharmacopoeial test method; that is, as a method whereby a microbiologist could determine whether a single article presented for analysis was sterile.

There was no indication in the pharmacopoeias until 1955 in the USP and until 1968 in the BP that the results of the Test should be or could be extended to apply to batches of product required to be certified as sterile. The USP initially required 10 units to be tested from each batch of autoclaved products and 20 units from each batch of other sterile products, the BP required 20 units. In the current pharmacopoeias, the sample size for the Test for Sterility is 20 units in all but a few exceptional circumstances.

However, with such a small sample size, successful results (no growth inferring with sterility or "passing" the Test for Sterility) provide little assurance that there is not a significant proportion of contaminated units in the batch. This has been recognized and debated for many years, even before the pharmacopoeial requirements were first published. In 1949, Knudsen (1) pointed out that when using a sample size of 20 units, batches containing 5% contaminated units would be "passed" as sterile on 35 of every 100 occasions. Brewer (2) elaborated further on the statistical limitations of sterility testing by showing that sample sizes of 20, 50, and even 100 units are hardly better than sample sizes of 10 units for detecting contamination in batches of product containing 0.1% contaminated units. The pharmacopoeial sampling requirements for the Test for Sterility are a compromise; they have been known to be, and shown to be, statistically unsound for decades. They are a compromise between the fact that the Test is destructive to the units sampled and the self-evident requirement for a very high level of assurance that batches of supposedly sterile product do not contain nonsterile units.

In practical terms a "pass" in the Test for Sterility should not be perceived to be of any more significance than any other successful measure of compliance with microbiological or physical standards or controls applicable to the manufacture of sterile products. A "pass" in the Test for Sterility must not be allowed to overrule any failure to comply with other environmental or control standard(s) because it is quite possible to "pass" the Test and still have a significant number of nonsterile units in the batch. On the other hand, a "failed" Test for Sterility is likely to be a good indicator of a genuine problem that has not been disclosed by some other microbiological or physical means.

Methods for sterility testing

The Test for Sterility may be performed in one of two ways, by direct inoculation (direct transfer) or by membrane filtration.

In direct inoculation, the product samples are put aseptically into the microbiological recovery medium and incubated. Clearly this approach is only suited to products that are not likely to be inhibitory to the growth of microorganisms in the recovery medium. An incubation period of 14 days is specified.

In the membrane filtration method, the product samples are put aseptically into a volume of noninhibitory diluent and then passed through a sterile 0.45-μm membrane filter (Fig. 1). The membrane is rinsed through with additional volumes of diluent, then aseptically cut in half. Half is

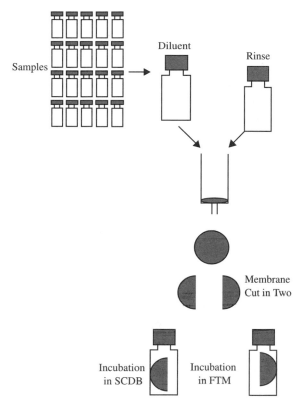

Fig. 1 Generalized scheme for the Test for Sterility by the membrane filtration method.

transferred to a container of soybean casein digest medium (SCDM) and the other to fluid thioglycollate medium (FTM).

A variation of membrane filtration is the use of "closed" systems such as the Millipore Steritest® system. At the heart of the Steritest system are two presterilized canisters, each with a membrane filter sealed into its base. The product under test is inoculated into its diluent and transferred via a peristaltic pump into the canisters and through the two membranes. During transfer the diluent is automatically split in two parts. After product filtration, the media are transferred into the canisters, SCDM to one canister and FTM to the other, by the same means. No manipulation of the membranes is required. The canisters are incubated at the temperatures specified in the pharmacopoeias.

Whichever variant of the membrane filtration method is used, SCDM is incubated at 20–25°C and the FTM at 30–35°C for 14 days.

Before 1999, the pharmacopoeias allowed incubation for only 7 days. Now the USP allows 7-day incubation only for terminally sterilized products. This extension of the incubation period from 7 to 14 days is a curious situation. The stimulus was an article published by the

Australian Regulatory Agency (3) indicating that it was possible for some drug products to be contaminated with microorganisms that would require more than 7 days of incubation to produce demonstrable growth under the conditions of the Test for Sterility. This was not, however, a remarkable new discovery. Brewer and Schmitt (4) observed (albeit with ethylene oxide sterilized medical devices) in 1966 that "slow growing" microorganisms (e.g., micrococci and diphtheroids) might take up to 4 weeks to produce demonstrable growth under the conditions of the USP Test for Sterility. There has been no actual evidence of patients having come to harm as a result of requiring only 7 days of incubation in the Test for Sterility. One can only suggest that some compromise was reached during the "harmonization" discussions, and the benefit must be for exporters to Australia where the "preharmonization" Test for Sterility (5) was far more demanding and restrictive.

Conditions for sterility testing

The Test for Sterility is vulnerable to false-positive and false-negative results. A false-positive means that a genuinely sterile product fails the test because of incidental contamination during the preparation of the sample or during the Test. A false-negative means that a nonsterile product passes the Test because viable contaminants fail to grow.

Both circumstances can have serious consequences, but false-positives are less likely to go unnoticed because high frequencies of false-positives have a commercial impact, at least delaying the release of product and at worst leading to suspension of manufacture.

The avoidance of false-negatives is addressed at length in the pharmacopoeias. Each batch of medium used in the Test for Sterility must have been shown to be capable of supporting the growth of low inocula of a specified array of microorganisms. Each Test for Sterility applicable to each specific product must be validated by repeated demonstration that the viabilities of low inocula of a specified array of microorganisms are not inhibited by product traces contained in the medium (direct inoculation) or on the membrane filter.

The pharmacopoeial attitude to false-positives changed in 1999, beginning in the 8th Supplement to USP 23 and in the 1999 Supplement of PhEur. An expectation of some level of false-positives had been tolerated in the Test for Sterility since its inception. This was in acknowledgement of there being a finite probability of the Test becoming contaminated as a result of the large number of aseptic manipulations required in its performance. However, times and technologies have changed.

When the Test for Sterility was first published in the 1930s, it was, at best, being done in glove boxes. The pharmacopoeias recognized the probability of incidental contamination and permitted, in the event of Test failure, an automatic right to retest without further ado. However, with the advent of HEPA filtration and laminar flow technology in the 1960s, the actual frequency of false-positive diminished, but the automatic right to retest remained. Isolation technology became available for doing the Test for Sterility in the last decade of the 20th century.

The automatic right to retest still remained in the pharmacopoeias until in the 1999 revisions, it was recognized that the testing technology was available whereby the probability of incidentally contaminating a Test for Sterility could be less than the probability of the sample actually being nonsterile. The current pharmacopoeial situation is therefore that retesting is only permitted when it can be unequivocally demonstrated that the contaminant in the Test arose incidentally during testing. Strictly, this is not a retest but a repeat Test because the first Test is at fault.

The consequence of this approach is that repeat testing is allowed only with a great deal of information about the microbiological conditions pertaining during the Test, and a large element of professional judgment by the functions held responsible for product release. Many companies have balanced the potential for the increased risk of commercial loss as a result of failures in the Test for Sterility with the potential for regulatory action in the event of disagreement over the judgment involved in repeat testing. They concluded that isolation technology is the only sensible future for the Test for Sterility.

Sterility assurance

Despite the attention, capital and resources given to the Test for Sterility, batches of product cannot be confirmed to be sterile by end-product testing. The Test for Sterility is in fact only a test for a specific broad range of microbial contaminants, and its sampling statistics are not capable of disclosing frequencies of contaminated units that would put patients at risk owing to nonsterility. This has been recognized by the pharmacopoeias, notably the PhEur, which for some years has carried a statement in Section 2.6.1 (formerly V.2.1.1):

> ... a satisfactory result only indicates that no contaminating microorganism has been found in the sample examined in the conditions of the test. .... The sterility test is ... the only analytical method available to the authorities who have to examine any product for sterility.

Then, how can sterility of batches of supposedly sterile products be confirmed by those functions within companies that are held responsible for product release? The answer is in the use of validated manufacturing processes based on sound scientific evidence that each product unit is most probably sterile.

This raises a second question of how much confidence must one have to claim sterility? The answer to this question, for terminally sterilized products, is that there must be no more than one chance in a million that viable contaminants survive in any one unit. This is called a sterility assurance level (SAL) of 10^{-6}. The answer for aseptically filled products is that the SAL must be as close to 10^{-6} as is technically possible, with the proviso that the degree of protection given to the process must afford no more than one chance in a thousand of any one unit becoming contaminated. This is called a contamination rate of 10^{-3}, and unlike the SAL it relates only to the protection given to the process and not to the potential for contaminants surviving or proliferating in actual products (6, 7).

The concept of the SAL is founded in academic studies of how microbial populations reduce in numbers in response to inimical treatments. In 1945 McCulloch (8) showed that for steam sterilization, a population of bacteria:

> exposed to a lethal degree of heat ... decreases in a fairly orderly manner. Thus if 90% of the viable population is killed during the first minute of exposure, approximately 90% of the survivors will

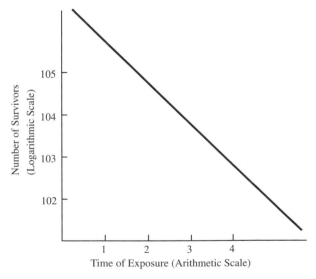

Fig. 2 Exponential inactivation of microorganisms (the survival curve).

be killed during each subsequent minute, which will continue until nearly all of the population is extinct.

This exponential order of inactivation of microbial populations (Fig. 2, the exponential survival curve) has subsequently been demonstrated to be a general characteristic of microorganisms in all processes of sterilization. The logarithmic axis of the exponential survival curve has no zero point. Thus, there can be no time of exposure at any temperature, no dose of radiation no matter how high, that can guarantee 100% inactivation of any microbial population.

Exponential inactivation is the basis of the concept of sterility assurance. If the behavior of microbial populations in response to a particular sterilizing procedure is regular and exponential over the region of the survival curve within which their response can be monitored, then the treatments required to achieve SALs of 10^{-6} can be extrapolated.

The aseptic filling process is not suited to the calculation of SALs in this way. This is because aseptic filling is not based on exponential inactivation and therefore provides no basis for extrapolation. The principle of aseptic manufacture is that, first of all, the drug product and its product-contact packaging components are sterilized to comply with SALs of 10^{-6}, and then they are brought together in ways that are intended to avoid further contamination (asepsis). Ideally, the finished product would still have an SAL of 10^{-6}. The short-fall from this ideal is primarily a function of the technology used in the aseptic filling process. Where sterile isolation technology is being used—this is a developing rather than an established technology at the time of writing in 2000—it is likely that there is very little shortfall. With standard technology, a level of process protection from microorganisms demonstrable through media fills offering a contamination rate of no more than 10^{-3} is nominally acceptable to regulatory bodies worldwide.

Microbiological GMP in the Manufacture of Sterile Drug Products

As far as manufacture is concerned, there are two broad categories of sterile products: those that are terminally sterilized (filled and hermetically sealed within their final containers before being exposed to a sterilization treatment), and those that are aseptically manufactured (the drug product and its product-contact packaging components are sterilized and then brought together in ways that are intended to avoid further contamination. Serious measures to protect the manufacture from microbiological contamination are necessary for both

categories but are clearly most critical in the poststerilization stages of aseptic manufacture.

There are several sources of standards and limits that may be applied to the manufacture of sterile products. They can be divided into sector-specific standards which are focused specifically on the manufacture of sterile pharmaceuticals and generic standards that are focused on particular technologies, irrespective of how the technologies are to be applied.

Sector-specific standards applying to manufacture of sterile drug products

There are five significant sources of sector-specific standards applying to the manufacture of sterile products. Two are mandatory, three are voluntary.

The two mandatory standards are Annex 1 of the European Union's GMPs (9) and the FDA's 1987 *Guideline on Sterile Drug Products Produced by Aseptic Processing* (10). The FDA document is under review at the time of writing this article.

The first of the two nonmandatory standards is contained in Section 1116 of the USP. It should be explained that this is a general chapter of the USP and is not therefore mandatory unless referenced in a USP monograph. At time of writing, Section 1116 is not referenced in any monographs.

The second of the voluntary standards is IS 13408 (11), applying to both medical devices and to pharmaceuticals according to the International Standards Organization (ISO) definition of "healthcare products." Here, it should be explained that the ISO is a voluntary body whose membership is drawn from national standards organizations. ISO standards have no legal authority in any country or territory unless the national standards body elects to adopt the ISO standard instead of publishing its own standards.

The third voluntary standard is The International Society of Pharmaceutical Engineer's (ISPE) *Baseline Pharmaceutical Engineering Guide* (12). This is one of a series of ISPE guidance documents that has limited endorsement by the FDA. It should be understood that only minimal standards are being endorsed and there are many reasons why specific sterile products and applications could be seen by the FDA to require compliance with higher standards.

Working with these five documents is not easy; they use different terminology and definitions and have different emphases that in part, may be a function of the 10-year span that encompasses publication dates. All of them are concerned with controlling microbiological contamination that may arise from the environment, from personnel, and from materials and equipment. Some individual standards within these documents may relate to microbial numbers, others to physical characteristics that relate to contamination control.

All of these documents stress a requirement for room classifications according to the concentration of nonviable airborne particles at 0.5 μm and larger. The EU GMPs (9) subordinate classification of the various areas applicable to sterile manufacture according a broader based grading system. Grades A to D are defined in terms of a range of independent characteristics such as the concentration of nonviable airborne particles at two sizes in operational and nonoperational conditions, the concentration of airborne viable particles in operational conditions, and several other indices of microbial contamination on surfaces and hands, etc. The inclusion of microbiological limits within this grading system is important in that it emphasizes that it is not solely the concentration of nonviable airborne particles in cleanrooms (room classification) that determines their suitability for manufacture of sterile products.

Generic standards for technologies used in the manufacture of sterile drug products

The most important generic standards applying to technologies used in the manufacture of sterile drug products relate to the protection of manufacture from contamination from the air. The air supply to facilities for sterile manufacture must be filtered, in some specific applications, it must be unidirectional, its velocity may have to be controlled within specified limits, and there must be pressure differentials between adjacent areas.

In the late 1990s, there had been a great deal of ISO activity in the harmonization of various standards applying to air quality (13). The first three parts address classification of air cleanliness, methods for testing and monitoring, and metrology. Parts 1 and 2 cover much of the ground but are not identical to FS 209 (14) (see below). The significant question emerging as these standards are published has to do with the reaction of the pharmaceutical regulatory agencies. Whereas we can with confidence be sure that the standards applying to the specifications of HEPA filter media and to the in situ HEPA filter integrity test will be accepted, there still are some doubts about the standard for room classification.

Both of the two mandatory sector-specific standards (9, 10) currently require room classification according to Federal Standard 209. This is a U.S. government standard; its current revision is FS 209E (14), and it will not be automatically replaced by IS 14644 (13). Thus, we are dependent on the next revision of Annex 1 of the EU GMPs (9) and of the FDA's *Guideline on Sterile Drug Products Produced by Aseptic Processing* (10) to

determine whether they will be adopted for the manufacture of sterile drug products.

Validation and Control of Sterilization Processes

Although there are many sterilization processes used in association with the manufacture of sterile drug products, the three primary processes are steam sterilization, dry heat sterilization, and sterile filtration. Dry heat sterilization is, in the context of the manufacture of sterile parenteral products, a subset of dry heat depyrogenation (see below).

Steam sterilization

Steam sterilization is widely used as a terminal process for drug products in glass ampules, vials, syringes, and plastic containers. It is also used for sterilizing closures, filters, manufacturing equipment, and cleaning equipment, etc.

Steam sterilization in autoclaves has a long and strong scientific basis (see above). The essence of validation of steam sterilization processes is to demonstrate that temperature and time conditions are being achieved uniformly through every item included the autoclave load and that the lethality being achieved in practical situations corresponds to that which would be expected from sterilization theory.

Thus, compliance with limits for temperature uniformity throughout empty autoclaves (heat distribution studies) is an index of the way in which the autoclaves are engineered. Compliance with limits for temperature uniformity within items loaded into the autoclaves (heat penetration) is an index of the way in which items are wrapped for sterilization (where applicable) and how they are loaded into the autoclaves in relation to the positions of steam inlets, drains, racks, trays, and thermal sensors.

With modern autoclaves, the major impediment of concern to successful sterilization is air in porous loads. Air may be present as a contaminant of the steam supply such that the temperatures theoretically achievable at particular steam pressures are depressed, or air may be present within the load, insulating it from the contact with the steam required for predictable lethality.

Pure steam generators are designed to deliver steam of satisfactory quality—standards are published in a UK document, Health Technical Memorandum (HTM) 2010 (15)—but noncondensable gas like air and nitrogen can accumulate in the steam through poorly insulated and trapped distribution systems and therefore should be tested periodically close to point of use. Autoclaves suited to sterilization of porous loads require some form of air removal, most often by deep pulsed vacuums, before the introduction of steam. The effectiveness of air removal is difficult to monitor by physical means; air entrapment may be a local phenomenon in particular locations in loads, in particular materials (e.g., in cartridge filters), or where items come into contact with one another (e.g., with rubber closures in bulk). Therefore, it is normal to use biological indicators to ensure that there is correspondence between theoretical and practical reality. Biovalidation of steam sterilization, although done extensively, is all very complex and, to an extent, a poorly understood. The basics are that a suitable biological indicator should be resistant to sterilization by steam (but not necessarily the most resistant microorganism known—spores *of Bacillus stearothermophilus*) are approved by the USP, PhEur, and others and are most often used. The biovalidation cycle must be of lower thermal lethality than the lowest thermal lethality allowable within the routine production-cycle specification. Some interesting reviews of biovalidation of steam sterilization have been published by Halls (16) and by Agalloco and colleagues (17).

Steam sterilization is not confined to autoclaves. Many items of manufacturing equipment, including some quite massive applications to vessels, pipe-work, filters, etc., are now sterilized in place with steam (SIP). It is essential that the equipment holds pressure, that air is removed, and that condensation does not accumulate in low points of the system. Biological validation is generally unsophisticated and is normally done by ensuring that the process inactivates several biological challenge test pieces, each carrying 10^6 spores of *Bacillus stearothermophilus* (D_{121}-values undefined but presumably meeting the pharmacopoeial criteria of equal to or greater than 1.5 min) placed at critical points. Academically, it is problematic to equate this approach with the sterility assurance level concept that applies to the sterilization of groups of items.

Steam sterilization processes are monitored for compliance with strict specifications of temperature, pressure, and time. Routine monitoring with biological indicators is not necessary. Indeed, any item of steam sterilizing equipment that is operating so erratically as to merit routine monitoring with biological indicators should be replaced.

Sterilization by filtration

Filtration is a means of sterilizing fluids by removing, rather than inactivating, microorganisms. The sterilization of liquids is used extensively in aseptic manufacture, sterilization of gases is used both in terminal sterilization and in aseptic manufacture. Most applications use cellulose esters, polyvinylidine fluoride, polytetrafluoroethylene, nylon, and other polymeric materials. The removal of microorganisms from fluids by passage through filters is very complex; sieving, or surface retention, is only one of a

series of mechanisms that depend on interactions among the chemistry and surface characteristics of the membrane, the microorganisms, and the suspending fluid (18).

The FDA (10) defines sterilizing filters as those that have pore-size ratings of 0.22 μm or smaller and relates this to a microbiological particle passage test using *Pseudomonas (Brevundimonas) diminuta*:

> A sterilizing filter is one which, when challenged with the microorganism *Pseudomonas diminuta*, at a minimum concentration of 10^7 organisms per cm^2 of filter surface will produce a sterile effluent.

It is essential that the microbiological particle passage test is performed as part of the development of new sterile formulations. Because of its very specialized nature, the test is normally performed only by the filter manufacturers, who then provide limits for secondary physical tests (e.g., bubble point, pressure decay, forward flow, etc.), which can be applied to verify the pore size rating and integrity of the membrane filters.

Maintenance of Sterility after Product Release

The sterility of a sterile dosage form can only be guaranteed while it is protected from the surrounding nonsterile environment within a container made from materials impermeable to microbial penetration.

Container and closure systems for sterile products must be capable of withstanding process conditions, storage, and transport without compromising the sterility of the product. This has been recently emphasized by the FDA, which has omitted a former obligation to provide data from the Test for Sterility in stability program for new sterile products in favor of verifying the microbial integrity of the container-closure system (19).

There are no standard methods for verifying microbiological integrity of container-closure systems. Documents such as that published by the Parenteral Society in 1992 (20) and the PDA in 1998 (21) may be helpful in relating microbiological integrity to secondary physical tests, but they do not specify detailed microbiological test methods.

There are two general approaches, wet tests and aerosol challenge tests. Wet tests consider penetration of microorganisms in liquid suspension into sealed containers usually previously filled with sterile medium. The basic assumption is that the most vulnerable route for penetration of liquid filled containers by microorganisms is in the event of a continuous liquid film or "bridge" forming between the outside and the inside of a container. Aerosol challenge tests are less critical than wet tests and should be applied only when total exclusion of moisture from the containment system can be ensured by secondary barriers.

No discussion of maintenance of sterility is complete without addressing multiple-dose ophthalmic presentations. The normal circumstances for sterile parenteral products are that they are unit dose or, if multiple dose, they are penetrated only by sterile transfer devices (syringes, giving sets, etc.) and used on one patient only. This is not the case for ophthalmic ointments and drops: unit-dose presentations are quite unusual and generally used only in hospital practice, for example, after eye surgery.

The multiple-dose presentation is the norm for ophthalmic products. The container is breached at first use and therefore has no further microbiological integrity over subsequent applications by the patient for an un-defined period possibly up to the expiration date of the product. Under these circumstances, contamination of the drug products can and must occur; the proliferation of the contaminating microorganisms the products is controlled by use of antimicrobial and preserved formulations. After opening they are, effectively, non-sterile products. Why, therefore, do we go to the trouble to manufacture ophthalmic ointments and drops as sterile products? There is no clear answer to this question; it is an anomaly. It has been a worldwide regulatory requirement "since the beginning of time" for ophthalmic products to be manufactured as sterile, and there is undoubtedly little point in contesting its logic or consistency. Another possible anomaly concerning sterility may be arising from the FDA's 1997 proposal (25) to require all aqueous inhalation products to be sterile. This example is anomalous because only in very exceptional circum-stances is the equipment used to administer inhalation products supplied and maintained sterile and, of course, neither are the nasopharyngeal and bronchial passages of the patient.

Pyrogens, Lipopolysaccharides, and Bacterial Endotoxins

Parenteral products are expected to be sterile because of the risk of infection. Another critical biological characteristic is that they should be free from pyrogens. Pyrogens are substances that, when injected in sufficient amounts into the human body, give rise to a variety of extremely unpleasant symptoms of which the most recognizable is a rise in body temperature. In extreme conditions, the rise in body temperature can be so rapid and to such an extent that the patient dies (endotoxic shock). In the pharmacopeias, pyrogenic products have

traditionally been defined in terms of the temperature rise induced in injected rabbits.

The causative agent of the pyrogenic response is lipopolysaccharide. This material is of microbiological origin, and although all bacteria appear to be capable of producing lipopolysaccharide, it is found primarily in the cell envelope of Gram-negative species. Naturally occurring lipopolysaccharide is referred to as bacterial endotoxin.

Bacterial endotoxin reacts with a high degree of specificity with a "clottable protein" contained in the amoebocyte cells of the horseshoe crab (*Limulus polyphemus*). This has allowed the development of in vitro testing of drug products and other substances for bacterial endotoxins. The pharmacopoeias are progress-ively replacing their former requirements for in vivo rabbit pyrogen testing of parenteral products with the in vitro Limulus Amoebocyte Lysate (LAL) test. There are a variety of test systems now marketed (gel clot, turbido-metric, chromogenic, etc.), but the pharmacopoeias regard the gel clot method as the reference test. In the gel clot method for the LAL test, a quantity of LAL reagent of defined sensitivity (λ), e.g., 0.03 EU (endotoxin units) per milliliter, is mixed with an equal quantity of the product under test (or a dilution thereof). The mixture is incubated for a defined period and then inverted. The production of a gel is evidence of bacterial endotoxin in the product sample at a concentration equal to or greater than the sensitivity of the LAL reagent.

Product endotoxin limits are based on dosage regimes (22) derived from a formula K/M, where K is the threshold dose for any substance capable of giving a pyrogenic response in humans. With some exceptions K has been given a fixed value of 5 EU/kg body weight of the patient, and adult patient body weight is standardized to 70 kg for calcualtion. M is the maximum dose of endotoxin per kilogram of body weight of a patient that is permitted to be given in a single 1-hr period.

Endotoxin limits are therefore unique to each dosage form. Because K is fixed, it is usually only necessary to determine M from the maximum human dosage indicated in the product instructions.

The validation and performance of the endotoxin test require rather elaborate and detailed attention to use of controls. These details are specified in Section 85 of the USP harmonized with Section 2.6.14 of the PhEur.

Control of bacterial endotoxins

Although bacterial endotoxins are of microbiological origin, they are not lost with loss of viability. Of the sterilization processes commonly used in the manufacture of sterile parenteral dosage forms (see above), only dry heat is capable of destroying bacterial endotoxins in a reasonable time frame (23). There is therefore no practical way of removing bacterial endotoxins from finished drug products; thus, they must be controlled at source.

The most likely source of bacterial endotoxins is water and product-contact packaging components that have been in contact with water. This is because bacterial endotoxins are most frequently found associated with Gram-negative bacteria, and Gram-negative bacteria have evolved to be primarily waterborne.

Water used in manufacture of sterile parenteral products must comply with pharmacopoeial limits for endotoxin of no more than 0.25 EU/ml (limits in the USP and PhEur for water for injection). In principle water complying with this limit can be produced by distillation, reverse osmosis, and ultrafiltration. PhEur allows only distillation to be used for the manufacture of ingredient water for parenteral products; the USP allows distillation and reverse osmosis (although reverse osmosis is rarely used in the United States, perhaps because of FDA pressure). Only the Japanese Pharmacopoeia allows water for injection to be manufactured using ultrafiltration.

Product-contact packaging components, such as glass vials, which are required to be sterile, are usually sterilized and depyrogenated by dry heat in ovens or tunnels. The standard required by the FDA for acceptable depyrogenation processes (10) is that they should be capable of reducing a bacterial endotoxin challenge by a factor of 10^{-3} (3 logs). Unfortunately, inactivation of bacterial endotoxins by dry heat is complex, and satisfactory process specifications are difficult to predict; inactivation of purified lipopolysaccharide may approximate to pseudo-second-order reaction kinetics (24). It appears that there may be a threshold temperature of approximately 160–170°C, below which a 3-log reduction of bacterial endotoxin cannot be achieved regardless of time of exposure.

MICROBIAL CONTROL OF NONSTERILE PRODUCTS

Nonsterile dosage forms are a diverse group of products. The microbiological risks that nonsterile products present to the patient arc equally diverse. A single microbiological standard cannot sensibly be applied to all nonsterile products, and this is well reflected by pharmacopoeial and regulatory requirements. Similarly, there can be no single standard applied to the microbiological control and prevention of contamination during the manufacture of nonsterile products.

The Microbial Limit Test

Microbial limit standards for some, but not all, nonsterile dosage forms are given in USP monographs. PhEur takes a slightly different approach. Section 5.1.4 lists microbiological criteria for two categories of nonsterile pharmaceutical products on the basis of usage. One of these categories is for products for topical and respiratory use, the other for product's for oral and rectal administration. Guidance to methods suited to testing products for compliance with these standards is given in Section 61 of USP and Section V.2.1.8 of the PhEur.

In setting appropriate limits for particular nonsterile products, both pharmacopoeias take account of the significance of microorganisms to different types of product, to the way in which the product is used, and to the potential hazard to the patient. For instance, 47 of 48 monographs defining microbial limits listed in USP 24 for oral dosage forms restrict microorganisms (*E. coli* and/or *Salmonella*) that are pathogenic by gastrointestinal ingestion. These are, of course, not the only microorganisms that could endanger a patient taking an oral dosage form. They have been selected as indicators of the general type because there are well defined methods for their recovery and they are easily recognizable in culture. Similarly, the USP typically (but not universally) restricts from topical products only those microorganisms (*Staphylococcus aureus, Pseudomonas aeruginosa*) that have the potential to cause skin infections. Sixty-seven of 68 monographs in the USP 24 require the absence of at least these two species, and of these 67 only 11 have additional requirements. These limits applying to the absence of specific indicator microorganisms appropriate to the product's usage may be supplemented by general hygiene restrictions on total numbers of microorganisms per gram or milliliter (typically to no more than 100 cfu per gram or milliliter). A very similar overall approach is taken by the PhEur.

Requirements are not specified in the pharmacopoeias for sample sizes appropriate to testing batches of nonsterile products for compliance with microbial limits. The test is destructive to the product, and it is extremely unlikely that statistically valid sampling plans are in use anywhere; samples composed of 10 1-g amounts taken from 10 separate 15-g tubes of cream, or of three 3.3-ml amounts taken from three separate 500-ml bottles of syrup, may be typical.

The Microbial Limit Test is, like the Test for Sterility, only confirmatory. It is not generally mandatory to test each batch of every nonsterile product for compliance with microbial limits. The exception is in the United States where it is mandatory to test every batch of nonsterile product. At the time of writing (early 2001), the FDA has proposed a relaxation of this rule for future registrations. However, in the case of tablets there is no requirement to register microbial limits, and therefore testing is not mandatory. The logic behind this is that the water content of tablets is too low to allow proliferation of micro-biological contaminants.

It should also be kept in mind that the major regulatory agencies (FDA, MCA) would not want to have the pharmacopoeial limits on numbers of microorganisms perceived as tolerance of microorganisms contaminating and proliferating in nonsterile products. The acceptance of these limits is only an acknowledgment of the reality that when products are not manufactured as sterile, some microbiological contamination is inevitable. Well for-mulated nonsterile products manufactured under micro-biologically controlled conditions are extremely unlikely to have bioburdens approaching the pharmacopoeial limits (typically 100 cfu per gram or milliliter). Most regulatory bodies now expect companies to set tighter microbial limits on their nonsterile products based on their typical results, these being seen as alert limits indicative of some loss of microbiological control if exceeded.

Microbiological GMP in the Manufacture of Nonsterile Drug Products

The extent to which the microbiological controls are required to be applied in the manufacture of nonsterile dosage forms is primarily a function of two factors: consequences of infection to the patients and probability of microorganisms proliferating in the product.

The seriousness of the risk to patients of infection from nonsterile dosage forms is primarily dictated by the route of administration of the dosage form. The probability of contaminating microorganisms surviving

and proliferating in a nonsterile dosage form is generally a function of its water content. Bearing these two concepts in mind, it is possible to classify the extent to which microbiological controls are required in the manufacture of nonsterile dosage forms according to a "good hotel guide" approach such as that given in Table 1. The precise allocation of "stars" is a matter of opinion, but at one extreme there is little doubt that aqueous inhalations merit "5-star" microbiological controls in manufacture, and possibly may soon be required to be sterile (25). Near the other extreme, the FDA, for example, does not require microbial limits to be registered for solid oral dosage forms.

There is little published guidance to microbiological controls for nonsterile manufacture. Equipment and facilities should be designed to minimize the opportunities for contact with air, personnel, and water.

Exposure to air is unavoidable, either as local atmospheric (environmental) air or as air from compres-sors used to operate manufacturing equipment and in fluid bed dryers, etc. Even for "1-star" nonsterile manufacture, the air supplied to areas used for manufacture and filling should be filtered. HEPA filters should be used in "5-star" nonsterile manufacture but are generally not necessary in "1-star," intermediate classifications of manufacture, requiring decisions on air filtration to be made from sensible risk assessments.

Personnel should be restricted from all areas of pharmaceutical manufacture to those who are necessary. Protection from contamination from personnel is by training in hygiene, enforcement of hygiene rules, and provision of protective clothing. Hair is the major source of contamination from personnel, and "street clothes" is the second most significant source. Hair-covers should be provided and worn properly in all areas of sterile manufacture; beards, moustaches, and other excessive facial hair should be covered. Overall sleeves should extend to the wrist and be elasticated or studded to provide a neat fit. Because dogs are still allowed to soil the streets,

Table 1 Classification of nonsterile manufacture according to the need for microbiological controls

Route of administration	Type of nonsterile dosage form		
	Aqueous liquids	Nonaqueous fluids	Solid dosage forms
Inhalation	☆☆☆☆☆	☆☆☆☆	☆☆☆☆
Intranasal, intrabuccal	☆☆☆☆	☆☆☆	☆☆☆
Topical	☆☆☆☆	☆☆	☆☆
Oral	☆☆☆	☆	☆
Anal	☆☆	☆	☆

protective footwear or shoe covers should be provided to all personnel allowed to enter pharmaceutical manufacturing areas.

Water is often the major ingredient in nonsterile products. When it is used as an ingredient, it must meet the pharmacopoeial limit for purified water of not more than 100 cfu/ml. Well designed and operated pharmaceutical purified water production and distribution set ups meet far tighter standards than these. Water is also often the principal cleaning fluid for equipment and facilities and is therefore unavoidable. It is a potent source of contamination because it usually contains sufficient nutrients to allow survival of metabolically versatile microorganisms, particularly *Pseudomonas spp.*

When water is left to stand, *Pseudomonas spp.* do not only survive, but increase in number. Water should not be permitted to stand on equipment (particularly in crannies and crevices), on floors, or in sinks and wash bays. Contamination spreads with water that forms films over surfaces and on the hands and clothing of personnel. Waterborne contaminants may be aerosolized by vibrations or when water falls more than a few centimeters.

To restrict the opportunity for contamination from water, there should be air breaks of approximately 5 cm installed between equipment drains and the tun dishes leading to foul drains.

The FDA has published guidances on the design and control of water systems (26).

Maintenance of Microbiological Quality of Nonsterile Products after Release

It is not desirable for those few microorganisms that may be present in nonsterile products at the time of release to increase to numbers to levels at which they may present a risk of infection to the patient or "spoil" the product.

Additional contamination in the period up to the first use by the patient or healthcare professional is provided by the packaging. It is neither necessary nor usual to find that nonsterile product packaging has been specifically designed or tested to be impermeable to microbiological contamination. On the other hand, many products are given good microbiological protection as a secondary consequence of the protection given to the stability of their active ingredients, etc. For instance, tablets packed individually in strips or foils are microbiologically protected until time of use. It is also unlikely for microorganisms to be able to contaminate pressurized metered-dose inhaler containers.

Microbiological protection of multiple-dose presentations such as liquid inhalations, nasal sprays, oral liquids, creams, and lotions is more complex. Once opened they are susceptible to microbiological contamination. If they are aqueous-based, they are in principle susceptible to proliferation of these "new" contaminants. To avoid this, they are formulated with antimicrobial agents or preservatives and are expected to be able to comply with preservative efficacy standards specified in the pharmacopoeias. Preservative efficacy tests (not harmonized) are described in Section 51 of the USP and Section VIII.14 of the PhEur (Fig. 3).

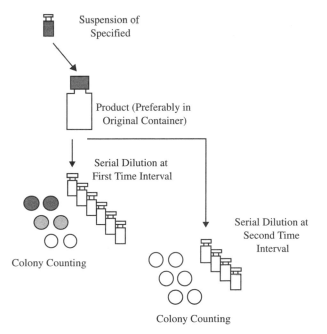

Fig. 3 Generalized scheme for preservative efficacy testing.

REFERENCES

1. Knudsen, L.F. Sample Size of Parenteral Solutions for Sterility Testing. J. Am. Pharmaceutical Assoc. **1949**, *38*, 332–337.
2. Brewer, J.H. Sterility Tests and Methods for Assuring Sterility. *Antiseptics, Disinfectants, Fungicides and Chemical and Physical Sterilization*; Reddish, G.F., Ed.; Henry Kimpton: London, NC, 1957.
3. Bathgate, H.; Lazzari, D.; Cameron, H.; McKay, D. The Incubation Period in Sterility Testing. PDA J. Pharm. Sci. Technol. **1993**, *47* (5).
4. Brewer J.H. Schmitt R.F. Special Problems in the Sterility Testing of Disposable Medical Devices. Annual General Meeting of the Parenteral Drug Association: New York, November, 2, 1966.
5. Commonwealth Department of Health, *Standard for Sterile Therapeutic Goods*; Therapeutic Goods Order No. 11, Australian Government Publishing Service: Canberra, 1984.

6. Bernuzzi, M.; Halls, N.A.; Raggi, P. Application of Statistical Models to Action Limits for Media Fill Trails. Eur. J. Parenteral Sci. **1997**, *2* (1), 3–11.

7. Pharmaceutical Drug Association. *Technical Report No 22. Process Simulation Testing for Aseptically Filled Products*; Pharmaceutical Drug Association Inc.: Bethesda, MD, 1996.

8. McCulloch, E.C. *Disinfection and Sterilization*; Lea and Ferbiger: New York, 1945.

9. Medicines Control Agency. *Rules and Guidance for Pharmaceutical Manufacturers and Distributors*; The Stationery Office: London, 1997.

10. Food and Drug Administration. *Guideline on Sterile Drug Products Produced by Aseptic Processing*; FDA: Rockville, MD, 1987.

11. *Aseptic Processing of Health Care Products. 1. General Requirements*; IS 13408-1, International Standards Organization: 1997.

12. ISPE Baseline Pharmaceutical Engineering Guide. *Sterile Manufacturing Facilities*; ISPE: 1998; 3.

13. Cleanrooms and Associated Controlled Environments I. Classification of Air Cleanliness; II. Specifications for Testing and Monitoring to Probe Continued Compliance with ISO 14644-1; III. Metrology and Test Methods. BS EN ISO 14644-1,2,3: , 1999.

14. *Airborne Particulate Cleanliness Classes in Cleanrooms and Clean Zones*; Federal Standard 209E. Federal Supply Service, General Services Administration: Washington. DC, 1998.

15. *Sterilization. III. Validation and Verification*; The Stationery Office: London, 1994; Health Technical Memorandum 2010.

16. Halls, N.A. Resistance "Creep" of Biological Indicators. *Sterilization of Medical Products*; Morrissey, R.F., Kowalski, J.B., Eds.; Polysciences Publications, Inc.: Champlain, NY, 1998.

17. Agalloco, J.P.; Akers, J.E.; Madsen, R.E. Moist Heat Sterilization—Myths and Realities. PDA J. Pharm. Sci. Technol. **1998**, *52* (6), 346–350.

18. Meltzer, T.H. *Filtration in the Pharmaceutical Industry*; Marcel Dekker, Inc.: New York, 1987.

19. Food and Drug Administration. *Guidance for Industry, Container-Closure Systems for Packaging Human Drugs and Biologics*; FDA Center for Drugs and Biologics: Rockville, MD, 1999.

20. *The Prevention and Detection of Leaks in Ampoules, Vials and other Parenteral Containers Parenteral Society Technical Monograph No. 3*; Parenteral Society: Swindon, UK, 1992.

21. *Pharmaceutical Package Integrity;* Technical Report No. 27 PDA: Bethesda, MD, 1998.

22. Weary, M.E. Understanding and Setting Endotoxin Limits. J. Parenteral Sci. Technol. **1990**, *44*, 16–17.

23. Ludwig, A.D.; Avis, K.E. Dry Heat Inactivation of Endotoxin on the Surface of Glass. J. Parenteral Sci. Technol. **1990**, *44*, 4–12.

24. Tsuji, K.; Harrison, S.J. Dry Heat Destruction of Lipopolysaccharide: Design and Construction of Dry Heat Destruction Apparatus. Appl. Environ. Microbiol **1978**, *36*, 710.

25. Federal Register. **September 23, 1997**, *62* (184).

26. *Food and Drug Administration Guide to Inspections of High Purity Water Systems*; FDA: Rockville, MI, 1993.

MICROBIOLOGIC MONITORING OF CONTROLLED PROCESSES

Gregory F. Peters
Marghi R. McKeon
Lab Safety Corp., Des Plaines, Illinois

INTRODUCTION

Microbiologic monitoring of controlled pharmaceutical and medical device manufacturing, and pharmacy compounding processes, is mandated in numerous standards and guidelines (1–3), although procedures, limits, and frequencies are not well defined (4). Because many characteristics of microbiologic sampling limit its value as a monitoring method (5), efforts to detect contamination in controlled environments require carefully developed and executed sampling plans to produce reliable data that confirm the acceptability of operating conditions.

Monitoring of any controlled process is a component of an outcome-producing, closed-loop system for assuring continued operation of critical processes in accordance with validated design conditions. To achieve this goal, a monitoring plan must be developed, conducted, and evaluated within the context of a Validation and Monitoring protocol. All results must be related to the original validated process, either as evidence that it continues to operate within acceptable limits, or as a means of detecting shifts in the process that might impinge on product quality. Ideally, monitoring results will also provide information that will be useful in determining the cause of such shifts.

The objectives of the monitoring plan within the validation and monitoring system for quality management must be clearly defined so that the information collected will be relevant to system goals. The limitations of sampling equipment and methods must be taken into consideration when developing the sampling plan and interpreting results. The underlying causes for shifts in various monitoring results must be understood in order to facilitate development of effective corrective action plans.

VALIDATION AND MONITORING RATIONALE

The regulatory requirements for validation of pharmaceutical aseptic processes are clear (6). Generally accepted quality assurance principles require initial demonstration of the efficacy of any process (*validation*), followed by regular, periodic observation to demonstrate that the process continues to operate in accordance with validation conditions (*monitoring*).

Validation usually consists of a series of "worst-case" process simulations, wherein a sterile growth medium is substituted for product to demonstrate that processing consistently yields products of acceptable quality (6). During this Process Qualification (PQ) phase, variable conditions that might effect product quality are carefully defined, controlled, monitored, and documented, and the assumption is reasonably made that the process will then yield the same product quality achieved during the PQ, so long as all variable factors are controlled to duplicate validation conditions. This assumption is based upon the results of monitoring data obtained from a variety of sources. The validity of the assumption of acceptable quality is, therefore, dependent upon the reliability of the monitoring data as a measure of control of process variables.

Validation Protocol

The validation protocol should define the manufacturing or compounding process, its purpose in terms of the desired positive impact on product quality, and how that impact will be demonstrated. The protocol should include the following components:

1. A description of the product, and applicable release criteria including AOQL/ROQL;
2. The facility design rationale for maintaining process integrity, including identification and elimination of inaccessible areas that may be difficult to decontaminate, enumeration of the clean-space engineering controls, and how these controls will be applied, tested, and monitored;
3. A schematic description of the aseptic process and the critical work surfaces, work zones, and support areas, including the designation of particulate cleanliness class (7), microbial target values (8, 9) (Table 1), and

Table 1 Process monitoring targets/frequency

Group headers: **Cleanliness class[a,b]** (Class 100[a], Class 10,000[a], Class 100,000[a], M 3.5, M 5.5, M 6.5) · **Monitoring frequency** (Each shift, Daily, Twice weekly, Weekly) · **C.F.U.[c] Target** (<0.1 Per Ft.[d], <0.5 Per M[d], <2.5 Per Ft.[d], <3.0 Per M[d], <20 Per M[d], <100 Per Ft.[d], 3 Per Contact plate, 5 Per Contact plate, 10 Per Contact plate, 20 Per Contact plate)

Function/Process	Class 100[a]	Class 10,000[a]	Class 100,000[a]	M 3.5	M 5.5	M 6.5	Each shift	Daily	Twice weekly	Weekly	<0.1 Per Ft.[d]	<0.5 Per M[d]	<2.5 Per Ft.[d]	<3.0 Per M[d]	<20 Per M[d]	<100 Per Ft.[d]	3 Per Contact plate	5 Per Contact plate	10 Per Contact plate	20 Per Contact plate
Critical worksurface[e]	•						•				A			A			S			
Support areas[e]		•					•					A			A			S		
Other support areas[e]			•	•					•			A			A					
Other potential prod./container contact[e]			•		•				•				A			A				
Other non-prod./container contact[e]			•		•					•			A			A				
Laminar airflow hoods	•						•				A			A			S[f]			
Biological safety cabs.	•						•				A			A			S[f]			
Host-cell culture	•[g]						•				A			A			S[f]			
Immediate Processing[g]	•[h]		•[h]				•		[h]	[h]	A[i]		A[h]	A[g]		A[h]	S[f,i]		S[h,i]	
Formulation		•					•					A		A				S		
Final Production	•						•				A			A			S[f]			
Equipment[e]	•	•		•			•										S[f]			
Equipment[e]		•			•		•											S		
Floor[e]	•			•			•										S			
Floor[e]			•		•		•											S		
Floor[e]		•				•	•												S[j]	
Personnel gloves[e]	•						•[g]										S			
Personnel gloves[k]		•							•[k]									S	S	
Personnel barriers[e]	•			•			•[k]		•									S		
Personnel barriers[e]		•		•			•		•[g]											S

[a]Federal Standard 209e U.S. Customary.

[b]SI. [c]Colony-forming units.

[d]Cubic valve.

[e]U.S.P. ⟨1116⟩.

[f]Including floor.

[g]Other support areas.

[h]Closed validated systems.

[i]Open systems.

[j]Recommended.

[k]Immediately adjacent to Class 100.

A. Aerobiologic; S. Surface.

Table courtesy of Lab Safety Corp., Des Plaines, Il.

engineering control equipment validation methods[a] (10);

4. The selection and justification of gowning and barrier techniques to ensure adequate isolation of personnel, based upon industry standards (3) and process requirements;

5. A definition of the aseptic techniques and work practices of operative personnel, and a report of findings based upon videotaped observation of the actual work stream during prequalification runs for identification and elimination of personnel-generated contamination sources, identification of susceptible areas including critical sites and steps, and indicator sites;

6. A description of sanitizing methods and sanitizing compound validation;

7. A definition of the equipment and methods to be used in assuring reliable test data; and

8. All test data, including instrument calibrations, testing and certification reports, and statistical justification.

Monitoring Plan

Following evaluation of all environmental monitoring data collected during the PQ, a monitoring plan (11) defining ongoing monitoring procedures, locations, and frequency should be implemented. The PQ data from product testing should be compared to environmental and process monitoring results to determine the monitoring sites and methods that best correlate with shifts in product quality. The plan should

1. Assure specified, periodic monitoring of critical manufacturing or compounding process parameters at critical points during periods of peak activity, and establish the circumstances and frequency with which monitoring is to be carried out to assure a reliable basis for claiming process control.

2. Provide for standardized, quantitative microbiologic sampling of process air, environmental surfaces, and personnel barriers, as well as sampling of other, related parameters.

3. Include sampling location maps, sample sizes, probe heights, methods, equipment, and frequency during

[a]Validation testing of HEPA filters requires an exacting aerosol challenge of 100% of the filtration media, frame, and locking device in accordance with Secs. 40 and 50 F.S. 209b (18). Successful testing in this manner establishes control of the "first air" emanating directly from the filter, as it approaches the entrance plane within the unidirectional slipstream, to better-than-Class I conditions. Monitoring of HEPA filters in accordance with F.S. 209e (7) involves an average of DPC readings derived from a number of representative locations to assure Class 10 or 100 conditions at the entrance plane of the unidirectional slipstream (10)

manufacturing operations, and a method for statistical justification of results.

4. Include alert and action limit criteria for acting upon ongoing monitoring information.

5. Include a system for evaluating and modifying the monitoring plan to assure collection of reliable, useful data, and

6. Include a corrective action plan, and methods of verifying the efficacy of any corrective actions taken.

Limitations of Microbiologic Monitoring

The minimum media-fill validation requirement of not more than one sterility failure per thousand units, representing the minimum sterility assurance level of 10^{-3} (>99.9%) is the only microbiologic limit in the validation and monitoring scheme that is based upon demonstrated product quality. Achievement of this sterility assurance level represents the aggregate impact of all process design and control factors, including sampling and attendant laboratory procedures. [This limit, however, probably does not reflect the true integrity of a valid aseptic process (12).] All other limits are indices, which are used indirectly to demonstrate that the process is under control as validated. Because all environmental monitoring is necessarily performed at some point downstream and apart from the product, no absolute evaluation of product quality is obtainable through monitoring procedures, however intensive. In addition, testing and monitoring methods do not always parallel or identify the pathways through which contaminants are introduced into the product.

Difficulty in validating microbiologic monitoring methods results from a lack of comprehensive testing standards, reliable test equipment, and reliable methods for correlating sample data to predictions of product quality. Several characteristics and qualities of both contamination events and sampling methods limit the usefulness of microbiologic monitoring as a method of determining the acceptability of a specific product batch:

1. Microbiologic contamination events in controlled facilities are usually not randomly distributed in time, space, or by type of organism;

2. No single sampling method repeatedly recovers a known and consistent percentage of all types of organisms;

3. For most types of contamination detected, there are usually many possible sources, not the least of which are the sampling personnel, equipment, and lab processing; and

4. An extended interval is required for development of results.

Perspectives

These considerations underscore recent concerns that regulatory groups may require that unreliable environmental monitoring data be used as release criteria (15). Current industry standards and regulatory guidelines do not, and should not be interpreted to condone the rejection of batches on the basis of absolute environmental counts alone. Microbiologic monitoring is employed for practical reasons, not because it is ideal or unique in detecting shifts in process conditions.

Regulatory agencies and auditors understandably seek easy-to-interpret data as a basis for decisions regarding product acceptability, and are becoming increasingly hesitant to accept product release in the absence of demonstrable levels of microbiologic control. Conversely, industry is justifiably reluctant to set microbiologic monitoring limits because regulators may misinterpret their meaning in a quality assurance (QA) context. The failure to meet process control limits is quite different from the failure to meet product specifications. Failure to meet a monitoring limit means only that monitoring data can no longer demonstrate validation conditions, and product quality *may* be adversely affected. Enhanced product testing or other corrective actions may be indicated, but batch rejection should not be extrapolated from QA monitoring results, alone.

Setting Limits

In the QA context, limits are established to trigger specific actions, or outcomes. The alert (warning) limit is the point at which the operator should become alerted to the possibility of a deteriorating trend. When an action limit is exceeded, the operator must take action to identify and correct the condition(s) that are causing a verified trend before a "fail" limit is reached and the data fail to indicate process control and support continued production. In a well-designed and executed process, however, such a fail limit should never be exceeded, except in the event of a sudden and catastrophic breakdown of a critical process control component.

Akers noted that values presented in the current U.S.P. ⟨1116⟩ (8) are target values (13). Given this designation, it is reasonable to consider these values to be *operational target levels,* rather than *product quality control limits.* There are several models for setting alert, action and fail limits, although many only establish alert and action limits (14) (other terminology may be used). Extending one current model (14), the alert limit might be considered to be the 95th percentile. Analysis and trending of actual data allow the calculation of this limit, as well as the 97th percentile for the action limit, and the 99th percentile as

the fail limit. Regardless of the model used initially to set limits, they should be based upon both historical data, and an evaluation of correlations between monitoring results and product quality. Data analysis should include a mechanism for evaluation and modification of the monitoring program and limits.

It is expected that results will fall within normally anticipated operating levels (8, 9) (Table 1) with 95% confidence, if randomness in critical environments and operations is sufficiently controlled. If data from successful PQ runs (when the process is demonstrated to be under control) do not meet this criterion, the monitoring methods may not measure a phenomenon that relates directly to process control, may not be sufficiently reproducible to provide useful information, or may have been incorrectly conducted. Every effort should be made to develop monitoring methods that comply with this performance expectation so that data will be useful.

Initial limits may be calculated and compared to results of any unsuccessful trials. These limits should eventually be adjusted based on historical data (see Fig. 1). When evaluating data to adjust limits, Wilson (14) noted, "Including data taken from a period of unusually high counts, where the process was out of control, will lead to inappropriately high alert/action limits."

Conduct of Sampling

Quality management and sampling personnel require both an in-depth understanding of the environmental sampling rationale, and a complete understanding of commonly available equipment, materials, sampling techniques, and development methods. Reporting forms should be carefully designed to convey all relevant information including identification of the technician, sample location (from a standardized sample map), date and time, media (including lot, expiration, and validation date), method, duration of sampling, and equipment (including calibration date and serial number). In addition, information such as the product batch, number and names of personnel, line throughput rate, number and nature of line interventions, and other available monitoring data such as room pressure and other engineering control status readings should be recorded. Any observed deviations from standard operating procedures (SOPs) should be noted and communicated to the individuals responsible for training and management of operative personnel. It is essential to repeat samples when such deviations occur in order to evaluate the impact they may have on results.

Sampling and laboratory personnel must be highly competent on both philosophical and functional levels, and

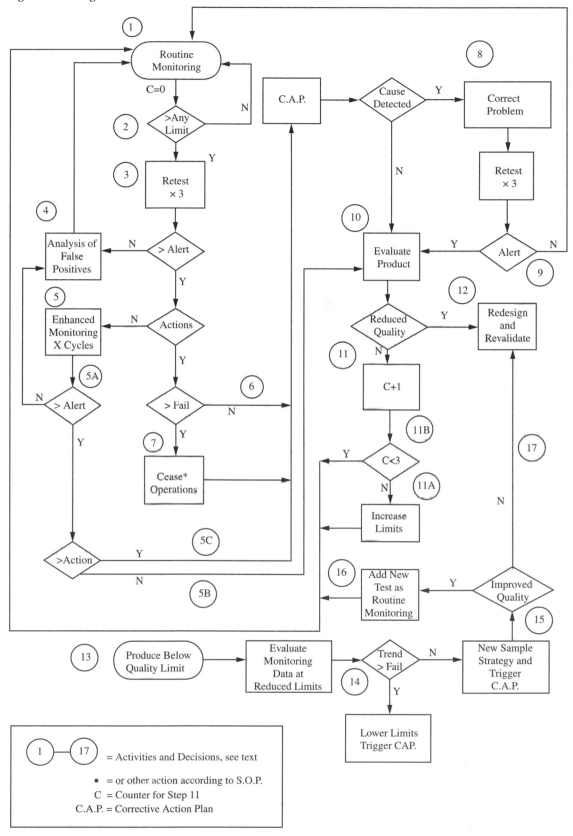

Fig. 1 Evaluation of monitoring plan and limits. (Courtesy of Lab Safety Corp., Des Plaines, IL.)

must develop and exercise *perfect* aseptic technique (13). A training program and operating procedures should be established defining all monitoring steps, including gowning, preparation of samplers, aseptic sampling techniques, sample recovery, handling and transport, and laboratory techniques for aseptic sample development. A laboratory QA program should assure that monitoring personnel conform to operating procedures and that technician skills are periodically tested and validated for high competence and flawless technique (13).

Sample Handling

Sampling, sample transport, and sample development should be conducted in a way that does not affect results. For example, if agar plates are improperly transported, condensate may form on the lid and drip onto the agar surface, redistributing microorganisms over the surface and around the edges of the plate, causing false readings. Agar plates should, therefore, be kept inverted and oriented horizontally during storage and transport. They should be handled gently, and transferred to the incubator as quickly as possible after exposure. With sieve impactors, false positives can usually be identified as colony forming units (CFUs) that fall outside the star pattern of jet indentations in the agar surface below the holes. Counts >20 CFUs may also be statistically corrected for increased accuracy by using the positive-hole correction table (15).

It is recommended that colony counts be made at several points in the incubation process, with separate tallies for bacterial and fungal colonies that tend to merge at a critical point during incubation, when fungal colonies may overgrow and obscure bacterial colonies. For this reason, any bacterial subcultures should be made prior to the onset of rapid fungal growth. Whenever possible, optical electronic colony counters with sufficient backlighting and magnification to enhance contrast and enumeration should be employed to increase accuracy. In the presence of known or potentially high counts, the microscope enumeration method should be used to closely differentiate and count microcolonies in impact areas on sample plates following a short incubation period.

DEVELOPING A MONITORING PLAN

Site Selection

A critical site is a point at which the product is exposed to the environment, when something is added to the product or product pathway, or a point at which unprotected product is manipulated. Any intervention into the process line increases the potential for contamination. (Examples of line interventions include the introduction, removal, or manipulation of materials and product, equipment adjustments, and sampling activities.) Particular attention should be given to these sites and events in the development of the monitoring plans (3).

Analysis of a videotape of repetitive prequalification should be studied for behavior and practices that may produce or harbor environmental contamination, leading to the refinement and optimization of work practices, and development of the formalized process to be instituted for the PQ validation run. The videotape may be used for identifying indicator sites, which should be incorporated into the monitoring plans, and intensively sampled during the validation run. These tapes should be retained and edited for both training and informational purposes.

For critical processes, it is important to select noninvasive sampling methods that have high collection efficiency for a broad range of organisms. To select the most suitable monitoring methods and equipment, the probable route of contamination for each critical site or process should be identified. For example, when the most likely route of potential contamination is touch, select surface sampling techniques for personnel barriers. When the most likely route is transfer from contaminated work surfaces, sampling of these surfaces is most useful. At sites where unprotected product is exposed to the environment, aerobiological monitoring is indicated, and, in unidirectional airflow, must be carried out isokinetically and isoaxially[b] in the manner of nonviable particle-count testing. Some processing steps may require multiple sampling methods.

Controlled support areas adjacent to critical areas are the essential interfaces in the transition from the general environment to the aseptic processing core. These areas should be adequately pressurized, facilitating a gradient flow of contaminants from cleaner to dirtier areas (10). Controlled staging, support, material storage areas, and work practices should be examined and indicator sites identified. Controlled areas should be maintained and monitored in accordance with guidelines and industry standards (Table 1).

---

[b]Isoaxial: A condition of sampling in which the direction (axis) of the airflow into the sampling probe inlet is the same as that of the unidirectional airflow being sampled (7). Isokinetic sampling: The condition of isoaxial sampling in which the mean velocity of the air entering the probe inlet is the same as that of the unidirectional airflow being sampled (7)

Personnel, Equipment, and Facility

Validation and monitoring of a process are normally divided into three main areas of concern: personnel, equipment, and facility.

The human factor is the greatest potential variable in any process. Uncontrolled variation in personal health and hygiene, barrier techniques, and aseptic technique may cause wide variation in contamination of controlled support areas and process materials during staging and preparation, as well as adventitious contamination of the aseptic process core and product. A suitable aseptic process, defining appropriate and standardized personal hygiene expectations, scrubbing and preparation techniques, barrier techniques, and operator techniques should be developed and challenged intensively during the PQ exercise. Personnel should periodically take both written and media-fill skill tests (3).

Ongoing monitoring for compliance with pertinent SOPs should then be conducted. Sampling of personnel barriers, such as gloves, shoe covers, hair cover, and gowns facilitates detection of potential "fallout" contaminants shed from personnel for evaluation of both barrier and aseptic techniques. This information may be useful in establishing required garb-change intervals, based upon measured garb-penetration times by endogenous contaminants. All accumulated data should be used periodically to develop a facility trend analysis which, in turn, modifies training and work practices as necessary.

All equipment used in controlled manufacturing or compounding processes should be designed, staged, and sanitized in a manner that facilitates unvarying routine operation, with minimal human intervention. This reduces the potential for random cross-contamination by operative personnel. Improperly sanitized or sterilized equipment or components are also a possible source of contamination.[c] Monitoring of representative surfaces of process equipment should be carried out and documented.

Facility sampling should be carried out under both as-built and at-rest (7) conditions during initial installation qualification (IQ) and operational qualification (OQ) of the facility, in order to baseline and "bracket" performance of the engineering controls, and to identify the normal background flora present in the manufacturing environment. Sampling should then be conducted in-process

under operational conditions (7) during the PQ, to identify the impact of the process and personnel on the product and environment. It is important to monitor the validation process during all shifts and throughout the shift. Sites should be standardized and selected by statistical models or grid profiling (16), based upon testing and monitoring requirements appropriate to the specific process (Table 1).

Surface sampling is useful in verifying the effectiveness of housekeeping and sanitizing procedures. It may also provide an alert to poor materials preparation prior to introduction into the controlled environment, or to lapses in personnel technique or barrier use. Aerobiologic sampling is most useful when conducted in conjunction with a complete program for testing of the engineering control system (10). Recommended tests include the following:

1. Facility pressurization, which should be routinely monitored at recommended intervals (20);
2. High efficiency particulate air (HEPA) filter velocity and uniformity testing for laminar airflow (21), and volume in cubic ft/min (CFM) for conventional flow, including a determination of room installation air changes (10);
3. HEPA filter leak-integrity testing (18);
4. Nonviable particulate cleanliness testing (7); and
5. Smoke-tracer visualization for establishing the integrity of unidirectional-flow areas (10).

Periodic retesting of challenges 1–4 is required by some regulatory groups, with the interval determined by the nature of the process and product in a given area (17). Repeating Test 5 may be useful in evaluating failures and can be an extremely valuable training tool. Concomitant particle count testing may be useful in identifying contamination indicator sites.

Monitoring of laminar airflow workstations (LAFWs) requires a complete understanding of HEPA filtration system performance, and is frequently conducted in ways that do not yield useful information. When properly validated in accordance with Federal Standard 209b [Appendix A, para. 40 and 50[a]], LAFWs provide air at the entrance plane which is far cleaner than Class 100 (10). Testing to this cleanliness level would permit particulate contamination levels two orders of magnitude greater than during filter OQ validation testing. More important, the use of any apparatus that samples discrete locations in a unidirectional slip stream is unlikely to detect filter leakage because isoaxial and isokinetic sampling at the exact point of leakage would be required. Therefore, placement of a sampling probe upstream from the product is unreliable and an unnecessary threat to sterility. The only practical, in-process use of these

---

[c]The sterilization process for any equipment or supplies that are sterilized prior to introduction into the controlled environment must be validated, with sterilization records and verifications included in all product batch histories. Validation of sterilization equipment, alone, is not sufficient to assure sterility. Because the types of materials being sterilized, and the arrangement of articles within the sterilizer can effect results, standardized load configurations must be developed and validated

instruments is to detect shifts in the amount of particles and microbiologic contaminants caused by the process at some point adjacent to or downstream from the product. Such a shift might signal a lapse in personnel technique, barrier use, or prestaging material preparation, or be caused by HEPA filter loading, which reduces airflow velocity.

Avoiding Sampling-Induced False Positives

Line interventions for sampling purposes must be balanced carefully against the total number of interventions necessary for production purposes. Sampling should present the minimum risk of contamination, which is theoretically the same for every line intervention. Because sampling-induced positives should not exceed 10% of total positives ($10^{-1}N_p$) (17), the number of sampling interventions should be significantly lower than the number of production line interventions. In isolators or other isolated critical processes, where no line interventions occur during production, not more than one, carefully controlled, aseptic sampling intervention is recommended.

Surface sampling the exterior of finished products, as indicator sites, assembled from purportedly sterile components as they exit the process while still under aseptic conditions, may be a more efficacious method of estimating microbiologic contamination potential than invading the critical production site. This method allows sampling the most critical site adjacen to the product, and more sites may be noninvasively sampled over a longer interval. In addition, this method may substantially reduce the incidence of sampling-induced contamination.

Monitoring Frequency

The frequency of monitoring should be determined by the maximum interval acceptable for an over-limit condition to remain undetected (19). This depends upon the critical nature of the process within the monitored area. In general, the minimum frequency should be consistent with applicable regulatory guidelines (Table 1). Although it has been suggested that monitoring frequency can be reduced if no over-limit condition is detected within a predetermined number of monitoring cycles, this practice is inconsistent with basic monitoring rationale. Monitoring is conducted to detect a breakdown in process controls, which may occur at any time. Even if no control component has failed for a prolonged period, it must be assumed that a failure will occur eventually and must be detected within the predetermined interval. In addition, lack of over-limit test results may be due to the fact that

monitoring method(s) are not sufficiently sensitive, or that limits are too high.

EVALUATION OF THE MONITORING PLAN AND LIMITS

Most discussions of microbiologic monitoring recommend that the monitoring plan and limits be based on historical data, but offer little guidance on how this can be accomplished. Figure 1 provides a guide for evaluation and revision of the monitoring plan and limits. An in-depth evaluation may be triggered by over-limit results from monitoring (Entry Point 1) or by adverse product testing results without detection of any over-limit condition through routine monitoring (Entry Point 2).

Entry Point 1:

1. Conduct routine monitoring. A counter (C) is used for Step 11. $C = 0$ at the beginning of the routine monitoring program.
2. If the results do not exceed any limit, then continue routine monitoring.
3. If the results exceed any limit, then perform retesting in triplicate to verify the accuracy of results. Retest under the same conditions noted on the sampling form (i.e., same time of day, same location and operator, same type of production).
4. If triplicate retest results are not over-limit, it is assumed that the original over-limit result was due to a nonassignable cause (*NAC*). Determine the probable cause of the over-limit count (i.e., unusual activities noted on test documentation, sampling, lab error, etc.). A record of positive NACs should be kept and analyzed to determine ways to improve affected processes and sampling procedures. Return to routine monitoring.
5. If results are over an alert limit, but not over the action limit, then enhance monitoring frequency for X cycles. (X is determined by the critical level of the area and process where the over-limit event occurred, but should provide an adequate interval to assure detection of a continued deterioration of process control.)

   a. If the alert limit is not exceeded again within X cycles, then return to Step 4.
   b. If the alert limit is exceeded but the action limit is not, then proceed to Step 10.
   c. If the action limit is exceeded, then go to the corrective action plan (CAP) (5).
6. If results following the triplicate retesting are over the action limit, but not the fail limit, then go to the CAP.

7. If the results following the triplicate resting are over the fail limit, traditional QA protocols usually require that operations cease. However, the appropriate action taken should depend on the critical nature of the monitored step and other conditions. An alternative to operation shut down may be to segregate and hold the product for enhanced testing for adverse effect; go to the CAP.

8. If implementation of the CAP results in the determination of the cause of the over-limit condition, then correct the condition, and retest in triplicate to verify that the problem was corrected. If no cause was found, then proceed to Step 10.

9. If test results following corrective action are within limits, then return to routine monitoring.

10. If test results following corrective action are still over-limit, or if no cause of the over-limit condition can be identified, then evaluate the product for adverse effects.

11. If no adverse impact on product quality can be detected, add 1 to the counter (C). The result may indicate that limits are too low, but one event is not sufficient to support a decision to increase limits.

    a. If $C = 3$, then the limits are too sensitive, and should be increased.
    b. If $C = <3$, return to routine monitoring, Because the results are over-limit at this point, a repeat investigation of the cause of over-limit results will be triggered. Limits should be increased judiciously, and it is important to be thorough in attempting to resolve any cause of over-limit testing with reasonable certainty before increasing limits. For example, if the cause of the over-limit result is sampling mistakes or lab error, there will be no detectable cause in the production facility, the process or engineering control evaluations, and probably no adverse effect on product quality. This should not, however, be interpreted to mean that limits are too sensitive.

12. If product is adversely affected, and no cause can be detected following implementation of the CAP, the monitoring plan and/or the process should be redesigned and revalidated.

Entry Point 2:
13. If product quality is below limits, but monitoring data did not detect the shift, then reevaluate monitoring data using lower limits to determine whether or not the process shift could have been detected. If the data have been graphically represented, this should be

quite simple; increasing the amplitude of the graph may be useful.

14. If lower limits would have detected the shift, then lower the limits and institute the CAP.

15. If lower limits would not have detected the shift, then evaluate the cause of the failure, and develop a new sampling strategy for the key step(s) where failure occurred. Institute the CAP and verify that corrective actions taken were effective in improving product quality.

16. If product quality improves, then add the new sampling method to the routine monitoring program.

17. If it does not, return to Step 12.

SELECTION OF MONITORING METHODS, MATERIALS, AND EQUIPMENT

Effective microbiologic monitoring of controlled processes usually includes sampling of process air for aerobiologic contamination, and facility, equipment, and operative personnel barriers for surface contamination. Equipment and methods used in monitoring procedures must be carefully considered for attributes and limitations and must be matched to sampling objectives to ensure that methods and techniques are noninvasive, and to facilitate development of well-organized sampling plans, techniques, data, and data trending analysis.

Surface Sampling

Surface sampling may be performed at the conclusion of critical operations to minimize disruption of these processes (8) and prior to sanitizing procedures (20) to estimate cumulative, inprocess contaminant burden (4). In addition, presanitization surface sampling is beneficial in detecting operations-induced bioburden and cross-contamination between environmental and equipment surfaces. Postsanitization surface sampling is useful for evaluating sanitizing methods and in retrieving sanitization-resistant isolates for identification and trend analysis in demonstrating sanitizing compound efficacy. The two most common types of surface sampling are swab-sampling, and surface contact sampling.

Swab-sampling

Swab-sampling is normally used for flat or irregular, nonabsorbent surfaces with qualitative development by inoculation of the swab matrix directly into nutrient broth, observed for growth/no growth. Quantitative development is also possible (5). The main advantage of the swab method is accessibility to difficult-to-reach equipment surfaces and areas of the production environment. Limitations are excessive time consumption, increased potential for adventitious contamination due to the cumbersome nature of the procedure, and failure of enumeration processes to correlate to full recovery of organisms.

Contact plates

Surface contact plates are normally used for sampling flat or irregular, absorbent or nonabsorbent surfaces. The surface contact plate consists of a clear plastic base housing a convex protrusion of nutrient agar with a plastic cover. Sampling is accomplished by pressing the agar against the site.

The covered plate is then incubated for development, and the CFUs per square centimeter enumerated (21). Advantages of surface contact plates are reproducibility, speed, simplicity of collection mechanism, and minimized potential for adventitious contamination; collection and correlation to recovery of organisms are superior to swab-sampling.

Aerobiologic Sampling

Aerobiologic sampling is conducted in critical and controlled areas to detect airborne viable contaminants present during manufacturing operations. Aerobiologic sampling procedures, frequency, and limits should be established based upon environmental conditions required to maintain product quality, and established for each processing step (4) (Table 1). Aerobiologic sampling employs two basic methodologies:

1. The gravity settle plate, which provides passive measurement of microorganisms likely to deposit by sedimentation at critical and controlled sites within a given period, and
2. The volumetric air sampler, which provides active measurement of viable contaminants by mechanical aspiration and dynamic inoculation of process air.

Gravity settle plates

The gravity settle plate measures microorganisms settling from the air onto a known surface area in a known time. Settle plates may be positioned within the critical area at indicator sites where the product may become exposed to airborne contamination, and in controlled areas at locations identified as likely sources or areas of "fallout" aerobiologic contamination. Settle plates are not appropriate aerobiologic sampling method for monitoring the efficiency of unidirectional (laminar)

airflow or other air-cleaning devices. This is based upon studies (22, 23), and the general assumption that "... the settling velocity of contaminants (in unidirectional airflow) is negligible, which implies that gravitation plays an inferior role. With the assumption of a constant value of the diffusion coefficient, the diffusion equation in a velocity field within rectangular coordinates becomes

$$\frac{\partial c}{\partial t} + v_x \frac{\partial c}{\partial X} + v_y \frac{\partial c}{\partial Y} + v_z \frac{\partial c}{\partial Z} = D\left(\frac{\partial^2 c}{\partial X^2} + \frac{\partial^2 c}{\partial Y^2} + \frac{\partial^2 c}{\partial Z^2}\right) \quad (1)$$

where c is concentration: v_x, v_y, v_z are velocities in the x, y, and z directions: and D is diffusion coefficient.

This gives the simplest possible mathematical model which describes a system with regard to transport of contaminants emitted in a source of an arbitrary position..." (23), demonstrating that particle dispersion in undisturbed streamlines is primarily a function of streamline uniformity and velocity. Disruptions of the parallel (laminar) airflow streamlines caused by equipment, personnel movement, and product result in turbulent flow, creating small and temporary vortices and eddies. It is only turbulent diffusion within the vortex that causes removal of entrained contaminants (23). Therefore settle plates, strategically placed, are reported to provide a superior method of predicting potential product contamination by mimicking the deposition of microbe-carrying particles (MCPs) into or onto the product[d] (24). They are inexpensive, may be used to continuously monitor the entire production interval, are less invasive of aseptic operations, and may usually be placed closer to exposed products than volumetric air samplers.

Settle plates cannot be used for quantitative measurement of airborne microorganisms because the sample volume of sedimentation air samples cannot be measured. Air turbulence around an open plate may also effect collection results, and smaller particles may not settle at all (22). In addition, extended exposure times may result in

[d]Regardless of placement of an aerobiological sampler in a laminar airflow work zone, it can at best measure the effect of the process at some point downstream from the product. For example, the mouth of a flask may be situated in "first air" issuing from the HEPA filter, while air impinging on the surface of a plate adjacent to it will be affected by disruptions of the airstream caused by the flask. Contamination found on the plate then results from a different set of conditions than those to which the product is subjected and does not exactly parallel the product contamination mechanism. Only a media-fill process simulation can fulfill this function. Aerobiologic sampling immediately downstream of the critical orifice can, however, detect downward shifts in the overall cleanliness of the critical process air, which in turn may indicate increased contamination potential near the product

some desiccation of the nutrient agar, resulting in poor microbial growth (25).

Volumetric air samplers

As an active sampling method, the volumetric air sampler aspirates a known volume of process air, capturing microorganisms into or onto a nutrient agar medium, a liquid, or a filter. Microorganisms are developed and quantified as an estimate of CFUs present in the sampled environment per cubic foot of air (or other volumetric measurement) (4). The quantitative principles of volumetric (active) air sampling may be expressed by

$$S(R_t)C = R_f \qquad (2)$$

where S is source intensity, R_t is transport rate, C is correction factor, and R_f is failure rate.

Volumetric air sampling is accomplished by a number of different methodologies, including impingement, impaction through single or multiple orifices, centrifugal impaction, and filtration. Each method has inherent advantages and disadvantages that affect the value of the data collected relative to the specific application. Table 2 presents a comparison of popular samplers based upon relative cost, difficulty of use, appropriate applications, and other factors.

Impingement: In an impinger, a known volume of air is drawn through fluid in a glass vessel (20, 30). Particles separate from the airstream by impinging at the flask bottom, where they are stopped and retained by the liquid as the air continues to flow out through the pump system. High air velocities passing through the impinger effectively break up bacterial/particulate aggregates, resulting in microbial counts, which more closely reflect the actual number of microorganisms, leading to recommendations that impingers be used as the standard reference method for monitoring aerobiologic contamination (26, 28). However, impingers may require the addition of antifoam agents and replacement of fluid, due to agitation and evaporation loss during longer sampling procedures.

These additional steps increase the possibility of adventitious contamination. It has been demonstrated that the sampling efficiency of an impinger is dependent upon both system design and the particle sizes being sampled (29). Accuracy and reproducibility of results have been reported to be difficult, and particles of <5.0 μm have been demonstrated to pass through the impingers tested (30).

Impaction: In slit-to-agar (STA) or sieve impactors, a known volume of air is aspirated through a single orifice (STA), or multiple orifices (sieve), and viable particles, due to their inertia, are forced out of inlet airflow streamlines and impacted onto perpendicular, target nutrient agars as the streamlines abruptly change direction to bypass the target stage. In the centrifugal impaction sampler, high centrifugal forces created by "spinning" air through an impeller turbine at sufficient velocities to cause separation of microorganisms from sample air streamlines result in their impaction onto a nutrient agar strip placed at the inner periphery of the sampling chamber, parallel to the inlet airflow axis.

Sieve impactors are available in single-stage or multistage designs that facilitate both enumeration and sizing of aerobiological contaminants. As the sample air transits the device, sample velocities increase at each stage, resulting in gradient deposition and accurate sizing of microorganisms of smaller diameters and lower mass. Microorganisms aspirated by sieve samplers through a matrix of multiple-inlet orifices impact directly onto an agar medium for development from a single agar plate for each vertically stacked stage, with no further subculture steps required for enumeration. Advantages of sieve samplers are generally high particle deposition rates, the ability to size particles and vary sampling time and volume, and superior collection efficiencies when compared to other methods of aerobiological testing. Single- and six-stage configurations have been reported to be two of the three sampling methods of choice (27).

Use of STA samplers in isolators and critical process zones should be accomplished using a sterile sampling hose and probe, facilitating remote location of the sampler in a noncritical area. In monitoring a unidirectional slipstream, this hose/probe configuration should be both isoaxially oriented, and isokinetic[b], in order to minimize disruption of the slipstream. Advantages of the STA include the ability to revolve the plate at varying rates so that the samples may demonstrate changes in aerobiological concentrations directly over time, and the ability to obtain multiple samples with a single petri dish (31). STA samplers have historically been the standard against which other air samplers are assessed (17, 32). Agar plates are easily removed from the sampler for development, with contamination enumerated as CFUs per unit of air sampled.

The STA is reported to be both unsuitable for use in the presence of high concentrations of organisms (33) and cumbersome to use (17). In addition, it has been demonstrated that a significantly higher percentage of particles sized 0.5–0.8 μm, and a significantly lower percentage of particles sized 3.0–25.0 μm, were present in sample air, which had passed through the slit of an STA,

Table 2 Relative cost/difficulty comparisons

Sampling method/sampler	Acquistion cost[a]	Cost of Use/Sample 1–6[b]	Ease of Use 1–6[b]	Sampling Speed 1–6[b]	Mobility 1–6[b]	Contamination Potential to Sample	Contamination Potential to Environment	Reproducibility 1–6[b]	Applications A-C	Isolators 1–6[b]
Swab Sample Typical	●	5	2	2	2	4	1	2	C	4
Contact Plate Typical	●	2	1	1	1	1	1	1	B	1
Gravity Settle Plate Typical	●	1	1	1	1	1	1	3	A	1
SAS Super 90 Air Sampler	5	2	2	2	2	2	2	2	A	3
STA New Brunswick	5	1	3	2	4	2	3	2	A	1[c]
Sieve Impactor Andersen 1-STAGE	2	1	3	2	2	2	3	1	A	3
Centrifugal Biotest RCS Plus	3	3	3	2	2	4	2	3	A	6
Sieve Impactor Anderson 6-STAGE	5	4	6	6	3	4	3	2	A	5
Gel Membrane Sartorius MD8	4	6	2	1	1	2	2	1	A	1[c]
SMA P200 Impactor	6	1	2	2	2	2	3	2	A	4
Glass Impinger All Glass	6	2	4	3	4	4	3	2	A	4

Table 2 Relative cost/difficulty comparisons

Sampling method/sampler	Laminar Airflow 1–6[b]	Critical Environments	Production Areas 1–6[b]	General Areas 1–6[b]	Flat Environmental Surfaces	Irregular Environ. Surfaces	Personnel Barriers 1–6[b]	Volumetric (SP) Y/N	Remote Probe Possible	External Power	Sample
Swab Sample Typical	4	2	2	1	2	1	4	N	●	●	S
Contact Plate Typical	1	1	1	1	1	4	1	N	●	●	S
Gravity Settle Plate Typical	1	1	1	1	●	●	●	N	●	●	S
SAS Super 90 Air Sampler	2	3	2	2	●	●	●	Y	N	Y	S
STA New Brunswick	1[d]	3	1	2	●	●	●	Y	Y	Y	S
Sieve Impactor Andersen 1-STAGE	2	2	1	1	●	●	●	Y	N	Y	S
Centrifugal Biotest RCS Plus	5	5	3	1	●	●	●	N	N	N	P
Sieve Impactor Anderson 6-STAGE	5	2	2	2	●	●	●	Y	N	Y	S
Gel Membrane Sartorius MD8	1[d]	1	1	1	●	●	●	Y	Y	Y	P
SMA P200 Impactor	3	3	2	1	●	●	●	Y	N	Y	S
Glass Impinger All Glass	4	3	2	2	●	●	●	Y	N	Y	S

[a]Acquisition cost in thousand dollars.
[b]Difficulty: 1–6 (easiest–hardest).
[c]With Hose/probe attachment.
[d]With Hose/isokinetic probe attachment.
A: Aerobiologic samples; B: Flat surface samples; C: Irregular surface samples; P: Proprietary media system; S: Standard Commercially-available system.
Table courtesy of Northview Biosciences Inc., Northbrook, IL.

than were found in ambient air (34). This was attributed to fragmentation of larger particles following passage through the slit of the STA.[e]

Due to dehydration of the agar reported to occur over long sampling periods, continuous sampling exceeding 30 min using an impaction sampler is not recommended. Areas of loss have been reported for sieve samplers (40), including *inlet loss* (the effect of cross-wind at the sample inlet point), *interstage loss* (deposition of particles on internal surfaces other than the impaction agar), and *particle re-entrainment* (particles reintroduced into the airstream due to particle "bounce," resulting from dehydration of the impaction agar).

Advantages of the centrifugal sampler are the capability of sampling large amounts of air (40 L/min) in a short time; it is quiet, lightweight, self-contained, and does not require cumbersome air pumps or external power for operation. Centrifugal samplers provide a good indication of environmental isolates (17).

Centrifugal sampling cannot be carried out isokinetically (23), and the accuracy of results is dependent upon the sizes of the particles being sampled. Since particulate sizes in the air volume being sampled are not routinely determined, the validity of the centrifugal sampler as a quantitative device has been called into question (36), especially for quantification of small particles (27, 37). Another recent study indicates that centrifugal sampling causes air to move in a turbulent, mixing manner, introducing heavily disturbed airflow patterns around the sampler which may, in turn, impart disturbances to any unidirectional airflow patterns being sampled (23). Reaspiration of sampled air is also a problem with earlier designs, creating difficulty in discriminating between incoming and outgoing airstreams, which is necessary to quantify microorganisms (38). Proprietary agar medium strips are specially designed and unique to this system, and require careful technique to insert and remove aseptically.

Membrane filtration: Membrane filtration (MF) sampling is accomplished by capturing aerobiological contamination as it passes through a cellulose membrane filter (CMF) or gelatin membrane filter (GMF). The mechanisms of MF particle removal are inertial impaction, diffusional interception, and direct interception. Following collection, the GMF may be plated aseptically onto an agar petri dish to dissolve, allowing microorganisms to grow directly on the nutrient medium. Dissolution of the membrane into a sterile solution is also possible (31).

[e]Interestingly, this attribute was reported by investigators to be an advantage of the all-glass Impinger (31, 32).

While MF sampling has been demonstrated to be the most effective means of retaining aerobiological contamination, CMF sampling exhibits a lower recovery rate than an impinger when tested against stress-sensitive microorganisms, such as *Serratia marcescens* (39) or *Escherichia coli* (27) due to desiccation on the CMF surface. Studies have indicated that gelatin foam filters incorporated into GMF gave significantly higher recovery rates than CMF over the same sampling period (40, 41). Recent comparisons of sampling systems indicate that GMF is equally as effective as the STA sampler, irrespective of particle size, and is significantly more effective than centrifugal sampling in the collection of microorganisms with sizes <5.0 μm (31). A recent study comparing the GMF system with centrifugal, sieve, and STA systems in sampling the unidirectional airflow slipstream in the presence of visual tracers indicates the GMF sampler to be the only sampling method capable of isokinetic and isoaxial sampling with no visual disturbance to the laminar airflow pattern (31). However, in this study, the STA was tested without the remote hose-isokinetic probe device.

Limitations of the GMF are an additional aseptic subculture step, which increases the probability of adventitious contamination, and a proprietary membrane filter, which results in a per-sample cost currently exceeding 12 times that of the one-stage sieve, SAS, STA, SMA, and glass impinger systems, and four times that of the centrifugal sampler.

Growth Media

Growth and collection media used in microbiologic monitoring should be selected on the basis of the target organisms, areas and surfaces sampled, and inhibitory residues that may remain on the sampled surfaces. Media commonly used for environmental monitoring are listed in Table 3. Under certain circumstances (e.g., when obligate anaerobes are recovered from the product), additional, specific media and methods should be selected by a qualified microbiologist (17).

Comparison of Aerobiologic Samplers

The different characteristics and operating principles of aerobiological samplers do not facilitate direct and simple comparisons. The user should, therefore, carefully evaluate the numerous advantages and disadvantages of each method in selecting a sampler for the intended application (42) (Table 2). Two studies that provide basic comparisons of aerobiological sampling systems may offer useful information:

Table 3 Media commonly used for environmental monitoring

Medium	Selective for	Sample application
Tryptic soy agar (TSA)[a,b]	Aerobes and facultative anerobes	Air and surface
Letheen agar[c]	Aerobes and facultative anerobes	Surface
DE neutralizing agar[d]	Aerobes and facultative anerobes	Surface
Sabouraud dextrose agar	Yeast and molds	Air and surface
Rose bengal agar	Yeast and molds	Air and surface
Buffer solution[e]		Surface

[a]Tryptic soy agar is also known as soybean casein digest agar.
[b]Unmodified general purpose medium use for culturing bacteria and/or fungi.
[c]Contains additives used to neutralize residuals of halogen-based disinfectants, such as sodium hypochlorite (bleach).
[d]Contains additives used to neutralize residuals of halogen and quaternary ammonium chloride-based disinfectants.
[e]Samples collected using sterile swabs and buffer solution must be transferred to media for culturing and enumeration.
(Courtesy of Northview Biosciences, Inc., Northbrook, IL.)

A study comparing eight bioaerosol samplers was carried out by Jensen et al. in 1992 (27). Results indicated that the Andersen 6-STG, I-STG, and Ace Glass AGI 30 samplers were the samplers of choice for recovering aerosols of free bacteria (i.e., mostly single cells of *E. coli* and *B. subtilis*, $d_{ae} \geq 2$ μm) under the controlled conditions of the study (43). Another study, comparing seven samplers commonly used in controlled environments, was conducted by Ljungqvist and Reinmiiller in 1998 (44). This study indicated widely varying results for the impaction samplers tested. The limited number of parallel tests performed prevented an evaluation of comparative collection efficiencies based upon statistical considerations. The salient recommendations of this study are that results should be seen more "... as an indication of a [contamination] level and not be taken as a true absolute value," and that aerobiological samplers be selected carefully, based on practicalities of using different types for different locations or situations. Furthermore, this study recommends the simultaneous use of a discrete particle counter (DPC) to measure the total number of airborne particles present in the area sampled.[f]

ANALYSIS AND INTERPRETATION OF MONITORING RESULTS

Effective interpretation of data from microbiologic monitoring of the environment can be the most difficult aspect of the monitoring process. Several factors complicate this process, including the inherently nonrandom distribution of most microbial contamination events, errors in sample handling, variation of sampling technique from one monitoring event to the next, and seasonal shifts in the type and level of contaminants likely to be present in the general environment.

The purpose of statistical evaluation of sample data is to extrapolate from a collection of individual events (e.g., 30 min of process time) to the entire population of events (e.g.,

[f]Because it is impossible to derive instantaneous results from microbiologic testing, the authors agree that such data should, where possible, be correlated with a DPC as an instantaneous data source, in developing useful historical data. Although "... no universal relationship has been established between the total concentration of airborne particles and the concentration of viable airborne particles..." (7), such a correlation may be possible under controlled operational conditions within a specific area or facility (determined by Ljungqvist and Reinmüller in two facilities) to be approximately 10^{-4} (10,000:1). Such a correlation would facilitate a "viability index" as a rational means of correlating shifts in instantly available particle count values with probable corresponding shifts in aerobiological contamination. This technique would be very useful in the instantaneous identification of contamination indicator sites. Similar correlations have been established on a facility-specific basis by the Lab Safety Corp. during the course of regular, periodic aerobiological sampling of three bone marrow transplant complexes over a period of several years. In all cases, a correlation of the total population of aerobiological contaminants to instantaneous DPC data (termed the "viability index") was used to trace the distribution and probable presence of the life-threatening organism *A. niger* in immunocompromised patient populations. Although it was found that in these highly controlled facilities (e.g., Class 1000 or better) the correlation was one to two orders of magnitude higher than that described by Ljungqvist and Reinmüller (42,44), the correlations were consistent, allowing facility managers to reliably detect possible life-threatening deteriorations of the critical patient environment through the use of instantaneous DPC data as an aerobiological contamination indicator. The data analyzed indicate that aerobiological contaminants appear to increase in proportion to nonviable contaminants as the cleanliness of a facility increases. This is probably due to the fact that, as general environmental contamination is eliminated, human activity becomes the principal source of contamination.

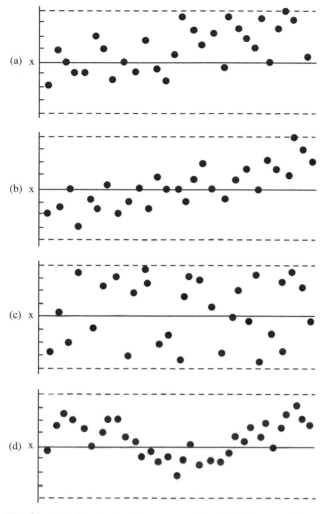

Fig. 2 Out-of-control pattern recognition. (a) Change or jump in level; (b) Trend or steady change in level; (c) Two populations; (d) Recurring cycles. (Chart courtesy of Prentice Hall, Inc., Upper Saddle River, NJ.)

8-h shift). Because microbial monitoring data usually measure the impact of human activity, which is not reproducible exactly from one event to the next, results usually do not fit standard statistical models for normal distributions. In spite of this limitation, it is necessary to summarize the data for comparison to limits. The best statistical methods of evaluation are determined by the nature of the data (14). Wilson suggests that microbial monitoring data histograms generally resemble Poisson or negative exponential distributions (14), whereas Akers points out that Poisson distributions may only be appropriate for systems with minimal human intervention (12). The formula for the Poisson distribution (45) is given by

$$P(C) = \frac{(np_o)^c}{C!} e^{-} np_o \tag{3}$$

where C is individual sample count, np_0 is average count, and $e = 2.718281$.

Trend analysis of results at individual sample locations may be more useful than statistical analysis of data summaries because each sampling location probably reflects a unique situation. Nontraditional groupings of data may also be valuable. For example, grouping all locations where a specific activity was noted on the sample collection form, grouping all data collected during a specific time frame (i.e., just after lunch, or near the end of a production cycle), or grouping all data for each operator may reveal specific problem areas.

The example control charts presented by Besterfield in Fig. 2 demonstrate four major types of out-of-control patterns (45). A fifth pattern is due to mistakes, which will usually show up as isolated, out-of-control points. All apply equally to production and sampling operations. All patterns may be observed on both range (R) charts and standard (or reference) process average charts (, but are usually more common to charts.

Likely causes for each type of pattern can be identified, and a checklist of assignable causes applicable to the particular process should be developed through cause and effect (C&E) analysis (45). Examples of likely causes for these patterns are:

a. A change or jump in pattern caused by an inexperienced operator, a change in raw materials, or a failure of an equipment part;
b. A trend or steady change in level due to a gradual change in the production environment, a gradual change in equipment performance (e.g. HEPA filter loading), or a gradual tendency toward lax observation of SOPs;
c. Two populations may be due to more than one process line or piece of critical equipment on the same chart, more than one operator on the same chart, or different samplers or sampling techniques; and
d. Recurring cycles may be caused by periodic operator rotation, operator fatigue and rejuvenation cycles, sanitizing and cleaning cycles, and seasonal shifts.

Recurring cycles may be missed if sampling intervals happen to coincide with the cycle frequency, in which case only the low or high range of the cycle may be detected. Out-of-limit trends near the lower limits of the R chart represent superior performance and should be analyzed to identify methods of maintaining these process levels (45). Whatever statistical methods are employed for summarizing data, graphic representations, such as histograms and process control charts can be extremely useful for detecting trends or cyclic patterns in test results.

There are two types of over-limit results: *Random* results are due to chance (unassignable) causes, whereas *nonrandom* results are due to assignable causes. For a controlled process and facility, the objective is to differentiate between individual data points that are assignable and those that are not. If the individual over-limit event is not repeated during subsequent, multiple retests, it is not assignable and does not represent a deteriorating trend. All statistical evaluation methods include mechanisms for "discarding" spurious data. There is, however, a cause for any unassignable result, and efforts should be made to identify and understand it. All data have meaning, and may be useful for improving the process or testing procedures.

Speciation

Speciation of microorganisms is indicated when product testing results detect the presence of a specific organism, when evaluating the efficacy of sanitizing compounds and routines, and when monitoring results trigger the corrective action plan. Speciation should be carried out and analyzed by a qualified microbiologist familiar with the sampling equipment, sampling methods employed, and the origins of organisms commonly found in cleanrooms (17,,46). Speciation should also be conducted periodically to identify isolates normally recovered when the process is operating within limits, and may be useful in identifying the probable cause(s) of any out-of-limit condition. During the initial phase of the corrective action plan, an analysis of probable contamination sources and routes should be made for all organisms identified (17). Information obtained by speciation may immediately indicate the most likely source. This information may also indicate less common contamination sources, such as perverted cleaning solutions.

Periodic re-evaluation of the monitoring plan should be carried out, and seasonal effects considered in trend analysis. Many sampling methods do not collect all organisms with equal efficiency, and organisms likely to be present may vary seasonally. Any seasonal shift (up or down) should be investigated by speciation, and sampler correction factors for the predominant organisms applied.

CORRECTIVE ACTION PLAN

The CAP should clearly define and document

1. The method of data analysis;
2. Alert, action, and fail limits;
3. Corrective actions to be employed in the event of detection of a deteriorating trend or an over-limit condition; and
4. A means of confirming the effectiveness of corrective action(s).

A verified trend above the action or fail limit should immediately trigger implementation of the CAP. Because human activity is the most likely source of process control failure, the investigative process normally begins with personnel, and proceeds through the various possible causes from most to least likely. An exception to this general plan is verification of room pressurization, which is a primary indication of engineering control equipment efficiency. Although routine monitoring of pressurization should detect any out-of-limit results, the simplicity of verifying proper pressurization suggests this as a first step.

In general, the cause of any deterioration in process or environmental control can be traced to one of three principle systems: a) personnel controls, b) process controls, or c) facility (engineering) controls. Increases in detected airborne microbiologic contamination levels may result from any of several conditions, and a simple set of logical challenges can be applied to the data to determine the most likely cause.

Challenge 1, *Is the increase real and reproducible?* If it is not reproducible, it may be due to sampling error, or NACs. If it is reproducible, it may be due to an actual increase in levels, or due to enhanced collection efficiency, due to changes in methods, materials, or seasonal or other shifts in the kinds of contaminants present (different organisms have different sampling efficiencies).; Challenge 2, *If the increase is real, is it due to an increase in source intensity, or to a decrease in the ability of engineering controls to maintain a clean air supply?* The easiest way to differentiate between these possibilities is to examine particle count data. There are several possible combinations of test results, each indicating a different cause for increased airborne contamination: a) If particle counts taken under operational conditions have not risen, but airborne microbiologic contamination has, it is most likely due to a breakdown in personnel discipline and/or gowning procedures. b) If operational particle counts have risen, but at-rest counts have not, it is again likely that the cause of elevated microbial contamination is personnel activity and that it represents an increase in source intensity (when human activity is eliminated, engineering controls are able to produce the same conditions that were present during the OQ validation phase). c) If at-rest particle counts have risen, the increase is probably due to a decrease in the efficiency of the engineering controls.

Similar logical tests can be applied to increases in surface contamination levels, which may be due to increases in source intensity, or decreases in the efficiency of barrier controls or cleaning and sanitizing procedures. Flow charts illustrating the logical evaluation of data, and investigation of out-of-limit results are useful as starting points in the development of corrective action plans (5).

REFERENCES

1. Code of Federal Regulation. *The Current Good Manufacturing Practices*; Title 21, Part 211, U.S. Government Printing Office: Washington, DC, 1992.

2. ASHP Technical Assistance Bulletin. Quality Assurance for Pharmacy-Prepared Sterile Products. AJHP **1993**, *50*, 2386–2398.

3. United States Pharmacopeial Convention, Inc. Sterile Drug Products for home use. USP **1998**, *23*, 1963–1975, ⟨1206⟩.

4. Roscioli, N. Environmental Monitoring Considerations for Biological Manufacturing. BioPharm **1996**, *9* (8), 32–38.

5. Peters, G.F.; McKeon, M.R. Microbiologic Monitoring of Aseptic and Controlled Processes. *Encyclopedia of Pharmaceutical Technology*; Swarbrick, J., Boylan, J.C., Eds.; Marcel Dekker, Inc.: New York, 2000; 19, 239–278.

6. Center for Drugs and Biologics and Office of Regulatory Affairs. *Guideline on Sterile Drug Products produced by Aseptic Processing*; FDA: Rockville, MD, 1987.

7. Institute of Environmental Science and Technology. In *Airborne Particulate Cleanliness Classes in Cleanrooms and Clean Zones*; Federal Standard U.S. Govt. Printing Office: Washington, DC, 1992.

8. United States Pharmacopeial Convention, Inc. Microbial Evaluation of Clean Room and other Controlled Environments. USP **1998**, *23*, 4426–4433, ⟨1116⟩.

9. National Aeronautics and Space Administration. In *NASA Standards for Clean Rooms and Work Stations for the Microbially Controlled Environment*; Publication NHB 5340.2; NASA: Washington, DC, 1967.

10. Peters, G. Laminar Airflow Equipment: Engineering Control of Aseptic Processing. *Encyclopedia of Pharmaceutical Technology*; Swarbrick, J., Boylan, J.C., Eds.; Marcel Dekker, Inc.: New York, 1993; 8, 317–359.

11. Satter, S. Biological and Physical Monitoring of a Controlled Environment. J. Am. Contam. Contr. **1998**, *1* (8), 27–31.

12. Akers, J.; Agalloco, J. Sterility and Sterility Assurance. PDA J. Pharm. Sci. Technol. **1997**, *51* (2), 72–77.

13. F.D.C. Reports, Inc. Quality Control Reports, The Gold Sheet September, 1998; 15–19.

14. Wilson, J. Setting Alert/Action Limits for Environmental Monitoring Programs. PDA J. Pharm. Sci. Technol. **1997**, *51* (4), 161–162.

15. Andersen Samplers, Inc.: Ed.; *Operating Manual TR# 76-900042*; Andersen Samplers, Inc. Atlanta, 1980; 23.

16. Parenteral Drug Association, Inc. Fundamentals of a Microbiological Monitoring Program. PDA J. Pharm. Sci. Technol. **1990**, *44* (S1), S3–S14.

17. BSI. *Guide to Operational Procedures and Disciplines Applicable to Clean Rooms and Clean Air Devices*; Part 1, British Standard 5295: London, 1989.

18. General Services Administration. In *Clean Room and Work Station Requirements, Controlled Environments*; Federal Standard 209b, U.S. Govt. Printing Office: Washington, DC, 1976.

19. Sanford, R. Cumulative Sum Control Charts for Admixture Quality Control. Am. J. Hosp. Pharm. **1980**, *37*, 655–659.

20. Akers, J. Environmental Monitoring and Control: Proposed Standards, Current Practices, and Future Directions. PDA J. Pharm. Sci. Technol. **1997**, *51* (1), 36–47.

21. Niskanen, A.; Pohja, M.S. Comparative Studies on the Sampling and Investigation of Microbial Contamination of Surfaces by the Contact Plate and Swab Method. J. Appl. Bacti. **1977**, *42*, 53–63.

22. Sayer, W.J.; MacKnight, N.M.; Wilson, H.W. Hospital Airborne Bacteria as estimated by the Andersen Sampler Versus the Gravity Settling Plate. Am. J. Clin. Path. **1972**, *58*, 558–562.

23. Ljungqvist, B.; Reinmüller, B. Interaction between Air Movements and the Dispersion of Contaminants: Clean Zones with unidirectional Air Flow. PDA J. Pharm. Sci. Technol. **1993**, *47* (2), 60–69.

24. Whyte, W. Support of Settle Plates. PDA J. Pharm. Sci. Technol. 50 (4), 201–204.

25. Kingston, D. Selective Media in Air Sampling: A Review. J. Appl. Bact. **1971**, *34* (1), 221–232.

26. Hering, S.V. Inertial and Gravitational Collectors. *Air Sampling Instruments for Evaluation of Atmospheric Contaminants*, 7th Ed.; Hering, S.V., Ed.; American Conference of Government Industrial Hygienists, Inc.: Cincinnati, 1989; 385.

27. Jensen, P.A.; Todd, W.F.; Davis, G.N.; Scarpino, P.V. Evaluation of Eight Bioaerosol Samplers Challenged with Aerosols of Free Bacteria. J. Am. Ind. Hyg. Assoc. **1992**, *53* (10), 557–660.

28. Brachman, P.S. Standard Sampler for Assay of Airborne Microorganisms. Science **1964**, *144*, 1295.

29. Macher, J.M.; First, M.W. Personal Air Samplers for Measuring Occupational Exposures to Biological Hazards. J. Am. Ind Hyg. Assoc. **1984**, *45* (2), 76–83.

30. Lyons, C. Sampling Efficiencies of all-glass Midget Impingers. J. Aerosol Sci. **1992**, *23* (S1), S599–S602.

31. Pickard, D.R.; Pendlebury, D.E. Examining Ways to Capture Airborne Microorganisms. Clean Rooms **1997**, *11* (6), 34–40.

32. Benbough, J.E.; Bennett, A.M.; Parks, S.R. Determination of the Collection Efficiency of a Microbial Air Sampler. J. Appl. Bacteri. **1993**, *74*, 170–173.

33. Decker, H.M.; Wilson, M.E. A Slit Sampler for Collecting Airborne Microorganisms. Appl. Environ. Microbiol. **1954**, *2*, 267–269.

34. Fields, N.; Oxbarrow, G.; Puleo, J.R.; Herring, G. Evaluation of Membrane Filter Field Monitors for Microbiological Air Sampling. Appl. Environ. Microbiol. **1974**, *27* (3), 17–520.

35. Marple, V.A.; Willeke, K. Impactor Design. Atmos. Environ. **1976**, *10*, 891–896.

36. Kaye, S. Efficiency of Biotest Rcs as a Sampler of Airborne Bacteria. PDA J. Parenter. Sci. Technol. **1988**, *42* (5), 147–152.

37. Trudeau, W.L.; Fernandez-Caldas, E. Identifying and Measuring Indoor Biologic Agents. J. Clin. Immunol. **1994**, *94* (2:2), 393–400.

38. Macher, J.M.; First, M.W. Reuter Centrifugal Air Sampler: Measurement of Effective Air-Flow Rate and Collection Efficiency. Appl. Environ. Microbiol. **1983**, *45*, 1960–1962.

39. Goetz, A. Application of the Molecular Filter Membrane to the Analysis of Aerosols. Am. J. Publ. Health. **1953**, *43*, 150–159.

40. Noller, E.; Spendlove, J.D. An Appraisal of the Gelatin Foam Filter as a Sampler for Bacterial Aerosols. Appl. Environ. Microbiol. **1956**, *4*, 300–306.

41. Mitchell, R.B.; Fulton, J.D.; Ellingson, H.V. A Soluble Gelatin Foam Filter for Airborne Microorganisms at Surface Levels. Am. J. Publ. Health **1954**, *44*, 1334–1339.

42. Ljungqvist, B.; Reinmüller, B. Active Sampling of Airborne Viable Particles in Controlled Environments: A Comparative Study of Common Instruments. Eur. J. Parenter. Sci. **1998**, *3* (3), 59–62.

43. CMF Only. GMF was not included in this study.

44. Ljungqvist, B.; Reinmüller, B. Hazard Analyses of Airborne Contamination in Clean Rooms: Application of a Method for Limitation of Risks. PDA J. Pharm. Sci. Technol. **1995**, *49*, 239–243.

45. Besterfield, D. *Quality Control*; Prentice-Hall, Inc.: Upper Saddle River, NJ, 1998.

46. Hyde, W. Origin of Bacteria in the Clean Room and their Growth Requirements. PDA J. Pharm. Sci. Technol. **1988**, *52* (4), 154–159.

MICROSPHERE TECHNOLOGY AND APPLICATIONS

Diane J. Burgess
University of Connecticut, Storrs, Connecticut

Anthony J. Hickey
The University of North Carolina, Chapel Hill, North Carolina

INTRODUCTION

The range of techniques for the preparation of microspheres offers a variety of opportunities to control aspects of drug administration. The term "control" includes phenomena such as protection and masking, reduced dissolution rate, facilitation of handling, and spatial targeting of the active ingredient. This approach facilitates accurate delivery of small quantities of potent drugs; reduced drug concentrations at sites other than the target organ or tissue; and protection of labile compounds before and after administration and prior to appearance at the site of action.

The characteristics of microspheres containing drug should be correlated with the required therapeutic action and are dictated by the materials and methods employed in the manufacture of the delivery systems.

The behavior of drugs in vivo can be manipulated by coupling the drug to a carrier particle. The clearance kinetics, tissue distribution, metabolism, and cellular interactions of the drug are strongly influenced by the behavior of the carrier. Exploitation of these changes in pharmacodynamic behavior may lead to enhanced therapeutic effect. However, an intelligent approach to therapeutics employing drug-carrier technology requires a detailed understanding of the carrier interaction with critical cellular and organ systems and of the limitations of the system with respect to formulation procedures and stability. A variety of agents have been used as drug carriers, including immunoglobulins, serum proteins, liposomes, microspheres, nanoparticles, microcapsules, and even cells such as erythrocytes.

Antineoplastic drugs (1–5), narcotic antagonists (6), steroid hormones (7, 8), luteinizing hormone releasing hormone analogs (9, 10), elastase (11), and other macromolecules (12) have been incorporated into microspheres. In addition, vaccines, living cells, and tissues have been encapsulated.

DEFINITION AND GENERAL DESCRIPTION

Microspheres can be defined as solid, approximately spherical particles ranging in size from 1 to 1000 μm. They are made of polymeric, waxy, or other protective materials, that is, biodegradable synthetic polymers and modified natural products such as starches, gums, proteins, fats, and waxes. The natural polymers include albumin and gelatin (13, 14); the synthetic polymers include polylactic acid and polyglycolic acid (15, 16).

The solvents used to dissolve the polymeric materials are chosen according to the polymer and drug solubilities and stabilities, process safety, and economic considerations. Substances can be incorporated within microspheres in the liquid or solid state during manufacture or subsequently by absorption. Fig. 1 shows two types of microspheres: Microcapsules, where the entrapped substance is completely surrounded by a distinct capsule wall, and micromatrices, where the entrapped substance is dispersed throughout the microsphere matrix.

Microspheres are small and have large surface-to-volume ratios. At the lower end of their size range they have colloidal properties (17). The interfacial properties of microspheres are extremely important, often dictating their activity. In fact, the principle of microsphere manufacture depends on the creation of an interfacial area, involving a polymeric material that will form an interfacial boundary and a method of cross-linking to impart permanency. The methods of manufacturing described later are by no means comprehensive and the reader should bear in mind that if the aforementioned criteria are adhered to, the only limitation to the manufacture of microspheres is the researcher's imagination.

HISTORICAL AND CONTEXTUAL PERSPECTIVE

The concept of packaging microscopic quantities of materials within microspheres dates back to the 1930s and

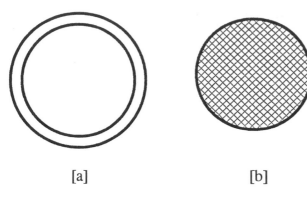

[a]   [b]

Fig. 1 Schematic diagram illustrating microspheres. (a) Microcapsule consisting of an encapsulated core particle, and (b) Micromatrix consisting of homogeneous dispersion of active ingredient in particle.

the work of Bungenberg de Jong and coworkers (18) on the entrapment of substances within coacervates. The first commercial application of encapsulation was by the National Cash Register Company for the manufacture of carbonless copying paper (19). The technology and applications have advanced over the last several decades. This technology is used by the agricultural, food, household products, medical, graphics, and cosmetics industries.

The potential use of microspheres in the pharmaceutical industry has been considered since the 1960s (20–22) for the following applications:

- Taste and odor masking
- Conversion of oils and other liquids to solids for ease of handling
- Protection of drugs against the environment (moisture, light, heat, and/or oxidation) and vice versa (prevention of pain on injection) (23)
- Delay of volatilization
- Separation of incompatible materials (other drugs or excipients such as buffers)
- Improvement of flow of powders
- Safe handling of toxic substances
- Aid in dispersion of water-insoluble substances in aqueous media, and
- Production of sustained-release, controlled-release, and targeted medications (24–27)
- Reduced dose dumping potential compared to large implantable devices

Microencapsulation has also been used medically for the encapsulation of live cells and vaccines. Biocompatibility can be improved by the encapsulation of artificial cells and biomolecules such as peptides, proteins, and

hormones (28, 29), which can prevent unwanted immunological reactions that would lead to inactivation or rejection. Microspheres are used for isolating materials until their activity is needed. The biotechnology industry employs microspheres to contain organisms and their recombinant products to aid in the isolation of these products (30).

PHARMACEUTICAL APPLICATIONS

A number of pharmaceutical microencapsulated products are currently on the market, such as aspirin, theophylline and its derivatives, vitamins, pancrelipase, antihypertensives, potassium chloride, progesterone, and contraceptive hormone combinations (31).

Microencapsulated KCl (Micro-K, R.H. Robins, Richmond, VA) is used to prevent gastrointestinal complications associated with potassium chloride. The dispersibility of the microcapsules and the controlled release of the ions minimize the possibility of local high salt concentrations, which could result in ulceration, hemorrhage, or perforation. Microspheres have also found potential applications as injection (32, 33) or inhalation (34–37) products. The number of commercially available products does not reflect the amount of research that has been carried out in this area, nor the benefits that can be achieved using this technology. Economic considerations have been a key factor in determining the number of pharmaceutical microencapsulated products. Most encapsulation processes are expensive and require significant capital investment for equipment. An exception is pan or spray coating and spray drying, since the necessary equipment may already be available within the company. An additional expense is due to the fact that most microencapsulation processes are patent protected.

OTHER APPLICATIONS

Applications of microencapsulation in other industries are numerous. The best known microencapsulated products are carbonless copying paper, photosensitive paper, microencapsulated fragrances, such as "scent-strips" (also known as "snap-n-burst"), and microencapsulated aromas ("scratch-n-sniff"). All of these products are usually prepared by gelatin–acacia complex coacervation. Scratch-n-sniff has been used in children's books and food and cosmetic aroma advertising (38). Microcapsules are also extensively used as diagnostics, for example, temperature-sensitive microcapsules for thermographic detection of tumors (39).

In the biotechnology industry microencapsulated microbial cells are being used for the production of recombinant proteins and peptides (30). The retention of the product within the microcapsule can be beneficial in the collection and isolation of the product. Encapsulation of microbial cells can also increase the cell-loading capacity and the rate of production in bioreactors. Smaller microcapsules are better for these purposes; they have a larger surface area that is important for the exchange of gases across the microcapsule membrane. Microcapsules with semipermeable membranes are being used in cell culture (40). A feline breast tumor line, which was difficult to grow in conventional culture, has been successfully grown in microcapsules (41). Microencapsulated activated charcoal has been used for hemoperfusion (29). Paramedical uses of microcapsules include bandages with microencapsulated antiinfective substances (25). A unique application of microencapsulation technology is for feeding organisms. Sea bass larvae have been fed with all-protein microcapsules or with microcapsules containing lipids to supplement their diet (42).

MICROSPHERE MANUFACTURE

The most important physicochemical characteristics that may be controlled in microsphere manufacture are:

- Particle size and distribution
- Polymer molecular weight
- Ratio of drug to polymer
- Total mass of drug and polymer

Each of these can be related to the manufacture and rate of drug release from the systems. The following discussion presents methods of manufacture of coated or encapsulated systems, referred to as microcapsules, and matrix systems containing homogeneously distributed drug, referred to as micromatrices.

Wax Coating and Hot Melt

Wax may be used to coat the core particles, encapsulating drug by dissolution or dispersion in the molten wax. The waxy solution or suspension is dispersed by high speed mixing into a cold solution, such as cold liquid paraffin. The mixture is agitated for at least one hour. The external phase (liquid paraffin) is then decanted and the microcapsules are suspended in a nonmiscible solvent, and allowed to air dry. Multiple emulsions may also be formed (43). For example,

a heated aqueous drug solution can be dispersed in molten wax to form a water-in-oil emulsion, which is emulsified in a heated external aqueous phase to form a water-in-oil-in-water emulsion. The system is cooled and the microcapsules collected. For highly aqueous soluble drugs, a nonaqueous phase can be used to prevent loss of drug to the external phase (44). Another alternative is to rapidly reduce the temperature when the primary emulsion is placed in the external aqueous phase.

Wax coated microcapsules, while inexpensive and often used, release drug more rapidly than polymeric microcapsules. Carnauba wax and beeswax can be used as the coating materials and these can be mixed in order to achieve desired characteristics (45). Wax-coated microcapsules have been successfully tableted. Small aerosol particles, 1–5 μm in diameter, have been condensation coated from a vapor of a fatty acid or paraffin wax (46, 47). These particles have been shown to exhibit reduced dissolution rates in vitro, corresponding to reduced absorption rates following deposition in the lungs of Beagle dogs.

Polyanhydrides (48) have been chosen for the preparation of microspheres because of their degradation by surface erosion into apparently nontoxic small molecules (49, 50). The mixture of polymer and active ingredient is suspended in a miscible solvent, heated 5°C above the melting point of the polymer and stirred continuously. The emulsion is stabilized by cooling below the melting point until the droplets solidify.

Spray Coating and Pan Coating

Spray coating and pan coating employ heat-jacketed coating pans in which the solid drug core particles are rotated and into which the coating material is sprayed. The core particles are in the size range of micrometers up to a few millimeters. The coating material is usually sprayed at an angle from the side into the pan. The process is continued until an even coating is completed. This is the process typically used to coat tablets and capsules.

Coating a large number of small particles may provide a safer and more consistent release pattern than coated tablets. In addition, several batches of microspheres can be prepared with different coating thicknesses and mixed to achieve specific controlled release patterns.

The Wurster process, a variation of the basic pan coating method, is an adaptation of the fluid-bed granulator (51, 52). The solid core particles are fluidized by air pressure and a spray of dissolved wall material is applied from the perforated bottom of the fluidization chamber parallel to the air stream and onto the solid core particles. Alternatively, the coating solution can be sprayed from the top or the sides into an upstream of fluidized particles. This adaptation allows the coating of small particles (53). The fluidized-bed technique produces a more uniform coating thickness than the pan-coating methodology. Problems can arise with inflammable organic solvents because of the high risk of explosion in the enclosed fluidizer chamber. Explosion proof units have been designed; however, over the past two decades aqueous coating solutions are being used more and more.

Examples of aqueous coating solutions include water-soluble low molecular weight cellulose ethers (54, 55), emulsion polymerization latexes of polymethacrylates (56), and dispersions of water-insoluble polymers such as ethylcellulose in the form of pseudolatex (57). These solvent-free coating solutions provide a range of different coatings from fast disintegrating isolating layers to enteric and sustained-release coatings. Lehmann has reviewed different commercial methods, the conditions required for coating, and various coating formulas including illustrations of the types of equipment used (58).

Coacervation

Coacervation is the simple separation of a macromolecular solution into two immiscible liquid phases, a dense coacervate phase, which is relatively concentrated in macromolecules, and a dilute equilibrium phase (18). Coacervates may be described as liquid crystals and mesophases. In the presence of only one macromolecule, this process is referred to as simple coacervation. When two or more macromolecules of opposite charge are present, it is referred to as complex coacervation (18). Simple coacervation is induced by a change in conditions, which results in dehydration of the macromolecules. This may be achieved by the addition of a nonsolvent, the addition of microions, or a temperature change, all of which promote polymer–polymer interactions over polymer–solvent interactions. Complex coacervation is driven by electrostatic interactive forces between two or more macromolecules (59).

Bungenberg de Jong et al. (60) first showed that solid particles could also be entrapped in coacervate systems. On phase separation by simple or complex methods tiny coacervate droplets are formed, which sediment or coalesce to form a separate coacervate phase. The coacervate forms around any core material that may be present, such as drug particles (Fig. 2). Agitation of the coacervate system can prevent coalescence and sedimentation of the droplets, which can be cross-linked to form stable microcapsules by addition of an agent, such as

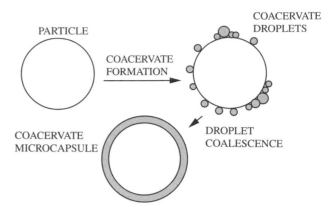

Fig. 2 Schematic diagram of the formation of a coacervate around a core material.

glutaraldehyde, or the application of heat (14, 24, 61, 62). Drug microencapsulation by coacervation has been reviewed by Madan (62) and by Nixon (24).

The large number of variables involved in complex coacervation (pH, ionic strength, macromolecule concentration, macromolecule ratio, and macromolecular weight) (18, 63) affect microcapsule production, resulting in a large number of controllable parameters. These can be manipulated to produce microcapsules with specific properties. Complex coacervate microcapsules have been formulated as suspensions or gels (64), and have been compounded within suppositories (65, 66) and tablets (66, 67).

Although many successful coacervate microencapsulation systems have been prepared, coacervate microcapsules have a number of limitations. They can be produced only at specific pH values, they require stabilization by cross-linking agents or heat, and the retention of the encapsulant depends on the extent of cross-linking. The pH limitation can be overcome to some extent by the addition of water-soluble nonionic polymers, such as polyethylene oxide or polyethylene glycol (68, 69). The presence of a small amount of these polymers allows microencapsulation to occur over an expanded pH range. For example, the pH range for coacervation of gelatin and acacia can be extended from pH 2.6–5.5 (63) to pH 2–9 (68). In addition, these polymers induce simple coacervation (68), as has been shown for macromolecules such as gelatin, carboxymethylcellulose, and ethylene–maleic anhydride copolymer. The pH range for simple coacervation is also expanded in the presence of these water-soluble nonionic polymers. For example, the pH range for simple coacervation of gelatin can be increased from only pH values close to the isoelectric point to the pH range of 5.5–9.5 (68).

Cross-linking of coacervates is necessary to stabilize coacervate emulsion droplets and hence form microcapsules. Both chemical cross-linking agents and the application of heat may be harmful to the encapsulant materials, such as thermolabile and chemically labile drugs and live cells. A stable coacervate system, formed without the use of chemical cross-linking agents or the application of heat, has been developed by Burgess and Singh (70, 71). This system is potentially useful for the delivery of protein and polypeptide drugs and other materials unable to withstand cross-linking procedures.

Calcium Alginate Microcapsules

Dropping or spraying a sodium alginate solution into a calcium chloride solution produces microcapsules. The divalent calcium ions cross-link the alginate, forming gelled droplets. These gel droplets can be permanently cross-linked by addition to a polylysine solution. Lim and Sun (72) developed this method for the encapsulation of live cells. Variations on this method with different polymers have been developed. Chitosan is a preferred polymer, because it has a better biocompatibility than alginate (73). Traditionally alginate beads were formed by dropping the alginate solution into the calcium chloride with a fine-bore pipette. However, the droplets were relatively large, because the drops do not fall until they reach a critical mass. Smaller droplets can be formed by using a pump to force the alginate through the pipette (72), a vibration system to help remove the drops from the end of the pipette (72), and an air atomization method (74).

Spray Drying

Spray drying is a single-step, closed-system process applicable to a wide variety of materials, including heat-sensitive materials. This process is often used commercially since the necessary equipment is frequently available at the manufacturing site. As a closed system, it is ideal for good manufacturing practice and the production of sterile materials. The drug and the polymer coating materials are dissolved in a suitable solvent (aqueous or nonaqueous) or the drug may be present as a suspension in the polymer solution. Alternatively, it may be dissolved or suspended within an emulsion or coacervate system. For example, biodegradable polylactide microcapsules can be prepared by dissolving the drug and polymer in methylene chloride (75). Methylcellulose and sodium carboxymethylcellulose spray-dried microspheres are prepared

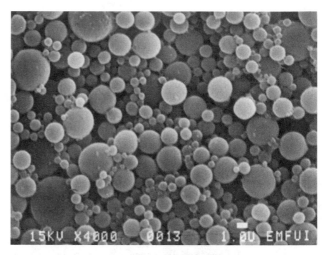

Fig. 3 Scanning electron micrograph of polylactic acid microspheres containing phenolphthalein prepared by the solvent evaporation method (77). Magnification × 4000.

by dissolving the polymers in aqueous systems. The microsphere size is controlled by the rate of spraying, the feed rate of the polymer drug solution, the nozzle size, the temperature in the drying and collecting chambers, and the size of these two chambers. The quality of spray-dried products is improved by the addition of plasticizers (76) that promote polymer coalescence and film formation and enhance the formation of spherical and smooth-surfaced microcapsules.

Solvent evaporation

This is one of the earliest methods of microsphere manufacture. The polymer and drug must be soluble in an organic solvent, frequently methylene chloride. The solution containing the polymer and the drug may be dispersed in an aqueous phase to form droplets. Continuous mixing and elevated temperatures may be employed to evaporate the more volatile organic solvent and leave the solid polymer–drug particles suspended in an aqueous medium. The particles are finally filtered from the suspension. Fig. 3 shows polylactic acid particles prepared in this manner (77).

Precipitation

Precipitation is a variation on the evaporation method. The emulsion consists of polar droplets dispersed in a nonpolar medium (78). Solvent may be removed from the droplets by the use of a cosolvent. The resulting increase in the polymer drug concentration causes precipitation forming a suspension of microspheres.

Freeze Drying

This technique involves the freezing of the emulsion (78); the relative freezing points of the continuous and dispersed phases are important. The continuous-phase solvent is usually organic and is removed by sublimation at low temperature and pressure. Finally, the dispersed phase solvent of the droplets is removed by sublimation, leaving polymer-drug particles.

Chemical and Thermal Cross-Linking

Microspheres made from natural polymers are prepared by a cross-linking process; polymers include gelatin, albumin, starch, and dextran. A water–oil emulsion is prepared, where the water phase is a solution of the polymer that contains the drug to be incorporated. The oil phase is a suitable vegetable oil or oil-organic solvent mixture containing an oil-soluble emulsifier. Once the desired water–oil emulsion is formed, the water soluble polymer is solidified by some kind of cross-linking process. This may involve thermal treatment (79) or the addition of a chemical cross-linking agent such as glutaraldehyde to form a stable chemical cross-link as in albumin (80). If chemical or heat cross-linking is used, the amount of chemical and the period and intensity of heating are critical in determining the release rates and swelling properties of the microspheres (79). If glutaraldehyde is the cross-linking agent, residual amounts can have toxic effects.

NANOPARTICLES

Nanoparticles, 10–1000 nm polymeric particles, are prepared from the same natural and synthetic biodegradable polymers as microspheres (81–83). Albumin nanoparticles are prepared by the cross-linking processes mentioned previously. For the preparation of particles from synthetic polymers, heterogeneous bulk polymerization techniques of suspension, emulsion, and micelle polymerization are often used.

Suspension polymerization of water-insoluble liquid monomer and drug may be achieved by agitating a dispersion of droplets, 10–1000 nm in diameter, in a continuous aqueous phase (84). The temperature must be carefully controlled. An initiator is frequently employed to increase the reaction rate in the droplets, and the aqueous phase may contain stabilizers to prevent coalescence and thickening agents to increase the viscosity. The polymer is formed by reaction of the functional groups of the monomer. This process has the advantage that the continuous phase absorbs the heat of the polymerization reaction and minimizes the temperature change within the droplets. However, aggregation of the particles may arise as the polymer molecules in suspended particles coalesce. Unfortunately, it is difficult to eliminate stabilizers and additives, used to prevent coalescence, from the final product.

Emulsion polymerization involves the dispersion of the monomer liquid in an aqueous phase to form droplets, 0.05–5 nm in diameter (85–88). An initiator and a surfactant, in a concentration higher than its critical micelle concentration, are present in the aqueous phase. Excess surfactant molecules form micelles whose hydrophobic interiors take up part of the available monomer, causing them to swell. Initiator radicals diffuse into these swollen micelles and begin the polymerization process. As the monomer is consumed, it is replaced by progressive diffusion of the remaining monomer from its location in the emulsified droplets to the interior of the micelles. The micelles continue to swell in size as polymerization proceeds. The enlarging surfaces compete for available surfactant, thus influencing the number of available micelles that can participate in the polymer formation. This method yields particles of very small size and predictable number at low temperatures. However, the particles usually have a high concentration of associated monomer, which may be toxic.

Micelle polymerization differs from emulsion polymerization in that all of the monomer and the drug is contained within micelles composed of surfactant. Diffusion of the monomer from the micelles is prevented by the nonsolvent properties of the outer phase. Therefore, the increase in particle size is negligible as the polymerization proceeds.

CHARACTERIZATION

Materials

The polymer employed to prepare microspheres must be characterized in terms of molecular weight and purity (89, 89–91), however this topic is beyond the scope of this article. Characterization of the materials may have implications for the formation of the microspheres. The viscosity and film-forming properties of the polymers used should be known. Viscosity can affect the tendency to form microspheres, their size, and even their shape. Burgess and coworkers (70, 92) have shown that albumin–acacia coacervates do not form microcapsules under certain conditions of pH and ionic strength, if the viscosity of the coacervate phase is too high. Burgess and Carless (63) developed a method to predict the optimum conditions for complex coacervation based on the charge carried by the two polymers involved.

Microspheres

Size characterization may be conducted by various methods including light microscopy, resistance blockage techniques (Coulter analysis), light blockage techniques, light scattering, laser diffraction analysis, and for particles less than 1 μm, photon correlation spectroscopy. Electron microscopy, scanning electron microscopy, and scanning tunneling microscopy are used for surface characterization of microspheres. Fourier transform Raman spectroscopy or X-ray photoelectron spectroscopy may be used to determine if any of the material which should have been entrapped is present on the surface and if any other contaminants are present (93, 94). Other surface characterization techniques include surface charge analysis using microelectrophoresis. Surface charge can provide information regarding microsphere aggregation (14, 95). Surface charge is an important parameter with respect to the interaction of microspheres within the body (96).

Surface forces are important in the entrapment, wetting, and adhesion of core material by the coating material. The wettability of solids by different liquids is usually assessed by contact-angle measurement (97, 98). When wetting of the core material is poor, it is difficult or impossible to form microcapsules. For example, Eudragit RS dissolved in THF-cyclohexane failed to encapsulate charcoal particles but was successful in ecapsulating potassium dichromate (99, 100). The surface hydrophobicity of oil droplets has been shown to affect their uptake into complex coacervate droplets (101). Oil uptake was directly related to the hydrophile–lipophile balance (HLB) value at the droplet interface. Additives, such as surfactants, which alter surface properties were shown to affect the uptake of core materials.

Biological Distribution

The disposition of microspheres upon entry to the body has been studied extensively. They are frequently labeled with a radionuclide to allow study by scintillation counting or scintigraphy (23). This work has largely focused on tissue distribution as a function of particle size, with the conclusion that particles below 7 μm tend to locate predominantly in the reticuloendothelial system of the liver, whereas particles 7–15 μm in size tend to be collected in the capillary system of the lung (77). The

acute toxicity (102), tissue interaction (103–105), cell interaction (106–108), and protein interaction (109) of various microspheres have been investigated. These studies demonstrated that the toxicity of microspheres is related to the number and size administered. Initial inflammatory responses to the administration of microspheres were consistent with observations that phagocytosis by neutrophils and macrophages may occur. The extent and nature of the cell and tissue affects of microspheres may be related to the surface characteristics of the polymer employed and to the particle size. For example, fibrinogen has been shown to associate with poly-DL-lactide microcapsules, affecting the surface-charge characteristics (104). This phenomenon is related to the hydrophobic nature of the surface. Indeed, hydrophilic coatings can reduce the uptake of microspheres by the liver and peritoneal macrophages (110–112).

THERAPEUTIC APPLICATIONS

Targeting

Drugs can be targeted to specific sites in the body using microspheres and other colloidal carrier systems. Targeting by colloid delivery systems is dealt with elsewhere in this encyclopedia (17). Targeting by microspheres may be passive, active, diversional, or physical. In passive targeting the microspheres follow their natural distribution in the body (which depends on particle size, shape, surface characteristics, particle deformation, and route of administration). In active targeting the natural distribution of the microspheres is altered (for example, by attachment of site-specific vectoring agents such as monoclonal antibodies and lectins). Diversional targeting means blocking the natural distribution of the microspheres, for example, partly or completely impairing the cells of the reticuloendothelial system, which would otherwise take up the microspheres. Physical targeting involves an external influence, such as a change in temperature or a magnetic field to direct the microspheres to the desired site.

Degrees of targeting can be achieved by localization of the drug to a specific area in the body, to a particular organ in the body (for example, the lungs), to a particular group of cells within the body (for example, the Kupffer cells), and even to intracellular structures (such as the lysosomes or the cell nucleus). The problems associated with directing microspheres to specific areas in the body following parenteral administration are discussed in the article Colloids and Colloid Drug Delivery in this encyclopedia (17).

Oral targeting can be achieved using microspheres; those less than 10 μm in diameter have been shown to target the Peyer's patch (113). Microspheres less than 5 μm were shown to be transported through the lymphatics within macrophages and those larger than 5 μm remained in the Peyer's patch (113). Toxoid vaccine microcapsules were effectively delivered and released in the gut-associated lymphoid tissue following oral administration (114).

Controlled Release

The rate of drug release from microspheres dictates their therapeutic action. Release is governed by the molecular structure of the drug and polymer, the resistance of the polymer to degradation, and the surface area and porosity of the microspheres (16, 115, 116). Reservoir delivery systems extend the residence time of drug within the systemic circulation and were originally focused on zero-order dissolution kinetics. This mathematical expression describes a linear relationship between rate of appearance in plasma and time. Ideally, the plasma drug concentration is independent of time for most of the dissolution period and is optimally maintained in the therapeutic window.

In nonporous polymeric systems the rate of drug release is dictated by the device surface area which is linked directly to its shape. Drug release from polymeric systems with a variety of geometries has been described (117). Zero-order release kinetics may be more easily achieved with slab or rod geometries than spheres. The rate of release from spheres may result from polymer diffusion or erosion (116, 118, 119). Diffusion-mediated release has been studied extensively and described mathematically (120, 121).

The internal structure of microspheres may vary as a function of the microencapsulation process employed (122). Reservoir microcapsules have a core of drug coated with a polymer. The drug is distributed homogeneously throughout the polymeric matrix in monolithic microspheres.

Controlled drug release from microspheres occurs by diffusion of drug through a polymeric excipient, diffusion of entrapped drug as the polymer erodes, and release of drug through pores in the polymeric microspheres. If the drug is released by diffusion through the polymer without erosion, the release depends on the surface area of the microspheres and the path length of the drug in transit to the surrounding environment. For example, increasing the surface area, by reducing particle size, results in an increased release rate. The path length of motion for the drug in the matrix can be controlled by manipulating the microsphere loading. Microspheres with a high drug content release the active ingredient more rapidly than those with a low load. Physicochemical properties of the drug and excipient such as permeability of one in the other, identity of the polymer, degree of crystallinity, inclusion of plasticizers and fillers, and thickness of the polymer influence the drug release rate.

Release from reservoir microcapsules

The factors affecting drug release may be elucidated by a study of drug release from the simplest system, a reservoir microcapsule. Diffusion of drug through such a structure may involve transport not only through an isotropic medium, such as the drug in solution, but also through a polymeric membrane. Transport of drug through such a membrane involves dissolution of the drug in the polymer at the high-concentration side of the membrane interface and diffusion across the membrane in the direction of decreasing concentration. In addition, the concentration difference across the membrane, which is taken as the driving force for drug transport, tends to decrease as the solubility of the drug on the upstream side of the membrane decreases. Therefore, the dissolution rate of poorly soluble drugs can be an important factor in limiting drug release.

Consider a spherical reservoir device where the thermodynamic activity of the core material is maintained constant within the device, and the coating is inert, homogeneous, and of uniform thickness. The steady-state release rate derived from Fick's law is

$$\frac{dM}{dt} = 4\,DKC\,\frac{r_o\,r_i}{r_o - r_i} \tag{1}$$

where r_o and r_i are the outside and inside radii, respectively, D is the diffusion coefficient of the drug molecule, K is the partition coefficient, and C is the concentration difference between either side of the coating. Assuming all parameters on the right side of Eq. 1 remain constant, consistent with no change in activity of the core material, C does not change. Integration of Eq. 1 over a finite period of the steady state would indicate that the drug release was zero-order. This is explained by the pathlength and surface area remaining constant since the membrane the drug has to traverse is of uniform thickness. If, however, the thermodynamic activity of the core material does not remain constant, then release is first-order.

It may be necessary to consider the effect of a boundary layer on the release rate. A boundary layer of appreciable drug concentration on the surface of the device would hinder drug release by diffusion. The effect of the layer is more marked with drugs of low solubility and with microparticles having irregular surfaces. From this simple example, it can be seen that various factors affect the release rate from reservoir microcapsules.

Release from monolithic micromatrices

In a monolithic microsphere the path length does not remain constant, since the drug in the center has a longer path to travel than the drug near the surface, and therefore the rate of release decreases exponentially with time.

Nevertheless, monolithic microspheres can be made to release drug at an approximately constant rate (117, 123). The core loading of these microspheres may be increased to create structures similar to those of reservoir microcapsules. An optimum combination of particle sizes (a size distribution), may be prepared to achieve a constant rate of drug release. Preparing microspheres with an erodible polymer in such a way that maximum erosion occurs in conjunction with minimum diffusion may establish a constant release rate. Although the principles described here appear simple, they are difficult to utilize because of their dependence on a number of factors, each of which can complicate the process.

Live-Cell Encapsulation

Microcapsules have been investigated as potential artificial cells [first demonstrated by Chang in 1964 (124)] and as a means to immobilize live cells (72). Potential medical applications of artificial cells have been investigated such as artificial liver, artificial kidney, and red blood cell substitutes. The encapsulation of living cells has been investigated as a means to transplant tissues without immune rejection. The capsule membrane must be semipermeable in order to be impermeable to high molecular weight antibodies, which would cause rejection or destruction of the transplanted cells, but be permeable to lower molecular weight species such as oxygen, nutrients, and internally generated therapeutic agents (for example, hormones such as insulin). The encapsulation process must not be harmful to the cells and therefore must not involve harsh conditions, such as those caused by the use of organic solvents and heat during processing. The finished microcapsules must be sterile, stable, and biocompatible. The encapsulation of mammalian cells is more difficult than that of microbial cells since their membranes are more fragile, and these must be preserved during encapsulation. The temperature, pH, ionic strength, and toxicity of solvent and reagent must be carefully controlled. A common method of microencapsulating live cells is to entrap the cells in a protective gel and form a permanent membrane around the gel droplets. A calcium alginate gel method was developed by Lim and Sun (72), has been successfully

applied to mammalian cells. A microencapsulation system combining the easy setting characteristics of alginate and the stability and biocompatibility of hydrogel polymers has been devised (125, 126); it involves an alginate-HEMA graft copolymer.

Immobilized islets of Langerhans are able to respond to external glucose concentrations and release insulin into the systemic circulation (72). A number of animal studies have shown that alginate-polylysine encapsulated pancreatic islets were successful in correcting the diabetic state in rats for periods of two to three weeks (127).

Immobilized cells are also used in biotechnology in the production of protein molecules. For example, entrapped hybridoma cells have been used for the production of monoclonal antibodies (30) which are secreted into the microcapsules. This allows for easier collection of the antibodies compared to growing the hybridoma cells directly in the culture medium. The microcapsules are easily separated from the culture medium and broken to collect the antibodies. Isolation of the antibodies from the culture medium involves numerous purification steps, and product is lost during each of these steps to an extent which depends on the efficiency of the process. Live vaccines have been encapsulated. For example. *Bacillus Calmette Guerin* has been encapsulated in an alginate polylysine-alginate system (74).

STERILIZATION

Microspheres that are administered parenterally must be sterile. Sterilization is usually achieved by aseptic processing. The final product may not be able to undergo terminal sterilization, which may be detrimental to the delivery system, altering the release pattern or destroying the targeting properties. In addition, the entrapped drug or biological substance may not be able to withstand the heat of sterilization. Although the exterior of the microspheres can be investigated for sterility by conventional plating methodology, it is difficult to determine whether the interiors of the microspheres are free from contamination. The microspheres can be broken, although this introduces the possibility of false positive or false negative results. A method has been developed whereby the presence of viable organisms in the interior of microsphere systems can be determined without breaking the microcapsules using a detection method for organism metabolism (128).

Sterilization is one of many aspects that must be addressed when considering microspheres for commercial purposes (129). The development of a product is achieved most effectively by parallel approaches to formulation and process design. Very little has been published with regard to industrial-scale manufacturing of microspheres for the delivery of pharmaceuticals.

REFERENCES

1. Fujimoto, S.; Miyazaki, M.; Endoh, F.; Takahashi, O.; Shrestha, R.D.; Okui, K.; Mori-moto, Y.; Terao, K. Cancer **1985**, *55*, 522–526.
2. Gupta, P.K.; Hung, C.T.; Perrier, D.G. Int. J. Pharm. **1986**, *33*, 137–146.
3. Gupta, P.K.; Hung, C.T.; Perrier, D.G. Int. J. Pharm. **1986**, *33*, 147–153.
4. Gupta, P.K.; Lam, F.C.; Hung, C.T. Int. J. Pharm. **1989**, *51*, 253–258.
5. Jones, C.; Burton, M.A.; Gray, B.N. J. Pharm. Pharmacol. **1989**, *41*, 813–816.
6. Schwope, A.D.; Wise, D.L.; Howes, J.F. Life Sci. **1968**, *17*, 1877–1886.
7. Gardner, D.L.; Patanus, A.J.; Fink, D.J. Steroid Release from Microcapsules. *Drug Delivery Systems*; Gabelnick, H.L., Ed.; DHEW Publ. No. (NIH), 77–1238. Department of Health, Education, and Welfare: Washington, 1977; 265–278.
8. Anderson, L.C.; Wise, D.L.; Howes, J.F. Contraception **1976**, *13*, 375–384.
9. Kent J.S.; Lewis D.H.; Sanders L.M.; Tice T.S. U.S. Patent 4,675,189 June 23, 1987.
10. Sanders, L.M.; Kent, J.S.; McRae, G.l.; Vickery, B.H.; Tice, T.R.; Lewis, D.H. J. Pharm. Sci. **1984**, *73*, 1294–1297.
11. Martodam, R.R.; Twumasi, D.Y.; Liener, l.E.; Powers, J.C.; Nishino, N.; Krejcarek, G. Proc. Natl. Acad. Sci. **1979**, *76*, 2128–2132.
12. Rhine, W.D.; Hsieh, D.S.T.; Langer, R. J. Pharm. Sci. **1980**, *69*, 265–270.
13. Yapel A.P. U.S. Patent, 4,147,767 Apr. 3., 1979.
14. Burgess, D.J.; Carless, J.E. Int. J. Pharm. **1986**, *32*, 207–212.
15. Redmon, M.P.; Hickey, A.J.; DeLuca, P.P. J. Contr. Rel. **1989**, *9*, 99–109.
16. Lzumikawa, S.; Yoshioka, S.; Aso, Y.; Takeda, J. J. Contr. Rel. **1991**, *15*, 133–140.
17. Burgess, D.J. Colloids and Colloid Drug Delivery Systems. *Encyclopedia of Pharmaceutical Technology*; Swarbrick, J., Boylan, J.C., Eds.; Marcel Dekker, Inc.: New York, 1990; 3, 31–63.
18. Bungenberg de Jong, H.G. Reversible Systems. *Colloid Science*; Kruyt, H.G., Ed.; Elsevier: New York, 1949; II, 335–432.
19. Green B.K.; Schleicher L. U.S. Patent, 2,800,458 1957.
20. Khalil, S.A.H.; Nixon, J.R.; Carless, J.E. J. Pharm. Pharmacol. **1968**, *20*, 215–225.
21. Luzzi, L.A.; Gerraughty, R.J. J. Pharm. Sci. **1964**, *53*, 429–431.
22. Phares, R.E.; Sperandio, G.J. J. Pharm. Sci. **1964**, *53*, 515–518.
23. Zhou, S.; Hickey, A.J.; Jay, M.; Warren, S.M.; Lord, M.; DeLuca, P.P. Pharm. Res. **1988**, *5*, S76.
24. Nixon, J.R. *Microencapsulation*; Marcel Dekker, Inc.: New York, 1976.
25. Gutcho, M.H. *Microcapsules and Other Capsules, Advanced Since 1975*; Noyes Data Corp.: Park Ridge, NJ, 1979.
26. Lim, F. *Biomedical Applications of Microencapsulation*; CRC Press Inc.: Boca Raton, FL, 1984.
27. Kondo, T. *Microencapsulation: New Techniques and Applications*; Techno Books: Tokyo, 1979.
28. Chang, T.M.S. *Artificial Liver and Artifical Cells*; Plenum Press: New York, 1978.
29. Chang, T.M.S. *Biomedical Applications of Microencapsulation*; Lim, F., Ed.; CRC Press: Boca Raton, FL, 1984; 85.
30. Jarvis, A.P.; Spriggs, T.A.; Chigura, W.R. In Vitro **1982**, *18*, 276.
31. Donbrow, M. *Microcapsules and Nanoparticles in Medicine and Pharmacy*; Donbrow, M., Ed.; CRC Press: London, 1991; 1–14.
32. Kissel, T.; Demirdere, A. *Controlled Drug Delivery*; Müller, B.W., Ed.; Wissen-Schaftliche Verlagsge-Sellschaft mbH: Stuttgart, 1984; 103–131.
33. Gurney, R.; Peppas, N.A.; Harrington, D.D.; Banks, G.S. Drug Dev. Ind. Pharm. **1981**, *7*, 1–25.
34. Gupta, P.K.; Hickey, A.J. J. Contr. Rel. **1991**, *17*, 129–148.
35. Masinde, L.E.; Hickey, A.J. Pharm. Res. **1991**, *8*, S120.
36. Masinde, L.E.; Hickey, A.J. Int. J. Pharm. *in press.*
37. Gupta, P.K.; Hickey, A.J.; Mehta, R.; DeLuca, P.P. Pharm. Res. **1990**, *7*, S82.
38. Versic, R.J. Drug Cosm. Ind. **1989**, *144*(6), 30, 32, 34, 75.
39. Maggi, G.C.; Di Roberto, F.M. *Microencapsulation*; Nixon, J.R., Ed.; Marcel Dekker, Inc.: New York, 1976; 103–111.
40. Lim, F.; Buchler, R.J. *Methods in Enzymology*; Langome, J.J., Van Vunakis, H., Eds.; Academic Press: New York, 1981; 73.
41. Lim, F. Adv. Biotechnol. Progr. **1988**, *7*, 185–197.
42. Walford, J.; Lim, T.M.; Lam, T.J. Aquaculture **1991**, *92*, 225–235.
43. Bodmeier, R.; Wang, J.; Bhagwatwar, H. J. Microencaps. **1992**, *9*, 99–107.
44. Benita, S.; Zonai, O.; Benoit, J.-P. J. Pharm. Sci. **1986**, *75*, 847–851.
45. Bodmeier, R.; Wang, J.; Bhagwaywar, H. J. Microencaps. **1992**, *9*, 89–98.
46. Hickey, A.J.; Fults, K.; Pillai, R.S. J. Biopharm. Sci. **1992**, *3*, 107–113.
47. Pillai, R.S.; Yeates, D.B.; Miller, 1.F.; Hickey, A.J. Proceed. Intern. Symp. Contr. Rel. Bioact. Mater. **1992**, *19*, 224–225.
48. Conix, A. Macromol. Synth. **1966**, *2*, 95–98.
49. Leong, K.W.; Brott, B.C.; Langer, R. J. Biomed. Mater. Res. **1985**, *19*, 945–955.
50. Mathiowitz, E.; Langer, R. J. Contr. Rel. **1987**, *5*, 13–22.
51. Wurster D.E. US Patent 2,648,609 1949.
52. Wurster, D.E. J. Am. Pharm. Assoc. Sci. Ed. **1959**, *48*, 451–454.
53. Robinson, N.J.; Gross, G.M.; Lantz, R.J. J. Pharm. Sci. **1968**, *57*, 1983–1988.
54. Porter, St.C. Pharm. Technol. **1979**, *3*, 54–59.
55. Porter, St.C. Pharm. Technol. **1980**, *4*, 66–75.

56. Lehmann, K.; Dreher, D. Pharm. Ind. **1972**, *34*, 894–903.
57. Banker, G.S. Pharm. Technol. **1981**, *5*, 54–62.
58. Lehmann, K. *Microcapsules and Nanoparticles in Medicine and Pharmacy*; Donbrow, M., Ed.; CRC Press: London, 1991; 73–97.
59. Burgess, D.J. J. Coll. Interface Sci. **1990**, *140*, 227–238.
60. Bungenberg de Jong, H.G.; Kruyt, H.R.; Lens, J. Kolloidchem. Beih. **1932**, *36*, 429–434.
61. Nixon, J.R.; Nouh, A. J. Pharm. Pharmacol. **1978**, *30*, 533–537.
62. Madan, P.L. Drug Dev. Ind. Pharm. **1978**, *4*(95).
63. Burgess, D.J.; Carless, J.E. J. Coil. Interface Sci. **1984**, *98*, 1–8.
64. Calanchi, M. *Microencapsulation*; Nixon, J.R., Ed.; Marcel Dekker, Inc.: New York, 1976; 93–101.
65. Urmeda, T.; Matsuzawa, A.; Yokoyama, T.; Kuroda, K.; Kuroda, T. Chem., Pharm. Bull. **1983**, *31*, 2793–2798.
66. Nakajima, T.; Takashima, Y.; Ilida, K.; Mitsuta, H.; Koishi, M. Chem. Pharm. Bull. **1987**, *35*, 1201–1206.
67. de Sabata, V. *Microencapsulation*; Nixon, J.R., Ed.; Marcel Dekker, Inc.: New York, 1976; 143–162.
68. Jizomoto, H. J. Pharm. Sci. **1984**, *73*, 879–882.
69. Jizomoto, H. J. Pharm. Sci. **1985**, *74*, 469–472.
70. Burgess, D.J.; Singh, O.N. J. Pharm. Pharmacol. **1993**, *45*, 586–591.
71. Singh, O.N.; Burgess, D.J. Pharm. Res. **1972**, *9*(S8).
72. Lim, F.; Sun, A.M. Science **1980**, *210*, 908–910.
73. Rha C.K.; Rodrigues-Sanches D. US Patent. 4,749,620, 1980.
74. Kwok, K.K.; Groves, M.J.; Burgess, D.J. Pharm. Res. **1991**, *8*, 341–344.
75. Bodmeier, R.; Chen, H. J. Pharm. Pharmacol. **1988**, *40*, 754–757.
76. Wan, L.S.C.; Heng, P.W.S.; Chia, C.G.H. J. Microencaps. **1992**, *9*, 53–62.
77. Hickey, A.J.; Tian, Y.; Parasrampuria, D.; Kanke, M. Biopharmaceut. Drug Dispos. **1933**, *14*, 181–186.
78. DeLuca, P.P.; Hickey, A.J.; Hazrati, A.M.; Wedlund, P.; Rypacek, F.; Kanke, M. *Topics in Pharmaceutical Sciences*; Breimer, D.D., Speiser, P., Eds.; Elsevier: New York, 1987; 429–442.
79. Burgess, D.J.; Davis, S.S.; Tomlinson, E. Int. J. Pharm. **1987**, *39*, 129–136.
80. Burgess, D.J.; Davis, S.S. Int. J. Pharm. **1988**, *46*, 69–76.
81. Couvreur, P.; Kante, B.; Lenaerts, V.; Scailteur, V.; Roland, M.; Speister, P. J. Pharm.Sci. **1980**, *69*, 199–202.
82. Couvreur, P.; Tulkens, P.; Roland, M.; Trouet, A.; Speiser, P. FEBS Letters **1977**, *84*, 323–326.
83. Couvreur, P.; Kante, B.; Roland, M.; Guiot, P.; Bauduin, P.; Speiser, P. J. Pharm. Pharmacol. **1979**, *31*(331).
84. Seymour, R.B.; Carraher, C.E. *Polymer Chemistry*; Marcel Dekker, Inc.: New York, 1988; 332–342.
85. Seymour, R.B. *Introduction to Polymer Chemistry*; McGraw-Hill: New York, 1971.
86. Harkins, W.D. J. Am. Chem. Soc. **1947**, *69*, 1429–1444.
87. Harkins, W.D. J. Polymer Sci. **1950**, *5*, 217–251.
88. Smith, W.V.; Ewart, R.H. J. Chem. Phys. **1948**, *16*, 592–599.
89. Kotliar, A.M.; McDonnell, M.E.; Walsh, E.K. *A Guide to Materials Characterization and Chemical Analysis*; Sibilia, J.P., Ed.; VCH Publishers, Inc.: New York, 1988; 229–249.
90. Hanrahan, J.M.; Gabriel, M.K.; Williams, R.J.; McDonnell, M.E. *A Guide to Materials Characterization and Chemical Analysis*; Sibilia, J.P., Ed.; VCH Publishers, Inc.: New York, 1988; 81–84.
91. Seymour, R.B.; Carraher, C.E. *Polymer Chemistry, An Introduction,* 2nd Ed.; Marcel Dekker, Inc.: New York, 1988; 156–169.
92. Burgess, D.J.; Kwok, K.K.; Megremis, P.T. J. Pharm. Pharmacol. **1991**, *43*, 232–236.
93. Binns, J.S.; Mella, C.D.; Davies, M.C. Proceed. Intern. Symp. Contr. Rel. Bioact. Mater. **1990**, *17*, 150–151.
94. Davies, M.C.; Lynn, R.A.P.; Khan, M.A.; Paul, A.; Domb, A.; Langer, R. Proceed. Intern. Symp. Contr. Rel. Bioact. Mater. **1990**, *17*, 232–233.
95. Labhasetwar, V.D.; Doric, A.K. J. Microencaps. **1991**, *8*, 83–85.
96. Tabata, Y.; Ikada, Y. Biomaterials **1988**, *9*, 356–362.
97. Wake, W.C. *Adhesion and the Formulation of Adhesives*; Applied Science: New York, 1982.
98. Kinlock, A.J. *Adhesion and Adhesives: Science and Technology*; Chapman and Hall: London, 1987.
99. Benita, S.; Hoffman, A.; Donbrow, M. J. Microencaps. **1985**, *2*, 207–215.
100. Donbrow, M.; Hoffman, A.; Benita, S. J. Microencaps. **1990**, *7*, 1–9.
101. Rabisková, M.; Opawale, F.O.; Burgess, D.J. Pharm. Res. **1991**, *9*, S-149.
102. Yokel, R.A.; Sabo, J.P.; Simmons, G.H.; DeLuca, P.P. Toxicol. Letters **1981**, *9*, 165–170.
103. Schoen, F.J.; Kintanar, E.B.; Osol, R.G.; Lee, E. J. Biomed. Mater. Res. **1986**, *20*, 709–721.
104. Vissher, G.E.; Robison, R.L.; Maulding, H.V.; Fong, J.W.; Pearson, J.E.; Argentieri, G.J. J. Biomed. Mater. Res. **1986**, *20*, 667–676.
105. Willmott, N.; Cummings, J. Biochem. Pharmacol. **1987**, *36*, 521–526.
106. Kanke, M.; Morlier, E.; Geissler, R.; Powell, D.; Kaplan, A.; DeLuca, P.P. J. Parent.Sci. Technol. **1986**, *40*, 114–18.
107. Scheffel, U.; Rhodes, B.A.; Natarajan, T.K.; Wagner, H.N. J. Nud. Mod. **1972**, *13*, 498–503.
108. Simon, S.I.; Schmid-Schonbein, G.W. Biophys. J. **1988**, *3*, 163–173.
109. Rolland, A.; Begue, J.-M.; Le Verge, R.; Guillouzo, A. Int. J. Pharm. **1989**, *53*, 67–73.
110. Makino, K.; Ohshima, H.; Kondo, T. J. Coil. Interf. Sci. **1987**, *115*, 65–72.
111. Illum, L.; Hunneyball, I.M.; Davis, S.S. Int. J. Pharm. **1986**, *29*, 53–65.
112. Illum, L.; Davis, S.S. J. Pharm. Sci. **1983**, *72*, 1086–1089.
113. Jani, P.; Florence, A.T.; Halbert, G.W.; Langridge, J. J. Pharm. Pharmacol. **1989**, *41*, 47.
114. Ritger, P.L.; Peppas, N.A. J. Contr. Rel. **1987**, *5*, 23–36.
115. Pitt, C.G.; Schindler, A. *Controlled Drug Delivery*; Bruck, S.D., Ed.; CRC Press: Boca Raton, FL, 1983; I, 53–80.
116. Pitt, C.G.; Gu, Z.-W. J. Contr. Rel. **1987**, *4*, 282–292.
117. Cheung, W.K.; Yakobi, A.; Silber, B.M. J. Contr. Rel. **1988**, *6*, 263–270.
118. Carstensen, J.T. *Controlled Drug Delivery*; Müller, B.W., Ed.; Wissenschaftliche Verlagsgesellschaft mbH: Stuttgart, 1984; 132–145.

119. Crank, J. *The Mechanics of Diffusion*, 2nd Ed.; Oxford Science Publications: Oxford, 1975.

120. Singh, S.K.; Fox, R.O.; Fan, L.T. Proceed. Intern. Symp. Contr. Rel. Bioact. Mater. **1987**, *14*, 65–66.

121. Redmon, M.P. *Physicochemical Characteristics of a Porous Polymer Matrix for Drug Delivery*; Ph.D. Thesis University of Kentucky: Lexington, KY, 1989.

122. Brannon-Peppas, L. Design and Mathematical Analysis of Controlled Release from Microsphere-Containing Polymeric Implants. J. Contr. Rel. **1992**, *20*, 201–207.

123. Chang, T.M.S. Science **1964**, *146*, 525–525.

124. Sefton, M.V.; Dawson, R.M.; Broughton, R.L.; Biysnink, J.; Sugamori, M.E. Biotechnol. Bioeng. **1987**, *29*, 1135–1143.

125. Lamberti, F.V.; Sefton, M.V. Biochim. Biophys. Acta. **1983**, *759*, 81–91.

126. Sun, A.M.; O'Shea, G.M.; Leung, Y. Artif. Organs **1983**, *5* (Suppl.), 69.

127. Sun, A.M.; O'Shea, G.M.; Goosen, M.F.A. Appl. Biochem. Biotechnol. **1984**, *10*, 87–100.

128. Kwok, K.K.; Burgess, D.J. Pharm. Res. **1992**, *9*, 410–413.

129. Floy, B.J.; Visor, G.C.; Sanders, L.M. Polymeric Delivery System: Properties and Applications. *ACS Symposium Series*; EI-Nokali, M.A., Piatt, D.N., Sharpentier, B.A., Eds.; American Chemical Society: Washington, DC, 1993; 520, 154–167.

130. Davis, S.S.; Illum, L.; McVie, J.G.; Tomlinson, E. *Microspheres and Drug Therapy: Pharmaceutical and Medical Aspects*; Elsevier: Amsterdam, 1984.

131. Donbrow, M. *Microcapsules and Nanoparticles in Medicine and Pharmacy*; CRC Press: London, 1991.

132. Goosen, M.F.A. *Fundamentals of Animal Cell Encapsulation and Immobilization*; CRC Press: London, 1992.

133. Guiot, P.; Couvreur, P. *Polymeric Nanoparticles and Microspheres*; CRC Press: Boca Raton, FL, 1986.

134. Gutcho, M.H. *Microcapsules and Other Capsules, Advanced Since 1975*; Noyes Data Corp.: Park Ridge, NJ, 1979.

135. Illum, L.; Davis, S.S. *Polymers in Controlled Drug Delivery*; Wright: Bristol, UK, 1987.

136. Kondo, T. *Microencapsulation: New Techniques and Applications*; Techno Books: Tokyo, 1979.

137. Lim, F. *Biomedical Applications of Microencapsulation*; CRC Press, Inc.: Boca Raton, FL, 1984.

138. Müller, R.H. *Colloidal Carriers for Controlled Drug Delivery and Targeting*; CRC Press: London, 1979.

139. Nixon, J.R. *Microencapsulation*; Marcel Dekker, Inc.: New York, 1976.

140. Tomlinson, E.; Davis, S.S. *Site-Specific Drug Delivery*; John Wiley & Sons: Chichester, UK, 1986.

141. Kreuter, J. *Colloidal Drug Delivery Systems*; Marcel Dekker, Inc.: New York, 1994.

142. Benita, S. *Microencapsulation*; Marcel Dekker, Inc.: New York, 1996.

143. Diederichs, J.E.; Muller, R.E. *Future Strategies for Drug Delivery with Particulate Systems*; CRC Press: Boca Raton, 1998.

144. Burgess, D.J. Colloids and Colloid Drug Delivery Systems. *Encyclopedia of Pharmaceutical Technology*; Swarbrick, J., Boylan, J.C., Eds.; Marcel Dekker, Inc.: New York, 1990; 3, 31–63.

145. Davis, S.S. Colloids and Drug Delivery Systems. Pharm. Technol. **1987**, *11*, 110–117.

146. Kaye, B.H. Microencapsulation: The Creation of Synthetic Fine Particles with Specified Properties. Kona **1992**, *10*, 65–82.

147. Morimoto, Y.; Fujimoto, S. CRC Crit. Rev. Ther. Drug Carrier Sys. **1985**, *2*, 119–163.

148. Oppenhein, R.C. Solid Colloidal Drug Delivery Systems: Nanoparticles. Int. J. Pharm. **1981**, *8*, 217–234.

149. Thies, C. Microencapsulation. *Encyclopedia of Polymer Science and Engineering*; Kroschwitz, J., Ed.; John Wiley & Sons, Inc.: New York, 1987; 9, 724–745.

150. Tomlinson, E. Theory and Practice of Site-Specific Drug Delivery. Adv. Drug Delivery Rev. **1987**, *1*, 87–198.

151. Torchilin, V.P. CRC Crit. Rev. Ther. Drug Carrier Systems **1985**, *2*, 119–163.

152. Yappel, A.F. Albumin Microspheres. Meth. Enzymol. **1985**, *112*, 3–67.

MIXING AND SEGREGATION IN TUMBLING BLENDERS

M

Troy Shinbrot
Fernando J. Muzzio
Rutgers University, Piscataway, New Jersey

MOTIVATION

Mixing of solids is essential to many industries, including pharmaceuticals, ceramics, metallurgy, chemicals, food, cosmetics, coal, and plastics. To give an idea of the magnitude of applications involving granular processes, U.S. worldwide production alone accounts for over a trillion kilograms of granular and powdered products annually, most of which must be uniformly blended to meet quality and performance goals. In this article, we present an example-oriented overview of current understanding of mixing and segregation mechanisms that are of importance to powder blending operations. We focus on industrial tumbler designs, which simultaneously comprise the bulk of solids blending operations and represent the systems for which predictive modeling appears to have the greatest potential. We direct the reader to existing literature sources (e.g., Harnby, 1997) for information on more specialized blending equipment. Numerous distinct mechanisms for both mixing and demixing of granular materials have been catalogued including convection, diffusion, shear, percolation, etc., and in most applications, several mechanisms act concurrently and interact in complex, and currently poorly understood, ways. Thus the mode by which powders are loaded into blenders of common design can alter the time needed to homogenize them by two orders of magnitude. Given that a certain blender can be designed to deliver acceptable performance in the laboratory, we have no consistent a priori mechanism to scale up the process and achieve the same performance in blenders of industrial size. Although comprehensive and predictive understanding of practical blending problems still remains a long-term goal, it has recently become possible to define models that generate respectable agreement with observations in practical granular devices (e.g., 3D tumblers), and methods have become sufficiently refined that systematic techniques to analyze new products and equipment are available, either off the shelf or as research-ready hardware.

FUNDAMENTALS

Research on granular flow and blending roughly can be divided chronologically: prior to about 1990, industrially usable results were mostly empirical (e.g., in experiments using a particular blend in a specific device), and fundamental research was largely analytic (e.g., using continuum approximations to the granular state applicable only to one phase of granular behavior). Although important progress was made into developing specialized engineering solutions and fundamental physical properties of granular systems, little generally applicable knowledge was attainable using either approach. Since that time, computational and methodological advances have permitted quantitative evaluations of granular flow, transport, and mixing at an unparalleled level of detail and accuracy. In this Section we have reviewed progress on tumbling flow and blending phenomenology that has led to the development of the best predictive models existing.

Definition of the "Granular State"

A chief limitation, and the principal area of opportunity for the future, in developing predictive understanding of granular flows is the coexistence of multiple, history-dependent, granular states. Within a device—be it a tumbler, a high shear intensifier, a mill, a fluidized bed, etc.—granular material can, and typically will, exhibit multiple rheologically different phases that vary nontrivially and often with profound consequences as a function of minor changes in material or environmental variables. This is a particular problem in the pharmaceutical industry, where products may be developed in dry, northern, latitudes and produced in wet, equatorial climates. Both hygroscopic excipients and actives behave very differently in these two environments, and blending regimens that work in one may fail in the other. Moreover, even within a single well-controlled bench-scale device, multiple phases are typically present. The tumbling blender is a case in point.

In Fig. 1, a deceptively common outcome of an attempt to blend dissimilar materials is shown, here of grains

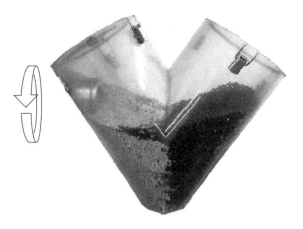

Fig. 1 "Left-right" segregated state, here in a transparent V-blender, between larger (dark) and smaller (light) grains. This state occurs spontaneously at high fill levels and fast tumbling speeds in many tumbler designs.

differing only in size and color. In this transparent 4-L capacity[a] V-blender, we have tumbled equal volumes of small light-gray and larger black grains at 6 rpm for 200 revolutions. The visibly segregated state is only one of several distinct segregated configurations that form spontaneously and reproducibly in all common blender geometries and scales, and persist despite the practitioner's best efforts at modification of process parameters. Developing cures for this type of problem demands a systematic understanding of why segregated states occur in the first place, so that the cause of segregation can be addressed directly. This understanding in turn requires an analysis of the different granular behaviors seen during the tumbling operation.

A first step in the analysis of granular behaviors is the characterization of the different granular phases that are inevitably present during flow. Grains, unlike common fluids, must "dilate" in order to flow, that is, grains in the static state are interlocked, and cannot move without separating. The locations and timing of dilation can be quite complex, but once dilation occurs, the overt granular behavior seen remains static and solid-like far from the regions of dilation, and becomes respectively glassy (disordered), fluid-like, or gas-like near the shear interface as the shear rate increases. The modifier, "like," is important to include, because a solid-like region is not truly elastic as it transmits stress along irregular compressive chains, undergoes slow creep and settling on time scales ranging from seconds to hours, and can solidify into a rigid "cake" over time scales of days to months. Likewise the fluid-like phase transmits shear discontinuously both in

space and time, and does not obey Navier–Stokes equations, and the gas-like phase is far from equilibrium and is not characterized by Maxwell–Boltzmann statistics. It is the differences between qualitative behaviors of different regions of a granular bed at different times and between any one of the behaviors and accepted models for flow and dispersion that make predictive understanding of even the simplest granular systems challenging.

Despite the intrinsic difficulties in developing an all-encompassing model for granular flow, important blending problems of practical interest have been effectively analyzed using model-based, computational, and semiempirical means. The current understanding of granular blending and demixing is summarized in subsequent sections.

Elementary Two-Dimensional Mixing Mechanisms

In tumbling applications, dilation and flow principally play out near the unconstrained upper surface of a granular bed, and the bulk of grains beneath are thought to remain nearly motionless during rotation of the blender. This simplified picture changes for some blender varieties (e.g., Fig. 2b), but predictive models for blending in most common blending geometries can be derived by disregarding all transport beneath the free surface. In the following sections, the best existing models and methods are summarized and their application to common tumbler designs is described.

Although it differs significantly from more complex practical blender geometries (see sections on Competitive Patterned Demixing and Examples), the horizontal drum tumbler has a simple geometry and therefore provides a useful environment for a first analysis of granular mixing and demixing. A horizontal drum mixer is the simplest form of a tumbling blender and it is used in many pharmaceutical, chemical, and metallurgical industries in the form of ball mills, dryers, rotary kilns, coating pans, and mixers.

Flow regimes

Flow in rotating drums has been described qualitatively in terms of regimes such as slipping, avalanching, rolling, cascading, cataracting, and centrifuging.

Slipping: The slipping regime occurs when the granular bed undergoes solid body rotation and then slides, usually intermittently, against the rotating tumbler walls. This most frequently occurs in simple drums that are only partially filled, and is often counteracted by including baffles of various designs along the inner walls of the tumbler. Although the slipping regime is not important for blending purposes per se, it is encountered even in effective blending systems, and an evaluation of the

[a]The reader should note that "capacity" customarily refers to a fraction (generally 60%) of the total interior volume of a blender.

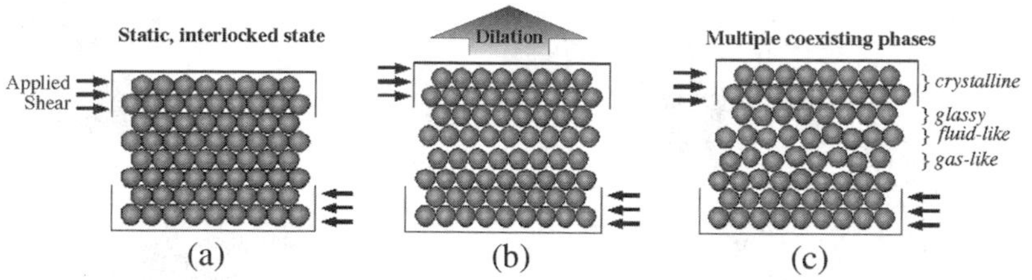

Static, interlocked state   **Dilation**   **Multiple coexisting phases**

Applied Shear

} *crystalline*
} *glassy*
} *fluid-like*
} *gas-like*

(a)   (b)   (c)

Fig. 2 Schematic of dilation mechanism that is a prerequisite for the flow of solids. (a) In undisturbed state, grains are interlocked and behave much like an ordinary solid. (b) A granular bed dilates in response to applied shear, and can then flow. (c) In the flowing state, the bed can form distinct crystalline, glassy, fluid-like and gas-like phases. The crystalline phase is regular and ordered, the glassy phase is disordered but static, the fluid-like state flows but exhibits enduring contacts, and the gas-like state is characterized by rapid and brief interparticle contacts.

number of times a bed is turned over per tumbler revolution will often reveal the presence of some slipping.

Avalanching: A second regime seen at slow tumbling speeds is the "avalanching" flow regime, also referred to as "slumping." In this regime, flow consists of discrete avalanches that occur as a grouping of grains travels down the free surface and comes to rest before a new grouping is released from above. The avalanching regime is not seen in large tumblers (larger than a few tens of centimeters in diameter), but is an instructive case because flow and mixing can be solved in closed form for simplified drum geometries, and lessons from this regime can, with due caution, be carried over to more realistic systems.

To analyze this problem, one only need observe that if the angle of repose at the free surface immediately before an avalanche is ϑ_i, and after an avalanche is ϑ_f, then the effect of an avalanche is to carry a wedge of material in the angle $\vartheta_f - \vartheta_i$, downhill, as sketched in Fig. 3a for an idealized 2D disk blender. The same caricature applies at

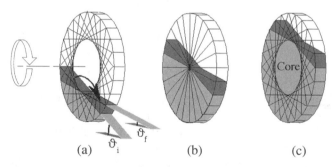

(a) ϑ_i ϑ_f (b)   (c)

Fig. 3 (a) Avalanching flow in an idealized disk tumbler transports grains from an uphill wedge to a downhill wedge as the free surface relaxes from an initial angle ϑ_i to a final angle ϑ_f. This implies that global mixing occurs in quadrilateral regions where grains within one wedge intersect with a second wedge. (b) Consequently, tumblers mix more efficiently at low fill levels than at high, and global mixing nearly stops at 50% fill. (c) At fill levels above 50%, a core develops that does not visit the avalanching surface and, therefore, does not experience transport or mixing.

all fill levels, and one can readily use this model to make several concrete predictions. First, mixing occurs during avalanches through two distinct mechanisms: one, particles within a wedge rearrange during a single avalanche, and two, particles rearrange globally between wedges during successive avalanches. Second, at 50% fill (Fig. 3b) no two avalanching wedges intersect, so no global mixing between separated regions can exist, and mixing must be slow. Third, since flow occurs only near the avalanching surface, at high fill levels a nonmixing core necessarily develops (Fig. 3c). Although this model is oversimplified and neglects material variations, boundary effects, and other important physics, these conclusions carry over to more realistic tumbling systems.

Rolling: At higher tumbling speeds, discrete avalanches give way to continuous flow at the surface of the blend. Grains beneath the cascading layer rotate nearly as a solid body with the blender until they reach the surface. One can solve for flow and transport subject to certain simplifying assumptions in this regime as well. For this solution, one assumes that the grains are so small as to be regarded as a continuum and one takes the free surface to be nearly flat, as sketched in Fig. 4a. The interface between the flowing layer and the supporting bed beneath has been determined experimentally and through detailed computations to be roughly parabolic in shape (1) and by demanding mass conservation at this interface one can construct continuum flow equations for this system (2). If one simulates the mixing in an idealized disk blender of mechanically identical grains initially separated by color to left and right of a vertical central plane, one obtains the results (for a particular fill level and flowing layer depth) as shown in Fig. 4b. Corresponding experimental results are shown in Fig. 4c.

Cascading, cataracting, and centrifuging: For larger tumblers, or for tumblers rotated at higher speeds, the surface is manifestly not flat, as shown in Fig. 5 in a 1 meter diameter disk tumbler (3). This flow, termed cascading, differs qualitatively from the rolling flow solution: here the flowing layer is thin and is nearly

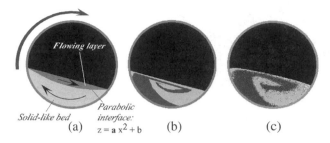

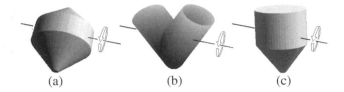

Fig. 6 Three common tumbler designs: (a) double-cone, (b) V-blender, and (c) tote, or bin blender.

Fig. 4 (a) In the rolling regime, the blend separates into a flowing layer near the surface and a solid-like supporting bed. (b) By establishing simple conditions such as mass conservation, one can generate an analytic model for the flow, producing mixing patterns between initially separated and colored, but otherwise identical, grains. (c) Comparison with experimental mixing patterns using freely flowing grains in a small drum tumbler reveals substantial agreement. The snapshot in (c) is obtained from the interior of the blend using the solidification technique described in the section on Solidification in this article.

uniform in speed and thickness, and has been modeled as depth averaged, plug-like flow. As the rotation speed of the tumbler is increased, the surface becomes increasingly sigmoidal until grains become airborne, and at higher speeds yet, the grains centrifuge against the tumbler wall. These regimes are termed cataracting and centrifuging, respectively, and have not been well analyzed.

MIXING MECHANISMS IN THREE-DIMENSIONAL TUMBLERS

Although drum blenders represent a convenient paradigm for the purpose of categorizing granular behaviors, most

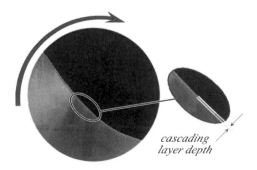

Fig. 5 Cascading flow occurs in large tumblers or during tumbling of fine, but freely flowing, grains. This snapshot shows a 1 m diameter transparent disk tumbler partially filled with colored ~500 μm irregular grains. The free surface is manifestly not flat, and the cascading layer is thin and nearly uniform with distance along the flowing surface.

blending operations occur in more complex tumbler geometries. Three of the most common geometries used in pharmaceutical operations are the double-cone, the V-blender, and the tote blender, sketched in Fig. 6. Each of these geometries have many variants, for example symmetry can be broken to introduce cross-flow by slanting the double-cone, by elongating one of the arms of the V-blender, or by inserting baffles in a tote.

To model flow and blending in complicated geometries, particle-dynamic simulations have been implemented. In these simulations, particles are treated as individual entities with physical properties (e.g., size, static and dynamic friction coefficients, coefficient of restitution, etc.) appropriate to the problem of interest, and Newton's laws of motion are integrated for each particle. Particle-dynamic simulations are similar in concept to molecular-dynamic simulations, but include features of importance to the flow of macroscopic particles (e.g., static and dynamic friction models) in place of microscopic properties (e.g., bond strengths and chemical potentials). Particle-dynamic simulations come in many different types depending on how they treat physical parameters such as rolling friction and particle shape or numerical issues such as search algorithms and routines to maintain computational stability. Results of distinct computational simulations can differ, sometimes significantly, and the importance of experimental validation of numerical results cannot be overemphasized.

Two of the most common classes of particle-dynamic simulations are termed "hard-particle" and "soft-particle" methods. Hard-particle methods calculate particle trajectories in response to instantaneous, binary collisions between particles and allow particles to travel ballistically between collisions. This class of simulation permits only instantaneous contacts, and is consequently often used in rapid flow situations as are found in chutes, fluidized beds, and energetically agitated systems. Soft-particle methods, on the other hand, allow each particle to deform elastoplastically and compute responses using standard models from elasticity and tribology theory. This approach permits enduring particle contacts and is therefore the method of choice for tumbler applications. The simulations described in this article use soft-particle methods that have been validated and found to agree in detail with comparison experiments (4, 5).

Convection

Mixing in all tumbling blenders consists of a fast convective stage, driven by the mean velocity of many particles, followed by a much slower dispersive stage, caused by velocity fluctuations leading to rearrangements of individual particles. Convection in grains (as in fluids) is by far the fastest and most efficient mixing mechanism, yet at the same time it suffers from the same mixing limitations known for fluids: convective flows can, and very often do, possess barriers to mixing (e.g., islands) that do not interact with surrounding material. Two pathologies are readily observed: overfilled mixers develop elliptic, nonchaotic, islands that rotate as a unit in the center of the granular bed (discussed earlier in Section on Flow Regimes), and symmetric blenders (seen in most standard designs) exhibit separatrices that divide the flow into noninteracting sectors. Beyond this, little is known currently of details of particle flow patterns and mixing barriers in practical, three-dimensional blender geometries. There is strong evidence, though, indicating that flow bifurcations analogous to those seen in fluids may be present in granular tumblers.

Convection in the context of granular blenders refers to transport associated with flow driven by gravity (in tumbling blenders) or impellers (in intensified, ribbon, or other blenders). Convection is observed in all functioning blender geometries, and can be visualized using particle-dynamic simulations. In Fig. 7 are shown successive front and side views taken a quarter revolution apart of 20,000

identical but colored spheres tumbled in a V-blender in the cascading regime. These snapshots illustrate the qualitative motion produced in this blender, which causes the bed to overturn from top to bottom. Mixing due to convective flow grows linearly with time insofar as the area of an interface between differently colored layers in these snapshots or in Fig. 4b and c, grows characteristically linearly with time. Although similar qualitative behaviors are seen in all tumbler geometries, the quantitative mixing seen can differ considerably between geometries (cf. Section. Mixing rates).

Dispersion

Dispersion, also referred to as diffusion, is contrasted with convection, which can effectively intersperse grains in a tumbler within tens to hundreds of revolutions. Dispersion also refers to the random relocation of individual grains due to collisions between adjacent particles and can take hundreds to thousands of revolutions to act. Thus particles cross a plane separating the two arms of the V-blender (or an equivalent symmetry plane in many other blender geometries) only as a result of occasional collisional happenstances and not as a result of an overall mean flow. Various stratagems, including the use of baffles, asymmetric cross-flow designs (referred to earlier), irregular rotation protocols, or axial rocking, have been introduced to mitigate this limitation. Notwithstanding these improvements, dispersion is the rate-limiting mechanism for mixing, and there is much potential for improvement of dispersive mixing.

Although convection is typically orders of magnitude more rapid than dispersion, as a practical matter the relative contribution of each mechanism to blending is strongly influenced by the initial distribution of species in the mixer. Thus ingredients loaded in horizontal layers (as in Fig. 7) can be mixed relatively rapidly, while ingredients layered side by side (either intentionally (as in Fig. 8) or inadvertently (as a result of careless loading of a tumbler) will typically mix enormously more slowly.

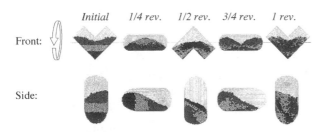

Fig. 7 Rapid, convective flow seen in particle-dynamic simulation of identical but colored spheres in V-blender. Top: view from front reveals that unlike in some designs, convection in this blender drives grains axially, alternately outward toward the tumbler arms and inward toward its center. This axial flow strongly influences mixing, as described in the section on Mixing Rates in this article. Bottom: view from side indicates that transport is dominated by a spiraling flow, seen also in drums and other blenders (cf. Fig. 4).

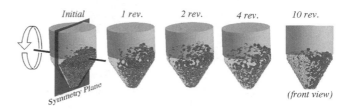

Fig. 8 Dispersive mixing is slow across the symmetry plane of a blender, here a tote design. After 10 revolutions, a front view reveals clear evidence of the initial left-right distribution of identical but colored spheres in this particle-dynamic simulation.

To visualize this effect, in Fig. 8 is shown the dispersive mixing of 8000 identical but colored grains loaded side by side, here in a tote blender. With each successive revolution, only a few particles cross the interface separating the two symmetric halves of the tumbler, and as a result, after 10 revolutions the original particle ordering is still unmistakable. Systematic assays obtained from experiments of blending of realistic pharmaceutical excipients and actives confirm that imperfectly loaded blends retain any initial asymmetry for many hundreds of tumbler revolutions.

Shear

A final class of mechanisms of granular and powder mixing is grouped under the category of shear. This includes a host of very different mechanisms that act in a shearing layer (cf. Fig. 2) or in a high-shear region as produced by an intensifier or related device. Grains rearrange during shearing and so disperse across a shear layer. In addition, large or irregular grains tend to be expelled from regions of high shear through a mechanism known in research on suspensions as "shear-induced migration." Finally, arrangements of adjacent grains become distorted through the influence of external strain. This is the most classic form of shear mixing, which itself admits several distinct subcategories.

First, there is the simple effect of shear on deforming a granular bed. In simple tumblers, this can manifest itself in a nearly continuous distribution of strain, resulting in regular and predictable mixing behavior such as is displayed in Fig. 4c. This figure was obtained using freely flowing grains, of mean size nearly 1 mm.

Second, a granular bed consisting of weakly cohesive materials (e.g., nontacky grains in the size range 50–300 μm) exhibits stick-slip motion so that flow becomes intermittent rather than continuous. This is a situation of practical importance because pharmaceutical blends, for example, use particles across a broad range of sizes and materials. As the size of grains diminishes or as interparticle cohesion grows, stick-slip flow transforms mixing interfaces from smooth, regular, patterns as shown in Fig. 9 (500- or 700-μm cases) to a complex, irregular pattern, shown in Fig. 9 (300- or 100-μm cases). In simple geometries, this response to shear can be accurately modeled: if we assume that the flowing surface of a bed periodically sticks and slips, then the mechanism displayed in Fig. 4a can be embellished by allowing the shear band between flowing layer and bed to deform periodically (2). This produces patterns of mixing between initially separated but identical grains that are substantially similar to experiment, as shown at the bottom of Fig. 9.

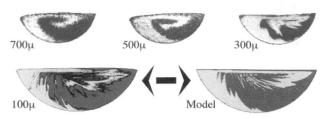

Fig. 9 Mixing patterns after 1 revolution in drum tumblers loaded with identical (except for color) grains in four experiments using successively finer grains, as well as in a model simulation of idealized stick-slip flow. At 700 and 500 μm, the mixing interface remains smooth and regular, while below about 300 μm, it becomes variegated due to intermittent slipping of the cascade. Each experimental snapshot shows a view from the interior of a blend using the solidification technique described in the section on Solidification in this article, and all cases began with light grains to the left of center and dark grains to the right.

This is important for blending because in smooth, regular flow, adjacent particles remain nearby for long periods of time, while in intermittent, stick-slip flow, particles can rapidly relocate across the blender. It is not difficult to show that periodic sticking and slipping results in an exponentially rapid growth of interfaces between separated regions of grains.

Third, for particles smaller than about 100 μm, cohesive forces (believed to be due to van der Waals interactions for intimate contacts, and to surface tension of adsorbed water layers for lubricated contacts) between particles becomes comparable to particle weights, and small particles can stick to one another in relatively rigid aggregates. Unless such aggregates are destroyed, the system will behave as if it had an effective particle size much larger than the primary particle size.

For strongly cohesive materials, it is typically necessary to fragment agglomerates through the introduction of high shear, "intensification," devices such as impellers or mills that energetically deform grains on the finest scale. Intensification is commonly performed in an early preblending stage using a fraction of the total desired excipient to avoid overblending the final product. Results of intensification are discussed in the section on Assays.

DEMIXING

Processing the blends of dissimilar grains almost invariably promotes demixing, also referred to as segregation, characterized by the spontaneous emergence of regions of nonuniform composition. Segregation due to differences in particle size in a blend has drawn the greatest attention in the literature, including studies of fluidized beds, chutes, hoppers, vibrated beds, and tumbling blender. Segregation due to particle density, shape, and triboelectric order have also been recorded. As a practical matter, segregation manifests itself in granular mixing that characteristically improves over a brief period (while convection generates large scale mixing) and then degrades, often dramatically (as slower segregational fluxes take over). Demixing should not be confused with the phenomenon of overblending, which is also frequently encountered in blending applications. Overblending is associated with physical degradation of material properties, as occurs for example when a waxy lubricant is excessively deformed causing it to coat pharmaceutical grains and reduce their bioavailability, or when coated granules are damaged through abrasion or fracture.

At the present time, mechanisms for segregation even in the simple tumbling drum remain obscure, and work on more complex and industrially common blender geometries is extremely limited. Three distinct types of demixing are moderately well characterized in tumblers. They are radial demixing, axial demixing, and competitive patterned demixing. We describe each of these in turn.

Radial Demixing

Segregation typically proceeds in two stages. First, large grains rapidly segregate radially, producing a central core of fine grains surrounded by larger grains, identified in Fig. 10 for a simple drum tumbler. Unlike the core seen in overfilled tumblers (Fig. 3c), this core appears at fill levels under 50% and is exclusively associated with migration of fine grains toward the center of an overturning blend. Radial segregation is seen in both quasi-2D and fully 3D blenders of various geometries. In simpler 3D geometries, such as the drum, double-cone or tote, the core is nearly always apparent when blending significantly dissimilar grains, while in more complicated geometries such as the V-blender or slant-cone the core becomes significantly distorted and may only be conspicuous for higher fill levels or in certain (e.g., upright) orientations of the blender. Even in the simplest case of the drum tumbler, however, the location and dynamics of the core remain somewhat enigmatic: as shown in Fig. 10, the core is actually located upstream of the geometric center of the granular cascade.

The core appears to form as a result of two cooperative influences. First, smaller grains percolate through the flowing layer to occupy successively lower strata each time the bed overturns. Second, once a sufficient volume of smaller grains has accumulated, the larger grains tend to roll increasingly freely over the (comparatively smooth)

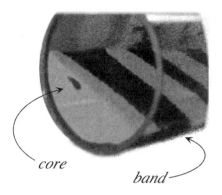

Fig. 10 Typical segregation pattern seen between fine (dark) and coarse (light) grains in small transparent drum tumbler. A core of fines extends along the entire length of the tumbler, connecting the bands that emerge at the surface in a single bulging tube. The coarse grains are constrained to flow within the confines defined by this tube. This constraint is important for understanding mechanisms of demixing in more complex geometries, as described in the section on Competitive Patterned Demixing in this article.

substrate of smaller grains. This higher speed surface flow reinforces the segregated state by expelling remaining slower small grains. These mechanisms are very robust, and cores are almost invariably found in tumbling of freely flowing grains with diameter ratios between about 1:1.5 and 1:7. As the diameter ratio approaches unity, the core becomes more diffused, while as the diameter ratio grows sufficiently large, fine grains can percolate increasingly freely through a matrix of larger grains or, if sufficiently fine, can coat the larger species.

Axial Demixing

A second stage of segregation occurs in drum tumblers as grains in the core migrate along the tumbling axis. Numerical and experimental investigations have attributed this migration to conflicting causes, e.g., a secondary flow within the core leading to a bulging of the core toward the surface versus different angles of repose of fine, mixed, and coarse grains. Whatever the ultimate cause, the result of this axial migration is the formation of a series of bands as shown in Fig. 10. In this final state, two pure phases of material are formed, divided by sharp boundaries with very little intermixing.

Competitive Patterned Demixing

In more complex, and more common, tumbler geometries, several distinct segregation patterns have been observed. These patterns are believed to arise from a competition between surface segregation of coarse grains flowing over

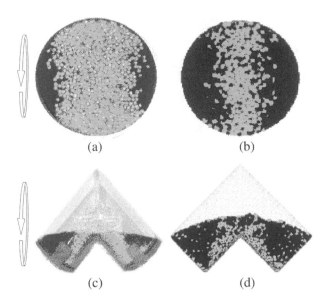

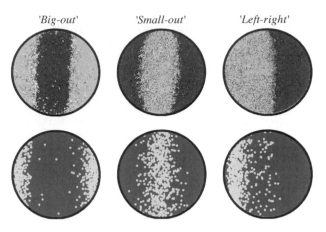

Fig. 12 Three common segregation patterns between large (light) and small (dark) grains seen in top views of double-cone blender. Top: experimental snapshots. Bottom: simplified continuum simulations.

Fig. 11 Axial segregation in top views of double-cone blender from (a) experiment and (b) particle-dynamic simulation using large (light) and small (dark) spherical grains. Similar patterns are seen in other tumbler designs, for example in the V-blender in (c) experiment and (d) simulation.

a radially segregated core of fine grains and interactions with the boundaries of the tumbler. Despite significant differences between common blender geometries, there is substantial commonality in the ultimate patterns seen. For example, mixing of large, light-gray and small, dark-gray grains in a double-cone and a V-blender generates similar patterns in both experiments and particle-dynamic simulations, as shown in Fig. 11.

As parameters such as fill level, tumbler speed, and concentrations of the different particle species are varied, the patterns observed though change significantly. Importantly, there appear to be a few dominant and recurring patterns that are seen both in experiments and in simulations in all blender geometries. Notably at high fill levels and tumbling speeds, the "left-right state" shown in Fig. 1 appears to dominate. This pattern and two other common variants are shown at the top of Fig. 12 in top views of the surface of a double-cone blender. Each of these patterns appears reproducibly and spontaneously whenever different size grains are tumbled in any of several blender geometries. Simulations shown beneath the experimental figures in Fig. 12 use a continuum model in which large particles are convected on the surface of an idealized convex bed of smaller grains. Container geometry is included by assuming that large particles rebound specularly when they reach the downstream boundary of the idealized blender. Correspondence

between experimental data and this simulation indicates that ongoing improvements in modeling show promise for unveiling the underlying mechanisms of demixing and permitting eventual accurate modeling of practical granular processing systems.

Scaling

An ultimate goal of granular research is to enable processing to be scaled up from bench to pilot to full-scale operations. Scale-up methods are well developed in other, (e.g., fluid) operations, but remain a distant objective in granular systems. Several alternative scale-up approaches have been suggested. For example, the natural dimensionless group associated with granular flow at a known speed, v, down a specified height incline, h, under gravity, g, is the Froude number, defined to be the ratio of kinetic to potential energies: $Fr = v^2/gh$. Experimental analysis reveals, however, that neither mixing nor segregation scale with Fr. Reasons for this are several: the competing mixing mechanisms of convection, diffusion, and shear each act on different characteristic time scales, and their interactions are therefore complex in the extreme. Additionally grains accelerate down a cascading surface, and therefore the resulting behavior changes qualitatively depending on whether they do or do not reach an asymptotic speed in the cascade (for example, compare Figs. 4c and 5). These and other influences make first-principles analysis of granular scale-up problematic.

Nevertheless, reproducible empirical scaling relations do appear to be attainable for specific blenders. As an example, in the drum blender it has been determined that dynamically similar convective flow occurs provided that

$R \cdot \Omega^{2/3}$ is held constant for lower tumbling speeds (where particles reach a terminal speed in the cascading layer) and provided that $R \cdot \Omega^{1/2}$ is held fixed for higher tumbling speeds (where particles do not reach a terminal speed), where R is the drum radius and Ω is the tumbler rotation speed. Likewise the demixing patterns shown in Figs. 1, 11 and 12 are found at all blender scales, and dynamical similarity relations have been obtained for transitions between these patterns. These encouraging findings indicate that scaling of a particular granular blending process in a specified geometry may be possible, but that scaling relations can be expected to vary quantitatively as process parameters (e.g., material properties, fill levels, tumbler geometries, etc.) are changed. As in any rapidly evolving field, the current state of understanding is not yet fully adequate for practical needs, but research trends show promise for the intermediate and longer terms.

MIXING MEASURES

A prerequisite to meaningful evaluation and interpretation of mixing is the use and understanding of a reliable measure of mixing. Though this concept may seem straightforward, some care needs to be exercised in its implementation. Any mixing measure is obtained by first evaluating a relevant quantity, typically concentration, in specified sample regions. Ideally, in order for the samples to be representative, they should be taken uniformly from a flowing stream that is itself uniform both in space and time. In tumblers, this is not practical, and very often sampling consists of extracting small aliquots of grains from a static bed. We discuss techniques, and limitations, of extracting such aliquots shortly, but first it is worthwhile to review what one would do if provided with complete access to concentration data throughout a granular bed. Such an idealized scenario is sketched in Fig. 13, where we display sequential snapshots of a 2D bed. Suppose we can subdivide the blender into identical boxes—elements of area in 2D, elements of volume in 3D. In each box, let us define a concentration, C_a, of a species of interest. Thus C_a might range from 0 in the black regions of Fig. 13, to 1 in the light-gray regions.

Data Interpretation

The first thing to notice is that not all boxes are completely occupied by grains, and boxes near the periphery of the bed can bias results strongly. For example, in the leftmost snapshot, partially filled boxes consist of anomalously high concentrations C_a, and an unweighted evaluation of

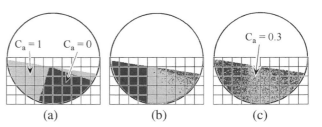

Fig. 13 (a) Subdivision of blend into sampling regions. By determining concentrations, C_a, of interest in each region, one can compute relevant statistics. (b) and (c) as time progresses, concentrations approach a mean value with standard error that diminishes as the number of sampled regions increases.

concentrations in all boxes would yield a mean concentration, for this particular case, of 60% light-gray grains. This is clearly wrong, and can be corrected either by reducing the box size (hence diminishing the fraction of boxes containing a boundary of the bed) and excluding boundary boxes or, preferably, by weighting each box based on its fractional fill level.

A second issue is that there is necessarily a trade-off between precision and resolution. That is, if the box sizes are reduced, one obtains more boxes and hence more values of C_a, and consequently any mixing measure will in principle have a lower standard error. On the other hand, this reduction has an obvious limit as the box size approaches the grain size, at which point any blend will statistically appear to be unmixed (because each box can only take on one of the two values, $C_a = 0$ or $C_a = 1$). In practice, a happy medium delivering both suitably low standard error and an adequate sample size[b] is easily achieved; nevertheless it is important to understand what it is that one is seeking to obtain before deciding on a sampling protocol.

A third issue is illustrated in Fig. 14, where we plot three schematic mixing states, each containing the same fraction of light and dark regions. Plainly the leftmost state is fully segregated, but most simple measures would provide the same evaluation of mixedness for the two other states. Moreover, the rightmost schematic represents a common outcome of shearing flows (cf. striated state in Fig. 9). For this reason, it may be desirable to customize one's mixing measure to accurately reflect the desired endpoint of measurement, and correspondingly innumerable different mixing measures have appeared in the literature. These many different measures unfortunately do little to advance the comprehensive understanding of granular blending or to permit comparisons between different data sources, and it is

---

[b]To compute a lower bound on box size, one typically assumes Poissonian statistics for the presence or absence of particles within a given box, so that uncertainties in a box containing n particles go as.

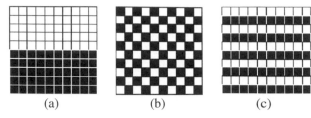

(a)   (b)   (c)

Fig. 14 Illustration of the importance of rational data interpretation. The state (b) intuitively looks well mixed, but has the same number of black and white boxes as states (a) and (c). Evidently a larger box size is required to make meaningful mixing measurements. States (b) and (c) have very different structures, but produce similar measures of mixing using common statistics. For this reason, many customized mixing measures have evolved in the literature.

consequently preferable, where feasible, to use a single set of mixing measures as suggested in the next section.

Intensity of Segregation

One of the most useful measures of mixedness is the intensity of segregation. This is little more than a normalized variance of concentration measurements. Intrinsic to the use of intensity of segregation, therefore, is the presumption that the mixing distribution is, at least to a first approximation, Gaussian. This raises two issues: first, it is not clear that granular mixing tends toward a Gaussian state, and second, in many practical applications a Gaussian is not the desired outcome. Indeed, in pharmaceutical processing, if a blend were Gaussian rather than uniform, then the unavoidable presence of exponential tails on a Gaussian distribution would guarantee that some small fraction of tablets made from the blend would be beyond any therapeutic range that one could specify. Fortunately, granular flows seem to scatter grains more uniformly than a simple Gaussian would predict, although the details and mechanisms for this behavior are not yet well understood.

With these caveats in mind, a definition of the intensity of segregation is:

$$I = \frac{\sigma^2 - \sigma_r^2}{\sigma_o^2 - \sigma_r^2},$$ (1)

where σ^2 is the variance of sampled data, σ_r^2 is the variance of the same number of randomly chosen concentration data, and σ_o^2 is the variance of an initial, typically fully segregated, state, again consisting of the same number of data points. Several forms of I appear in the literature; this form is useful because it is normalized so that $I = 1$ and $I = 0$ correspond to completely segregated and randomly mixed states, respectively.

Two other mixing measures of importance to pharmaceutical processing are, first, the relative standard deviation (RSD), defined to be:

$$\text{RSD} = \frac{\sigma}{\langle C_a \rangle}$$ (2)

where σ is the standard deviation and C_a is the mean concentration over all samples taken, and the mixing rate, k. The mixing rate is defined according to the relation:

$$I = I_o e^{-kt}$$ (3)

where I_o is an initial intensity and t is time. Many, though not all, mixing mechanisms produce an exponential approach to uniformity as presupposed by Equation (3). Deviations from Equation (3) are discussed in the next Section; for now, if we assume that the intensity of segregation decays according to Equation (3), we can extract a mixing rate from any given experiment and thereby evaluate and compare mixing efficiencies of different blenders, of blenders operated under different conditions, and of effects of changes in material or other properties of interest.

Examples

Mixing rates

To examine the behavior of mixing measures, it is useful to begin by considering systems free of experimental uncertainties. Particle dynamic simulations such as those discussed in the sections on Mixing mechanism in Three Dimensional Tumblers; and Demixing, represent such ideal systems: the presence and locations of all particles are known and are free of sampling errors (discussed in the section on Sampling Techniques).

The simplest of these simulations from the point of view of mixing measurement is the double-cone. Raw variances taken from volume elements initially separated axially in the blender are shown in Fig. 15a. The variances are color coded according to the initial locations sketched in the inset. Evidently, after the first or second revolution of the blender, variances decay nearly exponentially (i.e., linearly on this semi-log plot). Mixing is slowest, however, between particles initially near the axial center of the blender (light gray in Fig. 15a). This is to be expected because, as commented earlier, the rate limiting mixing process is dispersion across the symmetry plane of the blender, or looked at another way, grains starting further from the symmetry plane experience a secondary axial convective flow, that grains closer to this plane do not.

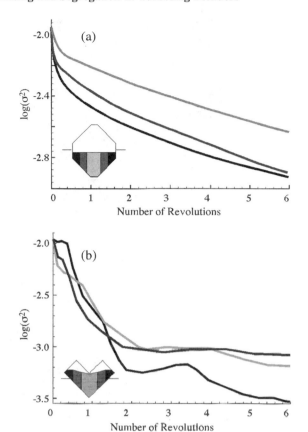

Fig. 15 Variance of concentrations of identical color-coded grains from particle-dynamic simulations of (a) a double-cone and (b) a V-blender. Notice that the smooth flow in the double-cone is reflected in a smooth, asymptotically exponential, reduction in variance with time, while the sloshing flow in the V-blender (cf. Fig. 7) produces periodic undulations in mixing response.

It is instructive to compare this simulation with its counterpart in the V-blender, shown in Fig. 15b, where mixing is much more irregular. This irregularity has been traced to periodic sloshing of grains to and from the arms of the blender. Again there is a barrier to mixing across the symmetry plane of the tumbler, but comparison of the scales of Figs. 15a and b reveals that the sloshing process accelerates mixing significantly. Thus as one would expect, the smooth flow seen in the double-cone is manifested in a smooth decay in variance shown in Fig. 15a and modeled by Equation (3), while the periodic sloshing of grains in the V-blender is poorly fit by such a simple relation. For all tumblers, it is notable that mixing evolves with each successive tumbler rotation and not with elapsed time, and all studies indicate that tumbler rotation rate (within a fixed regime) is nearly inconsequential.

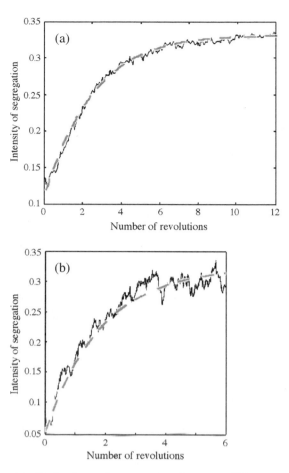

Fig. 16 Evaluation of segregation between different size particles in particle dynamic simulations in (a) double-cone and (b) V-blender.

Segregation rates

As its name suggests, the intensity of segregation is especially useful for analyzing segregating mixtures. For example, rather than evaluating I in a simulation of identical particles, as shown in Fig. 15, if we evaluate I for a simulation of the segregating mixture in the double-cone shown in Fig. 11b, we obtain the plot shown in Fig. 16a. Here the blend starts from an artificially mixed state, $I \ll 1$, and approaches an asymptotically segregated state, $I \cong 0.3$. The solid data points are obtained by dividing the total occupied volume into separate boxes and calculating the number of small grains within each box. The dashed gray curve is an exponential approach to an asymptote included for comparison, which indicates that segregation, as well as mixing, in simple geometry tumblers obeys a simple exponential relation. For more complex tumbler geometries, segregation approximately follows an exponential approach to an asymptotic segregated state, but is more erratic, as shown in Fig. 16b for the V-blender.

SAMPLING TECHNIQUES

Thieves

In practical blending processes, one cannot obtain arbitrary quantities of pristine data as one can using particle-dynamic simulations, and one must settle for sampling a static bed, as mentioned previously. In such a case, it is especially important to understand sampling limitations and systematic biases. A common means of obtaining samples in a tumbler is by the use of a scoop or thief sampler. These samplers are inserted into the bed and extract samples from its interior. In such an application, it is necessary to obtain a representative spatial distribution of samples throughout the bed, and for this purpose it is recommended that one build a jig above the tumbler opening into which one can insert samplers at fixed locations in the plane of the opening and to specified depths perpendicular to the plane.

The behaviors of two popular types of thief samplers are shown in Figs. 17 and 18. In Fig. 17 is shown the result of inserting a "side-sampling" thief, consisting of a tube with a slot in its side that can be opened to allow grains to flow into a cavity and closed to extract the sample. In the photograph of Fig. 17a, an interior section of a solidified bed (see section on Solidification) of light gray 200-μm and dark 60-μm grains is shown. The grains are initially layered, and from this snapshot it is clear that the act of inserting the thief causes grains to be entrained along the insertion route. This entrainment causes local particle rearrangements that typically result in the bed appearing to be anomalously well mixed. It is also significant that side-sampling thieves rely on particle flow into the sampling cavity to obtain grains, and consequently freely-flowing or smaller grains can penetrate the sampling slot more readily than cohesive or larger grains. These conclusions are borne out in quantitative tests: in Fig. 17b, we plot the fraction of smaller beads in samples obtained using a side-sampling thief in separate experiments in which 60-μm grains are initially arranged in a single thick layer over a bed of 200-μm grains. Evidently the thief obtains samples almost entirely consisting of the smaller species, irrespective of the genuine concentration originally in the sampling location.

The problem that side-sampling probes do not allow larger or more cohesive grains to enter the sampling cavity can be mitigated through the use of "end-sampling" thieves such as the one shown in Fig. 18. In these thieves, the sampling tube is inserted to a desired depth in the bed, an aperture at the distal end of the probe is opened, and then

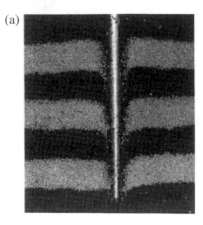

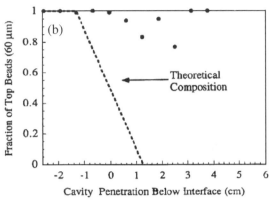

Fig. 17 Systematic sampling errors introduced by a side-sampling thief. (a) Initially layered configuration of large (light) and small (dark) grains are noticeably disturbed as this thief entrains grains during insertion. (b) This type of thief relies on free flow of grains to fill a cavity when a slot is opened in the side of the sampling tube. Consequently, fine and freely flowing grains are overrepresented by this probe, and fine grains are transported to regions where they were not originally placed.

the probe is pushed deeper into the bed and the aperture is closed again to allow extraction of the sample. Because grains are actively forced into the cavity, rather than passively flowing into it as in side-sampling thieves, this device is relatively free of differential sampling problems as can be caused by differences in particle flowability. However, as shown in Fig. 18a, these devices are typically bulky and consequently entrain considerable material during their insertion. The resulting sample concentration measurements (Fig. 18b) are therefore improved over those of the side-sampling thief, but remain very inaccurate and the data consistently overestimate a blend's mixedness.

Core Sampling

An alternative that is nearly free of either flow (e.g., Fig. 17b) or entrainment (e.g., Fig. 17a) anomalies is the

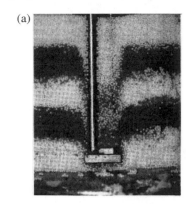

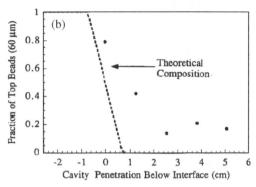

Fig. 18 Sampling errors introduced by an end-sampling thief differ from those of a side-sampling thief, but persist nonetheless. In this type of thief, a window is opened at the bottom of the sampling tube and grains are forced into a cavity by further insertion of the thief. This eliminates the bias toward grains that passively fill a cavity more easily than others, but on the other hand, (a) these thieves entrain more grains during insertion and (b) their performance again suffers from substantial systematic error.

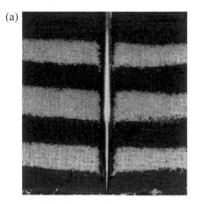

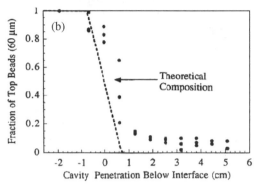

Fig. 19 Core sampler with end-cap can be used for freely-flowing (e.g., granulated) materials that would escape from the sampling tube during removal from the bed without the end-cap. (a) Very little entrainment is visible after insertion, and (b) systematic errors are reduced.

"core-sampler." This sampler extracts an entire contiguous core of grains throughout the depth of insertion. At its simplest, the probe consists of a thin walled tube that is inserted into a granular bed, together with a mechanized extrusion apparatus to permit samples to be extracted in a last-in, first-out manner after the tube has been removed from the bed. In the case of freely-flowing grains, which could otherwise flow out of the tube, the device is embellished by incorporating an end-cap that can be opened during insertion and then closed during extraction. Unlike the end-sampling thief, the end-cap mechanism here is internal to the sampling tube, and an entire core is extruded from the bed. The behavior of this device is demonstrated in Fig. 19. Using the end-cap (shown closed in Fig. 19a), the concentration data obtained compare favorably with other methods, as shown in Fig. 19b. Importantly, in the core sampler the core extends through the depth of the sampling tube and so sample sizes are large. Random uncertainties

are therefore small and corrections for systematic errors that remain can be predictably made.

Without the end-cap, agreement between experiment and theory is further improved. In Fig. 20 we display core sampling results for three different inner diameter sampling tubes using a two-layer bed of common pharmaceutical excipient powders: microcrystalline cellulose and lactose. For all sampler diameters, the experimental data are indistinguishable from ideal expected concentrations. In practice, we note that it is important that the walls of the sampling tubes be polished (to prevent excessive entrainment and difficulty filling the tube during insertion) and that a well-regulated extrusion device be employed.

Assays

Once samples have been obtained, one can use a variety of available chemical, optical, spectroscopic, chromatographic, or other assays to determine concentrations of interest. For example, data in Fig. 20 were obtained using a calibrated densitometric technique in which one

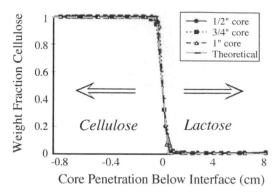

Fig. 20 Non-freely-flowing, powdered material can be extracted from a blend using a core sampler with an open end. In this case, measurement errors are virtually undetectable, here in a sampling experiment using a thick layer of microcrystalline cellulose above a bed of lactose.

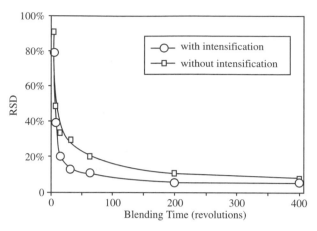

Fig. 21 Mixing rates in a V-blender tumbled at 24 rpm with and without shear induced by a high speed intensifier bar.

of the two species was colored in advance; identical results have been obtained using other assay techniques, e.g., reflection near-infrared spectroscopy used to evaluate distributions of magnesium stearate (a common pharmaceutical lubricant). One particularly useful technique for evaluating the effectiveness of tumbler design or process modifications involves the use of conductivity assays. For this technique, standard nonionic excipients are blended with mock-actives consisting of simple soluble salts (e.g., KCl or NaCl) granulated in the size of interest. Samples extracted from the interior of the blend using core-samplers (inserted at controlled locations using a jig as described previously) are then extruded in fixed weight aliquots and dissolved in a known quantity of solvent (typically just deionized water). The concentration of the solution is then measured using commercially available probes, and by comparing concentration data with calibration curves obtained separately, one can rapidly and accurately establish mixing statistics of the mock-active as a functions of operational parameters of interest.

As an example, we have mentioned that it is typically necessary to fragment cohesive agglomerates through the use of an intensifier bar (a high speed impeller) or similar device. To investigate the effectiveness of intensification during preblending, in Fig. 21 we show plots of RSD of mock active vs. blending time in a V-blender with and without intensification. Each data point is obtained from a separate experiment in which the blender is loaded in predefined layers and then tumbled for the specified time, after which multiple samples are taken (again always from the same locations in the bed) and assayed. Because the samples are taken using entire intact cores, large numbers of data are obtained throughout the depth of the bed.

Typically nine cores are taken, distributed uniformly in a grid around the blender opening; since the V-blender has two arms, in this set of experiments five cores were taken through openings at the end of each arm.

By solidifying an entire blend, one can obtain data in enormous quantities and in exceedingly high detail. For example, in Fig. 23, we show the interior of a blend in a double-cone solidified using a methacrylate solution and then sliced open through the tumbler symmetry plane. Here ~90-μm grains have been blended beginning with a segregated initial state, and the mixing structure, characteristic of stick-slip flow (described earlier), can be resolved down to the size of the grains themselves.

This type of sampling protocol permits the quantification of mixing under a variety of different conditions. As we have mentioned, because core sampling provides large quantities of bed material in a reproducible manner, one can assay some of the samples and retain others for later analysis—e.g., to perform dissolution or bioavailability tests or for archival purposes.

Solidification

Core sampling combined with calibrated assaying techniques represents the best available technology for quantification of mixing of industrial scale blenders. Other techniques are available, however, for laboratory scale studies. The gold standard for these is the solidification technique, described here. To solidify a granular bed, one performs a mixing experiment using colored or otherwise distinguishable grains and infiltrates the blend with a polymeric solution such as methacrylate copolymer, low viscosity epoxy, or heated gelatin. The polymer is allowed to set, and the solidified monolith is sliced open using a saw (for large samples solidified with methacrylate or epoxy) or a knife (for samples set in comparatively soft gelatin) to reveal internal mixing patterns. Separate experiments using structured (e.g. intentionally layered) blends confirm that the blend is not disturbed by infiltration provided that the infiltration is carried out slowly and from one end of the tumbler to the other (so as to avoid trapping bubbles). This technique is appropriate only for laboratory scale apparatus, in which setting times are short and it is feasible to handle and slice the entire frozen blend. Additionally, the technique typically involves sacrificing the blending vessel (which is obviously not always practical), although blends solidified in gelatin can be released from the blender by heating it from outside.

Typical results are shown in Fig. 22 using a segregating mixture of fine, dark, and coarse, light, grains in a drum tumbler solidified using gelatin. The slices displayed show clear evidence both of radial and axial segregation. These slices incidentally also reveal an evident shortcoming of attempting to visualize mixing only from the outside of the blend. This has been done many times in the literature, but without validating the results by examining the interior of the bed, such studies can be grossly misleading, as the differences between the exterior and interior slices shown in Fig. 22 illustrate.

Other Techniques

Other, more technologically involved, techniques have also been developed for visualizing the interior of granular beds. These include:

- Diffusing wave spectroscopy, used to measure statistics of fluctuations in relatively thin, Hele-Shaw configurations
- Positron emission tomography, in which a single radio-active grain is tracked during flow within a granular bed using an array of external photomultipliers
- Magnetic resonance imaging, in which magnetic moments of hydrogenated grains are aligned in structured configurations (e.g., stripes) and these structures are tracked for short periods of time
- X-ray tomography, in which a population of radio-opaque grains are tracked in a flow of interest.

These techniques are typically expensive and cumbersome to implement; nevertheless they reveal flows within an optically opaque bed and provide valuable information not attainable otherwise. For example, in Fig. 24, we display results of x-ray tomography experiments that show the evolution of the interior mixing structure within a double-cone blender using molybdenum-doped tracer particles (dark in Fig. 24). These experiments represent a

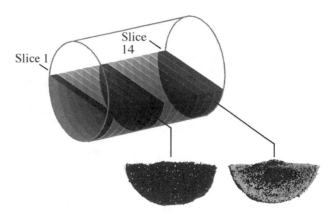

Fig. 22 Internal and external slices obtained by solidifying a blend, here of coarse (light) and fine (dark) grains in a drum tumbler. Segregation is evident, and the difference between internal and external slices highlights the importance of not relying on external appearances of tumbled blends.

scaled-up version of the solidification data shown in Fig. 23: the capacity is 8 times larger (~4.8 L vs. 0.6 L), and the particle diameter is 18 times larger (~1600 vs. 90 μm). Data of this kind reveal a complexity in flow and mixing evolution that simultaneously represents the cause

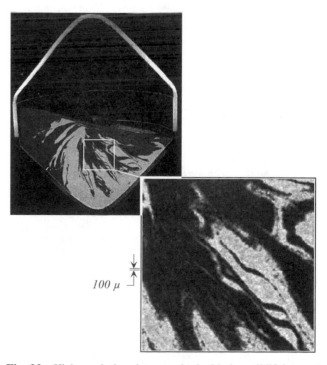

Fig. 23 High-resolution data are obtainable by solidifying and slicing an entire blend, here of identical but colored ~90-μm grains in a double-cone blender.

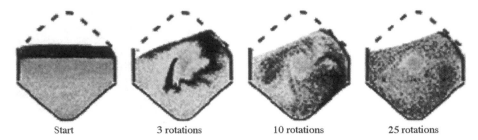

Start   3 rotations   10 rotations   25 rotations

Fig. 24 X-ray tomographic time series of blending of radio-opaque grains in double-cone blender is representative of several new techniques available for on-line and in situ assays of blending mechanisms.

of historical difficulty in understanding the subject and the opportunity for future developments.

ACKNOWLEDGMENTS

We thank Albert W. Alexander, Paulo Arratia, Osama Sudah and Erinn Martin for vital contributions and the National Science Foundation, the New Jersey Commission on Science and Technology, the Internationl Fine Particle Research Institute, Pfizer, Inc., Mobil, Technology, and Merck & Co., for financial support.

REFERENCES

1. Nakagawa, M.; Altobelli, S.A.; Caprihan, A.; Fukushima, E.; Jeong, E.K.; Non-Invasive Measurements of Granular Flows by Magnetic Resonance Imaging. Expt's in Fluids **1993**, *16*, 54–60.
2. Shinbrot, T.; Alexander, A.; Muzzio, F.J.; Spontaneous Chaotic Granular Mixing. Nature **1999**, *397, 67*, 5–8.
3. Lun, C.K.K.; Savage, S.B.; A Simple Kinetic Theory for Granular Flow of Rough, Inelastic, Spherical Particles. J. Appl. Mech. **1987**, *54*, 47–61.
4. Pöschel, T.; Buchholtz, V.; Static Friction Phenomena in Granular Materials: Coulomb Law vs. Particle Geometry. Phys. Rev. Lett. **1993**, *71, 396*, 3–6.
5. Müller, M.; Luding, S.; Herrmann, H.J.; Simulations of Vibrated Granular Media in 2D and 3D. *Friction, Arching and Contact Dynamics*; Wolf, D.E., Grassberger, P., Eds.; World Scientific: Singapore, 1997.

BIBLIOGRAPHY

Brone, D.; Wightman, C.; Connor, K.; Alexander, A.W.; Muzzio, F.J.; Robinson, P.; Using Flow Perturbations to Enhance Mixing of Dry Powders in V-Blenders. Powder Technol. **1997**, *91*, 165–172.

Chester, A.W.; Kowalski, J.A.; Coles, M.E.; Muegge, E.L.; Muzzio, F.J.; Brone, D.; Mixing Dynamics in Catalyst Impregnation in Double-Cone Blenders. Powder Technol. **1999**, *102*, 85–94.
Danckwerts, P.V.; The Definition and Measurement of Some Characteristics of Mixtures. Appl. Sci. Res. **1952**, *3*, 279–297.
DasGupta, S.; Khakhar, D.V.; Bhatia, S.K.; Axial Segregation of Particles in a Horizontal Rotating Cylinder. Chem. Eng. Sci. **1991**, *46* (5/6), 1513–1517.
Donald, M.B.; Roseman, B.; Mixing and Demixing of Solid Particles, Part I. Mechanisms in a Horizontal Drum Mixer. British Chemical Engineering, *7*, 749–753.
Harnby, N.; The Selection of Powder Mixers. *Mixing in the Process Industries, Butterworth Heinemann*; Oxford UK, 1997; 42–61.
Jaeger, H.M.; Nagel, S.R.; Behringer, R.P.; Granular Solids, Liquids, and Gases. Rev. Mod. Phys. **1996**, *68*, 1259–1273.
Lacey, P.M.C.; Developments in the Theory of Particle Mixing. J. Appl. Chem. **1954**, May 4, 257–268.
Moakher, M.; Shinbrot, T.; Muzzio, F.J.; Experimentally Validated Computations of Flow, Mixing and Segregation of Non-Cohesive Grains in 3D Tumbling Blenders. Powder Technology **2000**, *109*, 58–71.
Muzzio, F.J.; Robinson, P.; Wightman, C.; Brone, D.; Sampling Practices in Powder Blending. Int. J. Pharmaceutics **1997**, *155*, 153–178.
Muzzio, F.J.; Roddy, M.; Brone, D.; Alexander, A.W.; Sudah, O.; An Improved Powder-Sampling Tool. Pharm. Tech. **1999**, *23*, 92–110.
Reynolds, O.; On the Dilatancy of Media Composed of Rigid Particles in Contact with Experimental Illustrations. Philo. Mag. **1885**, *20, 46*, 9–82.
Ristow, G.H.; Simulating Granular Flow with Molecular Dynamics. J. Phys. I France **1992**, *2, 64*, 9–72.
Robinson, P.; Muzzio, F.J.; Wightman, C.; Brone, D.; Gleason, E.K. End-Sampling Thief Probe. US Patent 5,996,426, 1999.
Shinbrot, T.; Muzzio, F.J.; Nonequilibrium Patterns in Granular Mixing and Segregation. Physics Today, March, 2000; 25–30.
Walton, O.R.; Numerical Simulation of Inelastic, Frictional Particle-Particle Interactions. *Particulate Two-Phase Flow*; Roco, M.C., Ed.; Butterworth-Heinemann: Oxford UK, 1993; 884–911.
Williams, J.C.; Continuous Mixing of Solids—A Review. Powder Technol. **1976**, *15*, 237–243.

MOISTURE IN PHARMACEUTICAL PRODUCTS

R. Gary Hollenbeck

University of Maryland School of Pharmacy, Baltimore, Maryland

M

INTRODUCTION

The earth contains 75% water (1), some of it in pharmaceutical products. With regard to solid dosage forms, pharmaceutical scientists have struggled for years to answer questions on how much is there, in what form is it, afnd if, when, and how might it influence a product or manufacturing process.

The term moisture, usually defined as wetness conferred by an unidentified liquid (2), is assumed here to be due to water. Thus, the scope of this article is the characterization of and consequences due to relatively small amounts of water associated with solids of pharmaceutical interest. Chemical stability, crystal structure, powder flow, compaction, lubricity, dissolution rate, and polymer film permeability are some properties of pharmaceutical interest that have been demonstrated to be influenced by the presence of moisture. Wet granulation, extrusion, spheronization, tray drying, freeze drying, spray drying, fluid-bed drying, tableting, and aqueous film coating are some unit operations that obviously depend on the amount and state of water present.

Moisture can and does influence the properties of individual active ingredients and excipients, and it is essential, as a first step, to characterize the effect of moisture on these individual components. Indeed, most of this article examines the sorption behavior of specific chemicals. However, the behavior of a pharmaceutical formulation is a complicated function of the individual component attributes. The following is an example of heterogeneous moisture distribution: A powder blend containing 2% moisture has a 10% content of an hydrophilic binder. If one assumes that all the moisture is associated with the binder, the moisture content of the binder itself would be 20%. Photomicrographic evidence demonstrates dramatically how the presence of a disintegrant, for example, can dramatically alter the environment in which a moisture-sensitive drug may exist at a particular relative humidity (3). Even though at least one model has been developed that allows the prediction of component moisture contents in a blend (4), the distribution of water in complicated formulations is largely uncharted territory.

Historical Perspective

In the area of moisture in pharmaceutical products, it is possible to identify three stages in the scientific and regulatory history. The first stage dealt more or less exclusively with the amount of water present in pharmaceuticals, most of which were products of natural origin, with regard to issues of potency and commerce.

In the second stage, there was a realization that water could affect the chemical and physical properties of drugs and dosage forms. The fact that water might exist in different states was exemplified by partitioning the water into "bound" or "free" moisture. The implication was that the free, or solvent-like, moisture was responsible for most stability and production problems (5).

The third stage came with the realization that even small amounts of "bound" moisture could have a dramatic impact on properties and processes of pharmaceutical interest. In the evolution of this scientific pursuit, it is now evident that the state of moisture is as important as the amount present. Although sophisticated thermodynamic characterization of adsorbates has been the subject of research since the pioneering work of Gibbs (6), this stage has been enhanced by the ability to examine behavior at the molecular level by using powerful new analytical tools.

Over the years, only few studies linked a thorough characterization of moisture with physical and chemical stability and production problems. Recent interest indicates that the subject is still important, there are still questions to be answered, and the gap between thermodynamic characterization and technological application will continue to narrow.

Compendial Standards

The methods for moisture determination in USP 24/NF 19 (7) are at best, classical, addressing only the determination of moisture content (8). The specifications for most official articles are arbitrary and may be excessively restrictive or broad. They are not supported by the type of data referred to previously that relate moisture content to the stability or performance of the article.

A USP Advisory Panel on Moisture Specifications initiated a revision process (9) with the inclusion of background material in the general chapter ⟨1241⟩ "Water-Solid Interactions in Pharmaceutical Systems." However, this occurred over 10 years ago and it has not been followed by the inclusion of standard analytical tests that can be used to characterize the state of water.

The USP offers two methods for the determination of moisture content in solids: titrimetry (Karl Fisher titration) and gravimetry (e.g., thermal gravimetric analysis). Applications, advantages, and disadvantages of these methods are addressed later. Most articles listed in the official compendia contain specifications on "water" or "loss on Drying (LOD)." For chemicals, the gravimetric method is the same as the physical test in the general chapter ⟨731⟩ "Loss on Drying" (8). As volatile components other than water may be present, loss on drying is not a de facto moisture content determination. Inclusion of a "water" specification is an indication that the only volatile component present is water.

The nature of moisture content determinations is perhaps best exemplified by the fact that the *Handbook of Pharmaceutical Excipients* (10) lists 31 separate versions of laboratory tests to determine moisture content and one to determine equilibrium moisture content. These methods were used to assess the moisture content in the compilation of 148 monographs (10), many of which do not deal with solids.

BACKGROUND

Conventions, Definitions, and Terminology

The subjects of moisture and solids have not been distinguished by clear definitions and consistent usage. Table 1 clearly defines terms that are often misused.

Several conventions will be followed in this article. Moisture contents are expressed on a dry weight basis. When necessary, the subscript 1 is used for water, and the subscript 2 for the other component in the adsorbent; in the absence of a subscript, the property is to be attributed to water. Results of many routine tests conducted in my laboratory have been included here. Although the specific equipment used and all the experimental details are not provided, an effort has been made to include information that can substantially influence the results of the test (e.g., heating rate in thermal gravimetric analysis). These data should be taken as being representative of the substance tested and not necessarily as the results to be expected for a given lot of the substance examined with different instrumentation under different experimental conditions.

The sorption isotherm is the most widely used expression to quantify a substance's affinity for water. It is, as the term implies, a relationship at a constant temperature.

$$n = f(x) \tag{1}$$

where n, the number of moles of water sorbed, is a function of x, the partial pressure of water in the atmosphere at that temperature. The correspondence of n to moisture content and x to relative humidity, as defined in the Table 1, suggests that this functional relationship may be stated in numerous ways. Often, the graphical presentation of sorption isotherms is a plot of the dependent variable moisture content versus relative humidity, with both expressed on a percentage basis.

Idealized moisture isotherms are presented in this article for substances that sorb moisture in discrete stages (e.g., crystalline materials capable of forming a hydrates) and for substances that do not interact with water in discrete stages (11). These idealized isotherms form a basis for the discussion of deviations and unexpected effects of moisture sorption that can influence the physical or chemical properties of the solid.

Figure 1 is a sorption isotherm constructed for a hypothetical solid with a molecular weight of 180, which is capable of forming a monohydrate. In this case, the solubility of the substance in water is assumed to be 50 wt% and the critical humidity for the transition from anhydrous to monohydrate is assumed to be 60% RH. It is also assumed that a solution of the solid in water behaves ideally.

The stepwise character demonstrated in this profile is characteristic of a substance capable of forming a hydrate. At humidities below 60% RH, the moisture content of the solid remains virtually unchanged. When the activity of water reaches a critical relative humidity of 60%, water is sorbed by the solid as the anhydrous form converts to the monohydrate. For this example, the moisture content associated with the complete transition to the monohydrate is 10% (e.g., 1 mole of water = 18 g; 1 mole of the substance = 180 g).

Further increase of humidity has no appreciable effect on moisture content until a water activity is reached equal to that associated with a saturated solution of the substance in water at the temperature of the analysis. The relative humidity associated with this activity will be referred to as RH_s. In this case, $RH_s = 91\%$ relative humidity, as the solubility of 50 wt% is $x_2 = 0.09$. On a mole fraction basis, and, assuming ideal solution behavior, $x_1 = 1 - x_2 = P_1/P_1^o$. In this hypothetical case, the moisture content of the saturated solution when all the solid is dissolved is 100%; therefore, at 91% RH the monohydrate sorbs water from the atmosphere until dissolution is complete. The fact that constant humidity is produced by a saturated solution of a

Table 1 Definitions

Term	Symbol(s)	Definition
Sorption		The spontaneous acquisition of a component (water in this case) from the atmosphere by a system.
Adsorption		Sorption confined to the surface of the solid. The amount of water adsorbed is directly proportional to the surface area available.
Absorption		Sorption characterized by penetration of the sorbed component into the bulk structure of the solid. The amount of water absorbed does not depend on surface area.
Desorption		The spontaneous loss of the sorbed component (water) to the atmosphere.
Sorbent		The substance or system responsible for sorption.
Adsorbent		Ostensibly the substance responsible for adsorption. The term "absorbent" is not in common usage. Adsorbent is used without discriminating between adsorption or absorption.
Adsorbate		The substance being adsorbed (water in this case).
Moisture content	MC, W	The total amount of water present with the adsorbent.
Dry weight basis	W_D	An expression of moisture content related to the weight of dry solid. W_D = wt. water/wt. of dry solid
	$\%MC_D$	Amount of moisture present with 100 g of dry solid. $\%MC_D = 100 W_D$
Wet weight basis	W_W	An expression of moisture content referring to the total weight of the sample. W_W = wt. water/wt. of sample
	$\%MC_W$	Amount of moisture present in 100 g of sample. $\%MC_W = 100 W_W$
Equilibrium moisture content	EMC, %EMC, $W_{D.eq}$, $W_{W.eq}$	The moisture content (sometimes expressed on a percentage basis) at equilibrium under specified conditions of temperature, pressure, and vapor composition.
Partial pressure of water in the atmosphere	P/P_o	The vapor pressure of water in the atmosphere (P) expressed as a fraction of the saturation vapor pressure of pure liquid water (P_0) at the same temperature.

(Continued)

Table 1 Definitions (*Continued*)

Term	Symbol(s)	Definition
	x	As the behavior or water vapor is generally assumed to be ideal (fugacity = pressure), x is the activity of water.
Relative humidity	%RH, $100P/P_o$, $100x$	The vapor pressure of water in the atmosphere (P) usually expressed as a percentage of the saturation vapor pressure of pure liquid water (P_o) at the same temperature.
Term	Symbol(s)	Definition
Bound moisture		Water associated with a solid exhibiting a vapor pressure less than P.
Free moisture, unbound moisture		Water present in a solid exhibiting a vapor pressure greater that P. This water is sometimes referred to as "freezable" water.
Hygroscopicity		A term synonymous with sorption, implying an acquired amount or state of water sufficient to affect the physical or chemical properties of the substance.
Water of hydration		Water present in regular positions within a crystal lattice (3). (There is a specific stoichiometry with the other molecule.)
Efflorescence		Spontaneous loss of water of hydration (not thermally induced).
Deliquescence		Sorption sufficient to produce dissolution of the substance.
Monolayer capacity	V_m	Volume of water (STP) adsorbed at STP when the surface is covered.
	Y_m	Amount of water adsorbed when the surface is covered.

substance has been used as a basis for establishing controlled-humidity chambers.

At relative humidities above 91%, the colligative behavior of the solution results in absorption of water until the solution is in equilibrium with water vapor in the atmosphere. In Fig. 1, this region has been constructed based on Raoult's law.

Although some specific examples are given, several aspects of the sorption of water by crystalline substances deserve attention at this point. First, it is important to recognize that the large quantity of water that associates with these systems actually obscures small changes in moisture content that occur between hydrate transitions. It has been stated that lactose monohydrate, for example, "contains 5% water of crystallization and approximately 0.1% adsorbed water" (10), indicating that adsorption takes place on the hydrate.

Furthermore, this sorption isotherm is a thermodynamic relationship. Although it represents the equilibrium position, it does not provide any information about the rate at which the transitions take place. For example, the desiccant calcium sulfate goes through two stages of hydration, as shown in Eq. (2).

Stage 1: $CuSO_4 + \frac{1}{2}H_2O \rightarrow CuSO_4 + \frac{1}{2}H_2O$

Stage 2: $CuSO_4 + \frac{1}{2}H_2O + 1\frac{1}{2}H_2O \rightarrow CuSO_4 + 2H_2O$

$$(2)$$

The first stage where the hemihydrate is formed takes place instantaneously in the presence of water vapor,

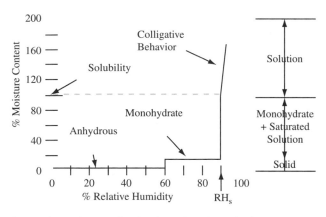

Fig. 1 Stepwise sorption isotherm for a hypothetical substance.

whereas the second stage requires a matter of weeks or months to reach completion, depending on the humidity at which the hemihydrate is stored (12).

Finally, the critical relative humidities are dependent on the nature of the solid. For example, the spontaneous dissolution process has been observed for many water-soluble substances at relative humidities significantly below that associated with a saturated solution of the substance in water (5). Van Campen et al. (13–15) have examined the moisture sorption kinetics of deliquescent solids at relative humidities above what they term the "critical relative humidity" (RH_o), where adsorbed water takes on the character of condensed water and serves as a solvent. It is important to recognize that a highly undesirable process such as deliquescence can occur when it may not be expected (e.g., when $RH_o < RH < RH_s$).

In all the previous examples, the process was absorption, and water ultimately had access to the entire solid; variations in particle size, and consequently, surface area, would not effect the profile. In many of the subsequent examples, not only is surface area a determinant of moisture content, but perturbation of the solid can occur during sorption to produce unexpected and dramatic effects.

Brunauer (16) organized the experimental isotherms observed for vapor sorption into the now classical five groups, Types I to V. Brunauer et al. (17) presented a unified theory of multilayer physical adsorption that was purported to describe all types of isotherms. Numerous texts present detailed discussion of the basis for this theory. In the context of this discussion, capillary condensation will not be considered and the focus will be Types I, II, and III behavior. Fig. 2 is a graphical representation of these three types, generated from Eqs. 3–5.

Type I isotherms, where sorption occurs on strong sorption sites, are characterized by a monotonic increase in the amount of vapor adsorbed, up to a maximum value assumed to represent a completed unimolecular layer. The Langmuir equation is generally a suitable functional relationship for $n = f(x)$, as given by

$$y = \frac{y_m B x}{1 + B x} \tag{3}$$

where y is the amount of water adsorbed at $x = P/P_o$, y_m is the monolayer capacity, and B is a constant, often referred to as the adsorption coefficient. Using the generally assumed value of 1250 nm^2 for the area occupied by a molecule of water on the adsorbent surface, the surface area can be estimated from y_m.

The characteristic inflection in Type II behavior occurs when multilayer sorption starts. The Brunauer, Emmett, Teller (BET) equation (17), shown as Eq. 4, can describe isotherms where multilayer sorption is evident:

$$\frac{y = y_m C x}{(1 - x)(1 + (C - 1)x)} \tag{4}$$

Based on the assumptions in the kinetic derivation of the BET equation, the constant C is related to the average heat of adsorption in the first layer. Type III isotherms occur when this value is low.

Application of the BET equation to experimental data has become the standard method for surface area determinations. The constants are determined from data

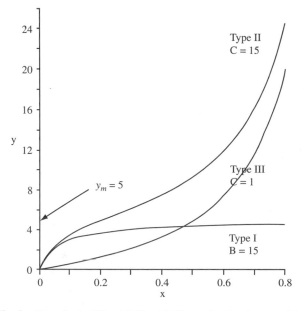

Fig. 2 Hypothetical Type I, II, and III sorption isotherms with a monolayer capacity of $y_m = 5$.

at low humidities (5–30% RH). Based on these parameters, the BET equation almost always over-estimates the amount of water associated with the solid at high humidity.

As 100% RH is approached, the BET theory predicts that the amount of water adsorbed will be infinite. As the influence of the solid surface does not extend indefinitely, it should be expected that a finite number of molecular layers would be adsorbed (presuming that the solid is not soluble.) Many authors attribute the "infinity catastrophe" of the BET theory to the lack of consideration of lateral adsorbate interactions (18–20).

Ostensibly the constant C relates to the state of water associated with the solid; however, the simplistic assumptions (all molecules in the second and higher layers are assumed to have the same character as bulk water and horizontal interactions between molecules are ignored for all layers) used in the derivation preclude really useful thermodynamic information.

Equation (5), a modification of the BET equation which assumes a third thermodynamic state for the adsorbate, was developed independently by Guggenheim et al. (21).

$$\frac{y = y_m C K x}{(1 - Kx)(1 + (C-1)Kx)} \tag{5}$$

where K is a constant that accounts for the intermediate state between tightly bound water in the first layer and bulk liquid. This model is also simplistic but it does fits data at high relative humidities better than the BET equation. Eq. 5 is termed the GAB equation (22).

All of the equations presented thus far are single-valued relationships between the amount adsorbed and the pressure of water in the atmosphere. However, hysteresis is frequently observed. When a sample that has reached a specific equilibrium moisture content is exposed to lower relative humidity, desorption occurs. In many cases, adsorption and desorption isotherms are not superimposable.

Fig. 3 is an example of a Type II sorption isotherm with hysteresis. Although the etiology of hysteresis has been the subject of many discussions (23–30), the phenomena usually can be attributed to

- Irreversible perturbation of the solid, that is, sorption can increase (swelling) or decrease (collapse of a freeze-dried cake) the surface area;
- Kinetic origin, that is, the new equilibrium position has actually not yet been reached; and
- An actual change in state of the adsorbate.

Most individuals recognize hysteresis in terms of a substance having different moisture contents at a specified

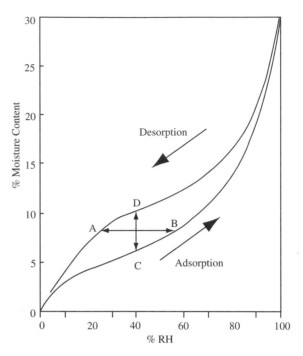

Fig. 3 Type II isotherm with hysteresis.

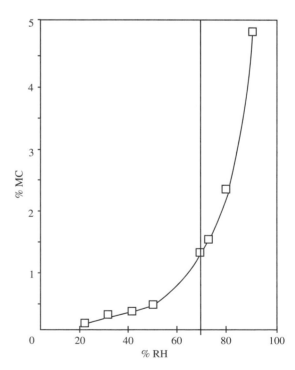

Fig. 4 Moisture sorption isotherm for lactose. (Adapted from Ref. 10.)

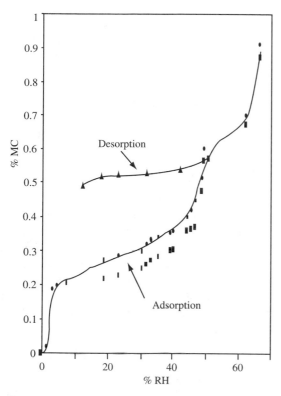

Fig. 5 Moisture sorption isotherm for compressible sugar. (Adapted from Ref. 31.)

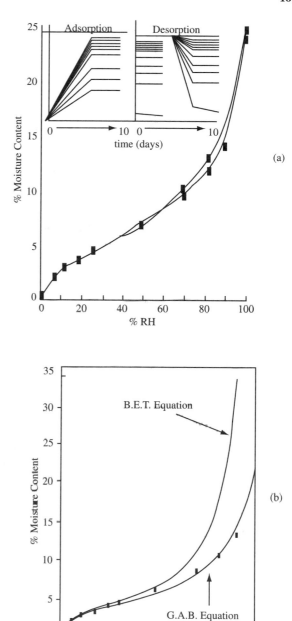

Fig. 6 (a) Moisture sorption isotherm for microcrystalline cellulose:adsorption and desorption. (Adapted from Ref. 22.) (b) BET and GAB equations describing the adsorption branch.

relative humidity (CD in Fig. 3). The implications of this situation are obvious: the moisture content of a material depends on its history of exposure to different relative humidity conditions. Controlling relative humidity can only insure that the moisture content lies within the range specified by the isotherm. The other aspect of hysteresis is that substances with equal moisture contents can have adsorbed water with different chemical activity (AB in Fig. 3).

Although the sorption isotherm is fundamental to the characterization of moisture interaction with water, it is generally not possible to make any judgments about the effect of water on the substrate from the isotherm alone. For example, it is not possible to determine if an increase in moisture content is due to multilayer adsorption, swelling of the substrate, or some combination of the two.

Sorption isotherms for lactose are shown in Fig. 4, compressible sugar in Fig. 5 (31), microcrystalline cellulose in Fig. 6 (32), and aspirin in Fig.7 (3). The isotherm for lactose has been adapted from data in the *Handbook of Pharmaceutical Excipients* (10); the step-wise isotherm expected is not evident. The dashed line in Fig. 4 is based on the statement that the monohydrate forms at 70% RH.

Compressible sugar NF is an example of a material that very slowly sorbs relatively small amounts of water, with a resulting isotherm that is not smooth. The adsorption isotherm was generated from a sample that had been carefully preconditioned to remove moisture. The dramatic difference between the desorption and adsorption branches of the isotherm indicates that water forms a

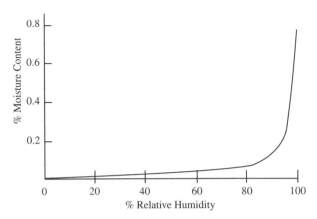

Fig. 7 Moisture sorption isotherm for aspirin. (Adapted from Ref. 3.)

hydrate-like phase (31). Zografi and Kontny (22) have demonstrated that almost all of the water taken up by compressible sugar is associated with the maltodextrin.

Moisture sorption of microcrystalline cellulose has been studied extensively (22, 32, 33). Fig. 6a includes the sorption and desorption studies for microcrystalline cellulose. The inserts are plots of moisture content versus time, which approximately represent the kinetics of sorption and desorption at each humidity. The equilibrium adsorption isotherm (Type II) has been fit to the BET equation ($C = 16.48$, $y_m = 0.033$ g/g solid) and this curve is presented in Fig.6b along with a curve described by the GAB equation by using the same monolayer capacity.

The isotherm for aspirin would be classified as Type III, indicating a low affinity for water followed by multilayer sorption. These four isotherms cover a broad range of moisture interaction with solids of pharmaceutical interest.

ANALYTICAL METHODS

There is no single analytical method that suffices in the characterization of moisture associated with solids. The best approach is a judicious combination of the following techniques.

In this era of automatic titrators, microprocessor-controlled thermal analysis, and definitive spectral techniques, one of the most powerful techniques, that is, optical microscopy, is frequently overlooked. The value of direct sample observation, preferably while it is exposed to different relative humidities, cannot be overstated. In the author's laboratory, a plexiglass chamber was constructed that can be placed on the stage of the microscope, through

which air of known humidity can be circulated. This simple technique has been very useful in examining the swelling (or lack) of disintegrants (34) and the influence of very hydrophilic excipients in combination with a moisture sensitive drug (3).

In a moisture determination by the physical separation of water from the solid, it is important to recognize that free and bound moisture must be dissociated from the solid by an applied stress, using

$$\text{Solid} \quad x\text{H}_2\text{O} \rightarrow \text{Solid.}y\text{H}_2\text{O} + (x - y)\text{H}_2\text{O} \qquad (6)$$

where x is the moles of water initially associated with the solid, Y the moles of water still associated with the solid, and $(x-y)$ the amount of water released as a consequence of the stress. The stresses used differ according to the conditions (e.g., high temperature, low vapor pressure, anhydrous solvent systems). Hence, the moisture contents determined by different methods may very well be different. There is no guarantee that $y = 0$, and no reason to expect that y has the same value for different methods.

An equally important consideration is the fact that these stresses are different than those that may be responsible for moisture release during manufacturing or within the product after manufacture. One should approach the determination of moisture content with the disconcerting realization that different methods can produce different results and that none of these results may be relevant.

Thermal Methods

Thermal gravimetric analysis (TGA) is undoubtedly the most widely used method of moisture content determination. The sensitivity and sophistication of TGA instruments ranges from the classical moisture balance (LOD) to specially designed microbalances enclosed in chambers that may be evacuated. Microprocessor control of the temperature increase has led to more reproducible and discriminating information.

The result of a TGA of dicalcium phosphate dihydrate is shown in Fig. 8. The profile represents the weight loss with increasing temperature (1.5°C/min) in an environment containing a desiccant. The total weight loss is the difference between the initial weight and the final constant weight of the dry solid. There are two regions in the profile, the first beginning at about 90°C and the second at about 170°C. Assuming that the only volatile component is water, calculations indicate $W_D = 0.228$ (22.8% MC), with W_D values of about 0.042 and 0.186 associated with Regions I and II, respectively.

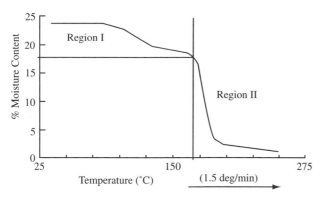

Fig. 8 Thermal gravimetric analysis of dicalcium phosphate dihydrate.

The profile in Fig. 8 is characteristic of a crystal hydrate, showing discrete regions of moisture loss occurring at relatively high temperature. This particular profile is consistent with the dehydration scheme shown in Eq. 7.

$$\text{Reaction 1} \quad CaHPO_2 \cdot 2H_2O \rightarrow CaHPO_4 \cdot 1\tfrac{1}{2}H_2O + \tfrac{1}{2}H_2O$$

$$\text{Reaction 2} \quad CaHPO_4 \cdot 1\tfrac{1}{2}H_2O \rightarrow CaHPO_4 + 1\tfrac{1}{2}H_2O$$

$$(7)$$

Differential scanning calorimetry (DSC) is a thermal method that measures the energy change accompanying a nonadiabatic process. A small sample of the moist solid contained in a metal sample container is exposed to a controlled increase in temperature. Water dissociated from the sample is swept out of the heating chamber by a nitrogen stream and the dynamic energy consumption (mcal/sec) required to keep the sample at the same temperature as an empty sample container is recorded. When the temperature is increased at a constant rate, the area under the DSC curve reflects the energy, in the form of heat, associated with the phase change.

The DSC profile for dicalcium phosphate dihydrate (Fig. 9 curve A) includes two endotherms consistent with the dehydration scheme shown in Eq. 7. (In all DSC plots reported here, endotherms are positive deflections from the base line.) It should also be noted that the energy change measured is not specific for water; it includes, for example, energy consumed or released because of changes in crystal structure. Thus, it is generally not appropriate to estimate moisture content from the enthalpy change for dehydration and the specific heat of vaporization of water.

A common error is to look at temperature profiles (TGA or DSC) and conclude, for example, that no water is released from dicalcium phosphate dihydrate at 50°C. It is important to recognize that this is a dynamic test with a large temperature increase examined over a relatively short time periods. Exposure of dicalcium phosphate dihydrate at 50°C may indeed drive off water of hydration; the system is not held at any particular temperature and the relative rate of moisture loss is slow.

Curve B in Fig. 9 is the result of an interesting test on a sample of anhydrous dicalcium phosphate that had been exposed to 100% RH for three months. Clearly, some of the moisture acquired by the solid was converted into water of hydration. However, the broad endotherm from about 50 to 130°C represents the energy consumed in the dissociation of water that is not part of the crystal structure. The existence of two states of water in the same solid raises a number of questions pertaining to the wisdom of using anhydrous dicalcium phosphate as an excipient for moisture-sensitive drugs.

The TGA profile for lactose is shown in Fig. 10. This profile is consistent with a monohydrate that loses its water of hydration in one step. DSC data for lactose are shown in

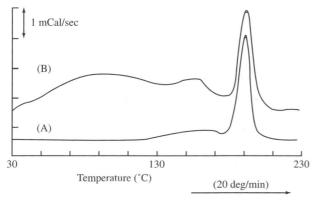

Fig. 9 Differential scanning calorimetry of dicalcium phosphate samples. (A) dicalcium phosphate dihydrate; (B) anhydrous dicalcium phosphate with adsorbed moisture.

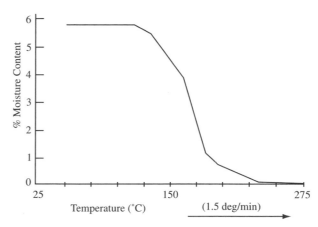

Fig. 10 Thermal gravimetric analysis of lactose monohydrate.

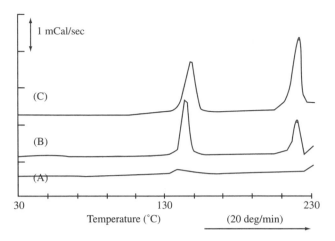

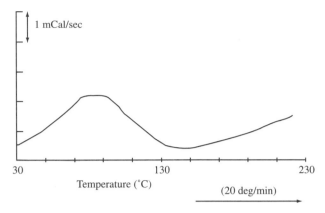

Fig. 11 Differential scanning calorimetry of lactose samples. (A) anhydrous lactose; (B) lactose monohydrate; (C) anhydrous lactose with adsorbed moisture.

Fig. 13 Differential scanning calorimetry of microcrystalline cellulose.

Fig. 11. Scan A for anhydrous lactose is rather uneventful, although comparison with the other scans seems to indicate the presence of a small quantity of water. Scan B is for lactose monohydrate; the single water of hydration is lost at approximately 135°C, with decomposition occurring at about 200°C. Scan C is for an anhydrous lactose sample that had been exposed to 100% RH for three days. Clearly, the water sorbed by anhydrous lactose was quickly and completely converted to water of hydration.

Thermal analyses of microcrystalline cellulose reveal distinctly different results. The TGA (Fig. 12) shows a loss of moisture at low temperature and a reasonably monotonic decrease that does not indicate discrete stages of hydration. The DSC (Fig. 13) shows a broad region of moisture loss at temperatures well below the boiling point of water.

The principal advantage of the thermal methods is convenience; however, these analyses are not specific for water, and exposure to high temperature may be an unrealistic stress or alter the sample. An acceptable determination of moisture content using a thermal method provides a result with minimal residual moisture and only minor alteration of the solid. Thermal methods can be combined with a specific titration of water by bubbling the evolved gas from TGA or DSC through the titration medium.

Karl Fisher Titration

For over 60 years, the specific titration of water has used a reagent developed by Karl Fisher, which consists of iodine, sulfur dioxide, and pyridine in methanol. The Karl Fisher titration of water is addressed in most analytical chemistry texts and is not presented here. A brief review with a pharmaceutical perspective has recently been published (35). However, the advantages and disadvantages of this method for the characterization of water associated with solids are discussed later.

In its simplest form, the Karl Fisher titration is a one-point determination of moisture content. The principal advantage is specificity for water. It is also a non-thermal method, which is very sensitive and can be easily automated. The main disadvantage is that the solid must dissolve in the titration medium to be sure that the total amount of moisture is released. If the analysis is carefully designed in such a way that moisture is "extracted" from the solid to the same degree each time, accurate and reproducible results can be obtained for solids that do not dissolve.

With automation, the Karl Fisher titration provides a titration kinetics profile (e.g., milliliters of titrant vs. time).

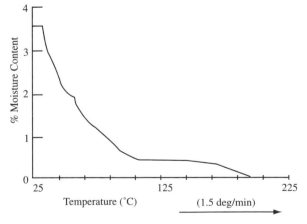

Fig. 12 Thermal gravimetric analysis of microcrystalline cellulose.

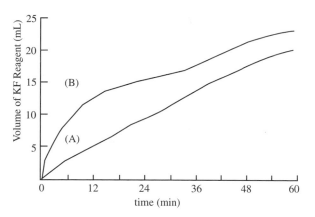

Fig. 14 Normalized Karl Fisher titrations of dicalcium phosphate dihydrate; (A) unmilled form; (B) milled form.

If the rate of water release from the solid is the rate-limiting step, the kinetics of the Karl Fisher titration profile can provide indirect information about the state of water associated with the solid. Fig. 14 shows the titrations of two different samples of dicalcium phosphate dihydrate. Here, and in the titration profiles in Fig. 15, the data have been normalized in such a way that each titration ultimately consumes 25 mL of reagent. This normalization is analogous to increasing the sample size in such a way that it contains an amount of available water which would require 25 mL of reagent to neutralize. Also, the direct titration of water can be finished in less than 90 s.

The titration profiles for dicalcium phosphate are not monotonic, but exhibit stages of dehydration consistent with the scheme shown in Eq. (7). It is also evident that the release of moisture is faster from the milled form (Fig. 14,

curve B) of the excipient. This is consistent with the increased total surface area and shorter diffusional path expected with smaller particle size.

In Fig. 15, Karl Fisher titration of anhydrous dicalcium phosphate, which had been exposed to 100% RH for 3 months (curve B), is compared to with that of milled dicalcium phosphate dihydrate (curve A). The adsorbed water, which was not incorporated into the crystal lattice, was released from the solid very rapidly.

Results of normalized Karl Fisher titrations for lactose monohydrate and microcrystalline cellulose both present profiles not significantly different from water, indicating a very rapid release of moisture.

Spectroscopic Methods

The most useful spectral methods for the characterization of water in solids are Fourier transform infrared spectroscopy (FTIR), nuclear magnetic resonance (NMR), and powder X-ray diffraction (XRD). A thorough treatment of these methods is not given here; instead the example of ampicillin presented by Brittan, et al. (36) is summarized.

Hydrates normally form crystal structures (pseudo-polymorphs) that differ from the anhydrous form. Different powder XRD patterns of ampicillin in the anhydrous and trihydrate forms are shown in Fig. 16,

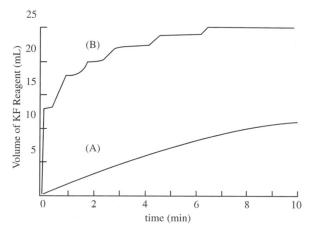

Fig. 15 Normalized Karl Fisher titration for dicalcium phosphate; (A) milled sample; (B) anhydrous sample with adsorbed moisture.

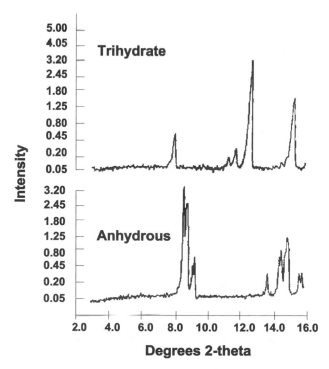

Fig. 16 Partial X-ray diffraction patterns of ampicillin samples. (Adapted from Ref. 36.)

Although moisture contents often present values that are close to being stoichiometric, X-ray confirmation of the differing crystal structure should be a requisite for designation as a hydrate.

The X-ray method is not just useful from the qualitative perspective. In samples that contain both anhydrous and hydrate forms, diagnostic regions of the pattern can be identified, and the relative areas of peaks in these regions may be used to establish the relative amounts of each phase (36).

Infrared analysis of water associated with a solid centers on an assessment of the degree to which the environment influences the stretching frequency associated with the —OH group. The —OH stretching mode for free water in the gaseous state has a characteristic energy of 3655 cm^{-1}. The frequency of this stretching is lowered when water is condensed and/or bound. Ice has a characteristic —OH stretching frequency of 3400 cm^{-1}. By comparison of the FTIR spectra for the anhydrous form with those of the sample with water, the —OH bands for water can be identified. The distinctive, sharp peak for crystalline water is shown in Fig. 17; when water is present in several states, multiple bands may be seen in the spectrum.

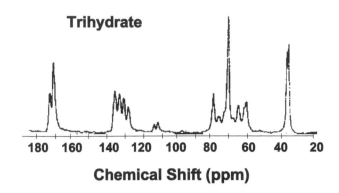
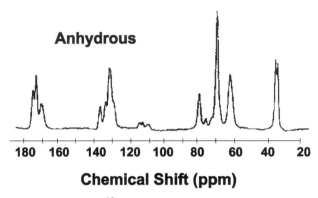

Fig. 18 Solid-state ^{13}C NMR spectra of ampicillin samples. (Adapted from Ref. 36.)

Solid-state NMR is a method that promises to increase the understanding of the state of water in solids and its specific influence on the chemicals of interest. In Fig. 18, for example, it is clear that the solid-state ^{13}C NMR spectra of ampicillin trihydrate is a very different form than that for the anhydrous form. Although three carbonyl resonances present in the anhydrous form (169.7, 172.7, and 174.6 ppm), it is interesting that only two (170.4 and 172.6 ppm) are fully resolved in the hydrate form (33). Thus, in the latter, two of the three carbonyls are equivalent. Evidence also exists for differences in carbons in the aromatic ring based on the presence of water of hydration.

INFLUENCE OF MOISTURE ON PRODUCT AND/OR PROCESS ATTRIBUTES

No attempt will be made to provide a comprehensive summary of the numerous studies that have been conducted and which show how water influences the processing and stability of pharmaceutical solids and dosage forms. For more information, the reader is referred

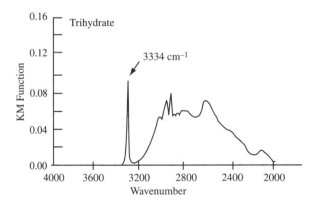
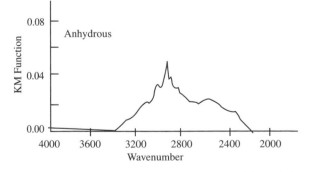

Fig. 17 Partial FTIR spectra of ampicillin. (Adapted from Ref. 36.)

to some classical texts (10, 27, 37, 40, 41), recent general articles on the subject (5, 11, 42, 43), and those with specific emphasis on the role of water on stability (44–47) or compaction properties (48–52).

In an earlier section, the potential for a water-soluble substance to deliquesce was discussed. The emphasis here is on less obvious effects of moisture on solid dosage forms, and three associated areas that link to information presented earlier in this article are discussed: 1) moisture-induced changes in the state of the solid, 2) the effect of moisture on the performance of excipients in the manufacture of compressed tablets, and 3) the chemical stability of bioactive agents alone and in combination with excipients.

Moisture-Induced Changes

That moisture can have a dramatic effect on the physical character of a substance has been demonstrated recently by Carstensen and Van Scoik (51). Amorphous sucrose spheres were prepared by lyophilization and placed in an environment at 33% RH. Lyophilization characteristically produces a highly porous, amorphous solid cake. As shown in Fig. 19, its moisture content increases considerably in the first few days of the study. However, the moisture absorbed by the porous amorphous sucrose phase eventually caused a collapse of the structure and a commensurate reduction in moisture content because of the dramatic decrease in available "surface." Not only did the physical structure change from a loose to a more dense

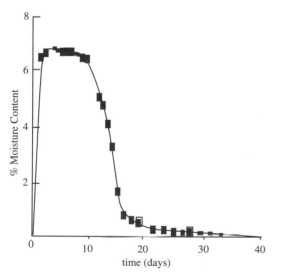

Fig. 19 Moisture uptake by amorphous sucrose at 23°C at 33%RH. (Adapted from Ref. 51.)

amorphous structure, but also the amorphous sucrose was shown to convert to the crystalline form at a rate that was dependent on relative humidity. This example is consistent with the increased emphasis being placed on changes in state of the solid as a result of sorption. One of the difficulties associated with a thermodynamic treatment of solids is the problem of dealing with changes in surface area as a continuous variable. An early thermodynamic treatment to address this problem was presented by Copeland and Young in 1961 (53). These authors considered a change in the number of moles of adsorbent as an addition or removal of particles with the same specific surface area, and, therefore, presented a basis for treating thermodynamic properties of powder systems as continuous functions. Wu and Copeland (54) used this approach in the characterization of barium sulfate. They found clear evidence to discount the "inert" adsorbent theory and stressed that even though thermodynamic variables of adsorbents are generally smaller than these for adsorbates, this can be misleading. Adsorbent properties are average properties of the respective component. When the adsorbed moisture is homogeneously distributed within the solid, this estimate is reasonable. However, if the process is adsorption and only the first few layers of the adsorbent are affected, the thermodynamic changes would be dramatically increased. Very few pharmaceutical studies involve the determination of thermodynamic properties of the adsorbent which is a promising area for further research.

The need to address changes in adsorbent is discussed by Zografi (5). He observes that water absorbed into the bulk structure of a solid can act as a plasticizer and depress the glass transition temperature. At temperatures above the glass transition point, the mobility of molecules or segments of molecules in the system increases (5). The change from the "glassy state" to the "rubbery state" can account for a number of physical chemical processes of pharmaceutical interest, including the collapse and subsequent crystallization of lyophilized cakes (see example previously), direct compaction properties, powder caking, permeability of coatings and packaging materials, and solid-state chemical stability (5). Recognition of this fact has been the single greatest recent advance in establishing a framework for understanding and predicting the impact of moisture.

Zografi and Kontny (22) corrected the experimentally determined monolayer capacities of microcrystalline cellulose for degree of crystallinity and found reasonably consistent values. This result supported the conclusion that water in microcrystalline cellulose is confined to the noncrystalline regions (22, 56).

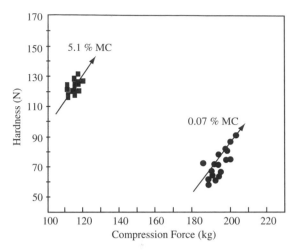

Fig. 20 Compression force vs. hardness plots for microcrystalline cellulose tablets with 0.07 and 5.1% MC. (The points represent individual tablets collected during manufacture.)

Effect of Moisture on Excipients and Tablet Manufacture

The bulk properties of celluloses are generally influenced by adsorbed moisture (58, 59). The effect of the change in bulk solid properties for microcrystalline cellulose has been demonstrated by a tableting operation in a very simplistic manner. Dry microcrystalline cellulose (%MC = 0.07) was compared with material with a moisture content above that associated with completion of the monolayer (%MC = 5.1). A thermodynamic picture of the character of water in these samples can be based on the adsorbate thermodynamic properties: $\Delta H > 3.5$ kcal/mole (14.65 kJ/mole), $\Delta G > 2.3$ kcal/mole (9.6 kJ/mole), $\Delta S < 4.12$ entropy units (e.u.) per mole with the dry solid, and $\Delta H = 1.5$ kcal/mole (6.27 kJ/mole, $\Delta G = 0.53$ kcal/mole (2.21 kJ/mole), $\Delta S = 3.35$ e.u./mole for moisture at the 5.1% level, or 1.5 times monolayer capacity. (The differential entropy goes through a maximum near the level where a monolayer is completed, and the large difference in free energy between the two states can be accounted for primarily in terms of the bonding of the water to the solid.)

In each case, preconditioned material was placed in the hopper of an instrumented tablet machine and the performance of these two materials was compared at constant machine settings. The sample with 5.1% MC produced tablets that weighed slightly less (an effect on flow and bulk density), and as a result were exposed to lower compression force. However, the moist microcrystalline cellulose resulted in harder tablets, even though it had been exposed to lower compression force. The loci of points on the compression force versus hardness profile (Fig. 20) for the tablets indicate a different fundamental behavior for the two materials.

In a similar, yet more extensive study, the compaction of compressible sugar was examined for materials preconditioned at different relative humidities. The hardness versus compression profiles (Fig. 21) for these samples show a group of lines whose slope appears to be a function of moisture content. This relationship is also demonstrated in Fig. 22, where the slope is used as a compressibility index. This index is a linear function of moisture content; samples with "desorbed" moisture did not differ from those with adsorbed moisture.

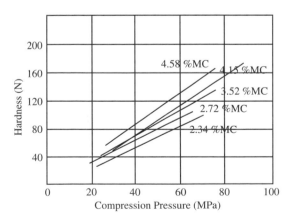

Fig. 21 Hardness vs. compression pressure for compressible sugar with different moisture contents. (Adapted from Ref. 31.)

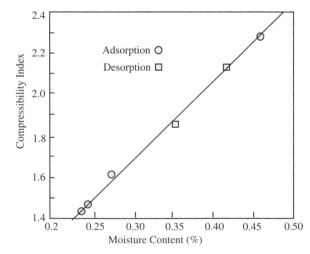

Fig. 22 Compressibility of compressible sugar as a function of moisture content. (Adapted from Ref. 31.)

Chemical Stability of Bioactive Agents

Despite recent advances in understanding the influence of moisture on the physical state of the solid, it is perhaps the effect of sorbed moisture on the chemical stability of moisture-sensitive drugs that is most important, particularly because many new bioactive agents are expensive moisture-sensitive proteins.

The literature related to the study of the influence of moisture on the properties and stability of proteins is extensive and growing rapidly. The examination of water associated with proteins and polymers is relevant to the pharmaceutical scientist dealing with the formulation and processing of small drug molecules as well because many excipients used belong in this large-molecule category. A review of protein stability from the pharmaceutical perspective has been presented by Hageman (44). He ascribes the effect of water content and activity on the solid-state stability of proteins to

- Changes in dynamic activity.
- Changes in conformational stability.
- Participation of water as a reactant or inhibitor, and
- Participation of water as a medium for mobilization of reactants.

Using an analysis of the hydration data of lysozyme and other proteins, Hageman (44) describes critical ranges of hydration based on certain properties of bound water (carboxylate absorbance at 1580 cm^{-1}, amide-1 shift at 1660 cm^{-1}, OD stretching frequency at 2570 cm$_{-1}$, specific heat capacity, diamagnetic susceptibility). Below monolayer capacity, these physical properties of water do not change significantly, and this water has very little

mobility. Between 6% and 25% water, the properties of bound water change dramatically, above 25% water, the properties of bound water are similar to bulk water.

In Fig. 23, the role of moisture in bimolecular reactions is classified by Hageman into three cases. The increases in reaction rate are attributed to a change in state of the water associated with the solid as reflected by a lower effective viscosity. In Case I, there is a continual increase in reaction rate with increasing water content above the monolayer. When all the reactant has been solubilized and further water dilutes the medium, Case II results. If the dilution is extensive, or if water is a product inhibitor of decomposition, a rate reduction can be observed (Case III). Case III behavior is an example of the effect of moisture on the progress of the Malliard reaction for the glucose-containing formulations of α-N-acetyl-L-lysine, poly-L-lysine, insulin, casein, and plasma proteins (43). The fact that there can be a maximum degradation rate at a humidity other than 100% RH is observed in other situations as well.

The presence of excipients in a formulation can influence product stability. The conceptually appealing strategy of including a "moisture scavenger" in a formulation is based on this. In glucose-containing systems, it was demonstrated that liquid and solid humectants can influence the mobility of water in the system. The location of the maximum rate of reaction was found to vary from 40% to 80% RH, depending on the additives (43). The addition of liquids such as glycerol or propylene glycol lowered the mobilization point and facilitated the reaction at lower humidities. The addition of the solid humectant sorbitol reduced the reaction rate dramatically by decreasing free water for mobilization of reactants.

Carstensen (11) has presented a summary of the effects of moisture on the stability of smaller molecules by addressing three cases: decomposition with nondepleting moisture, simultaneous decomposition in the solid and dissolved states, and decomposition with limited amounts of water. In the context of this discussion, emphasis here is placed on hydrolytic degradation processes.

The first case with abundant moisture was initially modeled by Leeson and Mattocks (55) by assuming that the solid particle was surrounded by a layer of moisture sufficiently mobile to permit dissolution of the drug substance. If the layer remains saturated with drug, this approach yields an apparent zero-order degradation process given

$$-\frac{dM}{dt} = kS[H_2O] \qquad (8)$$

where $-dM/dt$ is the rate of drug loss, k is a rate constant appropriate for the order of the reaction, S is the saturation

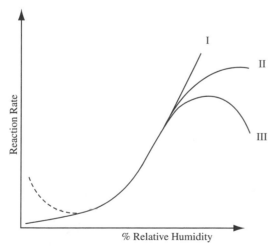

Fig. 23 Effect of sorbed water on the reaction rates of bimolecular reactions in the solid state. (Adapted from Ref. 43.)

concentration of the drug in the layer, and [H$_2$O] is the concentration of water. Although this simple approach often suffices in form to describe data observed in a stability study, it should not be expected to account for the effects of moisture present in the different states described previously.

The degradation of aspirin powder after 120 days at 100% RH and 25°C, for example, was found to be more than ten times greater than what would be expected based on suspension data (48). In addition, the actual rate of aspirin degradation has been found to increase with time (60,61). Carstensen presented a theory to describe this nonlinear behavior based on the fact that the formation of salicylic acid actually exposes moisture adsorption sites of higher energy on aspirin (61), thereby leading to the acquisition of more water. This explanation accounts for an increase in rate with time, but does not explain why the rate is higher for the powder than a suspension where the supply of water is in huge excess. This increased rate could be due to specific acid catalysis in a film of relatively small volume where the pH is dramatically affected by the hydrolysis itself (61).

Finally, the complicated situation faced when a moisture sensitive drug is combined with an hydrophilic excipient is shown in Fig. 24. In this study, aspirin was combined with 4% of the disintegrant and stored for 120 days at 25°C at the respective humidity. The moisture

contents stabilized within the first few days, and the degradation results are presented as moles of the degradation product salicylic acid per mole of water. Point A is the result for aspirin powder alone at 100% RH.

These results demonstrate many of the points presented here. At 100% RH, the reaction rate is lower than that expected for croscarmellose and sodium starch glycolate, because the disintegrants swelled and in doing so diminished the available moisture (crospovidone does not swell). Normalizing based on the total moisture present overstates the amount of water available to react and underestimates the actual reaction rate. At the other extreme (20% RH), the analysis is also biased by overstating the amount of water available, but for a different reason. The water associated with the system here is tightly bound to the disintegrant and not available. At intermediate humidities, depending on the excipient, the observed rate for degradation of the solid is higher than expected. This behavior may be a consequence of the activated sorption process and a specific acid catalysis described by Carstensen (61). Nevertheless, results of this sort are disconcerting for the product development pharmacist interested in making a stable tablet that disintegrates quickly.

SUMMARY

Real progress has been made in the last 10 years, providing pharmaceutical scientists with a solid basis for understanding the interaction of water with solids of pharmaceutical interest. Much of this progress has been the consequence of a paradigm shift: the model of the solid as an inert substrate is almost never valid. Further characterization of the state of water in solid–water systems may ultimately provide a basis for the design of stable formulations and permit the establishment of performance-based specifications for pharmaceutical excipients.

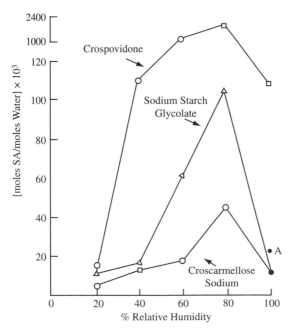

Fig. 24 Effect of humidity on the salicylic acid content in aspirin-disintegrant mixtures at 120 days and 25°C (A, aspirin powder). (Adapted from Ref. 60.)

REFERENCES

1. *Encyclopedia Americana*; Grolier: Danbury, CT, 1991; 28, 432.
2. *Webster's Ninth New Collegiate Dictionary*; Merriam-Webster Inc.: Springfield, MA, 1990; 763.
3. Mitrevej, A.; Hollenbeck, R.G. Int. J. Pharm. **1983**, *14*, 243.
4. Kontny, M.J. Drug Dev. Ind. Pharm. **1988**, *14*, 1991.
5. Zografi, G. Drug Dev. Ind. Pharm. **1988**, *14*, 1905.
6. Gibbs, J.W. *The Collected Works of J. Willard Gibbs*; Yale University Press: New Haven, 1948; 1.

7. *The United States Pharmacopeia 24th Rev., The National Formulary*, 19th Ed. United States Pharmacopeial Convention, Inc. Rockville MD, 2000.

8. Hollenbeck, R.G. Determination of Water: Compendial Viewpoint Proceedings of the Seventh Wisconsin Update Conference, Carstensen, J.T. Ed.; Extension Services in Pharmacy, University of Wisconsin, Madision ,1988; 77, 91.

9. Zografi, G. Pharmaceutical Forum, Nov–Dec: 3240 (1987).

10. *Handbook of Pharmaceutical Excipients*; American Pharmaceutical Association: Washington, DC, 1986.

11. Carstensen, J.T. Drug Dev. Ind. Pharm. **1988**, *14*, 1927.

12. Hammond, W.A. *Drierite and its Applications*; The Stoneman Press: Columbus, OH, 1958.

13. Van Campen, L.; Amidon, G.L.; Zografi, G.J. Pharm. Sci. **1983**, *72* (12), 1381.

14. Van Campen, L.; Amidon, G.L.; Zografi, G. J. Pharm. Sci. **1983**, *72* (12), 1388.

15. Van Campen, L.; Amidon, G.L.; Zografi, G. J. Pharm. Sci. **1983**, *72* (12), 1394.

16. Brunauer, S. *The Adsorption of Gases and Vapors*; Princeton University Press: Princeton NJ, 1943; 1.

17. Brunauer, S.; Emmett, P.H.; Teller, E. J. Am. Chem. Soc. **1938**, *60*, 309.

18. Hill, T.L. Adv. Catal. **1952**, *4*, 211.

19. Cassel, H.M. J. Chem. Phys. **1944**, *12*, 115.

20. Cassel, H.M. J. Phys. Chem. **1944**, *48*, 195.

21. Guggenheim, E.A. *Applications of Statistical Mechanics*; Clarendon Press: Oxford, 1986.

22. Zografi, G.; Kontny, M.J. Pharm. Res. **1986**, *3*, 187.

23. Dunford, H.B.; Morrison, J.L. Can. J. Chem. **1955**, *33*, 904.

24. Argue, G.H.; Maass, O. Can. J. Res. **1935**, *12*, 564.

25. Babbit, J.D. Can. J. Res. **1942**, *20*, 143.

26. Morrison, J.L.; Dzieciuch, M.A. Can. J. Chem. **1959**, *37*, 1379.

27. Gregg, S.J. *The Surface Chemistry of Solids*; Reinhold Publishing Co.: New York, 1951.

28. Young, J.H.; Nelson, G.L. Trans. Am. Agric. Eng. **1967**, *10*, 260.

29. Young, J.H.; Nelson, G.L. Trans. Am. Agric. Eng. **1967**, *10*, 756.

30. York, P. J. Pharm. Pharmacol. **1981**, *33*, 269.

31. Tabibi, S.E.; Hollenbeck, R.G. Int. J. Pharm. **1984**, *18*, 169.

32. Hollenbeck, R.G.; Peck, G.E.; Kildsig, D.O. J. Pharm. Sci. **1978**, *67*, 1599.

33. Marshall, K.; Sixsmith, D. Drug Dev. Commun. **1974–75**, *1*, 51.

34. Mitrevej, A.; Hollenbeck, R.G. Pharmaceut. Technol. **1982**, *6* (10), 48.

35. Connors, K.A. Drug Dev. Ind. Pharm. **1988**, *14*, 1891.

36. Brittan, H.G.; Bugay, D.E.; Bogdanowich, S.J.; DeVincentis, J. Drug Dev. Ind. Pharm. **1988**, *14*, 2029.

37. Adamson, A.A. *Physical Chemistry of Surfaces*, 4th Ed.; John Wiley &Sons: NY, 1982.

38. Harkins, W.D.; Jura, G. J. Am. Chem. Soc. **1944**, *66*, 919.

39. Franks, F. *Water: A Comprehensive Treatment*; Plenum Press: New York, 1972; 1 and 5, 1975.

40. Carstensen, J.T. *Pharmaceutics of Solids and Solid Dosage Forms*; Wiley: New York NY, 1977.

41. Conners, K.A.; Amidon, G.L.; Stella, V.J. *Chemical Stability of Pharmaceuticals*; Wiley-Interscience: New York, 1986.

42. York, P. Int. J. Pharm. **1983**, *14*, 1.

43. Umprayn, K.; Mendes, R.W. Drug Dev. Ind. Pharm. **1989**, *13* (4-5), 653.

44. Hageman, M.J. Drug Dev. Ind. Pharm. **1988**, *14*, 2047.

45. Plotkowiak, Z. Pharmazie **1989**, *44* (2), 837.

46. Fassihi, A.R.; Persicaner, P.H.R. Int. J. Pharm. **1987**, *37* (1-2), 167.

47. Hageman, M.J.; Water Sorption and Solid-State Stability of Proteins. *Stability of Protein Pharmaceuticals*; Ahern, T.J., Manning, M.C., Eds.; Plenum Press: New York, 1992.

48. Shukla, J.; Price, J.C. Pharm. Res. **1991**, *8* (3), 336.

49. Ahlneck, C.; Alderborn, G. Int. J. Pharm. **1989**, *56* (2), 143.

50. Teng, C.D.; Alkan, M.H.; Groves, M.J. Drug Dev. Ind. Pharm. **1986**, *12* (11-13), 2325.

51. Carstensen, J.T.; Van Scoik, K. Pharm. Res. **1990**, *7*, 1278.

52. Groves, M.J.; Teng, C.D.; The Effect of Compaction and Moisture on Some Physical and Biological Properties of Proteins. *Stability of Protein Pharmaceuticals*; Ahern, T.J., Manning, M.C., Eds.; Plenum Press: New York, 1992.

53. Copeland, L.E.; Young, T.F. Adv. Chem. Ser. **1961**, *33*, 348.

54. Wu, Y.C.; Copeland, L.E. Adv. Chem. Ser. **1961**, *33*, 357.

55. Leeson, L.J.; Mattocks, A.M. J. Am. Pharm. Assoc. Sci. Ed. **1958**, *47* (5), 329.

56. Zografi, G.; Kontny, M.J.; Yang, A.Y.S.; Brenner, G.S. Int. J. Pharm. **1984**, *18* (1–2), 99.

57. Ben-Rayana, E.; Seddas, A.; Ruelle, P.; Ho, N.T.; Kesselring, U.W. Mol. Cryst. Liq. Cryst. **1990**, *187*, 617.

58. Blair, T.C.; Buchton, G.; Breezer, A.E.; Bloomfield, S.K. Int. J. Pharm. **1990**, *63* (3), 257.

59. Sadeghnejad, G.R.; York, P.; Stanley-Wood, N.G.; Water Vapour Interaction with Pharmaceutical Cellulose Powders. *Pharmaceutical Technology: Drug Stability*; Rubenstein, M.H., Ed.; Ellis Horwood Limited: West Sussex, UK, 1989.

60. Mitrevej, A. *A Comprehensive Study of Water Vapor Sorption by Aspirin-Disintegrant Blends and its Relationship to Aspirin Stability*; Ph.D. Thesis, 1982.

61. Carstensen, J.T.; Attarchi, F. J. Pharm. Sci. **1988**, *74* (4), 314.

MONOCLONAL ANTIBODIES FOR DRUG DELIVERY

John B. Cannon
Ho-Wah Hui
Abbott Laboratories, Abbott Park, Illinois

Pramod K. Gupta
TAP Pharmaceuticals, Deerfield, Illinois

INTRODUCTION

The selective delivery of drugs to their site of action should increase their therapeutic effectiveness while minimizing unwanted side-effects. In the early 1900s, Paul Ehrlich proposed the potential use of antibodies as carriers of biological agents to the target sites, thus inventing the "magic bullet" concept. With the development of hybridoma technology, it is now possible to produce virtually unlimited quantities of homogenous antibodies having a defined specificity, that is, monoclonal antibodies (MoAbs), which have potential to fulfill Ehrlich's vision. While MoAbs have found use in sensitive diagnostic tests, the therapeutic use of MoAbs and their conjugates are only beginning to realize the promise that was predicted with the advent of the core technology (1–5).

Basic Terminology

In simplistic terms, an antibody is an immunoglobulin synthesized by the body's immune system in response to a foreign molecule (an antigen, i.e., an antibody generator), and is capable of binding the antigen with high specificity. In general, an antigen must have a relatively large molecular weight (>1000) to elicit an immune response; smaller molecules can be made to be antigenic by coupling it to a suitable macromolecule, e.g., albumin.

An antibody is a Y-shaped molecule (Fig. 1) (6), and contains two light chains and two heavy chains joined together by disulfide bonds. Each of the heavy chains also contains a carbohydrate residue. The bottom "trunk" portion of the antibody molecule is known as the constant (Fc) region because its amino acid sequence is often similar within a given animal species. The upper "arms", the antigen binding regions (Fab), are known as the variable regions because its amino acid sequence is determined by the antigen responsible for its formation.

The variable region, in turn, has several "hypervariable" regions, also known as the "complementarity determining regions" (CDR), which show greater variability than the rest of the variable region.

Antibodies can be classified in the following:

Polyclonal Antibodies: After an antigen is injected into an animal by a regimen designed to induce an optimal immune response, serum can be collected from the animal and the immunoglobulin fraction isolated. This "antisera" is enriched with antibodies specific for the original antigen. Because a large number of lymphocytes are involved in the production of the antisera, antibodies produced by this classical method are called polyclonal.

Monoclonal Antibodies: An antibody is called "monoclonal" when each immunoglobulin is produced by a single clone of cells and hence is identical to every other molecule in the preparation, in terms of heavy as well as light chain structure. Thus they are highly specific and offer more consistent efficacy and predictable toxicity in vivo than the polyclonal counterparts (7).

Antibody Fragments: The earliest MoAbs examined in animal and clinical studies were murine antibodies. Because of their nonhuman origin, they are immunogenic in humans, i.e., they have a tendency to elicit a human antimouse antibody (HAMA) response. They also have been shown to have much shorter clearance rates than human MoAb's. One approach to overcome these problems has been to cleave the antibody (e.g., by papain digestion) into its respective Fc and Fab fragments (Fig. 2a) (8). In general, the Fab fragments are less immunogenic than the corresponding intact antibodies, and their smaller molecular size may facilitate penetration into tumor tissue (9) and result in a longer half-life. However, they can lose some of their antigen binding capacity, and in some cases the

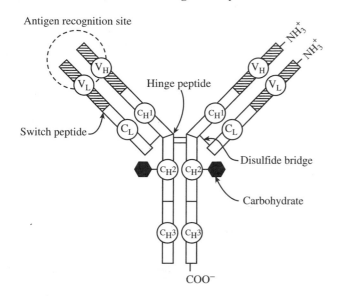

Fig. 1 Diagram of an monoclonal antibody molecule. (Adapted from Ref. 6.)

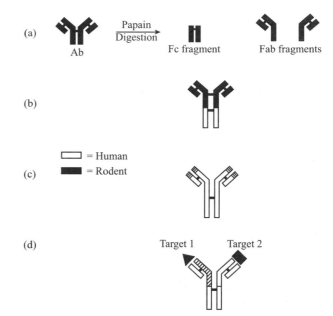

Fig. 2 Diagram of the most important MoAb constructs used clinically: a) antibody fragments; b) chimeric antibody; c) humanized antibody; d) bispecific antibody. (Adapted from Ref. 8.)

therapeutic effect may depend on the Fc portion of the antibody.

Chimeric Antibodies: The obvious solution to the problems encountered with murine antibodies would be to clone a fully human antibody. However, human hybridomas required for human MoAb production have been notoriously difficult to culture, and it may be impossible to obtain many of the appropriate antibodies. A strategy that has been devised to overcome the HAMA problem of murine MoAbs is by constructing a chimeric antibody (Fig. 2b), which contains the Fc region of human IgG, but the Fab regions are murine in origin. These can be made chemically by joining murine Fab fragments to the Human Fc fragment, but the preferred method is to use recombinant DNA technology, as detailed in a later section.

Humanized Antibodies: Although human studies have suggested that chimeric antibodies elicit less HAMA response than murine antibodies, they are still immunogenic due to their murine regions (generally about 30% of the total molecule). A major advance was achieved when it was recognized that only a small portion of an antibody molecule was actually responsible for antigen binding, in fact only the CDR regions. One can envision construction of a "humanized" antibody in which the majority of the antibody framework is human in origin, but the CDR's are murine (Fig. 2c). Synthesis of such humanized antibodies have been successfully achieved by recombinant DNA technology, and can have up to

95% homology with human antibodies. (Some confusion in the literature exists regarding the terminology for humanized and chimeric antibodies, in that some authors use the terms interchangeably.)

Bispecific Antibodies: Antibodies can be constructed using recombinant DNA technology in which each of the two arms are specific for two different antigens (Fig. 2d). For example, bispecific MoAbs reactive with CD15 antigen, and composed of Fab fragments of anti-CD64 MoAb 32 and a whole IgM antimyeloid cell MoAb, PM-81, have been investigated for the therapy of patients with CD15 positive tumors, e.g., acute myelogenous leukemia, small cell carcinoma of the lung, colorectal cancer, and breast carcinoma (10).

Immunoconjugate: For MoAb targeted drug delivery, a drug is bound covalently to an antibody that is chosen to target it to the desired site of action. The resulting immunoconjugate may contain a spacer between the drug and antibody, or a polymer to increase the number of drug molecules that can be bound to each antibody. Another possibility is a radioimmunoconjugate, which is designed to be concentrated at the target site by the targeting antibody, allowing the radiation from the bound radioisotope to exert its cytotoxic affect. Alternatively, the drug can be incorporated noncovalently into a liposome or microsphere to which the targeting antibody is bound to the surface, yielding an immunoliposome or immunomicrosphere, respectively.

PREPARATION AND MANUFACTURE OF ANTIBODIES AND ANTIBODY-BASED DELIVERY SYSTEMS

Manufacture

Every B-lymphocyte in an animal expresses an antibody of only one specificity. After it is triggered to differentiate, the B-cell turns into a plasma cell with the cytoplasmic machinery to synthesize and secrete large quantities of its own unique immunoglobulin. To prepare MoAbs, usually a mouse is immunized with the antigen of interest, e.g., human tumor cells. When an immune response ensues, B-lymphocytes from the spleen or lymph nodes of the animal are harvested in a single cell suspension. These cells are then fused with myeloma cells from the same species, using a fusogenic substance (e.g., polyethylene glycol) or electric current (11). Mutant myeloma cells are used which are deficient in an enzyme, hypoxanthine guanine phosphoribosyl transferase (HGPRT), which is needed for their survival in the presence of the folic acid antagonist, aminopterine. The resulting fused cells have the cytoplasmic machinery to promote cell division and produce large amounts of immunoglobulin. The cell suspension is then transferred to the wells of a microtiter plate in a medium such as hypoxanthine/aminopterine/thymidine. Only the hybridomas that have acquired the HGPRT from lymphocytes via cell fusion usually survive. The hybrids are cloned by limited dilution to one cell per well so that it is easy to identify an antibody of the desired titer, specificity, and avidity for propagation in mass culture. The cell supernatant is then purified by column or affinity chromatography to harvest the pure antibody.

For chimeric and humanized MoAb the above procedures are modified somewhat. The preferred method for the latter is to use recombinant DNA technology and construct a gene that expresses the chimeric or humanized antibody, by splicing the appropriate DNA sequences together in the plasmid of the hybridoma. Synthesis of such humanized antibodies have also been successfully achieved by recombinant DNA technology; the portions of gene encoding the murine CDR regions are spliced into the gene encoding the human antibody by transfection. Although these constructs proved to be much less immunogenic than murine or chimeric antibodies, early work indicated that they had lower antigen binding

capacity than the original murine MoAb. This was apparently because of the absence of certain residues in the human framework that while not directly involved in antigen binding, are required to retain the CDR regions in the correct conformation. Choice of human framework IgG, which is as homologous as possible with the murine antibody, will aid in this regard. In addition, sophisticated molecular modeling techniques based on X-ray crystallography and computer modeling has been used to identify these required residues, which has allowed introduction of the residues into the framework region by recombinant technology (12).

Due to the increased application of MoAbs in diagnostics and therapeutics, considerable effort has been made to develop technology for the large-scale production of MoAbs. Examples of the currently employed culture systems are hollow-fiber systems, suspensions, solid-phase cell immobilization, perfusion reactor, and encapsulation in semipermeable vesicles (13, 14). The system of choice is dependent on the cell line and on the desired characteristics and quantity of the final product. To increase the mixing efficiency of cell-culture equipments and to provide aeration, several different devices have been designed, e.g., vibromixer, marine propeller, turbine propeller, spinning magnetic bar, magnetic spinner, and airlift (14, 15).

Perfusion systems have also been used for successful scale-up of MoAb production. During the culture period, cell growth occurs exponentially until the cell density reaches a maximum. At that point, the medium needs a continuous supplementation of fresh nutrients and elimination of waste. In perfusion systems, fresh nutrients are supplied and wastes are removed continuously so that the medium meets the physiological needs of the cells. At steady state, the cell concentration is determined by space and other limitations. High cell densities have been achieved by immobilizing the cells in porous ceramic matrices or hollow fiber devices. Intermediate cell densities have been achieved by perfusion reactors with a spin filter, or in a fluidized bed reactor in which the cells are embedded in sponge-like microcarriers (14, 15).

Coupling Methods for Antibody Drug Conjugates

An important part of the design of an antibody-directed drug delivery system is the type of linkage and coupling method between antibody and drug. The drug can be covalently bound to the MoAb directly or through a short spacer, or the two can be conjugated through a linker such as a water-soluble polymer. Alternatively, a carrier such as a liposome or a polymeric microsphere can be used, wherein the drug is entrapped in or bound to the carrier, and the MoAb is bound to the surface of the carrier. Characteristics that would comprise an ideal antibody directed delivery system could include, preparation by a method that has high efficiency and yield, and is capable of scaleup; high stability of the conjugate, both under shelf storage conditions and in the circulation after injection; and retention of antigen-binding ability of the antibody while it is carrying the drug to the target tissue. Finally, upon reaching the target, either the immunoconjugate itself should have the desired pharmacological effect equivalent to the free drug, or must release free drug or a derivative that is fully efficacious. Although such a system is probably impossible to achieve for most therapeutic applications, a variety of coupling reagents are fortunately available that aid in optimizing the properties of an immunoconjugate.

Amino, sulfhydryl, and carboxyl groups are the most common functional groups on the antibody, carrier, and drug molecules used for coupling. If the drug lacks the desired group, it may be possible to introduce it. For example, as shown in Fig. 3, succinic anhydride (Fig. 3a) can convert an alcohol or amino group to a carboxyl group; 2-iminothiolane (Traut's reagent, Fig. 3b) can convert an amino group to a sulfhydryl.

For linkage of drug to antibody, "classical" protein cross-linking reagents have been used to prepare immunoconjugates. For example, carbodiimide reagents (e.g., dicyclohexyl carbodiimide, DCC, Fig. 3c, and its water soluble analogs) link amino groups with carboxyls via amide bonds. In an "active ester" method, carboxyl groups of the drug are linked to N-hydroxy succimide (NHS. Fig. 3d) in the presence of a carbodiimide to form an active ester derivative of the drug, which then reacts with the amino group of the antibody (16). Linkers such as dextran, allow conjugation of a much larger number of drug molecules with each antibody molecule. Thus, dextran and similar carbohydrate linkers are oxidized with periodic acid (Fig. 3e) to form aldehyde groups, which are then linked to amino groups of drug and antibody with formation of an imine. This product can be stabilized by reduction with sodium cyanoborohydride.

These simple reactions are often not specific enough for efficient immunoconjugate formation. More recently, a number of bifunctional reagents have been developed that are more specific in forming linkages of antibody to drug. Heterobifunctional reagents, which have two different reactive groups at the two ends of the molecule, have become the method of choice for preparation of immunoconjugates. Among the most widely used is

N-succimidyl 3-(pyridyldithio) propionate (SPDP, Fig. 3f). Generally, the reagent is used to derivatize the drug with a pyridyl disulfide group; reaction of this species with the antibody containing free sulfhydryl groups yields the immunoconjugate. N-[-6 maleimidocaproyl)oxy]succinimide (EMCS, Fig. 3g) is a reagent that reacts with amino groups at the succimide end and sulfhydryl groups at the maleimide end. A similar reagent, N-[-4 maleimidoethoxy succinyloxy]succinimide (MESS), has a metabolizable ester linker between the two active functionalities, thus providing a method to control release of free drug (17). Combinations of classical coupling methods with bifunctional reagents have also been used to advantage for preparation of immunoconjugates. For example, a 6 carbon spacer ending in a carboxyl group was introduced into dextran (MW 70,000), and then mitomycin C (MMC) was coupled to the spacer with a carbodiimide. The remaining carboxyl groups of the spacers were modified to amino groups, which were then coupled to MoAb A7 by means of SPDP, with a final MMC/MoAb ratio of 40. The antibody activity of the resulting conjugate was almost equivalent to native MoAb A7, and released free MMC by chemical hydrolysis to maintain cytoxicity (18). Similarly, Zara et al. modified an IgM against human carcinoma by oxidation of its carbohydrate residues, which were then coupled to a bifunctional reagent, S-(2-thiopyridyl)-L-cysteine hydrazide (TPCH) via the hydrazide. After Ricin A was coupled to the other end of the reagent by a disulfide bond, the immunoconjugate retained full toxin and antibody activity with up to 16 TPCH molecules incorporated per antibody, suggesting that carbohydrate residues of the antibody were not involved in the antigen-binding process (19).

Plasma or intracellular enzymes such as esterases or proteases can potentially degrade immunoconjugate linkages. Glutathione reductase and related enzymes are instrumental in cleavage of disulfide bonds of immunoconjugates. The local pH of the target tissue or of its intracellular environment (e.g., lysosomes) may also increase the rate of release of drug from the immunoconjugate. Thus it is important to consider the possible physiological destinations after injection of the immunoconjugate, and to monitor its degradation under conditions mimicing the biological milieu, which it may encounter. Ideally, an immunoconjugate should be sufficiently stable in the circulation to allow targeting to take place; once the antibody binds to its antigen on the target cell surface, the entire immunoconjugate should be internalized into the cell and be degraded to release free drug or an active derivative. However, for many cell types internalization of the immunoconjugate

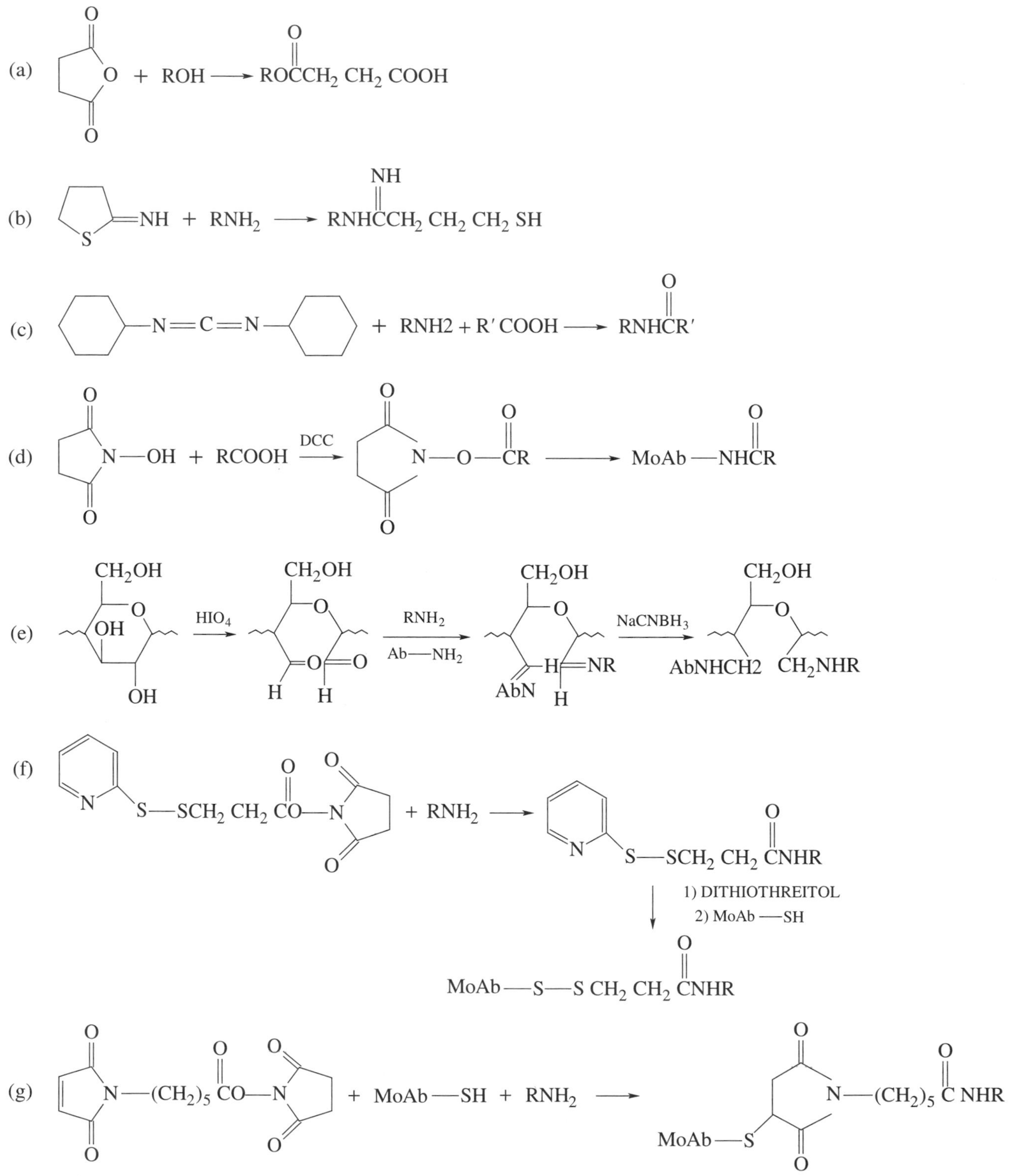

Fig. 3 Coupling reagents for conjugation of drugs to monoclonal antibodies, showing the reactions involved.

does not always occur in response to antibody binding. In that case, degradation of the immunoconjugate linkage should be sufficiently rapid to provide high local concentrations of free drug or active derivative for the desired pharmacological response. An advantage of bifunctional reagents is that they allow incorporation of a metabolizable linker into the immunoconjugate, thereby releasing free drug or an active derivative at a predictable rate.

A number of studies have explored coupling methods that allow control of the in vivo rate of release of active drug. Kaneko et al. (20) designed hydrazone linkers to release drug at lower pH: free doxorubicin was released from conjugated antibody within 6 h at 37°C at pH 4.5, conditions which mimic the environment of the lysosomes; the particular antibody used was known to be internalized. Similarly, Lavie et al. (21) constructed daunomycin conjugates linked to MoAb L6 via a polylysine and aconitate linkage, such that the conjugate releases free drug at pH 6. Although this antibody is not internalized, the lower pH of tumor tissue was suggested to lead to increased concentrations of free drug in tumors. New heterobifunctional reagents have been reported with greater versatility in release rate. The disulfide bond of SPDP conjugates has been shown to be labile in the circulation and release drug prematurely; an analog, NHS-ATMBA, is up to two orders of magnitude more stable than SPDP conjugates because of steric hindrance around the disulfide bond, and thus leads to more efficient targeting (22). Several new substituted 2-iminothiolane reagents, which exhibit increased stability of the disulfide bond of the resulting immunoconjugate, have also been synthesized (23).

Appropriate choice of spacer can also significantly improve the success of an immunoconjugate. For example, O'Neill and co-workers conjugated N,N-bis-(2-chloroethyl)-p-phenylenediamine (PDM) to the globulin fraction of rabbit anti-EL4 serum, which reduced the toxicity by as much as 20-fold relative to free drug. However, the conjugate was found to aggregate, making it difficult for clinical applications. Hence poly-L-glutamic acid (PGA) was tried as a spacer and it allowed preparation of a water-soluble PDM-PGA-Ig conjugate in molar ratio of 90:2:1 retaining 66% of the original antibody activity (24).

In the case of immunotoxins and other protein–antibody conjugates, a unique choice exists for their construction, viz. the conjugate can be made entirely by recombinant DNA techniques. This would require splicing the two genes together and expression of the chimeric gene in a monoclonal system. For example, the gene for angiogenin (a human toxin-like molecule) was fused to the gene for an antitransferrin receptor, and the chimeric gene was introduced into a transfectoma to clone cell lines that secrete the hybrid antibody-angiogenin protein. The conjugate was active as a cytotoxic agent, and the activity was mediated by the transferrin receptors (25). Similar techniques were used to construct a conjugate of urokinase-type plasminogen activator and a humanized antifibrin antibody, resulting in a 12-fold enhancement of fibrinolytic activity of the conjugate relative to the parent (unconjugated) urokinase (26). Construction of an immunoconjugate by this approach has the advantage that once the clones are expressed, the immunoconjugate can be made in one step without chemical modification. Also, a single species is generally produced by this method. It has the disadvantage that generally only a 1:1 or perhaps 2:1 ratio of drug to antibody can be accommodated by the immunoconjugate.

IMMUNOTHERAPY WITH UNCONJUGATED MONOCLONAL ANTIBODIES AND RADIOIMMUNOCONJUGATES

Within the last decade, several unconjugated MoAbs have come to market for treatment of cancer, renal transplantation, and other applications, as shown in Table 1. Results from the clinical trials of these and other MoAbs in development have shown that unconjugated MoAbs are able to kill cancer and other cells. When the circulating MoAb binds to its target antigen, several mechanisms may be initiated that are responsible for the therapeutic effect. One is antibody-dependent cellular toxicity (ADCC), wherein neutrophils, mononuclear phagocytes, eosinophils, natural killer, and T-cells, which have receptors for IgG (Fc), are triggered to mediate cell destruction (27). Also important is complement dependent cytotoxicity (CDC) wherein complement binds to the Fc portion of the MoAb after antigen binding and initiates the complement cascade ending in cell death. MoAb binding to the target antigens on cell surfaces can also act as "blocking" antibodies, interfering with the binding of certain peptides or growth factors needed for cell growth, or elicit a regulatory effect on the metabolism of the cell, especially for B-cell lymphocytes and B-cell lymphomas. The interaction of MoAbs with growth factor receptors (such as transferrin receptors) may also have an antitumor effect via a regulatory mechanism because transferrin is essential for the growth of cells and its receptors are predominantly present on proliferating cells (28).

Table 1 Therapeutic MoAb drug currently marketed

Generic name	Trade name (company)	Type of MoAb	Application(s)
Rituximab	Rituxan (IDEC/Genentech)	Chimeric anti-CD20	Non-Hodgkins lymphoma
Trasuzumab	Herceptin (Genentech)	Humanized anti-HER2	Metastatic breast cancer
Palivizumab	Synagis (Medimmune)	Humanized anti-RSV epitope	Antiviral (Pediatric lower respiratory tract disease)
Muromonab-CD3	Orthoclone OKT3 (Ortho)	Murine ant-CD3	Immunosuppressant (renal transplantation)
Daclizumab	Zenapax (Roche)	Humanized anti-CD25	Immunosuppressant (renal transplantation)
Abciximab	ReoPro (Centocor)	Fab fragment of chimeric anti-7E3	Platelet aggregation inhibitor (Coronary intervention)
Basiliximab	Simulect (Novartis)	Chimeric anti-CD25	Immunosuppressant (renal transplantation)

Among the most successful has been Rituximab (Rituxan). This MoAb binds to the CD20 antigen of B-lymphocytes, which is expressed on >90% of non-Hodgkin's lymphoma B-cells. Upon binding, the Fc region of the MoAb recruits immune effector functions to mediate B-cell lysis, possibly by both CDC and ADCC mechanisms. In a multicenter clinical trial with 166 non-Hodgkin's lymphoma patients, who received 375 mg/m^2 over 4 doses, the overall response rate was 48% (6% complete, 42% partial). A second study with 37 patients gave similar response rates, and single doses of up to 500 mg/m^2 were well-tolerated (29).

Tratsuzumab (Herceptin) binds to the extracellular domain of a transmembrane protein, human epidermal growth factor receptor 2 (HER2), which is overexpressed in 20–30% of primary breast cancer cells. It is thought to act primarily by ADCC. In a phase III trial, 222 breast cancer patients, who exhibited overexpressed HER2, were dosed weekly with 2 mg/kg tratsuzumab after a 4 mg/kg loading dose. There was a 14% overall response (2% complete response and 12% partial response), which appeared to be correlated to the degree of HER2 overexpression. Overall response was much better when tratsuzumab was combined with standard chemotherapy (viz., paclitaxel, doxorubicin + cyclophosphamide, or epiubicin + cyclophosphamide): 45% compared to chemotherapy alone (30). Similarly, tratsuzumab combined with cisplatin, either in pegylated liposomes or in saline/mannitol solution, was significantly better than either treatment alone in retarding tumor growth in a mouse xenograft tumor model (31).

Some workers have proposed use of anti-idiotypic antibodies as type of "tumor vaccine." In this approach, a MoAb is prepared against a given tumor antigen.

Rather than using it for immunotherapy directly, it is used to inoculate mice, which produces a second antibody against the idiotypic site of the original antibody (hence, the anti-idiotype). After cloning and administration to patients, this anti-idiotypic MoAb would mobilize the patient's own immune system to produce a third antibody (i.e., an anti-anti-idiotype), that would have the same idiotype of the first antibody and thus bind to the original antigen and lead to cytotoxicity (27). The perceived advantage of the approach is the multiplicative effect of the "vaccine," and it is believed to be more specific and safer than using the antigen itself as a vaccine. When 15 melanoma patients were treated with a mouse anti-idiotypic antibody homologous to a melanoma antigen, 7 patients developed the desired immune response, and there were 3 partial responses (32). Thus, although the approach may be promising, it has to be more fully evaluated to determine its utility.

Although MoAbs have many potential uses for tumor therapy, there are inherent problems associated with this approach: i) Cancer cells are heterogeneous, so those cells that are not recognized by the MoAb can escape and proliferate; ii) Some tumors contain semidead cores with poor circulation and thus cannot be reached by monoclonals; iii) MoAbs can interact with circulating target antigens before reaching their target; iv) Patients can experience possible immunogenic reactions. For these reasons, it has frequently proven more effective to combine MoAb treatment with standard chemotherapeutic agents.

Radioimmunoconjugates are MoAbs to which radionuclides have been conjugated, to provide cytotoxic radiation after the MoAb binds to its target antigen. The isotopes most commonly used are Iodine-131 and Yttrium-90, both of which are β^- emitters having half-lives of 8 and 2.5 days, respectively. The former is covalently bound to tyrosine residues of the MoAb by standard chemical techniques, whereas the latter is chelated to a ligand that has been conjugated to the MoAb by techniques described in the previous section (e.g., diethylenetriaminepentaacetic acid ligand coupled with a mixed anhydride method) (33,34). Radionuclide emissions from both ^{131}I and ^{90}Y can extend to 1–5 mm of their final location, corresponding to several cell diameters. Thus, their chief advantage resides in their ability to kill tumor cells that are poorly accessible and/or antigen-negative. Unlike conventional radiation therapy, radioimmunoconjugates provide continuous radiation from the decay of the radionuclide, which allows less opportunity for the tumor cells to repair sublethal damage (35). Depending on the type of MoAb, the antibody itself may trigger CDC and ADCC mechanisms that supplement the effect of the radionuclide.

Although no radioimmunoconjugates have progressed to the market, a number have been examined in clinical trials. Bexxar (^{131}I-tositumomab) is an anti-CD20 MoAb examined in Phase III trials for non-Hodgkin's lymphoma (36). In an early trial of this radioimmunoconjugate, 19 patients with non-Hodgkin's lymphoma, who had been prescreened for favorable biodistribution of the MoAb, received 234–777 mCi of the ^{31}I-anti-CD20 MoAb. Because this was considered a myeloablative dose, the patients received autologous marrow reinfusion following the therapy. Although adverse effects were substantial due to the high dose of radiation, the regimen resulted in a complete response in 16 patients and a partial response in 2 patients; the MTD in terms of tissue exposure was determined to be ≤2700 cGy (37, 38). A Phase II trial with a similar regimen in 21 patients achieved 17 complete responses, with an 81% progression-free survival at 12 months (35).

APPLICATIONS OF MONOCLONAL ANTIBODIES IN DRUG DELIVERY

Principle of Targeting

Several classes of drugs lack specificity for diseased cells; for example, the cytotoxic action of chemo-therapeutic agents is directed against any rapidly proliferating cell population. Due to this nonspecificity, many drugs have low therapeutic indices and often cause

serious side effects. One way of circumventing this problem is to deliver the drug in a manner such that it is preferentially localized at the desired site of action, or it predominantly attacks the diseased cells. This process is called targeting. Targeted drug delivery systems can be classified into three categories, viz. passive, physical, or active targeting (39). Passive targeting refers to the natural in vivo distribution pattern of the drug delivery system, which is determined by the inherent properties of the carrier (e.g., hydrophobic and hydrophilic surface characteristics, particle size and shape, surface charge, and particle number). For example, modulation of particle size makes it possible to passively target the lungs or reticuloendothelial system (RES) using particles >7 μm or 0.2–7 μm, respectively (40).

In physical targeting, some characteristics of the environment are utilized to guide the carrier to a specific site or to trigger selective release of its content at the site. Usually, it is accomplished via an external mechanism, such as induced local hyperthermia (e.g., using thermally sensitive liposomes) or a localized magnetic field (e.g., using magnetically responsive albumin microspheres). In active targeting, the natural disposition pattern of a carrier is modified to target it to specific organs, tissues, or cells. Athough cell-specific ligands have been used to target carriers to specific cell types, this approach is probably limited to a small number of tumor types. MoAbs would thus appear to be the more generally applicable mode of active targeting. While the field is less advanced than unconjugated MoAb and radioimmunoconjugates, there has been some success in targeting toxins (i.e., immunotoxins) and drugs (i.e., drug immunoconjugates) using MoAbs as targeting agents.

Toxin Conjugates

Over the last two decades, several toxin proteins like diphtheria toxin and ricin have been conjugated to tumor specific antibodies, with moderate to high degree of success in tumor drug delivery. There are several toxins produced by plants (e.g., ricin, abrin, saporin, and gelonin) or bacteria (e.g., diphtheria toxin and pseudomonas exotoxin) used to construct immunotox-ins. These toxins are highly potent, and generally a single toxin molecule is sufficient to lead to cell death (36). Most of the native toxins consist of two chains (e.g., Ricin A and B chains) one of which bind nonspecifically to cell surfaces and the other is responsible for the cytotoxicity. To construct an immunotoxin, the nonspecific binding chain (viz. Ricin B) must be removed or masked, and the cytotoxic chain (viz. Ricin A) conjugated to a MoAb chemically or by recombinant methods. Most toxins of plant origin exert their cytotoxicity by deactivating the ribosomal protein synthesis, and thus require internalization. A few others do not require internalization and are membrane-acting by a cytolytic mechanism; these include bacterial α-hemolysin, streptolysin, and the equinatoxin of sea anemone (41). In one of the first Phase I trials of an immunotoxin, an antiCD22 MoAb Fab' fragment was conjugated to Ricin A and administered to 15 patients. The MTD was 75 mg/m^2 and there was a 38% partial response (42, 43). Of the total of 200 patients in 9 clinical trials, which examined a variety of ricin-based immunotoxins, there was only a 3% complete response and a 12% partial response (43). This mediocre success may be due in part to the high inherent immunogenicity of immunotoxins. For ricin-based conjugates, the dose limiting toxicity arises from the vascular leak syndrome, a condition characterized by extravasation of fluid into interstitial space. Clinical trials have also indicated that poorly vascularized tumors are not suitable for immunotoxin therapy (43), perhaps because of their high molecular weight. To be more penetrating and to be less immunogenic, immunotoxins and similar targeting molecules need to be made smaller (44).

Drug Immunoconjugates

Over the last several decades, a number of antitumor agents, including chlorambucil, methotrexate, daunomycin, and doxorubicin conjugated to tumor specific antibodies, have been investigated, with varying degrees of success in tumor drug delivery. The most extensively studied has been a doxorubicin-BR96 immunoconjugate (BMS-182248-1). BR96 is a chimeric MoAb specific for a Lewis antigen found on the surface of tumor cells. The immunoconjugate is formed using an acid-labile hydrazone linkage attached through the thiol groups of the MoAb, with 8 moles of doxorubicin/mole of MoAb. After rapid internalization into antigen-bearing cells, the conjugate is designed to release free doxorubicin from the MoAb hydrazone linkage in the acidic environment of the lysosome (45). When tested in mice with xenografted human lung, breast, and colon carcinomas, there was an 89% and 72% cure rate (tumor reduction to nondetectable levels) in the lung and colon models, respectively. In breast carcinoma xenograft, results were less spectacular, with 10% complete response and 60% partial response. Doxorubicin or MoAb alone gave <1% cures in any of the models (46, 47). In a rat lung carcinoma xenograft model, there was a 94% cure rate, even though, unlike

mice, the Lewis antigen is expressed in normal tissue of rats (46, 47).

Because of the encouraging in vivo results, clinical development of this immunoconjugate was initiated. The pH-rate profile was determined using a stability-indicating size-exclusion HPLC assay, and exhibited a maximum stability at pH 7.5. The predominant route of degradation was hydrolysis at the hydrazone linkage to release free doxorubicin, with aggregation being a secondary pathway. This was supported by ELISA assay that demonstrated no loss of conjugate after 1 week of storage at 2–8°C. However, because the stability even at this temperature was insufficient for clinical development, a lyophilized formulation was developed. Formulations that remained amorphous due to the use of sucrose or lactose as lyoprotectant showed the greatest stability, with a shelf life of the lyophilized product of more than 12 months at 2–8°C. (48). In a Phase II study, the BR96 Doxorubicin conjugate (BMS182248-1) was administered to 14 metastatic breast cancer patients. However, there was only 1 partial response (7%), in contrast to doxorubicin alone, which gave 44% response. The toxicity profile of the two regimens was markedly different, with the doxorubicin showing the usual cardiotoxicity and hematologic toxicity, whereas the immunoconjugate showed GI associated toxicity, similar to the Phase I studies. It was proposed that the lack of correlation of the Phase II trial with the preclinical in vivo data could be because of the presence of the Lewis antigen at sites in the GI tract. This may act as an "antigen sink," preventing targeting to the tumor tissues and instead exacerbate the GI toxicity (49). Colon and lung cancer models showed better clinical responses than the breast cancer models (46), suggesting that clinical trials in these cancers may be more promising than breast cancer.

Another promising immunoconjugate is CMA-676, which is a conjugate of an anti-CD33 MoAb and calicheamicin, an anticancer drug shown to be 1000-fold more potent than doxorubicin in animal models. A Phase II trial of 39 acute myeloid leukemia patients resulted in 2 patients with complete remission and 7 patients who showed temporary removal of leukemia cells from the blood. CMA-676 is now in pivotol clinical studies in a number of centers in North America and Europe (36).

Preliminary clinical studies with chlorambucil-anti-melanoma globulin conjugates in patients with disseminated diseases have also indicated improvement in patient survival (50). The evaluation of vindesine-anti-CEA antibody conjugates in patients with advanced metastatic cancer (and probably expressing CEA) has demonstrated positive localization of the conjugate (51). In this study, 8 patients received escalating doses of antibody (1–42 mg) conjugated to 24–1800 μg vindesine, and no toxicity or hypersensitivity was noticed in any patient (51). However in most instances, the tumor versus normal tissue distribution ratio of antibodies approximated 2:1, and it rarely demonstrated specificity leading to a more desirable ratio like 10:1 (52).

Some studies have demonstrated synergism in antitumor response with drug–antibody conjugate. For example, a clinical trial with bronchial carcinoma patients compared chemotherapy with immunochemotherapy. The latter group received chemotherapy immediately prior to the administration of antibodies against a resected portion of the primary tumor. The group receiving chemotherapy alone demonstrated a 60% recurrence rate along with a 41% death rate; however, the immunochemotherapy group demonstrated only a 25% recurrence rate along with a 16% death rate (53).

Bispecific MoAbs composed of anti-CD3 or anti-CD2 MoAb, chemically conjugated to antitumor antibody and coated on lymphokine-activated killer (LAK) cells, have been clinically investigated for the treatment of malignant glioma, lymphoma, and ovarian cancer with encouraging results. In a trial involving malignant glioma therapy, bispecific MoAb-coated LAK cells were injected intracranially following surgical removal of tumor and whole brain irradiation and/or chemotherapy. This resulted in 76% of the patients being tumor-free after 2 years, as opposed to 33% of the patients tumorfree with LAK cell treatment alone (54).

Because of the ability to achieve higher drug–antibody ratios, various water-soluble polymeric carriers have been examined as linking agents in immunoconjugates. For example, encouraging results have been demonstrated with daunomycin conjugated to MoAbs via dextran bridge in rats bearing AH66 hepatoma cells (55). Similarly, MMC was conjugated to an anti-α-fetoprotein MoAb via a human serum albumin carrier in a molar ratio of 30:1:1. Full antibody activity was retained, and the conjugate was 20-fold more cytotoxic than free MMC in vitro and was also more effective than free MMC in tumor-bearing mice (56). Poly(lysine) has also been successfully used as a carrier, e.g., for targeting methotrexate (57) and muramyl dipeptide (58). N-(2-hydroxypropyl)-methacrylamide copolymers have been extensively examined as carriers for tumor targeted drug delivery (59, 60). Enzymatically cleavable spacers (e.g., oligopeptides) have been incorporated into these conjugates to allow release of active chemotherapeutic agent (59, 61).

Immunoliposomes

Generally, the antigens expressed by tumor cells are not specific but are merely present in higher ratio than on the normal cells. Hence, systems such as immunoliposomes have been developed to exploit these opportunities, as they are expected to bind to a greater extent to high antigen density tumor cells than to low antigen density normal cells. In immunoliposomes, the number of antibody molecules per liposome can be varied by as much as two orders of magnitude (62). Using egg phosphatidylcholine, cholesterol, phosphatidylserine, and N-4-nitrobenzo-2-oxa-1-1,3-diazole phosphatidylethanolamine in molar ratio of 56:33:10:1, unilamellar liposomes with 12–55 antibody molecules per vesicle have been investigated for binding with RDM-4 lymphoma cells with varying antigen density. The increase in the valency of liposomes (i.e. number of antibody molecules per liposome) increased their binding with low as well as high antigen density cells, and thus the low valency immunoliposomes were found to allow better discrimination between target and normal cells (62). An additional advantage of immunoliposomes is that a relatively high drug loading can potentially be accommodated, with the result that a small number of antibody molecules conjugated to the surface of an immunoliposome can deliver many more drug molecules to the target than is otherwise possible. Once the drug is released into the target cell, no further transformation is needed, because the entrapment process does not involve any chemical modification of the drug.

Heath et al. have proposed the use of immunoliposomes for the intracellular delivery of compounds that intrinsically do not enter diseased cells. These compounds are cytotoxic if they are transported intracellularly. Methotrexate-γ-aspartate, a good example of this type of compound, has been encapsulated in liposomes composed of phosphatidylcholine, cholesterol, and 4-(p-maleimido-phenyl)-butyryl-phosphatidylethanolamine in a molar ratio of 10:10:1. The liposomes were conjugated to either specific (anti-K2Kk IgG2A) or nonspecific MoAbs (antisheep erythrocyte IgG2A). The binding of targeted liposomes was found to be six fold higher to L929 fibroblasts (which express H2Kk protein) than nontargeted liposomes, whereas their binding was comparable in a nonspecific BALB/c 3T6 cell lines. The growth inhibition studies using L929 fibroblasts demonstrated the IC50 of free drug, targeted immunoliposomes, and nontargeted immunoliposomes to be 0.68, 0.066, and 1.2 μM, respectively (Fig. 4). Hence, the targeted immunoliposomes appeared to be 10 times more effective than free drug and 18 times more effective than nontargeted immunoliposomes, whereas targeted liposomes actually had the least efficacy in the nonspecific BALB/c 3T6 fibroblasts (63).

Extensive work is being pursued to assess the potential of immunoliposomes for the targeted drug delivery to CD4 positive cells in patients with HIV infection. The HIV infected cells possess CD4, which can be targeted by conjugating anti-Leu3A (CD4) MoAbs onto the surface of drug-loaded liposomes. Preliminary studies showed that immunoliposomes possessing surface-bound anti-Leu3A may be used to target antiviral agents to cells at risk from HIV infection (64). Cell adhesion molecules are glycoproteins expressed on cell surfaces during pathological inflammatory states such as rheumatoid arthritis, atopic dermatitis, and asthma; thus they also provide an opportunity for targeting. An F10.2 antibody against the cell adhesion molecule ICAM-1 was conjugated to liposomes; the immunoliposomes bound to human bronchial epithelial cells in a specific, dose-and time-dependent manner, correlating to the degree of ICAM-1 expression. Immunoliposomes of this type therefore have potential for targeted drug delivery in inflammatory disease states (65).

Heat-sensitive immunoliposomes have also been evaluated for the feasibility of drug delivery (66). These liposomes release the entrapped drug at temperatures above the phase transition temperature of the lipid(s). In vitro cell culture studies based on dipalmitoyl phosphatidylcholine liposomes with entrapped ^{3}H-uridine have demonstrated enhanced intracellular delivery of drug as compared to that observed with free drug and liposomes without MoAbs. Similarly, selection of appropriate lipids can also allow synthesis of pH-sensitive liposomes. Inclusion of target-cell specific immunogenic moieties in these colloidal particles leads to preparation of pH-sensitive immunoliposomes. Huang and co-workers have used 8:2 molar ratios of dioleoylphosphatidyl ethanolamine and oleic acid to develop pH-sensitive liposomes (67). Arabinofuranosylcytosine (ara-C) and methotrexate were encapsulated in the liposomes that were rendered immunospecific against L-929 cells by homing specific MoAbs. Compared to free drug, drug encapsulated in antibody-free liposomes and pH-insensitive immunoliposomes, the drug-encapsulated pH-sensitive immunoliposomes were found to significantly enhance the cytotoxic activity. Pretreatment of target cells with excess free MoAbs or placebo immunoliposomes was found to block the cytotoxic effect of the drug-loaded pH-sensitive immunoliposomes. In addition, it was shown that the drug release from these specific carrier particles occurs in cell endosomes (67).

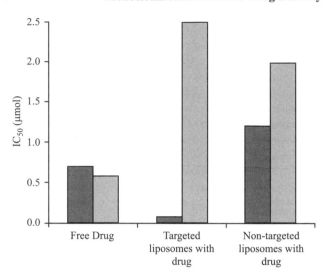

Fig. 4 Effect of treatment type on in vitro growth inhibition of (■) specific cell-line, L929 expressing H2Kk protein, and (▨) nonspecific cell-line, BALB/c3T6. The targeted and nontargeted liposomes were conjugated with "anti-H2Kk IgG2A" and "anti-sheep erythrocyte IgG2A," respectively. (Adapted in part from Ref. 63.)

Because of the complexities involved with distribution, uptake, and pharmacological effects of targeted drug delivery systems, in vitro results do not always adequately predict the efficacy of a proposed MoAb-targeted system such as an immunoliposome. In fact, there are only a few in vivo studies of immunoliposomes that clearly demonstrate the promise shown by in vitro studies. One encouraging example is a study by Onuma et al. that compared the in vivo efficacy of doxorubicin loaded immunoliposomes against free drug in cows. MoAb c143 against the antigen expressed by bovine leukemia cells was conjugated to liposomes containing doxorubicin. Two groups of antigen-positive cows received four i.v. injections of either 0.4 mg/kg free drug or an equivalent dose of drug via immunoliposomes at an interval of 4 days. Whereas the two animals receiving free drug demonstrated only a slight decrease in their antigen positive cells, the three animals receiving drug-immunoliposomes gradually became free of antigen-positive cells, and 2 of these animals became antigen-negative in 6- and 14-week periods after treatment, respectively (68). In another study, MoAbs against tumor-associated antigens expressed on bovine leukemia cells were conjugated with liposomes containing doxorubicin, and the formulation was administered intravenously to BALB/c nude mice inoculated with BLSC-KU cells on day 0, 3, and 7 after the initiation of treatment. The results were compared with untreated animals and the animals receiving doxorubicin liposomes conjugated to normal mouse IgG. The doxorubicin liposomes bearing target antigen specific antibodies significantly suppressed the tumor growth. The increase in tumor volume with this treatment, over 10 days after the initiation of therapy, was only 27% as opposed to 166% and 750% in the animals receiving nonspecific therapy and no therapy, respectively (see Fig. 5) (69). Histological screening of the tumors from animals receiving drug-loaded liposomes with specific antibody demonstrated scattered focal necrosis and marked proliferation of macrophages; however, in the untreated animals, active proliferation of tumor cells was observed with little involvement of macrophages (69).

A great deal of attention has been paid in recent years to long-circulating (also called sterically stabilized or "stealth") liposomes, in which polyethylene glycol (PEG) molecules have been grafted to the surface of the liposomes by covalent attachment of PEG to liposomal phospholipids (specifically phosphatidylethanolamine). These long-circulating liposomes have been shown to avoid the rapid uptake by the reticuloendothelial system (RES), which normally plagues conventional liposomes without PEG; the circulating half-life can be increased by an order of magnitude (70, 71). In fact, the presence of a MoAb on the surface of a conventional immunoliposome may actually increase the uptake by the RES system (72), suggesting that modification to insure long-circulation may be especially important for immunoliposomes. When designing PEG-modified immunoliposomes, the composition must be optimized for both antigen binding and extended circulating lifetimes. Antigen recognition by the liposomal antibody can be sterically hindered by the presence of the PEG. This can be overcome by either reducing the polymer size to 2000, or by moving the antibody out to the terminus of the PEG rather than the liposome surface (72).

Despite the extensive in vitro and in vivo research on immunoliposomes, these MoAb targeted systems have apparently not yet reached clinical trials. This may be because of a variety of factors, including the difficulty of clearly demonstrating efficacy in suitable animal models, and the obstacles associated with scaleup and manufacture of system as complex as a sterically stabilized MoAb-targeted liposome. Other potential problems of immunoliposomes are that they may not adequately penetrate the vasculature of solid tumors; they may not adequately release the loaded drug into the target cells; and they may demonstrate immunogenicity (73). Use of humanized antibodies may alleviate the latter effect to some extent. Recently, sterically stabilized liposomes

conjugated to Fab' fragments of a humanized anti-HER2 MoAb (similar to Herceptin) were studied in vitro using confocal microscopy techniques. The immunoliposomes bound selectively and were internalized by HER2-overexpressing breast cancer cells, reaching 8000–23,000 vesicles/cell at saturating liposome concentrations, which was at least two orders of magnitude greater than cells with low HER2 expression (74). These immunoliposomes, containing doxorubicin and optimized with respect to Fab'/lipid/PEG composition for intracellular tumor delivery, were subsequently examined in an in vivo human xenograft breast cancer model; they demonstrated significantly increased antitumor efficacy compared to free doxorubicin or non targeted doxorubicin liposomes, and less systemic toxicity than free doxorubicin (75). The studies demonstrate the importance of optimizing a delivery system with respect to binding to the target epitope as well as uptake and/or release of available drug at the target site. Such considerations are necessary before successful demonstration of efficacy of immunoliposomes in the clinic. An ideal immunoliposome system should allow efficient encapsulation of intended compound so as to protect its degradation prior to and during endothelial transfer, and hence minimize inherent toxicity; it should also allow controlled release of drug

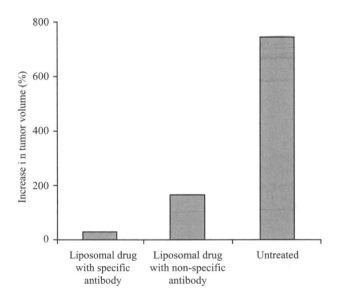

Fig. 5 Effect of treatment type on the increase in tumor volume in mice inoculated with BLSC-KU cells. The animals in treatment groups received i.v. doses of doxorubicin via tumor-specific or nonspecific liposomes on day 0, 3, and 7 after the initiation of treatment. The tumor-specific and nonspecific liposomes were conjugated with MoAbs against leukemia cells and normal mouse IgG, respectively. (Adapted in part from Ref. 69.)

in the extravascular compartment of target tissue. In this regard, it should be noted that the delivery systems based on particulate carriers may allow reversal of tumor cell drug resistance (Fig. 6) (76). Nevertheless, immunoliposomes fall short of meeting the above ideal criteria and much work remains to be done before they are clinically useful.

A related approach for lipophilic drugs is MoAb targeted emulsions. For example, a lung-targeted MoAb 34A was conjugated to the surface of a long-circulating emulsion composed of castor oil, phosphatidylcholine, and pegylated phosphatidylethanolamine. Upon intravenous injection into mice, 30% of the injected emulsion dose became preferentially associated with lung tissue within 30 min (77). A similar long-circulating emulsion conjugated to an anti-B-cell lymphoma MoAb LL2 was found to bind in vitro to three different Burkitt's lymphoma cell lines, and thus shows potential for delivery of anticancer drugs to B-cell malignancies (78).

Immunomicrospheres

In view of the availability of a wide variety of biocompatible and biodegradable polymers, and the ease of preparation of stable microparticles with predictable physicochemical characteristics, antibodies have been conjugated to polymeric microparticles for controlling their in vivo deposition.

Although a few in vitro studies have demonstrated promising results with immunomicrospheres (79, 80), limited information has been published on the in vivo efficacy of immunomicrospheres for drug delivery. In one case, following promising in vitro results, an in vivo study was conducted in mice bearing human tumor xenografts, using ^{14}C-polyhexylcyanoacrylate nanoparticles with adsorbed anti-osteogenic sarcoma MoAbs 971T/36. However, the particles were found to deposit predominantly in liver and spleen, and hence the study failed to demonstrate any appreciable improvements in drug delivery due to the immunocarrier (81). Lack of optimal particle size and/or tumor tissue permeability, lack of expression of sufficient Fab portions on the surface of particles, particle opsonization leading to a secondary non-interactive coating, distribution of specific antigens in the liver, and competitive displacement of the adsorbed MoAbs by serum components were suggested as possible reasons for this undesirable in vivo distribution of the immunoparticles. Another study has evaluated the in vivo drug delivery potential of albumin immunomicrospheres in mice (80). The microspheres bearing Lewis lung carcinoma MoAbs demonstrated slightly higher localization in lung carcinoma at 24 h after its administration.

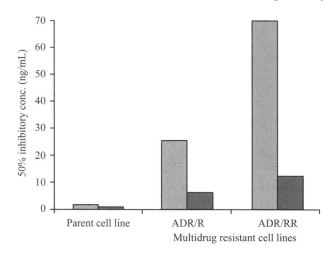

Fig. 6 A plot showing 50% inhibitory drug concentration in vitro, in normal and drug-resistant lines, following treatments with vinblastine solution (▢), or vinblastine encapsulated in liposomes (▪). The data suggest the possibility of the reversal of drug resistance by using carrier systems like liposomes. (Adapted in part from Ref. 76.)

REGULATORY CONCERNS

While a regulatory agency's prime concern remains the safety and efficacy of a new product in its proposed use, the technological issues concerning the manufacture of monoclonal-based therapeutics are not ignored. Indeed, because antibody-based systems involve specific immune reactions for their response, and they are comprised of components derived from biological origin, it is obvious that the proposed regulatory guidelines for the clinical use of these products are likely to be extremely strict. The technology for the development of antibodies and antibody-based delivery systems is relatively new and has been continuously expanding over the last several years. More and more practical changes in manufacturing process of these systems can therefore be expected over the next several years. Although most products are expected to be handled on a case-by-case basis, the following general guidelines should apply to all antibody-based systems: exhaustive characterization of the origin of cell lines, characterization of production procedures, product purification and characterization, quality control, and validation of processes involved during production and testings. For example, successful approval and use of a MoAb product will mandate declaration of the source, name and characteristics of the parent myeloma cell lines, and all pertinent details regarding the animal species used for hybridization. The rationale for selecting a particular cell line along with criterion for its acceptance, the genotype and husbandry of animals used for in vivo production, and steps taken to control contamination is expected to play a critical role. Once the product is made, extensive purification to reduce the level of contamination (using techniques like affinity, size exclusion or ion-exchange chromatography and/or ultracentrifugation) is likely to increase the probability of its approval. Measures would need to be undertaken to insure that the product does not contain any biological contaminant transferred from the original malignant hybridoma cell lines.

Once a bulk lot is in hand, its characterization for immunoglobulin and subimmunoglobulin class, and testings for potential aggregation, denaturation, fragmentation of immunoglobulin and immunologic specificity would be required. If a MoAb fragment is used, its degree of homogeneity would need to be confirmed. Finally, information on the sterility and polynucleotide contamination of the lot is likely to be required. It would be expected that the process validation allows rejection of lots with viral or nucleic acid contaminants. Additional tests may include determination of the product stability with respect to fragmentation, aggregation, and loss of potency. The preclinical toxicity testing with the final product would be required in at least one species bearing relevant antigen. Following the identification of an appropriate animal model, GLP-compliant pharmacokinetic evaluations involving in vivo distribution, metabolism and excretion, would be desired.

As mentioned earlier, in most instances the antigens are preferentially associated with the target site rather than specifically present there, i.e., small amounts of the same antigens are present in one or more nontarget organs. Because the probability of unacceptable levels of this cross-reactivity is reasonably high, regulatory guidelines recommend screening for cross-reactivity. For in vitro screening, blood cells, cell culture lines, fluorescent antibody tests, radioaudiography, and/or similar other techniques would be useful. If possible, tissues from unrelated human donors could be used to screen phenotypic expressions of potentially cross-reactive tissue antigens. If these tests demonstrate positive cross-reactivity, extensive in vivo testing in animals sharing similar phenomenon would be required to determine its frequency as well as intensity. Alternatively, an isolated perfused human organ system could be used. If these choices are not available, limited clinical testings may be advisable with particular emphasis on the quantitation of the product's biodistribution over a period of time.

It should be realized that the above guidelines, generally meant to assess and regulate the antibody or antibody-component of an overall product, would need to be expanded and/or modified according to the characteristics of the final product. For example, in antibody-based drug delivery systems, the effect of drug and antibody on the potency and biological activity of the final system would need to be assessed.

CONCLUSIONS

Problems and Possible Solutions

Despite the promise of MoAb-directed drug delivery, there are still a multitude of problems that need to be worked out before the technology makes a large impact on therapy. A MoAb is often not as specific in vivo as would be predicted from in vitro studies; i.e., tumor antibodies may bind to normal cells as well as target cells. Despite the fact that antigens associated with tumor tissue have been identified, antigens are rarely specific enough to allow quantitative drug targeting. For example, CA 19-9, BW 494, and DU-PAN-2 have been identified as pancreatic tumor associated antigens. However, MoAb based therapy of pancreatic tumors has not been encouraging (82). In some cases, peak drug concentrations with MoAbs, in tumor tissue, have been found to be only 2–3 times higher than the surrounding normal tissues (83). Current literature suggests that the availability of high affinity MoAbs, which recognize specific antigens without cross-interaction with normal cells, is still scarce. The only exception to this observation is the surface immunoglobin idiotype expressed by certain B-cell lymphomas (84).

The lack of genetic stability of antigens on tumor cell surfaces is another cause of low density of target antigen on the tumor cell. Antigenic modulation may result in nontumor specific antigen–antibody reaction, thus reversing the efficacy anticipated from the delivery system. Situations of low antigen density may readily saturate the MoAb-antigen binding. Quantitative evaluation of the localization of MoAbs in tumor tissue, at doses $<100\,\mu g$, have demonstrated a direct correlation between tumor mass and quantity of antibody localized, and at 2–3 days after administration only 8% of the dose could be detected in the tumor. However, the administration of larger doses of MoAbs have been shown to reduce the fraction localized in the tumor, with 1–2 mg doses almost saturating the tumor (83). The presence of circulating tumor-associated antigens is another factor that may decrease the overall efficacy of MoAb-directed delivery systems and complicate their evaluation. For example, the presence of circulating carcinoembryonic antigen has been shown to complicate the application of MoAbs against this antigen (85). In view of these problems, MoAb-directed delivery systems may ultimately be restricted to those few cases in which there are relatively high densities of known antigens in all cells of the target site.

The heterogeneity of tumor cells is another problem in targeting; i.e., a specific antigen may not be present in sufficient quantities in all cells of the target tissue to allow selection of suitable antibody. For example, it is now appreciated that multiple metastatic proliferation in a given host, and perhaps even in the same organ, can give rise to malignant tumors that contain heterogeneous subpopulation of cells with diverse biological characteristics, such as growth rate, antigenicity or immunogenicity, cell-surface receptors, response to individual and combined chemotherapeutic and immunological agents, invasiveness, and their overall metastatic potential (86). Trubetskoy et al. have proposed a method for MoAb-based drug delivery to target areas with heterogeneous antigens. The proposed method requires sequential administration of a mixture of modified antibodies against different antigens in the target area followed by administration of drug-carrier that recognizes and interacts with accumulated antibodies (Fig. 7) (87). The practical feasibility of this strategy was confirmed following administration of a mixture of biotinylated antibodies to target components followed by administration of biotinylated and avidin bearing liposomes. The binding of biotinylated liposomes via avidin was found to be higher than that achieved with liposomes bearing single antibody (87).

Solid tumors present special problems due to their frequent lack of vasculature; there is generally poor penetration of MoAbs, their fragments, and drug- or toxin-conjugates into solid tumor tissue. Because of the relatively intact microvascular barrier, and hence difficulties in carrier extravasation, the accumulation and uptake of immunoliposomes by solid tumor tissue is also generally low (88). On the other hand, the natural existence of increased transvascular permeability favors the use of MoAb-drug conjugates for the treatment of general lymphomas and leukemias.

The uptake of MoAb-based delivery systems by the reticulo-endothelial system (RES) is another drawback to these systems. It has been suggested that only 0.1–1% of the administered dose of antibody-based systems reaches nonRES sites, with ~8% dose reaching

non RES sites under optimal situations (89). However, a study comparing the in vivo tumor localization of anti-CEA MoAbs, and their F(ab')2 and Fab' fragments, to human colon carcinoma grafts in nude mice has demonstrated greater tumor uptake of F(ab')2 and Fab' fragments than the intact MoAbs (90), due to the smaller molecular size of the former. Often multiple intravenous injections, over a course of weeks, have been found to be more effective than single injections (91), and continuous infusion is more efficient than bolus regimen (43).

As mentioned earlier, the immunogenicity of "foreign" MoAbs has always been a major factor in the lack of success of MoAb-based therapeutic systems. It has been suggested that use of (Fab')2 fragments may improve drug delivery without sacrificing the specificity of antigen-MoAb binding because elimination of Fc portion would likely reduce immunogenicity and nonspecific binding to normal cells (92). Humanized antibodies probably hold the greatest promise in decreasing the immune response of MoAb-based therapies. While immunotherapy with these entities is promising and indicates greatly decreased immune responses, little work has been reported on humanized immunoconjugates. These entities may still be immunogenic due to the non-antibody portion of the conjugate. For example, rats injected with an unconjugated murine MoAb failed to elicit an antibody response, whereas rats injected with a MoAb-Vinca alkaloid conjugate mounted a strong antibody response directed against the linker portion of the conjugate (93).

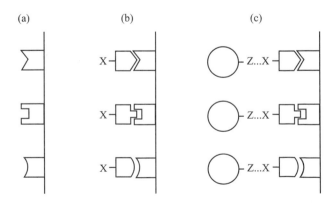

Fig. 7 A schematic representation of the unification of delivery systems to optimize therapeutic outcome with MoAbs: a) exposed target antigens; b) initial treatment with bridge molecules; c) specific binding of unified carrier systems. (Adapted in part from Ref. 87.)

Future Prospects

New applications in the field of antibody-directed drug delivery may be developed by combining the technology with another form of targeting or other means of optimization. For example, in photodynamic therapy a photosensitizing drug (e.g., a porphyrin, chlorin, purpurin, or phthalocyanine) is localized in a tumor, which is then irradiated to effect cell-killing (94). Several reports have described the use of MoAbs to further increase the localization. For example, Sn (IV) chlorin e6 was linked to the oligosaccharide moiety of an antimelanoma MoAb via a dextran carrier. In vitro studies indicated that phototoxicity was relatively specific for cells that exhibited the target antigen (95). Similarly, a chlorin derivative, meso chlorin e_6 mono(N-2-aminoethylamide), was linked via a tetrapeptide linker to an antibody directed against ovarian cancer cells. Targeted conjugates were taken up rapidly by cells and detected within the lysosomes, and the conjugate had higher photodynamic effects on ovarian carcinoma cells than nontargeted conjugates (IC_{50} of 0.38, 290, and 0.34 μM for MoAb-HPMA-e_6, HPMA-e_6, and free e_6, respectively) (96).

Another recent approach combines MoAb targeting with enzymatic prodrug activation. In this therapeutic method, called antibody-directed prodrug therapy (ADEPT), an enzyme–antibody conjugate is administered and allowed to accumulate in the target site (e.g., tumor). A latent, nontoxic prodrug is then injected, which on contact with the enzyme is converted into the active parent drug and subsequently kills the tumor cells (97). For example, a glutamic acid derivative of benzoic acid mustard was administered to choriocarcinoma-bearing mice, followed by a carboxypeptidase-antibody conjugate that cleaved glutamic acid from the active drug. Tumor contained the highest concentration of targeted enzyme conjugate, and was the only site in which all prodrug reaching the site was activated (98). The ADEPT technique has been tested clinically in colorectal cancer patients using para-N-(mono-2-chloroethyl monomesyl)-aminobenzoyl glutamic acid as the prodrug and an antibody conjugate of glutamate hydrolase as the activating enzyme, with temporary regression of disease in two out of five patients (99).

Despite the problems described in earlier sections, MoAbs should hold an important place in drug delivery and therapy in the future. Although the number of therapeutic applications that will eventually lend themselves to this technology may be small, the problems should not be insurmountable for these applications and may yield important advantages over other therapies. Proper attention to detail must be taken in the choice of antibody, coupling method, drug, route of administration, dose, and other factors in order to design an effective therapy for a particular disease; possible mechanisms of distribution, uptake, metabolism, and pharmacological effect must be properly understood to develop a rationale for a particular MoAb directed therapy. Humanized antibodies hold great promise to alleviate the immune response encountered in past clinical trials using murine derived antibodies. Many of the problems in the scaleup of MoAb manufacture have been solved, primarily because of the rapid growth of diagnostic applications of MoAbs and the coming to market of therapeutic MoAb's. Much work remains to be done, however, in the scaleup of immunoconjugates and complex systems such as immunoliposomes and immunomicrospheres. Nevertheless, it is likely that the next decade will see a number of MoAb-directed therapies reach extended clinical trials and perhaps come to the market.

REFERENCES

1. Ram, B.P.; Tyle, P. Immunoconjugates: Applications in Targeted Drug Delivery for Cancer Therapy. Pharm. Res. **1987**, *4*, 181–188.

2. Bodey, B.; Siegel, S.E.; Kaiser, H.E. Human Cancer Detection and Immunotherapy with Conjugated and Non-Conjugated Monoclonal Antibodies. Anticancer Res. **1996**, *16*, 661–674.

3. Panchagula, R.; Dey, C.S. Monoclonal Antibodies in Drug Targeting. J. Clin. Pharm. Ther. **1997**, *22*, 7–19.

4. Buske, C.; Feuring-Buske, M.; Unterhalt, M.; Hidderman, W. Monoclonal Antibody Therapy for B-Cell Non-Hodgkins's Lymphomas. Eur. J. Cancer **1999**, *35*, 549–557.

5. Multani, P.S.; Grossbard, M.L. Monoclonal Antibody-Based Therapies for Hematologic Malignancies. J. Clin. Oncol. **1998**, *16*, 3691–3710.

6. Devlin, T.M. *Textbook of Biochemistry with Clinical Correlations*; John Wiley & Sons: New York, 1982; 110.

7. Delmonico, F.L.; Cosimi, A.B. Monoclonal Antibody Treatment of Human Allograft Recipients. Surg. Gynecol. Obstet. **1988**, *166*, 89–98.

8. Myers, K.J.; Ron, Y. Current Approaches and Obstacles to Immunotherapy. Pharm. Technol. **1992**, *16*, 26–36.

9. Larson, S.M.; Carrasquillo, J.A.; Krohn, K.A.; Brown, J.P.; McGuffin, R.W.; Ferens, J.M.; Hill, L.D.; Beaumier, P.L.; Hellstrom, P.L.; Hellstrom, I. Localization of 131I-Labeled P97-Specific Fab Fragments in Human Melanoma as a Basis for Radiotherapy. J. Clin. Invest. **1983**, *72*, 2101–2107.

10. Ball, E.D.; Guyre, P.M.; Mills, L.; Fisher, J.; Dinces, N.B.; Fanger, M.W. Initial Trial of Bispecific Antibody-Mediated Immunotherapy of CD15-Bearing Tumors: Cytotoxicity of Human Tumor Cells Using a Bispecific Antibody Comprised of Anti-CD15 (MoAb PM81) and Anti-CD64/Fc Gamma RI (MoAb 32). J. Hematother. 1992, 1, 85–94.

11. Goding, J.W. *Monoclonal Antibodies: Principles and Practice*, 3rd Ed.; Academic Press: London, 1996; 153–160.

12. Kettleborough, C.A.; Saldanha, J.; Heath, V.J.; Morrison, C.J.; Bendig, M.M. Humanization of a Mouse Monoclonal Antibody by CDR Grafting. Protein Eng. 1991, 4, 773–783.

13. Randerson, D.H. Large-Scale Cultivation of Hybridoma Cells. J. Biotechnol. 1985, 2, 241–255.

14. Shepherd, P.; Dean, C. *Monoclonal Antibodies: A Practical Approach*; Oxford University Press: Oxford, 2000; 125–180.

15. King, D.J. *Applications and Engineering of Monoclonal Antibodies*; Taylor and Francis: London, 1998; 161–185.

16. Page, M.; Thibeault, D.; Noel, C.; Dumas, L. Coupling a Preactivated Daunorubicin Derivative to Antibody: A New Approach. Anticancer Res. 1990, 10, 353–357.

17. Arano, Y.; Matsushima, H.; Tagawa, M.; Koizumi, M.; Endo, K.; Konishi, J.; Yokoyama, A. A Novel Bifunctional Metabolizable Linker for the Conjugation of Antibodies with Radionuclides. Bioconjugate Chem. 1991, 2, 71–76.

18. Noguchi, A.; Takahashi, T.; Yamaguchi, T.; Kitamura, K.; Takakura, Y.; Hashida, M.; Sezaki, H. Preparation and Properties of the Immunoconjugate Composed of Anti-Human Colon Cancer Monoclonal Antibody and Mitomycin C-Dextran Conjugate. Bioconjugate Chem. 1992, 3, 132–137.

19. Zara, J.J.; Wood, R.D.; Boon, P.; Kim, C.-H.; Pomato, N.; Bredehorst, R.; Vogel, C.-W. A Carbohydrate-Directed Heterobifunctional Cross-Linking Reagent for the Synthesis of Immunoconjugates. Anal. Biochem. 1991, 194, 156–162.

20. Kaneko, T.; Willner, D.; Monkovic, I.; Knipe, J.O.; Braslawsky, G.R.; Greenfield, R.S.; Vyas, D.M. New Hydrazone Derivatives of Adriamycin and their Immuno-conjugates—A Correlation Between Acid Stability and Cytotoxicity. Bioconjugate Chem. 1991, 2, 133–141.

21. Lavie, E.; Hirschberg, D.L.; Schreiber, G.; Thor, K.; Hill, L.; Hellstrom, I.; Hellstrom, K.-E. Monoclonal Antibody L6-Daunomycin Conjugates Constructed to Release Free Drug at the Lower pH of Tumor Tissue. Cancer Immunol. Immunother. 1991, 33, 223–230.

22. Greenfield, L.; Bloch, W.; Moreland, M. Thiol Containing Cross-Linking Agent with Enhanced Steric Hindrance. Bioconjugate Chem. 1990, 1, 400–410.

23. Goff, D.A.; Carroll, S.F. Substituted 2-Iminothiolanes: Reagents for the Preparation of Disulfide Cross-Linked Conjugates with Increased Stability. Bioconjugate Chem. 1990, 1, 381–386.

24. Rowland, G.F.; O'Neill, G.J.; Davies, A.A. Suppression of Tumour Growth in Mice by a Drug-Antibody Conjugate Using a Novel Approach Linkage. Nature 1975, 255 (5508), 487–488.

25. Rybak, S.M.; Hoogenboom, H.R.; Meade, H.M.; Raus, J.C.M.; Schwartz, D.; Youle, R.J. Humanization of Immunotoxins. Proc. Nat. Acad. Sci. USA 1992, 89, 3165–3169.

26. Vandamme, A.; Dewerchin, M.; Lijnen, R.; Bernar, H.; Bulens, F.; Nelles, L.; Collen, D. Characterization of a Recombinant Chimeric Plasminogen Activator Composed of a Fibrin Fragment-D-Dimer-Specific Humanized Monoclonal Antibody and a Truncatred Single-Chain Urokinase. Eur. J. Biochem. 1992, 205, 139–146.

27. Weiner, L.M. An Overview of Monoclonal Antibody Therapy of Cancer. Semin. Oncol. 1999, 26 (4 Suppl. 12), 41–50.

28. Taetle, R.; Honeysett, J.M.; Trowbridge, I. Effects of Anti-Transferrin Receptor Antibodies on Growth of Normal and Malignant Myeloid Cells. Int. J. Cancer 1983, 32, 343–349.

29. *Physician's Desk Reference*, 53rd Ed.; Rituxan, Medical Economics Co.: Montvale, NJ, 1999; 1070–1072–1384–1386.

30. Cobleigh, M.A.; Vogel, C.L.; Tripathy, D.; Robert, N.J.; Scholl, S.; Fehrenbacher, L.; Wolter, J.M.; Paton, V.; Shak, S.; Lieberman, G.; Slamon, D.J. Multinational Study of the Efficacy and Safety of Humanized Anti-HER2 Monoclonal Antibody in Women Who Have HER2-Over-Expressing Metastatic Breast Cancer That has Progressed after Chemotherapy for Metastatic Disease. J. Clin. Oncol. 1999, 17, 2639–2648.

31. Colbern, G.T.; Hiller, A.J.; Musterer, R.S.; Working, P.K.; Henderson, I.C. Antitumor Activity of Herceptin in Combination with Stealth Liposomal Cisplatin or Nonliposomal Cisplatin in a HER2 Positive Human Breast Cancer Model. J. Inorg. Biochem. 1999, 77, 117–120.

32. Mittelman, A.; Chen, Z.J.; Kageshita, T.; Yang, H.; Yamada, M.; Baskind, P.; Goldbexy, N.; Puccio, C.; Ahmed, T.; Arlin, Z. et al. Active Specific Immunotherapy in Patients with Melanoma. J. Clin. Invest. 1990, 86, 2136–2144.

33. Magerstadt, M. *Antibody Conjugates and Malignant Disease*; CRC Press: Boca Raton, FL, 1991; 17–36, 79–110.

34. Preparation and Use of DTPA-Coupled Antitumor Antibodies Radiolabelled with Yttrium-90. In *Antibody-Mediated Delivery Sytems*; Hnatowich, D.J., Snook, D., Rowlinson, G., Stewart, S., Epentos, A.A., Eds.; Marcel Dekker, Inc.: New York, 1988; 353–374.

35. Corcoran, M.C.; Eary, J.; Bernstein, I.; Press, O.W. Radioimmunotherapy Strategies for Non-Hodgkin's Lymphomas. An. Oncol. 1997, 8 (Suppl. 1), 133–138.

36. Panousis, C.; Pietersz, G.A. Monoclonal Antibody-Directed Cytotoxic Therapy: Potential in Malignant Diseases of Aging. Drugs & Aging. **1999**, *1*, 1–15.

37. Press, O.W.; Eary, J.F.; Appelbaum, F.R.; Martin, P.J.; Badger, C.C.; Nelp, W.B.; Glenn, S.; Butchko, G.; Fisher, D.; Porter, B. Radiolabeled-Antibody Therapy of B-Cell Lymphoma with Autologous Bone Marrow Support. New Engl. J. Med. **1993**, *329*, 1219–1224.

38. Press, O.W. Radiolabeled Antibody Therapy of B-Cell Lymphomas. Semina. Oncol. **1999**, *26* (5 Suppl 14), 58–65.

39. Poste, G.; Kirsh, R. Site-Specific (Targeted) Drug Delivery in Cancer Therapy. Biotechnology **1983**, *1*, 869–878.

40. Alving, C.R. Delivery of Liposome-Encapsulated Drugs to Macrophages. Pharm. Ther. **1983**, *22*, 407–412.

41. Panchal, R.G. Novel Therapeutic Strategies to Selectively Kill Cancer Cells. Biochem. Pharmacol. **1998**, *55*, 247–252.

42. Vitetta, E.S.; Stone, M.; Amlot, P.; Fay, J.; May, R.; Till, M.; Newman, J.; Clark, P.; Collins, R.; Cunningham, D. et al. A Phase I Immunotoxin Trial in Patients with B-Cell Lymphoma. Cancer Res. **1991**, *15*, 4052–4058.

43. Winkler, U.; Barth, S.; Schnell, R.; Diehl, V.; Engert, A. The Emerging Role of Immunotoxins in Leukemia and Lymphoma. Ann. Oncol. **1997**, *8* (Suppl 1), 139–146.

44. Kreitman, R.J.; Pastan, I. Immunotoxins for Targeted Cancer Therapy. Adv. Drug Del. Rev. **1998**, *31*, 53–88.

45. Willner, D.; Trail, P.A.; Hofstead, S.J.; King, H.D.; Lasch, S.J.; Braslawsky, G.R.; Greenfield, R.S.; Kaneko, T.; Firestone, R.A. (6-Maleimidocaproyl)Hydrazone of Doxorubicin—A New Derivative for the Preparation of Immunoconjugates of Doxorubicin. Bioconjugate Chem. **1993**, *4*, 521–42.

46. Trail, P.A.; Willner, D.; Lasch, S.J.; Henderson, A.J.; Hofstead, S.; Casazza, A.M.; Firestone, R.A.; Hellstrom, I.; Hellstrom, K.E. Cure of Xenografted Human Carcinomas by BR96-Doxorubicin Immunoconjugates. Science **1993**, *261* (5118), 212–215.

47. Sjogren, H.O.; Isaksson, M.; Willner, D.; Hellstrom, I.; Hellstrom, K.E.; Trail, P.A. Antitumor Activity of Carcinoma-Reactive BR96-Doxorubicin Conjugate against Human Carcinomas in Athymic Mice and Rats and Syngeneic Rat Carcinomas in Immunocompetent Rats. Cancer Res. **1997**, *7*, 4530–4536.

48. Barbour, N.P.; Paborji, M.; Alexander, T.C.; Coppola, W.P.; Bogardus, J.B. Stabilization of Chimeric BR96-Doxorubicin Immunoconjugate. Pharm. Res. **1995**, *12*, 215–222.

49. Tolcher, A.W.; Sugarman, S.; Gelmon, K.A.; Cohen, R.; Saleh, M.; Isaacs, C.; Young, L.; Healey, D.; Onetto, N.; Slichenmyer, W. Randomized Phase II Study of BR96-Doxorubicin Conjugate in Patients with Metastatic Breast Cancer. J. Clin. Oncol. **1999**, *17* (2), 478–484.

50. Ghose, T.; Norvell, S.T.; Guclu, A.; Bodurtha, A.; Tai, J.; MacDonald, A.S. Immunochemotherapy of Malignant Melanoma with Chlorambucil-Bound Antimelanoma Globulins: Preliminary Results in Patients with Disseminated Disease. J. Natl. Cancer Inst. **1977**, *58*, 845–852.

51. Ford, C.H.J.; Newman, C.E.; Johnson, J.R.; Woodhouse, C.S.; Reeder, T.A.; Rowland, G.F.; Simmonds, R.G. Localisation and Toxicity Study of a Vindesine-Anti-CEA Conjugate in Patients with Advanced Cancer. Br. J. Cancer **1983**, *47*, 35–42.

52. Sezaki, H.; Hashida, M. Macromolecule-Drug Conjugates in Targeted Cancer Chemotherapy. CRC Crit. Rev. Ther. Drug Carrier Sys. **1984**, *1*, 1–38.

53. Newman, C.E.; Ford, C.H.J.; Davies, D.A.L.; O'Neill, G.J. Antibody Drug Synergism an Assessment of Specific Passive Immuno Therapy in Bronchial Carcinoma. Lancet **1977**, *2*, 163–164.

54. Nitta, T.; Sato, K.; Yagita, H.; Okumura, K.; Ishii, S. Preliminary Trial of Specific Targeting Therapy Against Malignant Glioma. Lancet **1990**, *335*, 368–371.

55. Tsukada, Y.; Hurwitz, E.; Kashi, R.; Sela, M.; Hibi, N.; Hara, A.; Hirai, H. Chemotherapy by Intravenous Administration of Conjugates of Daunomycin with Monoclonal and Conventional Anti-Rat Alpha-Fetoprotein Antibodies. Proc. Natl. Acad. Sci. USA **1982**, *79*, 7896–7899.

56. Ohkawa, K.; Tsukada, Y.; Hibi, N.; Umemoto, N.; Hara, T. Selective In Vitro and In Vivo Growth Inhibition against Human Yolk Sac Tumor Cell Lines by Purified Antibody against Human Alpha-Fetoprotein Conjugated with Mitomycin C Via Human Serum Albumin. Cancer Immunol. Immunother. **1986**, *23*, 81–86.

57. Shen, W.-C.; Dug, X.; Feener, E.P.; Ryser, H.J. The Intracellular Release of Methotrexate from a Synthetic Drug Carrier System Targeted to Fc Receptor-Bearing Cells. J. Contr. Rel. **1989**, *10*, 89–96.

58. Midoux, P.; Martin, A.; Collet, B.; Monsigny, M.; Roche, A.-C.; Toujas, L. Activation of Mouse Macrophages by Muramyl Dipeptide Coupled with an Anti-Macrophage Monoclonal Antibody. Bioconjugate Chem **1992**, *3*, 194–199.

59. Seymour, L.W.; Flanagan, P.A.; Al-Shamkhani, A.; Subr, V.; Ulbrich, K.; Cassidy, J.; Duncan, R. Synthetic Polymers Comjugated to Monoclonal Antibodies: Vehicles for Tumor-Targeted Drug Delivery. Sel. Cancer Thera. **1991**, *7*, 59–73.

60. Rihova, B.; Kopecek, J. Biological Properties of Targetable Poly[*N*-(2-Hydroxypropyl)-Methacrylamide]-Antibody Conjugates. J. Contr. Rel. **1985**, *2*, 289–310.

61. Duncan, R.; Hume, I.C.; Kopeckova, P.; Ulbrich, K.; Strohalm, J.; Kopecek, J. Anticancer Agents Coupled To *N*-(2-Hydroxypropyl)-Methacrylamide Copolymers. J. Contr. Rel. **1989**, *10*, 51–63.

62. Houck, K.S.; Huang, L. The Role of Multivalency in Antibody Mediated Liposome Targeting. Biochem. Biophys. Res. Commun. **1987**, *145*, 1205–1210.

63. Heath, T.D.; Montgomery, J.A.; Piper, J.R.; Paphadjopoulos, D. Antibody-Targeted Liposomes: Increase in Specific

Toxicity of Methotrexate-Gamma-Aspartate. Proc. Natl. Acad. Sci. USA **1983**, *80*, 1377–1381.

64. Phillips, N.C.; Tsoukas, C. Immunoliposome Targeting to CD4+ Cells in Human Blood. Cancer Detect. Prev. **1990**, *14*, 383–390.

65. Bloemen, P.G.M. Adhesion Molecules: A New Target for Immunoliposome-Mediated Drug Delivery. FEBS Letters **1995**, *357*, 140–144.

66. Sullivan, S.M.; Huang, L. Enhanced Delivery to Target Cells by Heat-Sensitive Immunoliposomes. Proc. Natl. Acad. Sci. USA **1986**, *83*, 6117–6121.

67. Connor, J.; Huang, L. pH-Sensitive Immunoliposomes as an Efficient and Target-Specific Carrier for Antitumor Drugs. Cancer Res. **1986**, *46*, 3431–3435.

68. Onuma, M.; Yasutomi, Y.; Yamamoto, M.; Watarai, S.; Yasuda, T.; Kawakami, Y. Antitumor Effect of Adriamycin Entrapped in Liposomes Conjugated with Anti-bovine Tumor Antigen Monoclonal Antibody in Leukemic Cows. Zentralbl. Veterinarmed. **1989**, *36*, 139–147.

69. Onuma, M.; Odawara, T.; Watarai, S.; Aida, Y.; Ochiai, K.; Syuto, B.; Matsumoto, K.; Yashuda, T.; Fujimoto, Y.; Izawa, H.; Kawakami, Y. Antitumor Effect of Adriamycin Entrapped in Liposomes Conjugated with Monoclonal Antibody against Tumor-Associated Antigen of Bovine Leukemia Cells. Jpn. J. Cancer Res. **1986**, *77*, 1161–1167.

70. Woodle, M.C. Sterically Stabilized Liposome Therapeutics. Adv. Drug Del. Rev. **1995**, *16*, 249–265.

71. Allen, T.M. Long-Circulating (Sterically Stabilized) Liposomes for Targeted Drug Delivery. Trends Pharmacol. Sci. **1994**, *15*, 215–20.

72. Maclean, A.L.; Symonds, G.; Ward, R. Immunoliposomes as Targeted Delivery Vehicles for Cancer Therapeutics. Int. J. Oncol. **1997**, *11*, 325–332.

73. Mastrobattista, E.; Koning, G.A.; Storm, G. Immunoliposomes for the Targeted Delivery of Antitumor Drugs. Adv. Drug Deliv. Reviews **1999**, *40*, 103–127.

74. Kirpotin, D.; Park, J.W.; Hong, K.; Zalipsky, S.; Li, W.L.; Carter, P.; Benz, C.C.; Papahadjopoulos, D. Sterically Stabilized Anti-HER2 Immunoliposomes: Design and Targeting to Human Breast Cancer Cells In Vitro. Biochemistry **1997**, *36* (1), 66–75.

75. Park, J.W.; Hong, K.; Kirpotin, D.B.; Meyer, O.; Papahadjopoulos, D.; Benz, C.C. Anti-HER2 Immunoliposomes for Targeted Therapy of Human Tumors. Cancer Lett. **1997**, *118*, 153–160.

76. Seid, C.A.; Fidler, I.J.; Clyne, R.K.; Earnest, L.E.; Fan, D. Overcoming Murine Tumor Cell Resistance to Vinblastine by Presentation of the Drug in Multi-lamellar Liposomes Consisting of Phosphatidylcholine and Phosphatidylserine. Sel. Cancer Thera. **1991**, *7*, 103–12.

77. Young, K.; Liu, D.; Maruyama, K.; Takizawa, T. Antibody Mediated Lung Targeting of Long-Circulating Emulsions. PDA J. of Pharm. Sci. Technol. **1996**, *50*, 372–377.

78. Lundberg, B.B.; Griffiths, G.; Hansen, H.J. Conjugation of an Anti-B-Cell Lymphoma Monoclonal Antibody, LL2, to Long-Circulating Drug-Carrier Lipid Emulsions. J. Pharm. Pharmacol. **1999**, *51*, 1099–1105.

79. Lee, K.C.; Lee, J.Y.; Kim, W.B.; Cha, C.Y. Monoclonal Antibody-Based Targeting of Methotrexate-Loaded Microspheres. Int. J. Pharm. **1990**, *59*, 27–33.

80. Akasaka, Y.; Ueda, H.; Takayama, K.; Machida, Y.; Nagai, T. Preparation and Evaluation of Bovine Serum Albumin Nanospheres Coated with Monoclonal Antibodies. Drug Design Del. **1988**, *3*, 85–97.

81. Illum, L.; Jones, P.D.; Baldwin, R.W.; Davis, S.S. Tissue Distribution of Poly(Hexyl 2-Cyanoacrylate) Nanoparticles Coated with Monoclonal Antibodies in Mice Bearing Human Tumor Xenografts. J. Pharmacol. Exp. Ther. **1984**, *230*, 733–736.

82. Bellet, D.; Bidart, J.M.; Rougier, P.; Bohuon, C. Use of Monoclonal Antibodies in the Treatment of Cancer of the Pancreas: Towards New Progress?. Bull. Cancer (Paris) **1990**, *77*, 283–238.

83. Pimm, M.V.; Baldwin, R.W. Quantitative Evaluation of the Localization of a Monoclonal Antibody (791T/36) in Human Osteogenic Sarcoma Xenografts. Eur. J. Clin. Oncol. **1984**, *20*, 515–524.

84. Thielemans, K.; Maloney, D.G.; Meeker, T.; Fujimoto, J.; Doss, C.; Warnke, R.A.; Bindl, J.; Gralow, J.; Miller, R.A.; Levy, R. Strategies for Production of Monoclonal Anti-Idiotype Antibodies against Human B-Cell Lymphomas. J. Immunol. **1984**, *133*, 495–501.

85. Mach, J.P.; Carrel, S.; Forni, M.; Ritschard, J.; Donath, A.; Alberto, P. Tumor Localization of Radiolabeled Antibodies against Carcinoembryonic Antigen in Patients with Carcinoma: A Critical Evaluation. N. Eng. J. Med. **1980**, *303*, 5–20.

86. Fidler, I.J. The Evolution of the Metastatic Phenotype. Proc. Am. Assoc. Cancer Res. **1991**, *32*, 486–487.

87. Trubetskoy, V.S.; Berdichevsky, V.R.; Efremov, E.E.; Torchilin, V.P. On the Possibility of the Unification of Drug Targeting Systems: Studies with Liposome Transport to the Mixtures of Target Antigens. Biochem. Pharmacol. **1987**, *36*, 839–842.

88. Matzku, S.; Krempel, H.; Weckenmann, H.P.; Schirrmacher, V.; Sinn, H.; Stricker, H. Tumour Targeting with Antibody-Coupled Liposomes: Failure to Achieve Accumulation in Xenografts and Spontaneous Liver Metastases. Cancer Immunol. Immunother. **1990**, *31*, 285–291.

89. Ranney, D.F. Drug Targeting to the Lungs. Biochem. Pharmacol. **1986**, *35*, 1063–1069.

90. Buchegger, F.; Haskell, C.M.; Schreyer, M.; Scazziga, B.R.; Randin, S.; Carrel, S.; Mach, J.-P. Radiolabeled Fragments of Monoclonal Antibodies against Carcinoembryonic Antigen for Localization of Human Colon Carcinoma Grafted into Nude Mice. J. Exp. Med. **1983**, *158*, 413–427.

91. Sivam, G.; Pearson, J.W.; Bohn, W.; Oldham, R.K.; Sadoff, J.C.; Morgan, A.C. Immunoconjugates to a

Human Melanoma-Associated Antigen. Cancer Res. **1987**, *47*, 3169.

92. Hurwitz, E.; Levy, R.; Maron, R.; Wilchek, M.; Arnon, R.; Sela, M. The Covalent Binding of Daunomycin and Adriamycin to Antibodies, with Retention of Both Drug and Antibody Activities. Cancer Res. **1975**, *35*, 1175–1181.

93. Johnson, D.A.; Barton, R.L.; Fix, D.V.; Scott, W.L.; Gutowski, M.C. Induction of Immunogenicity of Monoclonal Antibodies by Conjugation with Drugs. Cancer Res. **1991**, *51*, 5774–5776.

94. Dougherty, T.J. Photodynamic Therapy—New Approaches. Semin. Surg. Oncol. **1989**, *5*, 6–16.

95. Rakestraw, S.L.; Tompkins, R.G.; Yarmush, M.L. Antibody-Targeted Photolysis. In Vitro Studies with Sn(IV) Chlorine ^{6} Covalently Bound to Monoclonal Antibodies Using a Modified Dextran Carrier. Proc. Nat. Acad. Sci. USA **1990**, *87*, 4217–4221.

96. Omelyanenko, V.; Gentry, C.; Kopeckova, P.; Kopecek, J. HPMA Copolymer-Anticancer Drug-OV-TL16 Antibody Conjugates. II. Processing in Epithelial Ovarian Carcinoma Cells In Vitro. Int. J. Cancer **1998**, *75*, 600–608.

97. Bagshawe, K.D. Antibody-Directed Enzyme/Prodrug Therapy (ADEPT). Biochem. Soc. Trans **1990**, *18*, 750–752.

98. Antoniw, P.; Springer, C.J.; Bagshawe, K.D.; Searle, F.; Melton, R.G.; Rogers, G.T.; Burke, P.J.; Sherwood, R.F. Disposition of the Prodrug 4-(bis (2-Chloroethyl) Amino) Benzoyl-L-Glutamic Acid and its Active Parent Drug in Mice. Br. J. Cancer **1990**, *62*, 909–914.

99. Bagshawe, K.D.; Sharma, S.K.; Springer, C.J.; Antoniw, P.; Rogers, G.T.; Burke, P.J.; Melton, R.; Sherwood, R. Antibody-Enzyme Conjugates can Generate Cytotoxic Drugs from Inactive Precursors at Tumor Sites. Antibody Immunoconj. Radiopharm. **1991**, *4*, 915–922.

MUCOADHESIVE HYDROGELS IN DRUG DELIVERY

Hans E. Junginger
Maya Thanou
J. Coos Verhoef

Leiden/Amsterdam Center for Drug Research, Leiden University, The Netherlands

INTRODUCTION

This article focuses on defining the principles of bioadhesive delivery systems based on hydrogels to biological surfaces that are covered by mucus. An overview of the last decade's discoveries on mucoadhesion and applications of mucoadhesive hydrogels as drug carriers is given. Techniques that are frequently used to study the adhesion forces and physicochemical interactions between hydrogel, mucus, and the underlying mucosa are reviewed. Typical examples of applications of mucoadhesive hydrogels to mucosal routes of delivery are given. Finally, the perspectives of the application of these polymers in drug delivery are discussed.

Noninvasive drug delivery may require the administration of the drug delivery system (DDS) at an epithelium as a suitable site of absorption of the active compound. Such regions are usually called mucosae. In the human body several mucosal sites can be identified, the one mostly used for administration and absorption of therapeutics being the gastrointestinal route. In order to increase the residence time at these absorption sites, a so-called mucoadhesive delivery system has to be used. Generally, these systems consist of one or more types of hydrogels.

By definition, mucoadhesive hydrogels are a class of polymeric biomaterials that exhibit the basic characteristic of a hydrogel to swell by absorbing water and interacting by means of adhesion with the mucus that covers epithelia.

Bioadhesion has been defined as the attachment of synthetic or biological macromolecules to a biological tissue (1). The term mucoadhesion refers to the special case of bioadhesion where the biological tissue is an epithelium covered by mucus. Mucus is a thin blanket covering all epithelia that are in contact with the external environment in the gastrointestinal, respiratory, and urogenital tracts. The function of mucus is mainly the protection and lubrication of the underlying epithelium, but it may have additional functions dependent on the type of the covered epithelia. In each case of these mucosal routes, mucus characteristics (i.e., thickness) and functions are different. By this definition, the mucosal routes for drug delivery are:

- Buccal/oral route
- Nasal route
- Ocular route
- Vaginal route
- Gastrointestinal route

The concept of mucoadhesion in drug delivery was introduced in the field of controlled-release drug delivery systems in the early 1980s (2, 3). Thereafter, several researchers have focused on the investigations of the interfacial phenomena of mucoadhesive hydrogels (and of other type mucoadhesive compounds) with the mucus. Several techniques of studying these interactions were evaluated both in vitro and in vivo. These techniques have been recently reviewed by Harding et al. (4) and are given in Table 1.

A mucoadhesive hydrogel used as a drug delivery system should

1. Be loaded substantially by the active compound;
2. Not interact physicochemically with the active compound or create a hostile artificial environment that would lead to inactivation and degradation of the active compound;
3. Swell in the aqueous biological environment of the delivery–absorption site;
4. Interact with mucus or its components for adequate adhesion;
5. Allow, when swelled, controlled release of the active compound;
6. Be biocompatible (biomaterial) with the underlying epithelia by means of complete absence of cytotoxicity, ciliotoxicity, or other type of irreversible alterations of the cell membrane components;
7. Have the appropriate molecular size and conformation in order to escape systemic absorption from the administration site; and
8. Be excreted unaltered or biologically degraded to inactive, nontoxic oligomers/monomers that will be further subject of physical clearance.

Additionally, a mucoadhesive delivery system designed for controlled release of active compounds should be localized at specific sites of administration and absorption,

Table 1 Methods of studying mucoadhesion

Method	Comment
Direct assays	
Tensiometry	Force required to dislodge two surfaces, one coated with mucus, the other solid dosage form consisting of mucoadhesive hydrogel
Flow through	Flow rate dV/dt required to dislodge two surfaces; useful for microparticulate dosage forms
Colloidal gold staining	Measures the "adhesion number"
In vivo techniques	Endoscopy, gamma scintigraphy
Molecular mucin-based assays	
Viscometry and rheology	Intrinsic viscosity $[\eta]$ can be related to complex size via MHKS,[a] α coefficient
Dynamic light scattering	Diffusion coefficient, D, can be related to complex size via MHKS c. coefficient
Turbidity, light scattering	SEC MALLS[b] particularly useful for determining MW of mucin, turbidity, semiquantitative indicator
Analytical ultracentrifugation	Change in MW (sedimentation equilibrium), sedimentation coefficient ratio of complex to mucin
Surface plasmon resonance imaging methods	Needs mobile and immobile phase, atomic force microscopy (conventional and gold labeled), scanning tunneling microscopy

[a]Mark-Houwink-Kuhn-Sakurada.
[b]Size exclusion chromatography multiangle laser light scattering.
(Adapted from Ref. 4.)

and should prolong the residence time of the active compound at the site of administration to permit, if possible for one daily dosing.

The mucoadhesive delivery system, designed for the administration of macromolecular therapeutics like peptide or protein drugs, should have permeation-enhancing properties by means of alteration of the permeability properties of the underlying epithelium, and should protect the peptide drug from degradation by inhibiting the proteolytic enzymes usually present at the site of administration or by stabilizing the intrinsic environment of the delivery system by sustaining the suitable pH.

Solid dosage forms based on mucoadhesive polymers are used mainly for buccal delivery of drugs, whereas micro- or nanoparticulate formulations are preferred for the delivery of therapeutics in the nasal and intestinal tract (5).

During the last decade research was particularly focused on the delivery of mucoadhesive dosage forms in the gastrointestinal tract, which is the most favorable route of delivery with regard to patient compliance and ease of application. For this reason microparticulate formulations, consisting of mucoadhesive hydrogels, were designed and evaluated by different techniques (6, 7). However, solid dosage forms are more suitable for smaller cavities in the human body, like the oral cavity, either for systemic absorption of compounds or for local treatment of inflammatory diseases. In this case, monolithic devices

(tablets) made from mucoadhesive hydrogels were evaluated (8). Ocular and vaginal applications (for local or systemic absorption) of mucoadhesive hydrogels were also investigated.

The mucoadhesive properties of several classes of hydrogels have been identified, and two types of polymers have attracted special attention. Polyacrylates and their cross-linked modifications represent the anionic type, chitosan and its derivatives the cationic group. In addition, both types of polymers show a number of interesting characteristics beneficial for the administration of a wide range of therapeutics.

Specific type of mucoadhesive compounds, like lectins, have been evaluated to solve the difficulties presented by conventional mucoadhesive hydrogel systems, for instance in the gastrointestinal route. Since these compounds do not belong to the class of hydrogels, they are not extensively discussed here.

MUCUS

In higher organisms epithelia are covered by a protective gel layer defined as mucus. By weight, mucus consists mainly of water (95–99.5%) in which the mucous glycoprotein mucin (0.5–5%) is dispersed. Mucins are the major components responsible for the gel-like structure of the mucus. They possess a linear protein heavily glycosylated by oligosaccharide side chains. This protein core consists of a single polypeptide chain. One in every three residues is L-serine or L-threonine, in which the O-3 atoms provide the sites for glycosidic linkage. A mucus glycoprotein is composed typically of about 80% of carbohydrates, which for humans are restricted to five monosaccharides:

- L-Fucose
- *N*-Acetylglucosamine
- D-Galactose
- *N*-Acetylgalactosamine
- Sialic acid

The sialic acid residues are usually in a terminal position on the carbohydrate chain whereas the ester sulfate residues are in a more internal position; both contribute to give the molecule a net negative charge. The molecular weights of mucus glycoproteins range from 0.5 to 16×10^6 Da (4).

Mucins can be divided into two classes, membrane bound and secretory forms. Membrane-bound mucins are attached to cell surfaces and may affect immune responses or inflammation. It has been suggested that the high expression of cell-surface mucins, such as sialomucin MUC1, may result in cell–cell and cell–matrix interactions (10). Secretory mucins eminate from mucosal absorptive cells and specialized goblet cells. They constitute the major component of mucous gels in the gastrointestinal, ocular, respiratory, and urogenital epithelia. This type of mucus gel layer is functioning mainly as a physical barrier and lubricant. Important constituents in the mucus include growth factors and trefoil peptides, both secreted by the specialized cells located next to ulcerated mucosal tissue. This appears to be an adaptive phenomenon, important in maintaining the barrier function of the mucosal tissue, enhancing cell migration, and healing after injury. Other substances present in mucus include secretory immunoglobulin A (IgA), lysozyme, lactoferin, α_1-Antitrypsin, salts, and *N*-Glycosylated glycoproteins (10).

At present, nine different human epithelial mucin genes have been identified, each of which contains distinct sequences repeated in tandem that encode (apo)mucin core polypeptides (MUC) (10).

Leung and Robinson (11) defined four characteristics of the mucus layer related to mucoadhesion:

1. Mucus is a network of linear, flexible, and random-coil macromolecules.
2. Mucin is negatively charged due to sialic acid and sulfate residues.
3. Mucus is a cross-linked network connected by disulfide bonds between mucin molecules.
4. Mucin is heavily hydrated.

Several techniques have been used to estimate the rate of mucus secretion, but their accuracy seems to be doubtful. Nevertheless, it has been concluded that a slow baseline secretion of mucus is maintained by exocytosis from goblet cells in the gastrointestinal tract, which appears to be under cholinergic control (12). Rubinstein and Tirosh used carbachol (cholinergic agonist) at different doses to increase the mucus thickness in different parts of the gastrointestinal tract (13).

Attempts were also made to estimate the rate of turnover of the mucus gel. Lehr et al. (14) measured the amount of mucus produced per time unit, using an in situ perfused intestinal loop model in the rat. They found that this turnover time varies between 0.8 and 4.5 h.

MECHANISM AND THEORIES OF MUCOADHESION

The mechanistic processes involved in mucoadhesion between hydrogels and mucosa can be described in three steps:

1. Wetting and swelling of the polymer to allow for intimate contact with the biological tissue.
2. Interpenetration of the bioadhesive polymer chains and entanglement of polymer and mucin chains, and
3. Formation of weak chemical bonds between entangled chains (Fig. 1).

Several theories have been proposed to explain the biomucoadhesive phenomena (1, 15–17).

The electronic theory is based on the assumption that the mucoadhesive hydrogel and the target biological tissue have different electronic structures. When two materials come into contact with each other, electron transfer occurs, causing the formation of a double layer of electrical charge at the bioadhesive–biological interface. The bioadhesive force is believed to be due to attractive forces across this electrical double layer.

The adsorption theory states that the bioadhesive bond formed between an adhesive substrate and tissue or mucosae is due to van der Waals interactions, hydrogen bonds, and related forces. Alternatively, when mucus or saliva are interacting with a solid dosage form, the molecules of the liquid are adsorbed on the solid surface. This is an exothermic process. The free energy of adsorption is given by

$$\Delta G_{AD} = \Delta H_{AD} - T \Delta S_{AD} \qquad (1)$$

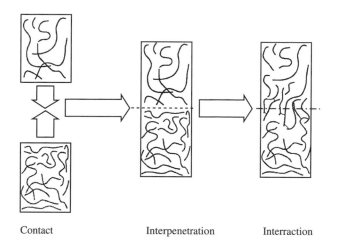

Contact   Interpenetration   Interraction

Fig. 1 Three stages in the interaction between a mucoadhesive polymer and mucin glycoprotein according to the interpenetration theory.

where ΔH_{AD} and ΔS_{AD} are the enthalpy and entropy changes, respectively. When adsorption takes place spontaneously, ΔG_{AD} is negative.

The contact angle θ of a liquid on a solid is the reflection of its wetting power. If $\theta = 0$, the liquid spreads freely on the solid surface and wets it. The relationship between the contact angle of a liquid on a solid and the surface tensions in the presence of saturated vapor of the liquid is given by the Young equation

$$\gamma_{sv} = \gamma_{sl} + \gamma_{lv} \cos\theta \qquad (2)$$

where γ_{sv} is the solid/vapor surface tension, γ_{sl} the solid/liquid surface tension, and γ_{lv} the liquid/vapor surface tension.

Another way to relate the interfacial tension γ_{sl} to the individual surface tensions of a liquid and solid is given by the Good equation.

$$\gamma_{sl} = \gamma_{sv} + \gamma_{lv} - 2\phi(\gamma_{sv}\gamma_{lv})^{1/2} \qquad (3)$$

Eq. 3 represents the reduction in interfacial tension resulting from molecular attraction between liquid and solid. The term ϕ is defined by

$$\phi = W_a / (W_{cl}W_{cs})^{1/2} \qquad (4)$$

where W_{cl} and W_{cs} are the work of cohesion of the liquid and the solid, respectively, and W_a is the work of adhesion.

The diffusion theory states that interpenetration and entanglement of polymer chains are additionally responsible for bioadhesion. The intimate contact of the two substrates is essential for diffusion to occur; that is, the driving force for the interdiffusion is the concentration gradient across the interface. The penetration of polymer chains into the mucus network, and vice versa, is dependent on concentration gradients and diffusion coefficients. It is believed that for an effective adhesion bond the interpenetration of the polymer chain should be in the range of 0.2–0.5 μm. It is possible to estimate the penetration depth (l) by

$$l = (tD_b)^{1/2} \qquad (5)$$

where t is the time of contact and D_b is the diffusion coefficient of the bioadhesive material in the mucus.

The fracture theory is the most widely applied theory in studying mucoadhesion mechanisms. It accounts for the forces required to separate two surfaces after adhesion. The maximum tensile stress (σ) produced during detachment can be determined by Eq. 6 by dividing the maximum force of detachment F_m by the total surface area (A_0) involved in the adhesive interaction:

$$\sigma = F_m / A_0 \qquad (6)$$

According to Duchêne and Ponchel (17), when tensiometry is used to measure the maximum detachment force as a function of the displacement of the upper support (function of the joint elongation), the work of bioadhesion can be defined as

$$W_b = F \times l \qquad (7)$$

Additionally, the fracture energy for a zero extension rate can be defined as the bioadhesion work to the initial surface between the bioadhesive material (in the form of a tablet or disk) and the biological support of a surface A_0, which allows for calculation of the fracture energy (ϵ) using

$$\epsilon = W_b / A_0 \qquad (8)$$

Thermodynamically, the fracture energy is the sum of the reversible work (W_r, representing the reversible molecular interactions at the interface) and irreversible work (W_i representing the irreversible deformation of the interfacial joint); both W_r and W_i are expressed per unit area of the fracture energy by.

$$\epsilon = W_r + W_i \qquad (9)$$

When a low extension rate is used for the measurements (for instance 1 mm/min), W_i can be considered as negligible and the fracture energy for zero extension rate (ϵ_0) is then equal to the reversible work of bioadhesion W_r, as shown by

$$\epsilon_0 = W_r = W_b / A_0 \qquad (10)$$

The fracture theory does not take into account biological phenomena such as stress caused, for example, by movement of the tissue.

THE STUDY OF MUCOADHESION OF HYDROGELS

During the last decade several methods to study mucoadhesion phenomena or mucoadhesive properties of hydrogels were used (Table 1). Tensiometry has already been reported as a suitable method during late 1980s and is still the most frequently used technique to study mucoadhesiveness of hydrogels. Peppas and coworkers developed a tensile technique for measurements of the bioadhesive strength of tablets containing polyacrylic acid to bovine mucosae (16, 18). A tensiometry setup for the investigation of solid devices is shown in Fig. 2. The system is better mimicking the in vivo conditions when the experiment is performed in an aqueous environment and the mucosa of interest is originating from freshly prepared biological tissue. It has been suggested that this system is most suitable for buccal or vaginal application, where biological liquid is controllable. Tensiometry has been shown to be very useful in comparing the mucoadhesive properties of different hydrogels (19).

Mikos and Peppas (20) described the flow channel to measure the bioadhesion of polymer microparticles on mucin gels. Later Lehr et al. (21) used an in situ loop model in the rat for the investigation of mucoadhesive microspheres (Fig. 3). They concluded that this approach allowed the study of the transit of particles. Another technique to study the mucoadhesive properties of microspheres is the electrobalance method, as described by Chickering et al. (22, 23). Environmental conditions

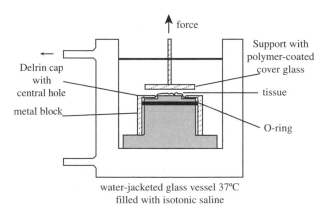

Fig. 2 Experimental setup to measure the force of detachment of mucoadhesive polymer films from mucosal tissue.

like temperature and pH can be easily controlled and several parameters can be obtained from one single experiment. The authors suggested that mucoadhesion in the bioerodible materials used to conduct the studies is not attributable to chain entanglement but to hydrogen bonding between hydrophilic functional groups (COOH) and mucus glycoproteins.

Colloidal gold staining has been introduced by Park (24) for studying the "adhesion number." The polymer in a form of strips is incubated with colloidal gold–mucin conjugates, and after a rinsing procedure the absorbance of strips is measured. Colloidal gold staining has also been used to investigate mucin–chitosan interactions (25).

Rheology measurements were used by Mortazavi et al. (26, 27) to investigate mucus–Carbopol 934P interactions at different pH values and the role of water movement in mucoadhesion. Similar rheological techniques were applied for studying four different types of polymers, and it was concluded that molecular interpenetration is an important factor in mucoadhesion by strengthening the mucus in the mucoadhesive–mucosal interface (28). Rheological methods were used to investigate the interpenetration between ion-sensitive polymers (Carbopol and deacetylated gellan gum, Gerlite) with two commercially available mucins: submaxillary gland mucin and porcine gastric mucin (29). It was suggested that the increase in the elastic modulus of a polymer–mucin mixture (compared to the elastic modulus of polymer alone) indicates a positive interaction caused by mucoadhesion. However, the concentration of the polymer, the type of the mucin used, and the quantity of ions present appeared to have a strong influence on the interactions between mucins and ion-sensitive polymers, indicating that the explanation of mucoadhesion by means of interpenetration should be applied only to interpret special cases of mucoadhesion between polymers and mucins.

Rossi et al. (30) evaluated rheologically mucins of different origin with polyacrylic acid and sodium carboxymethyl cellulose. The same group also reported a novel rheological approach based on a stationary viscoelastic test (creep test) to describe the interaction between mucoadhesive polymers and mucins (31, 32). Jabbari et al. (33) used attenuated total-reflection infrared spectroscopy to investigate the chain interpenetration of polyacrylic acid in the mucin interface.

Other techniques used for studying molecular interactions between polymers and mucus include ultracentrifugation, surface plasmon resonance, and electromagnetic transduction (4, 34). Illum and coworkers (35) investigated the interaction of chitosan microspheres, using turbidimetric measurements and adsorption studies of mucin to the microspheres.

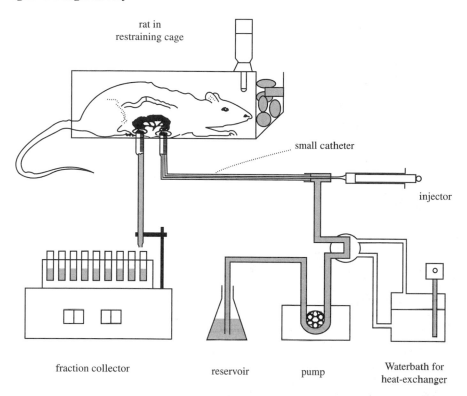

Fig. 3   Experimental setup to study the intestinal transit of mucoadhesive microspheres in a chronically isolated loop. (Adapted from Ref. 21.)

Microscopic visualization techniques have also been used to investigate mucus–polymer interactions (36–39). Transmission electron microscopy was used by Fiebrig et al. (36), whereas different microscopical techniques were used by Lehr et al. (37) for the visualization of mucoadhesive interfaces. Transmission electron microscopy in combination with near-field Fourier transform infrared microscopy (FTIR) has been shown to be suitable for investigating the adhesion-promoting effect of polyethyleneglycol added in a hydrogel (38). Moreover, scanning force microscopy may be a valuable approach to obtain information on mucoadhesion and specific adhesion phenomena (39).

THE MUCOSAL ROUTES OF DELIVERY

Buccal Route

The buccal route of drug administration is the most widely used method for application of mucoadhesive delivery systems. Both for local treatment of inflammation (i.e., apthae) and for rapid absorption of compounds (nitroglycerin), formulation technologies have employed the buccal route for over two decades, and sublingual or gingival

dosage forms are already established in the market (8) (Table 2).

Oral mucosae are composed of multiple layers of cells, which show various patterns of differentiation dependent on the functions of different regions in the oral cavity (40). The oral mucosa is covered by a stratified, squamous epithelium, and three different types of mucosa can be distinguished: the masticatory, the lining, and the specialized mucosa. Blood supply to the oral cavity tissues is delivered via the external carotid artery, which branches to the maxiliary lingual and facial artery. There are no mucus-secreting goblet cells in the oral mucosa, but mucins are found in human saliva. These mucins are water-soluble and form a gel of 10–200-μm thickness. Saliva, mainly composed of water (99%), is continuously secreted in the oral cavity and exists as a film with a thickness of 0.07–0.1 mm (40).

In the 1980s, Machida and Nagai (41) evaluated spray dosage forms based on hydroxypropyl cellulose (HPC) for the delivery of beclomethasone to treat recurrent and multiple apthae. Previously a double-layered tablet of HPC and Carbopol 934P was introduced in the market for the treatment of apthous stomatitis (41).

Bouckaert et al. (42) tested buccal tablets of miconazole based on modified starch–polyacrylic acid

Table 2 Drug products available for buccal and/or sublingual application using mucoadhesive polymers

Drug	Therapeutic area	Product names
Nitroglycerin	Angina pectoris	Suscard, Cardilate, Nitrobid, Nitromex, Nitrong
Isosorbide mononitrate	Angina pectoris	Imdur, Isordil, ISMO
Buprenorphine	Analgesia	Temgesic, Buprenex
Nicotine	Smoking cessation	Nicotinelle, Nicorette
Ergotamine	Migraine	Ergostat, Ergomar
Methyl testosterone	Hypogonadism, delayed puberty	Oroton Methyl, Testred, Virilon
Lorazepam	Anxiety, insomnia	Ativan

(Adapted from Ref. 8.)

mixtures. Although these tablets showed different mucoadhesion properties in vitro, no significant differences in the salivary content of miconazole could be observed in human volunteers.

Lee and Chien (43) evaluated mucoadhesive devices of a bilayer type, consisting of a fast-release layer containing polyvinylpyrrolidone (PVP) and a sustained-release layer of Carbopol 934P and PVP for prolonged delivery of luteinizing hormone-releasing hormone (LHRH) onto the porcine gingival and alveolar mucosa for 24 h. This device contained also an absorption enhancer (sodium cholate) and cetylpyridinium chloride to protect LHRH from degradation by microflora. The LHRH permeation appeared to increase by raising the loading of LHRH or enhancer in the fast-release layer. The formulation of the devices could be varied to achieve specific rates of transmucosal peptide drug permeation.

Nair and Chien (44) compared patches and tablets of different polymers (sodium carboxymethylcellulose, carbopol, polyethylene oxide, polymethyl vinyl ether–maleic anhydride, tragacanth) regarding their release characteristics of four drugs (chlorheximide, clotrimazole, benzocaine, and hydrocortisone). They observed sustained release of all four compounds from the mucoadhesive tablets, but only two of the active compounds, chlorheximide and clotrimazole, could be released in a controlled manner from the mucoadhesive patches.

Buccal bilayer devices (films and tablets) are comprised of a drug-containing mucoadhesive layer and a drug-free backing layer (45). The former consists of chitosan, free or cross-linked by an anionic polymer (polycarbophil, sodium alginate, gellan gum), and the latter of ethylcellulose. The in situ cross-linking of chitosan by polycarbophil gives tablets that exhibit controlled swelling, drug release, and adequate mucoadhesion to bovine sublingual mucosa.

The periodontal pocket is another site for drug delivery in the oral cavity. Needleman et al. (46) investigated three mucoadhesive polymers (cationic chitosan, anionic xanthan gum, neutral polyethylene oxide) in vitro, using organ cultures, and in vivo in patients on their periodontal and oral mucosa. Of the polymers studied, chitosan displayed the longest adhesion in vitro and on the periodontal pockets, and the shortest adhesion on oral mucosa.

Nasal Route

The nasal route of drug administration is the most suitable alternative of delivery for poorly absorbale compounds such as peptide or protein drugs. The nasal epithelium exhibits relatively high permeability, and only two cell layers separate the nasal lumen from the dense blood-vessel network in the lamina propria. The respiratory epithelium is the major lining of the human nasal cavity and is essential in the clearance of mucus by the mucociliary system. This epithelium is composed of ciliated and nonciliated columnar cells, goblet cells, and basal cells. The respiratory epithelium is covered by a mucus layer, which can be divided into two distinctive layers (the periciliary layer and a more gel-like upper layer). The periciliary layer consists of a liquid of lower viscosity. Mucus is secreted from goblet cells as highly condensed granules by exocytosis. The mucus layer is propelled by the cilia toward the nasopharynx, and the function of the mucociliary clearance is to remove foreign substances and particles from the nasal cavity, preventing them to reach the upper airways (47).

Various structurally different mucoadhesive polymers were tested for their ability to retard the nasal mucociliary clearance in rats (48). Methylcellulose, sodium carboxymethyl cellulose, hydroxypropyl methylcellulose, chitosan glutamate, Carbopol 934P, polyethylene oxide 600K, and Pluronic F127 were applied in gel form, and their clearance was measured using microspheres labeled with a fluorescent marker incorporated into the formulation. The clearance rate of each polymer gel was found to be lower than that of a control microsphere suspension, resulting in an increased residence time of the gel formulations in the nasal cavity. Methylcellulose (3%) gel gave the longest nasal residence time, whereas a Carbopol 934P (0.2%) aqueous gel was the least effective.

Illum et al. (49) evaluated chitosan solutions as delivery platforms for nasal administration of insulin to rats and sheep. They reported a concentration-dependent absorption-enhancing effect with minimal histological changes of the nasal mucosa in all concentrations applied.

Oechslein et al. (50) studied various powder formulations of mucoadhesive polymers for their efficacy to increase the nasal absorption of octreotide in rats. Although chitosan showed the highest water uptake (chitosan > microcrystalline cellulose > semicrystalline cellulose ≫ pectin = hydroxyethyl starch = alginic acid = Sephadex G25), the highest peptide drug bioavailability was found after coadministration of alginic acid and Sephadex G25 powders (4.1 and 5.56%, respectively). The authors concluded that the calcium-binding properties of the polymers used correlated better with the increased octreotide bioavailability.

Nakamura et al. (51) studied the adhesion of water-soluble and neutral polymers, hydroxypropyl cellulose (HPC), xanthan gum (XG), tamarind gum (TG), and polyvinyl alcohol (PVA)] to nasal mucosa in vitro and in vivo. The polymers, mixed with a dye, were applied as powders to the nasal cavity of rabbits, and the remaining dye residue was determined at 2, 4, and 6 h after nasal instillation with a thin fiberscope. The polymer XG showed the longest residence time of the dye in the cavity, followed by TG, HPC, and PVA in decreasing order. For the mixture XG and XG–PVA (2:8), some residue of dye could still be observed 6 h after administration. The order of adhesion of these polymers to agar plates in vitro agreed with that of their mucoadhesion in vivo. Illum et al. (52) introduced bioadhesive microspheres for nasal delivery of poorly absorbable drugs. Radiolabelled microspheres made from diethylaminoethyl (DEAE)-dextran, starch microspheres, and albumin microspheres were administered to human volunteers and appeared to be cleared significantly slower than solutions or nonmucoadhesive powder formulations. However, starch or hyaluronic acid microspheres significantly increased the absorption of peptide drugs from nasal mucosa (53).

Nakamura et al. (54) described a microparticulate dosage form of budesonide, consisting of novel bioadhesive and pH-dependent graft copolymers of polymethacrylic acid and polyethylene glycol, resulting in elevated and constant plasma levels of budesonide for 8 h after nasal administration in rabbits.

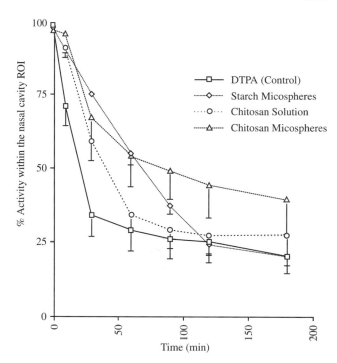

Fig. 4 The nasal clearance of bioadhesive formulations and a control in human volunteers. DTPA = diethylenetriaminepentaacetic acid. (From Ref. 55.)

Recently, starch and chitosan microspheres as well as chitosan solutions were tested for their clearance characteristics in human volunteers using gamma scintigraphy (55). The results revealed a 4-, 3-, and 2-times longer clearance half-life (compared to controls) for chitosan microspheres, starch microspheres, and chitosan solutions (Fig. 4). These observations support the hypothesis that chitosan delivery systems can reduce the rate of clearance from the nasal cavity, thereby increasing the contact time of the delivery system with the nasal mucosa and providing the potential for raising the bioavailability of drugs incorporated into these systems.

Ocular Route

The ocular route is used mainly for the local treatment of eye pathologies. Absorption of drugs administered by conventional eyedrops can result in poor ocular bioavailabilities (2–10%). This is due to the limited area of absorption, the lipophilic character of the corneal epithelium, and a series of elimination factors that reduce the contact time of the medication with the corneal surface, such as drainage of instilled solutions, lacrimation, and tear turnover and tear evaporation (56).

The first structure encountered by an ocular dosage form is the precorneal tear film, consisting of three layers:

Outer layer, oily and lipid, mainly prevents tear evaporation.
Middle layer, which is an aqueous salt solution layer, and
Inner layer, a mucus layer secreted by the conjuctiva goblet cells and the lacrymal gland. This layer is important for wetting the corneal and conjuctival epithelia. The ocular membranes comprise the cornea (not vascularized) and the conjuctiva (vascularized). The corneal epithelium consists of five or six layers of nonkeratinized squamous cells, and it is considered to be the major pathway for ocular drug penetration (57).

The following types of mucoadhesive preparations have been evaluated for ocular drug delivery: hydrogels, viscous liquids, solids (inserts), and particulate formulations (57). Hui and Robinson (58) introduced hydrogels consisting of cross-linked polyacrylic acid for ocular delivery of progesterone in rabbits. These preparations increased progesterone concentrations in the aqueous humor four times over aqueous suspensions.

Davies et al. (59) compared the precorneal clearance of Carbopol 934P to that of an equiviscous nonmucoadhesive PVA solution and phosphate buffered saline (PBS) using lacrimal dacryoscintigraphy in the rabbit. The precorneal retention of the Carbopol 934P was shown to be significantly longer than that of PVA, which, in turn, was significantly longer than that of PBS. In the same study, Carbopol 934P solution produced a significant increase in bioavailability of pilocarpine as compared to PVA and PBS. The same authors (60) described phospholipid vesicles coated with Carbopol 934P or Carbopol 1342 (a hydrophobic modified Carbopol resin). The mucoadhesive polymer-coated vesicles demonstrated substantially enhanced precorneal retention compared to noncoated vesicles at pH 5. However, the polymer-coated vesicles did not increase the ocular bioavailability of entrapped tropicamide compared to noncoated vesicles and aqueous solutions.

Lehr et al. (61) investigated two gentamicin formulations of polycarbophil (neutralized vs. nonneutralized) to pigmented rabbit eye. Both polymeric formulations doubled the uptake of gentamicin by the bulbar conjunctiva.

Saettone et al. (62) evaluated low viscosity polymers (polygalacturonic acid, hyaluronic acid, carboxymethylamylose, carboxymethylchitin, chondroitin sulfate, heparan sulfate, and mesoglycan) as potential mucoadhesive carriers for cyclopentolate and pilocarpine in a study of their influence on miotic activity in rabbits. Small but significant increases in bioavailability were observed and a correlation was found between the bioavailability of the two drugs and the mucoadhesive bond strength of the polymers investigated.

Calvo et al. (63) studied chitosan- and poly-L-Lysine (PLL)-coated poly-ε-Caprolactone (PECL) nanocapsules for ocular application. In comparison with commercial eyedrops, the systems investigated (uncoated, PLL-coated, and chitosan-coated nanocapsules) significantly increased the concentrations of indomethacin in the cornea and aqueous humor of rabbit eyes. The chitosan-coated formulation doubled the ocular bioavailability of indomethacin over the uncoated particles, whereas the PLL coating was ineffective. The authors concluded that the specific nature of chitosan was responsible for the enhanced indomethacin uptake and not the positive surface charge. Both the PLL- and chitosan-coated nanocapsules displayed good ocular tolerance (63).

A recent approach to ocular inserts was presented by Chetoni et al. (64) in a study of cylindrical devices for oxytetracycline, made from mixtures of silicone clastomer and grafted on the surface of the inserts with an interpenetrating mucoadhesive polymeric network of polyacrylic acid or polymethacrylic acid. The inserts were tested for drug release and retention at rabbit eyes. It was shown that some of the inserts are able to maintain prolonged oxytetracycline concentrations in the lacrimal fluid for 36 h.

Vaginal Route

The vaginal route is considered to be suitable for the local application and absorption of therapeutics like estrogens for hormone replacement therapy or contraception. Systemic absorption of peptide drugs such as LHRH agonists and calcitonin can also be achieved (65).

The vagina offers a substantial area for drug absorption because numerous folds in the epithelium increase the total surface area. A rich vascular network surrounds the vagina whereas the vaginal epithelium is covered by a film of moisture consisting mainly of cervical mucus and fluid secreted from the vaginal wall.

Conventional vaginal delivery systems include tablets, foam gels, suspensions, and pessaries. Mucoadhesive gel formulations based on polycarbophil have been reported to remain 3–4 days at the vaginal tissue, providing an excellent vehicle for the delivery of progesterone and nonoxynol-9 (66).

The benzyl ester of hyaluronic acid (HYAFF 11) is a highly mucoadhesive polymer which can be processed into microspheres. Such microspheres containing salmon calcitonin were intravaginally administered to rats as a dosage form for the prevention of ovariectomy osteopenia (65). In recent studies, HYAFF 11–salmon calcitonin microspheres were formulated as single-dose pessaries, resulting in sustained plasma concentrations of calcitonin (67).

Gastrointestinal Route

The peroral route represents the most convenient route of drug administration, being characterized by high patient compliance. The mucosal epithelium along the gastrointestinal tract varies. In the stomach the surface epithelium consists of a single layer of columnar cells whose apical membrane is covered by a conspicuous glycocalyx. A thick layer of mucus covers the surface to protect against aggressive luminal content. This site of the tract is of minor interest for drug delivery since the low pH and the presence of proteolytic enzymes make the stomach a rather hostile environment. However, there are examples of dosage forms specially designed to be retained in the stomach such as some gastroretentive systems consisting of mucoadhesive hydrogels (68). Akiyama et al. (69) evaluated microspheres for prolonged residence time in the gastrointestinal tract of rats. They prepared two types of polyglycerol fatty acid ester (PGEF)-based microspheres, Carbopol 934P-coated microspheres, and Carbopol 934P-dispersion microspheres. Significantly longer residence times were observed after administration of the dispersion-microspheres than with the coated ones. Additionally, it was shown that the microspheres were retained in the stomach of the animals.

The small intestine is characterized by an enormous surface area available for the absorption of nutrients and drugs. This large area is formed by crypts and villi. The intestinal epithelium consists of a single layer of three types of columnar cells: enterocytes, goblet cells, and enteroendocrine cells. The enterocytes are linked to each other by tight junctions and desmosomes. The goblet cells are mucin-producing unicellular glands intercalated between the enterocytes. The enteroendocrine cells are scattered between the enterocytes and goblet cells and release hormones that can modify the local environment or influence the intestinal motility. At the terminal ileum, the Peyer's patches, a particular specialization of the gut-immune system, are located. This domain contains the M cells, which are specialized in endocytosis and processing luminal antigens. The large intestine (colon) has the same cell populations as the small intestine, and its main function is the absorption of water and electrolytes. The role of mucus in the intestine is to facilitate the passage of food along the intestinal tract and to protect the gut from bacterial infections (70).

In the past decade several difficulties have been encountered in the design of successful mucoadhesive delivery systems for peroral applications. The reasons may be due to shortcomings of the mucoadhesive properties of the polymers or to the peculiar physiological limits of the digestive tract, soluble mucins, and shed-off mucus, food, or other contents of the intestinal lumen which would inactivate the mucoadhesive properties of the delivery system before having reached the absorbing membrane. Furthermore, the adhesion of the delivery system can last as long as the gel-state mucus itself remains attached to the intestinal mucosal tissue. Mucus turnover is continuously removing the mucus gel layer attached to the epithelium by a steady-state process (71).

The failure in increasing residence time of mucoadhesive systems in the human intestinal tract has led scientists to the evaluation of multifunctional mucoadhesive polymers. Research in the area of mucoadhesive drug delivery systems has shed light on other properties of some of the mucoadhesive polymers. One important class of mucoadhesive polymers, poly(acrylic acid) derivatives, has been identified as potent inhibitors of proteolytic enzymes (72–74). The interaction between various types of mucoadhesive polymers, and epithelial cells has a direct influence on the permeability of mucosal epithelia by means of changing the gating properties of the tight junctions. More than being only adhesives, some mucoadhesive polymers can therefore be considered as a novel class of "multifunctional macromolecules" with a number of desirable properties for their use as delivery adjuvants (72, 75).

Lueßen et al. (73, 74) evaluated the mucoadhesive polyacrylates, polycarbophil and Carbopol 934P, for their potency to inhibit intestinal proteases. These polymers are able to inhibit the activities of trypsin, α-chymotrypsin, and carboxypeptidase A and B as well as of cytosolic leucine aminopeptidase. Carbopol 934P was found to be more efficient in reducing proteolytic activity than polycarbophil (74). The pronounced binding properties of polycarbophil and Carbopol 934P for bivalent cations, such as zinc and calcium, were demonstrated to be a major reason for the observed inhibitory effect. These polymers have been shown to remove Ca^{2+} and Zn^{2+}, respectively, from the enzyme structures, thereby inhibiting their activities. Carboxypeptidase A and α-chymotrypsin activities were observed to be reversible upon the addition of Zn^{2+} and Ca^{2+} ions, respectively. Therefore, it was concluded that polyacrylates are promising excipients to protect peptide drugs from intestinal degradation. In vitro studies, using the Caco-2 cell intestinal epithelium model, showed that Carbopol 934P was able to substantially increase the transport of a macromolecular paracellular fluorescent marker (dextran) and the peptide drug 9-desglycinamide, 8-L-arginine vasopressin (76).

Carbopol 934P and chitosan gels were also tested in vivo for their ability to increase the absorption of the peptide analog buserelin when administered intraduodenally in rats (77). Both polymers increased the absorption of the peptide significantly, probably due to both permeation-enhancing and enzyme-inhibition properties; mucoadhesion played a secondary role. Chitosan was found to remarkably increase the peroral bioavailability of the peptide in comparison to Carbopol 934P (77), indicative of a more specific effect of chitosan with the tight junctions, than previously suggested by Artursson et al. (78).

Chitosan and chitosan salts, however, lack the advantage of good solubility at neutral pH values. They aggregate in solutions at pH values above 6.5, and recent studies have shown that only protonated chitosan (i.e., in its uncoiled configuration) can trigger the opening of the tight junctions, thereby facilitating the paracellular transport of hydrophilic compounds (79). This property implies that chitosan can be effective as an absorption enhancer only in a limited area of the intestinal lumen where the pH values are close to its pK_a. For this reason, chitosan and its salts may not be suitable carriers for targeted peptide drug delivery to specific sites of the intestine, for instance, the jejunum or ileum. To overcome this problem the chitosan derivative N,N,N-trimethylchitosan chloride (TMC) has been synthesized and characterized (80). This quaternized chitosan shows higher aqueous solubility than chitosan in a much broader pH range. Chitosan HCl and TMCs of different degrees of trimethylation were tested for enhancing the permeability of the radiolabelled marker ^{14}C-mannitol in Caco-2 intestinal epithelia at neutral pH values (for instance, pH 7.2). Chitosan HCl failed to increase the permeation of these monolayers and so did TMC with a degree of trimethylation of 12.8%. However, TMC with a degree of trimethylation of 60% significantly increased the permeability of the Caco-2 intestinal monolayers, indicating that a threshold value at the charge density of the polymer is necessary to trigger the opening of the tight junctions (81). Because of the absence of significant cyto- and ciliotoxicity, TMC polymers (particularly with a high degree of trimethylation) are expected to be safe absorption enhancers for improved transmucosal delivery of peptide drugs (82).

In recent studies, both in vitro (Caco-2 cells) and in vivo in rats, TMC with a degree of trimethylation of 60% was proven to be an excellent intestinal absorption enhancer of the peptide drugs buserelin and octreotide. The observed absolute bioavailability values were 13 and 16% for buserelin and octreotide, respectively (83)

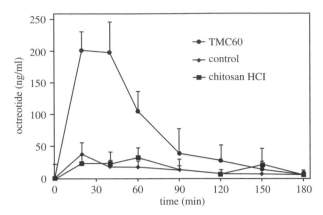

Fig. 5 Intestinal absorption of octreotide acetate in rats using mucoadhesive polymers. (From Thanou et al., unpublished data.)

(unpublished data; Fig. 5). Permeation-enhancing effects were more responsible for these increased bioavailabilities, rather than the mucoadhesive properties of the TMC polymers. Nevertheless, mucoadhesion is a prerequisite for these polymers in order to further act as absorption enhancers.

Mucus also appears to be a barrier to the permeation enhancing effect of polymeric or monomeric absorption enhancers. In the aforementioned TMC studies, the enhancement effect (enhancement ratio = permeation rate of the drug in the presence of polymer vs. permeation rate of the drug alone) was higher in vitro (Caco-2 cells; no mucus secretion) than the absorption enhancement in vivo. Meaney and O'Driscoll (84) studied the effect of mucus on the permeation properties of a micellar system consisting of sodium taurocholate in a coculture of Caco-2 and Ht29GlucH (mucin-secreting) cells. They found that the effect of bile salts on the permeation of hydrophilic paracellular markers was increased in the cocultures that were pretreated with the mucolytic compound N-acetylcysteine.

Bernkop-Schnürch (85) prepared a series of conjugates of protease inhibitors (pepstatin, Bowman-Birk, chymostatin, elastatinal, antipain bacitracin) and/or EDTA to three different types of polymers (carboxymethyl cellulose, polyacrylic acid, and chitosan). In addition to their mucoadhesive properties, most of these conjugates exhibited enzyme-inhibitory properties. Furthermore, the toxicity of these protease inhibitors was reduced by being covalently bound to the polymers. Chitosan–EDTA conjugates have proven to be potent inhibitors of the zinc-containing proteases as well as to be strong mucoadhesives (86).

In order to design highly mucoadhesive platforms for peroral drug delivery, Bernkop-Schnürch et al. (87) proposed thiol groups-bearing polycarbophil modifications, based on the mucolytic activity of thiols caused by disulfide exchange reactions between mucin glycoproteins and the mucolytic agent. Polycarbophil–cysteine conjugates appeared to exhibit superior mucoadhesiveness compared to polycarbophil itself, due to improved cohesion and rapid hydration of the gels. However, again mucus turnover is still the limiting factor of adhesion to the cell surfaces.

All the aforementioned polymers have been evaluated mainly for application in the intestine. Finally, the last part of the gastrointestinal tract, the rectum, should also be mentioned as a suitable site for delivery and fast absorption of therapeutics. Kim et al. (88) developed an in situ gelling and mucoadhesive acetaminophen liquid suppository prepared with poloxamers and sodium alginate. It was found that this particular formulation of acetaminophen in humans resulted in shorter T_{max} and higher maximum plasma concentrations of drug (C_{max}) than the conventional acetaminophen suppositories.

Suppositories are the preferable dosage form for patients that experience nausea. Yahagi et al. (89) evaluated a mucoadhesive suppository consisting of Witepsol H-15 and 2% Carbopol 934P for rectal delivery and absorption of the anti-emetic drug rumosclron hydrochloride (serotonin antagonist) in rabbits. These suppositories increased the $AUC_{(0-24h)}$ 2.5 times and prolonged the residence time compared to supposiories without mucoadhesive polymer. The anti-emetic effect of the formulation was tested in ferrets, and it was found that the Carbopol 934P-containing suppositories had the same effect as intravenous administration. This formulation was suggested as a once-a-day dosage form for the treatment of chemotherapy-induced nausea.

TRENDS AND PERSPECTIVES

In this article a number of polymer modifications have been described as novel drug delivery platforms, being second-generation mucoadhesive hydrogels. These polymers, both as safe absorption enhancers (75) or as improved mucoadhesive hydrogels, are the most recent developments in mucoadhesive delivery platforms for intestinal absorption of drugs.

Another trend observed during the past decade was the coating of liposomes with mucoadhesive polymers. Liposomes are coated with chitosan, long-chain PVA, and polyacrylates bearing a cholesteryl group (90). Chitosan-coated liposomes showed superior adhesion properties to rat intestine in vitro than the other polymer-coated liposomes. In vivo, chitosan-coated liposomes

containing insulin substantially reduced blood glucose levels after oral administration in rats, which were sustained up to 12 h after administration (90).

Another type of novel mucoadhesive formulations was suggested to be submicron emulsions (o/w), bearing droplets coated with Carbopol 940. These formulations have been shown to generate a 12-fold enhancement in rats in the oral bioavailability of the antidiuretic peptide drug desmopressin (91).

Specific adhesion approaches also show promise. The more specific bindings of plant lectins, mussel glue protein, and K99-fimbriae have been suggested as an alternative to the classical nonspecific mucoadhesive hydrogels. Tomato lectins were found to bind specifically onto both isolated porcine enterocytes and Caco-2 cells with the same affinity (92). However, lectin binding was inhibited in the presence of crude porcine gastric mucin, indicative of a marked cross-reactivity. Irache et al. (93) investigated three different plant lectins conjugated to latex, tomato lectin, *Asparagus pea* lectin, and *Mycoplasma gallisepticum* lectin. The extent of interactions of these three lectin–latex conjugates decreased from the duodenum to the ileum, when tested on rat intestinal mucosa without Peyer's patches. However, when mucosa containing Peyer's patches was used, a substantial increase in the interaction of the conjugates with the mucosa was found, which was more pronounced for the mycoplasma and asparagus lectins than for the tomato lectin (93).

A natural example of mucoadhesion can be the colonization of the small intestine by *Escherichia coli* strains mediated by cell-surface antigens called fimbriae (94). Fimbriae are long, thread-like protein polymers found on the surface of many bacterial strains. They enable bacteria to adhere to the brush border of epithelial cells. A special fimbriae antigen, K99-fimbriae, has been isolated from *E. coli* and bound to polyacrylic acid. The conjugate was tested by a hemagglutination assay for its ability to bind to equine erythrocytes, which have the same K-99-receptor structures as gastrointestinal epithelial cells. A 10-times stronger retention of erythrocytes was observed for the matrix-bound K-99 antigen than for the matrix-bound ovalbumin (94).

Mussel adhesive protein (MAP) is a 130-kDa protein produced by the blue mussel (*Mytilus edulis*), which provides strong adhesion to submerged surfaces. MAP films were prepared by drying and stored under nitrogen atmosphere. These films showed twice the adhesion strength of polycarbophil when tested on porcine duodenum in vitro (95).

All these examples of the applications of mucoadhesive polymers demonstrate that the use of mucoadhesive hydrogels is a powerful strategy to improve the absorption of therapeutics across mucosal epithelia. With respect to buccal, nasal, or ocular delivery of drugs, the use of such carriers has already been successfully established. However, the application of the mucoadhesive polymers in the gastrointestinal tract is still waiting for a breakthrough. Specific-binding principles may be applied in the near future to design a third generation of mucoadhesive polymers for application in the gastrointestinal tract.

REFERENCES

1. Peppas, N.A.; Buri, P. Surface, Interfacial and Molecular Aspects of Polymer Bioadhesion on Soft Tissue. J. Controlled Release **1985**, *2*, 257–275.
2. Smart, J.D.; Kellaway, I.W.; Worthington, H.E.C. An In Vitro Investigation of Mucosa Adhesive Materials for Use in Controlled Drug Delivery. J. Pharm. Pharmacol. **1984**, *36*, 295–299.
3. Park, K.; Robinson, J.R. Bioadhesive Polymers as Platforms for Oral Controlled Drug Delivery: Method to Study Bioadhesion. Int. J. Pharm. **1984**, *19*, 107–127.
4. Harding, S.E.; Davis, S.S.; Deacon, M.P.; Fiebrig, I. Biopolymer Mucoadhesives. Biotech. Gen. Engin. **1999**, *16*, 41–86.
5. Duchêne, D.; Ponchel, G. Bioadhesion of Solid Oral Dosage Forms, Why and How? Eur. J. Pharm. Biopharm. **1997**, *44*, 15–23.
6. Ponchel, G.; Irache, J.M. Specific and Non-Specific Bioadhesive Particulate Systems for Oral Delivery to the Gastrointestinal Tract. Adv. Drug Del. Rev. **1998**, *34*, 191–219.
7. Chen, H.M.; Langer, R. Oral Particulate Delivery: Status and Future Trends. Adv. Drug Del. Rev. **1998**, *34*, 339–350.
8. Hoogstraate, J.A.J.; Wertz, P.W. Drug Delivery via the Buccal Mucosa. Pharm. Sci. Tech. Today **1998**, *1*, 309–316.
9. Ahuja, A.; Khar, R.K.; Ali, J. Mucoadhesive Drug Delivery Systems. Drug Dev. Ind. Pharm. **1997**, *23*, 489–515.
10. Campbell, B.J. Biochemical and Functional Aspects of Mucus and Mucin-type Glycoproteins. *Bioadhesive Drug Delivery Systems*; Mathiowitz, E., Chickering, D.E., III, Lehr, C.-M., Eds.; Marcel Dekker, Inc.: New York, 1999; 85–103.
11. Leung, S.H.; Robinson, J.R. The Contribution of Anionic Polymer Structural Features to Mucoadhesion. J. Controlled Release **1988**, *5*, 223–231.
12. MacAdam, A. The Effect of Gastrointestinal Mucus on Drug Absorption. Adv. Drug Del. Rev. **1993**, *11*, 201–220.
13. Rubinstein, A.; Tirosh, B. Mucus Gel Thickness and Turnover in the Gastrointestinal Tract of the Rat: Response to Cholinergic Stimulus and Implication for Mucoadhesion. Pharm. Res. **1994**, *11*, 794–799.
14. Lehr, C.-M.; Poelma, F.G.J.; Junginger, H.E.; Tukker, J.J. An Estimate of Turnover Time of Intestinal Mucus Gel Layer in the Rat In Situ Loop. Int. J. Pharm. **1991**, *70*, 235–240.
15. Baier, R.E.; Shafrin, E.G.; Zisman, W.A. Adhesion: Mechanisms that Assist or Impede It. Science **1968**, *162*, 1360–1368.
16. Ponchel, G.; Touchard, D.; Duchêne, D.; Peppas, N.A. Bioadhesive Analysis of Controlled-Release Systems. I. Fracture and Interpenetration Analysis in Poly(acrylic acid) Containing Systems. J. Controlled Release **1987**, *5*, 129–141.
17. Duchêne, D.; Ponchel, G. Principle and Investigation of the Bioadhesion Mechanism of Solid Dosage Forms. Biomaterials **1991**, *13*, 709–714.
18. Peppas, N.A.; Ponchel, G.; Duchêne, D. Bioadhesive Analysis of Controlled-Release Systems. II. Time-Dependent Bioadhesive Stress in Poly(acrylic acid)-Containing Systems. J. Controlled Release **1987**, *5*, 143–150.
19. Lehr, C.-M.; Bouwstra, J.A.; Schacht, E.H.; Junginger, H.E. In Vitro Evaluation of Mucoadhesive Properties of Chitosan and Some Other Natural Polymers. Int. J. Pharm. **1992**, *78*, 43–48.
20. Mikos, A.; Peppas, N.A. Bioadhesive Analysis of Controlled-Release Systems. IV. An Experimental Method for Testing the Adhesion of Microparticles with Mucus. J. Controlled Release **1990**, *12*, 31–37.
21. Lehr, C.-M.; Bouwstra, J.A.; Tukker, J.J.; Junginger, H.E. Intestinal Transit of Bioadhesive Microspheres in an In Situ Loop in the Rat—A Comparative Study with Copolymers and Blends based on Poly(acrylic acid). J. Controlled Release **1990**, *13*, 51–62.
22. Chickering, D.E., III; Mathiowitz, E. Bioadhesive Microspheres. I. A Novel Electrobalance-Based Method to Study Adhesive Interactions between Individual Microspheres and Intestinal Mucosa. J. Controlled Release **1995**, *34*, 251–262.
23. Chickering, D.E., III; Jacob, J.S.; Mathiowitz, E. Bioadhesive Microspheres. 2. Characterization and Evaluation of Bioadhesion Involving Hard, Bioerodible Polymers and Soft Tissue. Reactive Polymers **1995**, *25*, 189–206.
24. Park, K. A New Approach to Study Mucoadhesion: Colloidal Gold Staining. Int. J. Pharm. **1989**, *53*, 209–217.
25. Fiebrig, I.; Várum, K.M.; Harding, S.E.; Davis, S.S.; Stoke, B.T. Colloidal Gold and Colloidal Gold Labelled Wheat Germ Agglutinin as Molecular Probes for Identification in Mucin/Chitosan Complexes. Carbohydr. Polym. **1997**, *33*, 91–99.
26. Mortazavi, S.A.; Carpenter, B.G.; Smart, J.D. An Investigation of the Rheological Behavior of the Mucoadhesive/Mucosal Interface. Int. J. Pharm. **1992**, *83*, 221–225.
27. Mortazavi, S.A.; Smart, J.D. An Investigation into the Role of Water Movement and Mucus Gel Dehydration in Mucoadhesion. J. Controlled Release **1993**, *25*, 197–203.
28. Madsen, F.; Eberth, K.; Smart, J.D. A Rheological Assessment of the Nature of Interactions between Mucoadhesive Polymers and a Homogenised Mucus Gel. Biomaterials **1998**, *19*, 1083–1092.
29. Hägerström, H.; Paulsson, M.; Edsman, K. Evaluation of Mucoadhesion for Two Polyelectrolyte Gels in Simulated Physiological Conditions Using a Rheological Method. Eur. J. Pharm. Biopharm. **2000**, *9*, 301–309.
30. Rossi, S.; Bonferoni, M.C.; Lippoli, G.; Bertoni, M.; Ferrari, F.; Caramella, C.; Conte, U. Influence of Mucin Type on Polymer–Mucin Rheological Interactions. Biomaterials **1995**, *16*, 1073–1079.

31. Rossi, S.; Bonferoni, M.C.; Caramella, C.; Ironi, L.; Tentoni, S. Model-Based Interpretation of Creep Profiles for the Assessment of Polymer–Mucin Interaction. Pharm. Res. **1999**, *16*, 1456–1463.

32. Caramella, C.M.; Rossi, S.; Bonferoni, M.C. A Rheological Approach to Explain the Mucoadhesive Behavior of Polymer Hydrogels. *Bioadhesive Drug Delivery Systems*; Mathiowitz, E., Chickering, D.E., III, Lehr, C.-M., Eds.; Marcel Dekker, Inc.: New York, 1999; 25–65.

33. Jabbari, E.; Wisniewski, N.; Peppas, N.A. Evidence of Mucoadhesion by Chain Interpenetration at a Poly(acrylic acid)/Mucin Interface Using ATR-FTIR Spectroscopy. J. Controlled Release **1993**, *26*, 99–108.

34. Hertzog, B.A.; Mathiowitz, E. Novel Magnetic Technique to Measure Bioadhesion. *Bioadhesive Drug Delivery Systems*; Mathiowitz, E., Chickering, D.E., III, Lehr, C.-M., Eds.; Marcel Dekker, Inc.: New York, 1999; 147–173.

35. He, P.; Davis, S.S.; Illum, L. In Vitro Evaluation of the Mucoadhesive Properties of Chitosan Microspheres. Int. J. Pharm. **1998**, *166*, 75–88.

36. Fiebrig, I.; Harding, S.E.; Rowe, A.J.; Hyman, S.C.; Davis, S.S. Transmission Electron Microscopy Studies on Pig Gastric Mucin and its Interactions with Chitosan. Carbohydr. Polym. **1995**, *28*, 239–244.

37. Lehr, C.-M.; Bouwstra, J.A.; Spies, F.; Onderwater, J.; Van het Noordeinde, J.; Vermeÿ-Keers, C.; Van Munsteren, C.J.; Junginger, H.E. Visualization Studies of the Mucoadhesive Interface. J. Controlled Release **1992**, *18*, 249–260.

38. Sahlin, J.J.; Peppas, N.A. Enhanced Hydrogel Adhesion by Polymer Interdiffusion: Use of Linear Poly(ethylene glycol) as an Adhesion Promoter. J. Biomater. Sci. Polym. Ed. **1997**, *8*, 421–436.

39. Zur Mühlen, E.; Koschinski, P.; Gehring, S.; Ros, R.; Tiefenauer, L.; Haltner, E.; Lehr, C.-M.; Hartmann, U.; Schwesinger, F.; Plückthun, A. Force Microscopy of Cells to Measure Bioadhesion. *Bioadhesive Drug Delivery Systems*; Mathiowitz, E., Chickering, D.E., III, Lehr, C.-M., Eds.; Marcel Dekker, Inc.: New York, 1999; 197–221.

40. Squier, C.A.; Wertz, P.W. Structure and Function of the Oral Mucosa and Implications for Drug Delivery. *Oral Mucosal Drug Delivery*; Rathbone, M.J., Ed.; Marcel Dekker, Inc.: New York, 1996; 1–26.

41. Machida, Y.; Nagai, T. Bioadhesive Preparations as Topical Dosage Forms. *Bioadhesive Drug Delivery Systems*; Mathiowitz, E., Chickering, D.E., III, Lehr, C.-M., Eds.; Marcel Dekker, Inc.: New York, 1999; 641–657.

42. Bouckaert, S.; Lefebvre, R.; Remon, J.-P. In Vitro/In Vivo Correlation of the Bioadhesive Properties of a Buccal Bioadhesive Miconasole Tablet. Pharm. Res. **1993**, *10*, 853–856.

43. Lee, Y.L.; Chien, Y.W. Oral Mucosa Controlled Delivery of LHRH by Bilayer Mucoadhesive Polymer Systems. J. Controlled Release **1995**, *37*, 251–261.

44. Nair, M.K.; Chien, Y.W. Development of Anticandidal Delivery Systems. 2. Mucoadhesive Devices for Prolonged Drug Delivery in the Oral Cavity. Drug Dev. Ind. Pharm. **1996**, *22*, 243–253.

45. Remunan-Lopez, C.; Portero, A.; VilaJato, J.L.; Alonso, M.J. Design and Evaluation of Chitosan/Ethylcellulose Mucoadhesive Bilayered Devices for Buccal Drug Delivery. J. Controlled Release **1998**, *55*, 143–152.

46. Needleman, I.G.; Martin, G.P.; Smales, F.C. Characterisation of Bioadhesives for Periodontal and Oral Mucosal Drug Delivery. J. Clin. Periodontol. **1998**, *25*, 74–82.

47. Martin, E.; Schipper, N.G.M.; Verhoef, J.C.; Merkus, F.W.H.M. Nasal Mucociliary Clearance as a Factor in Nasal Drug Delivery. Adv. Drug Del. Rev. **1998**, *29*, 13–38.

48. Zhou, M.P.; Donovan, M.D. Intranasal Mucociliary Clearance of Putative Bioadhesive Polymer Gels. Int. J. Pharm. **1996**, *135*, 115–125.

49. Illum, L.; Farraj, N.F.; Davis, S.S. Chitosan as a Novel Nasal Delivery System for Peptide Drugs. Pharm. Res. **1994**, *11*, 1186–1189.

50. Oechslein, C.R.; Fricker, G.; Kissel, T. Nasal Delivery of Octreotide: Absorption Enhancement by Particulate Carrier Systems. Int. J. Pharm. **1996**, *139*, 25–32.

51. Nakamura, F.; Ohta, R.; Machida, Y.; Nagai, T. In Vitro and In Vivo Nasal Mucoadhesion of Some Water-Soluble Polymers. Int. J. Pharm. **1996**, *134*, 173–181.

52. Illum, L.; Jorgensen, H.; Bisgaard, H.; Krogsgaard, O.; Rossing, N. Bioadhesive Microspheres as a Potential Nasal Drug Delivery System. Int. J. Pharm. **1987**, *39*, 189–199.

53. Illum, L. Bioadhesive Formulations for Nasal Peptide Delivery. *Bioadhesive Drug Delivery Systems*; Mathiowitz, E., Chickering, D.E., III, Lehr, C.-M., Eds.; Marcel Dekker, Inc.: New York, 1999; 507–539.

54. Nakamura, K.; Maltani, Y.; Lowman, A.M.; Takayama, K.; Peppas, N.A.; Nagal, T. Uptake and Release of Budesonide from Mucoadhesive, pH-Sensitive Copolymers and their Application to Nasal Delivery. J. Controlled Release **1999**, *61*, 329–335.

55. Soane, R.J.; Frier, M.; Perkins, A.C.; Jones, N.S.; Davis, S.S.; Illum, L. Evaluation of the Clearance Characteristics of Bioadhesive Systems in Humans. Int. J. Pharm. **1999**, *178*, 55–65.

56. Saettone, M.F.; Burgalassi, S.; Chetoni, P. Ocular Bioadhesive Drug Delivery Systems. *Bioadhesive Drug Delivery Systems*; Mathiowitz, E., Chickering, D.E., III, Lehr, C.-M., Eds.; Marcel Dekker, Inc.: New York, 1999; 601–640.

57. Joshi, A. Microparticulates for Ophthalmic Drug Delivery. J. Ocul. Pharmacol. **1994**, *10*, 29–45.

58. Hui, H.W.; Robinson, J.R. Ocular Delivery of Progesterone Using a Bioadhesive Polymer. Int. J. Pharm. **1985**, *26*, 203–213.

59. Davies, N.M.; Farr, S.J.; Hadgraft, J.; Kellaway, I.W. Evaluation of Mucoadhesive Polymers in Ocular Drug Delivery. J. Viscous Solutions. Pharm. Res. **1991**, *8*, 1039–1043.

60. Davies, N.M.; Farr, S.J.; Hadgraft, J.; Kellaway, I.W. Evaluation of Mucoadhesive Polymers in Ocular Drug Delivery. II. Polymer-Coated Vesicles. Pharm. Res. **1992**, *9*, 1137–1144.

61. Lehr, C.-M.; Lee, Y.H.; Lee, V.H. Improved Ocular Penetration of Gentamicin by Mucoadhesive Polymer Polycarbophil in the Pigmented Rabbit. Invest. Ophthalmol. Vis. Sci. **1994**, *35*, 2809–2814.

62. Saettone, M.F.; Monti, D.; Torracca, M.T.; Chetoni, P. Mucoadhesive Ophthalmic Vehicles: Evaluation of Polymeric Low-Viscosity Formulations. J. Ocul. Pharmacol. **1994**, *10*, 83–92.

63. Calvo, P.; VilaJato, J.L.; Alonso, M.J. Evaluation of Cationic Polymer-Coated Nanocapsules as Ocular Drug Carriers. Int. J. Pharm. **1997**, *153*, 41–50.

64. Chetoni, P.; Di-Colo, G.; Grandi, M.; Morelli, M.; Sacttone, M.F.; Darougar, S. Silicone Rubber/Hydrogel Composite Ophthalmic Inserts: Preparation and Preliminary In Vitro/In Vivo Evaluation. Eur. J. Pharm. Biopharm. **1998**, *46*, 125–132.

65. Bonucci, E.; Ballanti, P.; Ramires, P.A.; Richardson, J.L.; Benedetti, L.M. Prevention of Ovariectomy Osteopenia in Rats after Vaginal Administration of Hyaff 11 Microspheres Containing Salmon Calcitonin. Calcif. Tissue Int. **1995**, *56*, 274–279.

66. Robinson, J.R.; Bologna, W.J. Vaginal and Reproductive-System Treatments Using Bioadhesive Polymer. J. Controlled Release **1994**, *28*, 87–94.

67. Richardson, J.L.; Armstrong, T.I. Vaginal Delivery of Calcitonin by Hyaluronic Acid Formulations. *Bioadhesive Drug Delivery Systems*; Mathiowitz, E., Chickering, D.E., III, Lehr, C.-M., Eds.; Marcel Dekker, Inc.: New York, 1999; 563–599.

68. Hwang, S.J.; Park, H.; Park, K. Gastric Retentive Drug-Delivery Systems. Crit. Rev. Ther. Drug Carr. Syst. **1998**, *15*, 243–284.

69. Akiyama, Y.; Nagahara, N.; Kashihara, T.; Hirai, S.; Toguchi, H. In Vitro and In Vivo Evaluation of Mucoadhesive Microspheres Prepared for the Gastrointestinal Tract Using Polyglycerol Esters of Fatty Acids and a Poly(acrylic acid) Derivative. Pharm. Res. **1995**, *12*, 397–405.

70. Schumacher, U.; Schumacher, D. Functional Histology of Epithelia Relevant for Drug Delivery. *Bioadhesive Drug Delivery Systems*; Mathiowitz, E., Chickering, D.E., III, Lehr, C.-M., Eds.; Marcel Dekker, Inc.: New York, 1999; 67–83.

71. Lehr, C.-M. From Sticky Stuff to Sweet Receptors—Achievements, Limits and Novel Approaches to Bioadhesion. Eur. J. Drug Metab. Pharmacokinet. **1996**, *21*, 139–148.

72. Lehr, C.-M. Bioadhesion technologies for the Delivery of Peptide and Protein Drugs to the Gastrointestinal Tract. Crit. Rev. Ther. Drug Carr. Syst. **1994**, *11*, 119–160.

73. Lueßen, H.L.; De Leeuw, B.J.; Pérard, D.; Lehr, C.-M.; De Boer, A.G.; Verhoef, J.C.; Junginger, H.E. Mucoadhesive Polymers in Peroral Peptide Drug Delivery. 1. Influence of Mucoadhesive Excipients on the Proteolytic Activity of Intestinal Enzymes. Eur. J. Pharm. Sci. **1996**, *4*, 117–128.

74. Lueßen, H.L.; Verhoef, J.C.; Borchard, G.; Lehr, C.-M.; De Boer, A.G.; Junginger, H.E. Mucoadhesive Polymers in Peroral Peptide Drug Delivery. II. Carbomer and Polycarbophil are Potent Inhibitors of the Intestinal Proteolytic Enzyme Trypsin. Pharm. Res. **1995**, *12*, 1293–1298.

75. Junginger, H.E.; Verhoef, J.C. Macromolecules as Safe Penetration Enhancers for Hydrophilic Drugs—A Fiction? Pharm. Sci. Tech. Today **1998**, *1*, 370–376.

76. Lueßen, H.L.; Rentel, C.O.; Kotze, A.F.; Lehr, C.-M.; De Boer, A.G.; Verhoef, J.C.; Junginger, H.E. Mucoadhesive Polymers in Peroral Peptide Drug Delivery. 4. Polycarbophil and Chitosan are Potent Enhancers of Peptide Transport across Intestinal Mucosae In Vitro. J. Controlled Release **1997**, *45*, 15–23.

77. Lueßen, H.L.; De Leeuw, B.J.; Langemeyer, M.W.; De Boer, A.G.; Verhoef, J.C.; Junginger, H.E. Mucoadhesive Polymers in Peroral Peptide Drug Delivery. VI. Carbomer and Chitosan Improve the Intestinal Absorption of the Peptide Drug Buserelin In Vivo. Pharm. Res. **1996**, *13*, 1668–1672.

78. Artursson, P.; Lindmark, T.; Davis, S.S.; Illum, L. Effect of Chitosan on the Permeability of Monolayers of Intestinal Epithelial Cells (Caco-2). Pharm. Res. **1994**, *11*, 1358–1361.

79. Kotzé, A.F.; Lueßen, H.L.; De Boer, A.G.; Verhoef, J.C.; Junginger, H.E. Chitosan for Enhanced Intestinal Permeability: Prospects for Derivatives Soluble in Neutral and Basic Environments. Eur. J. Pharm. Sci. **1999**, *7*, 145–151.

80. Sieval, A.B.; Thanou, M.; Kotzé, A.F.; Verhoef, J.C.; Brussee, J.; Junginger, H.E. Preparation and NMR Characterization of Highly Substituted *N*-Trimethylchitosan Chloride. Carbohydr. Polym. **1998**, *36*, 157–165.

81. Kotzé, A.F.; Thanou, M.M.; Lueßen, H.L.; De Boer, A.G.; Verhoef, J.C.; Junginger, H.E. Enhancement of Paracellular Drug Transport with Highly Quaternized *N*-trimethylchitosan Chloride in Neutral Environments: In Vitro Evaluation in Intestinal Epithelial Cells (Caco-2). J. Pharm. Sci. **1999**, *88*, 253–257.

82. Thanou, M.M.; Verhoef, J.C.; Romeijn, S.G.; Merkus, F.W.H.M.; Nagelkerke, J.F.; Junginger, H.E. Effects of *N*-trimethylchitosan Chloride, A Novel Absorption Enhancer, on Caco-2 Intestinal Epithelia and the Ciliary Beat Frequency of Chicken Embryo Trachea. Int. J. Pharm. **1999**, *185*, 73–82.

83. Thanou, M.; Florea, B.I.; Langermeÿer, M.W.E.; Verhoef, J.C.; Junginger, H.E. *N*-Trimethylated Chitosan Chloride (TMC) Improves the Intestinal Permeation of the Peptide Drug Buserelin In Vitro (Caco-2 Cells) and In Vivo (Rats). Pharm. Res. **2000**, *17*, 27–31.

84. Meaney, C.; O'Driscoll, C. Mucus as a Barrier to the Permeability of Hydrophilic and Lipophilic Compounds in the Absence and Presence of Sodium Taurocholate Micellar Systems Using Cell Culture Models. Eur. J. Pharm. Sci. **1999**, *8*, 167–175.

85. Bernkop-Schnürch, A. The Use of Inhibitory Agents to Overcome the Enzymatic Barrier to Perorally Administered Therapeutic Peptides and Proteins. J. Controlled Release **1998**, *52*, 1–16.

86. Bernkop-Schnürch, A.; Krajicek, M.E. Mucoadhesive Polymers as Platforms for Peroral Peptide Delivery and Absorption: Synthesis and Evaluation of Different Chitosan-EDTA Conjugates. J. Controlled Release **1998**, *50*, 215–223.

87. Bernkop-Schnürch, S.A.; Schwarz, V.; Steininger, S. Polymers with Thiol Groups: A New Generation of Mucoadhesive Polymers? Pharm. Res. **1999**, *16*, 876–881.

88. Kim, C.K.; Lee, S.W.; Choi, H.G.; Lee, M.K.; Gao, Z.G.; Kim, I.S.; Park, K.M. Trials of In Situ Gelling and

Mucoadhesive Acetaminophen Liquid Suppository in Human Subjects. Int. J. Pharm. **1998**, *174*, 201–207.

89. Yahagi, R.; Machida, Y.; Onishi, H. Mucoadhesive Suppositories of Ramosetron Hydrochloride Utilizing Carbopol. Int. J. Pharm. **2000**, *193*, 205–212.

90. Takeuchi, H.; Yamamoto, H.; Niwa, T.; Hino, T.; Kawashima, Y. Enteral Absorption of Insulin in Rats from Mucoadhesive Chitosan-Coated Liposomes. Pharm. Res. **1996**, *13*, 896–901.

91. Han, E.; Amselem, S.; Weisspapir, M.; Schwarz, J.; Yogev, A.; Zawoznik, E.; Friedman, D. Improved Oral Delivery of Desmopressin via a Novel Vehicle: Mucoadhesive Submicron Emulsion. Pharm. Res. **1996**, *13*, 1083–1087.

92. Lehr, C.-M.A.; Bouwstra, J.A.; Kok, W. Bioadhesion by Means of Specific Binding to Tomato Lectin. Pharm. Res. **1992**, *9*, 547–553.

93. Irache, J.M.; Durrer, C.; Duchêne, D.; Ponchel, G. Bioadhesion of Lectin–Latex Conjugates to Rat Intestinal Mucosa. Pharm. Res. **1996**, *13*, 1716–1719.

94. Bernkop-Schnürch, A.; Gabor, F.; Szostak, M.P.; Lubitz, W. An Adhesive Drug Delivery System based on K99-fimbriae. Eur. J. Pharm. Sci. **1995**, *3*, 293–299.

95. Schnurrer, J.; Lehr, C.-M. Mucoadhesive Properties of the Mussel Adhesive Protein. Int. J. Pharm. **1996**, *141*, 251–256.

NANOPARTICLES AS DRUG DELIVERY SYSTEMS

Elias Fattal
Christine Vauthier
University of Paris XI, Châtenay-Malabry, France

INTRODUCTION

Nanoparticles are small colloidal particles which are made of non biodegradable and biodegradable polymers. Their diameter is generally around 200 nm. One can distinguish two types of nanoparticles (Fig. 1): nanospheres, which are matrix systems; and nanocapsules, which are reservoir systems composed of a polymer membrane surrounding an oily or aqueous core. These systems were developed in the early 1970s. This approach was attractive because the methods of preparation of particles were simple and easy to scale-up. The particles formed were stable and easily freeze-dried. Due to these reasons, nanoparticles made of biodegradable polymers were developed for drug delivery. Indeed, nanoparticles were able to achieve with success tissue targeting of many drugs (antibiotics, cytostatics, peptides and proteins, nucleic acids, etc.). In addition, nanoparticles were able to protect drugs against chemical and enzymatic degradation and were also able to reduce side effects of some active drugs. This review focuses on the preparation and characterization methods of nanoparticles. The main applications of these systems are also described.

PREPARATION OF NANOPARTICLES

Polymer nanoparticles including nanospheres and nanocapsules (Fig. 1) can be prepared according to numerous methods that have been developed over the last 30 years. The development of these methods occurred in several steps. Historically, the first nanoparticles proposed as carriers for therapeutic applications were made of gelatin and cross-linked albumin (1, 2). Then, to avoid the use of proteins that may stimulate the immune system and to limit the toxicity of the cross-linking agents, nanoparticles made from synthetic polymers were developed. At first, the nanoparticles were made by emulsion polymerization of acrylamide and by dispersion polymerization of methyl-methacrylate (3, 4). These nanoparticles were proposed as adjuvants for vaccines. However, since they were made of nonbiodegradable polymers, these nanoparticles were

rapidly substituted by particles made of biodegradable synthetic polymers. Couvreur et al. (5) proposed to make nanoparticles by polymerization of monomers from the family of alkylcyanoacrylates already used in vivo as surgical glue. They succeeded in making nanoparticles by polymerization of the monomers in oil-in-water type emulsions prepared with an acidified aqueous phase. During the same period of time, Gurny et al. (6) proposed a method based on the use of another biodegradable polymer consisting of poly(lactic acid) used as surgical sutures in humans. In this method, nanoparticles were formed directly from the polymer. Based on these initial investigations, several groups improved and modified the original processes mainly by reducing the amount of surfactant and organic solvents. At that time, the methods developed were only able to produce nanospheres (Fig. 1A). A breakthrough in the development of nanoparticles occurred in 1986 with the development of methods allowing the preparation of nanocapsules corresponding to particles displaying a core-shell structure with a liquid core surrounded by a polymer shell (7–9) (Fig. 1B). From 1986, there was also an acceleration in the development of new methodologies for the preparation of all types of nanoparticles. The nanoprecipitation technique was proposed (10) as well as the first method of interfacial polymerization in inverse microemulsion (11). In the following years, the methods based on salting-out (12), emulsion–diffusion (13, 14), and double emulsion (15) were described. Finally, during the last decade, new approaches were considered to develop nanoparticles made from polysaccharides based on the gelation properties of these natural macromolecules (16). These nanoparticles were developed for peptides and nucleic acid delivery. Another goal was the development of surface modified nanoparticles to produce long circulating particles able to avoid the capture by the macrophages of the mononuclear phagocyte system after intravenous administration (17).

All the methods can be classified into two groups depending on whether the nanoparticles are formed at the same time than the polymer itself requiring a polymerization reaction or are directly obtained from a polymer. There are numerous valuable reviews on the subject (9, 18–21). The general principles of the methods leading

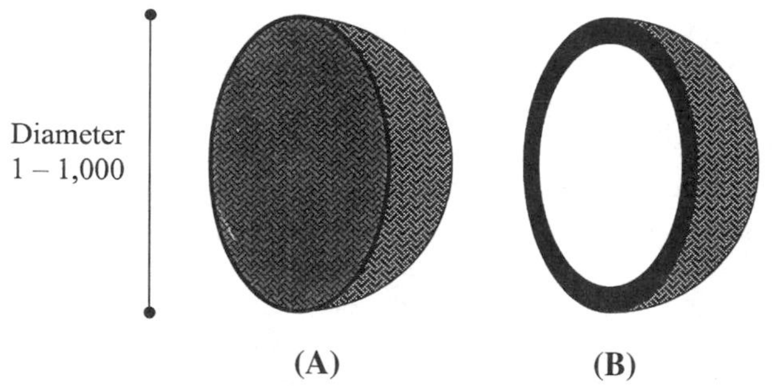

Diameter
1 – 1,000

(A)   **(B)**

Fig. 1 Schematic representation of a nanosphere (A) and of a nanocapsule (B). In nanospheres, the whole particle consists of a continuous polymer network. Nanocapsules present a core-shell structure with a liquid core surrounded by a polymer shell.

to nanoparticle preparation are described and details of the most representative over are given.

Preparation of Nanoparticles by Polymerization

Nanospheres are mostly prepared by emulsion polymerization whereas nanocapsules are obtained by interfacial polymerization performed in emulsion or in microemulsion. In emulsion polymerization, the monomer itself, if liquid, is dispersed under agitation in a continuous phase in which it is nonmiscible. The polymerization is usually initiated by the reaction of the initiators with the monomer molecules that are dissolved in the continuous phase of the emulsion. The polymerization continues by further addition of monomer molecules that diffuse toward the growing polymer chain through the continuous phase. The growing polymer chain remains soluble until it reaches a certain molecular weight for which it becomes insoluble.

Therefore, phase separation occurs leading to the nucleation of the polymer particles and the formation of the tyndall scattering effect. Further growth of the nucleated particles occurs according to a mechanism that depends on the stability conditions of the whole system. This includes capture of new growing polymer chains, fusion or collision between nucleated particles (22). Throughout the polymerization, the monomer input in the continuous phase of the emulsion takes place by diffusion from the monomer droplets, which play the role of monomer reservoirs. When the reaction is completed, the particles formed contains a large number of polymer chains (19, 22). Emulsion polymerization can be performed in emulsifier free systems and in both oil-in-water and water-in-oil emulsions.

The poly(alkylcyanoacrylate) nanospheres, widely used as drug carriers, are prepared by emulsion polymerization according to a method initially introduced by Couvreur et al. (5). The monomers (isobutylcyano-acrylate, isohexylcyanoacrylate, n-butylcyanoacrylate) are dispersed in a continuous acidified aqueous phase under magnetic agitation. The anionic polymerization of the alkylcyanoacrylate is rapidly and spontaneously initiated by the remaining OH^- ions of the acidified water and is completed within 3–4 h depending on the monomer type (Fig. 2). The preparation is performed at low pH (pH ~2.5) to slow down the anionic polymerization of the alkylcyanoacrylate, therefore allowing the polymer to arrange as colloidal particles. Dextran 70 or Pluronic® F68 are usually dissolved in the aqueous phase to ensure the stability of the polymer particles. The size of the nanospheres can be controlled by the amount of Pluronic® F68 from a diameter of 40–250 nm for

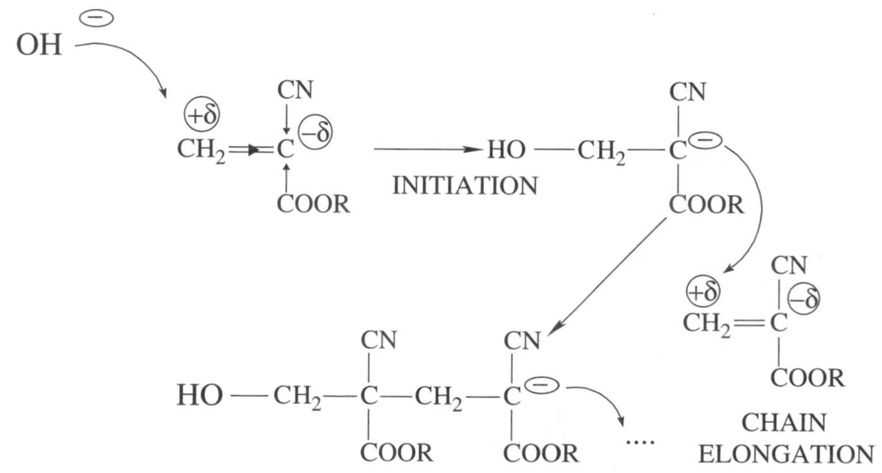

Fig. 2 Anionic polymerization of alkylcyanoacrylate initiated by the OH^- from the dissociation of the water molecule.

concentrations ranging from 3 to 0%, respectively (23). Numerous drugs have been associated with these nanospheres including doxorubicin, an anticancer agent, a peptide growth hormone, and several antibiotics. Antisense oligonucleotides were adsorbed on the nanosphere surface via the formation of an ion-pair with a cationic surfactant, cethyltrimethylammonium bromide. Finally, it should be mentioned that some drugs can lose their biological activity during the preparation of poly(alkylcyanoacrylate) nanospheres. Generally, these molecules contain chemical functions that are able to initiate the polymerization of alkylcyanoacrylates and be covalently attached to the polymer constituting the nanospheres. The mode of such an interaction has been elucidated for two molecules including phenylbutazone (an anti-inflammatory drug) and vidarabine (an antiviral molecule). In contrast, the side reactions can be used to achieve the covalent linkage of defined compounds to give specific properties to the nanospheres. This has been used with poly(ethylene glycol) that initiated the polymerization of isobutylcyanoacrylate to give poly(ethylene glycol)-coated nanospheres, therefore presenting a more hydrophilic surface than those prepared according to the original method (24).

Methylidene malonates are other monomers that give biodegradable polymers and polymerize according to a similar mechanism than alkylcyanoacrylates. These monomers were also used to make nanospheres by emulsion polymerization for drug delivery (25).

Nanocapsules can be prepared by interfacial polymerization of alkylcyanoacrylates (7). The main advantage of using these monomers is their very fast polymerization rate when they come into contact with water. Oil containing nanocapsules were prepared by the rapid dispersion of an ethanol phase including ethanol, the oil, the monomer, and the molecule to be encapsulated in an aqueous solution of surfactant. When the ethanol diffuses in the aqueous phase, tiny individual oil droplets form, and because of the contact with water at the oil/water interface, the polymerization of the alkylcyanoacrylate takes place on the droplet surface (26). This method is mainly adapted for the encapsulation of oily soluble substances (9). However, surprisingly, highly water-soluble molecules such as insulin could be entrapped in these nanocapsules with high encapsulation yields (up to 97%) (27).

Water containing nanocapsules were prepared by interfacial polymerization of the alkylcyanoacrylate in water-in-oil microemulsions. In these systems, water swollen micelles of surfactants of small and uniform sizes are dispersed in an organic phase. To prepare nanocapsules, the monomer is added to the oily phase of the already prepared microemulsion. The anionic polymerization of the alkylcyanoacrylate is initiated at the surface of the water swollen micelles and the polymer formed locally to make the shells of the nanocapsules. In the method first introduced by Gasco and Trotta (11), the microemulsions were prepared with hexane as the organic phase and Aerosol-OT as the surfactant. Both of these constituents are not compatible for the development of an acceptable drug carrier system. Thus, the method was recently adapted to microemulsions formulated with more biocompatible compounds, but still quite high concentrations of surfactant (up to 14 wt%) are required for their preparation (28). The nanocapsules obtained by this method are dispersed in an organic medium and can mainly be used for oral administration. Indeed, for intravenous administrations, it is necessary to transfer the nanocapsules into an aqueous continuous phase. Such a transfer still remained a problem until recently, since the total elimination of the organic phase and the redispersion of the nanocapsules, in water is a difficult task to achieve avoiding the aggregation of the nanocapsules. Recently, Lambert et al. (29) proposed to perform this operation by ultracentrifugation of the nanocapsule dispersion over a layer of pure water. Using this simple approach, the nanocapsules transferred from the organic phase to the aqueous phase without any aggregation problem during the centrifugation. In addition, this technique allows the elimination of the excess surfactant, which remains in the organic phase. This nanoencapsulation method has special interest for the encapsulation of water soluble molecules such as peptides (28) and nucleic acids including antisense oligonucleotides (29).

Preparation of Nanoparticles Using a Polymer

In this group of methods, the nanoparticles are obtained from a polymer, which was prepared according to a totally independent method. This approach presents the major advantage that the polymers entering the composition of the nanoparticles are well characterized and their intrinsic physicochemical characteristics will not depend on the conditions encountered during the preparation of the nanoparticles as it can be the case with the previously described methods. Most methods starting from polymers have taken advantages of the physicochemical properties of the polymer used in terms of its solubility or its faculty to form a gel under certain conditions. Basically, two approaches are followed. One is based on the spontaneous formation of colloidal particles of the polymer that are then stabilized in a second step of the procedure. The second approach is based on the adaptation of methods initially developed to make microparticles. In this case, the goal is to reduce the size of the particles formed with these methods. A third approach leading to the formation of very specific particles named SupraMolecular BioVectors by their authors (30) is described separately. The different ways to produce nanoparticles from a polymer is summarized in Fig. 3.

Methods based on the spontaneous formation of the nanoparticles

Spontaneous formation of nanoparticles can be achieved by taking advantage of the solubility and gelling properties of a dissolved polymer. Usually, the step allowing polymer colloidal particles to form is reversible, and it is necessary to complete the procedure by a second step required to stabilize the particles.

Based on the solubility properties of a polymer, the general principle is to prepare a solution of the polymer and to induce a phase separation by the addition of a nonsolvent of the polymer (10) or by a salting-out effect (2). The occurrence of the phase separation can be followed by turbidimetric measurements (2) or investigated using ternary phase diagrams (31). Phase separations leading to polymer colloid particles are usually obtained with diluted solutions of polymers. In a ternary phase

diagram, it corresponds to a small domain. Using higher polymer concentrations in the solvent, the colloidal particles formed at the limit of the phase separation as followed by turbidimetric measurements in the case of proteins. To facilitate the formation of colloidal dispersion of polymer particles, it is better to induce the phase separation in totally miscible solvent–nonsolvent systems. At that stage, the particles form spontaneously and quasi-instantaneously.

Once the proper conditions to obtain the polymer colloidal nanoparticles are identified, the particles must be stabilized. This is usually achieved either by the elimination of the polymer solvent by evaporation or by chemical cross-linking of the polymer as it is the case with proteins (32).

This method, also known as the nanoprecipitation method, can be applied to numerous synthetic polymers (10, 31). In general, the polymer is dissolved in acetone and the polymer solution is added into water. The acetone is then evaporated to complete the formation of the particles. Surface active agents are usually added to water to ensure the stability of the polymer particles. This easy technique of nanoparticle preparation was scaled up for large batch production. It leads to the formation of

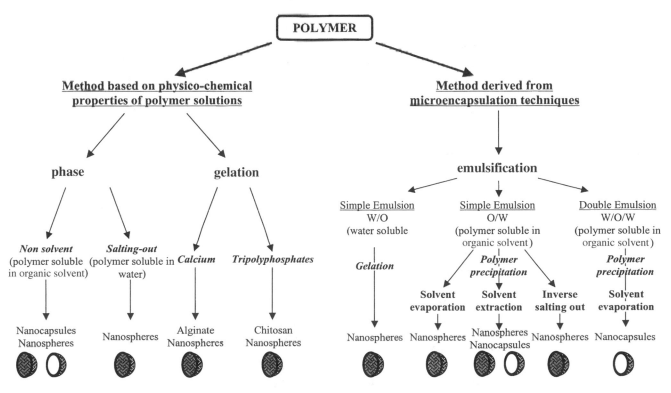

Fig. 3 Summary of the different methods to prepare nanospheres and nanocapsules from a polymer. W/O: water-in-oil, O/W: oil-in-water, W/O/W: water-in-oil-in-water.

nanospheres. Nanocapsules can easily be prepared by the same method just by adding a small amount of an organic oil in the polymer solution (8, 9). When the polymer solution is poured into the water phase, the oil is dispersed as tiny droplets in the solvent–nonsolvent mixture and the polymer precipitates on the oil droplet surface. This method leads to the preparation of oil-containing nanocapsules and can be valuably used for the encapsulation of liposoluble drugs.

Techniques based on the use of proteins are much more adapted to the encapsulation of hydrosoluble compounds and were recently developed to produce gelatin nanospheres as carrier systems for gene delivery (33, 34).

Based on the gelation properties displayed by certain polymers, nanoparticles are formed spontaneously by controlling the gelation process. This approach has been developed with alginate and chitosan that form highly water-swollen gels. The gelling agents for these two natural polysaccharides are respectively calcium and tripolyphosphate. Nanoparticles are formed in a certain domain of concentrations of the polysaccharide and of the gelling agent (35, 36). With the alginate, it has been shown that nanoparticles can be prepared when the respective concentrations of alginate and calcium are comprised in the domain of the pregel stage of the alginate gelling process (alginate 0.6 wt%, calcium chloride 0.9 mM). At this composition, tiny particles of gels form resulting from inter and intramolecular aggregations of alginate molecules caused by the interaction with calcium. These aggregates are stabilized by the formation of a polyelectrolyte complex with polylysine. Alginate and chitosan nanoparticles are interested for nucleic acid and protein delivery as recently reviewed by Vauthier and Couvreur (16).

Methods derived from microencapsulation techniques

Methods derived from microencapsulation techniques require the formation of an emulsion as a first step of the procedure. To produce nanometer-scale-sized particles, the size of the emulsion droplets must be small enough. This can be achieved by the use of special equipments such as high pressure homogenizers and microfluidizers. The energy input produced by these apparatus is important and is mainly due to high turbulence and cavitation forces. It allows an efficient dispersion of the polymer solution in the continuous phase. Once the desired emulsion is prepared, the formation of the nanoparticles can be induced according to two routes including the gelation of the polymer and the precipitation of the polymer either by solvent displacement or by solvent evaporation. Gelation can be induced by increasing the pH, adding calcium, or decreasing the temperature of emulsions containing

respectively, chitosan, alginate, and agarose (16). In the solvent displacement technique, the emulsion is formed with a solvent of the polymer, which is partially soluble in water and with an aqueous phase saturated with the solvent. Once the emulsion is formed with ethylacetate as an example, it is diluted by the further addition of water to displace the solvent from the dispersed phase inducing the polymer precipitation (14). This principle was also developed on the base of an inverse salting-out method (12). In this procedure, a solution of polymer in acetone is dispersed in an aqueous phase containing a high concentration of salt to keep the acetone nonmiscible with water. Just by diluting the emulsion with a large amount of pure water, the acetone is then extracted from the dispersed phase inducing the polymer precipitation. The total elimination of the acetone can be achieved by evaporation. Finally, precipitation of the polymer solubilized in the dispersed phase can also be induced by the removal of the solvent by evaporation (6, 37). In this method named emulsification-solvent evaporation, the polymer solvent diffuses through the aqueous continuous phase and evaporates at the air/water interface. The emulsion should remain under agitation during the time required for the total evaporation of the solvent. These methods produce nanospheres. To make nanocapsules, small amounts of oil can be added in the dispersed phase of the emulsion that will form the nanocapsules by solvent displacement (13). Nanocapsules can also be prepared with the solvent evaporation technique from a double water-in-oil-in-water emulsion (15). The removal of the organic solvent of the intermediate phase of this double emulsion by evaporation causes the polymer to precipitate at the surface of the inner aqueous phase. Whereas nanocapsules made by the solvent displacement method is more adapted for the encapsulation of lipophilic compounds, this last method allows the encapsulation of hydrosoluble compounds.

Preparation of SupraMolecular BioVector

SupraMolecular BioVector consists of polysaccharide nanospheres surrounded by a bilayer of phospholipids (30). At the origin, these systems were developed to mimic the low density lipoproteins that are natural colloidal structures encountered in the blood circulation and designed for the transport of cholesterol and cholesterol esters in vivo. SupraMolecular BioVector are prepared in several steps including the functionnalization and chemical cross-linking of a polysaccharide (starch or dextran), the purification and the drying of the modified polysaccharide followed by the fragmentation of the resulted powder under high pressure to produce small polysaccharide nanoparticles. Finally, a lipid bilayer is adsorbed on the surface of the nanoparticles. The chemical modification of the polysaccharide forming the core of the SupraMolecular BioVector lead to various possibilities in terms of the type of molecules that can be associated with such a carrier system. Indeed, the polysaccharide core can be either negatively or positively charged or even neutral opening large application potential.

Preparation of Surface Modified Nanoparticles

Once intravenously administered, the body distribution of the nanoparticles is controlled by their surface properties. Indeed, despite their small size, nanoparticles display an enormous specific surface area that makes the interaction with the surrounding medium very important especially for their fate in vivo. Thus, the preparation of surface modified nanoparticles received much attention during the last decade to produce nanoparticles that are able to circulate for a long period of time in the blood stream at first and, more recently, to achieve an effective targeting of the device or to improve their bioadhesivity to mucosae.

Nanoparticles that are able to circulate for a long time in the blood stream should not be recognized by macrophages of the mononuclear phagocyte system. To achieve this goal, at least one of the two major known mechanisms involved in the recognition of foreign particles by macrophages should be avoided. These two mechanisms include the particle opsonization and the complement activation, which consists in protein adsorption and subsequent recognition by macrophages. A barrier to protein adsorption could be achieved by creating an efficient barrier of steric hindrance, therefore, by coating or adsorbing hydrophilic polymers to nanoparticle surface.

Nanospheres coated with poly(ethylene glycol) were first obtained by the simple adsorption of triblock copolymers of poly(ethylene glycol)–poly(propylene glycol)–poly(ethylene glycol) on the surface of already prepared nanospheres (38). To improve the stability of the poly(ethylene glycol) coating, nanospheres were prepared by nanoprecipitation or by emulsification-solvent evaporation using copolymers of poly(lactic acid)–co-poly (ethylene glycol) or of poly(alkylcyanoacrylate)–co-poly(ethylene glycol) (17, 39–41). Finally, poly(ethylene glycol) can initiate the polymerization of alkylcyanoacrylate to produce poly(ethylene glycol)-coated poly-(alkylcyanoacrylate) nanoparticles by emulsion polymerization (24, 41).

To make nanoparticles able to escape complement activation, Passirani et al. (42) proposed to coat nanospheres with heparin. This compound, which is a polysaccharide, is a physiological inhibitor of complement activation in vivo. Heparin-coated poly(methylmethacrylate) nanoparticles were prepared by emulsion polymerization. In the method, the radical polymerization of methylmethacrylate was initiated by heparin according to an original method involving cerium ions and allowing heparin to covalently attach to poly(methylmethacrylate).

The next step now is the development of targeted nanoparticles toward a specific cell type. This has recently been investigated by Stella et al. (43) who prepared poly(alkylcyanoacrylate) nanoparticles showing residues of folic acid on their surface. These nanoparticles will be used to target cancer cells overexpressing a membrane receptor for the folic acid. The targeting moiety, consisting on the folic acid, was grafted on the surface of poly(aminopoly(ethylene glycol) cyano-co-hexadecylcyanoacrylate) nanoparticles that were obtained by nanoprecipitation.

In another way, chitosan was used as a coating agent for nanoparticles to improve their bioadhesive properties after oral and nasal administration (44). Indeed, chitosan is known to have bioadhesive properties as well as an interesting absorption enhancing capacity.

CHARACTERIZATION OF NANOPARTICULATE DRUG CARRIERS

Nanoparticles can be characterized by all the different physico chemical techniques that apply for polymer colloids (45). Concerning the development procedure of nanoparticles as drug carriers, the main physico chemical parameters that are investigated are the shape, the size, the surface properties, the density, and the concentration of the particles (19). The size as well as the size distribution are important parameters to be determined to achieve safe intravenous administration. Surface properties are also important to consider as nanoparticles display considerable specific surface area responsible for the interactions with the surrounding medium. Finally, the density and the concentration are required to deduce the specific surface area of the particles together with the size.

Nanoparticles can be visualized using different microscopy techniques. Transmission electron microscopy is usually applied to nanoparticles after negative staining with phosphotungstate acid or with uranyl acetate after it has been checked that the staining agents do not modify the particles. Recent progress in transmission electron microscopy now allows direct observations of the nanoparticles without the use of any staining agent that may cause artefacts in some cases. In particular, direct observations of the nanoparticles after a sample of the nanoparticle dispersion has been freezing at very low temperature can be carried out by cryotransmission electron microscopy. Scanning electron microscopy is performed on samples coated with a thin layer of gold metal to produce the contrast. These techniques as well as those based on atomic force microscopy give useful images of the nanoparticles showing their shape. Measurements of the size and of the size distribution require determination of the diameters number of individual nanoparticles that may be assisted by the use of valuable image analysis softwares. The internal structure of the nanoparticles can be observed by freeze fracture and cryotransmission electron microscopy.

Generally, mean size and size distribution of nanoparticles are evaluated by quasi-elastic light scattering also named photocorrelation spectroscopy. This method is based on the evaluation of the translation diffusion coefficient, D, characterizing the Brownian motion of the nanoparticles. The nanoparticle hydrodynamic diameter, d_H is then deduced from this parameter from the Stokes Einstein law.

Other techniques can be used to determine the size and the size distribution of the nanoparticles. The field flow fractionation method is based on the separation of particles according to their size in a thin glass channel in which the flow carrying on the nanoparticles is submitted to an external perpendicular force produced either by a crossed flow or a sedimentation (46, 47). This technique, which can be applied for particles in a wide range of size (10 nm to several hundred μm), will gain more attention in the future for size determination and also for nanoparticle surface analysis (48). Size and size distribution of nanoparticles can also be determined by size exclusion chromatography performed on appropriate gels. This approach, requiring less equipment than the previous methods, presents the main limitation that only particles having a diameter lower than 120 nm can be characterized by this method (49).

As mentioned earlier, surface characteristics of the nanoparticles are of primary importance for the interaction of the nanoparticles with the surrounding medium. The main nanoparticle surface characteristics that are considered are the charge, the hydrophilicity, the chemical composition and the capacity to adsorb proteins and to induce complement activation.

The charge of the nanoparticle surface is usually evaluated by the measurement of their zeta potential, which gives information about the overall surface charge of the particles and how it is affected by changes in the environment (50). Zeta potential is affected by the surface composition of the nanoparticles, the presence or the absence of adsorbed compounds, and the composition of the dispersing phase, mainly the ionic strength and the pH.

The hydrophilicity of the nanoparticle surface can be evaluated by hydrophobic interaction chromatography (51). This technique, based on affinity chromatography, allows a very rapid discrimination between hydrophilic and hydrophobic nanoparticles. The nanoparticles are passed through a column containing a hydrophobic interaction chromatography gel. The nanoparticles that are retained by the gel and only eluted after the addition of a surfactant are considered as hydrophobic, whereas the nanoparticles that do not interact with the gel and that are directly eluted from the column are considered as hydrophilic. Apart from the hydrophobic interaction chromatography, the field flow fractionation techniques recently appeared to present interesting potential for the characterization of nanoparticles with different surface characteristics (48).

X-ray photoelectron spectroscopy (ESCA) can be use to determine the chemical composition of the nanoparticle surface. This technique is a very useful tool for the development of surface modified nanoparticles providing a direct evidence of the presence of the components that are believed to be on the nanoparticle surface (38, 41).

The capacity of the nanoparticles to adsorb proteins and to activate the complement in vivo after intravenous administration will influence the fate of the carrier and its body distribution. To approach this aspect, in vitro tests have been developed to investigate the profile of the type of serum proteins that adsorbed onto the nanoparticle surface after incubation in serum and to evaluate the capacity of the nanoparticles to induce complement activation. The analysis of the protein adsorbed onto the nanoparticle surface can be performed by 2D-polyacrylamide gel electrophoresis. This technique allows the identification of the proteins that adsorbed onto the nanoparticle surface (52). To evaluate modifications of the composition of the adsorbed protein with time, a faster method based on capillary electrophoresis can also be used (53). Finally, the activation of the complement produced by nanoparticles can be evaluated either by a global technique or by a specific method measuring the specific activation of the component C3. In the global technique, nanoparticles are incubated with serum and, after the incubation, the remaining nonactivated complement in the serum is evaluated using a red blood cell lysis test (54, 55).

The concentration of nanoparticle in the dispersion can be deduced from gravimetric determination or by turbidimetric measurements based on the application of the Mie's law (48, 56). Density of the nanoparticles is evaluated either by pycnometry (57) or by isopycnic centrifugation (13, 58).

PHARMACEUTICAL APPLICATIONS OF NANOPARTICLES

Nanoparticles were first developed in the mid-seventies by Birrenbach and Speiser (3). Later on, their application for the design of drug delivery systems was made available by the use of biodegradable polymers that were considered to be highly suitable for human applications (5). At that time, the research on colloidal carriers was mainly focusing on liposomes, but no one was able to produce stable lipid vesicles suitable for clinical applications. In some cases, nanoparticles have been shown to be more active than liposomes due to their better stability (59). This is the reason why in the last decades many drugs (e.g., antibiotics, antiviral and antiparasitic drugs, cytostatics, protein and peptides) were associated to nanoparticles.

Intravenous Administration

Fate of nanoparticles and their content after intravenous administration

The main interest of nanoparticles is their ability to achieve tissue targeting and enhance the intracellular penetration of drugs. After intravenous administration, nanoparticules are taken up by the liver, spleen and to a lower extent the bone marrow (60). Within these tissues, nanoparticles are mainly taken up by cells of the mononuclear phagocyte system (MPS) (61). The uptake occurs through an endocytosis process after which the particles end up in the lysosomal compartment (61) where they are degraded producing low molecular weight soluble compounds that are eliminated from the body by renal excretion (62). As a result of the MPS site specific targeting, avoidance of some organs was made possible, thus reducing the side effects and toxicity of some active compounds. Due to their strong lysosomal localization, one could imagine that nanoparticles are not suitable to target to the cytoplasm. To avoid their trapping within the lysosomal compartment, several compounds able to destabilize the lysosomal membrane were added to the nanoparticulate systems (e.g., cationic surfactant) (63) allowing some drugs to be delivered to the cytoplasm. Recently, to avoid MPS uptake, several groups have developed a strategy consisting of the linkage to the nanoparticles of poly(ethylene glycol) derivatives (39, 64, 65). This linkage results in a lower uptake of nanoparticles by the MPS and in a longer circulation

time. As a consequence, these so-called stealth® nanoparticles would be able to extravasate across endothelium that becomes permeable due to the presence of solid tumors.

Application to the treatment of intracellular infections

Intracellular infections were found to be a field of interest for drug delivery by means of nanospheres. Indeed, infected cells may constitute a "reservoir" for micro organisms, which are protected from antibiotics inside lysosomes. The resistance of intracellular infections to chemotherapy is often related to the low uptake of commonly used antibiotics or to their reduced activity at the acidic pH of lysosomes. To overcome these effects, the use of ampicillin, a β lactam antibiotic, bound to nanospheres was proposed as endocytozable formulation (66). The effectiveness of polyisohexylcyanoacrylate (PIHCA) nanospheres was tested in the treatment of two experimental intracellular infections.

Firstly, ampicillin-loaded nanospheres were tested in the treatment of experimental *Listeria monocytogenes* infection in congenitally athymic nude mice, a model involving a chronic infection of both liver and spleen macrophages (67). After adsorption of ampicillin onto nanospheres, the therapeutic activity of ampicillin was found to increase dramatically over that of the free drug. Bacterial counts in the liver were at least 20-fold reduced after linkage of ampicillin to PIHCA nanospheres. In addition, nanoparticulate ampicillin was capable of ensuring liver sterilization after two injections of 0.8 mg of nanospheres bound drug, whereas no such sterilization was ever observed with any of other regimens tested. Reappearance of living bacteria in the liver after the end of the treatment was probably due to a secondary infection derived from other organs such as the spleen, which was not completely sterilized by the treatment (67).

Secondly, nanosphere-bound ampicillin was tested in the treatment of experimental salmonellosis in C57/BL6 mice, a model involving an acute fatal infection (66). All mice treated with a single injection of nanoparticle-bound ampicillin survived, whereas all control mice and all those treated with unloaded nanospheres died within 10 days postinfection. With free ampicillin, an effective-curative effect required three doses of 32 mg each. Lower doses (3×0.8 mg and 3×16 mg) delayed but did not reduce mortality. Thus, the therapeutic index of ampicillin, calculated on the basis of mice mortality, was increased by 120-fold when the drug was bound to nanospheres.

In order to clarify the mechanism by which nanospheres improved the antimicrobial efficacy of ampicillin, Forestier et al. (68) have compared in vitro the efficacy of ampicillin bound to poly(isobutylcyanoacrylate) (PIBCA) nanospheres with that of free ampicillin in terms of survival of *L. monocytogenes* in mouse peritoneal macrophages. After 30 h of incubation, nanospheres-bound ampicillin decreased the number of viable bacteria by 99% as compared to the controls whereas with free ampicillin, the number of bacteria was slightly lower than in the controls. Nanoparticle-ampicillin thus appeared to be much more effective than free ampicillin for inhibiting intracellular growth of *L. monocytogenes*. With in vitro *Salmonella typhimurium* infected macrophages, the situation was a little bit more complicated since the bactericidal effect of ampicillin-bound PIHCA nanospheres was poor although the intracellular capture of ampicillin was dramatically increased and its efflux in the extracellular medium reduced (69). In another study, confocal microscopy and transmission electron microscopy were used to establish the intracellular traffic of ampicillin-bound PIHCA nanospheres and its relation with the bacteria within the subcellular compartments (70). The data obtained clearly demonstrated the active uptake by phagocytosis of ampicillin-bound PIHCA nanospheres by murine macrophages and their localization in the same vacuoles as the infecting bacteria, but in a restrictive way (70). Thus, it was difficult to understand the limited bactericidal effect of ampicillin-bound nanospheres. The most probable explanation is to be found in the resistance mechanism of *S. typhimurium* involving the inhibition of the phagosome–lysosome fusion (71), which lets some bacteria in phagosomes free of nanospheres. If this proposed hypothesis (inhibition of phagosome–lysosome fusion) is correct, the dramatic efficiency observed in vivo should rather be due to the specific targeting of the infected tissues (rich in reticuloendothelial cells), than to an efficient intracellular targeting as it could be supposed.

In order to eliminate both dividing and nondividing bacteria, a fluoroquinolone antibiotic, ciprofloxacin, has been associated with PIBCA and PIHCA nanospheres. In an animal model of persisting Salmonella infection, although an effect on the early phase of the infection was observed, neither free nor nanosphere-bound ciprofloxacin was able to eradicate truly persisting bacteria (72).

Since they accumulate in the MPS, nanospheres hold promise as drug carriers for the treatment of visceral leishmaniosis (73). Thus, it has been shown that PIHCA nanospheres can be used as a carrier of primaquine whose activity was increased 21-fold against intracellular *Leishmania donovani* when associated with nanospheres (74). A part of the activity was attributed to the fact that phagocytosis of nanospheres led to the induction of a respiratory burst, which was more pronounced in infected than in noninfected macrophages (74). Dehydroemetine is

also one of the drug candidates for this treatment but has some side effects involving the heart, which were reduced after linkage with nanospheres (75).

Application to the treatment of cancer

When given intravenously, anticancer drugs are distributed throughout the body as a function of the physicochemical properties of the molecule. A pharmacologically active concentration is reached in the tumor tissue at the expense of massive contamination of the rest of the body. For cytostatic compounds, this poor specificity raises a toxicological problem, which presents a serious obstacle to effective therapy. The use of colloidal drug carriers could represent a more rational approach to specific cancer therapy. In addition, the possibility of overcoming multidrug resistance might be achieved by using cytostatics-loaded nanospheres.

The antitumor efficacy of doxorubicin-loaded nanospheres was first tested using the lymphoid leukemia L-1210 as a tumor model. In this study, one intravenous injection of doxorubicin-loaded PIBCA nanospheres was found to be more effective against L1210 leukemia than when the drug was administered in its free form following the same dosing schedule (76). Although the increased life span (ILS %) of mice injected with doxorubicin-loaded PIBCA nanospheres was twice as high as the ILS % for free doxorubicin, there were no long-term survivors.

The effectiveness of doxorubicin-loaded PIHCA nanospheres against L1210 leukemia was even more pronounced than that of doxorubicin loaded onto PIBCA nanospheres. The drug toxicity was markedly decreased when it was bound to this sort of nanospheres, so that impressive results were obtained with this formulation at doses for which the therapeutic efficiency of free doxorubicin was completely masked by the overpowering toxicity of the drug (76). Furthermore, preliminary experiments suggested that one i.v. bolus injection of doxorubicin-loaded nanospheres was more active, in L1210-bearing mice, than perfusion of the free drug for 24 h.

The superiority of doxorubicin targeted with the aid of poly(alkylcyanoacrylate) nanospheres was later confirmed in a murine hepatic metastases model (M5076 reticulosarcoma) (77). Irrespective of the dose and the administration schedule, the reduction in the number of metastases was much greater with doxorubicin-loaded nanospheres than with free doxorubicin, particularly if treatment was given only when the metastases were well established. The improved efficacy of the targeted drug, as clearly confirmed by histological examinations, shows that both the number and the size of the tumor nodules were lower when doxorubicin was administered in its nanoparticulate form (77). Furthermore, liver biopsies of animals treated with the nanosphere-targeted drug showed a lower cancer cell density inside tumor tissue. Necrosis was often less widespread with the nanosphere-associated drug than in the control group and the group treated with free doxorubicin.

Studies performed on total homogenates of livers from both healthy and metastases-bearing mice showed extensive capture of nanoparticulate doxorubicin by the liver; no difference in hepatic concentrations was noted between healthy and tumor-bearing animals (77). In order to elucidate the mechanism behind the enhanced efficiency of doxorubicin-loaded nanospheres, doxorubicin measurements were made in both metastatic nodules and neighboring healthy hepatic tissue. This provided quantitative information concerning the drug distribution within these tissues (78). During the first 6 h after administration, the exposure of the liver to doxorubicin was 18 times greater for nanosphere-associated doxorubicin. However, no special affinity for the tumor tissue was detected and the nanospheres were seen by electron microscopy to be located within Kupffer cells (macrophages). However, at later time-points, the amount of drug in the tumor tissue increased in nanosphere-treated animals to 2.5 times the level found in animals given free doxorubicin. Since uptake of nanospheres by neoplastic tissue is unlikely, this increase in the doxorubicin concentration in tumor tissue probably resulted from doxorubicin released from healthy tissue, in particular Kupffer cells. Hepatic tissue could play the role of drug reservoir from which prolonged diffusion of the free drug (from nanospheres entrapped in Küpffer cell lysosomes) toward the neighboring malignant cells occurs.

This hypothesis raises the question of the long-term effect of an 18-fold increase of doxorubicin concentration in the liver. Although toxicological data have shown that doxorubicin-loaded nanospheres were not significantly or unexpectedly toxic to the liver in terms of survival rate at high doses, body weight loss, and histological appearance (79), this possibility should be borne in mind, especially since a temporary depletion in the number of Kupffer cells, and hence the ability to clear bacteria, was observed in rats treated with doxorubicin-loaded liposomes (80). A systematic study using unloaded poly(alkylcyanoacrylate) nanoparticles confirmed a reversible decline in the phagocytic capacity of the liver after repeated dosing, as well as a slight inflammatory response (81, 82). Nanoparticle-associated doxorubicin also accumulated in bone marrow, leading to a myelosuppressive effect (83). However, this tropism of carriers might be useful to deliver myelostimulating compounds such as granulocyte colony stimulating factor to reverse the suppressive effects

of intense chemotherapy (84). Nanospheres are also captured by splenic macrophages (85). In this study, the spleen architecture was shown to play a role in the localization of the nanospheres: in mice, uptake was mainly observed in metallophilic macrophages of the marginal zone whereas in rats, which have sinusoidal spleens similar to that of humans, particles were found in the red pulp macrophages.

On the other hand, alteration of the drug distribution profile by linkage to nanospheres can, in some cases, considerably reduce the toxicity of a drug because of reduced accumulation in organs where the most acute toxic effects are exerted. This concept was indeed illustrated with doxorubicin, which displays severe acute and chronic cardiomyopathy. After intravenous administration to mice, plasma levels of doxorubicin were higher when the drug was adsorbed onto nanospheres and at the same time the cardiac concentration of the drug was dramatically reduced (86). In accordance with the observed distribution profile, doxorubicin associated with nanospheres was found to be less toxic than free doxorubicin (78).

The ability of tumor cells to develop simultaneous resistance to multiple lipophilic compounds represents a major problem in cancer chemotherapy. Cellular resistance to anthracyclines has been attributed to an active drug efflux from resistant cells linked to the presence of transmembrane P-glycoprotein, which was not detectable in the parental drug-sensitive cell line. Drugs, such as doxorubicin, appear to enter the cell by passive diffusion through the lipid bilayer. Upon entering the cell, these drugs bind to P-glycoprotein, which forms transmembrane channels and uses energy from ATP hydrolysis to pump these compounds out of the cell (87). To solve this problem, many authors have proposed the use of competitive P-glycoprotein inhibitors, such as the calcium channel blocker verapamil, which are able to bind to P-glycoprotein and to overcome pleiotropic resistance. However, since the adverse effects of verapamil are serious, its clinical use to overcome multidrug resistance is limited.

During the past few years, many studies have been devoted to evaluating the antitumor potential of carrier-drug complexes (88). The effect of nanospheres loaded with doxorubicin, resistance to which is known to be related to the presence of P-glycoprotein, was evaluated. The cytotoxicity of free-doxorubicin, doxorubicin-loaded PIHCA nanospheres (NP-Doxorubicin) (mean diameter 300 nm), and nanospheres without drug (NP), against sensitive (MCF7) and multidrug resistant (Doxorubicin R MCF7) human breast cancer cell lines was compared (89). MCF7 cells were more sensitive to free-doxorubicin than

Doxorubicin R MCF7 cells with a 150-fold difference in the IC_{50}. No significant difference was observed in the survival rate of MCF7 treated with free-Doxorubicin or NP-doxorubicin. In contrast, for doxorubicin R MCF7, the IC_{50} for doxorubicin was 130-fold lower when NP-doxorubicin were used instead of free-doxorubicin (89). These results indicated that nanospheres provided an effective carrier for introducing a cytotoxic dose of doxorubicin into the pleiotropic resistant human cancer cell line Doxorubicin R MCF7.

Complementary experiments, conducted with other sensitive and resistant cell lines, have confirmed this efficacy of nanospheres (90, 91). Doxorubicin resistance was circumvented in the majority of the cell lines tested, and some encouraging results were obtained in vivo in a P388 model growing as ascites (90). Further studies were undertaken to elucidate the mechanism of action of polyalkylcyanoacrylate nanospheres. The incubation time and number of particles per cell were important factors (92) and, when PIBCA nanospheres were used, doxorubicin accumulation within P388/ADR resistant leukemic cells was increased compared with free drug, although no endocytosis of nanospheres occurred (93). On the other hand, when the less rapidly degradable PIHCA nanospheres were used, reversion was observed in the absence of increased intracellular drug (94). The degradation products of poly(alkylcyanoacrylate) nanospheres [mainly poly(cyanoacrylic acid)] were also able to increase both accumulation and cytotoxicity of doxorubicin, although they were soluble in the culture medium. Hence, the reversion of resistance seems to be due both to the adsorption of nanospheres on the cell surface and to the formation of a doxorubicin-poly(cyanoacrylic acid) ion pair, which facilitates the transport of the drug across the cell membrane (94).

In the light of the results obtained with doxorubicin-loaded nanospheres in the liver metastases model described earlier (77), the role of macrophages as a reservoir for doxorubicin was tested in a two-compartment coculture system in vitro with both resistant and sensitive P388 cells (95). Even after prior uptake by macrophages, doxorubicin-loaded PIBCA nanospheres were able to overcome resistance. However, this reversion was only partial. It was decided to take advantage of the particulate drug carrier offers to associate an anticancer drug and a compound capable of inhibiting the P-glycoprotein. This approach was tested with doxorubicin and cyclosporin A bound to the same nanospheres and was found to be extremely effective in reversing P388 resistance (95). The association of cyclosporin A with nanospheres would ensure that it reaches the same sites as the anticancer drug at the same time and would also reduce its toxic side effects.

As early as 1986, Al Khouri et al. (96) observed that like other colloidal carriers, nanocapsules, administered by the IV route in rabbits, were taken up rapidly by organs of the mononuclear phagocyte system. One application that takes advantage of this uptake concerns nanocapsules of (muramyl tripeptide cholesterol) (MTP-Chol). This immunostimulating agent is able to activate macrophages and induce toxicity toward tumor cells, and would therefore be a useful agent to treat metastatic cancer. The mechanisms by which activated macrophages arrest tumor proliferation include production of nitric oxide and TNF-α. It was showed in in vitro models of rat alveolar macrophages and RAW 264.7 mouse monocyte macrophage line that nanocapsules based on poly(D,L-lactide) containing MTP-Chol are more efficient activators than the free drug (97, 98). This action could be due to an intracellular delivery of the immunomodulator encapsulated in nanocapsules after phagocytosis and to an intermediate transfer of the drug to serum proteins (99). This system has also demonstrated its efficiency in vivo; in fact, Barratt et al. (100) reported that antimetastatic effects of nanocapsules contained MTP-Chol in a model of liver metastases. Some antimetastatic activity was also seen after oral administration.

Nanospheres for oligonucleotide delivery

Oligodeoxynucleotides are potentially powerful new drugs because of their selectivity for particular gene products in both sense and antisense strategies. However, using antisense oligonucleotides in therapeutics is a challenge to pharmaceutical technology because of their susceptibility to enzymatic degradation and their poor penetration across biological membranes. Nanoparticulate preparations might be an interesting alternative because of better stability in the presence of biological fluids. In the case of nanospheres made of synthetic polymers [poly(alkylcyanoacrylate), poly(lactic acid)], since oligonucleotides have no affinity for the polymeric matrix, association with nanoparticles has been achieved by ion pairing with a cationic surfactant, cetyltimethylammonium bromide (CTAB) adsorbed onto the nanoparticle surface (101). Oligonucleotides bound to poly(alkylcyanoacrylate) nanospheres in this way were protected from nucleases in vitro (63) and their intracellular uptake was increased (102). In addition, nanospheres were able to concentrate intact oligonucleotides in the liver and in the spleen (103). Antisense oligonucleotides formulated in this way were able to specifically inhibit mutated Ha-*ras*-mediated cell proliferation and tumorigenicity in nude mice (104).

This approach has recently been applied to the association of a phosphodiester antisense oligonucleotide directed against the 3' nontranslated region of the PKCα

gene with nanospheres prepared from PIBCA. These nanospheres were able to inhibit PKCα neo-expression in cultured Hep G6 cells (105).

Nanospheres containing oligonucleotides have also been formulated from a naturally occurring polysaccharide, alginate, which forms a gel in the presence of calcium ions. In this case, the oligonucleotides penetrate into the gel matrix by reptation, thus providing a high loading yield and good protection against nucleases (106).

Subcutaneous/Intramuscular Administration

Subcutaneous administration of nanoparticles was achieved mainly for the delivery of peptides and vaccines. It allows slow release of the entrapped drugs therefore reducing the number of administrations, increasing blood half-life of the active drug, and finally, in some cases, reducing side effects.

PIBCA nanospheres were injected subcutaneously to rats. Autoradiographic pictures obtained after using radiolabelled polymer have shown a progressive staining reduction in the muscular tissue suggesting that nanospheres were slowly biodegraded (107). In the same study, nanospheres were found to release a peptide (GRF) in a sustained manner. Comparison of the AUC of free GRF and GRF-loaded nanospheres showed that in addition to the slow release process nanospheres were able to improve the bioavailability of the peptide. This improvement could be attributed to the fact that free administered GRF is very quickly metabolized at the injection site, whereas it is partly protected from massive enzymatic degradation when it is administered associated with nanospheres (107).

A few examples of the use of nanospheres as adjuvant for antigens/allergens delivery were described in the literature. The main advantage of this approach is to design single shot vaccine. In this case the drug carrier has to remain at the site of administration and deliver either continuously or pulsatively the antigen. The use of slowly degradable polymers (PLA, PMMA) is suitable for this application, since peptide or protein release is more adequate. Poly(methyl methacrylate) were first investigated as adjuvants for injectable vaccines (108,109). These nanospheres were claimed to be biodegradable after subcutaneous or intramuscular injection and shown to exhibit very powerful adjuvant properties for a number of antigens. However, the adjuvant properties were shown to be better when the antigen was incorporated during the polymerization process than when adsorbed onto nanospheres (110). When comparing the effect of PMMA with other polymers (polystyrene and 2-hydroxyethyl methacrylate/methyl methacrylate copolymer, HEMA:

MMA), it was also demonstrated that a decrease in particle size and an increase in the hydrophobicity of nanospheres increased the antibody response after immunization against influenza whole and split virus, bovine serum albumin, and HIV2 split virus (111–113).

Oral Route

There are numerous reports showing that uptake and translocation of nanoparticles and microparticles take place after oral administration to animals (114–116). Different mechanisms have been proposed to explain the translocation of particulate material across the intestine: i) uptake via Peyer's patches or isolated lymphoid follicles; ii) intracellular uptake, and iii) intracellular/paracellular passage. The uptake of poly(alkylcyanoacrylate) nanocapsules by Peyer's patches has been shown by Damgé et al. (116). When administered in the lumen of an isolated ileal segment of the rat, polylalkylcyanoacrylate nanocapsules were found preferentially over Peyer's patches through which they passed massively and rapidly (116). Nanocapsules were clearly visible in M-cells and in intercellular spaces around the lymph cells. Intracellular uptake of nanospheres has been proposed by Kreuter et al. (117) based on electron-microscopic autoradiographic investigations showing radioactivity into epithelial and goblet cells after oral administration of poly(hexylcyanoacrylate) (PHCA) nanospheres labeled with ^{14}C. The translocation of particles by a paracellular pathway has been evidenced in a study done by Aprahamian et al. (118) using PIBCA nanocapsules. Nanocapsules were filled with an iodinized oil (lipiodol) in order to render them detectable using a scanning electron microscope equipped with an energy-dispersive X-ray spectrometer. When they were administered in an isolated segment of a dog jejunum, they appeared as vesicles associated with intraluminal mucus. Subsequently, they were observed in intravillus capillaries in close contact with red cells or adsorbed to the inner wall of endothelial cells. Among these three mechanisms and according to many studies involving nanoparticles made of other biodegradable and nondegradable polymers, translocation via the uptake in Peyer's patches seems to be the major pathway for a rapid and substantial passage after oral administration of nanoparticles. Although it might exist in certain situations, the passage of particles between the absorptive cells is rather less likely if the barrier of tight junctions has not been disrupted. Although there are abundant reports from various independent workers showing evidence of absorption of particulate systems by the gastrointestinal tract, the oral absorption of nanoparticles remains a controversial issue. However, even if a more clear estimation of the quantity of absorbed particles is needed as well as a better understanding of the factors affecting particles uptake, it must be concluded that translocation of small sized particles like poly(alkylcyanoacrylate) nanoparticles is possible. The question remains if the extent of particle translocation is compatible with a strategy of drug administration with therapeutic perspectives. This will be discussed below.

Oral Delivery of Peptides and Proteins and Vaccines

Poly(isobutylcyanoacrylate) nanocapsules were shown 10 years ago to be able to encapsulate insulin and to increase its activity as assessed by a reduction of glycemia (119). Several aspects of this phenomenon are surprising: encapsulation of a hydrophilic drug in the oily core of nanocapsules; reduction of glycemia was only obtained with diabetic animals; hypoglycemia appeared two days after a single administration and was maintained for up to 20 days depending on the insulin doses, although the amplitude of the pharmacological effect (minimum level of blood glucose) did not depend on the insulin dose. Damgé et al. (116) and Lowe and Temple (120) suggested that nanocapsules could protect insulin from proteolytic degradation in intestinal fluids, based on the protection of encapsulated insulin, observed in the presence of different enzymes in vitro. Later studies showed that insulin did not react with the alkylcyanoacrylate monomer during the formation of nanocapsules and was located within the oily core rather than adsorbed on their surface (27, 121)

The capacity of insulin nanocapsules to reduce glycemia could be explained by their translocation through the intestinal barrier, as suggested by Damgé et al. (116); for example by paracellular pathway or via M cells in Peyer's patches (122). Recently, the use of Texas Red®-labeled insulin allowed this translocation to be visualized more readily (123). One hour after oral administration, nanocapsules reached the ileum. The presence of fluorescent areas within the mucosa and even in the lamina propria suggested that insulin-loaded nanocapsules could cross the intestinal epithelium. Although this passage is certainly an important factor, it does not explain the duration of the hypoglycemia. This prolonged action could be due to the retention of a part of the colloidal system in the gastrointestinal tract.

Interestingly, a prolonged hypoglycemic effect was also observed with insulin entrapped in poly(alkylcyanoacrylate) nanospheres when these were dispersed in an oily phase containing surfactant (124). This suggests that some components of nanocapsules could act as promoters of absorption.

Recently, Damgé et al. (125) showed that the incorporation of octreotide, a somatostatin analogue, in poly(alkylcyanoacrylate) nanocapsules also improved and prolonged the therapeutic effect of this peptide, after administration by the oral route.

Even if the main limitation to oral administration of poly(alkylcyanoacrylate) nanoparticles is that their passage through the intestinal barrier is probably restricted and sometimes erratic, they represent an interesting tool for oral delivery of antigens. Indeed, M-cells appear to be the main site for the uptake of poly(alkylcyanoacrylate) nanoparticles after oral administration (116) and, furthermore, it is generally accepted that limited doses of antigen are sufficient for a mucous immunization. In fact, oral delivery of antigens may be considered as the most convenient means of producing an IgA antibody response. However, it is importantly limited by enzymatic degradation of antigens in the GI tract and, additionally by their poor absorption. Thus, it has been postulated that the use of micro- or nanoparticles for the oral delivery of antigens should be efficient if those systems are able to achieve the protection of the antigenic molecule. Poly(alkylcyanoacrylate) nanoparticles have been shown to enhance the secretory immune response after their oral administration in association with ovalbumin (126). This result was not fully reproduced in the case of poly(acrylamide) nanoparticles loaded with the same antigen. It was postulated that in the case of poly(acrylamide) nanospheres, much of the antigen was located at the surface of the polymer and could have been degraded during its passage through the gut. The relatively high surface concentration of ovalbumin adsorbed onto poly(butylcyanoacrylate) nanospheres may have reduced the ability of the proteolytic enzymes in the gut to gain access to and to degrade the antigen, resulting in a greater antigen availability.

Ocular Delivery

The anatomical structure and the protective physiological process of the eye exert a strong defense against ocular drug delivery. This is the reason why conventional ocular dosage forms exhibit extremely low bioavailability. Limited absorption of the drug through the lipophilic corneal barrier is mainly because of short precorneal residence time due to the tear turn-over, rapid nasolacrimal drainage of instilled drug from the tear fluid, and nonproductive absorption through the conjonctiva. Only a small proportion (1–3%) of the applied drug penetrates the cornea and reaches intraocular tissues. For these reasons, it is necessary to develop efficient and more acceptable ocular therapeutic systems.

Different strategies can be carried out to improve the precorneal residence time and/or penetration ability of the active ingredient. Among them, one approach consists of using colloidal drug delivery systems such as nanoparticles. Initial studies carried out with nanocapsules, as ocular drug carriers, attempted to increase the penetration of lipophilic drugs into the eye by prolonging the precorneal residence time, as observed with other colloidal systems, liposomes and nanospheres. These studies, which concerned antiglaucomatous agents, such as betaxolol, carteolol, and metipranolol encapsulated in nanocapsules, only showed a reduction of the noncorneal absorption (systemic circulation) leading to reduced side-effects as compared with the free drug (127–129). These systemic side-effects are due to a poor ocular retention of drugs that are directly absorbed into the systemic circulation by conjunctival and nasal blood vessels. In two cases (carteolol and betaxolol), encapsulation in nanocapsules produced an improved pharmacological effect (reduction of intraocular pressure) than produced by free drug and nanospheres (although the penetration of nanocapsules was not tested) and reduced cardiovascular systemic side-effects (127,128). Metipranolol showed the same activity alone and associated with nanocapsules but, as in the case of carteolol and betaxolol, its side-effects were reduced. When betaxolol was used, the nature of the polymer making up the nanocapsule wall was found to be important, and poly(ε-caprolactone) was more efficient than PIBCA or poly(lactic-co-glycolic acid) (127).

Calvo et al. (130) explored the mechanisms of interaction of nanocapsules with ocular tissues to better understand the pharmacological responses obtained with antiglaucomatous agents. By confocal microscopy, they showed that poly(ε-caprolactone) nanocapsules could specifically penetrate the corneal epithelium by an endocytic process without causing any damage to the cells, in contrast with PIBCA nanoparticles, the uptake of which was associated with cellular lysis (131). These results explained the improved therapeutic effect and the reduction of systemic side-effects as a result of drug loss through the conjunctiva provided by poly(ε-caprolactone) nanocapsules by increasing corneal epithelium penetration of lipophilic drugs. Calvo et al. (132) also excluded the influence of the oily inner structure in the activity of the nanocapsules, in the light of the absence of differences in penetration between nanospheres and nanocapsules, in contrast with Marchal Heussler et al. (128) who observed a better therapeutic effect with nanocapsules than with nanospheres. Moreover, Calvo et al. (132) demonstrated with indomethacin-loaded nanocapsules that the colloidal

nature of the carrier was the main factor influencing its ocular bioavailability. The same authors were also interested in the influence of the nature and the charge of the surface of nanocapsules on their physical stability and on their ocular bioavailability (133, 134). They found that coating the negatively charged surface of poly(ε-caprolactone) nanocapsules with cationic polymers could prevent their degradation caused by the adsorption of lysozyme, a positively charged enzyme found in tear fluid (133). Moreover, they noticed that a cationic polymer, chitosan, adsorbed on the surface of nanocapsules was able to provide the best corneal drug penetration without any local intolerance as compared to another positively charged polymer. This was achieved by a combination of effects: Penetration of particles into the corneal epithelial cells, mucoadhesion of positively charged particles onto negatively charged membranes, and a specific effect on the tight junctions (134).

This effect of improvement of ocular absorption was also reported by Calvo et al. (135) with the immunosuppressive peptide cyclosporin A. The corneal level of the drug was increased fivefold as compared with an oily solution of the drug owing to a highly loaded nanocapsule preparation, also containing poly(ε-caprolactone). The efficacy of this topical formulation has also been observed on a penetrating keratoplasty rejection model in the rat (136). Le Bourlais et al. (137) also proposed an alternative preparation of cyclosporin nanocapsules based on poly (alkylcyanoacrylate) dispersed in poly(acrylic acid) gel able to drastically reduce toxicity of poly(alkylcyanocrylates) on the cornea and to promote absorption of the drug.

REFERENCES

1. Scheffel, U.; Rhodes, B.A.; Natarajan, T.K.; Wagner, H.N. Albumin Microspheres for the Study of the Reticulo-Endothelial System. J. Nucl. Med. **1972**, *13*, 498–503.
2. Marty, J.J.; Oppenheim, R.C.; Speiser, P. Nanoparticles: A New Colloidal Drug Delivery Systems. Pharm. Acta Helv. **1978**, *53*, 17–23.
3. Birrenbach, G.; Speiser, P. Polymerized Micelles and their use as Adjuvants in Immunology. J. Pharm. Sci. **1976**, *65*, 1763–1766.
4. Kreuter, J.; Speiser, P. New Adjuvants on a Poly(methylmethacrylate) Base. Infec. Immunol. **1976**, *13*, 204–210.
5. Couvreur, P.; Kante, B.; Roland, M.; Guiot, P.; Baudhuin, P.; Speiser, P. Poly(cyanoacrylate) Nanoparticles as Potential Lysosomotropic Carriers: Preparation, Morphological and Sorptive Properties. J. Pharm. Pharmacol. **1979**, *31*, 331–332.
6. Gurny, R.; Peppas, N.A.; Harrington, D.D.; Banker, G.S. Development of Biodegradable and Injectable Lattices for

Controlled Release Potent Drugs. Drug Dev. Ind. Pharm. **1981**, *7*, 1–25.

7. Al Khoury-Fallouh, N.; Roblot-Treupel, L.; Fessi, H.; Devissaguet, J.P.; Puisieux, F. Development of a New Process for the Manufacture of Poly(isobutylcyanoacrylate) Nanocapsules. Int. J. Pharm. **1986**, *28*, 125–136.

8. Fessi, H.; Devissaguet, J.P.; Puisieux, F. Procédé De Préparation Des Systèmes Colloïdaux Dispersibles Sous Forme De Nanocapsules, French Patent 86.18.444, 1986.

9. Legrand, P.; Barratt, G.; Mosqueira, V.; Fessi, H.; Devissaguet, J.P. Polymeric Nanocapsules as Drug Delivery Systems: A Review. S.T.P. Pharma Sci. **1999**, *9*, 411–418.

10. Fessi, H.; Devissaguet, J.P.; Puisieux, F. Procédé De Préparation De Systèmes Colloïdaux Dispersibles D'une Substance Sous Forme De Nanoparticules, French Patent 2.608.988, 1986.

11. Gasco, M.; Trotta, M. Nanoparticles from Microemulsions. Int. J. Pharm. **1986**, *29*, 267–268.

12. Alléman, E.; Doelker, E.; Gurny, R. Preparation of Aqueous Polymeric Nanodispersions by a Reversible Salting-Out Process, Influence of Process Parameters on Particle Size. Int. J. Pharm. **1992**, *87*, 247–253.

13. Quintanar-Guerrero, D.; Alléman, E.; Doelker, E.; Fessi, H. Preparation and Characterization of Nanocapsules from Preformed Polymers by a New Process Based on Emulsification–Diffusion Technique. Pharm. Res. **1998**, *15*, 1056–1062.

14. Quintanar-Guerrero, D.; Alléman, E.; Fessi, H.; Doelker, E. Pseudolatex Preparation Using a Novel Emulsion–Diffusion Process Involving Direct Displacement of Partially Water-Miscible Solvents by Distillation. Int. J. Pharm. **1999**, *188*, 155–164.

15. Zambaux, M.F.; Bonneauz, F.; Gref, R.; Maincent, P.; Dellacherie, E.; Alonso, M.J.; Labrude, P.; Vigneron, C. Influence of Experimental Parameters on the Characteristics of Poly(lactic acid) Nanoparticles Prepared by a Double Emulsion Method. J. Controlled. Release **1998**, *50*, 31–40.

16. Vauthier, C.; Couvreur, P. Development of Polysaccharide Nanoparticles as Novel Drug Carrier Systems. *Handbook of Pharmaceutical Controlled Release Technology*; Wise, Trantolo, Cichon, Inyang, Stottmeister, Eds.; Chap. 21, Marcel Dekker, Inc.: New York, 2000; 413–429.

17. Gref, R.; Minamitake, Y.; Peracchia, M.T.; Domb, A.; Trubetskoy, V.; Torchilin, V.; Langer, R. Poly(ethylene Glycol)-Coated Nanospheres: Potential Carriers for Intravenous Drug Administration. Pharm. Biotechnol. **1997**, *10*, 167–198.

18. Vauthier-Holtzscherer, C.; Benabbou, S.; Spenlehauer, G.; Veillard, M.; Couvreur, P. Methodology for the Preparation of Ultradispersed Polymer Systems. S.T.P. Pharma Sci. **1991**, *1*, 109–116.

19. Kreuter, J. Nanoparticles. *Colloidal Drug Delivery Systems*; Kreuter, J., Ed.; Marcel Dekker, Inc.: New York, 1994; 219–342.

20. Quintanar-Guerrero, D.; Alléman, E.; Fessi, H.; Doelker, E. Preparation Techniques and Mechanisms of Formation of Biodegradable Nanoparticles from Preformed Polymers. Drug Dev. Ind. Pharm. **1998**, *24*, 1113–1128.

21. De Jaeghere, F.; et al. Nanoparticles. *The Encyclopedia of Controlled Drug Delivery*; Mathiowitz, E., Ed.; Wiley and Sons, Inc.: New York, 1999; 641–664.

22. Lowell, P.A., El-Aasser, M.S. Eds.; *Emulsion Polymerization and Emulsion Polymers,* Wiley: New York, 1997; 801.

23. Seijo, B.; Fattal, E.; Roblot-Treupel, L.; Couvreur, P. Design of Nanoparticles of Less than 50 nm in Diameter. Preparation, Characterization and Drug Loading. Int. J. Pharm. **1990**, *62*, 1–7.

24. Peracchia, M.T.; Vauthier, C.; Popa, M.; Puisieux, F.; Couvreur, P. Investigation of the Formation of Sterically Stabilized Poly(ethyleneglycol/isobutylcyanoacrylate) Nanoparticles by Chemical Grafting of Poly(ethylene glycol) During Polymerization of Isobutylcyanoacrylate. S.T.P. Pharma Sci. **1997**, *7*, 513–520.

25. De Keyser, J.L.; Poupaert, J.H.; Dumont, P. Poly(diethyl methylidenemalonate) Nanoparticles as a Potential Drug Carrier: Preparation, Distribution and Elimination After Intravenous and Peroral Administration to Mice. J. Pharm. Sci. **1991**, *80*, 67–70.

26. Gallardo, M.M.; Couarraze, G.; Denizot, B.; Treupel, L.; Couvreur, P.; Puisieux, F. Preparation and Purification of Isohexylcyanoacrylate Nanocapsules. Int. J. Pharm. **1993**, *100*, 55–64.

27. Aboubakar, M.; Puisieux, F.; Couvreur, P.; Deyme, M.; Vauthier, C. Study of the Mechanism of Insulin Encapsulation in Poly(isobutylcyanoacrylate) Nanocapsules Obtained by Interfacial Polymerization. J. Biomed. Mater. Res. **1999**, *47*, 568–576.

28. Watnasirichaikul, S.; Rades, R.; Tucker, I.G.; Davies, N.M. Manipulating the Release of Insulin from Nanocapsules Prepared by Interfacial Polymerization of Microemulsions, Proceedings of the 27th International Symposium on Controlled Release of Bioactive Materials of the Controlled Release Society, Inc.: Paris France July 9–13 2000, Abstract # 6138.

29. Lambert, G.; Fattal, E.; Pinto-Alphandary, H.; Gulik, A.; Couvreur, P. Polyisobutylcyanoacrylate Nanocapsules Containing an Aqueous Core as a Novel Colloidal Carrier for the Delivery of Oligonucleotides. Biochimie **1998**, *80*, 969–976.

30. De Miguel, I.; Ioualalen, K.; Bonnefous, M.; Peyrot, M.; Nguyen, F.; Cervilla, M.; Soulet, N.; Dirson, R.; Rieumajou, V.; Imbertie, L.; Solers, C.; Cazes, S.; Favre, G.; Samain, D. Synthesis and Characterization of Supramolecular Biovector (SMBV) Specifically Designed for the Entrapment of Ionic Molecules. Biochim. Biophys. Acta. **1995**, *1237*, 49–58.

31. Stainmesse, S. *Etude galénique D'un Nouveau Procédé D'obtention De Vecteurs Colloïdaux Submicroniques à Partir D'une Protéine Ou D'un Polymère Synthétique*; Thesis Université De Paris Sud, 1990.

32. Weber, C.; Coester, C.; Kreuter, J.; Langer, K. Dessolvation Process and Surface Characterization of Protein Nanoparticles. Int. J. Pharm. **2000**, *194*, 94–102.

33. Leong, K.W.; Mao, H.Q.; Truong-Le, V.L.; Roy, K.; Walsh, S.M.; August, J.T. DNA-Polycation Nanospheres as Non-Viral Gene Delivery Vehicles. J. Control. Rel. **1998**, *53*, 183–193.

34. Truong-Le, V.L.; Walsh, S.M.; Schweibert, E.; Mao, H.Q.; Guggino, W.B.; August, J.T.; Leong, K.W. Gene

Transfer by DNA-Gelatin Nanospheres. Arch. Biochem. Biophys. **1999**, *361*, 47–56.

35. Rajaonarivony, M.; Vauthier, C.; Couarraze, G.; Puisieux, F.; Couvreur, P. Development of a New Drug Carrier Made from Alginate. J. Pharm. Sci. **1993**, *82*, 912–918.

36. Calvo, P.; Remunan-Lopez, C.; Vila-Jato, J.L.; Alonso, M.J. Novel Hydrophilic Chitosan-Polyethylene Oxide Nanoparticles as Protein Carriers. J. Appl. Polym. Sci. **1997**, *63*, 125–132.

37. Vanderhoff, J.W.; El-Aasser, M.S.; Ugelstad, J. Polymer Emulsification Process, U.S. Patent 4.177.177, 1979.

38. Illum, L.; Davis, S.S. The Organ Uptake of Intravenously Administered Colloidal Particles can be Altered Using Non-Ionic Surfactant (Poloxamer 338). FEBS Let. **1984**, *167*, 79–82.

39. Gref, R.; Minamitake, Y.; Peracchia, M.T.; Trubeskoy, V.; Torchilin, V.; Langer, R. Biodegradable Long-Circulating Nanospheres. Science **1994**, *263*, 1600–1603.

40. Peracchia, M.T.; Desmaële, D.; Couvreur, P.; D'Angelo, J. Synthesis of a Novel Poly(PEG-Cyanoacrylate-co-Alkylcyanoacrylate) Amphiphilic Copolymer for the Development of "Stealth" PEG-Coated Nanoparticles. Macromolecules **1997**, *30*, 846–851.

41. Peracchia, M.T.; Desmaële, D.; Vauthier, C.; Labarre, D.; Fattal, E.; D'Angelo, J.; Couvreur, P. Development of Novel Technologies for the Synthesis of Biodegradable Pegylated Nanoparticles. *Targeting of Drugs 6: Strategies for Stealth Therapeutic Systems*; Gregoriadis, B., McCormack, B., Eds.; Plenum Press: New York, 1998; 225–239.

42. Passirani, C.; Ferrarini, L.; Barratt, G.; Devissaguet, J.P.; Labarre, D. Preparation and Characterization of Nanoparticles Bearing Heparin or Dextran Covalently-Linked to Poly(methylmethacrylate). J. Biomater. Sci. Polym. Ed.; **1999**, *10*, 47–62.

43. Stella, B.; Arpicco, S.; Peracchia, M.T.; Desmaële, D.; Hoebeke, J.; Renoir, M.; D'Angelo, J.; Cattel, L.; Couvreur, P. Characterization of Folic Acid-nanoparticles Conjugates for Tumoral Targeting Proceedings of the 27th International Symposium on Controlled Release of Bioactive Materials of the Controlled Release Society, Inc.: Paris France July 9–13, 2000; Abstract # 6307

44. Kawashima, Y.; Yamamoto, H.; Takeuchi, H.; Kuno, Y. Mucoadhesive DL-Lactide/Glycolide Copolymer Nanospheres Coated with Chitosan to Improve Oral Delivery of Elcatonin. Pharm. Dev. Technol. **2000**, *5*, 77–85.

45. Candau, F., Ottewill, R.H., Eds.; *An Introduction to Polymer Colloids;* Kluwer Academic Publishers: Dordrecht, The Netherlands, 1989; 240.

46. Giddings, J.C. Field-Flow Fractionation: Analysis of Macromolecular, Colloidal and Particular Materials. Science **1993**, *260*, 1456–1465.

47. Anger, S.; Caldwell, K.; Niehus, H.; Muller, R.H. High Resolution Size Determination of 20 nm Colloidal Gold Particles by SedFFF. Pharm. Res. **1999**, *16*, 1743–1747.

48. Tan, J.S.; Butterfield, D.E.; Voycheck, C.L.; Caldwell, K.D.; Li, J.T. Surface Modification of Nanoparticles by PEO/PPO Block Copolymers to Minimize Interactions with Blood Components and Prolong Blood Circulation in Rats. Biomaterials **1993**, *14*, 823–833.

49. Huve, P.; Verrecchia, T.; Bazile, D.; Vauthier, C.; Couvreur, P. Simultaneous Use of Size Exclusion Chromatography and Photon Correlation Spectroscopy for Poly(lactic Acid) Nanoparticle Characterization. Chromatographia **1994**, *675*, 129–139.

50. Barratt, G. Characterization of Colloidal Drug Carrier Systems with Zeta Potential Measurements. Pharmaceutical Technology Europe **1999**, *25–32*.

51. Cartensen, H.; Muller, B.W.; Muller, R.H. Adsorption of Ethoxylated Surfactants on Nanoparticles. I. Characterization by Hydrophobic Interaction Chromatography. Int. J. Pharm. **1991**, *67*, 29–37.

52. Blunk, T.; Hochstrasser, D.F.; Sanchez, J.C.; Muller, B.W.; Muller, R.H. Colloidal Carriers for IV Drug Targeting: Plasma Protein Adsorption Patterns on Surface Modified Latex Particles Evaluated by Two-Dimensional Polyacrylamide Gel Electrophoresis. Electrophoresis **1993**, *14*, 1382–1387.

53. Olivier, J.C.; Vauthier, C.; Taverna, M.; Puisieux, F.; Ferrier, D.; Couvreur, P. Stability of Orosomucoid-Coated Poly(isobutylcyanoacrylate) Nanoparticles in the Presence of Serum. J. Controlled Release **1996**, *40*, 157–168.

54. Vittaz, M.; Bazile, D.; Spenlehauer, G.; Verrecchia, T.; Veillard, M.; Puisieux, F.; Couvreur, P. Effect of PEO Surface Density on Long Circulating PLA-PEO Nano-Particles which Are Very Low Complement Activators. Biomaterials **1996**, *17*, 1575–1581.

55. Passirani, C.; Barratt, G.; Devissaguet, J.P.; Labarre, D. Interactions of Nanoparticles Bearing Heparin or Dextran Covalently Bound to Poly(methylmethacrylate) with the Complement System. Life Sci. **1998**, *62*, 775–785.

56. Irache, J.; Durrer, C.; Ponchel, G.; Duchene, D. Determination of Nanoparticle Concentration in Latexes by Turbidimetry. Int. J. Pharm. **1993**, *90*, R9–R12.

57. Kreuter, J. Physico-Chemical Characterization of Polyacrylic Nanoparticles. Int. J. Pharm. **1983**, *14*, 43–58.

58. Vauthier, C.; Schmidt, C.; Couvreur, P. Measurement of the Density of Polymeric Nanoparticulate Drug Carriers Made of Poly(alkylcyanoacrylate) and Poly(lactic Acid) Derivatives. J. Nanoparticle Res. **1999**, *1*, 411–418.

59. Fattal, E.; Rojas, J.; Youssef, M.; Couvreur, P.; Andremont, A. Liposome-Entrapped Ampicillin in the Treatment of Experimental Murine Listeriosis and Salmonellosis. Antimicrob Agents Chemother **1991**, *35*, 770–772.

60. Grislain, L.; Couvreur, P.; Lenaerts, V.; Roland, M.; Deprez-Decampeneere, D.; Speiser, P. Pharmacokinetics and Distribution of a Biodegradable Drug-Carrier. Int. J. Pharm. **1983**, *15*, 335–345.

61. Lenaerts, V.; Nagelkerke, J.F.; Van Berkel, T.J.; Couvreur, P.; Grislain, L.; Roland, M.; Speiser, P. In Vivo Uptake of Polyisobutyl Cyanoacrylate Nanoparticles by Rat Liver Kupffer, Endothelial, and Parenchymal Cells. J. Pharm. Sci. **1984**, *73*, 980–982.

62. Lenaerts, V.; Couvreur, P.; Christiaens-Leyh, D.; Joiris, E.; Roland, M.; Rollman, B.; Speiser, P. Degradation of Poly(Isobutyl cyanoacrylate) Nanoparticles. Biomaterials **1984**, *5*, 65–68.

63. Chavany, C.; Ledoan, T.; Couvreur, P.; Puisieux, F.; Helene, C. Polyalkylcyanoacrylate Nanoparticles as Polymeric Carriers for Antisense Oligonucleotides. Pharm. Res. **1992**, *9*, 441–449.

64. Peracchia, M.T.; Fattal, E.; Desmaele, D.; Besnard, M.; Noel, J.P.; Gomis, J.M.; Appel, M.; d'Angelo, J.;

Couvreur, P. Stealth PEGylated Polycyanoacrylate Nanoparticles for Intravenous Administration and Splenic Targeting. J. Controlled Release **1999**, *60*, 121–128.

65. Bazile, D.; Prud'homme, C.; Bassoullet, M.T.; Marlard, M.; Spenlehauer, G.; Veillard, M. Stealth Me.PEG-PLA Nanoparticles Avoid Uptake by the Mononuclear Phagocytes System. J. Pharm. Sci. **1995**, *84*, 493–498.

66. Fattal, E.; Youssef, M.; Couvreur, P.; Andremont, A. Treatment of Experimental Salmonellosis in Mice with Ampicillin-Bound Nanoparticles. Antimicrob. Agents Chemother. **1989**, *33*, 1540–1543.

67. Youssef, M.; Fattal, E.; Alonso, M.J.; Roblot-Treupel, L.; Sauzieres, J.; Tancrede, C.; Omnes, A.; Couvreur, P.; Andremont, A. Effectiveness of Nanoparticle-Bound Ampicillin in the Treatment of Listeria Monocytogenes Infection in Athymic Nude Mice. Antimicrob. Agents Chemother. **1988**, *32*, 1204–1207.

68. Forestier, F.; Gerrier, P.; Chaumard, C.; Quero, A.M.; Couvreur, P.; Labarre, C. Effect of Nanoparticle-Bound Ampicillin on the Survival of Listeria Monocytogenes in Mouse Peritoneal Macrophages. J. Antimicrob. Chemother. **1992**, *30*, 173–179.

69. Balland, O.; Pinto-Alphandary, H.; Pecquet, S.; Andremont, A.; Couvreur, P. The Uptake of Ampicillin-Loaded Nanoparticles by Murine Macrophages Infected with Salmonella Typhimurium. J. Antimicrob. Chemother. **1994**, *33*, 509–522.

70. Pinto-Alphandary, H.; Balland, O.; Laurent, M.; Andremont, A.; Puisieux, F.; Couvreur, P. Intracellular Visualization of Ampicillin-Loaded Nanoparticles in Peritoneal Macrophages Infected in Vitro with Salmonella Typhimurium. Pharm. Res. **1994**, *11*, 38–46.

71. Buchmeier, N.A.; Heffron, F. Inhibition of Macrophage Phagosome–Lysosome Fusion by Salmonella Typhimurium. Infect. Immun. **1991**, *59*, 2232–2238.

72. Page-Clisson, M.E.; Pinto-Alphandary, H.; Chachaty, E.; Couvreur, P.; Andremont, A. Drug Targeting by Polyalkylcyanoacrylate Nanoparticles is Not Efficient Against Persistent Salmonella. Pharm. Res. **1998**, *15*, 544–549.

73. Gaspar, R.; Opperdoes, F.R.; Preat, V.; Roland, M. Drug Targeting with Polyalkylcyanoacrylate Nanoparticles — In Vitro Activity of Primaquine-Loaded Nanoparticles Against Intracellular Leishmania-Donovani. Ann. Trop. Med. Parasitol. **1992**, *86*, 41–49.

74. Gaspar, R.; Preat, V.; Opperdoes, F.R.; Roland, M. Macrophage Activation by Polymeric Nanoparticles of Polyalkylcyanoacrylates: Activity Against Intracellular Leishmania Donovani Associated with Hydrogen Peroxide Production. Pharm. Res. **1992**, *9*, 782–787.

75. Fouarge, M.; Dewulf, M.; Couvreur, P.; Roland, M.; Vranckx, H. Development of Dehydroemetine Nanoparticles for the Treatment of Visceral Leishmaniasis. J. Microencapsul. **1989**, *6*, 29–34.

76. Brasseur, F.; Verdun, C.; Couvreur, P.; Deckers, C.; Roland, M. Evaluation Expérimentale De L'efficacité Thérapeutique De La Doxorubicine Associée Aux Nanoparticules De Polyalkylcyanoacrylate. *Proceedings of the 4th International Conference on Pharmaceutical Technology,* Paris, France, June, 3–5, 1986; 177–186.

77. Chiannilkulchai, N.; Driouich, Z.; Benoit, J.P.; Parodi, A.L.; Couvreur, P. Doxorubicin-loaded Nanoparticles:

Increased Efficiency in Murine Hepatic Metastases. Sel. Cancer Ther. **1989**, *5*, 1–11.

78. Chiannilkulchai, N.; Ammoury, N.; Caillou, B.; Devissaguet, J.P.; Couvreur, P. Hepatic Tissue Distribution of Doxorubicin-Loaded Nanoparticles After I.V. Administration in Reticulosarcoma M 5076 Metastasis-Bearing Mice. Cancer Chemother. Pharmacol. **1990**, *26*, 122–126.

79. Couvreur, P.; Grislain, L.; Lenaerts, V.; Brasseur, F.; Guiot, P.; Biornacki, A. Biodegradable Polymeric Nanoparticles as Drug Carrier for Antitumor Agents. *Polymeric Nanoparticles and Microparticles*; Guiot, P., Couvreur, P., Eds.; CRC Press, Inc.: Boca Raton, FL, 1986; 27–93.

80. Daemen, T.; Hofstede, G.; Ten Kate, M.T.; Bakker-Woudenberg, I.A.; Scherphof, G.L. Liposomal Doxorubicin-Induced Toxicity: Depletion and Impairment of Phagocytic Activity of Liver Macrophages. Int. J. Cancer. **1995**, *61*, 716–721.

81. Fernandez-Urrusuno, R.; Fattal, E.; Porquet, D.; Feger, J.; Couvreur, P. Evaluation of Liver Toxicological Effects Induced by Polyalkylcyanoacrylate Nanoparticles. Toxicol. Appl. Pharmacol. **1995**, *130*, 272–279.

82. Fernandez-Urrusuno, R.; Fattal, E.; Rodrigues, J.M., Jr.; Feger, J.; Bedossa, P.; Couvreur, P. Effect of Polymeric Nanoparticle Administration on the Clearance Activity of the Mononuclear Phagocyte System in Mice. J. Biomed. Mater. Res. **1996**, *31*, 401–408.

83. Gibaud, S.; Andreux, J.P.; Weingarten, C.; Renard, M.; Couvreur, P. Increased Bone Marrow Toxicity of Doxorubicin Bound to Nanoparticles. Eur. J. Cancer **1994**, *6*, 820–826.

84. Gibaud, S.; Rousseau, C.; Weingarten, C.; Favier, R.; Douay, L.; Andreux, J.P.; Couvreur, P. Polyalkylcyano acrylate Nanoparticles as Carriers for Granulocyte-Colony Stimulating Factor (G-CSF). J. Controlled Release **1998**, *52*, 131–139.

85. Demoy, M.; Gibaud, S.; Andreux, J.P.; Weingarten, C.; Gouritin, B.; Couvreur, P. Splenic Trapping of Nanoparticles: Complementary Approaches for In Situ Studies. Pharm. Res. **1997**, *14*, 463–468.

86. Verdun, C.; Brasseur, F.; Vranckx, H.; Couvreur, P.; Roland, M. Tissue Distribution of Doxorubicin Associated with PIHCA Nanoparticles. Cancer Chemother. Pharmacol. **1990**, *26*, 13–18.

87. Kartner, N.; Evernden-Porelle, D.; Bradley, G.; Ling, V. Detection of P-glycoprotein in Multidrug-Resistant Cell Lines by Monoclonal Antibodies. Nature **1985**, *316*, 820–823.

88. Brasseur, F.; Couvreur, P.; Kante, B.; Deckers-Passau, L.; Roland, M.; Deckers, C.; Speiser, P. Actinomycin D Absorbed on Polymethylcyanoacrylate Nanoparticles: Increased Efficiency Against an Experimental Tumor. Eur. J. Cancer **1980**, *16*, 1441–1445.

89. Treupel, L.; Poupon, M.F.; Couvreur, P.; Puisieux, F. Vectorisation of Doxorubicin in Nanospheres and Reversion of Pleiotropic Resistance of Tumor Cells. C. R. Acad. Sci. III **1991**, *313*, 171–174.

90. Cuvier, C.; Roblot-Treupel, L.; Millot, J.M.; Lizard, G.; Chevillard, S.; Manfait, M.; Couvreur, P.; Poupon, M.F. Doxorubicin-Loaded Nanospheres Bypass Tumor Cell Multidrug Resistance. Biochem. Pharmacol. **1992**, *44*, 509–517.

91. Bennis, S.; Chapey, C.; Couvreur, P.; Robert, J. Enhanced Cytotoxicity of Doxorubicin Encapsulated in Poly-isohexylcyanoacrylate Nanospheres Against Multidrug-Resistant Tumour Cells in Culture. Eur. J. Cancer **1994**, *1*, 89–93.

92. Nemati, F.; Dubernet, C.; Colin de Verdière, A.; Poupon, M.F.; Treupel Acar, L.; Puisieux, F.; Couvreur, P. Some Parameters Influencing Cytotoxicity of Free Doxorubicin Loaded Nanoparticles in Sensitive and Multidrug Resistant Leucemic Murine Cells: Incubation Time, Number of Particles Per Cell. Int. J. Pharm. **1994**, *102*, 55–62.

93. Colin de Verdiere, A.; Dubernet, C.; Nemati, F.; Poupon, M.F.; Puisieux, F.; Couvreur, P. Uptake of Doxorubicin from Loaded Nanoparticles in Multidrug-Resistant Leukemic Murine Cells. Cancer Chemother. Pharmacol. **1994**, *33*, 504–508.

94. Colin de Verdiere, A.C.; Dubernet, C.; Nemati, F.; Soma, E.; Appel, M.; Ferte, J.; Bernard, S.; Puisieux, F.; Couvreur, P. Reversion of Multidrug Resistance with Polyalkylcyanoacrylate Nanoparticles: Towards a Mechanism of Action. Br. J. Cancer **1997**, *76*, 198–205.

95. Soma, C.E.; Dubernet, C.; Barratt, G.; Nemati, F.; Appel, M.; Benita, S.; Couvreur, P. Ability of Doxorubicin-Loaded Nanoparticles to Overcome Multidrug Resistance of Tumor Cells After Their Capture by Macrophages. Pharm. Res. **1999**, *16*, 1710–1716.

96. al Khouri, N.; Fessi, H.; Roblot-Treupel, L.; Devissaguet, J.P.; Puisieux, F. An Original Procedure for Preparing Nanocapsules of Polyalkylcyanoacrylates for Interfacial Polymerization. Pharm. Acta Helv. **1986**, *61*, 274–281.

97. Morin, C.; Barratt, G.; Fessi, H.; Devissaguet, J.P.; Puisieux, F. Improved Intracellular Delivery of a Muramyl Dipeptide Analog by Means of Nanocapsules. Int. J. Immunopharmacol. **1994**, *16*, 451–456.

98. Seyler, I.; Appel, M.; Devissaguet, J.P.; Legrand, P.; Barratt, G. Relationship Between NO-Synthase Activity and TNF-Alpha Secretion in Mouse Macrophage Lines Stimulated by a Muramyl Peptide Entrapped in Nanocapsules. Int. J. Immunopharmacol. **1996**, *18*, 385–392.

99. Seyler, I.; Appel, M.; Devissaguet, J.P.; Legrand, P.; Barratt, G. Macrophage Activation by a Lipophilic Derivative of Muramyldipeptide. J. Nanoparticle Res. **1999**, *1*, 91–97.

100. Barratt, G.; Puisieux, F.; Yu, W.P.; Foucher, C.; Fessi, H.; Devissaguet, J.P. Anti-Metastatic Activity of MDP-L-Alanyl-Cholesterol Incorporated into Various Types of Nanocapsules. Int. J. Immunopharmacol. **1994**, *16*, 457–461.

101. Fattal, E.; Vauthier, C.; Aynie, I.; Nakada, Y.; Lambert, G.; Malvy, C.; Couvreur, P. Biodegradable Polyalkylcyanoacrylate Nanoparticles for the Delivery of Oligonucleotides. J. Controlled. Rel. **1998**, *53*, 137–143.

102. Chavany, C.; Saison-Behmoaras, T.; Le Doan, T.; Puisieux, F.; Couvreur, P.; Helene, C. Adsorption of Oligonucleotides Onto Polyisohexylcyanoacrylate Nanoparticles Protects them Against Nucleases and Increases Their Cellular Uptake. Pharm. Res. **1994**, *11*, 1370–1378.

103. Nakada, Y.; Fattal, E.; Foulquier, M.; Couvreur, P. Pharmacokinetics and Biodistribution of Oligonucleotide Adsorbed onto Poly(isobutylcyanoacrylate) Nanoparticles

104. After Intravenous Administration in Mice. Pharm. Res. **1996**, *13*, 38–43.

104. Schwab, G.; Duroux, I.; Chavany, C.; Helene, C.; Saison-Behmoaras, E. An Approach for New Anticancer Drugs: Oncogene-Targeted Antisense DNA. Ann. Oncol. **1994**, *5*, 55–58.

105. Lambert, G.; Fattal, E.; Brehier, A.; Feger, J.; Couvreur, P. Effect of Polyisobutylcyanoacrylate Nanoparticles and Lipofectin Loaded with Oligonucleotides on Cell Viability and PKCa Neosynthesis in HepG2 Cells. Biochimie, **in press**.

106. Aynie, I.; Vauthier, C.; Chacun, H.; Fattal, E.; Couvreur, P. Spongelike Alginate Nanoparticles as a New Potential System for the Delivery of Antisense Oligonucleotides. Antisense. Nucleic Acid Drug Dev. **1999**, *9*, 301–312.

107. Gautier, J.C.; Grangier, J.L.; Barbier, A.; Dupont, P.; Dussosoy, D.; Pastor, G.; Couvreur, P. Biodegradable Nanoparticles for Subcutaneous Administration of Growth Hormone Releasing Factor (hGRF). J. Controlled. Rel. **1992**, *3*, 205–210.

108. Kreuter, J.; Speiser, P.P. In Vitro Studies of Poly(methyl methacrylate) Adjuvants. J. Pharm. Sci. **1976**, *65*, 1624–1627.

109. Kreuter, J. Possibilities of Using Nanoparticles as Carriers for Drugs and Vaccines. J. Microencapsul **1988**, *5*, 115–127.

110. Kreuter, J.; Liehl, E. Long-Term Studies of Microencapsulated and Adsorbed Influenza Vaccine Nanoparticles. J. Pharm. Sci. **1981**, *70*, 367–371.

111. Kreuter, J.; Haenzel, I. Mode of Action of Immunological Adjuvants: Some Physicochemical Factors Influencing the Effectivity of Polyacrylic Adjuvants. Infect Immun **1978**, *19*, 667–675.

112. Kreuter, J.; Berg, U.; Liehl, E.; Soliva, M.; Speiser, P.P. Influence of the Particle Size on the Adjuvant Effect of Particulate Polymeric Adjuvants. Vaccine **1986**, *4*, 125–129.

113. Kreuter, J.; Liehl, E.; Berg, U.; Soliva, M.; Speiser, P.P. Influence of Hydrophobicity on the Adjuvant Effect of Particulate Polymeric Adjuvants. Vaccine **1988**, *6*, 253–256.

114. Jani, P.; Halbert, G.W.; Langridge, J.; Florence, A.T. The Uptake and Translocation of Latex Nanospheres and Microspheres After Oral Administration to Rats. J. Pharm. Pharmacol. **1989**, *41*, 809–812.

115. Le Fevre, H.E.; Joel, D.D.; Shidlousky, G. Retention of Ingested Latex Particles in Peyers Patches of Gerinfree and Conventional Mice. Soc. Exp. Biol. Med. **1985**, *179*, 522–528.

116. Damge, C.; Michel, C.; Aprahamian, M.; Couvreur, P.; Devissaguet, J.P. Nanocapsules as Carriers for Oral Peptide Delivery. J. Control. Rel. **1990**, *13*, 233–239.

117. Kreuter, J.; Muller, V.; Munz, K. Quantitative and Microautoradiographic Study on Mouse Intestinal Distribution of Polycyanoacrylate Nanoparticles. Int. J. Pharm. **1989**, *55*, 39–45.

118. Aprahamian, M.; Michel, C.; Humbert, W.; Devissaguet, J.P.; Damge, C. Transmucosal Passage of Polyalkylcyanoacrylate Nanocapsules as a New Drug Carrier in the Small Intestine. Biol. Cell **1987**, *61*, 69–76.

119. Damge, C.; Michel, C.; Aprahamian, M.; Couvreur, P. New Approach for Oral Administration of Insulin with

Polyalkylcyanoacrylate Nanocapsules as Drug Carrier. Diabetes **1988**, *37*, 246–251.

120. Lowe, P.J.; Temple, C.S. Calcitonin and Insulin in Isobutylcyanoacrylate Nanocapsules: Protection Against Proteases and Effect on Intestinal Absorption in Rats. J. Pharm. Pharmacol. **1994**, *46*, 547–552.

121. Aboubakar, M.; Puisieux, F.; Couvreur, P.; Vauthier, C. Physico-Chemical Characterization of Insulin-Loaded Poly(isobutylcyanoacrylate) Nanocapsules Obtained by Interfacial Polymerization. Int. J. Pharm. **1999**, *183*, 63–66.

122. Michel, C.; Aprahamian, M.; Defontaine, L.; Couvreur, P.; Damge, C. The Effect of Site of Administration in the Gastrointestinal Tract on the Absorption of Insulin from Nanocapsules in Diabetic Rats. J. Pharm. Pharmacol. **1991**, *43*, 1–5.

123. Aboubakar, M.; Couvreur, P.; Pinto-Alphandary, H.; Gouritin, B.; Lacour, B.; Farinotti, R.; Puisieux, F.; Vauthier, C. Insulin-Loaded Nanocapsules for Oral Administration: In Vitro and In Vivo Investigation. Drug Devel. Res. **2000**, *49*, 109–117.

124. Damge, C.; Vranckx, H.; Balschmidt, P.; Couvreur, P. Poly(alkyl cyanoacrylate) Nanospheres for Oral Administration of Insulin. J. Pharm. Sci. **1997**, *86*, 1403–1409.

125. Damge, C.; Vonderscher, J.; Marbach, P.; Pinget, M. Poly(alkyl cyanoacrylate) Nanocapsules as a Delivery System in the Rat for Octreotide, A Long-Acting Somatostatin Analogue. J. Pharm. Pharmacol. **1997**, *49*, 949–954.

126. O'Hagan, D.T.; Palin, K.; Davis, S.S. Poly(butyl2cyano acrylate) Particles as Adjuvant for Oral Immunization. Vaccine **1989**, *7*, 213–216.

127. Marchal-Heussler, L.; Sirbat, D.; Hoffman, M.; Maincent, P. Poly(epsilon-caprolactone) Nanocapsules in Carteolol Ophthalmic Delivery. Pharm. Res. **1993**, *10*, 386–390.

128. Marchal-Heussler, L.; Fessi, H.; Devissaguet, J.P.; Hoffman, M.; Maincent, P. Colloidal Drug Delivery Systems for the Eye. A Comparison of the Efficacy of Three Different Polymers: Polyisobutylcyanoacrylate, Poly(lac-tic-co-glycolic Acid, Poly-Epsilon Caprolactone. S.T.P. Pharma **1992**, *2*, 98–104.

129. Losa, C.; Marchal-Heussler, L.; Orallo, F.; Vila Jato, J.L.; Alonso, M.J. Design of New Formulations for Topical Ocular Administration: Polymeric Nanocapsules Containing Metipranolol. Pharm. Res. **1993**, *10*, 80–87.

130. Calvo, P.; Thomas, C.; Alonso, M.J.; Vila Jato, J.L.; Robinson, J.R. Study of the Mechanism of Interaction of Poly(epsilon caprolactone) Nanocapsules with the Cornea by Confocal Laser Scanning Microscopy. Int. J. Pharm. **1994**, *103*, 283–291.

131. Zimmer, A.; Kreuter, J.; Robinson, J.R. Studies on the Transport Pathway of PBCA Nanoparticles in Ocular Tissues. J. Microencapsul **1991**, *8*, 497–504.

132. Calvo, P.; Alonso, M.J.; Vila-Jato, J.L.; Robinson, J.R. Improved Ocular Bioavailability of Indomethacin by Novel Ocular Drug Carriers. J. Pharm. Pharmacol. **1996**, *48*, 1147–1152.

133. Calvo, P.; Vila-Jato, J.L.; Alonso, M.J. Effect of Lysozyme on the Stability of Polyester Nanocapsules and Nanoparticles: Stabilization Approaches. Biomaterials **1997**, *18*, 1305–1310.

134. Calvo, P.; Vila-Jato, J.L.; Alonso, M.J. Evaluation of Cationic Polymer-Coated Nanocapsules as Ocular Drug Carriers. Int. J. Pharm. **1997**, *153*, 41–50.

135. Calvo, P.; Sanchez, A.; Martinez, J.; Lopez, M.I.; Calonge, M.; Pastor, J.C.; Alonso, M.J. Polyester Nanocapsules as New Topical Ocular Delivery Systems for Cyclosporin. A. Pharm. Res. **1996**, *13*, 311–315.

136. Juberias, J.R.; Calonge, M.; Gomez, S.; Lopez, M.I.; Calvo, P.; Herreras, J.M.; Alonso, M.J. Efficacy of Topical Cyclosporine-Loaded Nanocapsules on Keratoplasty Rejection in the Rat. Curr. Eye Res. **1998**, *17*, 39–46.

137. Le Bourlais, C.A.; Chevanne, F.; Turlin, B.; Acar, L.; Zia, H.; Sado, P.A.; Needham, T.E.; Leverge, R. Effect of Cyclosporine a Formulations on Bovine Corneal Absorption: Ex-Vivo Study. J. Microencapsul **1997**, *14*, 457–467.

NON-INVASIVE PEPTIDE AND PROTEIN DELIVERY

Patrick J. Sinko
Gerald Scucci
Rutgers University, Piscataway, New Jersey

Yong-Hee Lee
Trega Biosciences, Inc., San Diego, California

OVERVIEW

Peptide and protein drugs have been increasingly utilized in the treatment of various diseases since recent dramatic advances in recombinant DNA and modern synthetic technologies have allowed for the cost-effective production of considerable quantities of protein pharmaceuticals. For the past several decades, major efforts have been directed toward developing effective means for the nonparental (i.e., noninvasive) delivery of protein pharmaceuticals. However, low bioavailability has limited the success of noninvasive delivery attempts (1–5). The primary reasons for low bioavailability include unfavorable physicochemical characteristics such as large molecular weight, charge, hydrophilicity, and physicochemical instability, and biological limitations such as poor membrane permeability, and presystemic enzymatic metabolism. Administration via these routes often requires specialized delivery systems, absorption enhancers, and/or proteolytic enzyme inhibitors to improve bioavailability. Various noninvasive routes of administration have been investigated and reviewed to deliver protein pharmaceuticals, including oral, mucosal-membrane, pulmonary, and transdermal routes (6, 7). To date, nearly all therapeutic proteins are administered by intravenous (IV), subcutaneous (SC), or intramuscular (IM) injection. A partial listing of protein pharmaceuticals in clinical use is shown in Table 1.

The only notable success in the noninvasive delivery of peptides or protein pharmaceuticals has been the oral delivery of small peptide drug analogs such as the penicillins, cephalosporins, ACE inhibitors, and renin inhibitors (8, 9). The intestinal absorption pathways of small peptides differ significantly from those for larger peptides and proteins. Smaller peptide drugs undergo carrier-mediated absorption by means of the human intestinal peptide transporters (hPepT1 and hpt1) (8–10). Peptides analogs with greater than three amino acid residues are not typically transported via the peptide

carriers, although the exact mechanisms of absorption have not yet been fully elucidated. The focus of this chapter is on the noninvasive delivery of larger peptide and protein pharmaceuticals. Some success has been achieved in the noninvasive delivery of protein pharmaceuticals, most notably in nasal delivery. Several examples of systemic protein delivery via noninvasive routes are described in this chapter. The chapter concludes with a focused discussion on strategies for the oral delivery of protein pharmaceuticals using a model small protein drug, salmon calcitonin (sCT).

NONINVASIVE ROUTES

Oral Delivery

The mucosal surface of the digestive tract is a vast area covered by a monolayer of epithelial cells joined by tight junctions that provide an effective barrier to absorption. The potential convenience and improved patient compliance associated with oral delivery have led to considerable research in this area. Some protein drugs have surprisingly good absorption characteristics. For example, the cyclic 11-amino acid compound cyclosporine has a relatively high bioavailability when properly formulated. Compared with the standard formulation (Sandimmune, Novartis, NJ), the microemulsion formulation (Neoral) increases the AUC and C_{max}, and reduces t_{max}, intrapatient variability, and the effect of bile on cyclosporine absorption (11, 12). Oral absorption of cyclosporine from the Sandimmune formulation is shown in Fig. 1. With the exception of cyclosporine, very limited success has been achieved in delivering protein pharmaceuticals orally (Table 1). Detectable quantities of growth hormone, insulin, and calcitonin can be found in the systemic circulation after oral administration. However, the absorption of these drugs is highly inefficient. Typically, upward of 1000 times more drug is required

Table 1 Therapeutic polypeptide drugs and their clinical application

Therapeutics	Molecular weight (in Daltons)	Indications	Route of administration[a]
Alglucerase	59,300	Gaucher's disease	IV infusion
α-1 Antitrypsin	52,000	Congenital α-1 antitrypsin deficiency	IV infusion
Calcitonin	4500	Paget's disease, postmenopausal osteoporosis, hypercalcemia	IM, SC, intranasal
Cyclosporine	1200	Prophylaxis for allogeneic organ rejection	Oral, IV infusion
Desmopressin	1183	Intranasal: primary nocturnal enuresis	Intranasal, SC, IV infusion
		IV Infusion: hemophilia A and von Willebrand's disease	
Dornase alfa	37,000	Cystic fibrosis	Inhalation
Erythropoietin	30,400	Treatment of anemia	SC, IV infusion
Etanercept	150,000	Rheumatoid arthritis	SC
Factor IX	55,000	Christmas disease	IV infusion
Filgrastim	18,800	Severe chronic neutropenia	SC
Glatiramer acetate	Average: 4,700–11,000	Multiple sclerosis	SC
Imiglucerase	60,430	Gaucher's disease	IV infusion
Insulin	Varies: minimum; 6000	Diabetes mellitus	SC, IV infusion
Interferon alfacon-1	19,434	Hepatitis C infection	SC
α-Interferon	19,271	Hairy cell leukemia	IM, SC
β-Interferon	22,500	Multiple sclerosis	SC
γ-Interferon	16,000–25,000	Reduce frequency of infections associated with chronic granulomatous disease	SC
Oxytocin	1007.2	Labor induction	IV infusion
Proleukin	15,300	Carcinoma	IV infusion
Reteplase	39,571	Management of acute myocardial infarction	IV infusion
Sargramostim	Varies: 19,500, 16,800; and 15,500	Myeloid reconstitution	SC, IV infusion
Somatrem	22,000	Growth hormone	SC, IM
Streptokinase	47,000	Fibrinolytic	IV infusion
Thymosin α1 (Thymalfasin)	3108	Chronic hepatitis B	SC (currently in phase 3 studies)
Tissue plasminogen activator	70,000	Fibrinolytic	IV infusion

[a] SC, subcutaneous; IM, intramuscular; IV, intravenous.

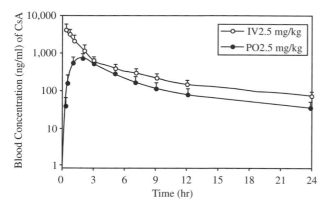

Fig. 1 Mean blood cyclosporine A (CsA) concentration (ng/ml)-time curves in 22 psoriatic patients (mean ± SD) after a single IV administration of 2.5 mg/kg (IV infusion over 2 h with 0.5% solution of CsA in 0.9% NaCl) and after 1 week, oral administration of the same dose (Sandimmune, oral solution 100 mg/ml). The mean bioavailibility was 44% (range, 22–63%). (From Galla, F.; Marzocchi, V.; Croattino, L.; Poz, D.; Baraldo, M.; Furlanut, M. Oral and Intravenous Disposition of Cyclosporine in Psoriatic Patients. Ther. Drug Monitor. **1995**, *17*, 302–304.)

to achieve the same effect after oral administration than when given by IV or SC injection. The oral delivery of protein drugs is critical for keeping health care costs low owing to enhanced compliance, reduced expenses compared with inpatient therapies, etc. The primary problems encountered with the oral delivery of protein pharmaceuticals include the poor intrinsic permeability owing to their hydrophilic nature and large molecular size, presystemic enzymatic metabolism by intestinal proteases and peptidases, chemical instability including tendencies to aggregate, and/or nonspecific binding to a variety of physical and biological surfaces. Because protein drugs are highly susceptible to all these factors, protein-delivery systems will have to simultaneously address all the issues to achieve higher bioavailability (13).

Although several approaches can be taken toward solving an oral bioavailability problem, the causes of incomplete bioavailability must first be understood. When poor membrane permeability is identified as a probable cause, approaches to formulate the drug with absorption enhancers that transiently modify biological membranes are used. Potential approaches to reduce presystemic metabolism include the transient modulation of the intestinal environment by limiting the activity of intestinal enzymes through the use of protease inhibitors (14); adjusting the local pH to values that correspond to the pH minima of specific enzymes present in the gut (15–17); maintaining high local drug concentrations to saturate

enzymes; regiospecific targeting because of regional differences in the activity of intestinal proteolytic enzymes, dilution, and spreading patterns; and surface area differences (18, 19). Other potential oral delivery approaches are chemical modification of proteins to produce prodrugs and analogs (20–22), substitution of D-amino acids to reduce hydrolysis (23, 24), and use of bioadhesive polymers that have a variety of mechanisms for enhancing protein drug absorption including inhibition of proteolytic enzymes or reducing the resistance of tight junctions (25).

Several attempts have been made to facilitate intestinal protein drug absorption by targeting specific absorptive transporter systems, such as the monosaccharide or bile acid transporters, or by modulating the secretory transport activity of *P*-glycoprotein (Pgp) (9). The coupling of unstable peptides with sugars has been demonstrated to improve hydrolytic stability and membrane permeability (26). Insulin has been modified with *p*-nitrophenyl-α-D-glucopyranoside and *p*-nitrophenyl-α-D-mannopyranoside. The coupling of these agents enhanced membrane permeation by an unknown mechanism and reduced the potential for enzymatic hydrolysis (27). In terms of modulating secretory transport, the intestinal absorption of some peptides that interact with Pgp, such as cyclosporine, tends to increase to some extent when efflux transporter inhibitors are used (28). Another delivery strategy includes the utilization of macromolacular ligands. Recently, the cellular and molecular mechanisms whereby macromolecules and particles are internalized have been studied (10). Although the use of endocytic pathways is currently highly inefficient, the mechanisms are being studied in cell culture models such as Caco-2 and Madin-Darby canine kidney (MDCK) cells in the hope of improving efficiency. By gaining a better understanding of how to target membrane transport mechanisms or modulate biological barriers, the oral bioavailability of protein drugs may be enhanced. Until then, the oral delivery of protein drugs will remain a considerable challenge for the foreseeable future, given the multiple biological obstacles that must be overcome to achieve therapeutic blood concentrations.

Mucosal Delivery

The high vascularity and accessibility of the mucosal membranes have made this tissue a potential route of protein delivery. Mucous membranes include the nasal, buccal, ocular, rectal, and vaginal membranes (29). Advantages of mucosal routes are that they bypass hepatic first-pass metabolism and are readily accessible, and locally acting agents such as penetration enhancers, enzyme inhibitors, and mucus-suppressing agents can be used.

Mucus is a highly viscous product that forms a protective coating over the lining of organs in contact with external media. Mucus is a mixture of large glycoproteins (mucins), water, electrolytes, sloughed epithelial cells, enzymes, bacteria and bacterial products, and various other materials, depending on the source and location of the mucus (30). Mucins are synthesized either by goblet cells lining the mucosal epithelium or by special exocrine glands with mucus cell acini. Mucoadhesive polymers have received considerable attention as platforms for protein drug delivery. Advantages include the ability to deliver drugs locally, prolong the residence time, and optimize contact with the absorbing surface to permit modification of tissue permeability to inhibit enzyme activity or to suppress mucus production (25–30). Bioadhesive bonds may be physical or mechanical bonds, secondary chemical bonds, or primary chemical bonds. Other approaches for mucosal protein delivery are formulating proteins in liposomes (7), microemulsions, and small particles (e.g., nanoparticles) (31, 32). The common rationale in all three cases is the protection of proteins from the local environment before to absorption and localization of the protein at or near the cellular membrane to optimize the driving force for passive permeation.

Nasal delivery

The nasal route has been intensively investigated because of its convenience (33). It presents a large surface area ($\sim$200 cm^2) that is lined by a single layer of columnar epithelial and goblet cells overlaying a rich blood supply. The extensive network of blood capillaries underneath the nasal mucosa provides an important part of the driving force required for the systemic delivery of proteins. Because the mucosal surface is covered by mucin that is cleared on a 15–30 min cycle, the residence time of solutions in the nasal mucosa is short. Therefore, mucoadhesive polymer solutions are typically required to increase the residence time. This route has been shown to be acceptable for peptides with 10 or fewer residues, whereas satisfactory bioavailability is obtained for proteins of 20 or more residues only when permeation enhancers are used (33).

The nasal mucosa contains enzymes capable of hydrolyzing peptides. The predominant enzyme appears to be aminopeptidase, among other exopeptidases and endopeptidases. The cytochrome P-450 activity in the olfactory region of the nasal epithelium is higher than in the liver (34). Phase II enzyme activity has also been found in the nasal epithelium (34). The metabolic cleavage of thyrotropin-releasing hormone (TRH) and met-enkephalin has been demonstrated in human nasal epithelial cell

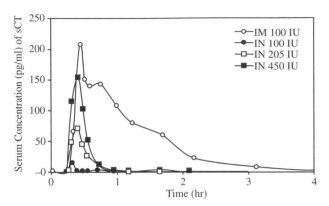

Fig. 2 Mean serum salmon calcitonin (sCT) concentration (pg/mL)-time curve after intramuscular (IM) administration of 100 IU of sCT and intranasal (IN) administration of 100, 205, and 450 IU of sCT with 0.5% sodium tauro-24,25-dihydrofusidate (STDHF) in 10 healthy subjects (7 males, 3 females). Relative to the i.m. dose, the bioavailabilities of the i.n. formulations containing 0.5% STDHF were 3.9, 7.9, and 7.4%, respectively. The nasal calcitonin doses were administered as one 100-μl spray per nostril using two single-dose spray units. sCT-STDHF formulations were prepared by reconstitution of solid sCT with a sterile isotonic (NaCl) solution of 0.5% STDHF in 20 mM acetate buffer, pH 5.0, and used immediately. (From Lee, W.A.; Ennis, R.D.; Longenecker, J.P.; Bengtsson, P. The Bioavailability of Intranasal Salmom Calcitonin in Healthy Volunteers with and without a Permeation Enhancer. Pharm. Res. **1994**, *11*, 747–750.)

monolayers, suggesting that the nasal mucosa may be a significant metabolic barrier to the systemic delivery of protein drugs (35). Permeation enhancers and protease inhibitors are usually coadministered to achieve successful delivery of proteins by this route. Intranasal absorption of salmon calcitonin is demonstrated in Fig. 2. Relative to the IM dose, the bioavailability of intranasal (IN) administration of sCT was low, 3.9–7.9%. When eel calcitonin (eCT) was coadministered with nafamostat mesilate, a protease inhibitor, or with sodium decanoate, the sodium salt of fatty acid, the nasal absorption of eCT was significant, and serum calcium (Ca^{2+}) concentration was effectively decreased (36). Several nasal products have been available clinically including buserelin, desmopressin, oxytocin, and calcitonin (29).

Buccal delivery

Delivery of protein drugs through the buccal mucosa has also received considerable attention (37). Despite its apparent disadvantages, such as limited absorptive surface area and moderate mucosal permeability, the buccal route might be acceptable for small-or medium-sized peptide drugs. Potential advantages for buccal delivery are the avoidance of gastrointestinal (GI) or hepatic first-pass metabolism, the feasibility of locally controlled absorption enhancement, the ease of administration and removal of an administered device, and the possibility of prolonged drug delivery and action. The buccal epithelium has an average thickness of 500–600 μm. The epithelial cells at the outer surface are continuously peeled off because of abrasion that occurs during mastication. Therefore, starting from nondifferentiated cells located above the basal membrane, fresh epithelial cells are produced by mitosis. During their 5- to 8-day passage from the basal membrane to the outer surface, the epithelial cells undergo maturation resulting in a change in form and size.

The buccal cavity exhibits greater proteolytic enzyme activity than does the nasal or vaginal mucosa. The metabolic activity is shown to reside primarily in the epithelium (38). A mucoadhesive buccal patch was evaluated in rabbits for transmucosal delivery of oxytocin (OT) after incorporation into custom coformulations of Carbopol 974P and silicone polymer (39). It was observed that plasma OT concentrations remained 20- to 28-fold greater from 0.5 to 3.0 h than concentrations in control animals administered placebo patches. Several transmucosal therapeutic systems (TmTs) were also investigated to study the enhanced/controlled delivery of leuteinizing hormone-releasing hormone (LHRH) in dogs (40). The TmTs is a track field-shaped bilayer mucoadhesive device consisting of fast- and sustained-release layers. A stream of 0.5–2 L of saliva constantly washes the oral cavity daily. The resulting salivary layer covering all oral epithelia can interfere with the penetration of drugs as well as with the adhesion of buccally administered delivery devices. Therefore, several factors must be considered in designing buccal dosage forms—the taste of drugs and excipients, the size of the dosage form, and the mechanism for fixing the dosage form onto the oral mucosa. Nevertheless, even under optimized conditions, the buccal delivery of proteins may not allow for bioavailabilities as high as that with other mucosal sites. Thus, the chances for buccal protein delivery, if any, will be restricted to special cases and for special proteins of high permeability. In this instance, however, buccal delivery might be a preferred route of administration, mainly owing to the undisputed acceptance and compliance of oral dosage forms and to the unmatched robustness of the epithelium.

Ocular delivery

The ocular route has been investigated for the systemic delivery of protein drugs (41, 42). Systemic absorption of proteins after topical administration to the eye results through contact with the conjunctival and nasal mucosa, the latter occurring as a result of the drainage through the nasolacrimal duct. When systemic absorption is desired, absorption through the conjunctival and nasal mucosa needs to be maximized. The systemic delivery of proteins through the ocular route has several advantages including convenience, rapid absorption/onset, and avoidance of hepatic first-pass metabolism, and it is amenable to controlled-release delivery. However, this route typically yields low bioavailability, although it is well accepted by patients. As with other delivery routes, the size, charge, and hydrophilic nature of proteins are the primary determinants that limit their extent of absorption. Because the systemic delivery of proteins depends on their transport mechanisms and contact time with mucosal membrane of the conjunctiva and the nasolacrimal system (43), the following factors need to be considered: 1) precorneal factors such as tear drainage, instilled volume, viscosity, pH, and tonicity; 2) that the eye formulations used must avoid the potential for local irritation and/or side effects; and 3) that inclusion of permeation enhancers may be necessary when dealing with agents with a molecular weight higher than 10,000 Da.

Systemic delivery of insulin and glucagon through the ocular route was demonstrated as a feasible alternative to parental injection, particularly when permeation enhancers were added (44).

Rectal delivery

The rectal epithelium is columnar or cuboidal, with numerous goblet cells. However, unlike the small intestine, the rectal epithelium does not contain villi. The human rectum has a length of 5 inches and a surface area of only approximately 200–400 cm^2, compared with 2,000,000 cm^2 for the small intestine. Consequently, absorption from the rectum could be much lower than from the remainder of the GI tract (45). The lower venous drainage system (inferior and middle hemorrhoidal veins) is connected directly to the systemic circulation by the ileac vein and vena cava, whereas the upper venous drainage system (superior hemorrhoidal vein) is connected to the portal vein system. Thus, an opportunity to reduce the extent of hepatic first-pass elimination exists in the rectum. The rectum also has a large number of lymphatic vessels that offer an opportunity to target drug delivery to the lymphatic circulation.

Extensive studies have been conducted regarding the rectal absorption of proteins, especially insulin. However, the rectal absorption of this drug is low, probably owing to a combination of poor membrane permeability and metabolism at the absorption site (46). Therefore, it is generally believed that absorption enhancers are required to achieve therapeutic plasma levels of rectally administered proteins. The rectal route can be an extremely useful route for the delivery of drugs to infants and young children in whom difficulties can arise using per oral administration. Historically, the rectum has not been an accepted site of drug delivery. Its principal applications have been for local therapy, e.g., hemorrhoids, and for systemic delivery of drugs to populations presenting practical problems for parenteral or oral dosing (e.g., the elderly, infants, patients with epilepsy, etc.). Even though the systemic delivery of peptide can occur by this route, it is not widely accepted among the populations of the world.

Vaginal delivery

The vaginal wall consists of an epithelial layer (epithelial lamina and lamina propria), muscle layer, and tunica adventitia. It is regulated by cyclic alteration of the reproductive system, which is directly controlled by hormones such as estrogen, progesterone, leuteinizing hormone (LH), and FSH (45). Before puberty, the epithelium is very thin, but after puberty, it increases in thickness with estrogen activity. In the adult stage, the vaginal surface during the follicular phase appears homogeneous with large superficial polygonal cells with a high degree of proliferation caused by estrogen stimulation and the presence of cornification. This proliferation of cells concomitantly increases the epithelial thickness and number of layers. The lamina propria specialized supporting structure of the epithelial cells contains a blood supply, a lymphatic drainage system, and a network of nerve fibers. The vaginal epithelium is aglandular but is usually covered with a surface film of moisture. The pH of the vaginal lumen is controlled mainly by the lactic acid produced from cellular glycogen by the action of the normal microflora, Doderlein's bacilli. The arterial blood supply in the vagina is derived from the visceral branches of the internal iliac artery, and venous drainage occurs mainly via the uterine vein to the internal iliac vein.

It is known that several peptide hormones and antigenic proteins are absorbed intact through the vaginal membrane and that the bioavailability is greater than that by the oral route because of higher intercellular permeability and reduced first-pass metabolism. The amount and duration of the hypoglycemic and hypocalcemic effects induced by intrauterine delivery of insulin and calcitonin, respectively, were equivalent to those obtained after s.c. injections in intact and ovariectomized rats (47). Regarding the enzymatic barrier, few enzymes have been found in the vaginal epithelium and in the peptidase activity against enkephalins, substance P, insulin, and proinsulin in the absorptive mucous membranes in the rabbit. In fact, supernatants of homogenates of the vaginal, nasal, buccal, rectal, and ileal mucous membranes of

rabbit exhibit similar proteolytic activity (46). Vaginal delivery of sCT was demonstrated effectively in ovariectomized rats using the highly mucoadhesive polymer, the benzyl ester of hyaluronic acid (Hyaff 11), by closely adhering to the mucosal surface and by protecting the drug from enzymatic inactivation (48). Most of the vaginal preparations on the market are used for local action on the vaginal membrane, using antibacterial, antifungal, or antiviral agents.

Pulmonary Delivery

Pulmonary delivery provides an attractive route of administration for systemic protein delivery. Of all the noninvasive routes for protein delivery, the pulmonary route has provided the most encouraging data and has recently generated great interest in the biotechnology industry (49, 50). Advantages of the pulmonary route include the fact that the walls of the alveoli are thinner than are other epithelial/mucosal membranes, that the surface area of the lung is much greater, and that the lungs receive the entire blood supply from the heart. Of course, the lungs are rich in enzymes, and overcoming this barrier is no easy task. Peptide hydrolases, peptidases, and a wide variety of proteinases are present in lung cells. The respiratory tract has several unique features (51): 1) a large surface area that can be exposed to drug almost simultaneously as opposed to the intestine, which has a similar total surface area but does not allow for simultaneous exposure; 2) a high blood flow that does not directly expose absorbed drug to the clearance mechanisms present in the liver; and 3) relatively less metabolic activity.

The upper respiratory tract, including the trachea and large bronchi, has a relatively limited surface area for absorption compared with the alveolar region, which provides more than 95% of the surface area of the lung. The respiratory tract is lined on its luminal surface by a layer of columnar epithelial cells that become progressively less columnar in the smaller airways and alveolar region. The surface of the airway epithelial cells in the larger conducting airways is covered with cilia that aid in the clearance of material from the lung. Two types of epithelial cells are present in the alveolar region of the lung: the type I and the type II pneumocytes. Type I cells are flat cells with broad, thin extensions covering up to 95% of the alveolar surface, whereas type II cells are cuboidal cells without extensions that can differentiate into type I cells and participate in the repair of the epithelial cell surface after damage. The alveolar epithelium is assumed to be the site of protein delivery, based on surface area considerations. The passages leading to the lower lung from the nasal region are narrower than the oral passages. This allows for much more efficient filtration and much less efficient delivery after nasal administration and has led to the development of a variety of devices that deliver aerosols via the mouth. Dry and liquid particles can be prepared and inhaled with the aid of dry powder dispensers, liquid aerosol generators, and nebulizers. These devices produce particles that range from 1 to 5 μm, which may penetrate deeply into the alveoli of the lung. Once deposited deep in the lung, the alveoli provide a large surface area (80–140 m^2) for rapid transfer into the pulmonary circulation.

In the literature, molecules ranging to greater than 100,000 Da have been demonstrated to be appropriate candidates for pulmonary delivery. Several proteins are currently under investigation for systemic delivery, including insulin, calcitonin, leuteinizing-hormone-releasing hormone (LHRH) analogs, granulocyte colony-stimulating factor (gCSF), and human growth hormone (hGH). Inhalation of regular insulin for meal time (i.e., postprandial) glucose control has been found to be safe, efficacious, and reliable in type I and type II diabetes patients (52). Compared directly with s.c. injection, inhaled insulin provides equivalent glucose control. A potential advantage of aerosol insulin is that it is more rapidly absorbed (serum peak at 5–60 min) and cleared than SC injection (peak at 60–150 min), which provides a more relevant and convenient therapy for mealtime glucose control. Deftos et al. (53) have evaluated the intrapulmonary (IP) delivery of sCT in normal subjects with a dry powder inhaler. Compared by dose, i.p. sCT had 66% of the bioactivity and 28% of the bioavailability of intramuscular (IM) sCT (Fig. 3).

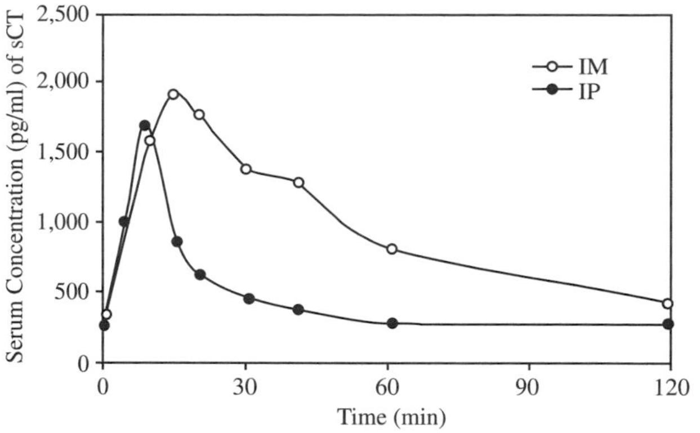

Transdermal Delivery

Considerable effort has been given to the transdermal delivery of pharmaceutical proteins, but clinical applications have thus far been limited to nonprotein drugs (54). The skin is impermeable to molecules as large as proteins. The physical (stratum corneum) and proteolytic enzymatic barriers create a formidable barrier against any permeation under normal circumstances. A molecular size of approximately 1000 Da is generally believed the molecular size limit for transdermal delivery, but there are some reports on the permeation of macromolecules across the stratum corneum by passive diffusion. In addition to molecular size, the lipid-protein partition coefficient of the penetrant is very important. The skin also consists of an enzymatic barrier capable of metabolizing proteins. The composition of enzymes and the spectrum of metabolic reactions in the skin are similar to those in the liver, although the skin

Fig. 3 Mean serum salmon calcitonin (sCT) concentration (pg/ml)-time curves after intramuscular (IM) administration of 100 IU of sCT and intrapulmonary (IP) administration of 160 or 320 IU of sCT in 10 normal males. sCT was administered with a dry powder-delivery inhaler. Dosage adjustments were made by dividing serum sCT concentrations by dose units. The apparent concentration of sCT at time zero represents assay blank in an RIA method. There were no additional substantial changes in sCT after 120 min. Compared by dose, IP sCT had 66% of the bioactivity and 28% of the bioavailability of IM sCT. (From Ref. 53.)

has significantly less metabolic activity than does the liver (55).

Various strategies have been attempted to surmount these barriers. These include the use of protease inhibitors to suppress enzymatic activity and the use of penetration enhancers to reversibly reduce the barrier resistance of the stratum corneum. Other alternatives include forced delivery under an electric field (iontophoresis) and ultrasonic energy (phonophoresis), but their efficacy has been limited by the large size and relatively low electrical charge of proteins. Green et al. (56) and Singh et al. (57) review iontophoresis.

Iontophoresis generates an electrical potential gradient that facilitates the movement of solute ions across the membrane and has been used with the greatest success in the treatment of hyperhidrosis. However, iontophoresis is capable of delivering large hydrophilic proteins in a continuous manner over a prolonged period because of their charged nature. Human studies have been performed to demonstrate the safe, effective, and reproducible delivery of a positively charged calcitonin analog with a molecular weight of approximately 3000 to the systemic circulation (Fig. 4). Some success has been reported in delivering peptides such as antiflammin 1 by iontophoresis (58). It has also been reported recently that proteins as large as insulin (~6000 Da), interferon γ (~17,000 Da), and erythropoeitin (~30,400 Da) could be delivered

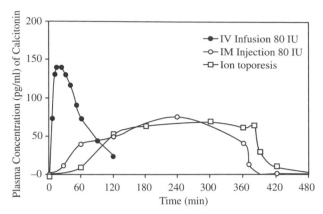

Fig. 4 Mean plasma calcitonin concentration (pg/ml)-time curve resulting from 6-h iontophoretic delivery ($n = 12$) of a calcitonin analog peptide in healthy male volunteers. Plasma levels obtained from IV infusion for 6 h (80 IU, $n = 8$) and IM injection (80 IU, $n = 11$) of the peptide are also shown. Plasma concentration time-profiles indicate that steady-state plasma levels are achieved rapidly, and the decline in plasma levels appears to be absorption-limited rather like an i.m. injection. However, short lag times are observed, which are consistent with diffusion across the outermost layers of the skin but shorter than those typically associated with passive transdermal diffusion. The active and placebo iontophoretic treatment patches were applied at a current density of 200 $\mu A/cm^2$ for a 6-h period. Blood samples were removed for pharmacokinetic assessment at the start of dosing and at regular intervals during and after treatment. Plasma samples were assayed using an RIA method. (From Ref. 56.)

across the skin at therapeutic concentrations with the aid of low-frequency ultrasound (58).

ORAL DELIVERY STRATEGIES

The remainder of this chapter focuses on strategies for improving the oral bioavailability of protein pharmaceuticals and, in particular, describing our experiences with salmon calcitonin. sCT is an endogenous polypeptide hormone composed of 32 amino acids that plays a crucial role in both calcium homeostasis and bone remodeling (59, 60). Four forms of CT are used clinically, namely synthetic human CT, synthetic salmon CT, natural porcine CT, and a synthetic analog of eel calcitonin. Currently, CT is administered parenterally or nasally (61, 62). To effectively inhibit the manifestations of metabolic bone disorders such as Paget's disease and osteoporosis, a frequent and relatively high dosage of CT is administered (63). The oral route is a preferred route of administration, considering the chronic nature of CT therapy. However,

because of extensive proteolytic degradation in the GI lumen and low intrinsic intestinal membrane permeability, insufficient oral bioavailability (BA) of CT necessitates the use of high doses (4000 to 6000 IU/mg) of sCT, even though sCT is 20–30 times more potent than hCT (150–200 IU/mg) (64–66). The unique structure of sCT protects it against its sequestration and metabolism in the liver (67). In this chapter, several approaches for enhancing the oral absorption of sCT are presented. sCT delivery systems for the treatment of osteoporosis are reviewed for many routes including nasal, transdermal, ocular, oral, bronchial, rectal, and vaginal administration (68).

Permeation Enhancement

The poor intrinsic permeability of proteins across biological membranes is well documented (1, 2, 4, 69) and can generally be attributed to their hydrophilic nature and large molecular size. Membrane carrier systems that facilitate the absorption of small peptides (di- and tripeptides) are not efficient at transporting larger peptides and proteins. Permeation enhancers have received considerable attention in attempts to modify the basic barrier properties of the intestinal epithelial cell membrane. Various classes of formulation additives including bile acids, salicylates, fatty acids, acylcarnitines, surfactants, medium chain glycerides, and chelating agents have been studied as absorption enhancers. Each of these agents exerts its enhancing effects by different mechanisms, and each has been associated with adverse effects (70).

Recently, we published in vitro and in vivo results of the evaluation of the performance of formulation additives to enhance the intestinal uptake of sCT (71). The effect of formulation additives on sCT effective permeability (P_{eff}) and transepithelial electrical resistance (TEER) was evaluated in side-by-side diffusion chambers using rat intestinal segments. Various additives such as sodium taurodeoxycholate (TDC), sodium taurocholate, sucrose sterate, sucrose ester-15, Tween 80, lauroyl carnitine chloride (LCC), myristoyl carnitine chloride, cetyl pyridinium chloride, and cetrimide were evaluated in rat jejunum at concentrations ranging from 0.01 to 1%. The effective permeability of sCT was greatest in the presence of TDC (2.73 ± 0.54 E-5 cm/s), increasing up to 14 times over the control (1.91 ± 0.45 E-6 cm/s) in a concentration dependent manner (Fig. 5A). The permeability enhancement relative to control was 5 times for LCC, 3.9 times for Tween 80, 3.2 times for sodium taurocholate, 2.6 times for myristoyl carnitine chloride, 2.3 times for sucrose stearate, 2.0 times for cetyl pyridinium chloride, 1.7 times for sucrose ester-15, and 1.3 times for cetrimide at 1% additives. The order of enhancement on the basis of

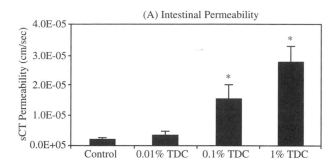

(A) Intestinal Permeability

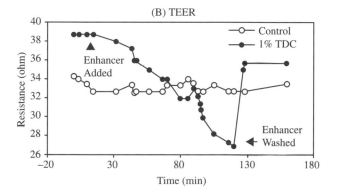

(B) TEER

◀**Fig. 5** (A) Plot of effective permeability (sm/s) of sCT in rat jejunum (mean ± SD; $n = 3$). Effect of TDC was investigated at various concentrations ranging from 0.01 to 1%. * indicates the significant difference from control by $P < 0.05$. Side-by-side diffusion chambers were used. The exposed tissue surface area was 0.636 cm,^{2} and the volume of each half-chamber was 1.7 ml. Mixing in the chambers was controlled using a gas lift mechanism. The temperature was maintained at 37°C throughout the experiment. A 1.5- to 2-cm strip of rat intestinal tissue was excised from the animals, rinsed free of luminal contents using Ringer's buffer (pH 7.4), and mounted onto a diffusion half-chamber maintained at 37°C. Tissues were bathed in 15 mM Mes Ringer's buffer containing 50 μM of sCT with or without formulation additives on the mucosal side (pH 5, 290 mOsm/kg) and Ringer's buffer without additives on the serosal side (pH 7.4, 290 mOsm/kg). Small aliquots (0.5 ml) were taken from the serosal chamber at 30, 45, 60, 75, 90, and 105 min and analyzed by RIA. The effective permeabilities were calculated from the experimental data using the following equation based on Fick's First Law: $P_{eff} = (V_r/A \, ^* C_0)^* dC/dt$ where V_r is the volume of the receiver chamber, A is the absorbing surface, C_0 is the initial drug concentration in the donor (mucosal) phase, and dC/dt is the change in drug concentration in the receptor (basolateral) phase per unit of time. In the presence of TDC, the effective permeability of sCT (2.73 ± 0.54 E-5 cm/s) was increasing up to 14 times over the control (1.91 ± 0.45 E-6 cm/s) in a concentration-dependent manner. (B) Transepithelial electrical resistance (TEER, ohm) versus time curves with or without 1% TDC in rat jejunum. Chambers connected to a voltage-current clamp for measuring transepithelial electrical resistance (TEER) of the intact tissue. The exposed tissue surface area was 1.5 cm^2, and the volume of each half-chamber was 7 ml. Rat intestinal tissue was mounted in chambers, and then two sets of Ag/AgCl electrodes were connected to the voltage-clamp system to pass the current through the membrane. Tissues mounted in chambers usually required approximately 20 min for reaching temperature and TEER equilibrium. Experiments with formulation additives were not initiated until this time. The mucosal strips were then exposed to formulation additives at concentrations ranging from 0.01 to 1% at pH 4 Mes Ringer's buffer. After the initial equilibrium period, TEER was measured and subsequently recorded at regular time intervals. To determine the reversibility of additive effects on TEER, the buffer was replaced with fresh buffer without additives, and the TEER was monitored until a stable reading was observed. When 1% formulation additives were washed after an approximate 100-min exposure, the TEER was returned to 92% of initial value for TDC. (From Ref. 71.)

EC_{50} values (concentration of enhancer for 50% enhancement) was TDC, LCC > sodium taurocholate > tween 80 > myristoyl carnitine chloride > sucrose stearate > sucrose ester-15 > cetyl pyridinium chloride > cetrimide. After the exposure to various additives such as TDC, LCC, and cetrimide at concentration ranging from 0.1 to 1%, the TEER was reduced in a concentration- and contact time-dependent manner for all additives, whereas the TEER increased when the tissue was washed free of additives (Fig. 5B). When 1% formulation additives were washed after approximately 100 min exposure, the TEER returned to 92% of the initial value for TDC and approximately 80% of initial value for the others. As demonstrated during the in vitro and in vivo evaluation of formulation additives, the oral absorption of protein drugs can be maximized by balancing permeability increases and the toxic effects associated with the use of enhancers.

The effect of formulations on the intestinal bioavailability of sCT was studied in an intestinal and vascular access port (IVAP) dog model (71). A schematic representation of the IVAP dog with four ports in the duodenum (ID), ileum (IL), colon (IC), and portal vein (PV) is shown in Fig. 6. The regional (jejunal and ileal) bioavailabilities from formulations DDS1 and DDS2 [DDS1 and DDS2 contained sCT, citric acid (CA), and lauroyl carnitine chloride (LCC) or sodium taurodeoxycholate (TDC), respectively] were significantly greater than their respective controls. Bioavailability enhancement ranged from 98 to 337% for all treatments and regions studied. Compared which sCT alone (without CA), bioavailability enhancement ranged from 1220 to 3070% for DDS1 or DDS2. The in vivo augmentation of sCT absorption by DDS1 or DDS2 correlated well to the in vitro permeation enhancement (Fig. 7).

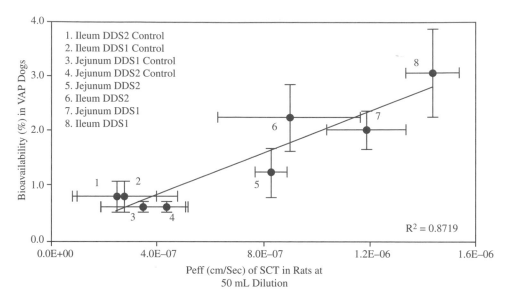

Fig. 7 The plot of in vitro effective permeability (P_{eff}) of sCT in rats (mean $\pm$ SD; $n = 3$) versus in vivo absolute bioavailability of sCT formulation in intestinal and vascular access port (IVAP) dogs (mean $\pm$ SD; $n = 5$ to 6). The in vitro diffusion study was carried out in side-by-side diffusion chambers at concentrations equivalent to the dilution of sCT control and DDS formulation ingredients in 50 ml of buffer solution. DDS1 contains sCT, CA, and LCC, and DDS2 contains sCT, CA, and TDC. The in vivo intestinal bioavailability experiment of formulations was carried out in an IVAP dog model at concentrations of sCT and DDS additives in 5 ml of buffer solution. The ports for IVAP infusions were accessed transcutaneously with a 22-G Huber needle. It was observed that formulations containing TDC or LCC had a significantly higher effective permeability compared with their respective controls. The enhancement in the ileal segment was significantly higher than in the jejunal segment for DDS1 and DDS2. Bioavailability enhancement ranged from 98 to 337% for all treatments and regions studied. The in vivo augmentation of sCT absorption by DDS1 or DDS2 correlated well to the in vitro permeation enhancement. (Reproduced from Ref. 71.)

Protection from Enzymatic Degradation

The susceptibility of proteins to enzymatic attack is well known and remains a major challenge of oral delivery (1, 3, 4, 72–73). Yamamoto et al. (74) reported that various protease inhibitors, including sodium glycocholate, camostat mesilate, and bacitracin, can increase the glucose-lowering activity of insulin administered to rat intestine and colon, apparently by inhibiting protease activity in the lumen and mucous layer of the intestinal tissue. The degradation of calcitonin is also decreased in the presence of protease inhibitors such as camostat and aprotinin (75). The mucoadhesive polymers polycarbophil and carbomer, approved by the U.S. FDA, may have potential for protecting peptides from tryptic degradation by immobilizing trypsin under the depletion of Ca^{2+} (76).

Another potential approach to minimize the activity of intestinal enzymes includes adjusting the pH of the intestinal contents to the corresponding pH minima for proteolytic enzyme activity. Several laboratories have shown that proteolytic activity against insulin, calcitonin, and insulin-like growth factor-I was completely inhibited by pH-lowering mechanisms using polyacrylic acid

polymer (16, 17). We recently used traditional pharmacokinetic techniques combined with radiotelemetric measurement of intestinal pH to elucidate the effect of pH modulation on the oral absorption properties of sCT (77). Studies were performed to characterize the disintegration of the formulation, intestinal pH changes, and the appearance of the peptide in the blood. Enteric-coated formulations containing sCT and various amounts of citric acid (CA) were tethered to a Heidelberg capsule (HC) and given orally to normal beagle dogs (Table 2).

Table 2 The composition of sCT enteric capsules tested in beagle dogs

Formulations	sCT (mg)	CA (mg)	LCC (mg)	Talc (mg)	Dextrose (mg)
97B	1.11	0	55.2	55.2	552.4
97C	1.20	145.7	54.7	54.7	400.7
97D	1.15	260.2	51.9	52.2	260.5
97E	1.19	565.1	56.3	56.3	0

CA; citric acid; LCC, lauroyl carnitine chloride.

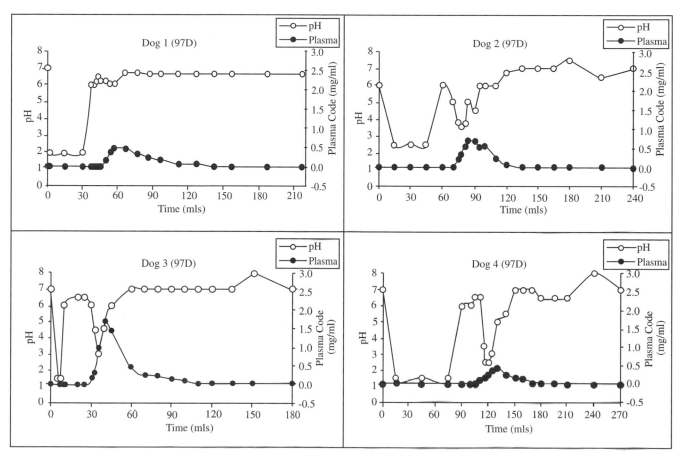

Fig. 8 The pH and plasma sCT concentration-time profiles after oral administration of formulation 97D (containing 1.15 mg of sCT, 260.2 mg of CA, 51.9 mg of LCC, 52.2 mg of Talc, and 260.5 mg of dextrose) (Table 2) tethered to a Heidelberg capsule in normal beagle dogs. Continuous determination of pH was accomplished using a radiotelemetric device, the Heidelberg capsule (HC). The device consists of a battery-operated, high-frequency radio transmitter and a pH electrode housed in a nondigestible acrylic capsule 7 mm in diameter and 20 mm in length. The dogs wore an antenna strapped around the body to receive the radio signal that was then recorded on a chart recorder. The capsule battery was activated with normal saline and calibrated in pH 1 and pH 7 buffer solutions maintained at 37°C. The HC was then tethered to the drug capsule using surgical thread (3-0 vicryl) and administered orally to dogs. Because pH values change with location within the gut and the drug capsule dissolution, alterations in pH were interpreted to be indicative of the movement of the HC-drug capsule through the different segments until the drug capsule dissolves. Generally, Heidelberg capsules provide readings with ±0.5 pH unit accuracy and excellent in vivo reproducibility in the pH range of 1–8 for 22 h after activation. Four male beagle dogs were used to monitor the disintegration and oral absorption of sCT formulation 97D. An HC tethered to an enteric capsule was given orally with 10 ml of water to each dog. Two baseline blood samples were drawn before to dosing and another immediately after gastric emptying (GE). From the time the capsules enter the small intestine, blood samples were taken every 10 min until the HC showed a drop in pH, which signified the disintegration of the test capsule. More frequent blood sampling was performed from the time that disintegration was first detected, with blood samples taken at 3, 6, 9, 12, 15, 20, 30, 45, 60, 75, 90, 120, 150, and 180 min. The peak plasma concentrations of sCT were always observed when the intestinal pH declined. (Reproduced from Ref. 77.)

Blood samples were collected and analyzed using radioimmunoassay (RIA). Intestinal pH was continuously monitored using the HC system. The intraindividual variation in gastric emptying (GE) of the delivery system was large. There were large interindividual differences in the disintegration and absorption properties. However, the peak plasma concentrations of sCT were always observed when the intestinal pH declined (Fig. 8). The intestinal pH decrease was not observed when CA was not included, but an intestinal pH decrease was obvious in all formulations that included CA. The intestinal pH was significantly affected by the amount of CA in the formulations. Plasma concentrations of sCT were observed in all formulations that included CA, but plasma concentrations of sCT were

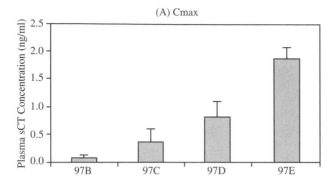

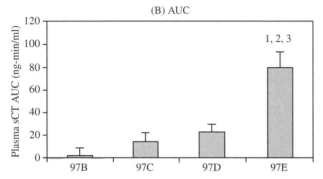

Fig. 9 The plasma C_{max} (**A**) and AUC (**B**) of sCT after oral administration of various formulations (Table 2) in normal beagle dogs. Data are expressed mean ± SEM ($n = 3$ to 4). Formulation 97E was significantly different from 97B(1), 97C(2), and 97D(3) by $P < 0.05$ using one-way ANOVA. By increasing the amount of CA in the formulation, the oral absorption of sCT increased gradually. (Reproduced from Ref. 77.)

not observed in formulation 97B in which CA was not included (Table 2). There was a good correlation between the time to reach the trough intestinal pH ($t_{pH,min}$) and time to reach the peak plasma concentration ($t_{conc,max}$) of sCT ($t_{conc,max} = 0.95 \times t_{pH,min} + 14.1, n = 11, r^2 = 0.91$). As a consequence, the intestinal pH decrease caused by CA appears to be critical for the oral absorption of sCT. By increasing the amount of CA in the formulation, the oral absorption (C_{max} and AUC) of sCT increased gradually (Fig. 9). These results indicate that the oral absorption/or enhancement of sCT absorption is directly related to the stabilization of sCT by a reduction in intestinal pH. The pH stability of pancreatic trypsin (human) is optimal at pH 5–6. At pH 4.0, approximately 45% of the activity remained, where as 15% of activity was retained at pH 3.5 (78). As evidenced in this study, reducing intestinal pH resulted in a significant improvement in sCT absorption.

Another approach to providing protection against proteolytic attack, rather than enzyme inhibition, has been to protect proteins in the physical environment

of the formulation itself. In recent years, significant efforts have been directed toward formulating proteins in microemulsions, small particles (e.g., nanoparticles), and bioadhesive particles (31, 32). The rationale in all three cases is often similar: protection of proteins from the intestinal environment before absorption and localization of the protein at or near the cellular membrane to optimize the driving force for passive permeation. Pegylation of a therapeutic protein may be a suitable form of the protein

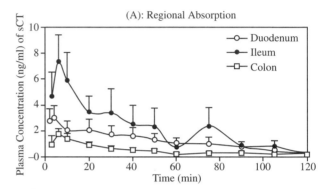

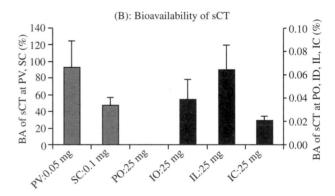

Fig. 10 (A) Plasma concentration (mean ± SEM) of sCT versus time curves after bolus duodenal, ileal, and colonal administration in intestinal and vascular Access port (IVAP) dogs ($n = 5$ to 6). The ports for IVAP infusions were accessed transcutaneously with a 22-G Huber needle. The sCT formulation (25 mg/5 ml/dog) was infused rapidly (12 ml/min), and the port was cleared with a final flush of 1 ml of sterile water. Blood samples were drawn at 1, 3, 6, 9, 12, 15, 20, 30, 45, 60, 75, 90, 120, 150, 180, and 240 min. Absorption of sCT from the ileum was better than from the other regions studied. (Reproduced. from Ref. 71.) (B) Bioavailability of sCT (mean ± SEM) after portal venous (pv 50 μg), subcutaneous (sc 100 μg), and oral (po), duodenal (ID), ileal (IL), and colonic (IC) administration of 25 mg sCT in IVAP dogs ($n = 4$ to 6). The BA (mean ± SD) of unformulated sCT was 92.8 ± 32.0% for portal vein, 47.5 ± 9.3% for subcutaneous, 0% for oral, 0.039 ± 0.017% for duodenal, 0.064 ± 0.022% for ileal, and 0.021 ± 0.004% for colon. The hepatic extraction of sCT is negligible in IVAP dogs.

in an oral-delivery formulation (79). Recombinant human granulocyte colony stimulating factor (PEG–gCSF) resulted in an increase in stability and in retention of in vivo bioactivity when administered by the intraduodenal route. Another reported approach uses mucoadhesion of nanoparticles having surface hydrophilic polymeric chains (80). In that report, it was observed that there was a good correlation between mucoadhesion and enhancement of sCT absorption in rats. The GI transit rates of nanoparticles having surface poly(*N*-isopropylacrylamide), poly(vinylamine), and poly(methacrylic acid) chains were reduced, and sCT absorption was improved. Temperature and pH-sensitive polymers for hCT delivery are also reported (81). Stimuli-sensitive polymers are suitable candidates for oral delivery vehicles because they will prevent gastric degradation in the stomach while providing a controlled release of a peptide drug. The beads made of the polymers with a high content of acrylic acid (most hydrophilic) provided better loading, stability, and release of hCT. In vivo biological activity of the released hCT was preserved.

Maintaining High Local Drug Concentrations

The extent of protein degradation by intestinal enzymatic attack is concentration-dependent following Michaelis–Menten kinetics. Because regional drug concentrations of orally administered proteins depend on intestinal spreading and dilution patterns (19), modulating regional drug concentrations may alter the oral absorption of proteins. Because sCT is an excellent substrate for the pancreatic serine protease trypsin, the rate of degradation of sCT in the GI lumen is dependent on the concentration of sCT in the intestinal lumen. If degradation was the controlling factor, sCT absorption would be much more affected at low sCT concentrations (i.e., the kinetics are in the first-order region of the Michaelis–Menten curve). To evaluate the intestinal dilution and spreading on oral sCT BA, slow infusion (2 ml/min) and high dilution (25 mg/20 ml/dog) treatments were evaluated in dogs in vivo (71). In IVAP studies, the slower and larger infusion volume resulted in significantly lower sCT absorption, demonstrating that intestinal dilution and spreading significantly affected the oral BA of sCT. Scott-Moncrieff et al. (82) reported increased insulin absorption after direct jejunal administration in dogs of a 30-mM sodium glycocholate and 40-mM linoleic acid mixed micelle formulation, although the apparent bioavailability was only 1.8%. This same formulation approach elicited 41% insulin bioavailability in a rat loop model, and the researchers proposed that the much-reduced effect in dogs was possibly attributable to

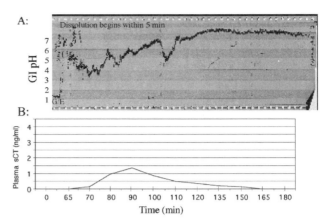

Fig. 11 Duodenal pH recovery (A) and sCT absorption (B) profiles when enteric capsule disintegrated at the duodenum after oral administration of an sCT formulation containing 565 mg of citric acid and 1.2 mg of sCT into the normal dogs. An enteric coated capsule was tethered to a HC with a 3-0 silk suture and given orally to normal dogs with 10 ml of water. Two baseline samples were drawn before dosing and another immediately after gastric emptying. From the time the capsules enter the small intestine (SI), blood samples were taken every 10 min. When the HC showed a drop in pH, indicating the disintegration of the test capsule, more frequent blood sampling was performed (3, 6, 9, 12, 15, 20, 30, 45, 60, 75, 90, 120, 150, and 180 min). Transit time was used to estimate the SI location being monitored. Capsule disintegration in the duodenum begins 5 min after gastric emptying (GE) at 65 min. The initially variable pH momentarily reached pH 3 and soon rose above pH 5. (Reproduced from Ref. 88.)

dilution and spreading of the formulation, resulting in a reduced concentration of insulin, which increased exposure of insulin to proteolytic enzymes.

Regiospecific Targeting

The regiospecific difference of intrinsic permeability of proteins and proteolytic enzymatic activity is well documented (18). Insulin absorption was greater in the ileum and large intestine than in the jejunum using an in situ loop method (83). Several studies have indicated reduced enzymatic activity in the distal intestine (72). It has been hypothesized that the colon could be an optimal site for the absorption of peptides and proteins from the GI tract. This hypothesis is based on the fact that the colon contains little or no digestive enzymes, therefore, the inherent stability of polypeptide materials should be higher. Although the distal small intestine has less lumenal and apical proteolytic activity, it has high activities of some apical peptidases (84). Colonic contents showed high degradation of insulin and calcitonin with high chymotrypsin activity, which suggests that care should be

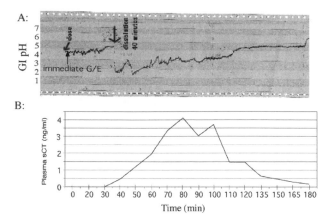

Fig. 12 Late jejunal/or ileal pH recovery (**A**) and sCT absorption (**B**) profiles when enteric capsule disintegrated at late jejunum after oral administration of an sCT formulation containing 565 mg of citric acid and 1.2 mg of sCT into the normal dogs. This figure shows a 40-min delay between GE (less than 5 min) and disintegration. The observed pH drop was sharper and steadier, with the pH remaining below 5 for nearly 90 min. The better absorption profile occurs when disintegration begins in the lower small intestine (LSI). (Reproduced from Ref. 88.)

taken when administering protein drugs to the large intestine for colon-specific drug delivery (75).

Recently, our group published baseline PK information on the regional dependence of unformulated sCT oral absorption evaluated by direct administration into the PO, ID, IL, and IC by means of surgically implanted, chronic catheters (71) (Fig. 6). The plasma concentration and bioavailability values of sCT in dogs are shown and compared with p.v. and s.c. routes in Fig. 10. Plasma sCT concentrations after a p.o. dose were below the LOQ (80 pg/ml), and this may be attributed to the extensive gastric and/or intestinal enzymatic degradation. Absorption of sCT after ID administration was rapid, with peak concentrations occurring within approximately 10 min. BA of sCT was 0.039 ± 0.017%, 0.064 ± 0.022%, and 0.021 ± 0.004% for ID, IL, and IC administration, respectively, in IVAP dogs. Compared with that in other regions, the low BA of sCT in the colon is probably related to the combined effects of poor membrane permeability and/or proteolytic degradation by microorganisms specifically residing in the colon. The colonic results in dogs suggest that additional formulation efforts may be required to successfully deliver sCT to the colon. Calcitonin was rapidly degraded in cecal supernatants by microorganisms (85). Interestingly, the rational design of colon-specific protein/peptide delivery systems has been based on two premises: 1) that the colon compartment has decreased pancreatic proteolytic activity, and/or 2) the colon

possesses bacterial activities with unique specificities for polymer targeting (86, 87).

The successful oral delivery of sCT also depends on intestinal spreading and dilution patterns (19). As a consequence, modulating regional sCT concentrations and/or pH using a formulation approach may alter the oral absorption of CT. To understand the oral absorption process, there is a need to define both the location of release of the delivery system's contents and its effective transit time through the gut. Recently, our group published results using a radiotelemetric measurement of intestinal pH, radiographic visualization of intestinal tract, and pharmacokinetics to investigate how upper small intestine (USI) and lower small intestine (LSI) react differently in intestinal spreading and pH recovery in conscious IVAP beagle dogs (88). Regional intestinal differences of spreading and pH recovery were studied. One port was placed in the duodenum and a second port in the ileum. Fluoroscopy and Heidelberg studies were performed to characterize the intestinal spreading and pH recovery. A radiopaque dye and CA were infused into the ports, and a radiopaque powder capsule containing CA was given orally. Fluoroscopy clearly showed that when the radiopaque dye was infused into the duodenum and capsule disintegration occurred early, there was significant dilution and spreading of the excipients throughout a large section of upper small intestine. Once mixed, the contents moved slowly down the GI tract. However, when the radiopaque dye was infused into the ileum and capsule disintegration occurred lower down, the excipients moved along as a bolus (i.e., a plug). Hence, the local exposure of the intestinal wall was more concentrated in the lower small intestine. The results of the pH monitoring concurred with those of the fluoroscopy studies. In the duodenum, the pH dropped only momentarily then rose quickly. However, steady pH lowering and slower recovery were recorded in the lower small intestine. To investigate the regional intestinal differences of spreading and pH recovery and their impact on sCT oral absorption, normal male beagle dogs were dosed with an enteric capsule containing 565 mg of CA and 1.2 mg of sCT (88). Regular blood samples were collected and analyzed using RIA to determine the absorption characteristics of sCT. Figs. 11 and 12 show two extreme cases demonstrating how the same formulation can produce different results depending on where it begins to disintegrate. Because sCT is protected by low pH conditions (78) and is readily absorbed when concentrations are high, the best absorption occurs when disintegration begins lower in the small intestine. Fig. 11 depicts the disintegration of the delivery system in the duodenum, beginning 5 min after GE (65 min). The initially variable pH momentarily reaches pH 3 and soon rises above pH 5. Fig. 12 shows a 40-min delay between GE (less than 5 min) and disintegration. The pH drop was sharper and more steady. The pH remained below 5 for nearly 90 min. The C_{max} and AUC were 1.3 ng/ml and 47 ng·min/ml, respectively, for duodenal disintegration (Fig. 11), whereas the values were 4.1 ng/ml and 234 ng·min/ml, respectively, for late jejunal/or ileal disintegration (Fig. 12). These results show the regiospecific intestinal absorption of sCT and how it relates to the effective transit time (i.e., disintegration time after GE) of the delivery system in the small intestine. Plasma levels of sCT were optimal when disintegration occurred in the mid to lower SI.

Chemical Modification

Peptide and proteins often possess physical and/or chemical properties that present significant stability problems not encountered with many small, organic drug molecules. Because of the complex nature of proteins, self-aggregation is always a concern in formulation efforts. The tendency of insulin to form hexamers is well documented, and the absorption of hexamers will most likely be very different from monomer absorption. Hovgaad et al. (89) reported the use of alkyl saccharide surfactants (e.g., dodecyl maltoside) to minimize insulin aggregate. The insulin–dodecyl maltoside complex also afforded some protection against enzymatic degradation. Human calcitonin is also known to self-organize into fibrillar structures with reduced biologic activity (90). The use of various surfactant approaches to maximize monomer concentration during protein release may afford advantages in minimizing the size of the complex that must cross epithelial cell layers. Another potential oral delivery approach is the chemical modification of proteins to produce prodrugs and analogs. It is plausible that this approach may protect protein against degradation by proteases and other enzymes present at the mucosal barrier and renders protein more lipophilic, resulting in increased BA. Using chemical modification with fatty acids (20, 21) or N-acylated α-amino acids (22), a significant increase in CT intestinal absorption was observed in comparison with the native CT. The stability and permeability of peptides were improved by acylation with fatty acids and the derivatized amino acids only weakly inhibited by trypsin or leucine aminopeptidase. The stability of peptides in gastrointestinal fluids and serum was improved by substituting D-amino acids (23, 24). As exemplified by cyclosporine, the cyclic 11-amino acid compound has a surprisingly high bioavailability by chemical modification to improve its stability within the GI tract and to make it more lipophilic to enhance membrane permeability. When

administered in the microemulsion formulation, 50% or more of this molecule can be absorbed from the GI tract (11, 12, 91). Chemical modification of small peptides has been successful in protecting certain peptide structures from enzymatic attack without significant loss of biological activity, but less success has been achieved with larger polypeptides.

CONCLUDING REMARKS

Establishing an oral delivery system for peptides and protein drugs is of great importance because parenteral administration results in poor patient compliance during chronic treatment, resulting in limited clinical utility. The advantages of oral delivery systems in terms of patient compliance and acceptability are further augmented by the potential cost savings because noninvasive delivery routes do not require sterile manufacturing, and administration can be effected without direct involvement of a healthcare provider. The clinical development of protein pharmaceuticals, however, has been impeded because of poor absorption across bioilogical membranes and rapid proteolytic degradation that typically result in low bioavailabilities. Although only very limited success (e.g., cyclosporine) has been achieved in developing and marketing oral peptide delivery systems, interest remains extremely high. It is clear that a well controlled and rational formulation design process is necessary. The problems with protein delivery are not trivial and will not be overcome by trivial solutions. Because the barriers to protein absorption (permeability, enzymatic degradation, presystemic hepatic degradation, and chemical and physical stability) will likely exhibit significant protein specificity, delivery systems will have to be investigated and developed for efficacy and safely on a case-by-case basis. In this chapter, we focused on enhancing oral absorption using several approaches. Potential approaches to modulate the intestinal environment include modulating intestinal permeability, limiting the activity of intestinal enzymes, maintaining high local drug concentrations, and regiospecific targeting. Using these strategies, sCT oral delivery systems have been fabricated and successfully tested in humans.

REFERENCES

1. Zhou, X.H. Overcoming Enzymatic and Absorption Barriers to Non-Parenterally Administered Protein and Peptide Drugs. J. Controlled Release **1994**, *29*, 239–252.

2. Amidon, G.L.; Lee, H.J. Absorption of Peptide and Peptidomimetic Drugs. Annu. Rev. Pharmacol. Toxicol. **1994**, *34*, 321–341.

3. Lagguth, P.; Bohner, V.; Heizmann, J.; Merckle, H.P.; Wolffram, S.; Amidon, G.L.; Yamashita, S. The Challenge of Proteolytic Enzymes in Intestinal Peptide Delivery. J. Controlled Release **1997**, *46*, 39–57.

4. Lee, V.H.L.; Yamamoto, A. Penetration and Enzymatic Barriers to Peptide and Protein Absorption. Adv. Drug Delivery Rev. **1990**, *4*, 171–207.

5. Bai, J.P.; Amidon, G.L. Structural Specificity of Mucosal-Cell Transport and Metabolism of Peptide Drugs: Implications for Oral Peptide Drug Delivery. Pharm. Res. **1992**, *9*, 969–978.

6. Pettit, D.K.; Gombotz, W.R. The Development of Site-Specific Drug-Delivery Systems for Protein and Peptide Biopharmaceuticals. Trends Biotechnol. **1998**, *16*, 343–349.

7. Wearley, L.L. Recent Progress in Protein and Peptide Delivery by Noninvasive Routes. Crit. Rev. Ther. Carrier Syst. **1991**, *8*, 331–394.

8. Dantzig, A.H. Oral Absorption of β-Lactams by Intestinal Peptide Transport Proteins. Adv. Drug Delivery Rev. **1997**, *23*, 63–76.

9. Tsuji, A.; Tamai, I. Carrier-Mediated Intestinal Transport of Drugs. Pharm. Res. **1996**, *13*, 963–977.

10. Lee, V.H.; Chu, C.; Mahlin, E.D.; Basu, S.K.; Ann, D.K.; Bolger, M.B.; Haworth, I.S.; Yeung, A.K.; Wu, S.K.; Hamm-Alvarez, S.; Okamoto, C.T.J. Biopharmaceutics of Transmucosal Peptide and Protein Drug Administration: Role of Transport Mechanisms with a Focus on the Involvement of PepT1. J. Controlled Release **1999**, *62*, 129–140.

11. Noble, S.; Markham, A. Cyclosporin. A Review of the Pharmacokinetic Properties, Clinical Efficacy and Tolerability of a Microemulsion-Based Formulation (Neoral). Drugs **1995**, *50*, 924–941.

12. Schroeder, T.J.; Cho, M.J.; Pollack, G.M.; Floc'h, R.; Moran, H.B.; Levy, R.; Moore, L.W.; Pouletty, P. Comparison of Two Cyclosporine Formulations in Healthy Volunteers: Bioequivalence of the New Sang-35 Formulation and Neoral. J. Clin. Pharmacol. **1998**, *38*, 807–814.

13. Neutra, M.R.; Kraehenbuhl, J.P. Transepithelial Transport of Proteins by Intestinal Epithelial Cells. *Biological Barriers to Protein Delivery*; Audus, K.L., Raub, T.J., Eds.; Plenum Press: New York, 1993; 107–129.

14. Bernkop-Schnurch, A. The Use of Inhibitory Agents to Overcome the Enzymatic Barrier to Preorally Administered Therapeutic Peptides and Proteins. J. Controlled Release **1998**, *52*, 1–16.

15. Friedman, D.I.; Amidon, G.L. Oral Absorption of Peptides: Influence of pH And Inhibitors on the Intestinal Hydrolysis of Leu-Enkephalin and Analogues. Pharm. Res. **1991**, *8*, 93–96.

16. Bai, J.P.; Chang, L.L.; Guo, J.H. Effects of Polyacrylic Polymers on the Luminal Proteolysis of Peptide Drugs in the Colon. J. Pharm. Sci. **1995**, *84*, 1291–1294.

17. Bai, J.P.; Chang, L.L.; Guo, J.H. Effects of Polyacrylic Polymers on the Degradation of Insulin and Peptide Drugs by Chymotrypsin and Trypsin. J. Pharm. Pharmacol. **1996**, *48*, 17–21.

18. Woodley, J.F. Enzymatic Barriers for GI Peptide and Protein Delivery. Crit. Rev. Ther. Drug Carrier Syst. **1994**, *11*, 61–95.

19. Grundy, D. *Gastrointestinal Motility*; MTD Press Limited: 1985.

20. Yamamoto, A. Improvement of Intestinal Absorption of Peptide and Protein Drugs by Chemical Modification with Fatty Acids. Nippon Rinsho **1998**, *56*, 601–607.

21. Muranishi, S. Delivery System Design for Improvement of Intestinal Absorption of Peptide Drugs. Yakugaku Zassshi **1997**, *117*, 394–414.

22. Leone-Bay, A.; Santiago, N.; Achan, D.; Chaudhary, K.; DeMorin, F.; Falzarano, L.; Haas, S.; Kalbag, S.; Kaplan, D.; Leipold, H.; Lercara, C.; O'Toole, D.; Rivera, C.; Rosado, C.; Sarubb, D.; Vuocolo, E.; Wana, N.; Milstein, S.; Baughman, R.A. *N*-acylated Alpha-Amino Acids as Novel Oral Delivery Agents for Proteins. J. Med. Chem. **1995**, *38*, 4263–4269.

23. Krondahl, E.; Orzechowski, A.; Ekstrom, G.; Lennernas, H. Rat Jejunal Permeability and Metabolism of Mu-Selective Tetrapeptides in Gastrointestinal Fluids from Humans and Rats. Pharm. Res. **1997**, *14*, 1780–1785.

24. Hong, S.Y.; Oh, J.E.; Lee, K.H. Effect of D-Amino Acid Substitution on the Stability, the Secondary Structure, and the Activity of Membrane-Active Peptide. Biochem. Pharmacol. **1999**, *58*, 1775–1780.

25. Lehr, C.M. Bioadhesion Technologies for the Delivery of Peptide and Protein Drugs to the Gastrointestinal Tract. Crit. Rev. Ther. Drug. Carrier Syst. **1994**, *11*, 119–160.

26. Mizuma, T.; Sakai, N.; Awazu, S. Na$^+$-Dependent Transport of Aminopeptidase-Resistant Sugar-Coupled Tripeptides in Rat Intestine. Biochem. Biophys. Res. Commun. **1994**, *203*, 1412–1416.

27. Haga, M.; Saito, K.; Shimaya, T.; Maezawa, Y.; Kato, Y.; Kim, S.W. Hypoglycemic Effect of Intestinally Administered Monosaccharide-Modified Insulin Derivatives in Rats. Chem. Pharm. Bull. **1990**, *38*, 1983–1986.

28. Gan, L.-S.L.; Thakker, D.R. Applications of the Caco-2 Model in the Design and Development of Orally Active Drugs: Elucidation of Biochemical and Physical Barriers Posed by the Intestinal Epithelium. Adv. Drug Delivery Rev. **1997**, *23*, 77–98.

29. Sayani, A.P.; Chien, Y.W. Systemic Delivery of Peptides and Proteins across Absorptive Mucosa. Crit. Rev. Ther. Drug Carrier Syst. **1996**, *13*, 85–184.

30. Junginger, H.E. Bioadhesive Polymer Systems for Peptide Delivery. Acta Pharm. Technol. **1990**, *36*, 110–126.

31. Fix, J.A. Oral Controlled Release Technology for Peptides: Status and Future Prospects. Pharm. Res. **1996**, *13*, 1760–1764.

32. Bernkop-Schnurch, A.; Pasta, M. Intestinal Peptide and Protein Delivery: Novel Bioadhesive Drug-Carrier Matrix Shielding from Enzymatic Attack. J. Pharm. Sci. **1998**, *87*, 430–434.

33. Su, K.S.E. Nasal Route Delivery of Peptide and Protein Drug Delivery. *Peptide and Protein Drug Delivery*; Lee, V.H.L., Ed.; Marcel Dekker, Inc. : New York, Chap. 13.

34. Sarkar, M.A. Drug Metabolism in the Nasal Mucosa. Pharm. Res. **1992**, *9*, 1–9.

35. Kissel, T.; Werner, U. Nasal Delivery of Peptides: An in Vitro Cell Culture Model for the Investigation of Transport

and Metabolism in Human Nasal Epithelium. J. Controlled Release **1998**, *53*, 195–203.

36. Watanabe, Y.; Mizufune, Y.; Utoguchi, N.; Endo, K.; Matsumoto, M. Studies of Drug Delivery Systems for a Therapeutic Agent Used in Osteoporosis. II. Enhanced Absorption of Elcatonin from Nasal Mucosa in Rabbits. Biol. Pharm. Bull. **1998**, *21*, 1191–1194.

37. Merkle, H.P.; Wolany, G.J.M. Intraoral Peptide Absorption. *Biological Barriers to Protein Delivery*; Audus, K.L., Raub, T.J., Eds.; Plenum Press: New York, 1993; 131–160.

38. Garren, K.W.; Repta, A.J. Buccal Absorption. III. Simultaneous Diffusion and Metabolism of an Aminopeptidase Substrate in the Hamster Cheek Pouch. Pharm. Res. **1989**, *6*, 966–970.

39. Li, C.; Bhatt, P.P.; Johnston, T.P. Transmucosal Delivery of Oxytocin to Rabbits Using a Mucoadhesive Buccal Patch. Pharm. Dev. Technol. **1997**, *2*, 265–274.

40. Nakane, S.; Kakumoto, M.; Yukimatsu, H.; Chien, Y.W. Oramucosal Delivery of LHRH: Pharmacokinetic Studies of Controlled and Enhanced Transmucosal Permeation. Pharm. Dev. Technol. **1996**, *1*, 251–259.

41. Krishnamoorthy, R.; Mitra, A.K. Ocular Delivery of Peptides and Proteins. *Ophthalmic Drug Delivery Systems*; Mitra, A.K., Ed.; Marcel Dekker, Inc.: New York; 1993, 455–469.

42. Chiou, G.C. Systemic Delivery of Polypeptide Drugs Through Ocular Route. J. Ocul. Pharmacol. **1994**, *10*, 93–99.

43. Lee, V.H.L. Precorneal, Corneal, and Postcorneal Factors. *Ophthalmic Drug Delivery Systems*; Mitra, A.K., Ed.; Marcel Dekker, Inc.: New York, 1993; 59–81.

44. Chiou, G.C.; Shen, Z.F.; Zheng, Y.Q. Adjustment of Blood Sugar Levels with Insulin and Glucagon Eyedrops in Normal and Diabetic Rabbits. J. Ocul. Pharmacol. **1990**, *6*, 233–241.

45. Muranishi, S.; Yamamoto, A.; Okada, H. Rectal and Vaginal Absorption of Peptides and Proteins. *Biological Barriers to Protein Delivery*; Audus, K.L., Raub, T.J., Eds.; Plenum Press: New York, 1993; 199–227.

46. Lee, V.H.L.; Yamamoto, A. Presentation and Enzymatic Barriers to Peptide and Protein Absorption. Adv. Drug Delivery Rev. **1990**, *4*, 171–207.

47. Golomb, G.; Avramoff, A.; Hoffman, A. A New Route of Drug Administration: Intrauterine Delivery of Insulin and Calcitonin. Pharm. Res. **1993**, *10*, 828–833.

48. Bonucci, E.; Ballanti, P.; Ramires, P.A.; Richardson, J.L.; Benedetti, L.M. Prevention of Ovariectomy Osteopenia in Rats After Vaginal Administration of Hyaff 11 Microspheres Containing Salmon Calcitonin. Calcif. Tissue Int. **1995**, *56*, 272–279.

49. Johnson, L.G.; Boucher, R.C. Macromolecular Transport Across Nasal and Respiratory Epithelia. *Biological Barriers to Protein Delivery*; Audus, K.L., Raub, T.J., Eds.; Plenum Press: New York, 1993; 161–178.

50. Yu, J.; Chien, Y.W. Pulmonary Drug Delivery: Physiologic and Mechanistic Aspects. Crit. Rev. Ther. Drug Carrier Syst. **1997**, *14*, 395–453.

51. Smith, P.L. Peptide Delivery Via the Pulmonary Route: A Valid Approach for Local and Systemic Delivery. J. Control. Release **1997**, *46*, 99–106.

52. Patton, J.S.; Bukar, J.; Nagarajan, S. Inhaled Insulin. Adv. Drug Delivery Rev. **1999**, *35*, 235–247.

53. Deftos, L.J.; Nolan, J.J.; Seely, B.L.; Clopton, P.L.; Cote, G.J.; Whitham, C.L.; Florek, L.J.; Christensen, T.A.; Hill, M.R. Intrapulmonary Drug Delivery of Salmon Calcitonin. Calcif. Tissue Int. **1997**, *61*, 345–347.

54. Banga, A.K.; Chien, Y.W. Dermal Absorption of Peptides and Proteins. *Biological Barriers to Protein Delivery*; Audus, K.L., Raub, T.J., Eds.; Plenum Press: New York, 1993; 179–197.

55. Merkle, H.P. Transdermal Delivery Systems. Methods Funds Exp. Clinical Pharmacol. **1989**, *11*, 135–153.

56. Green, P.G. Iontophoretic Delivery of Peptide Drugs. J. Controlled Release **1996**, *41*, 33–48.

57. Singh, P.; Maibach, H.I. Iontophoresis in Drug Delivery: Basic Principles and Applications. Crit. Rev. Ther. Drug Carrier Syst. **1994**, *11*, 161–213.

58. Mitragotn, S.; Blankschtein, D.; Langer, R. Ultrasound-Mediated Transdermal Protein Delivery. *Science*; Wash, DC, 1995; 269, 850–853.

59. McDermott, M.T.; Kidd, G.S. The Role of Calcitonin in the Development and Treatment of Osteoporosis. Endocr. Rev. **1987**, *8*, 377–390.

60. Patel, S.; Lyons, A.R.; Hosking, D.J. Drugs Used in the Treatment of Metabolic Bone Diseases. Drugs **1993**, *46*, 594–617.

61. Stevenson, J.C.; Evans, I.M. Pharmacology and Therapeutic Use of Calcitonin. Drugs **1981**, *21*, 257–272.

62. Reginster, J.Y.; Jeugmans-Huynen, A.M.; Sarlet, N.; McIntyre, H.D.; Franchimont, P. The Effect of Nasal hCT on Bone Turnover in Paget's Disease of Bone—Implications for the Treatment of Other Metabolic Bone Diseases. Br. J. Rheumatol. **1992**, *31*, 35–39.

63. Schneyer, C.R. Calcitonin and the Treatment of Osteoporosis. MD Med. J. **1991**, *40*, 469–473.

64. Sinko, P.J.; Hu, P.; Wagner, E.; Sturmer, A.; Gilligan, J.P.; Stern, W. Determination of the Intestinal Permeability of Recombinant Salmon Calcitonin. Pharm. Res. **1993**, *10*, (suppl.) S293.

65. Yu, H.; Jiang, F.; Stern, W.; Sinko, P.J. Intestinal Binding and Degradation of Recombinant Salmon Calcitonin. Pharm. Res. **1994**, *11*, (suppl.) S254.

66. Heintz, M.L.; Flanigan, E.; Orlowski, R.C.; Regnier, F.E. Correlation of Calcitonin Structure with Chromatographic Retention in High-Performance Liquid Chromatography. J. Chromatogr. **1988**, *443*, 229–245.

67. Singer, F.; Habener, J.F.; Greene, E.; Godin, P.; Pottisjun, J.T. Inactivation of Calcitonin by Specific Organs. Nature New Biology **1972**, *237*, 269–270.

68. Satoh, T.; Yoshida, G.; Orito, Y.; Koike, T. Drug Delivery System for the Treatment of Osteoporosis. Nippon Rinsho **1998**, *65*, 742–747.

69. Humphrey, M.J. The Oral Bioavailability of Peptides and Related Drugs. *Delivery Systems for Peptide Drugs*; Davis, S.S., Illum, L., Thomlinson, E., Eds.; Plenum Press: New York, 1986; 139–151.

70. LeCluyse, E.L.; Sutton, S.C. In Vitro Models for Selection of Development Candidates. Permeability Studies to Define Mechanisms of Absorption Enhancement. Adv. Drug Delivery. Rev. **1997**, *23*, 163–183.

71. Sinko, P.J.; Lee, Y.H.; Makhey, V.; Leesman, G.D.; Sutyak, J.P.; Yu, H.; Perry, B.; Smith, C.T.; Hu, P.;

Wagner, E.J.; Falzone, L.M.; McWhorter, L.T.; Gilligan, J.P.; Stern, W. Biopharmaceutical Approaches for Developing and Assessing Oral Peptide Delivery Strategies and Systems: In Vitro Permeability and in Vivo Oral Absorption of Salmon Calcitonin (sCT). Pharm. Res. **1999**, *16*, 527–533.

72. Lee, V.H.L. Enzymatic Barriers to Peptide and Protein Absorption. Crit. Rev. Ther. Drug Carrier Sys. **1988**, *5*, 69–97.

73. Bai, J.P.F.; Amidon, G.L. Degradation of Insulin by Trypsin and α-Chymotrypsin. Pharm. Res. **1992**, *9*, 969–978.

74. Yamamoto, A.; Taniguchi, T.; Rikyuu, K.; Tsuji, T.; Fujita, T.; Murakami, M.; Muranishi, J. Effects of Various Protease Inhibitors on the Intestinal Absorption and Degradation of Insulin in Rats. Pharm. Res. **1994**, *11*, 1496–1500.

75. Tozaki, H.; Emi, Y.; Horisaka, E.; Fujita, T.; Yamamoto, A.; Muranishi, S. Degradation of Insulin and Calcitonin and Their Protection by Various Protease Inhibitors in Rat Caecal Contents: Implications in Peptide Delivery to the Colon. J. Pharm. Pharmacol. **1997**, *49*, 164–168.

76. Luessen, H.L.; Verhoef, J.C.; Borchard, G.; Lehr, C.M.; de Boer, A.G.; Junginger, H.E. Mucoadhesive Polymers in Peroral Peptide Drug Delivery. II. Carbomer and Polycarbophil are Potent Inhibitors of the Intestinal Proteolytic Enzyme Trypsin. Pharm. Res. **1995**, *12*, 1293–1298.

77. Lee, Y.H.; Perry, B.A.; Labruno, S.; Lee, H.S.; Stern, W.; Falzone, L.M.; Sinko, P.J. Impact of Regional Intestinal pH Modulation on Absorption of Peptide Drugs: Oral Absorption Studies of Salmon Calcitonin in Beagle Dogs. Pharm. Res. **1999**, *16*, 1233–1239.

78. Legg, E.F.; Spencer, A.M. Studies on the Stability of Pancreatic Enzymes in Duodenal Fluid to Storage Temperature and pH. Clin. Chim. Acta **1975**, *65*, 175–179.

79. Jensen-Pippo, K.E.; Whitcomb, K.L.; DePrince, R.B.; Ralph, L.; Habberfield, A.D. Enteral Bioactivity of Human Granulocyte Colony Stimulating Factor Conjugated with Poly(ethylene Glycol). Pharm. Res. **1996**, *13*, 102–107.

80. Sakuma, S.; Sudo, R.; Suzuki, N.; Kikuchi, H.; Akashi, M.; Hayashi, M. Mucoadhesion of Polystyrene Nanoparticles Having Surface Hydrophilic Polymeric Chains in the Gastrointestinal Tract. Int. J. Pharm. **1999**, *177*, 161–172.

81. Serres, A.; Baudys, M.; Kim, S.W. Temperature and pH-Sensitive Polymers for Human Calcitonin Delivery. Pharm. Res. **1996**, *13*, 196–201.

82. Scott-Moncrieff, J.C.; Shao, Z.; Mitra, A.K. Enhancement of Intestinal Insulin Absorption by Bile Salt-Fatty Acid Mixed Micelles in Dogs. J. Pharm. Sci. **1994**, *83*, 1465–1469.

83. Kimura, T.; Sato, K.; Sugimoto, K.; Tao, R.; Murakami, T.; Kurosaki, Y.; Nakayama, T. Oral Administration of Insulin As Poly(vinyl Alcohol)-Gel Spheres in Diabetic Rats. Biol. Pharm. Bull. **1996**, *19*, 897–900.

84. Bai, J.P.; Chang, L.L.; Guo, J.H. Targeting of Peptide and Protein Drugs to Specific Sites in the Oral Route. Crit. Rev. Ther. Drug Carrier Syst. **1995**, *12*, 339–371.

85. Tozaki, H.; Emi, Y.; Horisaka, E.; Fujita, T.; Yamamoto, A.; Muranishi, S. Metabolism of Peptide Drugs by the Microorganisms in Rat Cecal Contents. Biol. Pharm. Bull. **1995**, *18*, 929–931.

86. Saffran, M.; Kumar, G.S.; Savariar, C.; Burnham, J.C.; Williams, F.; Neckers, D.C. A New Approach to the Oral Administration of Insulin and Other Peptide Drugs. Science Wash **1986**, *233*, 1081–1084.

87. Mrsny, R.N. The Colon As a Site for Drug Delivery. J. Controlled Release **1992**, *22*, 15–34.

88. Lee, Y.H.; Perry, B.A.; Sutyak, J.P.; Stern, W.; Sinko, P.J. Regional Differences in Intestinal Spreading and pH Recovery on the Effectiveness of Pharmaceutical Excipients and the Impact on Salmon Calcitonin Absorption in Beagle Dogs. Pharm. Res. **2000**, *17*, 284–290.

89. Hovgaad, L.; Mack, E.J.; Kim, S.W. Insulin Stabilization and GI Absorption. J. Controlled Release **1992**, *19*, 99–108.

90. Merkle, H.P. New Aspects of Pharmaceutical Dosage Forms for Controlled Drug Delivery of Peptides and Proteins. Eur. J. Pharm. Sci. **1994**, *2*, 19–21.

91. Senel, F.M.; Yildirim, S.; Karakayali, H.; Moray, G.; Haberal, M. Comparison of Neoral and Sandimmune for Induction and Maintenance Immunosuppression After Kidney Transplantation. Transpl. Int. **1997**, *10*, 357–361.

NUCLEAR MAGNETIC RESONANCE SPECTROSCOPY IN PHARMACEUTICAL TECHNOLOGY

Kevin L. Facchine
Thomas M. O'Connell
GlaxoSmithKline, Research Triangle Park, North Carolina

INTRODUCTION

Nuclear magnetic resonance spectroscopy plays a vital role in essentially all aspects of pharmaceutical development. In the early stages of lead development, NMR is used as a high throughput tool in the analysis of combinatorial libraries and in screening large numbers of compounds for receptor binding. In the synthesis and development of a lead compound, NMR is applied in all manner of structural analyses, including low-level synthetic impurities, degradation products, and metabolites. Advances in sensitivity and experimental design have enabled its use in the analysis of ever more complicated molecules at concentrations down to the nanomolar range. The coupling of NMR with HPLC systems has facilitated the characterization of trace compounds in complex mixtures. Further in-line coupling of NMR with MS systems has provided unprecedented amounts of structural information from a single analysis. In the final stage of drug development, solid-state NMR has been applied to the analysis of bulk drug properties such as polymorphic forms present in drug substances and formulations. The goal of this review is to introduce the reader to the basic principles of NMR and its application to the various stages of drug development. The references are not exhaustive, but have been selected to highlight the key principles and discoveries and point the interested reader toward further study.

PRINCIPLES OF MAGNETIC RESONANCE

The NMR Phenomenon

The nuclear magnetic resonance phenomenon occurs for certain nuclei that possess a magnetic moment μ. When placed in a magnetic field, nuclear moments will align themselves in a discrete number of orientations. The number of orientations is determined by the nuclear spin I, which is a fundamental property of certain nuclei and has values of 0, 1/2, 1, 3/2, etc. The number of allowed orientations of a nucleus is given by 2I + 1. The most commonly observed nuclei in NMR, for example, ^{1}H and ^{13}C, possess a spin equal to $\frac{1}{2}$ and therefore have only two allowed orientations. These two states can be thought of as having the nuclear dipole aligned either with the external magnetic field ($+\frac{1}{2}$, lower energy state) or against the field ($-\frac{1}{2}$, higher energy state). Nuclei such as ^{12}C and ^{16}O, have spin equal to 0 and therefore do not align in a magnetic field and cannot be observed using NMR.

The relationship between the magnetic moment and the nuclear spin is shown in Eq. 1. The proportionality constant γ is known as the gyromagnetic ratio.

$$\gamma = 2\pi\mu/hI \tag{1}$$

The gyromagnetic ratio is directly related to the sensitivity of detection of a particular nucleus. Nuclei with large γ values are more sensitive, that is, easier to detect than those with low values.

NMR experiments involve the application of pulses of radiofrequency (rf) radiation in order to excite nuclei from one energy state to another. The energy separation between these states is given by

$$\Delta E = h\nu = \gamma B_0/2\pi \tag{2}$$

where B_0 is the strength of the applied magnetic field. For the hydrogen nucleus (^{1}H), or proton as it is commonly referred to, the energy difference corresponds to a radio frequency of around 500 MHz with an external magnetic field of 11.7 T (1 T = 10^4 G). (Often the magnet strength is referred to in terms of the proton resonance frequency, hence an 11.7 T magnet is called a 500 MHz magnet.) Note also from Eq. 2 that γ for a given nucleus determines the relationship between the static magnetic field B_0 and the nuclear magnetic resonance frequency ν. NMR is typically considered to be one of the more insensitive spectroscopic methods due to the fact that the population difference between spin states is about 1 in 10,000 for protons in a 10 T magnetic field. This means that only about 0.01% of the

Table 1   Properties of nuclides important in the study of pharmaceuticals

Nuclide	Spin	% Natural abundance	Relative sensitivity[a]	Absolute sensitivity[b]	Gyromagnetic ratio $(10^7 \text{ rad s}^{-1} \text{ T}^{-1})$	NMR frequency at 11.7436 T (MHz)
^{1}H	1/2	99.985	1.00000	1.00	26.7515	500.000
^{2}H	1	0.015	0.00965	1.45E-06	4.1065	76.753
^{3}H[c]	1/2	0	1.21354	0	28.5343	533.320
^{13}C	1/2	1.108	0.01591	1.76E-04	6.7281	125.752
^{15}N	1/2	0.366	0.00104	3.81E-06	−2.7126	50.699
^{19}F	1/2	100	0.83400	8.34E-01	25.1808	470.642
^{31}P	1/2	100	0.06652	6.65E-02	10.8391	202.589

[a]Expressed relative to ^{1}H = 1 for constant field and equal number of nuclei.
[b]Absolute sensitivity = relative sensitivity × natural abundance.
[c]^{3}H is radioactive with a half life of 12.3 years.
(From Lide, D. R. Ed. *CRC Handbook of Chemistry and Physics*, 81st Ed.; CRC Press: New York, 2000, 2001; 9–92.)

sample gives rise to a signal in contrast to other spectroscopies such as IR and UV. Recent advances in commercially available superconducting magnets up to 21.1 T (900 MHz) have greatly increased the sensitivity of NMR experiments.

Table 1 lists some of the important properties of several commonly observed nuclides in the study of pharmaceuticals. Notice that some elements such as hydrogen, have several magnetically active isotopes with very different properties. Interestingly, ^{3}H has the highest sensitivity to detection of any nucleus, but its use is limited by the added complexity of working with a radioactive isotope. The absolute sensitivity listed in the table takes into account the natural abundance of the isotope. Sensitivity can be improved in some studies by the chemical incorporation of magnetically active isotopes such as ^{13}C and ^{15}N.

The basic NMR experiment is most simply described using the vector model shown in Fig. 1. In this model, the bulk magnetization vector represents the slightly greater proportion of the nuclei aligned with the external magnetic field designated as the z-axis. The effect of an rf pulse generated perpendicular to the magnetic field is to tip this vector into the transverse (x, y) plane. In the transverse plane the nuclear spin imparts a precession frequency on each nucleus that is a function of its chemical environment, that is, each chemically distinct type of nucleus has a characteristic precession frequency. The detected signal is the sum of the cosine-modulated amplitudes of each of the precessing spins. Fourier transformation of this signal yields the familiar NMR spectrum. The spectrum contains valuable structural information in the form of chemical shifts, scalar couplings, relative intensities, and linewidths.

Each of these properties will be discussed in the next sections.

Chemical Shifts

When a molecule is placed in a magnetic field, electrons within the molecule shield the nuclei from the magnetic field. The actual magnetic field experienced by a given nucleus is therefore due to both the large external magnetic field, B_o and the effects of nuclear shielding. The chemical shift is defined as the nuclear shielding divided by the applied field. It is always measured from a suitable reference, which is commonly a known compound added directly to the sample. The chemical shift is expressed in parts per million of the resonance frequency of the reference and calculated using Eq. 3

$$\delta(\text{ppm}) = [(\nu_{\text{sample}} - \nu_{\text{ref}}) \times 10^6]/\nu_{\text{ref}} \qquad (3)$$

For proton and carbon NMR in organic solvents, the most common reference is tetramethylsilane (TMS), with four sets of equivalent methyl groups whose signal is assigned a value of 0 ppm. For aqueous solutions, trimethylsilylpropionate (TSP) is commonly used, and the trimethyl proton signal is also assigned a value of 0 ppm. The range of chemical shifts experienced by different nuclei is quite variable. The chemical shift range for ^{1}H is approximately 10 ppm. In contrast, several of the other nuclei listed in Table 1 have much great spectral dispersion. The ^{13}C resonances typically cover a spectral window of approximately 250 ppm. For ^{15}N and ^{19}F, typical chemical shift ranges are greater than 400 ppm. The wide spectral dispersion experienced by the latter nuclei is very valuable in reducing spectral crowding.

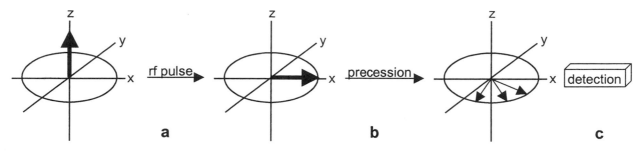

Fig. 1 The basic NMR experiment a) the rf pulse tips the bulk magnetization vector in the the x–y plane; b) the individual spins start to precess according to the frequency determined by their chemical environment; c) the precessing spins are detected along the x-axis as a set of cosine-modulated signals. Fourier transformation of these signals leads to the final spectrum.

Scalar Coupling

Signals in an NMR spectrum can present a characteristic pattern based on through bond interactions with neighboring nuclei. This phenomenon is known as scalar coupling. The proton spectrum of ibuprofen, shown in Fig. 2 has six chemically distinct sets of protons. At each chemical shift, the signals are split into multiple lines due to scalar coupling. This splitting arises from the interactions between neighboring magnetic dipoles (spins). For example, the methyl protons at C_3 of ibuprofen are next to the methine proton at C_2. At any given time, some of the methine protons will be aligned either with or against the magnetic field. The two orientations of this nucleus result in two contributions to the effective field of the methyl group that leads to the presence of the doublet for the methyl group. The separation between the peaks is known as the coupling constant. The general rule for scalar coupling is that the number of peaks in a multiplet equals $2n\mathrm{I} + 1$, where n is the number of neighboring equivalent nuclei and I is the nuclear spin. Thus, the methine proton at C_2 yields a quartet due to coupling to the three equivalent methyl protons. The intensities of each component of a multiplet follow the pattern of Pascal's triangle. This yields peak ratios of 1:1 for a doublet, 1:2:1 for a triplet, 1:3:3:1 for a quartet and so on. In highly crowded spectra the simple $2n\mathrm{I} + 1$ rule can break down and more complicated patterns are seen. For more details on the interpretation of these patterns see Chapter 4 of the book by Friebolin (1). The effects of scalar coupling that bring about the multiplicity of a signal provides very useful information regarding the chemical structure.

Scalar coupling data can also yield valuable stereochemical information. The Karplus equation shown below provides a quantitative relationship between the three-bond scalar coupling constant J and the dihedral angle ϕ between two protons (2).

$$J_{\mathrm{vicinal}} = 4.22 - 0.5\cos\phi + 4.5\cos^2\phi \qquad (4)$$

In this example, the coefficients above have been empirically optimized for H–C–C–H couplings. It should be noted that the form of Eq. 4 results in two possible dihedral angles for each coupling constant, but stereochemical arguments are often enough to determine a single conformation.

Integration

Another important characteristic of a signal in an NMR spectrum is its integral. Unlike other spectroscopic methods, the detected signal in NMR is directly proportional to the number of nuclei producing it. This

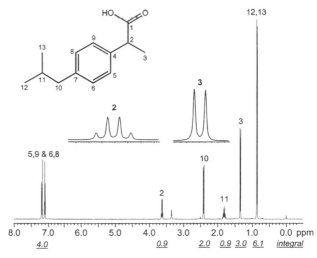

Fig. 2 One-dimensional ^{1}H spectrum of ibuprofen (5 mg in 600 μl DMSO-d_6, 25°C, 400 MHz). Peak assignments are given above each set of signals. Expansions of the multiplets for the protons attached to C_2 and C_3 demonstrate the $2n\mathrm{I} + 1$ rule of scalar coupling. The integral values are given below the chemical shift axis. Note that the peak for the hydroxyl proton at 11.1 ppm is not shown. Small peaks at 3.3, 2.5, and 0 ppm are from H_2O, DMSO-d_5, and TMS, respectively.

feature is very useful in the interpretation of NMR spectra since the relative integrals of the signals directly correlate to the relative numbers of nuclei in the molecule giving rise to those signals. The integral values of the ibuprofen signals are displayed below the chemical shift axis in Fig. 2. A caveat in the quantitative interpretation of integrals is that different nuclei require different amounts of time to relax back to equilibrium between pulses. When a signal is not fully relaxed between pulses the amount of magnetization that will be tipped into the $x-y$ plane by the subsequent pulse will be reduced thereby diminishing the integral value. These effects are seen in the slight deviations from the expected integer values in the ibuprofen spectrum. Precise and reliable quantitation of NMR signals therefore requires long delays between pulses. More details of relaxation follow.

Relaxation

After the rf pulse has tipped the magnetization into the transverse plane and the spins begin to precess, nuclear relaxation also begins to bring the signals back to equilibrium along the z-axis. The mechanisms by which energy is transferred to effect relaxation and the rates at which these mechanisms occur are very useful parameters and can be measured experimentally. There are several different relaxation mechanisms, which are more or less important under particular sets of conditions. In solution state studies, the dipole–dipole relaxation mechanism is by far the most important. Any given nucleus in a molecule is surrounded by other dipolar nuclei which are in motion. This motion leads to fluctuating magnetic fields, which can cause nuclear transitions and hence relaxation. Dipolar relaxation is therefore highly dependent upon the molecular motion. The three main forms of relaxation that are important for solution state structural studies are spin–lattice (T_1), spin–spin (T_2), and the nuclear Overhauser effect (nOe). These three mechanisms and their impact on molecular structure analysis are described below.

Spin-lattice relaxation is a process by which the excited spins give up energy to the surroundings (the lattice). This type of relaxation is most efficient when the molecule tumbles at a rate that is very close to the resonance frequency of the nucleus being studied. The rate of tumbling of a molecule is described by the correlation time τ_c. The correlation time can be approximated by

$$\tau_c = 4\pi \eta a^3 / 3kT \qquad (5)$$

where η is the viscosity of the solution and a is the radius of the molecule. An approximation of the correlation time

in a typical organic solvent can be derived from the molecular weight (MW), using

$$t_c \approx \mathrm{MW} \times 10^{-12} \qquad (6)$$

For a proton in an 11.7 T magnet, T_1 relaxation will be fastest when the correlation time is on the order of 500×10^{-6} s. The dependence of T_1 upon correlation time is given in Fig. 3. In typical organic solvents the T_1 minimum is reached for molecules with a molecular weight in the neighborhood of 1–2 kDa.

The T_1 relaxation time is the critical relaxation parameter in obtaining quantitative integrations. For essentially complete relaxation to occur after application of a 90° pulse, a delay time of about $5 \times T_1$ between pulses is recommended, but for nonquantitative analyses, the time can be closer to $1 \times T_1$. In practice, pulses much less than 90° are often used, which allows for more quantitative spectra in less time. For protons on small molecules (MW < 1000), typical ^{1}H T_1 relaxation times range from less than one to several seconds. For ^{13}C, the relaxation times are much longer, in some cases greater than 60 s. The extremely long delays required for accurate ^{13}C integration limit the practical application of quantitative ^{13}C NMR. T_1 times can be readily measured using the inversion-recovery experiment in which the signal intensities are modulated by a series of pulses and delays (1). Curve fitting of the signal intensities as a function of the delays yields the T_1 values.

Spin–spin relaxation is a process in which there is no net loss or gain of energy, but the spins lose phase coherence. The basis of this type of relaxation is the

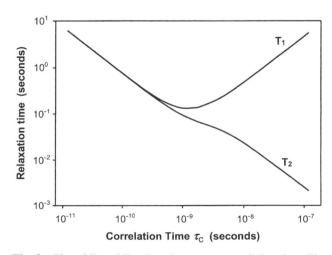

Fig. 3 Plot of T_1 and T_2 relaxation versus correlation time. The curves have been computed for the dipolar relaxation between two protons separated by 2.0 Å in a magnetic field of 11.7 T.

transfer of energy from one nucleus to another via the fluctuation magnetic fields. As one spin is excited to a higher state, another is relaxed back to the lower state. The net result of these transitions is that the phases of particular types of spins spread out or dephase. As the spins continue to dephase, they will eventually cancel one another resulting in the loss of the signal.

The T_2 time has a critical relationship to the linewidth of the NMR signal at half height ($\Delta\nu$) given by

$$\Delta\nu_{12} = 1\pi T_2{}^* \tag{7}$$

The term $T_2{}^*$ is used to denote inclusion of the contributions to T_2 from magnetic field inhomogeneities. When the magnetic field is not totally homogeneous, the small differences in the magnetic field experienced by the same nucleus at different locations in the sample gives rise to slight differences in the precessional frequencies. This leads to the same type of phase coherence loss as the inherent T_2 processes. T_2 relaxation times can be measured using spin-echo experiments designed to eliminate the contributions of field inhomogeneities. These experiments are well described in the book by Friebolin (1).

As with T_1 relaxation, T_2 relaxation has a strong dependence upon the molecular correlation time. Unlike T_1 relaxation, T_2 relaxation does not reach a minimum and then increase, but continues to decrease, as shown in Fig. 3. Therefore large, slowly tumbling molecules have very short T_2 times. This poses a great challenge in the study of large molecules or molecules in the solid state since the lifetime of the signal is very short and the linewidths are very broad.

The nuclear Overhauser effect is the most widely measured of the relaxation phenomena in structural studies. The nOe experiments directly measure the dipole–dipole relaxation between nuclei. The great utility of the nOe is its potential to determine internuclear distances. The magnitude of the nOe is proportional to $(r_{IS})^{-6}$ where r_{IS} is the distance between spins I and S. The nOe effects an increase or decrease in the intensity of a particular signal, based on the spacial proximity of its neighbors and the dynamics of the molecule. For a more rigorous description of the physical basis of the nOe the reader is referred to the excellent text by Neuhaus and Williamson (3).

The dependence of the nOe upon molecular motion is shown in Fig. 4. Notice that both the sign and magnitude of the nOe are a function of the correlation time. An important feature of the nOe is that for molecules in a particular tumbling regime, the nOe passes through zero. This is important for many pharmaceutically relevant compounds since for some molecules with molecular

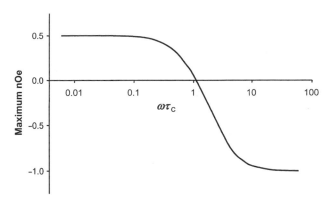

Fig. 4 Plot of maximum nOe versus $\omega\tau_c$ where ω ($= 2\,\pi\nu$) is the precessional frequency of the nuclei and τ_c is the correlation time. The curve has been computed for a pair of protons separated by 2.0 Å in a magnetic field of 11.7 T.

weights around 1–2 kDa in a viscous solvent like DMSO the tumbling rate can result in nOes very near zero. In this situation no nOe will be observed, irrespective of molecular structure. For these studies, another form of the nOe is more useful. The rotating frame Overhauser effect (rOe) is also function of dipolar relaxation, but occurs under a different set of experimental conditions (4, 5). The advantage of the rOe is that the effect does not pass through zero. The rOe experiments are somewhat more difficult to setup than nOe experiments and quantitative interpretation is more difficult, but they have proven very valuable in the structural analysis of many pharmaceuticals.

NMR TECHNIQUES

NMR has been an integral part of the chemist's analytical toolbox for decades. The most common and fundamental experiment is the one-dimensional (1D) ^{1}H experiment. The relatively high sensitivity of the ^{1}H nucleus makes this a very useful start, but for a complex molecule the 1D spectrum can be crowded and often uninterpretable. In these cases more advanced techniques can be used to provide increased resolution and specific types of structural information. In this section we will describe a range of NMR techniques from the simplest 1D experiments to complex multidimensional, multinuclear experiments. The focus of this section will be on the general principles underlying these experiments and their applications to molecules of pharmaceutical interest. Further details on these experiments can be found in the references.

One-Dimensional Experiments

A one-dimensional NMR spectrum provides a wealth of information, which for simple molecules may yield enough detail for complete structural characterization. The ^{1}H spectrum of a 5 mg sample of ibuprofen shown in Fig. 2 was taken in less than 1 min. Given the relative simplicity of this molecule, all of the ^{1}H resonances can be assigned by inspection. Full characterization of pharmaceutical molecules often requires that the ^{13}C chemical shifts be assigned as well. However, ^{13}C NMR spectra require much longer acquisition times than ^{1}H spectra due to the relative sensitivity and low natural abundance (see Table 1). Fig. 5 shows the 1D ^{13}C spectrum of the same 5-mg sample of ibuprofen taken in about 30 min. The broad chemical shift range for ^{13}C yields spectra with typically well-resolved peaks. This spectrum was acquired with the proton decoupler on throughout the experiment, which collapses all of the ^{13}C multiplets into singlets. Additionally the ^{1}H decoupling provides a signal enhancement of up to 200% due to the ^{1}H–^{13}C nOe. [Further details on heteronuclear nOes can be found in Chapter 2 of Ref. (3)]. For relatively simple compounds in which there are ample amounts of sample, the 1D ^{1}H and ^{13}C spectra can yield unequivocal assignments.

For samples such as natural products, metabolites, and degradation products, the sample amounts are typically far less than the 5 mg used in the example above. In these cases the ^{1}H spectrum is still a necessity, but it may be impractical to acquire a ^{13}C spectrum. The signal to noise ratio (S/N) for NMR spectra is a linear function of sample concentration, but builds up as the square root of the number of scans. Therefore, if the sample concentration is reduced by a factor of 100, it will take 100^2 times the number of scans to achieve a spectrum with the same S/N.

Spin Polarization Transfer

Several methods of signal enhancement have been developed to help overcome the inherently low sensitivity of important nuclei such as ^{13}C and ^{15}N. These experiments rely on the principle of spin polarization transfer where magnetization on the more sensitive nuclei, usually ^{1}H, is transferred to the attached nuclei of interest through a specific sequence of pulses and delays. The signal enhancement achievable through polarization transfer is proportional to γ_I/γ_S, where I and S represent the abundant and rare spins, respectively. This corresponds to a factor of 4 for ^{13}C and a factor of 10 for ^{15}N (see Table 1) and can yield dramatic savings in

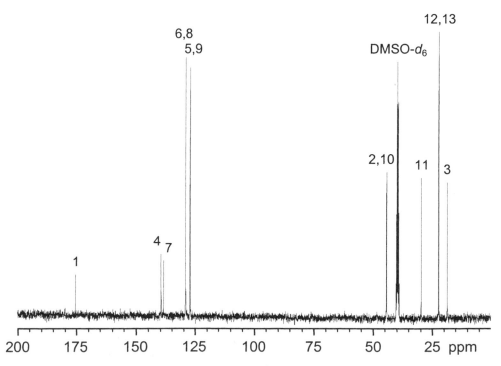

Fig. 5 ^{13}C NMR spectrum of ibuprofen (5 mg in 600 µl DMSO-d_6, 25°C, 100 MHz). Peak assignments are given above the signals and refer to the chemical numbering shown in Fig. 2. Note the overlap between C$_2$ and C$_{10}$.

acquisition time. Polarization transfer experiments also enable use of faster repetition rates based on the typically shorter T_1 relaxation rates of the protons thereby providing an additional gain in overall sensitivity. Two methods of polarization transfer used in solution NMR are the INEPT (Insensitive Nuclei Enhanced by Polarization Transfer) experiment (6) and the DEPT (Distortionless Enhancement by Polarization Transfer) experiment (7). The latter experiment provides the added feature of spectral editing such that subspectra containing different types of carbons can be obtained or a single spectrum generated where methyl and methine carbon resonances are phased positive and methylene carbon resonances are negative. Quaternary carbons are not observed in these experiments since the signals rely on the transfer of polarization from attached protons.

Two-Dimensional Experiments

As the size and complexity of a molecule increases, the proton NMR spectrum can easily become crowded and very difficult to interpret. Steroids are a common class of compounds of pharmaceutical interest and provide a very good example of spectral crowding. Steroid ^{1}H NMR spectra typically contain a region between approximately 1 and 4 ppm known as the methylene envelope in which a large proportion of the proton signals reside (8). In this situation, two-dimensional (2D) NMR can be used to spread the signals out into a second dimension providing an invaluable increase in resolution. The simplest of the 2D experiments is the COSY (COrrelation SpectroscopY) experiment. COSY spectra are characterized by two types of peaks, those along the diagonal and crosspeaks located off of the diagonal. The diagonal is effectively a 1D spectrum, and the crosspeaks indicate a scalar coupling relationship between the two resonances at coordinate chemical shifts of the crosspeak. Fig. 6 shows an expansion of the double quantum filtered COSY spectrum of the highly crowed region of dutasteride. The double quantum filtered COSY is a simple modification of the COSY experiment, which, among other benefits, yields narrower diagonal peaks allowing for crosspeaks close to the diagonal to be better resolved (9). Notice that the crosspeaks in the spectrum are characterized by a specific pattern, which contains the scalar coupling information between the correlated protons. COSY spectra can provide both connectivity and scalar coupling constants from highly crowded spectra, although the latter is not always straightforward.

TOCSY (TOtal Correlation Spectroscopy) is another important homonuclear 2D correlation experiment where correlations arise due to the presence of homonuclear scalar coupling (10). In the standard COSY experiment, crosspeaks appear for spins in which the scalar coupling occurs over typically two to four bonds. In the TOCSY experiment crosspeaks can appear for spins separated by many more bonds as long as they are part of a contiguous network of coupled spins. The correlations are effected by the application of a series of low-power rf pulses termed the spin-lock. The duration of the spin-lock period determines the extent to which the correlations are propagated through the spin system. The TOCSY experiment is a useful complement to the COSY methods for the elucidation of complex structures.

The 2D nOe experiment NOESY (Nuclear Overhauser Enhancement SpectroscopY) provides correlations between nuclei that are close in space. While nOe experiments can be carried out using selective excitation of individual signals, one at a time, to determine the identity of protons proximal to the selected peak, the NOESY experiment enables the determination of nOe information between all spins in one experiment. Cross peaks in a NOESY experiment indicate which protons are close to one another. Typically nOe crosspeaks can be observed for protons less than 5 Å apart in the molecule. Fig. 7 shows the NOESY spectrum of dutasteride with several key correlations highlighted. The results of this experiment enable complete stereochemical assignment of all the protons in the molecule.

Two dimensional experiments can also show correlations between different types of nuclei. These heteronuclear experiments have the advantage that nuclei such as ^{13}C and ^{15}N have much wider chemical shift ranges, and therefore the 2D experiments achieve a tremendous reduction in spectral crowding. The HETCOR (HETeronuclear CORrelation) experiment was the first 2D experiment developed to provide correlations between ^{1}H and ^{13}C. In this experiment, the magnetization is transferred from a proton to its attached carbon via the one bond scalar coupling in a manner similar to the DEPT experiment. The acquisition parameters can be modified to allow for the correlation of protons to carbons several bonds away by optimizing for the smaller multiple bond heteronulcear scalar coupling constants. The multiple bond correlations can be combined with the single bond correlations to put together the pieces of a molecule for complete structure elucidation or spectral assignment. While it provides important C–H connectivity information, the HETCOR experiment suffers from relatively poor sensitivity resulting from the detection of the carbon signals.

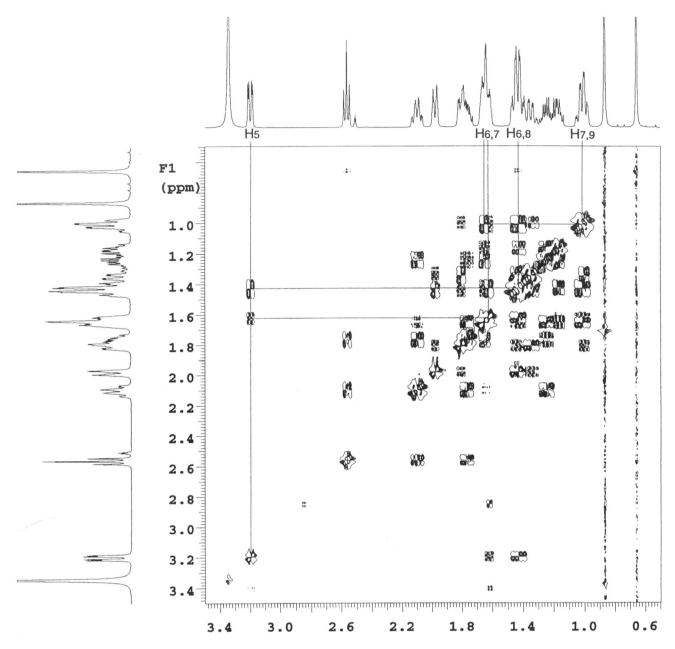

Fig. 6 Aliphatic region of a DQF–COSY spectrum of dutasteride in DMSO-d_6. Correlations show scalar connectivities between neighboring protons and facilitate proton resonance assignments, which begin with H_5 and are traced throughout the spin system. (See Fig. 10 for structure and numbering scheme.) Complete analysis is complicated by overlapping resonances.

Inverse Detection Experiments

Inverse detection experiments consist of a sequence of pulses and delays that transfer the magnetization from ^1H to the attached X nuclei (typically ^{13}C or ^{15}N) and then back to ^1H for detection. In this way, the experiments maintain a sensitivity level much closer to

a standard ^1H experiment and represent a marked improvement over the HETCOR experiments. The first of these types of experiments was the HMQC (Heteronuclear Multiple Quantum Coherence) experiment (11). Fig. 8 shows the HMQC spectrum of dutasteride. The utility of this experiment is the ability to resolve overlapping proton resonances by spreading

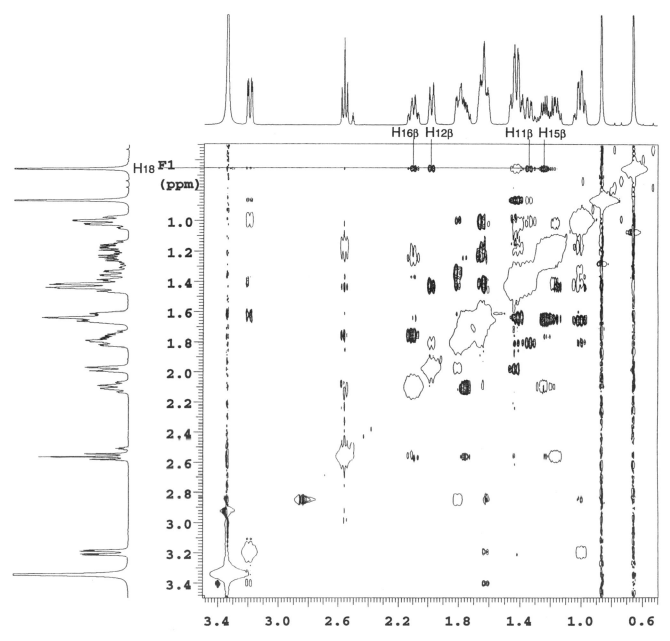

Fig. 7 Aliphatic region of a NOESY spectrum of dutasteride in DMSO-d_6. Correlations show through space interactions between neighboring nuclei and are used to make relative stereochemical assignments for proton resonances. Correlations between the H_{18} methyl group and nearby protons on the same side of the steroid ring system are highlighted. (See Fig. 10 for structure and numbering scheme.)

them out over the carbon chemical shift dimension and assign carbon resonances from known proton assignments or vice versa. Some key correlations are highlighted. Note that inequivalent methylene protons are readily identified as they show correlations to the same carbon. This experiment contains exactly the same type of information as the HETCOR, but spectra of

equivalent S/N can be acquired in about one-fourth the time for $^1H-^{13}C$ correlations and one tenth the time for $^1H-^{15}N$ correlations. Given the inherently low sensitivity of ^{15}N, direct observation of ^{15}N is rarely done, but inverse detection methods have made $^1H-^{15}N$ correlations much more facile. A recent review by Martin describes the utility of the $^1H-^{15}N$ inverse

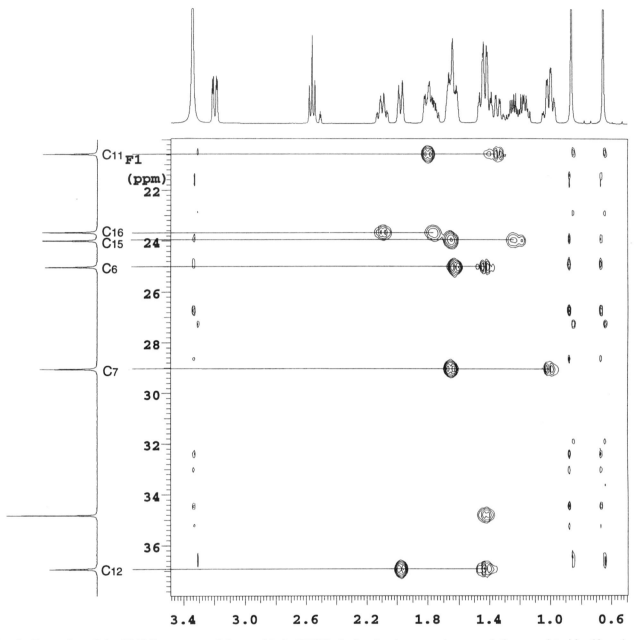

Fig. 8 Expansion of the HMQC spectrum of dutasteride in DMSO-d_6 showing heteronuclear correlations used to identify pairs of methylene protons and assign carbon resonances based on proton assignments. The six methylene proton pairs highlighted are readily identified since there are two protons with different chemical shifts correlated to each carbon. (See Fig. 10 for structure and numbering scheme.)

detection experiments in the structural determination of natural products (12).

The HSQC (Heteronuclear Single Quantum Coherence) experiment is another widely used inverse detection experiment (13, 14). It provides essentially the same information as HMQC, but relies on a different sequence

of pulses to effect the transfer of magnetization between ^{1}H and the heteronucleus. A direct comparison of HMQC and HSQC in the study of a natural product has indicated some advantages of the latter-sequence, which may provide improved sensitivity and narrower crosspeaks for improved resolution (15).

Long range proton connectivities to heteronuclei can also be obtained from inverse detection experiments. A modification of the HMQC referred to as the HMBC (Heteronuclear Multiple Bond Coherence) experiment can be optimized for transfer through multiple bonds based on the value of the multiple bond couplings (16), which is typically about 8 Hz for a three-bond $^1H-^{13}C$ coupling. The HMBC spectrum of dutasteride shown in Fig. 9 illustrates the utility of this experiment for assigning quaternary carbons, connecting isolated spin systems (e.g., H_{18} and H_{19}) to other spin systems in the molecule, and confirming assignments made from the COSY and HMQC spectra.

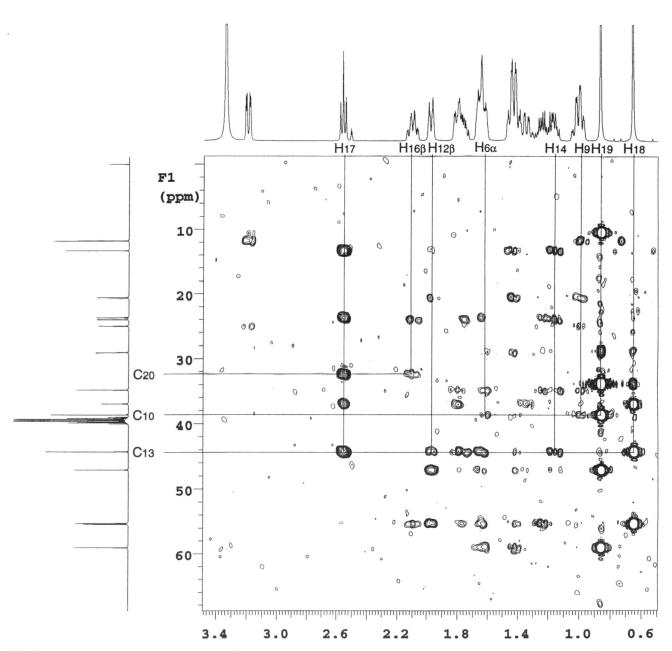

Fig. 9 Expansion of the HMBC spectrum of dutasteride in DMSO-d_6 showing multiple bond correlations used to assign quaternary carbon resonances. Highlighted are correlations used to assign C_{10}, C_{13}, and the carbonyl resonance C_{20}, which is folded over in the ^{13}C dimension. Other correlations in the spectrum serve to confirm resonance assignments made based on results from the other experiments. (See Fig. 10 for structure and numbering scheme.)

Recent years have seen a great deal of activity in the improvement of HMBC sequences including the accordion type experiments. These experiments are optimized for transfer through a wide range of heteronuclear couplings (e.g., 2–25 Hz) and can provide H–C correlations over two to four bonds. Accordian experiments have found great utility in the assignment of some complex natural products. The details and specific advantages of these experiments has been recently reviewed (17).

For small molecules of pharmaceutical interest, the foregoing array of NMR experiments yield most if not all of the information required to fully interpret the ^{1}H and ^{13}C NMR spectra and to completely characterize the structure of a molecule. The results of this type of analysis are summarized in Figs. 10 and 11, typical of what is often required for regulatory submissions.

Higher-Dimensional Experiments

There is no limit to the complexity of molecular structures and thus, it is clear that NMR spectra can become ever more complicated. In large molecules such as proteins, the second dimension is often not enough to provide the necessary resolution for facile interpretation. This has lead to the development of three-dimensional (3D) experiments (18). In these experiments the resonances are spread out into a third dimension with the spectrum taking the form of a cube. Examples of a heteronuclear 3D experiment include HMQC–COSY and HMQC–NOESY in which the crosspeaks of a COSY or NOESY spectrum are further separated in the third dimension by their respective carbon chemical shifts (19). Four-dimensional (4D) experiments are also frequently used in the study of proteins in which correlations can be made between ^{1}H, ^{13}C, and ^{15}N in a single (triple-resonance) experiment. These spectra can be visualized as a cube in which each slice through the cube can be expanded into another cube. Protein studies often involve the incorporation of ^{13}C and ^{15}N isotopes into the protein, which greatly increases the sensitivity of the highly time consuming 3D and 4D experiments. An excellent description of higher dimensional experiments and their applications to protein structure elucidation is given in the review by Clore and Gronenborn (20).

Pulsed Field Gradients

One of the most important developments in NMR in recent years has been the application of pulsed field gradients (PFGs) (21). PFGs have long been used in magnetic resonance imaging methods, but only in the last decade has the technology been developed for routine use in high resolution NMR. PFGs consist of an extra magnetic field applied across the sample in a spacially dependent manner. This imparts a phase shift to a given signal which is correlated to its position in the sample. PFGs have many utilities in high resolution NMR. They can be used to eliminate certain undesired signals by selectively dephasing them. Alternatively, signals can be selected using pairs of gradients in which the first gradient dephases all spins and a second gradient is optimized to refocus only selected spins. The judicious implementation of PFGs in pulse sequences has lead to much cleaner spectra with fewer artifacts.

Another important use of PFGs is in the study of diffusion processes. A pair of PFGs of opposite sign separated by a delay time can be used to analyze the diffusion of molecules. If a molecule migrates significantly during the diffusion period, the second gradient will not effectively refocus those spins and the signals for that molecule will become attenuated. The use of PFG diffusion studies in high throughput screening studies will be discussed ahead.

APPLICATIONS OF NMR

The NMR techniques described in the last section provide the foundation for many of the advanced applications of NMR in the pharmaceutical industry. The challenges of this industry have lead to the optimization of hardware and experimental design to answer specific questions. Some of the most important questions and the NMR applications that have been developed to answer them will be described in the next sections.

Analysis of Small Sample Quantities

Small volume NMR probes

Samples such as metabolites, degradation products, and natural products may be very laborious to isolate and purify and are often available in only extremely small quantities. The sensitivity of NMR is considered low *vis a vis* other structural methods such as UV, IR, and MS, but the high information content has made increasing the limits of detection a very active and worthwhile pursuit. Sensitivity increases have traditionally been achieved by increasing the sample concentration or the magnetic field strength, but in recent years, optimization of the NMR probe has yielded significant gains. The NMR probe houses the hardware for the delivery of rf pulses and the detection of the NMR signal. Until recently, 5 mm sample tubes with a sample volume of 500–600 μl was the

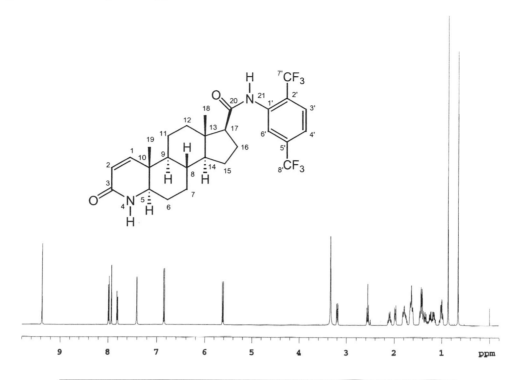

Chemical shift (δ)[a]	Multiplicity[b]	Integration	Assignment
9.38	s	1	21
7.99	d	1	3'
7.93	brs	1	6'
7.81	d	1	4'
7.40	d	1	4
6.85	d	1	1
5.62	dd	1	2
3.20	dd	1	5
2.56	t	1	17
2.10	m	1	16β
1.98	m	1	12β
1.80	m	1	11α
1.76	m	1	16α
1.65	m	2	7β, 15α
1.26	m	1	6α
1.43	m	2	8, 12α
1.42	m	1	6β
1.34	m	1	11β
1.24	m	1	15β
1.17	m	1	14
1.01	m	1	7α
0.99	m	1	9
0.87	s	3	19
0.66	s	3	18

[a] ppm downfield from TMS =0.00 ppm: DMSO-d_5 and H_2O appear at 2.51 and 3.34 ppm, respectively.
[b] s=singlet: d=doublet: t=triplet: q=quartet m=multiplet: br=broad.

Fig. 10 ^{1}H NMR spectrum and characterization of dutasteride in DMSO-d_6.

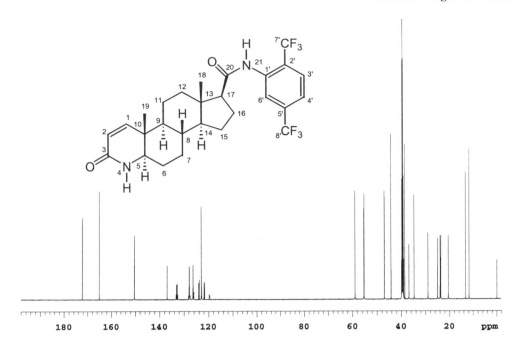

Chemical shift(δ)[a]	Multiplicity[b]	$J^{19}\text{F-}^{13}\text{C}$(Hz)	Assignment
172.33	s	–	20
165.07	s	–	3
150.38	s	–	1
136.95	q	1.7	1'
132.89	q	32.6	5'
127.85	q	5.2	3'
127.83	q	29.6	2'
126.37	q	3.5	6'
123.09	q	273.1	8'
123.07	s	–	2
122.97	q	3.4	4'
122.77	q	273.9	7'
59.02	s	–	5
55.37	s	–	17
55.23	s	–	14
47.04	s	–	9
44.25	s	–	13
38.58	s	–	10
36.91	s	–	12
34.80	s	–	8
29.03	s	–	7
25.01	s	–	6
23.98	s	–	15
23.66	s	–	16
20.56	s	–	11
13.29	s	–	18
11.77	s	–	19

[a]ppm downfield from TMS = 0.00 ppm: DMSO-d_6 appears at 39.47 ppm.
[b]Arising from ^{19}F coupling: s = singlet: q = quartet.

Fig. 11 ^{13}C NMR spectrum and characterization of dutasteride in DMSO-d_6.

standard for solution NMR studies. With very small sample amounts this results in a very dilute sample. Commercial NMR probes are now available for sample tubes as small as 1.7 mm with sample volumes down to 30μl. Efficient coupling of the NMR detector coil to physically smaller samples has resulted in a more than eightfold decrease in acquisition time over the standard 5-mm NMR sample tube configuration (22). The decrease in sample volumes has been taken even further by Sweedler and coworkers who have recently designed microcoil probes with a 200-nl sample volume (23). Reductions in sample volume provide an effective means to increase sensitivity, but further reductions may be less effective due to difficulties in routinely handing such small samples.

Low temperature probes

Increases in sensitivity can be also achieved by reducing the temperature of the detection coil. This was first demonstrated by Styles and coworkers who obtained substantial increases by operating the coil at cryogenic temperatures (24, 25). Recently an application of high resolution NMR on a natural product has been reported using a probe with rf coils made of high-temperature superconducting (HTS) materials operating at 25 K (26) where an enhancement in signal to noise of 3.5 was obtained over conventional probes. Currently, the HTS probes appear to have limited utility because the geometry of the coils cannot be optimized for standard cylindrical NMR tubes. Using the same idea of reduced temperature rf coil detection, cold probes are now being developed in which standard probe coil materials are cooled. This probe cooling combined with optimization for small sample volumes provides further sensitivity enhancements.

Flow NMR Methods

High-throughput NMR

Advances in parallel synthesis and combinatorial chemistry have given pharmaceutical companies the ability to generate an unprecedented number of compounds. In lead compound optimization efforts, libraries containing hundreds of compounds are often made for which structure validation is often necessary. For the synthetic chemist, high resolution NMR would be the tool of choice for this effort, but the standard method of preparing hundreds of individual NMR tubes for analysis would be prohibitively time consuming. This hurdle has been overcome by the development of flow NMR systems (27), which utilize a specialized flow cell in the probe so that samples can be injected into the NMR without the preparation of individual sample tubes. HPLC type autosamplers connected to an injector system deliver the sample directly to the flow cell of the probe. In this way, samples in microtiter plates can be analyzed in an automated fashion. After the spectrum is taken, the flow can be reversed and the sample returned to its original location in the plate or diverted to waste. These probes have been optimized in terms of sensitivity to detect small sample quantities from micrograms down to hundreds of nanograms.

LC–NMR

Many of the most important chemical questions in the pharmaceutical industry involve the analysis of complex mixtures. Identification of low-level metabolites and drug substance impurities usually requires high-performance liquid chromatography for the separation of these mixtures or isolation of a compound of interest from a sample matrix. In these analyses, the structural information obtainable for the low-level compounds is limited by the type of detection used. The coupling of HPLC and mass spectrometry has become routine and provides useful molecular weight and fragmentation information, but this is often not enough for complete structure elucidation.

Recently, NMR spectrometers directly coupled with LC systems have become commercially available (28, 29). Spectra can be acquired in either of two modes, continuous or stopped flow. In continuous flow mode the spectrum is acquired as the analyte flows through the cell. This method suffers from low sensitivity since the analyte may be present in the cell for only a brief period of time, but it has the advantage of continuous monitoring of the LC peaks without interruption. Fig. 12a shows a contour plot of the continuous flow NMR analysis of a mixture of vitamin A acetate isomers (30). Fig. 12b shows the spectra taken from slices through the contour plot. These plots highlight the olefinic region of the spectra which provided ample information for the identification of each of the isomers. With very limited sample quantities, the more common method of LC–NMR analysis is stopped flow. Here the analyte peak is parked in the flow cell so any of the standard NMR experiments can be run.

A problem with the coupling of HPLC to NMR is that typical LC solvents give rise to very large background signals. The simplest way to avoid this is by using deuterated solvents, but given the relatively large volumes of solvent necessary, this can be very expensive. Recently developed solvent suppression methods have provided excellent means of reducing the signals from fully protonated solvents. These methods utilize a series of selective pulses along with pulsed field gradients and can simultaneously suppress several solvent signals in the spectrum (31). Another problem can arise when gradient elution methods

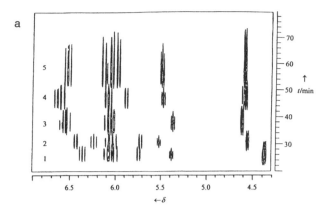

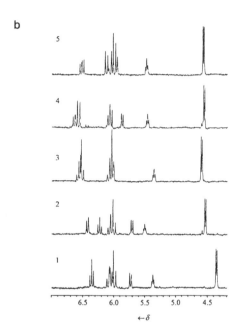

Fig. 12 a) Contour plot of the LC-NMR analysis of a mixture of vitamin A acetate isomers (400 MHz). b) Slices taken through the contour plot showing spectra of the individual components of the mixture. (From Ref. 30.)

are used in the LC separation because the chemical shifts of the solvent resonances can change as the gradient mixture changes. This is addressed by software that can dynamically modify the solvent suppression scheme to keep up with the chemical shift changes of the solvent resonances. Even with fully deuterated solvents for all mobile phase components solvent supression methods are often still required for the residual protonated solvent signals.

LC–NMR–MS

The combination of LC with analytical methods has been taken a step further with in-line coupling of LC, NMR, and

MS systems to provide maximum information with minimal sample handing (32, 33). This setup yields both structural and molecular mass information from a single HPLC injection. The practical issues of running a mass spectrometer in close proximity to the magnetic field of the NMR provided somewhat of a hurdle to the technique, but this has been recently addressed by actively shielded magnets in which the stray magnetic fields are greatly attenuated by counter acting fields engineered into the magnet. The NMR and MS are typically setup in parallel with the flow split such that a small amount of the sample is sent to the MS and the rest to the NMR flow cell. This provides two sets of synchronized datasets, which facilitates interpretation. This also avoids potential issues of back pressure from the flow at the interface between the NMR and the MS.

NMR Based Screening Methods

Affinity NMR

One of the challenges that arises from the synthesis of combinatorial libraries is the screening of huge numbers of molecules for a desired biological activity. Mixtures of molecules are often screened in a single test which can lead to erroneous results. In some assays the sum of multiple small interactions can lead the screen to give a positive result when in fact no single molecule in the mixture is suitable for further study. A variety of experiments based on NMR have been developed recently that allow for the screening of complex mixtures with no need for physical separation and no risk of false positives from the additive effects of weak interactions. One of the methods for screening mixtures referred to as affinity NMR or diffusion edited NMR can be used to selectively observe only those ligands in a mixture that bind to a receptor molecule (34). The selection process is based on the changes in the diffusion rate of a ligand that occurs upon binding.

Affinity NMR experiments exploit the fact that the diffusion rate of molecules that bind to a receptor molecule will be greatly reduced. As described earlier, a PFG is applied to dephase all of the NMR signals. An equal but opposite PFG is applied after a delay time to refocus only those spins involved in binding to the receptor. Molecules not involved in binding will rapidly diffuse during the delay period between gradients, and their signals will be greatly attenuated. A qualitative ranking of ligand binding can be made based on the observed signal intensities. Although there are certain factors such as exchange phenomena that can complicate the interpretation of diffusion studies [see

Ref. (34)], the relative simplicity and nondestructive nature of diffusion based NMR screening make it a very valuable tool in drug discovery.

Transferred nOe screening

Another form of affinity NMR relies on the transferred nOe (35). As discussed earlier, small rapidly tumbling molecules display positive nOes and large slowly tumbling molecules display negative nOes. Upon binding to a large receptor, a small molecule assumes the correlation time of the receptor and large negative nOes develop. After the molecule dissociates from the receptor, the intensities of the signals remain perturbed by the large negative nOes, but the rapid small molecule tumbling rate yields narrow linewidths. The NOESY sequence can be used in these studies, and the negative nOe signals can be selectively displayed. The sensitivity of this method can be adjusted by varying the ratio of ligand to receptor. Typically, studies have observed the ligand in a 10–20-fold excess that allows these experiments to be carried out with very small amounts of receptor. This is a great advantage of transferred nOe based screening, especially with receptors that are difficult to produce and isolate.

Biomolecular NMR Studies

Protein structure studies

Due to their size and spectral complexity, proteins are among the most challenging molecules for NMR spectroscopy. As discussed earlier, a large number of sophisticated multidimensonal, multinuclear NMR methods have been developed for the complete structural determination of proteins. The general procedure for protein structure determination can be summarized as four basic steps. The first step is sequential assignment of all amino acid resonances, using through-bond or through-space experiments. The second step is torsion angle determination using three-bond scalar coupling information. The third step is identification of through space interactions, using nOes. And the fourth step is calculation of the structure based on the structural restraints (nOes and torsion angles) using one or more computational refinement tools (20). This process requires large amounts of data to be acquired for a complete structure elucidation, which can be very time-consuming. Advances in molecular biology have made the incorporation of isotope labels in proteins using microbial systems relatively routine. With ^{15}N and ^{13}C labels the requisite 3D and 4D experiments can often be acquired in a matter of hours

rather than days. Currently it is possible to determine the structures of proteins in the 15–35 kDa range at a resolution comparable to ~2.5 Å resolution crystal structures.

Protein–ligand interactions

Solution state NMR experiments that probe the interactions between ligands and receptors have become an important part of the drug development process. When the structure of a protein has been completely determined by NMR, small changes in the chemical shifts of residues in the binding site will occur upon addition of an active ligand. These chemical shift changes are readily observed in ^{1}H{^{15}N} HSQC spectra acquired using ^{15}N labeled proteins. This method, known as chemical shift mapping, has been used to identify the binding sites of proteins, screen for active ligands, and design and optimize lead compounds.

High-throughput chemical shift mapping studies to screen for active ligands has recently been demonstrated using cryoprobe technology. The increased sensitivity of the cryoprobes enables protein ^{1}H{^{15}N} HSQC spectra to be acquired using very low protein concentrations. Since the total concentration of added molecules in these studies must be kept at a reasonable level (~5–10 mM), the use of lower protein concentrations allows for higher ligand concentrations. Hadjuk and coworkers analyzed mixtures of 100 compounds for the presence of tight binding molecules (36). The authors suggest that libraries of more than 200,000 compounds can be tested in less than one month using this strategy.

Structure–activity relationships (SAR) by NMR

A fundamental part of the drug design process is the development of structure–activity relationships. Recently an NMR method has been developed to produce SARs (37). In this method ligands are constructed from building blocks that have been optimized for binding to individual protein sub-sites. In the first step, a library of small organic molecules is screened for binding to a labeled protein. The binding event is detected by the observation of ^{15}N or ^{1}H chemical shift changes in the ^{1}H{^{15}N} HSQC spectra for resonances near the binding site. Once a lead molecule is identified, analogs are synthesized to optimize the binding. The process is then repeated to identify ligands that bind to a proximal binding site. Finally the separately optimized ligands are linked together to form a single high affinity ligand. This method was used to design a ligand to the immunosuppressant protein FK506 with an affinity of 19 nM.

SOLID-STATE NMR

A large proportion of pharmaceuticals end up in a solid formulation, so there is a clear need to characterize drugs in the solid state. Many different methods are available to study solid-state drug substances, including IR, Raman and X-ray diffraction, each with its own advantages and disadvantages (38). As in the solution state, solid-state NMR offers a potentially high level of structural information compared to other methods. In this section, a brief review of some of the fundamental differences between solid and liquid state NMR will be given along with some illustrative examples of the role of solid state NMR in pharmaceutical development.

Anisotropy in the Solid State

Simply placing a pellet of solid drug substance in an NMR tube and acquiring a 1D ^1H or ^{13}C spectrum will yield very poor results. The resulting spectrum would typically appear as a collection of highly overlapping signals with linewidths in the thousands of Hertz. The basis for this extreme line broadening is the presence of anisotropic (orientation dependent) effects that are averaged out in solution, but become dominant in the solid state. The most important of these anisotropic effects are the dipole–dipole interactions. The local field, B_{loc} of any nucleus is influenced by the presence of neighboring dipoles. The effect on a given nucleus, I is described in Equation (8), where μ_s is the magnetic moment of a neighboring nucleus S, r_{IS} is the distance between nuclei I and S, and θ is the angle between the internuclear vector and the static B_o field.

$$B_{loc} = \pm \mu_S r_{IS}^{-3}(3 \cos^2 \theta_{IS} - 1) \qquad (8)$$

In solution, the rapid tumbling causes an averaging of the local field over all orientations that yields a net local field of zero. In the solid state, this averaging process does not occur, and the sum of all of the dipolar interactions yields linewidths on the order of kilohertz.

The other important contribution to broad overlapping lines in solid state NMR spectra is chemical shift anisotropy (CSA). As discussed earlier, the chemical shift is affected by electrons that shield the nucleus from the applied magnetic field. The magnitude of this shielding is a function of the particular orientation of the molecule in the magnetic field. Like the dipolar interactions, the effects of CSA averages out to zero in solution, but not in the solid state. The angular dependence of the CSA also takes the form $(3 \cos^2 \theta - 1)$

where θ is the angle between the B_o field and the principle axis of the chemical shift (e.g., the C–O bond for a carbonyl carbon). The combined effects of dipolar coupling and CSA yield the tremendously broad lines observed in solid-state NMR.

Magic Angle Spinning and Cross-Polarization

The challenge of solid state NMR is to narrow the linewidths to an extent that the spectrum can be interpreted in a manner similar to a solution NMR spectrum. This challenge was met by noting that the $(3 \cos^2 \theta - 1)$ dependence of the dipolar interactions and CSA goes to zero when the angle θ is set to 54.7°, the magic angle. If a sample is spun about an axis oriented at the magic angle relative to B_o, the average orientation of the crystal axes will be equal to the magic angle and the anisotropic effects will be greatly diminished. The very strong dipolar interactions between ^{13}C and the attached protons may still yield broadened lines, therefore ^1H decoupling is often used in addition to magic angle spinning to achieve narrow lines in ^{13}C spectra.

The most widely studied nucleus in solid state NMR of pharmaceuticals is ^{13}C. As in solution, observation of ^{13}C suffers from inherently low sensitivity. Additionally, ^{13}C nuclei in the solid state have very long relaxation times, which limits the number of scans that can be acquired in a given amount of time. To enhance the sensitivity and allow for faster repetition rate, cross-polarization (CP) methods have been developed. CP is very analogous to spin polarization transfer. A train of simultaneous rf pulses on both the ^1H and ^{13}C is used to transfer the ^1H magnetization to the ^{13}C. In this way, the intensity of the ^{13}C line is greatly increased and the pulse repetition rate is dependent upon the ^1H and not the ^{13}C relaxation. Cross-polarization magic angle spinning (CP–MAS) experiments constitute the majority of solid state NMR studies in the pharmaceutical industry and provide the foundation for many of the more advanced techniques.

Applications of Solid State NMR

Gel-phase NMR

The synthesis of combinatorial libraries relies heavily on solid phase synthetic methods. Previously the analysis of these libraries, using high throughput flow NMR methods was discussed. These analyses relied on the cleavage of the product from the solid phase support. In some cases, the cleavage reaction can be very harsh, and it is often desirable to analyze the solid phase reaction product with the compound still attached to the bead. Given the macromolecular

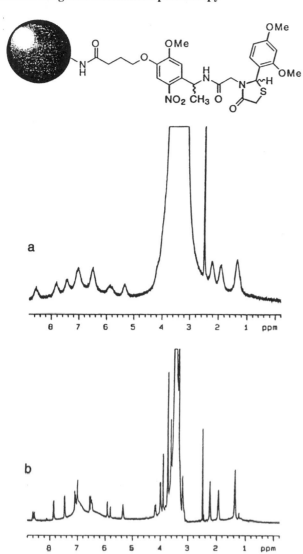

Fig. 13 a) ^{1}H spectrum of the "gel-phase" compound shown taken using a conventional 5-mm liquids probe. (100 mg sample suspended in 600 μl DMSO-d_6, 500 MHz) b) ^{1}H spectrum of the same sample taken using the Varian Nano-probe (Varian NMR Instruments Palo Alto, CA, USA) probe with magic angle spinning (10-mg sample suspended in 30 μl of DMSO-d_6, 500 MHz). (From Ref. 40.)

size of the bead, simply placing a sample of the solid phase material into an NMR tube would give spectra with broad overlapping lines. Magic angle spinning has been applied in order to narrow the lines of solid phase combinatorial samples (39). As the solid phase supports are swollen by solvents and therefore have properties that are neither distinctly solution phase nor solid phase, the term "gel-phase" NMR is used. This technique was used by Fitch and coworkers to generate 500 MHz spectra of organic

compounds bound to SPS resins with linewidths as narrow as 4 Hz (40). Fig. 13 shows the spectra of a "gel-phase" sample taken with conventional NMR methods and with magic angle spinning.

Polymorph studies

It has been estimated that approximately 30% of organic compounds crystallize in two or more forms that differ in the conformation and/or arrangement of molecules in the crystal lattice (41, 42). The crystalline form of a drug can have profound effects on the physicochemical properties. The density, melting point, dissolution rate, bioavailablity, and ease of formulation are all influenced to some degree by the crystal form. Polymorphism is defined as the ability of a compound to exist in more than one solid-state form with identical chemical structures, but different crystal lattices. Solvates are an important form of polymorphism in which the crystal lattice changes by the inclusion of solvent. Given the influence of polymorphic forms on physicochemical properties, characterization of all polymorphic forms present in a drug substance is becoming a requirement of the relevant regulatory agencies.

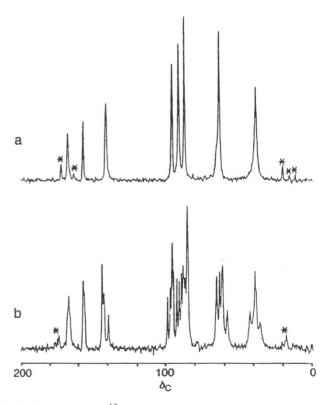

Fig. 14 Solid-state ^{13}C CP–MAS spectra of two polymorphic forms of lamivudine recorded at 125 MHz a) Form II, b) Form I. Signals indicated by asterisks are spinning sidebands. (From Ref. 43.)

Nuclear Magnetic Resonance Spectroscopy

Solid-state NMR has emerged as a powerful tool in the analysis of polymorphic drug forms. ^{13}C CP–MAS spectroscopy can be used to identify the number of crystallographically inequivalent sites in a unit cell and to understand the molecular structure on the basis of the chemical shifts. Fig. 14 shows the solid-state ^{13}C spectra of two forms of lamivudine (43). Form II shows a relatively simple spectrum in which there is only one molecule in the crystallographic asymmetric unit. The spectrum of Form I is much more complex, especially in the region from 80 to 100 ppm. Analysis of this spectrum indicates that there are five distinct molecules in the unit cell. This rare phenomenon was subsequently confirmed by X-ray diffraction.

Solid-state structural studies

Standard 1D ^{13}C CP–MAS spectra provide highly valuable data in terms of characterizing a single polymorph or determining the number of polymorphs in a sample, but high resolution structural data on solid materials requires more sophisticated methods. These methods include CP–MAS variants of some of the 2D methods described earlier that can yield through-bond and through-space connectivities (44) and typically require the use of selective or uniform isotopic labeling. A detailed study of the polymorphic forms of cimetidine was carried out using selective ^{13}C labeling. The distance constraints obtained in this study were used in molecular modeling studies to determine the possible conformations of cimetidine present in the different polymorphs (45).

FUTURE DIRECTIONS—SMALLER, FASTER, EASIER

The challenge of NMR in the pharmaceutical industry is to provide the intrinsically high information content of NMR spectra on smaller sample amounts, more rapidly, and with less time-intensive interpretation. Currently, each of these areas are the focus of intensive research efforts. Sensitivity gains can be expected with further innovations in probe design and with higher magnetic fields. Advances in experimental design will continue to provide more detailed information for both the qualitative and quantitative analyses of pharmaceutical compounds. The rapid analysis and interpretation of NMR data is being addressed with advances in computational methods (46). Improvements in spectral prediction and automated structure elucidation will greatly reduce the interpretation bottleneck in NMR applications. These advances, along with those yet uncovered, will insure that NMR assumes an even greater role in essentially all aspects of pharmaceutical research and development in the future.

REFERENCES

1. Friebolin, H. *Basic One- and Two-Dimensional NMR Spectroscopy*; VCH Publishers: New York, 1993.
2. Karplus, M. Vicinal Proton Coupling in Nuclear Magnetic Resonance. J. Am. Chem. Soc. **1963**, *85*, 2870–2871.
3. Neuhaus, D.; Williamson, M. *The Nuclear Overhauser Effect in Structural and Conformational Analysis*; VCH Publishers: Cambridge, UK, 1989.
4. Bothner-By, A.A.; Stephens, R.L.; Lee, J.-M. Structure Determination of a Tetrasaccharide: Transient Nuclear Overhauser Effects in the Rotating Frame. J. Am. Chem. Soc. **1984**, *106*, 811–813.
5. Bax, A.; Davis, D.G. J. Magn. Reson. **1985**, *63*, 760–762.
6. Morris, G.A.; Freeman, R. Enhancement of Nuclear Magnetic Resonance Signals by Polarization Transfer. J. Am. Chem. Soc. **1979**, *101*, 760–762.
7. Doddrell, D.M.; Pegg, D.T.; Bendall, M.R. Distortionless Enhancement of NMR Signals by Polarization Transfer. J. Magn. Reson **1982**, *48*, 323–327.
8. Kirk, D.N.; Toms, H.C.; Douglas, C.; White, K.A.; Smith, K.E.; Latif, S.; Hubbard, R.W.P. A Survey of the High Field ^{1}H NMR Spectra of the Steroid Hormones, Their Hydroxylated Derivatives and Related Compounds. J. Chem. Soc., Perkin Trans. 2 **1990**, 1567–1594.
9. Piatini, U.; Sørensen, O.W.; Ernst, R.R. Multiple Quantum Filters for Elucidating NMR Coupling Networks. J. Am. Chem. Soc. **1982**, *104*, 6800–6801.
10. Davis, D.G.; Bax, A. Assignment of Complex ^{1}H NMR Spectra Via Two-Dimensional Homonuclear Hartmann-Hahn Spectroscopy. J. Am. Chem. Soc. **1985**, *107*, 2821–2822.
11. Bax, A.; Griffey, R.H.; Hawkins, B.L. Sensitivity-Enhanced Correlation of ^{15}N and ^{1}H Chemical Shifts in Natural-Abundance Samples Via Multiple Quantum Coherence. J. Am. Chem. Soc. **1983**, *105*, 7188–7190.
12. Martin, G.E.; Hadden, C.E. Long-Range ^{1}H–^{15}N Heteronuclear Shift Correlation at Natural Abundance. J. Nat. Prod. **2000**, *63* (4), 543–585.
13. Bodenhausen, G.; Ruben, D. Nature Abundance Nitrogen-15 NMR by Enhanced Heteronuclear Spectroscopy. J. Chem. Phys. Lett. **1980**, *69*, 185–189.
14. Brüehwiler, D.; Wagner, G. Selective Excitation of ^{1}H Resonances Coupled to ^{13}C. Hetero COSY And RELAY Experiments with ^{1}H Detection for a Protein. J. Magn. Reson. **1986**, *69*, 546–551.
15. Reynolds, W.F.; McLean, S.; Tay, L.-L.; Yu, M.; Enriquez, R.G.; Estwick, D.M.; Pascoe, K.O. Comparison of ^{13}C Resolution and Sensitivity of HSQC and HMQC Sequences and Application of HSQC-Based Sequences to the Total ^{1}H and ^{13}C Spectral Assignment of Clionasterol. Magn. Reson. Chem. **1997**, *35*, 45–462.
16. Summers, M.F.; Marzilli, L.G.; Bax, A. Complete ^{1}H and ^{13}C Assignments of Coenzyme B$_{12}$ Through the Use of

New Two-Dimensional NMR Experiments. J. Am. Chem. Soc. **1986**, *108*, 4285–4294.

17. Martin, G.E.; Hadden, C.E.; Crouch, R.C.; Krishnamurthy, V.V. ACCORD-HMBC: Advantages and Disadvantages of Static Versus Accordion Excitation. Magn. Reson. Chem. **1999**, *37*, 517–528.

18. Griesinger, C.; Sørensen, O.W.; Ernst, R.R. A Practical Approach to Three-Dimensional NMR Spectroscopy. J. Magn. Reson. **1987**, *73*, 574–579.

19. Fesik, S.W.; Zuiderweg, E.R.P. Heteronuclear Three-Dimensional NMR Spectroscopy. A Strategy for the Simplification of Homonuclear Two-Dimensional NMR Spectra. J. Magn. Reson. **1988**, *78*, 588–593.

20. Clore, G.M.; Gronenborn, A.M. NMR Structures of Proteins and Protein Complexes Beyond 20,000 Mr. Nat. Struct. Biol. **1997**, 849–853.

21. Keeler, J.; Clowes, R.T.; Davis, A.L.; Laue, E.D. Pulsed Field Gradients: Theory and Practice. Methods Enzymol. **1994**, *239*, 145–207.

22. Martin, G.E.; Hadden, C.E. Comparison of 1.7 mm Submicro and 3 mm Micro Gradient NMR Probes for the Acquisition of ^1H–^{13}C and ^1H–^{15}N Heteronuclear Shift Correlation Data. Magn. Reson. Chem. **1999**, *37*, 721–729.

23. Olson, D.L.; Lacy, M.E.; Sweedler, J.V. High Resolution Microcoil NMR for Analysis of Mass-Limited, Nanoliter Samples. Anal. Chem. **1998**, *70*, 645–650.

24. Styles, P.; Soffe, N.F.; Scott, C.A. An Improved Cryogenically Cooled Probe for High-Resolution NMR. J. Magn. Reson. **1989**, *84*, 376–378.

25. Styles, P.; Soffe, N.F.; Scott, C.A.; Gragg, D.A.; Row, F.; White, D.J.; White, P.C.J. A High-Resolution NMR Probe in which the Coil and Preamplifier are Cooled with Liquid Helium. J. Magn. Reson. **1983**, *60*, 397–404.

26. Logan, T.M.; Murali, N.; Wang, G.; Jolivet, C. Application of a High Resolution Superconducting NMR Probe in Natural Product Structure Determination. Magn. Reson. Chem. **1999**, *37*, 512–515.

27. Keifer, P.A.; Smallcombe, S.H.; Williams, E.H.; Salomon, K.E.; Mendez, G.; Belletire, J.L.; Moore, C.D. Direct-Injection NMR (DI-NMR): A Flow NMR Technique for the Analysis of Combinatorial Libraries. J. Comb. Chem. **2000**, *2*, 151–171.

28. Albert, K. On-Line Use of NMR Detection in Separation Chemistry. J. Chromatogr. A **1995**, *703*, 123–147.

29. Lindon, J.C.; Nicholson, J.K.; Sidelmann, U.G.; Wilson, I.D. Directly Coupled HPLC-NMR and its Application to Drug Metabolism. Drug Metab. Rev. **1997**, *29*, 705–746.

30. Albert, K.; Schlotterbeck, G.; Braumann, U.; Händel, H.; Spraul, M.; Krack, G. Structure Determination of Vitamin A Acetate Isomers through Coupled HPLC and ^1H NMR Spectroscopy. Angew. Chem., Int. Ed. **1995**, *34* (9), 1014–1016.

31. Smallcombe, S.H.; Patt, S.L.; Keifer, P.A. WET Solvent Suppression and its Applications to LC-NMR and High-Resolution NMR Spectroscopy. J. Magn. Reson., Ser. A **1995**, *117*, 295–303.

32. Pullen, F.S.; Swanson, A.G.; Newman, M.J.; Richards, D.S. Online Liquid Chromatography/Nuclear Magnetic Resonance/Mass Spectrometry—A Powerful Spectroscopic Tool for the Analysis of Mixtures of Pharmaceutical Interest. Rapid Commun. Mass Spectrom. **1995**, *9*, 1003–1006.

33. Holt, R.M.; Newman, M.J.; Pullen, F.S.; Richards, D.S.; Swanson, A.G. High Performance Liquid Chromatography/NMR Spectrometry/Mass Spectrometry: Further Advances in Hyphenated Technology. J. Mass Spectrom. **1997**, *32*, 64–70.

34. Chen, A.; Shapiro, M.J. Affinity NMR. Anal. Chem. **1999**, *669A–675A*.

35. Henrichsen, D.; Ernst, B.; Magnani, J.L.; Wang, W.-T.; Meyer, B.; Peters, T. Bioaffinity NMR Spectroscopy: Identification of an E-Selectin Antagonist in a Substance Mixture by Transfer NOE. Angew. Chem., Int., Ed. **1999**, *38*, 98–102.

36. Hajduk, P.J.; Gerfin, T.; Boehlen, J.-M.; Häberli, M.; Marek, D.; Fesik, S.W. High-Throughput Nuclear Magnetic Resonance Based Screening. J. Med. Chem. **1999**, *42*, 2315–2317.

37. Shuker, S.B.; Hajduk, P.J.; Meadows, R.P.; Fesik, S.W. Discovering High-Affinity Ligands for Proteins: SAR by NMR. Science **1996**, *274*, 1531–1534.

38. Britton, H.G. *Physical Characterization of Pharmaceutical Solids*; Marcel Dekker, Inc.: New York, 1995.

39. Keifer, P.A. High-Resolution NMR Techniques for Solid-Phase Synthesis and Combinatorial Chemistry. Drug Discovery Today **1997**, *11*, 468–478.

40. Fitch, W.L.; Detre, G.; Holmes, C.P.; Shoolery, J.N.; Keifer, P.A. High-Resolution ^1H NMR In Solid-Phase Organic Synthesis. J. Org. Chem. **1994**, *59* (26), 7955–7956.

41. Kuhnert-Brandstatter, M.; Riedmann, M. Thermal Analysis and Infrared Spectroscopy Investigation on Polymorphic Organic Compounds-I. Mikrochim. Acta **1987**, *2*, 107–120.

42. Haleblian, J.; McCrone, W. Pharmaceutical Applications of Polymorphism. J. Pharm. Sci. **1969**, *58* (8), 911–929.

43. Harris, R.K.; Yeung, R.R.; Lamont, R.B.; Lancaster, R.W.; Lynn, S.M.; Staniforth, S.E. 'Polymorphism' in a Novel Anti-Viral Agent: Lamivudine. J. Chem. Soc., Perkin Trans. 2 **1997**, 2653–2659.

44. Blümich, B.; Spiess, H.W. Two-Dimensional Solid State NMR Spectroscopy: New Possibilities for the Investigation of the Structure and Dynamics of Solid Polymers. Angew. Chem. Int. Ed. **1988**, *27* (12), 1655–1672.

45. Middleton, D.A.; Le Duff, C.S.; Peng, X.; Reid, D.G.; Saunders, D. Molecular Conformations of the Polymorphic Forms of Cimetidine from ^{13}C Solid State NMR Distance and Angle Measurements. J. Am. Chem. Soc. **2000**, *122*, 1161–1170.

46. Williams, A. Recent Advances in NMR Prediction and Automated Structure Elucidation Software. Curr. Opin. Drug Discovery Dev. **2000**, *3* (3), 298–305.

OPTIMIZATION METHODS

Gareth A. Lewis

Sanofi-Synthelabo, Chilly Mazarin, France

INTRODUCTION

What Is Optimization?

Optimization of a formulation or process is finding the best possible composition or operating conditions. Determining such a composition or set of conditions is an enormous task, probably impossible, certainly unnecessary, and in practice, optimization may be considered as the search for a result that is satisfactory and at the same time the best possible within a limited field of search. Thus, the type and components of a formulation may be selected, according to previous experience, by expert knowledge (possibly using an expert system), or by systematic screening as described later. Then the relative and/or total proportions of the excipients are varied to obtain the best endpoint, or a process is chosen, and a study is carried out to determine the best operating conditions to obtain the desired formulation properties. Both of these are optimization studies. This article concentrates on statistical experimental design-based optimization.

Screening, Factor Studies, and Optimization

Systematic screening and factor influence studies are closely related to optimization, being often sequential stages in the development process and involving statistical experimental design methods. Screening methods are used to identify important and critical effects, for example, in the manufacturing process. Factor studies are quantitative studies of the effects of changing potentially critical process and formulation parameters. They involve factorial design and are also quite often referred to as screening studies; however, the resulting relationships have just as often been used for optimization.

The type of study carried out will depend on the stage of the project. In particular, experimental design may be carried out in stages, and the experiments of a factor study may be augmented by further experiments to a design giving the detailed information needed for true optimization. It cannot be stressed to highly that the quality of a statistically designed experiment depends on the choice of experimental run with respect to an a priori model, and

this quality can and must be assessed before starting the experiments.

Brief Historical Review

Statistical methods for screening, factor studies, and optimization have been available for a long time: factorial designs since 1926 (1); screening designs since 1946 (2); and the central composite design for response surface optimization, was introduced by Box and Wilson, in 1951 (3). Their use started to be described in the pharmaceutical literature from the early 1970s, but it was only from approximately 1988 that there was a sudden increase in the number of published articles, and the numbers have continued to rise. A conception or presupposition of the difficulty or complexity of experimental design had to be overcome. The change has been attributed of course to a great extent to the availability of computing power and of relatively inexpensive high-performance software that allows previously difficult or advanced methods to be applied. In particular, much attention is now being given to robust processes and formulation, and there are developments in treating nonlinear and highly correlated responses (4).

Methods for Optimization

There are four primary methods. First, there is the statistically designed experiment, in which experiments are set up in a (normally regular) matrix to estimate the coefficients in a mathematical model that predicts responses within the limits of formulation or operating conditions being studied. This is generally the most powerful method, provided the experimentation zone has been correctly identified, and is the subject of most of this article.

Second, the direct optimization method, the best known being the sequential simplex, is a rapid and powerful method for determining an experimental domain, best combined with experimental design for the optimization itself.

Third, there is the one-factor-at-a-time method in which the experimenter varies first one factor to find the best value, then another. Its disadvantages are that it cannot be used for multiple responses and that it will not work when there are strong interactions between factors.

Finally, the nonsystematic approach in which the knowledge and intuition of the developer allow him to improve results, changing a number of factors at the same time is often surprisingly successful in the hands of a skilled worker. Where he is less skilled or less lucky, he can waste a remarkable amount of time and resources.

The use of artificial intelligence and expert systems is treated elsewhere in this work.

SCREENING

Obtaining a Formulation Suitable for Optimization

Once the dosage form has been selected, the excipients must be identified, their choice often limited by practical considerations of time and resources determined by patents, company practice, or according to expert knowledge. However, it may be possible or necessary to test a number of different excipients for each function, for example, several diluents, lubricants, binders. This approach has proved useful in drug–excipient compatibility testing in which protoformulations are set up according to a statistical screening design to assess stability and compatibility.

Here the *factor* is the excipient's function. This can be set at different levels, the level being the excipient itself. So the factor may be "binder," and the levels are, for example, HPMC, povidone, polyvinylacetate, and no disintegrant present. A mathematical model relates the response (in this case, degradation) to composition. It includes variables corresponding to each factor with

(qualitative) levels corresponding to each excipient. Plackett and Burman (5) described designs suitable for treating this kind of problem. Designs with the factors at only two levels are widely used. However, there are other designs at 3, 4, and 5 levels as well as asymmetric designs derived from them in which the various factors take a different number of levels (5, 6).

It is assumed that there are no *interactions* between factors; that is to say, the effect of a given excipient on stability does not depend on what other excipients are found in the formulation. (The same reasoning applies to other kinds of factors or responses.) This can only be an approximation; however, if it should be necessary to take interactions into account, many more experiments would be needed, and it would probably be necessary to limit the number of levels for each factor to two for the number of experiments to be manageable.

The choice of excipients may be considered a qualitative optimization, their quantitative compositions not having yet been optimized. This and the fact that the process used will most likely be on a small laboratory scale may affect the affect the choice of excipients. However, it is in most circumstances an unavoidable limitation.

An example of such a qualitative screening is shown in Table 1. This is an experimental design for testing the compatibilities of experimental drug (at two concentrations) with a number of number of excipients. The samples, which were wet granulated, were stored for 3 weeks at 50°C/50% relative humidity. The results are also given in Table 1. The mean degradation level was high, at 6.2%, indicating a fairly unstable drug. The effects of each excipient were calculated by linear regression, or, because the design is *orthogonal*, by linear combinations of the responses, and plotted in Fig. 1. There, the

Table 1 Experimental design and plan for granulated protoformulations

Number	Diluent	Disintegrant	Lubricant	Binder	Dose (%)	Degradation
1	Lactose	CCNa[a]	Mg stearate	Povidone	0.25	12.26
2	Cellulose[b]	CCNa	Mg stearate	HPMC	1.0	7.27
3	Phosphate[c]	CCNa	Glyceryl behenate	Povidone	1.0	11.43
4	Mannitol	CCNa	Glyceryl behenate	HPMC	0.25	4.94
5	Lactose	NaSG[d]	Glyceryl behenate	HPMC	1.0	1.63
6	Cellulose	NaSG	Glyceryl behenate	Povidone	0.25	4.56
7	Phosphate	NaSG	Mg stearate	HPMC	0.25	2.49
8	Mannitol	NaSG	Mg stearate	Povidone	1.0	4.79

[a]Croscarmellose sodium.
[b]Microcrystalline cellulose.
[c]Calcium hydrogen phosphate.
[d]Sodium starch glycolate.

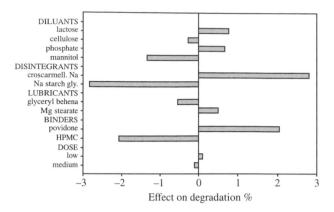

Fig. 1 Compatibility study—effects of excipients calculated from data of Table 1, relative to a hypothetical ("mean") reference state.

degradation for each excipient is calculated in each excipient type (e.g., disintegrant), setting the excipients in the remaining type to a hypothetical mean value. Thus, the value for magnesium is the mean response for all mixtures containing magnesium stearate, and the effect of stearate on the response is the difference between this figure and the global mean.

Inspecting the results shows that the disintegrant and binder have major effects, and mixtures containing sodium starch glycolate and HPMC are more stable than those containing croscarmellose sodium and povidone, respectively. Diluents had only small effects here, however, these were much greater in the mixtures stored at low humidity, where mixtures containing microcrystalline cellulose or, especially, calcium phosphate were less stable than those containing lactose or mannitol. Thus, a capsule based on lactose, sodium starch glycolate, HPMC, and magnesium

stearate (the last being selected for reasons of feasibility, there being no difference in stability between it and glyceryl behenate) was formulated and gave satisfactory stability.

Before Optimizing a Process

The major choice to be made here is that of equipment, and that will depend on what is available in the laboratory and also in the factory. There may be a very large number of factors to be studied, and it will probably be necessary to identify the critical factors before optimizing the process. This stage will probably be at the laboratory scale, whereas the optimization proper is carried out at pilot scale.

Because process factors are usually quantitative and continuous, two levels only, at minimum and maximum values, are often tested in screening and factor influence studies. Thus, the highly efficient, two-level Plackett–Burman designs and two-level factorial designs may be used for screening. For example, in screening (assuming no interactions), up to 11 factors, (continuous or discrete or qualitative with two levels) may be tested by means of 12 experimental runs (Table 2). The difference between minimum and maximum for each factor is generally quite large. Such a test clears the ground for optimization process.

Methods for screening factors

Because a large number of factors may need to be screened, the postulated model must be simple. It is usually assumed that the response(s) y depends only on the level (value or state) of each factor x_i separately and not on combinations of levels. The model is thus first-order, for example:

$$y = \beta_0 + \beta_1 x_1 + \beta_2 x_2 + \beta_3 x_3 + \beta_4 x_4 + \beta_5 x_5 + \varepsilon$$

Table 2 A Plackett–Burman design of 12 experiments

Experiment	X_1	X_2	X_3	X_4	X_5	X_6	X_7	X_8	X_9	X_{10}	X_{11}
1	+1	+1	−1	+1	+1	+1	−1	−1	−1	+1	−1
2	−1	+1	+1	−1	+1	+1	+1	−1	−1	−1	+1
3	+1	−1	+1	+1	−1	+1	+1	+1	−1	−1	−1
4	−1	+1	−1	+1	+1	−1	+1	+1	+1	−1	−1
5	−1	−1	+1	−1	+1	+1	−1	+1	+1	+1	−1
6	−1	−1	−1	+1	−1	+1	+1	−1	+1	+1	+1
7	+1	−1	−1	−1	+1	−1	+1	+1	−1	+1	+1
8	+1	+1	−1	−1	−1	+1	−1	+1	+1	−1	+1
9	+1	+1	+1	−1	−1	−1	+1	−1	+1	+1	−1
10	−1	+1	+1	+1	−1	−1	−1	+1	−1	+1	+1
11	+1	−1	+1	+1	+1	−1	−1	−1	+1	−1	+1
12	−1	−1	−1	−1	−1	−1	−1	−1	−1	−1	−1

If the factors are quantitative, they are set at their extreme values. Thus, if the factor is *granulation time*, and the possible range is 1.5–7 min, the normal values tested are 1.5 min and 7 min. They are expressed in terms of dimensionless *coded variables*, normally taking values −1 and +1. Thus, on transformation to the coded variable x_1, 1.5 min corresponds to $x_1 = -1$, and 7 min corresponds to $x_1 = +1$.

If the factors are quantitative, they may take any number of levels. Only two-level designs are described here. Qualitative levels are set arbitrarily at the coded levels. If, for example, the screening method was one of the factors tested, wet screening could be set at −1 and dry screening at +1 (or vice versa).

Quite wide limits are generally chosen for screening quantitative factors. They are then often narrowed for more detailed quantitative study of the influence of factors where interactions between factors them are taken into account and for determining a predictive model for optimization.

The designs, proposed by Plackett and Burman in 1946 (2), comprise experiments in multiples of four. They will allow screening of up to one less factor than the number of experiments. Those with 2^n experiments (4, 8, 16, 32 H) are also fractional factorial designs. The nonfactorial designs have particular properties and complex *aliasing*, which has been held to make their interpretation difficult but also gives them certain advantages over the fractional factorial designs. The 12-experiment design, shown in coded variables (Table 2), is such a design, and is useful for about 7–11 factors.

The structure of the design is shown clearly in the table because the experiments are in their standard order. However, they should be carried out in a random order, as should all the designs described here, as much as is practicable.

The coefficient β_i is the *effect of the factor X_i*, and is equal to half the average change in the response y when the level of the factor is changed from $x_i = -1$ to $x_i = +1$. It is estimated (as b_i) in the Plackett–Burman design by subtracting the sum of the responses for experiments for which $x_i = -1$ from those for which $x_i = +1$ and dividing by the number of experiments. Important and unimportant effects can then be identified according to their absolute values. (Determining active factors from the results of a factorial design are shown later.)

Use of results of a screening design

Estimation of the effects allows influential or possibly influential factors to be identified. Noninfluential factors (small effects) will not require further study. They may be set at their midpoints, at their most economical values (e.g., a short mixing time), or at their apparently best value even if the measured effect is apparently nonsignificant.

After elimination of these noninfluential factors, there may still be too many factors to optimize in terms of the resources available (time, raw material, operators, availability of equipment, etc.). Generally, these less influential factors are kept constant, equal to their best level and the remainder optimized. In more complex situations, it is advisable to carry out a more detailed study between the screening and optimization (response surface studies). This could be a completion of the screening study by means of a complementary foldover design (3, 7) or by a separate quantitative study to allow individual effects of the factors and/or their binary interactions to be calculated separately (shown in factorial designs, later).

All these studies on the process are generally done after the optimization of the formulation. However, because the effects of formulation and process changes are not generally independent, it may become necessary to carry out some sort of process study at the same time as the formulation optimization.

QUANTITATIVE PROCESS STUDIES USING FACTORIAL DESIGNS

Purpose

Whereas the purpose of a screening study is to determine which of a large number of factors have an influence on the formulation or process, that of a factor study is to determine quantitatively the influence of the different factors together on the response variables. The number of levels is usually again limited to two, but sufficient experiments are carried out to allow for *interactions* between factors.

Two-level full factorial designs

The simplest such designs are the 2^k full factorial designs, in which the experiments are all the 2^k possible combinations of two levels of k factors variables. Therefore, they consist of 4, 8, 16, 32, 64 H experiments for 2, 3, 4, 5, 6 H factors. Examples are given in Table 3 of the 2^2, 2^3, and 2^4 designs (each enclosed at the right and below by the solid lines). Thus, lines 1–4 of columns 1 and 2 show a 2^2 design for two factors, and lines 1–16 of columns 1–4 a 2^4 design for four factors.

The design is transformed into an experimental plan (with the natural or experimental values of the factor variable at each level −/+1. The mathematical model associated with the design consists of the *main effects* of each variable plus all the possible *interaction effects*,

Table 3 Some full and fractional factorial designs for two to five factors[a]

	X_1	X_2	X_3	X_4	X_5	Response
1	-1	-1	-1	-1	1	189
2	1	-1	-1	-1	-1	56
3	-1	1	-1	-1	-1	94
4	1	1	-1	-1	1	80
5	-1	-1	1	-1	-1	212
6	1	-1	1	-1	1	212
7	-1	1	1	-1	1	76
8	1	1	1	-1	-1	125
9	-1	-1	-1	1	-1	351
10	1	-1	-1	1	1	534
11	-1	1	-1	1	1	275
12	1	1	-1	1	-1	219
13	-1	-1	1	1	1	154
14	1	-1	1	1	-1	752
15	-1	1	1	1	-1	374
16	1	1	1	1	1	478

[a]The response particle size (μm) in for the 2^{5-1} fractional factorial design. (From Ref. 8.)

interactions between two variables, but also between three and four factors and, in fact, between as many as there are in the model. However, although two-factor interactions are important, three-factor interactions are normally far less so. Higher-order interactions are invariably ignored and the values determined for them attributed to the random variation of the experimental system.

Determining Active Factors from the Results of a Factorial Design

We take the four-factor model as an example. The complete synergistic mathematical model consists of the constant term, four main variables ($\beta_1 x_1$ H $\beta_1 x_4$), six interactions between two factors ($\beta_{12} x_1 x_2$, etc.), four interactions between three factors ($\beta_{123} x_1 x_2 x_3$, etc.) and one between four factors. The last five of these are not generally expected to be important. The model is thus:

$$y = \beta_0 + \beta_1 x_1 \ldots + \beta_{12} x_1 x_2 \ldots + \beta_{123} x_1 x_2 x_3 \ldots$$
$$+ \beta_{1234} x_1 x_2 x_3 x_4 + \varepsilon$$

The effects (coefficients) βi_i in the model are estimated, usually by multilinear regression. The values obtained b_i are estimates because of the random experimental error (represented by ε in the equation). The next step is to decide which of the 15 effects calculated are *active* or important.

The are a number of ways of doing this. If the experiments have been replicated, ANOVA will reveal which effects are statistically significant. Otherwise, we rely on the fact that most of the effects are probably small and distributed randomly about zero. Thus, we look for the effects with the largest absolute values that stand out from the others (6). Making a normal probability plot of the distribution of their values is a widely used method.

The responses are usually treated separately; however, when there are a number of more or less correlated responses being studied, appropriate combinations (principal components) may be analyzed instead of the original responses (9).

Once the important effects have been identified, a simplified model can be written. If an interaction term has been identified, the corresponding main effects should also be included in the model even if they are not all found active. Thus, if the interactions between the factors X_1 and X_2 and the main effect of the factor X_1 are active, $b_2 x_2$ should be included in the model as well as $b_1 x_1$ and $b_{12} x_1 x_2$.

Two-Level Fractional Factorial Designs

The number of experiments needed to study five or more factors in a full factorial design is large, and to determine the main effects and their interactions, a fraction of the full design is often sufficient. These are $2k-r$ fractional factorial designs, where $r = 1$, 2, H for the half, quarter, etc. fractions. An example of a half-factorial design for five factors (2^{5-1}) is given in Table 2 (the entire table). Note that the first four columns are the same as the four factor, full-factorial design, and the column for the fifth factor is constructed by multiplying the first four columns together. Methods for constructing such designs and their limitations are described in many textbooks (5–7).

Evidently, for the 2^{5-1} design, the 16 triple and higher interactions are not determined. In fact, they are confounded with the calculated effects. Thus, the estimate of the interaction between factors one and two includes the triple interaction between the other three factors. Because the latter is assumed negligible, this does not usually matter.

Menon et al. studied the formation of pellets by fluid-bed granulation using this design (8). The five factors investigated were (X_1), the binder concentration; (X_2), the method of introducing it (dry or solution); (X_3), the atomization pressure; (X_4), the spray rate; and (X_5), the inlet temperature. Particle sizes of the resulting particles are shown in Table 3.

The coefficients of the model are calculated by linear regression (the logarithm of the particle size was used

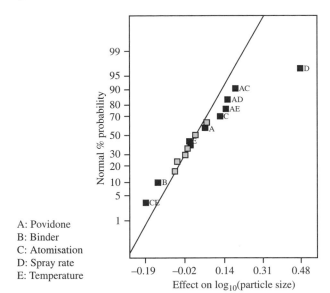

A: Povidone
B: Binder
C: Atomisation
D: Spray rate
E: Temperature

Fig. 2 Calculated effects form a two-level factorial design. Those to the left and right of the line are considered active. (From Ref. 8.)

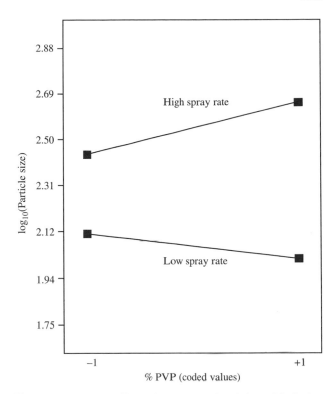

Fig. 3 Calculated effects from a two-level factorial design. Interaction diagram for spray rate and % povidone on particle size (logarithmic scale).

here) and then plotted as a cumulative distribution of a normal plot (Fig. 2). The important coefficients are those that are strongly positive or negative, for example, the spray rate b_4 and the interaction between atomization pressure and inlet temperature b_{35}. Others not identified on the diagram are not considered significant and could well be representative mainly of experimental error. The equation can thus be simplified to include only the important terms. However, if interactions are included, their main effects should be included also, even if they are small. Here, we have:

$$y = \beta_0 + \beta_1 x_1 + \beta_2 x_2 + \beta_3 x_3 + \beta_4 x_4 + \beta_5 x_5$$
$$+ \beta_{13} x_1 x_3 + \beta_{14} x_1 x_4 + \beta_{15} x_1 x_5 + \beta_{35} x_3 x_5$$

Information That Can Be Obtained

The significant main effects are identified and also quantified. Thus, increasing the spray rate over the range studied will give an increase in the log(particle size of twice 0.24, representing a more than threefold increase. However, it can be seen that there is an interaction with the binder concentration; that is, the effect of spray rate depends on the amount of binder in the formulation. The effects of increasing spray rate are shown in Fig. 3 for both high and low levels of binder; the effect of spray rate is much greater at high levels of binder.

However, the effect of binder also interacts with two other factors, the atomization pressure and the inlet temperature. Thus, the individual variables cannot be considered separately.

Note also that there is a great deal of information often hidden in large designs (16 or more experiments), and, in particular, indications on factors affecting the robustness of a process may sometimes be extracted (see the last section).

Use of Center Points

In both screening and factor-influence studies in which the factor is quantitative, it is tempting to interpolate between the upper and lower limits. This is useful if only to find a more restricted zone for further study. However, in the case of a screening study, the limits studied are often so wide that it would be most unlikely for the estimated model to be accurate enough for prediction, and there is also likely to be curvature of the response surface over the experimental domain. Such attempts are less risky for the more detailed factorial studies, but even then, they should be used with caution.

Adding center points (experiments at the center of the domain, coded co-ordinates 0, 0, H 0 is useful for factorial and screening experiments), even though they do not enter into the calculation of the model equation because:

1. They are often a priori at or near the most interesting conditions;
2. They allow identification of curvature in the responses (by comparing calculated with measured responses);
3. If they are replicated, the experimental reproducibility may be assessed; and
4. They may allow extension of the experiment at a subsequent stage to a central composite design for modeling of response surfaces (shown later).

EXPERIMENTAL DESIGNS FOR PROCESS OPTIMIZATION (INDEPENDENT VARIABLES)

In this section, we look at methods of obtaining a mathematical model that can be used for qualitative predictions of a response over the whole of the experimental domain. If the model depends on two factors, the response may be considered a topographical surface, drawn as contours or in 3D (Fig. 4). For more factors, we can visualize the surface by taking "slices" at constant values of all but two factors. These methods allow both process and formulation optimization.

Mathematical Models

The design used is a function of the model proposed. Thus, if it is expected that the important responses vary relatively

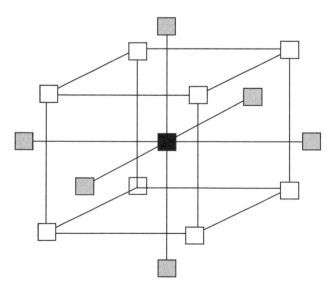

Fig. 4 Central composite design for three factors. The factorial points are shaded, the axial points unshaded, and the center point(s) filled.

little over the domain, a first-order polynomial will be selected. This will also be the case if the experimenter wishes to perform rather a few experiments at first to check initial assumptions. He may then change to a second-order (quadratic) polynomial model. Second-order polynomials are those most commonly used for response surface modeling and process optimization for up to five variables.

Examples of polynomial models are a first order model for five factors:

$$y = \beta_0 + \beta_1 x_1 + \beta_2 x_2 + \beta_3 x_3$$
$$+ \beta_4 x_4 + \beta_5 x_5 + \varepsilon$$

and a second-order model for two factors:

$$y = \beta_0 + \beta_1 x_1 + \beta_2 x_2 + \beta_{12} x_1 x_2$$
$$+ \beta_{11} x_1{}^2 + \beta_{22} x_2{}^2 + \varepsilon$$

The coefficients in the models are estimated by multilinear least-squares regression of the data.

Third-order models are very rarely used in the case of process studies and, in any case, third-order terms are only added for those variables where they can be shown to be necessary (i.e., augmentation of a second-order model and the corresponding design). This does not mean that second-order designs are always sufficient, and other methods of constructing response surfaces may sometimes be useful.

Statistical Experimental Designs for First-Order Models

The design must enable estimation of the first-order effects, preferably free from interference by the interactions between factors other variables. It should also allow testing for the fit of the model and, in particular, for the existence of curvature of the response surface (center points). Two-level factorial designs may be used for this (shown earlier).

Important points to note when using a first-order model, with or without interactions, are that:

1. Maximum and minimum values of responses are of necessity predicted at the edge of the experimental domain;
2. The first-order model should normally be used only in the absence of curvature of the response surface. If the experimental values of the center points are different from the calculate values (i.e., there is lack of fit), then the response surface is curved and a second-order design and model should be used; and
3. The experimenter should test for interaction terms between two factors in the model. If interactions seem to be important he should make sure that they are properly identified.

Statistical Experimental Designs for Second-Order Models

The central composite design (Box–Wilson design)

This is the design most often used for response surfaces. It is a combination of a factorial with an axial design (3, 10) with experiments at a distance of $\pm\alpha$ along each axis (thus, the name). It requires a relatively large number of experimental runs, which can be a disadvantage if resources are limited. However, it can be carried out in two stages: the factorial design first then the axial design if the results are satisfactory.

If we wish to study the system by varying the parameters around a point of interest, the domain is a sphere, and the coordinates of axial experiments are outside those of the factorial ones. α is chosen to give the best statistical properties (e.g., constant prediction precision) and lies between 2 and approximately 2.4. The design for three factors, where α is set at 1.682, is shown in Fig. 5 and Table 4.

Center-point experiments must be done as part of both stages. Another advantage is that each factor is at five levels, thus allowing testing of lack of fit and for the possible need for cubic terms in the model.

Fig. 4 shows response surfaces calculated from the data of Senderak et al. (11) obtained using such a design at a constant value of the third factor.

Other standard designs

The central composite design is most often used, however, there are others whose particular properties make them particularly useful. One of these is the Doehlert design, which is part of a continuous hexagonal network (12). It requires slightly fewer experiments than does the central composite design but cannot be set up by augmenting a factorial design.

The design for three factors is shown in Table 5. It can be seen that the hexagonal design for two factors is the first seven rows and the first two columns. Thus, it possible to add a factor to a design. Another advantage is that because it is part of a continuous network, it allows the experimental domain to be shifted in any direction by adding experiments at one side of the domain and eliminating them at the other (Fig. 6). Vojnovic et al. (13) give an example of its use in granulation.

Hybrid designs are saturated or almost saturated designs; that is, they have only enough experimental

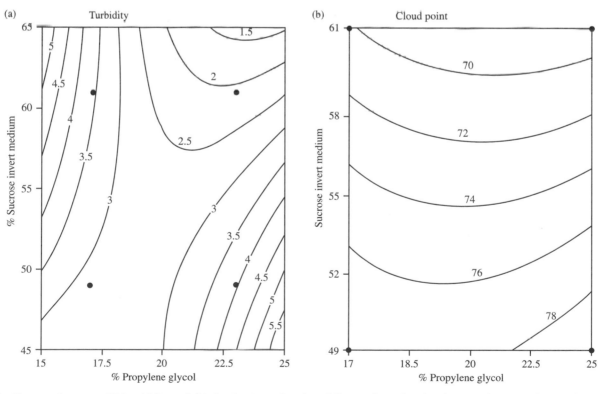

Fig. 5 Contour diagrams of (a) turbidity and (b) cloud point as function of % propylene glycol and sucrose invert medium. (slice taken at constant value of 4.3% polysorbate 80). (From Ref. 11.)

Table 4 A central composite design for three factors

Number	X_1	X_2	X_3	
1	−1	−1	−1	Factorial design 2^3
2	+1	−1	−1	
3	−1	+1	−1	
4	+1	+1	−1	
5	−1	−1	+1	
6	+1	−1	+1	
7	−1	+1	+1	
8	+1	+1	+1	
9	−1.682	0	0	Axial design
10	+1.682	0	0	
11	0	1.682	0	
12	0	+1.682	0	
13	0	0	−1.682	
14	0	0	+1.682	
15	0	0	0	Center points[a] (number of replicates flexible)
16	0	0	0	
17	0	0	0	

[a]To be included with both axial and factorial designs if carried out separately.

runs to calculate the coefficients of the quadratic model (10 runs for 3 factors 16 runs, for 4 factors, and 28 runs, for 6 factors). They are useful when the responses are not expected to vary enormously but where the quadratic model is esteemed necessary and resources (in possible numbers of experiments) are low (6, 14).

If the experimental region is defined by maximum and minimum values of each factor, then the domain is "cubic." The central composite design can be applied to such a situation, the axial points being set then at ±1, coded values corresponding to the minimum and maximum allowed values. Other designs for the cubic domain are reviewed in Ref. 6.

Mixed and Irregular Domains—D-Optimal Designs

If the experimental domain is cubic and spherical or spherical, the standard experimental designs can normally be used. However, the domain may be irregular in shape as certain combinations of values variable may be excluded a priori for technical reasons or may even have been tried and failed to give a result, or certain factors may be forced to take either fixed discrete but numerical values or may even be qualitative in nature.

There are no classic experimental designs that exist for such circumstances, and a purely empirical approach is required: 1) to postulate a mathematical model that is expected to describe the response, and 2) to then select

from among the many possible experiments a design that will determine the model coefficients with maximum efficiency.

There are various ways of obtaining such a design, by far the most common being based on the exchange algorithm of Fedorov. There are also a number of criteria for describing how good the design is, the D-optimal criterion being the most usual, based on optimization of the overall precision of estimation of the coefficients of the model (6, 15, 16). This method and type of design is extremely flexible because:

Table 5 Doehlert design for three factors

k	X_1	X_2	X_3
1	0	0	0
2	1	0	0
3	0.5	0.866	0
4	−0.5	−0.866	0
5	0.5	−0.866	0
6	−0.5	0.866	0
7	−1	0	0
8	0.5	0.289	0.816
9	−0.5	0.289	0.816
10	0	0.577	0.816
11	0.5	−0.289	−0.816
12	−0.5	−0.289	−0.816
13	0	0.577	−0.816

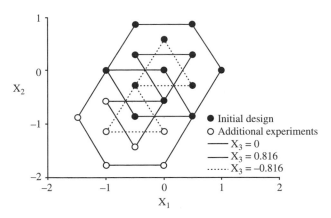

Fig. 6 Doehlert design in three dimensions (factors) showing extension to a new experimental domain.

1. It allows experiments within irregular experimental domains;
2. Previous experiments carried out within the experimental domain may be taken into account;
3. Classical designs in which experiments have failed to give a result may be repaired by redefining the domain and finding the best experiments (according to the D-optimal criterion) to replace the experiment(s) which failed;
4. The models may be polynomials with missing coefficients, or even nonpolynomials;
5. The experiments may be carried out in two or more stages, with models of increasing complexity;
6. Further experiments may be added to a D-optimal design to validate the model (lack of fit); and
7. They can be used for mixture models with constraints (see below).

In conclusion, a wide variety of experimental designs is available, allowing the design to be selected according to the problem in question, rather than adapting the experiment to the design.

EXPERIMENTAL DESIGNS FOR FORMULATION OPTIMIZATION (MIXTURE DESIGNS)

Formulations almost invariably consist of mixtures of a drug substance and excipients. Their properties usually depend not so much on the quantity of each substance present as on their proportions. The total comes to 100%, so the number of independent variables is one less than the number of components. This has the effect that the models and the designs have particular properties, and the designs

described above (screening, factor studies, and response surfaces) normally cannot be used. The entire topic of mixture designs is fully described by Cornell (17).

Mathematical Models for Mixtures

Because there is one less independent variables than the number of components, the polynomials take a particular form. For example, for three components, where the response y has a first-order dependence on the fractions x_1, x_2, x_3, because $x_1 + x_2 + x_3 = 1$,

$$y = \alpha_0 + \alpha_1 x_1 + \alpha_2 x_2 + \alpha_3 x_3 + \varepsilon$$

becomes

$$y = \beta_1 x_1 + \beta_2 x_2 + \beta_3 x_3 + \varepsilon$$

The variables cannot be varied independently. If there are no upper and lower restraints on the proportions of the components, the domain for three factors can be described as a equilateral triangle whose apices represent the pure components. A four-component mixture is described by a regular tetrahedron. For five components, the equivalent 4D figure must be imagined.

Just as the first-order mixture model has a different form from that for independent variables, so does the second-order design:

$$y = \beta_0 + \beta_1 x_1 + \beta_2 x_2 + \beta_3 x_3 + \beta_{12} x_1 x_2$$
$$+ \beta_{13} x_1 x_3 + \beta_{23} x_2 x_3 + \varepsilon$$

The special cubic model describes a certain third-order curvature in the response surface:

$$y = \beta_0 + \beta_1 x_1 + \beta_2 x_2 + \beta_3 x_3 + \beta_{12} x_1 x_2$$
$$+ \beta_{13} x_1 x_3 + \beta_{23} x_2 x_3 + \beta_{123} x_1 x_2 x_3 + \varepsilon$$

Mixture Designs and the Simplex Experimental Domain

The equilateral triangle and regular tetrahedron are described above as the domain of a mixture where all possible compositions of the components are allowed for are regular simplexes. (In the remainder of the section, they are referred to as simplexes.) Such circumstances in which there are no composition restraints are rare in formulation. However, if each component is present at a minimum level, and no other constraints are imposed, then the domain is also a simplex.

Designs in this case, primarily attributed to Scheffé (18), are derived very simply. That shown in Fig. 7 for three components is suitable for first-, second,- and partial

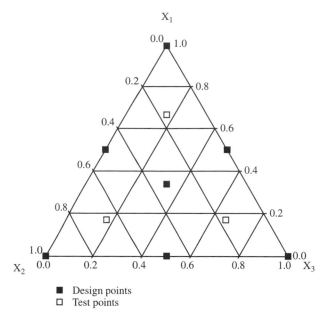

Fig. 7 Scheffé central composite design for three factors. Open squares are test points.

third-order models. The latter is the central composite design and is quite commonly used. Test points for checking model fit are also shown.

Constrained Systems and Pseudocomponents

Simplex designs are quite rarely used because such circumstances in which there are no composition restraints are rare in formulation. However, if each component is present at a minimum level, and no other constraints are imposed, then the domain is also a simplex. An example could be of the solubility of a drug being tested in ternary or quaternary mixtures of pharmaceutically acceptable solvents. The single constraint might be that a minimum percentage of water is required. In any case, the experimental domain would be a regular simplex, and standard designs may be used. In the case of solid dosage forms, simplex domains are rarer still. A possible example might be a study of the optimum composition of a diluent in a tablet formulation, the proportions of the active substance and other excipients being held constant. The diluent might consist of a mixture of lactose, microcrystalline cellulose, and starch, and its composition might then be adjusted to obtain optimum tableting properties as well as rapid disintegration and dissolution (for rapid action of the drug after the patient swallows the tablet). Again, standard experimental designs such as the simplex–centroid design may be used.

Constrained Systems and Nonsimplex Designs

Limits in the amounts of excipients present normally lead to the domain taking on an irregular shape. Each component must be present within a given concentration range to fulfill its function. For example, lactose or cellulose may make up most of the amount of a tablet or capsule, whereas magnesium stearate is limited to between 0.5 and 2%. In particular, when there are both upper and lower limits, the space is almost invariably nonsimplex.

Mixture models (such as those of Scheffé) are still useful, especially when there are three or more such excipients with fairly large ranges of variation. In solid formulations, this is often the case for diluents (or fillers) and also for the polymers or waxes incorporated into controlled-release tablets to form a matrix through which the drug diffuses slowly out when immersed in aqueous fluid, i.e., in the gastrointestinal tract.

The experimental designs of nonsimplex experimental regions are D-optimal for the selected model, obtained by an exchange algorithm (19).

Thus, we have the example of the optimization of a sustained-release tablet for which the release rate of a highly water-soluble drug was limited by its diffusion though a matrix. The matrix-forming substance is a cellulose derivative swelling in water (hydroxypropyl-methylcellulose) but the diluents microcrystalline cellulose, lactose, and calcium phosphate also have a role. These four components were varied as well as the percentage of drug substance (to have two doses at constant tablet mass), and the experimental domain defined. A D-optimal design was then obtained for a second-order mixture model (using an exchange algorithm), the experiments performed, and the results analyzed by multilinear regression to give response surfaces as contour plots (Fig. 8). The formulation could thus be optimized to give the required drug release profile (6).

It is interesting to note that the work was done in two stages. Initially, experiments were chosen for a first-order mathematical model from the projected second-order design. These were carried out first, to check that there was no problem and that the experimental domain was adequate, before doing the remaining experiments for a predictive model that could be used for optimizing.

Conditions for Independent Variable Designs

If one of the components (for example, a diluent or solvent) is in considerable excess, and the limits for all other components are narrow in comparison, then it can be eliminated from the analysis because its concentration changes little. The concentrations of the remaining

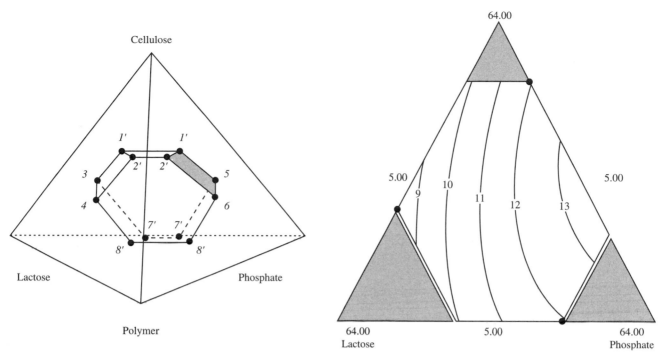

Fig. 8 D-optimal mixture design. (Left) definition of the design space. (Right) Contour plot of mean dissolution time at 25% polymer content. (From Ref. 6.)

components can then be treated as independent variables, and the methods described previously can be applied without using the special considerations for mixtures.

OPTIMIZATION METHODS USING RESPONSE SURFACE METHODOLOGY

Graphical Methods

It is usually relatively simple to find the optimum conditions for a single response that does not depend on more than four factors once the coefficients of the model equations have been estimated, provided, of course, that the model is correct. Real problems are usually more complex. In the case of pellet formation, it is not only the yield of pellets that is important but also their shape (how near to spherical), friability, smoothness, and ease of production. The optimum is a combination of all these.

One possible approach is to select the most important response, the one that should be optimized, such as the yield of pellets. For the remaining responses, we can choose acceptable upper and lower limits. Response surfaces are plotted with only these limits, with unacceptable values shaded. The unshaded area is the acceptable zone. Within that acceptable zone, we may

either select the center for maximum ruggedness of formulation or process or look for a maximum (or minimum or target value) of the key response.

Graphical Optimization of Two Opposing Responses

When there are only two independent factors (including the case of three mixture components), the responses may be plotted on a single graph. Graphics programs that allow plotting of upper and lower allowed limits of the responses, with portions of the diagram where there the responses are outside the limits shaded, are useful because they allow an acceptable zone to be identified very rapidly. An example of graphical analysis for formulation of an oral solution (11) is shown in Fig. 9. The objective was to reduce the turbidity as much as possible and to obtain a solution with a cloud point less than 70°C. A level of invert sucrose as high as possible was preferred (in spite of its deleterious effect on the cloud point). Slices were taken in the propylene glycol, sucrose plane (X_2, X_3) at different levels of polysorbate, that at 4.3% being shown in the Fig. 9. This can to be compared with the response surface in Fig. 5. An optimum compromise formulation is found at approximately 58% sucrose medium, 4.3% polysorbate 80, and 23% polyethylene glycol.

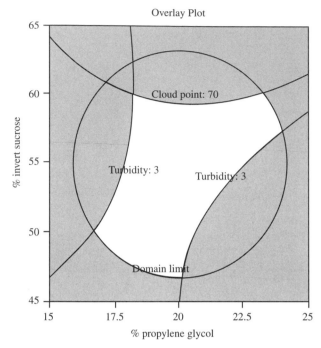

Fig. 9 Superposition of contour plots for turbidity <3 ppm and cloud point <70° to determine an optimum region ("slice" at 4.3% polysorbate 80). Compare with Fig. 5 (From Ref. 11.)

The method becomes difficult with four independent continuous factors, and for five or more variables, the method is totally impracticable despite its simplicity. The number of "slices" to be examined is simply too high—up to 125 diagrams to be displayed or plotted. Under such circumstances, the desirability method must be used.

Desirability

Derringer and Suich (6, 20) described a way of overcoming the difficulty of multiple, sometimes opposing, responses. Each response is associated with its own partial *desirability function*. If the value of the response is optimum, its desirability equals 1, and if it is totally unacceptable, its value is zero. Thus, the desirability for each response can be calculated at a given point in the experimental domain. An overall desirability function can be calculated by multiplying all of the r partial functions together and taking the rth root. Evidently, if the desirability for any response is zero at a point, the overall desirability there is also zero. The optimum is the point with the highest value for the desirability. The experimenter should study the contour plot of the desirability surface around the optimum and combine this with contour plots of the most important responses. A

large area or volume of high desirability will indicate a robust formulation or set of processing conditions.

A number of different forms, linear, convex, concave, unilateral, bilateral, are available for the dependence of the partial desirability on the value of the response. Weighting of responses is also possible. The method requires appropriate computer software, but it is a very powerful method of optimization, and with practice, it is relatively easy. It is especially appropriate for four or more factors. McLeod et al. give an example (21).

Limitations of Response Surface Methodology

The approach of using a mathematical model to map responses predictively and then to use these models to optimize is limited to cases in which the relatively simple, normally quadratic model describes the phenomenon in the optimum region with sufficient accuracy. When this is not the case, one possibility is to reduce the size of the domain. Another is to use a more complex model or a nonpolynomial model better suited to the phenomenon in question. The D-optimal designs and exchange algorithms are useful here as in all cases of change of experimental zone or mathematical model. In any case, response surface methodology in optimization is only applicable to continuous functions.

Lately, there has been a great deal of interest in the use of artificial neural networks in many fields, including that of prediction and expert systems, and they are of interest here for the description of response surfaces that have a nonlinear relation to the factor variables (22, 23). In such cases, the response surface may well fit the data better than that calculated from the model estimated by least-squares regression (24).

However, the choice of experiments is still important for the artificial neural network approach, and it is best selected in a regular pattern. The central composite design, in which each factor takes five levels, is a generally a good compromise (24). Great care must be taken not to "overfit," and, in general, more experiments are required than for the classic RSM approach.

SEARCHING FOR A NEW DOMAIN

The Steepest Ascent Method and Optimum Path Methods

Screening and factor studies will sometimes indicate whether, and if so, where we should search for an optimum within the domain being studied. However, if the optimum (we are considering a single "key" variable here) lies outside the present experiment, then the steepest ascent method comes into its own. The direction of steepest increase of the response in terms of the coded variables is determined, and then experiments are carried out along this line. If a maximum or minimum value (according to the target) is found along this line, the point at which it is found could be the center of a new experimental design for optimization (7). The optimum path method (6, 13) is similar and is used for extrapolating from a second-order design along a curved trajectory.

Sequential Simplex Optimization

Introduction

Unlike the other optimization methods described here, the sequential simplex method for optimization neither assumes nor determines a mathematical model for the phenomena studied.

A simplex is a convex geometric figure of $k+1$ nonplanar vertices in k dimensional space, the number of dimensions corresponding to the number of independent factors. Thus, for two factors, it is a triangle, and for three factors, it is a tetrahedron. The method is sequential because the experiments are analyzed one by one as each is carried out. The basic method used a constant step size (25), allowing the region of experimentation to move at a constant rate toward the optimum. However, a modification that allows the simplex to expand and contract, proposed by Nelder and Mead (26) in 1965, is more generally used. It has been reviewed recently by Waters (27).

Optimization by the extended simplex method

Assume that we wish to optimize a response depending on three to five factors without assuming any model for the dependence other than the domain being continuous. We choose an initial domain and place a regular simplex in it. The experiments for the initial simplex are then carried out and the response measured. In the basic simplex method, an experiment is done outside the simplex in a direction directly opposite to the "worst" point of the simplex. The worst point is discarded, and a new simplex is obtained, the process being repeated. The simplex therefore moves away from the "poor" regions toward the optimum. In the extended simplex method, if the optimum is outside the initial experimental domain, we may leave it rapidly while expanding the simplex for a region with an improved response. As the simplex approaches the optimum, it is contracted rapidly.

Of the experiments of a given simplex let W, N, and B be the "worst" (W), "next worst" (N), and "best" (B) points

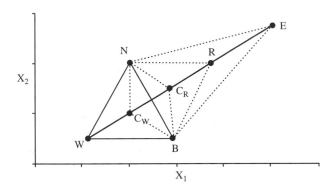

Fig. 10 Summary of the expanded simplex method of Nelder and Mead.

of the initial simplex. A new experiment R is carried out opposite point W to give a new simplex reflecting the original one. Depending on the value of the response at R relative to that at W, N, and B, the step size may be expanded to arrive quickly at the region of the optimum, and then be contracted around the optimum. The various possibilities are shown in Fig. 10 for two factors. "$R > W$" means that point R is better than point W, etc.

R replaces W	if :	$N \leq R \leq B$	Reflection
	or:	$R > B$ and $E \leq B$	
E replaces W	if :	$R > B$ and $E \leq B$	Expansion
C_R replaces W	if :	$W < R \leq N$	Contraction (exterior)
C_W replaces W	if :	$W > R$	Contraction (interior)

At the end of the sequential simplex, if more detailed information is needed, the experimenter may carry out a response surface study around the supposed optimum.

DESIGNING ROBUST PROCESSES AND FORMULATIONS

Until now, optimization and improvement have been taken as being equal or closer to what is considered most desirable with respect to the mean responses. However, it is also necessary that all units of all batches manufactured fall within those specifications. Apart from variation in the measurement method, all variation is attributed to the manufacturing process and the manufacturing and storage environment.

Taking the traditional quality control approach, any product that is within the specifications will pass and is considered equally good. However, one might still normally consider that the nearer the response to the target, the better the product. Therefore, the key is to choose a formulation and/or condition that gives a product not only as close as possible to the target, but with as little variability as possible.

The basic concepts and seminal work in this field are from Taguchi (28), who stated that any product whose performance characteristics are different from the target values suffers a loss in quality, which he quantified by a parabolic function. He then classified factors as: 1) *control factors*, which can be controlled under normal operating conditions; and 2) *noise factors*, which are difficult, impossible, or very expensive to control.

The effects and interactions of control and noise factors could be measured by means of an experimental design, and then settings of the control factors would be determined that would minimize the effects of the noise factors.

One problem in such an approach, apart from the difficulty of controlling noise factors, is to know what they are. Examples of possible noise factors are the drug substance and excipient batches, the ambient temperature and humidity, the machine used, the exact granulation time, and the rate at which liquid is added.

The simplest approach in many cases would be to set up an experimental design in the control factors and repeat each experiment many times, hoping for enough natural variation in the noise factors to be able to find conditions to minimize variation. This requires a very large number of experiments, but it is sometimes the only possible way.

Taguchi's solution was to vary the noise factors artificially (28). A design is set up in the control factors, another (factorial) design in the noise factors, and the two multiplied together. The effect of changes in the noise factors can thus be assessed at each point and the variability minimized. This method is preferred to the previous method, but nonetheless, the number of experiments required using Taguchi's *orthogonal networks* is extremely high. Now it is more usual to set up designs in which the number of experiments, although still high, is minimized (29–31) and to find regions where the response is equal to the target value and is at the same time highly insensitive to the noise factors. The design must allow interactions among noise factors, and not only the control factors themselves, but preferably all the terms in the control factor model.

It should be noted that there is a great deal of information "hidden" in large factorial designs ($n = 16$). When analysis shows that only a few factors are significant, the residuals (differences between calculated and measured values) may be analyzed (32). A small spread of residuals under certain conditions as opposed to others *may* indicates better reproducibility of the process or formulation under these conditions. An example of its pharmaceutical use is presented in the example of Menon et al. (8).

REFERENCES

1. Fisher, R.A. *The Design of Experiments*; Oliver and Boyd: London, 1926.
2. Plackett, R.L.; Burman, J.P. The Design of Optimum Multifactorial Experiments. Biometrica **1946**, *33*, 305–325.
3. Box, G.E.P.; Wilson, K.B. On the Experimental Attainment of Optimum Conditions. J. Royal Stat. Soc. Ser. B **1951**, *13*, 1–45.
4. Myers, R.H. Response Surface Methodology—Current Status and Future Directions. J. Qual. Technol. **1999**, *31* (1), 30–44.
5. Montgomery, D.C. *Design and Analysis of Experiments*; 2nd Ed.; Wiley: New York, 1984.
6. Lewis, G.A.; Mathieu, D.; Phan-Tan-Luu, R. *Pharmaceutical Experimental Design;* Marcel Dekker, Inc.: New York, 1999.
7. Box, G.E.P.; Hunter, W.G.; Hunter, J.S. *Statistics for Experimenters*; Wiley: New York, 1978.
8. Menon, A.; Dhodi, N.; Mandella, W.; Chakrabarti, S. Identifying Fluid-Bed Parameters Affecting Product Variability. Int. J. Pharm. **1996**, *140* (2), 207–218.
9. Carlson, R.; Nordahl, A.; Barth, T.; Myklebust, R. An Approach to Evaluating Screening Experiments when Several Responses are Measured. Chemom. Intell. Lab. Syst. **1992**, *12*, 237–255.
10. Box, G.E.P.; Draper, N.R. *Empirical Model-Building and Response Surface Analysis*; Wiley: New York, 1987.
11. Senderak, E.; Bonsignore, H.; Mungan, D. Response Surface Methodology as an Approach to the Optimization of an Oral Solution. Drug Dev. Ind. Pharm. **1993**, *19*, 405–424.
12. Doehlert, D.H. Uniform Shell Designs. Appl. Stat. **1970**, *19*, 231–239.
13. Vojnovic, D.; Rupena, P.; Moneghini, M.; Rubessa, F.; Coslovich, S.; Phan-Tan-Luu, R.; Sergent, M. Experimental Research Methodology Applied to Wet Pelletization in a High-Shear Mixer. Part 1. S.T.P. Pharma Sci. **1993**, *3*, 130–135.
14. Roquemore, K.G. Hybrid Designs for Quadratic Response Surfaces. Technometrics **1976**, *18*, 419–424.
15. de Aguiar, P.F.; Bourguignon, B.; Khots, M.S.; Massart, D.L.; Phan-Tan-Luu, R. D-optimal Designs. Chemom. Intell. Lab. Syst. **1995**, *30*, 199–210.
16. Atkinson, A.C. The Usefulness of Optimum Experimental Designs. J. Royal Stat. Soc. Ser. B. **1996**, *58* (1), 58–76.
17. Cornell, J.A. *Experiments with Mixtures*; 2nd Ed.; J. Wiley: New York, 1990.

18. Scheffé, H. Experiments with Mixtures. J. Royal Statist. Soc. Ser. B **1958**, *20*, 344–360.

19. Snee, R.D. Computer-Aided Design of Experiments—Some Practical Examples. J. Qual. Technol. **1985**, *17* (4), 222–236.

20. Derringer, G.; Suich, R. Simultaneous Optimization of Several Response Variables. J. Qual. Technol. **1980**, *12*, 214–219.

21. McLeod, A.D.; Lam, F.C.; Gupta, P.K.; Hung, C.T. Optimized Synthesis of Polyglutaraldehyde Nanoparticles Using Central Composite Design. J. Pharm. Sci. **1988**, *77*, 704–710.

22. Bourquin, J.; Schmidli, H.; van Hoogevest, P.; Leuenberger, H. Basic Concepts of Artificial Neural Networks (ANN) Modeling in the Application to Pharmaceutical Development. Pharm. Dev. Technol. **1997**, *2* (2), 95–109.

23. Bourquin, J.; Schmidli, H.; van Hoogevest, P.; Leuenberger, H. Application of Artificial Neural Networks (ANN) in the Development of Solid Dosage Forms. Pharm. Dev. Technol. **1997**, *2* (2), 111–121.

24. Takahara, J.; Takayama, K.; Nagai, T. Multi-Objective Simultaneous Optimization Technique Based on an Artificial Neural Network in Sustained Release Formulations. J. Control. Rel. **1997**, *49* (1), 11–20.

25. Spendley, W.; Hext, G.R.; Himsworth, F.R. Sequential Application of Simplex Designs in Optimization and Evolutionary Operation. Technometrics **1962**, *4*, 441.

26. Nelder, J.A.; Mead, R. A Simplex Method for Function Minimization. Comput. J. **1965**, *1*, 308.

27. Walters, F. Sequential Simplex Optimization—An Update. Anal. Lett. **1999**, *32* (2), 193.

28. Taguchi, G. *System of Experimental Design: Engineering Methods to Optimize Quality and Minimize Cost*, UNIPUB/Fraus International White Plain, 1987.

29. Nair, V. Taguchi 's Parameter Design: A Panel Discussion. Technometrics **1992**, *34*, 127–161.

30. Shoemaker, A.C.; Kwok, L.; Wu, C.F.J. Economical Experimentation Methods for Robust Design. Technometrics **1991**, *33* (4), 415–427.

31. Montgomery, D.C. Using Fractional Factorial Designs for Robust Process Development. Qual. Eng. **1990**, *3*, 193–205.

32. Box, G.E.P.; Meyer, R.D. Dispersion Effects from Fractional Designs. Technometrics **1986**, *28*, 19–27.

33. Anderson, V.L.; McLean, R.A. *Design of Experiments: A Realistic Approach*; Marcel Dekker, Inc.: New York, 1974.

34. Haaland, P.D. *Experimental Design in Biotechnology*; Marcel Dekker, Inc.: New York, 1989.

35. Myers, R.H.; Montgomery, D.C. *Response Surface Methodology*; Wiley-Interscience: New York, 1995.

36. Grove, D.M.; Davis, T.P. *Engineering Quality and Experimental Design*; Longman Scientific and Technical: Harlow, UK, 1992.

37. Schmidt, S.R.; Launsby, R.L. *Understanding Industrial Designed Experiments*, 3rd Ed.; Air Academic Press: Colorado Springs, 1993.

ORPHAN DRUGS

Carolyn H. Asbury

University of Pennsylvania, Philadelphia, Pennsylvania

INTRODUCTION

As drug development costs began to rise in the late 1960s and 1970s with new Food and Drug Administration (FDA) requirements for demonstrating relative safety and efficacy, manufacturers of drugs, biologicals, and diagnostic agents faced a dilemma. How could they consider developing drugs that were important medically but not likely to be profitable? Drugs for diseases and conditions that were rare in the United States were one of several—and the most visible—of such drug types. Rarity meant few patients would be available to participate in clinical trials of safety and efficacy under the sponsor's Investigational Exemption of a New Drug (IND) application. Slow patient recruitment into trials increased development time, with the 17-year patent-protection clock ticking. And once the pharmaceutical sponsor received approval for the New Drug Application (NDA) required for interstate marketing, there would be few customers. This generally translated into a low return on investment (ROI). Moreover, the time devoted to testing and gaining approval for a drug for a rare disease was an opportunity cost. Manufacturers would otherwise have devoted the time and resources to products with more favorable market returns.

Six other drug categories were of limited commercial interest. They included products for (1):

1. Chronic diseases, requiring extended testing phases to assess long-term effects, using up critical patent-protection time;
2. Single administration, such as vaccines, requiring separate production facilities, used by many but on a one-time basis, and carrying high liability risks; and diagnostic agents that had relatively low sales volume;
3. Women of childbearing age, presenting unparalleled liability risks;
4. Children and the elderly, both of whom were excluded from clinical testing at the time. Children presented high liability risks and could be difficult to enroll in clinical trials. Elderly people, who often had multiple conditions, were excluded from trials by the FDA because the multiple conditions and drugs used to treat them would confound trial results. (Once a drug was marketed, physicians could prescribe it for these two populations. However, optimal dosing had not been determined, and likely drug interactions in elderly patients had not been identified);
5. Diseases, rare or common, for which the intended drugs were not patentable including shelf chemicals, drugs known to exist, natural chemicals, and drugs for which the patent had expired;
6. Substance abuse or relapse prevention, intended for a population considered to be a high liability risk, uncooperative with treatment trials, and requiring extensive records once marketed; and
7. Developing countries, with the related problems of distributing and paying for products.

Observing that certain drugs could be in common use but were not potentially profitable enough to invite commercial introduction, Provost referred to them in the *American Journal of Hospital Pharmacy* in 1968 as homeless or "orphan" drugs (2). This chapter focuses on orphan drugs for rare diseases. It provides background on the issues and on attempts to deal with them—a description of the Orphan Drug Law, enacted in 1983, to address these issues—and an accounting of progress and problems to date emanating from the law.

BACKGROUND

The 1938 Food, Drug and Cosmetics Act and the 1962 Kefauver-Harris Amendments to it substantially altered drug development in this country. They strengthened the safety and efficacy determinations of drugs, but at cost, one of which was industry disinterest in drugs for rare diseases. The 1938 law required proof of safety after diethylene glycol, used as a sulfanilamide vehicle was found to form lethal quantities of oxalic acid in the body. This resulted in 100 fatalities, mostly children (3). The law required manufacturers to provide evidence that the drugs were relatively safe. For the FDA to keep a drug off the market, however, the onus was on the *agency* to prove that the drug was not safe. The thalidomide disaster changed that situation. Tragic birth defects were reported

Encyclopedia of Pharmaceutical Technology

in infants born to women in Europe and Canada who had taken the drug while pregnant. At the time the news broke, Congress was working on amendments to the 1938 law that required sponsors to provide proof of drug efficacy before receiving market approval. The thalidomide catastrophe propelled Congress to require sponsors also to show proof of safety. To implement these two requirements, the FDA created the IND process requiring sponsors to test for and establish relative safety before embarking on clinical trials to determine drug efficacy. The FDA set up the NDA approval process for ruling on safety and efficacy before the drug could be marketed interstate (4).

An essential interplay developed between patent protection and regulatory requirements. Patent protection became essential for emerging products developed by research-intensive, vertically integrated firms that looked to a few major market winners to survive in this era of increased development costs (5). Patent time used in the IND and NDA premarket stages reduced the time remaining for manufacturers to protect their products, once marketed, against less costly generic drug competition. Drug development also became more expensive. Development costs in the late 1960s and early 1970s, before the FDA amendments became operationally implemented, were estimated to range from a low of $2.7 million to a high of $16.9 million per new chemical entity (NCE) (6, 7). By the late 1970s, the estimate had risen to $54 million (8). Since then, estimates have continued to leap upward: $124 million in the late 1980s, $231 million in 1991, and $500 million today (9, 10).

By the late 1960s and early 1970s, market winners generated most of a company's profits and also helped encourage brand loyalties by prescribing physicians. Other drugs needed to at least break even. Although not blockbusters, these drugs generally were for large markets. Drugs for rare diseases usually did not break even and became therapeutic orphans. They became wards of government and university-sponsored development efforts.

Cancer treatment drugs were among the first wards of government. Even before the 1962 amendments to the Food, Drug and Cosmetics Act, the federal government had developed and maintained a role in stimulating the development of cancer drug treatment that was not being addressed by industry. The National Cancer Institute (NCI) created the Cancer Chemotherapy Program in 1955 with a $5 million Congressional authorization. Congress decided that the NCI should take on the challenge. Impressed with industry's spectacular antibiotics development, Congress recognized that a low ROI was precluding industry's interest in exploiting the early successes in antitumor drugs (antifol aminopterin for acute childhood leukemia and

methotrexate for uterine choriocarcinoma). Beginning as a small grant-oriented program to develop antileukemia agents, the program was based on the use of transplantable tumors in syngeneic rodents as a system for testing new drugs. After the NCI drafted an agreement allowing for the trade secret status of data, industry submitted compounds for screening of bioactivity. Within three years, the Cancer Chemotherapy Program had grown into a $35 million industrial contract effort. After a few missteps, when the FDA would not accept the cancer-funded research results as provided, the FDA and NCI developed a clear understanding of how data needed to be provided. From that point until at least the early 1980s, the NCI was involved in the development and/or clinical testing of every antineoplastic drug available in the United States (11–13).

In 1966, the National Institute of Neurological and Communicative Disorders and Stroke, as it was then named, established the Antiepileptic Drug Development Program to develop clinical trial methodologies and then to conduct clinical trials of antiepileptic agents already available in other countries. The program later developed a screening program similar to that of the NCI. The Institute filed INDs for drugs that entered clinical testing, and by 1981, four drugs had commercial sponsorship by the NDA stage (14, 15).

Although most of the federal funding for drug programs by the National Institutes of Health (NIH) was for the development of drugs for rare diseases—cancers and epilepsy—the NIH also devoted funding to development of other categories of orphan drugs. These included drugs to prevent and treat substance addiction and relapse, contraceptives for women of childbearing age, and some vaccines being developed by NIH and by the Centers for Disease Control (now the Centers for Disease Control and Prevention). Before 1983, when the Orphan Drug Act was signed into law, NIH drug development programs and grant-supported research had resulted in 13 drugs for the treatment of rare diseases being approved and on the market. In the 17 years before the Orphan Drug Law, the pharmaceutical industry had developed and marketed 34 drugs or biologicals for use in rare diseases or conditions (16). Ten of these marketed orphan drugs and biologicals had been developed solely by industry without government or university support (17).

The Gathering Storm

Nonetheless, several articles published in medical journals by academic researchers chronicled their plight in formulating new dosages for available drugs or encapsulating chemical ingredients for clinical tests in patients with rare diseases, because no pharmaceutical sponsor had come to their rescue (18–20). One of these researchers, Cambridge University's John Walshe, proclaimed that this "do-it-yourself" problem had gone far enough and should be placed on a sound commercial basis (21). The FDA published a list of potentially promising therapeutic agents that were under development primarily by academic or government-based scientists who had failed to find commercial sponsors to undertake the costly phase III clinical trials for efficacy, file the NDA, and market the product (22). In 1979, the FDA convened a Task Force on Drugs of Little Commercial Value to determine how to find commercial sponsors. That same year, Louis Lasagna, who was then at the University of Rochester, invoked Provost's notion in an article in the journal *Regulation* by asking who will adopt the orphan drugs (23)?

NIH-funded academic researchers were reporting failed attempts to interest industry in taking on and securing NDA approval for drugs it had not developed. Industry had cited three major problems. First, NIH-funded scientists may not have gathered and analyzed data according to FDA requirements. Second, the trade secret status of data could not be preserved if the researcher had previously published information in the scientific literature. And third, many of the NIH-funded studies were of drugs that were not (or no longer) patentable. The FDA task force recommended that incentives be provided to industry to develop drugs of limited commercial value, but that any profits made from those incentives be returned, in whole or in part, to the government. (24). This arbitration-type approach was based on the assumption that industry would be willing to make trade-offs with the FDA on behalf of these drugs. But this assumption was made in the absence of any indication from industry that this was the case (25).

Although the task force was the first official policy response to the orphan drug situation (apart from the NIH-sponsored research responses), there were several private-sector efforts underway to promote the development and availability of orphan products. The Pharmaceutical Manufacturers Association (PMA, now called the Pharmaceutical Research and Manufacturers of America, or PhRMA) had been seeking sponsors among its member companies for promising orphan therapeutics. And a consumer group, the National Organization for Rare Disorders (NORD), was growing in number (now representing more than 20 million patients and their families) and undertaking efforts to raise public awareness and to help link patients to researchers conducting clinical studies of their diseases or conditions.

Lightning Strikes

A researcher at the Mount Sinai School of Medicine New York, who was seeking a pharmaceutical company sponsor for the drug L-5HTP for myoclonus, appealed to his Congressperson, Elizabeth Holtzman (D-New York) for a legislative remedy to the plight of orphan drug research. She introduced a bill in 1980 to establish the Office of Drugs of Limited Commercial Value to assist the NIH in developing drugs for the treatment of rare diseases (26). Although no action was taken on the bill, the committee heard testimony from a young California man suffering from Tourette's syndrome, a genetically determined neurological condition causing its victims to twitch, tic, and have uncontrollable verbal (and often abusive) outbursts. When haloperidol proved unsuccessful in controlling his symptoms, the patient had tried desperately to obtain and try pimozide, a drug available for the condition in Canada and Europe, but not in the United States.

A Los Angeles newspaper carried an account of the testimony, which caught the eye of the producer of the television series *Quincy*. Before long, a *Quincy* episode was devoted to dramatizing the conundrum of patients trying to cope with Tourette's syndrome and of industry trying to contend with the commercial disincentives to develop drugs to treat these patients. The episode demonstrated that there were no villains and no remedies. In a compelling scene before a Congressional committee, *Quincy* delivered an impassioned appeal to Congress to find a remedy. Shortly thereafter, *Quincy* star Jack Klugman was asked by Congressman Henry Waxman (D-California) to appear at a hearing on an orphan drug bill that was similar to Holtzman's, introduced by her colleague Representative Ted Weiss (D-New York). Klugman testified at the hearing, using the identical appeal he had delivered on the show (27). A *Wall Street Journal* editorial, entitled "Leave of Reality," likened Klugman's appearance before the Waxman subcommittee as an orphan drug expert to having Leonard Nimoy (Mr. Spock on *Star Trek*) testify as an expert on the nation's space program (28). By the end of 1981, Congressman Waxman had introduced H.R. 5238, the Orphan Drug Act.

The orphan drug survey

To find out the current status of development of drugs for the treatment of rare diseases, the subcommittee surveyed the industry, the NIH, and the FDA on three groups of drugs:

1. Products listed by PMA (now PhRMA) member companies as drugs for the treatment of rare diseases

that industry sponsors had marketed or had made available on a compassionate basis to specialists;

2. Drugs and biologicals listed by the FDA as under development, but needing a commercial sponsor for FDA approval and marketing; and
3. Drugs under development by NIH scientists or grantees.

From this survey, the Subcommittee learned that industry had marketed 34 drugs for the treatment of rare diseases extending back to 1965 and had made an additional 24 drugs (under development) available to physicians on a compassionate basis for treating patients with rare diseases. Most (82%) of the marketed drugs were for conditions affecting fewer than 100,000 people in the United States; 10% were for 100,000 to 500,000 people, and the remaining 8% were for up to 1 million people. Industry respondents indicated that substantial federal funding had been provided for research and/or development (R&D) for all but 10 of these marketed drugs.

The picture of disincentives confirmed claims by industry spokespeople sponsors indicated that the ROI for 83% of the drugs was lower than the sponsors' average return for marketed drugs, whereas development costs were higher than average for 12% of these drugs. Other issues cited by industry were the lack of clarity of FDA clinical testing guidelines when small numbers of patients were available and involved. This further eroded the sponsors' ability to estimate the length of clinical testing, and therefore the length of remaining patent protection time, once the drug was approved. Survey data indicated that industry-sponsored marketed orphan drugs took an average of 5.75 years for clinical testing (from filing the IND to filing the NDA). Unpatented orphan products were increasingly unlikely to be submitted for NDA approval, suggesting the importance of having at least some period of market protection. Whereas nearly two-fifths (39%) of industry-sponsored drugs for the treatment of rare diseases had been marketed in the 1960s, even though they were not protected by patent, this fell to 29% by the 1970s. Liability claims had been filed against the manufacturers of one-fifth of the marketed orphan drugs. The promising finding was that one in four industry-sponsored marketed orphan drugs also had a common indication. This suggested that orphan drugs were a relatively good market gamble (29).

Orphan Drug Act's Passage Provides Market Incentives and Regulatory Assistance

Based primarily on Congressional testimony marshaled by NORD revealing that millions of people and their families were profoundly affected by rare diseases and conditions, and on survey data revealing market and regulatory disincentives to therapeutic progress, Congress passed the Orphan Drug Act during a lame duck session in December 1992. Called "the golden egg of the lame duck Congress" by the head of the Generic Pharmaceutical Industry Association (GPIA), the bill was signed into law the first week of January 1983 (30). The act (Public Law 97–414) was supported initially by the GPIA, which had begun seeking sponsors for developed orphan products, and eventually by the PMA after certain provisions were deleted or modified. Provisions in the law, and in subsequent amendments in 1984, 1985, and 1988, addressed market and regulatory issues and provided incentives for pharmaceutical industry development of drugs for the treatment of rare diseases.

The law, as amended, defines a rare disease or condition as one that affects fewer than 200,000 persons in the United States. Alternatively, the disease or condition can affect more than 200,000 persons in the United States, if there is no reasonable expectation that the cost of developing and making a drug available for such disease or condition in the United States will be recovered from U.S. sales of the drug. Therefore, a drug can be designated by the FDA as an orphan by demonstrating applicability of the law's financial criteria, regardless of the total number of people affected in the United States. Major provisions are the availability of two market incentives and the reduction of regulatory barriers. The FDA Office of Orphan Products Development administers nearly all the law's provisions.

One incentive is seven years of market exclusivity granted by the FDA for a specific indication of a product. Exclusivity begins on the date the FDA approves the marketing application for the designated orphan drug and applies only to the indication for which the drug has been designated and approved. An application for designation as an orphan drug for a specific indication must be made before submission of the NDA (or biologic product license application, PLA) for market approval (31). Other sponsors can receive approval for a different drug to treat the same rare disease or can receive approval to market an identical drug for some other orphan or common indication. Market exclusivity, therefore, only precludes a second sponsor from obtaining approval to provide an identical drug for the identical orphan indication for which the first sponsor received exclusive market approval. Initially, market exclusivity pertained only to unpatented products. A 1985 amendment allowed exclusive approval for all orphan drugs, whether patented or not. This change was designed to provide incentives for sponsors of products for the treatment of rare diseases whose patents would expire before or soon after approval, or in cases in which prior publication (usually by an academic or government scientist) had precluded issuance of a patent.

A second incentive provides tax credits equal to 50% of the costs of human clinical testing undertaken in any given year by a sponsor to generate data required for obtaining FDA market approval through successful completion of the NDA process. The Internal Revenue Service administers the tax credit provisions.

The act provides for the FDA to award grants to support clinical studies of designated orphan products under-development. FDA grant funding as of March 2000 from the FDA totaled $126.3 million. From initial funding in 1983 of $500,000 in grants, the grant program peaked in 1994 at $12.3 million and has declined slightly but steadily thereafter, totaling $11.1 million in 1999 (32). Applications are reviewed by outside experts and are funded according to a priority score. The FDA Office of Orphan Product Development provides information at its website (www.fda.gov/orphan/GRANTS/patients) on investigators seeking research subjects. Listed by the name of the disease or condition, information includes a description of the study, criteria for inclusion in clinical trials (such as age, stage of disease, etc.), and contact information on the clinical investigator seeking participants for clinical trials. Patients, their families, or their physicians are able to follow up with the clinical investigator.

To address regulatory barriers the FDA also provides formal protocol assistance when requested by the sponsor of an orphan drug. Although formal review of a request for protocol assistance is the direct responsibility of the FDA Centers for Evaluation and Research (one for drugs, the other for biologicals), the Office of Orphan Products Development is responsible for ensuring that the request qualifies for consideration. A sponsor need not have obtained orphan drug designation to receive protocol assistance.

Table 1 Designated and approved orphan drug products

	Pre-1983	1989	1991	3/2000
Cumulative total approved orphan products	34[a]	36	54	235
Total sponsors of approved orphan drugs[b]	17			110

[a]At the time, these were called drugs for rare diseases, not orphan drugs.
[b]Sponsors identified only for the two endpoints.

Finally, the FDA is required to encourage sponsors to design open protocols for drug availability to patients not included in clinical trials.

The Current Status of Orphan Drugs

The FDA approved 201 orphan products between 1983 and March 2000 (33). In the 17 years since passage of the act, therefore, the number of approved orphan drugs has increased sixfold from the number approved in the 17 years before the act (Table 1). The drugs are classified within 16 therapeutic categories, primarily for the treatment of cancer, infectious disease, AIDS and related conditions, and central nervous system conditions (Table 2). Included in the 201 approved drugs are 24 (12%) that received FDA grant support for clinical trials (34). A list of these grant-supported products is available at the FDA Office of Orphan Products Development website (www.fda.gov/orphan/GRANTS).

The number of sponsors of approved orphan drugs (nearly all of them produced at pharmaceutical or biotechnology companies) has increased from 17 (for the 34 drugs marketed before the act) to 110 as of March 2000. The number of approved drugs per sponsor ranges from one to eight, with a preponderance of one-drug sponsors (Table 3). A total of 813 products have received orphan designations as of March 2000. Sponsors of approximately 25% of these designated products have filed INDs for the products, indicating that they are under active development (35).

Many of the designated and approved orphan products are developed at biotechnology companies. Beginning in the 1970s, molecular biology had begun to spur the creation of biotechnology research companies. These companies reportedly recognized early on that market exclusivity, and lack of competition to develop products for the treatment of rare diseases, provided protection essential to raising venture capital. As a result, orphan drugs are now among biotechnology's most prevalent, and, according to some, most lucrative products. Between 1988 and 1992, biotechnology product designations increased by 31%, from 8 to 39% of total orphan designations (36). In addition to industry, however, sponsors have included a university, an individual researcher, and a state public health unit, which in aggregate sponsored six orphan drugs at the time of approval. Lists of approved and designated orphan drugs can be obtained from the FDA Office of Orphan Products Development. These data suggest that orphan drug development has consistently risen over the years since the law was enacted. Aggregate sales of

Table 2 Approved orphan drugs: Number per therapeutic category[a]

Category	Number of approved orphan products N = 201
Cancer	49
Infectious disease	23
Central nervous system	22
Hematopoetic	21
AIDS, AIDS-related	21
Endocrine	18
Inborn errors of metabolism	12
Renal	8
Cardiovascular disease	7
Respiratory	5
Gastrointestinal	5
Bone	3
Immunological	2
Dermatological	2
Antidote	2
Urinary tract	1

[a]Does not include drugs for rare diseases marketed before the 1983 Orphan Drug Law.

orphan drugs have been reported to be more than $1 billion a year (37).

A Resulting Issue: High Pricing for Some Products

By the early 1990s, U.S. sales data collected for 41 of the approved orphan drugs that had been on the market for a year or more indicated that 75% of the products had generated earnings of less than $10 million per drug. Three products had earnings between $10 and $25 million, six

Table 3 Approved orphan drugs per sponsor, March 2000[a]

Drugs per sponsor	Sponsors
1	69
2	19
3	6
4	2
5	5
6	2
7	1
8	2

[a]Does not include sponsors of drugs for rare diseases approved before the Orphan Drug Act of 1983.

drugs between $26 and $100 million, and two products more than $100 million. Biotechnology firms produced four of the 11 drugs with relatively high sales.

Those orphan drugs that command high prices have generated intense controversy over whether the market exclusivity provision is creating an unnecessary monopoly, keeping prices artificially high. One example is recombinant human erythropoietin (r-EPO), intended for patients with chronic renal failure-related anemia. EPO eliminates the need for frequent blood transfusions by patients with end-stage renal disease who are undergoing kidney dialysis. These patients are covered under the federally financed Medicare program. Both Amgen Inc. and Genetics Institute applied to the FDA for market exclusivity for their r-EPO products. Amgen was the first to receive FDA approval and market exclusivity. Genetics Institute was the first to receive a patent. On appeal, the court ruled that Amgen had exclusive marketing rights. Sales of r-EPO exceeded $100 million in the first six months of marketing, paid for by Medicare. By 1991, sales totaled $400 million (38).

Human growth hormone (r-hGH), another example, generated sales of $150 million in 1991. Intended to treat approximately 12,000 children in the United States with retarded growth caused by a lack of endogenous pituitary hormone, two companies provide r-hGH. Genentech received FDA market exclusivity in 1985. Eli Lilly received market approval two years later, based on the determination that the two products differed by one amino acid (39,40). But the shared market did not lead to price competition: each company was earning approximately $20,000 per child annually, depending on the dosage needed.

A third example, aerosol pentamidine, generated sales of $130 million in 1991. Helping to prevent *Pneumocystis carinii* pneumonia associated with the human immunodeficiency virus (HIV), the increasing number of users resulting from a rapidly escalating HIV prevalence rate was expected to soon exceed the 200,000 population figure specified in the law. This example, along with the other two, prompted efforts to seek a legislative remedy. A series of amendments were introduced and passed by Congress in 1990 that sought to eliminate orphan status for products intended for use in epidemics and to allow shared market access for identical products developed simultaneously for the same indication, in the hope that this would lead to price competition. The amendments were vetoed (41). As Arno, Bonuck, and Davis present in *Milbank Quarterly*, AIDS treatment drugs exemplify the policy dilemma of how to use the Act to meet the legislative intent of stimulating development of drugs for small patient populations without resulting in prices that make such drugs inaccessible (42).

Another, more recent, example is enzyme therapy for Gaucher's disease, an inborn error of metabolism, treated with Ceredase. The therapy, which requires more than a ton of placenta annually to extract and make the drug, can cost as much as $500,000 per year per person, depending on the dosage needed. A 1996 National Institutes of Health technology assessment panel addressed issues in diagnosis and treatment of the disease and concluded that despite the success of enzyme therapy, treatment is limited by the cost. The panel reported that it was imperative to define the appropriate clinical indications for treatment and to determine the lowest effective initial and maintenance doses (43).

Although the survey undertaken prior to the Act found that retail costs of drugs for the treatment of rare diseases were reportedly higher than the manufacturer's average for 60% of the products marketed before the act, the pricing for some orphan drugs after the act, as exemplified by these examples, is a critically important consequence of the law. This consequence merits continued public scrutiny. It is a sign of progress that for some orphan drugs, accessibility rather than availability is now the challenge requiring creative solutions.

REFERENCES

1. Asbury, C.H. Medical Drugs of Limited Commercial Interest: Profit Alone is a Bitter Pill. Intern. J. Health Serv. **1981**, *11* (3), 451–462.
2. Provost, G.P. Homeless or Orphan Drugs. Am. J. Hosp. Pharm. **1968**, *25*, 609.
3. Silverman, M.; Lee, P.R. *Pills, Profits and Politics*; University of California Press: Berkeley, 1974; 2.
4. Harris, R. *The Real Voice*; Macmillan: New York, 1964; 21–25.
5. Temin, P. Technology, Regulation and Market Structure in the Modern Pharmaceutical Industry. Bell J. Econ. **1979**, *10* (2), 427–446.
6. Report of the Panel on Chemicals and Health of the President's Science Advisory Committee, 73–500, NSF, U.S. Government Printing Office: Washington, DC, 1973.
7. Schwartzman, D. *Innovation in the Pharmaceutical Industry*; Johns Hopkins University Press: Baltimore, 1976; 106–107.
8. Hansen, R.W. The Pharmaceutical Development Process: Estimates of Development Costs and Times and Effects of Proposed Regulatory Changes. *Issues in Pharmaceutical Economics*; Chien, R., Ed.; Lexington Books: Lexington, MA, 1980; 151–181.
9. DiMasi, J.; Hanson, R.; Grabowski, H.; Lasagna, L. The Cost of Innovation in the Pharmaceutical Industry and Health Economics. J. Health Econ. **1991**, *10*, 107–142.
10. Rosenbaum, D.E. The Gathering Storm Over Prescription Drugs. The New York Times **Nov. 14, 1999**, *1*, Section 4 (Week in Review).
11. Devita, V.; Oliverio, V.T.; Muggia, F.M.; Wiernick, P.W.; Ziegler, J.; Goldin, A.; Rubin, D.; Henney, J.; Schepartz, S. The Drug Development and Clinical Trials Programs of the Division of Cancer Treatment, National Cancer Institute. Cancer Clin. Trials **1979**, *2*, 195–216.
12. Zubrod, C.G.; Schepartz, S.; Leiten, J.; Endicott, K.M.; Carrese, L.M.; Baker, C.E. *Cancer Chemotherapy Reports October 1996, 50 (7)*; DHEW: Washington, DC, 1968.
13. Rate of Development of Anticancer Drugs by the National Cancer Institute and the U.S. Pharmaceutical Industry and the Impact of Regulation. *Final Report for the National Cancer Institute*; University of Rochester Medical Center: New York, 1981; 40.
14. Krall, R.A. Anti-Epileptic Drug Development. I. History and a Program for Progress. Epilepsia **1978**, *19* (4), 398–408.
15. Program Performance Summary. *National Institute of Neurological and Communicative Disorders and Stroke Antiepileptic Drug Development Program*; NINCDS: Washington, DC, 1982.
16. Orphan Drugs in Development, 1992 Annual Survey. Pharmaceutical Manufacturers Association: Washington, DC, 1992.
17. Orphan Drug Act Report, 97th Congress, 2nd Session. Washington, DC, Sept 17; 1982.
18. Van Woert, M. Profitable and Non-Profitable Drugs. N. Engl. J. Med. **1978**, *298* (16), 903–906.
19. Rawlins, M. No Utopia Yet. Br. Med. J. **1977**, *2*, 1076.
20. Rawlins, M. Editorial. Lancet **1976**, *2*(7970), 835–836.
21. Walshe, J.M. Treatment of Wilson's Disease with Trientine (Triethylene Tetramine) Dihhydrochloride. Lancet **1982**, *1*, 643–647.
22. Asbury, C.H. *Medical Drugs of Limited Commercial Interest: The Development of Federal Policy*; Johns Hopkins School of Hygiene and Public Health Thesis, Baltimore, 1981; 157–175.
23. Lasagna, L. Who Will Adopt the Orphan Drugs? Regulation **1979**, *3* (6), 27–32.
24. U.S. Food and Drug Administration Report. *Interagency Task Force Report to the Secretary of DHEW*; FDA: Washington, DC, 1979;, 1–82.
25. Asbury, C.H.; Stolley, P. Orphan Drugs: Creating Federal Policy. Ann. Intern. Med. **1981**, *95* (2), 221–224.
26. Holtzman, E. Rep. H.R. 7089, 96th Congress, 2nd Session. Washington, DC, April 17, 1980.
27. Klugman, J.; Seligman, A. Testimony, Serial No. 97–17, U.S. Government Printing Office: Washington, DC, 1981; 10–16.
28. Leave of Reality (Editorial). The Wall Street Journal **March 12, 1981**, .
29. Asbury, C.H. *Orphan Drugs: Medical vs. Market Value*; D.C. Heath: Lexington, MA, 1985; 136–155.
30. Waxman, H.R. Rep. H.R. 5328, 97th Congress, 1st Session. Washington, DC, 1981.
31. FDA Office of Orphan Products Development, www.fed.gov/orphan/about/progovw.htm (accessed Feb 2000).
32. Personal Communication, *FDA OOPD*, March 2000.
33. *FDA List of Approved Orphan Products through 02/24/2000*, FDA: Washington, DC, 2000; Provided on Request from the FDA OOPD.

34. Grant-Supported Products with Marketing Approval, *FDA OOPD*, Washington, DC, www.fda.gov/orphan/grants/magrants (accessed Feb 2000).

35. Personal Communication, *FDA OOPD*, March 2000.

36. Schuman, S.R. Implementation of the Orphan Drug Act. Food Drug Law J. **1992**, *47* (4), 363–403.

37. Grady, D. In Quest to Cure Rare Diseases, Some Get Left Out. *The New York Times*; Nov. 16, 1999.

38. Coster, J.M. Recombinant Erythropoietin: Orphan Product with a Silver Spoon. Intern. J. Technol. Assess. Health Care **1992**, *8* (4), 635–646.

39. Hilts, P.J. Seeking Limits to a Drug Monopoly. *The New York Times*; May 14, 1992, D1; 7.

40. Asbury, C.H. Evolution and Current Status of the Orphan Drug Act. Intern. J. Technol. Assess. Health Care **1992**, *8* (4), 573–582.

41. Asbury, C.H. The Orphan Drug Act: The first 7 years. J. Am. Med. Assoc. **1991**, *265*, 893–897.

42. Arno, P.S.; Bonuck, K.; Davis, M. Rare Disease Drug Development and AIDS: The Impact of the Orphan Drug Act. Milbank Q. **1995**, *73* (2), 231–252.

43. NIH Technology Panel on Gaucher Disease. Gaucher Disease. Current Issues in Diagnosis and Treatment. J. Am. Med. Assoc. **1996**, *275* (7), 548–553.

44. Asbury, C. *Orphan Drugs: Medical vs Market Value*; D.C Heath and Company: Lexington, MA, 1985.

45. Scheinberg, I.H., Walshe, J.M. Eds. *Orphan Diseases and Orphan Drugs;* Manchester University Press: Manchester, UK, 1986.

46. Wagner, J. Orphan Technologies. Int. J. Technol. Assessment **1992**, *8* (4), www.fda.gov/orphan.

47. Arno, P.S.; Bonuck, K.; Davis, M. Rare Diseases, Drug Development, and AIDS: The Impact of the Orphan Drug Act. Milbank Q. **1995**, *73* (2), 241–252.

48. Henkel, J. Orphan Drug Law Matures into Medical Mainstay. FDA Consumer **1999**, *33* (3), 29–32.

OTIC PREPARATIONS

William H. Slattery III

House Ear Institute, Los Angeles, California

INTRODUCTION

Otic preparations are commonly used to treat diseases of the external ear and occasionally of the middle ear. Diseases of the ear include cerumen impaction, dermatitis of the external ear canal, and infectious processes. External otitis (swimmers' ear) and chronic otitis media constitute the majority of infectious diseases of the ear. This article gives an overview of otic preparations, their uses, current availability, and the area of future development.

Anatomy and Physiology of the Ear

Figure 1 is a diagram of the normal ear, which comprises the external ear canal, middle ear space, and hearing canal, or cochlea. The outer two-thirds of the external ear canal is formed by a cartilage framework. The medial or inner one-third of the external ear canal has its framework composed of bone. There is a thin layer of skin covering this bone on the medial one-third. The outer two-thirds is also covered with skin but also has a thick soft tissue lining containing the apopilosebaceous unit. External sounds travel through the external ear canal to reach the tympanic membrane. Vibration of the tympanic membrane transmits a sound wave to the three middle ear ossicles. These, in turn, send the sound wave to the inner ear (cochlea), where it is transformed into a nerve impulse. This impulse is sent to the brain, where the perception of hearing occurs.

The normal external auditory canal has several mechanisms that protect if from infections. The S-shaped anatomy of the external auditory canal provides protection from foreign bodies under normal circumstances. The tragus provides protection anteriorly, and hair from follicles found just inside the meatus prevent airborne debris from entering.

The external auditory canal skin is normally acidic, with a pH level between 4 and 5. Keratin, which consists of desquamated epithelial cells, is produced by the epithelial (skin) lining of the external ear canal; it has an isoelectric point of pH 5. Any increase above this value causes hydration of the keratin layer, increasing susceptibility to pathogenic organisms. Because as most organisms responsible for otitis externa and chronic superlative otitis grow best at an alkaline pH level of 7.2–7.6, the acidic pH of the external ear canal is bactericidal or bacteriostatic to many of these pathogenic organisms. The natural low pH level is therefore helpful in preventing ear infections. Anything that alters the pH balance such as swimming may increase the risk of bacterial infections.

Enzymes produced by sweat and sebaceous glands provide antimicrobial activity. Muramidase, a lysozyme excreted by the sweat glands, may be effective in lysing *Staphylococcus epidermidis* and other gram-positive organisms found on the surface of the ear canal skin. Unsaturated fatty acids, resulting from the breakdown of lipids secreted from sebaceous glands, exert antimicrobial activity against gram-negative organisms and fungi (1).

An intact tympanic membrane protects the normal sterile middle ear space from bacterial pathogens. A ruptured tympanic membrane or tympanostomy tube allows external bacteria access to the middle ear space.

Cerumen, or earwax, is produced in the outer third of the external ear canal. It consists of keratin from the epithelial lining and the enzymes and unsaturated fatty acids produced by the sweat and sebaceous glands. It exerts a protective role by forming an oily, mechanical barrier, considered bacteriostatic and fungistatic, over the skin of the external ear canal. A cerumen plug consists mainly of sheets of keratin. It also contains hair and the secretions of both the sebaceous and ceruminous glands of the external ear canal. Contained within these secretions are glycopeptides, lipids, hyaluronic acid, sialic acid, heparin sulfate, lysosomal enzymes, and immunoglobulin (2). The overall chemical composition of cerumen consists of saturated and unsaturated long-chain fatty acids, alcohols, squalene, and cholesterol (3).

Pathology and Bacteriology of Otitis

Development of new drugs and devices to treat diseases of the external ear requires an understanding of pathophysiology and knowledge about the most common organisms responsible for ear inflammation and infections.

Acute otitis external (swimmers' ear) is an inflammatory condition of the external ear canal, most commonly precipitated by local trauma, that is, Q-tips, fingernails, or

Encyclopedia of Pharmaceutical Technology

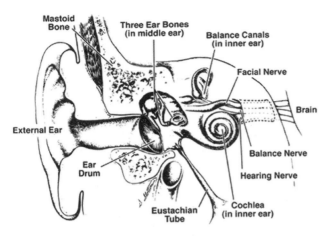

Fig. 1   Diagram of the ear.

other foreign objects that abrade the external ear canal skin. Other predisposing factors include (4):

- Maceration of the epithelial tissue in the ear canal from prolonged exposure to water or moisture;
- Plugging of sebaceous gland ducts, which lowers resistance to infection;
- Moisture absorption by the stratum corneum layer of the epithelium at humidity levels at approximately 80%;
- Elevated ambient temperature against a background of high relative humidity;
- Invasion of exogenous organisms through breaches in a damaged epithelial surface;
- An absence of cerumen; and
- The presence of an alkaline secretion.

Clinical manifestations of the preinflammatory stage of external otitis include itching of the external ear canal and congestion of the apopilosebaceous unit. This is thought to result from the loss of lipids in the external auditory canal that, in turn, results in an increase in the aqueous content of the stratum corneum, causing intracellular edema. The acute inflammatory stage is seen with trauma induced by scratching. By this means, bacteria are allowed access to the dermis. A spectrum of clinical manifestations occurs, ranging from mild edema of the ear canal skin with a clear serous discharge to a severe form characterized by intense pain, a grossly edematous ear canal, and a purulent discharge. A chronic inflammatory stage has also been described. It is characterized by the thickening of the skin, eczematization, lichenification, and superficial skin ulceration (4).

Otomycosis is the result of a superficial fungal infection in the external ear canal. This may commonly result from an underlying bacterial infection or occur in the presence of moist cerumen. Fungi initially implant into the stratum

corneum, where they lie dormant for several days to weeks. They then grow in the superficial layer of the skin, causing inflammation. Initially, the patient usually complains of itching. In the earliest stages, mild edema may be the only clinical symptom. Later, the patient may present with a fungal mass consisting of waxy debris surrounded by a velvety gray membrane with small black spores (5).

Chronic suppurative otitis media is an inflammatory condition of the middle ear. The presence of a tympanic membrane perforation or a tympanostomy tube allows drainage into the external ear canal. Increased vascularity of the mucosa and submucosa, combined with acute and chronic inflammatory cells, is its hallmark. Granulation tissue, fibrosis, and osteoneogenesis are also commonly present. The granulation tissue contains neutrophils and plasma cells associated with small blood vessels and fibroblasts (6).

Pseudomonas aeruginosa and *Staphylococcus aureus* are the most common organisms responsible for acute otitis externa. *Proteus* species are though to be responsible for the chronic inflammatory stage associated with it. *Aspergillus niger* and *Candida albicans* are the most common organisms responsible for otomycosis. *Mucormycosis*, yeast-like fungi, dermatophytes, and *Actinomyces* may also be seen (5).

Cultures from patients with chronic suppurative otitis media demonstrate that the most common responsible organisms are *P. aeruginosa* and *S. aureus*. These are usually mixed infections with a variety of organisms present (7, 8), and they exhibit a higher resistance to antibiotics.

In a study of 119 cases of chronic suppurative otitis media, Papstavros (9) noted a large number (81%) of gentamicin-resistant organisms in patients previously treated with topical gentamicin. Brook (7) cultured drainage from 54 children with chronic suppurative otitis media and showed that 70% of these patients harbored β-Lactamase-producing bacteria. Of 37 patients with β-Lactamase-producing bacteria, 21 had been treated previously with an oral penicillin or cephalosporin. No child in this study had received prior ototopical drops. In 39% of the children with bilateral-draining ears, a different organism predominated on each side. Both of these studies demonstrate the potential for encountering resistant organisms in chronic otitis media after previous oral or topical antibiotic therapy.

Cerumen Preparations

Normal desquamation of the epithelial layer of the external ear canal results in migration of cerumen toward the meatus. Any interference with this normal self-cleaning mechanism results in cerumen impaction. An in vitro study has demonstrated that cerumenolysis occurs as the keratin cells, the major constituents of a cerumen plug, are hydrated, resulting in lysis of these cells (2). Consistent with this finding, aqueous preparations have been demonstrated to be better cerumenolytic products than organic, nonaqueous preparations (2, 10, 11). Before using any cerumenolytic agent, the presence of an intact tympanic membrane must be confirmed to prevent two possible complications. Introduction of these compounds into the middle ear is often painful, and the irrigation of cerumen with its keratin cells into the middle ear space may result in a cholesteatoma, a benign but destructive skin growth that requires surgical treatment.

Impacted cerumen can be simply removed by instillation of mineral oil or glycerin into the ear canal. These solutions soften the cerumen, facilitating the separation of the keratin plug from the epithelium, and thus assist the normal migration of cerumen toward the external meatus. Irrigation of the ear canal with hydrogen peroxide is another simple method. The release of oxygen provides a mechanical means for both softening the cerumen and separating it from canal skin. Hydrogen peroxide also increases the moisture within the ear canal, because the breakdown of hydrogen peroxide is water and oxygen. This may predispose to acute otitis externa by increasing the amount of moisture within the ear canal.

Unfortunately, these simple methods are not always successful, and cerumenolytics have been developed to help dissolve cerumen and facilitate its removal. In severe cases, flushing the ear canal with a rinsing solution or physical extraction is still required.

Over the years, numerous cerumenolytic agents composed of aqueous solutions or organic solvents have been tested (Table 1) (12). Currently, the most common over-the-counter products consist of carbamide peroxide in glycerin. The latter softens the wax, whereas the oxygen

released from the peroxide helps to loosen tissue debris. Usually, this agent has to be applied repeatedly over several days for the wax to soften. The softened wax may be removed with gentle irrigation or by blowing air into the external canal.

Triethanolamine polypeptide oleate condensate in propylene glycol (Cerumenex) requires a prescription. Its mechanism of action is thought to result from softening of the cerumen plug and lubrication of the ear canal (2), which is usually achieved in 15–20 min; however, mechanical removal of the cerumen plug may still be necessary. Application of this agent is best confined to a physician's office because severe allergic skin reactions occur occasionally.

Although not marketed as a cerumenolytic, docusate sodium has been found to be a very effective agent (13). Most commonly used as an aqueous fecal softener, its action on cerumen results in keratin cell expansion and lysis. The preparation is alkaline and in solution releases free hydroxyl ions (2). Drops placed in the ear canal for 10–15 min usually result in cerumen disimpaction. The plug may then be easily rinsed out of the ear canal or mechanically removed.

The ideal cerumenolytic preparation (a hypo-osmolar, alkaline, aqueous solution) has not yet been developed. It should be able to lyse the keratin cells of cerumen and allow for easy disimpaction (2).

In contrast to the use of cerumenolytic agents, cerumen replacement products for conditions such as dry skin, eczema, psoriasis, and chronic otitis of the external ear canal are occasionally required for some patients Unfortunately, there is no product available currently to meet this need.

Antiseptics

Antiseptic agents are often used for the treatment of external ear canal disease. As with cerumenolytics, the

Table 1 Cerumenolytic products

Product	Cerumenolytic agent	Other ingredients
Cerumenex	Triethanolamine polypeptide oleate condensate	Propylene glycol Chlorbutanol (0.5%)
Debrox drops	Carbamide peroxide (6.5%)	Glycerin Propylene glycol Citric acid
Murine ear drops	Carbamide peroxide (6.5%)	Alcohol (6.3%) Glycerin

presence of an intact tympanic membrane must be confirmed before their use. Some antiseptics are commonly used for otologic surgical prophylaxis. Antiseptic otologic preparations are marketed only as the acetic acid solutions.

Acetic acid preparations (usually 2–5% solutions) have both antibacterial and antifungal activities. They are particularly useful against *P. aeruginosa Staphylococci,* β-hemolytic *Streptococci, Candida* species, and *Aspergillus.* No organisms are resistant to these preparations (14). Acetic acid solutions placed in the external ear are generally well tolerated and nonsensitizing; however, instillation into the middle ear cavity is associated with pain. The primary drawback of these agents is the vinegar-like smell associated with the instillation. Acetic acid solutions may be combined with aluminum acetate or a steroid compound for anti-inflammatory and antipruritic properties (15). There is a tendency for acetic acid solutions to induce proliferation of the keratin layer, thus increasing the amount of debris within the ear canal associated with theses infections. This may complicate the infection, making it slower to resolve.

General antiseptics such as povidine iodine (Betadine®), chlorhexidine gluconate (Hibiclens®), and hexachlorophene (pHisohex®) may be used ototopically for surgical prophylaxis. Povidine iodine is the most common preparation used because of its broad spectrum of activity against microflora, microzoa, and viruses. It must be prevented from entering the middle ear during surgical prophylaxis because it inhibits fibroblast migration during the healing process. Either chlorhexidine or hexachlorophene may be used for surgical prophylaxis in patients who are allergic to iodine. Chlorhexidine is the preferred agent in the iodine-allergic patient because it has a broad spectrum of antimicrobial activity against both gram-positive and gram-negative organisms. Hexachlorophene's bacteriostatic activity is more effective against gram-positive than gram-negative organisms, and suppuration decreases its activity (15, 16).

Isopropyl alcohol is used to rinse the ear canal in patients prone to the development of external otitis. It is commonly applied after swimming as a prophylactic measure. Although isopropyl alcohol has broad bactericidal activity, it is widely used as a drying agent for the external ear canal. It displaces water left in the ear canal after swimming. Application into the middle ear space causes severe pain, and it should not be used in the presence of a perforated tympanic membrane.

Gentian violet and thimerosal (Merthiolate) are used for the treatment of fungal infections and are discussed later.

Antifungal Preparations

Most otomycotic infections are the consequence of treatment with antibiotics. Simple cleaning of the external ear canal and discontinuation of the medication will usually suffice to clear up the infection. However, primary and persistent infections require ototopical antifungal medications (Table 2).

Clotrimazole, as a 1% solution, is the most effective topical fungicide for the treatment of otomycosis. It is active against *Aspergillus* and *Candida* species, the most common pathogens responsible for these infections. It acts by interfering with the biosynthesis of ergosterol and is very effective for refractory or chronic cases caused by the dermatophytes or *Candida* species (17).

Amphotericin B is also an effective ototopical preparation. It may be used as a lotion or in a powder form (shown later). Its spectrum of activity covers a variety of fungi, including those responsible for otomycosis. Topical therapy is well tolerated with only rare minor side effects of local skin irritation reported. It is poorly absorbed through the skin (18).

Nystatin and miconazole have a spectrum of activity similar to that of amphotericin B against the common yeast and fungi responsible for otomycosis (17). Nystatin is occasionally used in solution as an ototopic drop. Miconazole is rarely used because it is readily available only as a cream. Application into the ear canal is difficult without impairing the hearing.

m-Cresyl acetate (Cresylate), a derivative of cresol, is marketed as an ototopical antifungal preparation. It is highly active against *Candida* and *Aspergillus.* The ear canal may be painted with *m*-Cresyl acetate on a cotton-tipped applicator, or the compound may be used in solution as an ototopical drop. It is considered the antiseptic of choice for the treatment of otomycosis because it is easily used in the outpatient setting, and, in contrast to gentian violet and thimerosal, no staining is associated with its use. However, eczematization may occur if applied to the concha, and therefore its application should be limited to the external ear canal (16, 19).

Gentian violet is used regularly in the office setting for the treatment of fungal infections. It also has bacteriostatic and bactericidal activity against most gram-positive organisms. The external ear canal is painted with the gentian violet on a cotton-tipped applicator under direct vision using an operating microscope. This compound is a strong dye, and blind application into the external ear canal is difficult without staining. For this reason, self-application by the patient is rarely performed (16).

Thimerosal (Merthiolate) may also be used topically for the treatment of otomycosis. Considered bacteriostat, it is

Table 2   Otomycotic preparations

Product	Antifungal agent	Other ingredients
Otic Domeboro solution	Acetic acid (2%)	Aluminum sulfate Boric acid
VoSol Otic solution	Acetic acid (2%)	Propylene glycol (3%) Benzethonium chloride
VoSol HC Otic solution	Acetic acid (2%)	Hydrocortisone (1%) Propylene glycol (3%) Benzethonium chloride
Fungizone lotion	Amphotericin B (3%) Thimerosal	Propylene glycol
Lotrimin solution	Clotrimazole	Polyethylene glycol
Mycelex solution	Clotrimazole	Polyethylene glycol
Cresylate solution	*m*-Cresyl acetate (25%)	Propylene glycol Isopropanol (25%)
Gentian violet solution	Gentian violet (1%)	Ethanol (10%)
Merthiolate	Thimerosal 1:1000	
Monistat-Derm lotion	Miconazole (2%)	Pegoxol 7 stearate Mineral oil Benxoic acid
Nystatin suspension	Nystatin (100,000 U/mL)	None

an excellent antiseptic agent in vitro against the common yeast and fungi responsible for otomycosis (16, 17).

Fungal cultures may be required in refractory or persistent cases of otomycosis, in which less common fungi may be responsible; the appropriate ototopical agent may be selected based on culture results. Systemic antifungal medications are rarely indicated for the treatment of otomycosis, unless associated with systemic fungal infections.

Topical preparations for the treatment of otomycosis should not be used in the presence of a perforated tympanic membrane.

Antimicrobial Drops

As a group, antimicrobial otic drops are the most commonly prescribed ototopical medication (Table 3). Most of the preparations listed in Table 3 contain a mixture of antibiotics in combination with a steroid agent. Acetic acid or an alcohol may be added for bactericidal activity. Some of these preparations contain acetic acid as the primary antibacterial agent. Most of these compounds have a low pH, between 3 and 5, similar to that of the normal external ear canal.

Antimicrobial otic drops should be used with caution in the presence of a tympanic membrane perforation because of the potential for ototoxicity. In the case of suppuration, the ear canal should be cleaned before drop instillation.

Purulence within the ear canal will not allow ototopical drops to penetrate the skin, and it is thus prevented from treating the ear infection. Ear cleaning is extremely important when suppuration occurs.

Neomycin and Polymyxin B are the two most common antibiotic agents found in ototopical preparations. Neomycin is bactericidal to many gram-positive and gram-negative organisms, including those responsible for external and chronic otitis such as *S. aureus*, *C. diphtheriae, Escherichia coli, Proteus, Enterobacter, Klebsiella, and Haemophilus influenzae.* It has no activity against anaerobes, and many strains of *Pseudomonas* are resistant. Cutaneous hypersensitivity is estimated to occur in 6–8% of patients who receive topical treatment (20).

Polymyxin B and Colistin (polymyxin E), first discovered in 1947, have similar antibiotic spectrums limited to gram-negative organisms. *P. aeruginosa* is particularly sensitive to these medications. Other sensitive gram-negative organisms include *Enterobacter, E. coli, Klebsiella*, and *Haemophilus*. These agents interact with the cell-membrane phospholipids to disrupt the bacterial cells; hypersensitivity is very rare. These antibiotics are poorly absorbed, even when applied to denuded skin (21).

Chloramphenicol may be used ototopically for selective cases of chronic otitis. Despite its relative lack of activity against *P. aeruginosa*, it is bacteriostatic against the other common organisms responsible for chronic otitis,

Table 3 Otic antimicrobial preparations

Product	Antimicrobial	Ingredients			
		Anti-inflammatory	Acid	Antiseptic	Others
Chloromycetin Otic Cipro HC Otic	Chloramphenicol Ciprofloxacin	Hydrocortisone (1%)	Hydrochloric acetic	Alcohol	Propylene glycol Polyvinyl alcohol Sodium acetate Phospholipon 90HB Polysorbate
Coly-Mycin S Otic	Colistin Neomycin	Hydrocortisone (1%)	Acetic	Thimerosal[a]	Thonzonium Polysorbate 80 Sodium acetate
Cortisporin Otic solution	Polymyxin B Neomycin	Hydrocortisone (1%)	Hydrochloric		Glycerin Propylene glycol
Cortisporin Otic suspension	Polymyxin B Neomycin	Hydrocortisone (1%)	Sulfuric[b]	Alcohol Thimerosal[a]	Propylene glycol Polysorbate 80
Cortisporin-TC Otic suspension	Colistin Neomycin	Hydrocortisone (1%)	Acetic	Thimerosal	Thonzonium Bromide Polysorbate 80
Floxin Otic Lazersporin-C solution	Ofloxacin Polymyxin B Neomycin	Hydrocortisone (1%)	Hydrochloric		Benzethonium chloride
Otic Domeboro solution			Acetic Boric		Aluminum sulfate Calcium carbonate
Otobiotic	Polymyxin B	Hydrocortisone (0.5%)	Sulfuric[b]		Propylene glycol Glycerin
Pedi-Otic suspension	Polymyxin B Neomycin	Hydrocortisone (1%)	Sulfuric[b]	Alcohol Thiomerosal[a]	Glyceryl monostearate Mineral oil Polyoxyl 40 stearate Propylene glycol
Pyocidin-Otic	Polymyxin B	Hydrocortisone (0.5%)	Hydrochloric[b]		Propylene glycol
Star-Otic solution			Acetic Boric		Propylene glycol
Tridesilon Otic solution		Desonide (0.05%)	Acetic Citric		Propylene glycol Sodium acetate
VoSol Otic solution			Acetic		Propylene glycol Benzethonium chloride
VoSol HC Otic solution		Hydrocortisone (1%)	Acetic		Propylene glycol Benzethonium chloride

[a] Preservative.
[b] To adjust pH.

including *E. coli, Clostridium* species, *S. aureus, H. influenzae, Bacteroides fragilis, Klebsiella* species, and certain strains of *Proteus* (15, 22). However, blood dyscrasias and death have been reported after local application, and local skin hypersensitivity may occur with topical therapy (12). Although rarely used for primary therapy, it is used for refractory chronic otitis, especially when a susceptible organism is cultured.

Despite similar antibacterial composition, ototopical preparations may differ in delivery vehicle and pH level. Cortisporin Otic Solution is the most acidic, whereas Coly-Mycin S Otic has a pH of 5, the highest of the group (12, 23). The low pH of these compounds and the alcohol used as an antiseptic agent cause a burning sensation when in contact with the middle ear.

Otobiotic and Pyocidin-Otic contain only the antibiotic polymyxin B. These compounds are useful for the patient allergic to neomycin but should be used only in certain cases because polymyxin B does not act against gram-positive organisms such as *Staphylococcus* and the gram-negative organisms *Proteus* and *B. fragilis*.

Two new fluoroquinolone otic preparations have recently been introduced. Floxic Otic and Cipro HC have recently been approved by the FDA for treatment of external ear disease. Ciprofloxacin and ofloxacin are the active ingredients in these two preparations. Both antimicrobials have a broad spectrum of activity, especially against organisms commonly responsible for otitis externa, including *Pseudomonas, S. aureus, P. mirabilis, Streptococcal* species, and various gram-negative enteric *Bacilli*. In addition, Cipro HC contains hydrocortisone, which adds to the anti-inflammatory properties of this agent. Cipro HC has a low pH level, which makes it ideal for treating external otitis. Floxin Otic has a buffered pH and is FDA-approved for installation into the middle ear space. One difficulty with these newly introduced medications is that many insurance health plans do not cover the cost. These medications are ideally suited for first-line therapy.

The ototopical antimicrobial preparations stated earlier suffice for most cases of otitis externa and selected cases of chronic suppurative otitis. However, these compounds have a limited effect in certain patients with resistant strains of bacteria, drug-induced allergies, or a tympanic membrane perforation that requires administration into the middle ear space. In the last case, ototopical preparations may cause pain because of the acidic pH or the presence of alcohol. Ototoxicity of neomycin, polymyxin B, and colistin is also of concern, and many otolaryngologists prefer topical ophthalmic preparations (23). Ophthalmic preparations are discussed in the article *Ocular Drug Formulation and Delivery* in this volume.

Ophthalmic compounds that may be used as ototopical remedies are given in Table 4 (12). Generally, these products differ from the otic preparations in a neutral pH and the absence of alcohol. For example, in contrast to its otic counterpart, Chloromycetin Ophthalmic has a buffered pH and offers a preparation with hydrocortisone. Likewise, the primary difference between Cortisporin Ophthalmic and the otic preparation is the neutral pH.

Compared with the otic antimicrobial preparations, ophthalmic antimicrobial preparations offer the physician a broader range of antibiotics to treat the difficult ear infection. Gentamicin, tobramycin, and sulfonamides are the most common antibiotics used.

Gentamicin and tobramycin ophthalmic preparations are commonly used to treat difficult ear infections. The latter is less toxic than gentamicin, and its activity against *Pseudomonas* is higher. These antibacterial agents also have a wide spectrum of activity including *Proteus, Klebsiella, E. coli*, and *Staphylococcus* (20). As stated earlier, resistance to gentamicin develops after topical use (9). Although both of these drugs are known to be ototoxic, the clinical significance is thought to be minimal.

Sulfonamides are bacteriostatic against a wide range of gram-positive and gram-negative organisms. In chronic otitis, ophthalmic preparations are used for their activity against *P. aeruginosa, Proteus* species, *Streptococcus, Corynebacterium, Diphteriae*, and *H. influenzae*.

Ciprofloxacin is well known for its wide range of bactericidal activity, especially against *S. aureus, Staphylococcus epidermidis*, and *P. aeruginosa* (24). This preparation has the ideal antimicrobial spectrum for refractory otitis; however topical therapy should not be considered alone for more serious infections such as those with underlying osteomyelitis.

The ophthalmic preparations should only be used in refractory cases of otitis because organism resistance may develop with widespread use. Ophthalmic preparations are also not improved by the FDA for use in the ear canal, but treating physicians may use their discretion for refractory cases. The recent introduction of Floxin and Cipro Otic drops have decreased the use of ophthalmic preparations for the treatment of refractory ear canal conditions.

Powder Preparations

Powdered preparations have been used for many years in otology. These were originally applied as dusting powders for chronic otitis and were especially useful for a mastoid cavity. Before the advent of antibiotics, antiseptic and acid powders were insufflated into mastoid cavities. Unlike many other otic preparations, powders do not cause pain on administration.

Table 4 Ophthalmologic antimicrobial preparations commonly used ototopically

Product	Antimicrobial	Anti-Inflammatory	Acid	Antiseptic	Others
				Ingredients	
Chloromycetin ophthalmic solution	Chloramphenicol		Boric		Buffer
Chloromycetin hydrocortisone	Chloramphenicol	Hydrocortisone (2.5%)	Boric		Buffer; Chloesterol; Methycellulose; Benzethonium chloride[a]
Ciloxan	Ciprofloxacin		Acetic, Hydrochloric[b]		Benzethonium chloride[a]; Sodium acetate; Mannitol Edetate disodium
Cortisporin ophthalmic solution	Polymyxin B, Neomycin	Hydrocortisone (1%)	Sulfuric[b]	Cetyl alcohol	Mineral oil; Propylene glycol; Polyoxyl 40 sterate; Glyceryl monostearate; Phenylmercuric nitrate; Disodium phosphate; Monosodium phosphate; Benzalkonium chloride[a]
Gantrisin ophthalmic solution	Sulfisoxazole				
Garamycin ophthalmic solution	Gentamycin				Sodium phosphate; Tyloxapol; Edetate disodium; Benzalkonium chloride[a]
Metimyd ophthalmic solution	Sulfacetamide	Prednisolone		Thiosulfate, Alcohol	
Neosporin ophthalmic solution	Polymyin B, Neomycin, Gramicidin			Alcohol, Thimerosal[a]	Propylene glycol; Polyoxyethylene-polyoxypropylene compound
Polytrim ophthalmic solution	Trimethoprim sulfate, Polymyxin B		Sulfuric[b]		Benzalkonium chloride[a]; Sodium hydroxide
Sulamyd ophthalmic solution	Sulfacetamide			Thiosulfate	Methylcellulose; Methylparaben; Propylparaben
Terra-Cortril ophthalmic solution	Oxytetracycline	Hydrocortisone (1.5%)			Mineral oil; Aluminum tristearate
Tobradex ophthalmic solution	Tobramycin	Dexamethasone	Sulfuric[b]		Benzalkonium chloride[a]; Tyloxapol; Edetate disodium; Hydroxyethyl cellulose
Tobrex ophthalmic solution	Tobramycin		Boric, Sulfuric[b]		Sodium sulfate; Tyloxapol

[a]To adjust pH
[b]Preservative

Table 5 Ototopical powder preparations[a]

Ingredients	Amount per dosage (mg)
Chloromycetin	50
Sulfanilamide	50
Fungizone	5
Chloromycetin	50
Sulfanilamide	50
Fungizone	5
Hydrocortisone	1

[a]For patients who are allergic to sulfanilamide, these preparations are available without sulfanilamide.

A powder insufflator can be used for the instillation of antimicrobial agents into the external ear canal or mastoid cavity (25). Current antibiotic preparations suitable for the insufflator device are shown in Table 5 (26). They are packaged into capsules that fit into the insufflator. The patient can easily blow the powder into the ear canal without spreading it around. The activity of these antibiotics against organisms responsible for chronic otitis has already been stated. Other common antibiotics or antiseptics may be applied in powder form in an otolaryngologist's office; boric acid is the most common example (Fig. 2).

Anesthetic Preparations

Anesthetic agents (Table 6) are used to eliminate the pain associated with infections such as external otitis, otitis media, and bullous myringitis. They may also be used locally before surgical manipulation, most commonly during myringotomy. These agents are only recommended for patients with an intact tympanic membrane.

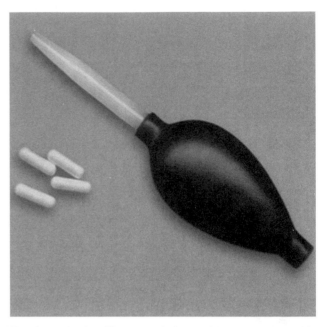

Fig. 2 Bulb insufflator used for antibiotic powders. The capsules contain the antibiotic powder and are placed inside the bulb insufflator.

Most local anesthetic preparations contain benzocaine. Because benzocaine is poorly absorbed through the skin, it remains localized for a long time; however, its effectiveness is unpredictable. Benzocaine has also been known to produce local hypersensitivity reactions (15).

EMLA is a new anesthetic ointment that anesthetizes the external ear canal and eardrum. After keeping the ointment in the external ear canal for 15–20, min it is removed. The surgical procedure may then be completed. This product has been used for myringotomy under local anesthesia.

Phenol is the common topical anesthetic for myringotomies. It is applied over the specific area of the tympanic membrane where the myringotomy is to be performed. It

Table 6 Otic anesthetic preparations

Product	Anesthetic agent	Other ingredients
Americaine Otic	Benzocaine (20%)	Glycerin Polyethylene glycol Benzethonium chloride
Auralgan Otic solution	Benzocaine Antipyrine	Glycerin
EMLA	Lidocaine Prilocaine	Polyoxyethylene Carboxypolyethylene Sodium hydroxide
Phenol	Carbolic acid	

acts by causing instant epidermal destruction. The section of the tympanic membrane in contact with the phenol turns white owing to the anticipated proteins, indicating an anesthetic effect. Healing occurs by hyperplasia of the epithelium and connective tissue but may take some time after applications (16).

Other Preparations

Propylene glycol is a good base for many of the combination antibiotic drops. It acts as a dehydrating agent to fungi and enhances the effectiveness of other antifungal medications. Occasionally, a patient may develop a contact dermatitis from this agent.

Corticosteroids are added to many ototopical combination drops to reduce the inflammation and puritis associated with the acutely infected ear. Corticosteroids may also be used primarily to treat dermatoses found in the external ear canal, primarily psoriasis and seborrheic dermatitis. These compounds may reduce the scaling, itching, and inflammation.

Silver nitrate, as a solution or as a powder on a stick applicator, is occasionally used in the external ear canal as a cauterizing agent. It may be applied to granulation tissue or to the site of a superficial infection. Generally, it is well tolerated; however, if it is excessively applied and bone is exposed, the area does not heal, and surgical correction may be required.

Ototoxicity

The subject of ototoxicity must be addressed whenever discussing the development of new ototopical preparations. It is an important topic from a clinical standpoint and a medicolegal point of view.

In the presence of an intact tympanic membrane, ototoxicity is less important, because the preparation has to be systemically absorbed for an ototoxic effect to occur. This issue is most relevant in cases of chronic suppurative otitis media with a perforated tympanic membrane for which the ototopical medication has the potential to reach the inner ear via the middle ear. Placed within the middle ear, ototopical medication may diffuse across the oval or round window, resulting in inner ear absorption. These windows consist of a thin membrane separating the middle ear space from the inner ear fluids. There is controversy regarding the clinical relevance of ototoxicity in cases of chronic suppurative otitis media.

A comprehensive review of the ototoxicity of the various ototopical preparations has been published (28). Table 7 lists the agents in which ototoxicity has been demonstrated in animal models. There is no antiseptic that is thought to be free of ototoxicity. The antifungal medications nystatin, amphotericin B, clotrimazole, and tolnaftate have been tested in animal models and found to be free of ototoxicity. The antibiotic found in common otic compounds (Polymyxin B and Neomycin) has demonstrated ototoxicity. Chloramphenicol and Colistin are also ototoxic. The new quinolone otic preparations (Floxin and Cipro) have not demonstrated ototoxicity. The antibiotic Sulfacetamide present in ophthalmic preparations has not demonstrated ototoxicity. No evaluation of the ototoxic effects of topical Tobramycin has been published, although it is thought to be similar to gentamicin in this respect. Although hydrocortisone has demonstrated ototoxicity in animal models, other corticosteroids such as triamcinolone and dexamethasone have not. Desonide has not been tested.

Numerous animal studies have been undertaken to evaluate the ototoxic effects of these different medications; however, the results must be examined with caution because of the differences between the animal models and the human temporal bone. The small mammals used in these studies, usually chinchillas or guinea pigs, have a round window that is easily exposed and very thin compared with the human ear. The human round window is more deeply recessed in bone and is six times thicker than that in the chinchilla. Some temporal bones may actually demonstrate a thin shelf of bone or a thick fibrous plug covering the round window. (29) Further studies must be completed to determine the significance of these

Table 7 Ototoxic otic preparations

Solvent	Antifungal	Antiseptics	Antimicrobials	Anti-Inflammatory
Propylene glycol	Cresylate	Acetic acid Alcohol Benzalkonium chloride Iodochlorhydroxyquinolone Chlorhexidene acetate	Chloramphenicol Colistin Gentamycin Neomycin Polymyxin B	Hydrocortisone
				Povidone-iodine

differences with respect to ototoxicity and ototopical preparations.

A 1992 survey of otolaryngologists revealed that 80% believed that the risk of sensorineural hearing loss resulting from otitis media was higher than the risk of sensorineural hearing loss from using an ototopical agent known to be ototoxic (30). As McCabe noted in his editorial comment (31):

> In 30 years of practice, I have not recognized a single ear damaged in hearing from any antibiotic ear drop, however long term. This total experience has not changed since then.

This comment is important not only for patient care, but also for medicolegal reasons.

SUMMARY

A variety of otic preparations have been reviewed here, including indications, side effects, and limitations. The ideal cerumenolytic compound has not yet been developed, nor has a cerumen replacement product. Antiseptics enjoy wide application but are limited when used in the presence of a perforated tympanic membrane. Available antifungal medications appear to be adequate for the treatment of otomycosis, although none have been approved as otic preparations. The limitations of the otic antimicrobial drops have been stated, including the potential both for organism resistance and for ototoxicity. The recent introduction of Floxin and Cipro HC products make available better otic antimicrobial drops for treatment of otitis externa and chronic otitis media. These drops have generated renewed interest in the development of ototopical preparations. Powder preparations are not widely available and must be specifically prepared by a pharmacist each time they are dispensed.

The current practice of some otolaryngologists using medications that have not been approved by the FDA for ototopical use demonstrates the need for new otic preparations. It is hoped that this article will lay the foundation that to enable the development of these new products.

REFERENCES

1. Cassisi, N.; Cohn, A.; Davidson, T.; Witten, B.R. Diffuse Otitis Externa, Clinical and Microbiologic Findings in the Course of a Multicenter Study on a New Otic Solution. Ann. Otolaryngol. Rhinol. Laryngol. **1977**, *86* (Suppl 39).
2. Robinson, A.C.; Hawke, M.; MacKay, A.; Ekem, J.K.; Stratis, M. The Mechanisms of Cerumenolysis. J. Otolaryngol. **1989**, *18* (6), 268–273.
3. Okuda, I.; Binghan, B.; Stoney, P.; Hawke, M. The Organic Composition of Earwax. J. Otolaryngol. **1991**, *20*(3), 212–215.
4. Senturia, B.H.; Marcus, M.D.; Lucente, F.E. *Disease of the External Ear*; Grune & Stratton: Orlando, 1980; 31–36.
5. Lucente, F.E.; Smith, P.G.; Thomas, J.R. Disease of the External Ear. *Otologic Medicine and Surgery*; Alberti, P.W., Rube, R.J., Eds.; Churchill Livingstone: New York, 1988; 1073–1092.
6. Meyerhoff, W.L. Pathology of Chronic Suppurative Otitis Media. Ann. Otolaryngol. Rhinol. Laryngol. **1998**, (Suppl. *131*), 21.
7. Brook, I.; Yocum, P. Quantitative Bacterial Cultures and β-Lactamase Activity in Chronic Suppurative Otitis Media. Ann. Otolaryngol. Rhinol. Laryngol. **1989**, *98*, 293–297.
8. Kenna, M.A.; Rosane, B.A.; Bluestone, C.D. Medical Management of Chronic Suppurative Otitis Media Without Cholesteatoma in Children—Update 1992. Am. J. Otol. **1993**, *14* (5), 469–473.
9. Papstavros, T.; Giamarellou, H.; Varlejides, S. Role of Aerobic and Anaerobic Microorganisms in Chronic Otitis Media. Laryngoscope **1986**, *96*, 438–442.
10. Robinson, A.C.; Hawke, M. The Efficacy of Cerumenolytics: Everything Old is New Again. J. Otolaryngol. **1989**, *18*(6), 263–267.
11. Bellini, M.F.; Terry, R.M.; Lewis, F.A. An Evaluation of Common Cerumenolytis Agents: An In-Vitro Study. Clin. Otolaryngol. **1989**, *14*, 23–25.
12. *Physicians Desk Reference;* Medical Economics Company: Oradell, NJ, 1993.
13. Chen, D.A.; Caparosa, R.J. A Nonprescription Cerumenolytic. Am. J. Otolaryngol. **1991**, *12* (6), 475–476.
14. Jones, E.H. *External Otitis. Diagnosis and Treatment*; Charles C. Thomas, Publisher: Springfield, IL, 1965.
15. *Drug Evaluations Annual 1992*; American Medical Association: Washington, DC, 1992; 1479–1515.
16. Harvey, S.C. Antiseptic and Disinfectants: Fungicides; Ectoparasiticides. *The Pharmacological Basis of Therapeutics*, 5th Ed.; Goodman, L.S., Gilman, A., Eds.; Macmillan Publishing Co.: New York, 1975; 987–1017.
17. Stern, J.C.; Shah, M.K.; Lucente, F.E. In Vitro Effectiveness of 13 Agents in Otomycosis and Review of the Literature. Laryngoscope **1998**, *98*, 1173–1177.
18. Lopez, L.; Evens, R.P. Drug Therapy of Aspergillus Otitis Externa. Otolaryngol. Head Neck Surg. **1980**, *88*, 649–651.
19. *Personal communication*; The Recsei Laboratories: Goleta, CA, 1991.
20. Sande, M.A.; Mandell, G.L. Antimicrobial Agents: The Aminoglycosides. *Pharmacological Basis of Therapeutics*; 8th Ed.; Gilman, A.G., Rail, T.W., Nies, A.S., Taylor, P., Eds.; Pergamon Press: New York, 1991; 1098–1116.

21. Sande, M.A.; Mandell, G.L. Antimicrobial Agents: Tetracyline, Chloramphenicol, Erythromycin, and Miscellaneous Antibacterial Agents. *Pharmacological Basis of Therapeutics*, 8th Ed.; Gilman, A.G., Rall, T.W., Nies, A.S., Taylor, P., Eds.; Pergamon Press: New York, 1991; 1117–1145.

22. Fairbanks DNF Otic Topical Agents. Otolaryngol. Head Neck Surg. **1980**, *88*, 327–331.

23. Hoffman, R.A.; Goldofsky, E. Topical Ophthalmologics in Otology. Ear Nose Throat J. **1991**, *70* (4), 201–205.

24. Mandell, G.L.; Sande, M.A. Antimicrobial Agents: Sulfonamides, Trimethoprim, Sulfamethoxazole, Quinolones, and Agents for Urinary Tract Infections. *Pharmacological Basis of Therapeutics*, 8th Ed.; Gilman, A.G., Rall, T.W., Nies, A.S., Taylor, P., Pergamon Press: New York, 1991; 1047–1064.

25. House, J.W.; Sheehy, J.L. Powder Insufflator for the Ear. Otolaryngol. Head Neck Surg. **1983**, *91* (4), 461–462.

26. Personal communication, Medical Square Pharmacy: Los Angeles, CA, 1992.

27. Hickey, S.A.; Buckley, J.F.; O'Connon, A.F.F. Ventilation Tube Insertion Under Local Anesthesia. Am. J. Otolaryngol. **1991**, *12* (2), 142–143.

28. Rohn, G.N.; Meyerhoff, W.L.; Wright, C.G. Ototoxicity of Topical Agents. Otolaryngol. Clin. North. Am. **1993**, *26* (4), 747–758.

29. Alzamil, K.S.; Linthicum, F.H., Jr. Extranious Round Window Membranes and Plugs: Possible Effect on Intratympanic Therapy. Ann. Otol. Rhinol. Laryngol. **2000**, *109* (1), 30–32.

30. Lundy L.B.; Graham M.D. Ototoxicity and Ototopical Medications: A Survey of Otolaryngologists Presented at the Ninth Shambaugh-Shea Weekend of Otology Chicago, IL, March 6–8, 1992.

31. McCabe, B.F. Editorial Comment. Ann. Otolaryngol. Rhinol. Laryngol. **1990**, *99*, 41.

OUTSOURCING OF PHARMACEUTICALS

Duane B. Lakings

Drug Safety Evaluation Consulting, Inc.,
Birmingham, Alabama

INTRODUCTION

Outsourcing of pharmaceutical development is big business and getting bigger. Of the over $40 billion per year research and development budget of pharmaceutical companies, about one-fifth, or $8 billion, is presently expended at contract service organizations (CSO), and the amount is projected to increase at a rate of about 10% per year in the future. The term CSO includes contract research organizations (CRO), contract manufacturing organizations (CMO), site management organizations (SMO), and any other organization that provides the pharmaceutical industry, or client, with a contract service. Most of this outsourced effort is being expended on the nonclinical drug development, clinical trials, and manufacturing aspects of the drug development process. However, many clients are now using CSOs for drug discovery and potential for development characterization support to generate novel compounds with biological activity against a given target system and then to identify those discovery leads that have the desired attributes with a minimum of detrimental effects needed to become successful preclinical drug candidates. The purposes of this article are to:

1. Describe the history and present status of CSOs;
2. Discuss how clients and CSOs interact;
3. Summarize the services CSOs provide clients;
4. Outline how virtual organizations and consultants interface with clients and CSOs; and
5. Present emerging trends for CSOs.

A complete listing of all the CSOs that offer clients support in one or more of the drug discovery and development processes is beyond the scope of this article. A number of reports are available that provide detailed information on CSOs and the services they provide. Some of these reports are listed in the References. Another common source of information on the services offered by CSOs is the Internet, where most CSOs maintain detailed, up-to-date websites.

HISTORY OF OUTSOURCING

CSOs have been around since the 1940s but have only been major participants in the drug development process for the past 30 years or so and in drug discovery for 10 years or less. The first firms to offer drug development services were not-for-profit research institutes such as Stanford Research Institute, now SRI International, and Midwest Research Institute. With the regulatory requirement that nonclinical safety studies, primarily in toxicology, be conducted according to Good Laboratory Practices (GLP) regulations, for-profit CSOs started to offer chronic toxicity and carcinogenicity study support. At about the same time, the clinical testing requirements needed to characterize the safety and efficacy of a novel chemical entity (NCE) increased dramatically, and Good Clinical Practices (GCP) regulations were issued. Monitoring and auditing of clinical trials to ensure that the data captured on Case Report Forms (CRFs) and other documents accurately reflected information in the raw data were initially accomplished by Clinical Research Associates (CRAs) of the clinical trial sponsor. First independent CRAs and then CSOs were employed by pharmaceutical firms to provide independent auditing of the clinical trial investigational sites.

In the 1980s, a new player came onto the field, biotechnology, with the intent to make macromolecules into therapeutic products. Although many of the new firms had excellent biology and pharmacology expertise, they knew little about the regulatory-driven nonclinical and clinical research and manufacturing requirements necessary to develop a discovery idea into a therapeutic product. Thus, these new companies turned to CSOs. However, most, if not all, of these service providers also did not know how to effectively characterize and develop macromolecules. Thus, the biotechnology companies, the regulatory agencies, and the CSOs rapidly learned how to solve the major problems associated with macromolecule research. After submitting an IND, the biotechnology companies turned to CSOs for assistance in conducting

Encyclopedia of Pharmaceutical Technology

clinical trials, which required the CSOs to expand services to include protocol development, CRF design, investigator and site selection, data management and statistical evaluation, and report writing. With the increased level of outsourcing, the number of clinical CSOs grew rapidly.

In the 1990s, a group of major events again changed the CSO playing field. The ability to generate libraries of compounds using combinatorial chemistry techniques, high-throughput screening (HTS) techniques to rapidly evaluate the biological activity of these libraries, and bioinformatics to manage and evaluate the large amount of data being generated changed the drug discovery process. The mapping of the human genome will produce a dramatic increase in the number of therapeutic targets available, with the number projected to grow from the few hundreds of targets available today to many thousands in the next few years. Drug discovery groups have been charged to expeditiously find new drug candidates to fill the drug development pipeline. Some companies have developed, or are developing, in-house groups to meet this challenge, whereas others formed partnerships with small biotechnology firms, and still others combined these approaches. In addition, a number of new CSOs were started to provide research services in these relatively novel areas of genomics, proteomics, combinatorial chemistry, HTS, and bioinformatics.

PRESENT STATUS OF OUTSOURCING

CSOs are rapidly adapting to meet the needs of their clients. These changes appear to take one of two avenues. Some CSOs, such as MDS and Quintiles Transnational, are attempting to become full-service, or almost full-service, CSOs by providing research services in drug discovery, potential for development characterization, nonclinical drug development, clinical trial research, and manufacturing. Other CSOs specialize in a given area, such as animal pharmacology studies or phase II to IV clinical trial support. Many pharmaceutical industry observers think that the midsize CSOs will disappear over the next few years, either through mergers with other CSOs or by acquisition by larger CSOs or companies that desire to enter this rapidly growing, but highly competitive, business.

Only a few years ago, drug discovery research was never, or only very infrequently, outsourced to CSOs. Grants to university groups were used to develop models and at times to test discovery leads in these newly defined models. Now, many pharmaceutical companies use CSOs in addition to university groups to support some aspects of their drug discovery efforts. The transition from drug discovery to drug development has also undergone substantial change in the last decade. A number of CSOs now support this rapidly growing area to assist clients in determining whether a discovery lead(s) has the necessary attributes for further development. The greatest consolidation in the CSO industry has been in nonclinical and clinical drug development, in which contractors that had offered services in one of these areas are adding the other so that they can better serve clients. These additions are frequently accomplished by acquisition of other CSOs that are already offering the desired services, but some CSOs are developing and increasing their own capabilities. A similar trend is occurring in CSOs offering manufacturing support, in which capabilities to produce Good Manufacturing Practice (GMP)-quality drug substances and drug products are being augmented with services such as shelf-life stability studies and impurity profiling.

With consolidation and expansion, large CSOs are becoming bigger and are now being called mega-CSOs. Since 1996, the eight largest CSOs have made more than 40 acquisitions, suggesting that the market is shifting from small CSOs to larger firms. Some recent highly publicized acquisitions include Quintiles' purchase of Innovex and Medical Action Communications and Bulter Clinical Recruitment Service. For Phoenix International Life Sciences, which was acquired by MDS in 2000 and is now called MDS Pharm Services, expansion started in 1995 with the acquisition of I.T.E.M. Holding S.A, IBRD-Rostrum Global, Institute for Pharmacodynamic Research, Anawa Holding, McKnight, and Clinserve to provide multinational capability in clinical research and Chrysalis International to supplement services in nonclinical development. PPD, Inc. has purchased Wisconsin Analytical and Research Service, Gabbay Group, Ltd., Applied Bioscience International, Inc., Belmont Research, SARCO, Inc., GSX Technology, and ATP. Numerous other mergers and acquisitions have taken place, and the trend is expected to continue. However, for each CSO that combines with or is acquired by another CSO, a new player, usually offering a novel service such as genomics or in vitro metabolism, comes onto the field. Whether to use a mega-CSO or a number of smaller, but specialized, CSOs to support outsourcing needs is a question to be addressed by pharmaceutical clients. Another way of asking the question is whether "one-stop" shopping is better than looking at a number of "specialty houses" that offer only a limited line.

As pharmaceutical clients develop drug candidates for the global market, CSOs have expanded their services, primarily clinical trial support services, to include not only

North America, Europe, and Japan, but also a number of emerging markets. A major reason that pharmaceutical companies can enter the foreign markets and that CSOs can offer support services in these markets is the harmonization of the drug development processes through the efforts of the International Conference on Harmonisation (ICH) and the ICH guidelines. Even through ICH guidelines currently apply only to U.S., European, and Japanese research efforts, most other countries are adopting these guidelines. The presently issued ICH guidelines primarily deal with the quality of drug substances and drug products, nonclinical safety, and clinical trials. CSOs, although not a major participant in the definition of the ICH guidelines, are an influential group for their implementation.

CLIENT AND CONTRACTOR INTERACTIONS

Outsourcing is now a common practice of almost all pharmaceutical companies. For example, the use of CSOs to support some aspect of clinical trial research has grown from approximately 30% of the clinical studies conducted in 1993 to over 60% in 1997. The processes that a client uses to select a CSO and how a client interacts with the CSO ensure contracted research studies are monitored appropriately and completed on time and within budget.

A pharmaceutical company identifies a lead candidate that mediates a human disease. For a variety of reasons, corporate management decides to have some or all regulated nonclinical and clinical studies or the manufacturing aspects of drug development performed by a CSO(s). The drug development project team is commonly responsible for coordinating the outsourcing program and for ensuring that the development program stays on time, on track, and on budget. For a small company, this may be the responsibility of two or three researchers who need to have a good understanding of each of the scientific disciplines for which outsourced studies are being considered. A common practice for many firms is to use a consultant or a consulting firm to assist in outsourcing.

The first requirement for a successful research program at CSOs is to identify which aspects of the drug development program are to be conducted at a CSO and the projected timeline for when these studies need to be initiated and completed so that the results are available for decision making and regulatory agency submissions. A well constructed drug development logic plan provides much of this information. The client needs

to identify and then select the appropriate CSO(s) to conduct the desired research studies. The client also needs to monitor the CSO(s) to ensure that the studies are conducted as described in the study protocol and that the results generated are appropriately recorded first in the study records and then in a study report.

CSO Selection

The steps a client should take to identify and select CSOs include but are not be limited to:

- Preparing detailed study designs for each of the research projects to be contracted
- Determining which CSOs are to be considered
- Soliciting cost and time proposals for each study design from each CSO selected
- Evaluating the proposals and selecting those CSOs to be considered further
- Conducting site visits to ensure that the CSOs are qualified to conduct the research studies
- Negotiating time and cost for completion of the research studies
- Selecting the CSOs and awarding the contracts for each study to be outsourced.

The number of person-hours required for the identification and selection process depends on the size of the research program to be contracted. Normally, a minimum of 1 to 2 person-weeks is necessary to effectively evaluate three to four CSOs for each research study to be outsourced. Many clients use consultants to assist in the CSO selection process. However, these clients need to ensure that the consultant has the necessary expertise and knowledge of how CSOs operate. A common mistake is to hire a consultant with expertise in a disease area but not in the research process, such as toxicology or drug metabolism, or in regulatory compliance but not in the science necessary to characterize a drug candidate successfully.

Clients commonly use one of three strategies to identify CSOs. These strategies can be designated virtual, preselected, and special study. The virtual strategy is favored by clients who do not have the resources to conduct GLP-, GCP-, or GMP-regulated research studies. A primary benefit is that the various types of expertise and the infrastructure needed to support regulated studies can be devoted to completing research studies without the client having to build the in-house groups and facilities and thus experiencing costly time delays. A primary limitation is that the client can be vulnerable to poor CSO selection or to mismanagement by the CSO. In the preselected strategy, a limited number of CSOs are prequalified to support a client's possible outsourcing needs. The qualification process usually includes a detailed site visit to determine which types of research studies can be placed at the CSO. This strategy can provide a synergistic working relationship between the client and the CSO. A major drawback is the unnecessary limitation of outsourcing. If a number of CSOs have the desired expertise but the client's prequalified list contains only a couple of those CSOs, other possibly better qualified CSOs are not even considered. The final strategy, special study, is used by some clients to place single or a few research studies with a contractor. This strategy allows a critical study to be completed to meet the timeline on a drug development plan. However, some companies use this strategy for all of their outsourcing needs and then attempt to integrate the results for the independently conducted studies into a drug development story. For a client with substantial drug development expertise, this strategy may work but requires considerable effort in identifying and selecting CSOs, monitoring the various CSOs, and synthesizing the results from the various research studies. CSOs are generally not in favor of this strategy because they become only "a pair of hands," and have little understanding of the overall development program and thus cannot provide the client with their considerable expertise. Whichever selection strategy is used, the client needs to select the CSO carefully. One poorly conducted study can effectively delay the drug development process until the study has been repeated and the results integrated into the overall story. If this delay is for a research study on the drug development critical path, the projected time for regulatory agency submission has to be changed, thus delaying approval for marketing and resulting in lost revenue for the client.

What are some of the items clients look for when evaluating and selecting CSOs? That list could be quite long, and only a few of the many criteria are presented here.

- *Project management skills*: The CSO project manager ensures that the contracted activities are completed in a timely and cost-effective manner. This individual needs to be identified early so that an acceptable working arrangement can be established.
- *Research area and therapeutic experience*: A CSO with expertise in a variety of scientific disciplines and therapeutic areas will have a pool of experts available as a knowledge resource as results become available for evaluation.
- *Flexibility and adaptability*: The ability to adapt to changes in research study parameters and timelines is

important to understanding the dynamic nature of the drug discovery and development process. A CSO needs to be able to interact effectively with a client to modify a study design or an ongoing research study.
- *Timeliness*: A CSO needs to be able to provide the contract service(s) agreed on in the desired time frame.
- *Integrity*: The results to be generated need to be accurate, complete, and unbiased. Previous performance or references from other clients can assist in ascertaining how the CSO will perform in providing "good" as well as "bad" news.
- *Quality assurance (QA) awareness*: The CSO's established procedures ensure both quality work and that current regulations are followed. A review of the CSO's standard operating procedure (SOP) manual and discussions with the QA manager will provide this information. Also, results from recently conducted regulatory agency audits should be reviewed.
- *Training*: The documented training process ensures that all research study personnel have the necessary skills for conducting their aspect of the contracted study.
- *Services offered*: The CSO offers a sufficiently broad scope of services for conducting the contracted research study in the shortest time possible. The services offered anticipate contract project demands and respond quickly to project dynamics.
- *Communication*: The CSO provides information in an acceptable format and on a timely basis. A constant open line of communication should exist between the client and the CSO.
- *Partnership*: The CSO considers itself a partner with the client and is service-oriented. The CSO creates a team environment to perform as an extension of the client's project team.

One item not listed above is cost. Most clients use cost as an evaluation criteria, at times the only criteria. Although important, cost needs to be evaluated in conjunction with other CSO selection items. A CSO offering the lowest price may not:

- Fully understand the research objectives;
- Be able to conduct the studies on the timeline desired;
- Include all the tests or evaluations necessary to support a regulatory submission; or
- Provide a complete evaluation of the study results.

If all other selection criteria among CSOs are equal, then cost can and should be used to select the contractor. Once a CSO has been selected, time and cost negotiating is justifiable to ensure that the client receives the best quality study for the best price.

CSO Monitoring

The identification and selection process is only the first step. The second aspect involves monitoring the CSOs to ensure that the research studies are conducted according to the research protocol, that the results are obtained using appropriate techniques and procedures, and that the data generated are correctly recorded and documented in the study report. Many clients hire firms, such as other CSOs or consultants, to monitor outsourced research studies, particularly clinical trials and manufacturing projects. In doing so, the clients should use the same techniques to select and evaluate the monitors as they use to identify a CSO. Monitoring studies at CSOs should include but are not be limited to:

- Reviewing and approving the protocols, which should provide information on all aspects of the study, and detailing the procedures to be followed to successfully complete the study
- Monitoring various aspects of each study to ensure that the data collected do not contain "surprises" that can prevent the results from being used to support submissions to regulatory agencies
- Assisting in the evaluation and interpretation of results to ensure that the data are analytically acceptable and correctly correlated to tell the story of the experimental results
- Reviewing study reports to ensure that they accurately reflect the generated results, document any deviation from the study protocols, and give appropriate conclusions.

The number of person-hours required to appropriately monitor a research study conducted by a CSO again depends on the size of the research program. Normally, a minimum of 1 person-week for each in-life or inpatient phase month of a research study is required and includes the time necessary to review and approve the study report.

OUTSOURCING OF DRUG DISCOVERY

Drug discovery strives to find new ways to discover novel compounds and to identify new targets for treating the various disorders affecting humans. After years of first synthesizing individual compounds, then purifying and obtaining physical and chemical characterization of the new chemicals, and finally testing the NCEs in pharmacological models of a particular human disease, the pharmaceutical industry has embraced combinatorial chemistry as a way to generate large numbers of structurally unique compounds, HTS to test these

chemicals for biological activity against a target, genomics to identify the genetic code for enzymes and proteins that might be new drug targets, proteomics to produce the newly identified natural proteins and to characterize their functions in the body, and bioinformatics to organize and evaluate the enormous amounts of data generated. Once a lead or, more likely, a group of leads is identified, the biological activity in other in vitro and in vivo pharmacology models is explored further, and structural activity relationship (SAR) techniques are used to further modify the molecular structures of the leads to identify NCEs with very high potency and specificity, which means the leads have minimal or acceptable adverse effects or interference with other physiological functions or organ systems.

The present cost and time estimate for the drug discovery and development process is approximately $500 million and 12 to 14 years, respectively, for each new therapeutic agent that reaches the market. The time and cost profile is shown in Fig. 1. The drug discovery and preclinical phases, or the first few years, are relatively inexpensive relative to the clinical, nonclinical, and manufacturing phases, in which over 80% of the cost and more than half the time are expended. The $500 million cost includes the money spent on the losers, those compounds that were identified as having biological activity against a target but that do not successfully complete the process. Because only approximately 2% of discovery leads selected for preclinical development enter into clinical studies and only an estimated 5% of these

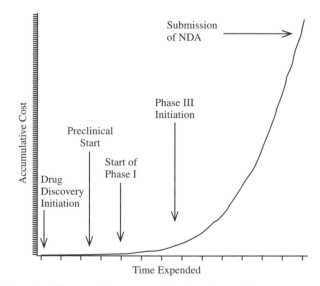

Fig. 1 Time and cost profile for drug discovery and development.

drug candidates result in New Drug Application (NDA) submissions (for an overall success rate of about 0.1%), finding and gleaning the losers probably uses more than 80% of the cost and half the time needed to put a novel therapeutic agent on the market. By identifying the losers early in the process and thereby reserving precious resources for discovering compounds that have a better chance of success, companies could substantially reduce the overall cost for each new therapeutic agent and use precious resources on discovering and developing compounds with a higher probability of being a winner and thus also shorten the time required for drug discovery and development.

All successful pharmaceutical firms understand this problem and are constantly searching for novel approaches to expedite the process and to reduce the cost. One approach used more and more is to outsource some or all of the drug discovery and pharmacology aspects to CSOs that have particular expertise that are not available in a pharmaceutical company and that would be costly in time and resources to establish. This section summarizes the present scientific disciplines involved in the drug discovery process. Because the techniques and procedures used in this rapidly evolving area are changing so quickly, only summary information can be presented. A few CSOs that provide services in more than one discovery area are listed in Table 1.

The entire human genome is projected to be sequenced by 2002 or shortly thereafter. The human genome contains 60,000 to 80,000 genes that code for proteins, many of which could be new targets of mediating human diseases, and many others that have little potential as targets for drug therapy. Present projections suggest that 5000 to 10,000 of the genes, or approximately 10%, may be involved in regulating some aspect of cellular function or in producing signals to simulate or inhibit extracellular events or other cells. In combination with chemical libraries and HTS techniques, these new targets are expected to identify many novel ways of treating diseases. A major problem is determining which of these genes are important in a disease process and which are not. Proteomics is the science that will help in these determinations. The newly discovered genes can be transfected into bacterial or mammalian cell lines to produce sufficient quantities of the protein for further characterization and study.

Combinatorial chemistry technology and the merging of automated library synthesis with the traditional medicinal chemistry principles to provide a more rational approach to library generation are providing pharmaceutical companies with millions of novel compounds. Advantages of generating these diverse libraries include acting as a synthetic substitute for natural samples in random discovery screening programs and providing a

Table 1   Various drug discovery services provided by CSOs

CSO	Gene[a]	Prot[b]	Chem[c]	Screen[d]	Bioinf[e]	Pharm[f]
Axiom Biotechnologies				X	X	X
Cellomics				X	X	X
Commonwealth Biotechnologies, Inc.	X	X	X			
Genespan	X	X		X		X
Jerini Bio Tools			X	X		
Marin Biologic	X	X	X		X	X
MDS		X	X	X		X
MRI	X	X	X			X
PPD, Inc.	X		X	X	X	X
SRA Life Sciences	X			X		X
SRI International			X	X		X
THETAGEN	X		X		X	
TNO Pharma Institute	X	X		X		X

[a]Genomic research including sequencing, cloning, and analysis.
[b]Proteomic research including expression and analysis.
[c]Chemical synthesis of compounds including combinatorial chemistry to synthesize libraries of small organic molecules, peptides, and oligonucleotides.
[d]Screening of drug discovery leads for pharmacological activity including HTS and assay development.
[e]Bioinformatic techniques for genomic, chemistry, and pharmacology research efforts.
[f]Pharmacology evaluation in either in vitro and in vivo models.

systematic approach for SAR studies to assist chemists and pharmacologists in defining the pharmacophore and other chemical structure attributes that can be important for metabolic stability, aqueous solubility, and lipid membrane penetration. A key aspect is molecular modeling, which is critical to understanding the chemical reactions and can be used to model structures, provide conformational analysis, and develop the pharmacophore or other structural attributes. To support these efforts, a number of CSOs offer combinatorial chemistry services and classical synthetic capabilities for small organic molecules and for macromolecules.

The library or other source of chemicals is screened for biological activity, usually employing an in vitro system in which a known biochemical process is agonized or antagonized. The identification and characterization of the target system can be a rate-limited step, especially for a newly discovered, genomic-defined target. The increased number of compounds to be tested has required pharmacologists to devise novel techniques to rapidly screen for biological activity. With a number of new targets becoming available, many pharmaceutical companies are turning to CSOs for assistance in developing and implementing HTS assay systems to evaluate the biological activity of the novel compounds in libraries.

Bioinformatics assists in understanding information content and flow in biological systems and processes and is becoming more and more important because of the unprecedented growth in quantity and diversity of these data. Applications for bioinformatic techniques include understanding biological processes and how they may malfunction, thus having an important place in drug discovery and development processes. At present, the role and function of most proteins are at best incomplete and often nonexistent. Bioinformatics can assist researchers in understanding what protein each gene produces and in determining the physiological role and function of each of these proteins. Bioinformatics can facilitate the selection of drug targets, biological pathways, receptor functions, gene regulation, and intercellular communication and the impact that each of these has on the others and on normal and disease states. A number of CSOs have developed bioinformatics tools and techniques and offer these services to clients. Because this area is growing so rapidly and new players are continuously entering the field, any list of CSOs involved in bioinformatics would be outdated before publication.

After a biologically active compound(s) has been identified, additional, experiments are conducted to further study the pharmacological activity. These studies are frequently conducted in in vivo models, and analogs of the lead are also tested to further characterize the mechanism of action and to ensure that a compound with high potency and specificity is identified. This more classic in vivo approach to evaluating the biological potency is a more rigorous SAR assessment than one that uses in vitro systems because the discovery lead(s):

- Has to be administered to the animal model and be delivered to the site of action
- Is subjected to drug metabolizing enzymes
- May cause unexpected responses that describe a novel activity or an unwanted adverse effect
- Has to prevent the normal clearance processes from eliminating the lead before it reaches the target in sufficient concentration to elicit the desired biological response.

For these and other reasons, most pharmacologists still consider the use of in vivo animal models to evaluate the pharmacology of a discovery lead(s) to be the gold standard for assessing biological potency and specificity. An important requirement in SAR determination is having or developing an animal model that correlates with a disease in humans. Developing these animal models can be time-consuming and expensive, and many important human diseases do not yet have predictive animal models. Research to develop acceptable models for these diseases is a high priority at pharmaceutical companies. Many CSOs are also involved in the definition and characterization of novel in vivo models and, once available, offer these novel models to clients.

OUTSOURCING OF POTENTIAL FOR DEVELOPMENT CHARACTERIZATION

Completed drug discovery studies indicate that a lead(s) mediates a disease process and has potential as a therapeutic agent in humans. Is this lead now ready to be transferred to the preclinical drug development group? Or should additional, nondefinitive experiments be conducted to characterize more fully the properties of the lead(s)? If more studies are necessary, what experiments should be done? This section describes some of the experiments that could be conducted to evaluate the potential of a discovery lead to become a development candidate and provides information on CSOs that offer services in this relatively new and rapidly evolving field. These nondefinitive studies may also uncover problems that have to be resolved before starting the definitive preclinical development studies and designing the clinical trial protocols to evaluate safety and efficacy in humans. A number of questions should be answered to effectively plan the research studies needed to assess the potential for development of a discovery lead. These questions include but are not limited to the following:

- What is the human disease indication for the potential drug candidate?
- What are the proposed route of delivery and frequency of dosing in human clinical studies?
- How long does the lead need to be in the body to elicit the desired pharmacological response?
- Will the physical and chemical properties of the lead allow delivery to the site of action?
- Can the lead be synthesized in sufficient quantity to support a drug development program?

Six scientific disciplines, shown in Fig. 2, are involved in the potential for development characterization of a lead or the assessment of which lead from a group has more development attributes and fewer drawbacks. The classic approach to discover lead optimization has been to turn the actives over to the pharmacology group. The lead with the highest potency is then selected for further development. During the past few years, a major strategic change has been the addition of screening for bioavailability or delivery, chemical and metabolic stability, and, in some cases, pharmacokinetics and toxicity to complement the pharmacology testing. A drug delivery group assesses which leads are effectively delivered by the proposed clinical route of administration. A solubility and stability group defines which leads are easily degraded and are thus not good prospects for formulation development or have insufficient aqueous solubility to first dissolve and then stay in solution after administration. The physiological distribution and disposition of these leads are studied by the pharmacokinetics group. The potential for the leads to be metabolized to inactive or active metabolites is ascertained by a drug metabolism group, which can also

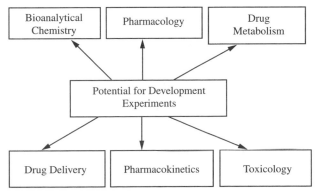

Fig. 2 Scientific disciplines involved in potential for development characterization evaluations.

conduct the drug–drug interaction studies recommended as part of the drug development process (1). An in vitro toxicology group evaluates the leads for cellular, genetic, and immunotoxicity. Finally, an acute toxicity study in animals may be conducted to select the lead with the optimal chance of successful development. This acute toxicity study is not an LD_{50} study, which is not needed for overall risk assessment (2). If the pharmacologically defined actives do not meet the potential for development requirements, a pharmaceutical company has at least two choices. The first is to select the compound with the "best" overall profile and enter formal development, which will most likely result in the selected candidate being one of the preclinical or clinical losers. The other is to start the discovery process over, hoping that the next time an acceptable lead will be found and that the lost time does not result in a competitor discovering an acceptable compound that becomes first on the market.

Safety pharmacology evaluations are commonly considered to be part of the toxicology program but are in reality pharmacology studies at exaggerated doses designed to reveal the potential of an identified discovery lead(s) or drug candidate to produce adverse effects or secondary pharmacological effects on major organ systems. Safety pharmacology is commonly conducted shortly after a discovery lead has been selected for further development, and the results are used to assist in determining whether continued development is warranted, to support regulatory agency submissions, and to identify potential adverse effects. An ICH guideline (3) indicates that safety pharmacology studies include assessment of effects on vital functions such as the cardiovascular, central nervous, and respiratory systems and that these tests should be conducted before human exposure. In keeping with the current regulatory climate, most pharmaceutical companies conduct, or have a CSO conduct, a battery of tests and, at times, subdivide these tests into groups to first determine specific properties of compounds and then to more fully characterize those areas where a response is observed.

During the past few years, techniques to rapidly evaluate potential for development parameters of a large number of leads have been developed and are now offered to clients as a service by a number of CSOs. These screening methods use small amounts of each lead and, in some cases, can evaluate more than one lead simultaneously in a given sample. A few of the CSOs that offer clients more than one service in potential for development characterization and the scientific disciplines for which they have expertise are given in Table 2.

Table 2 CSOs providing potential for development-assessment services

CSO	Tox[a]	SafPh[b]	DM[c]	PK[d]	DDel[e]	Bioan[f]
CEDRA			X			X
Genespan	X			X		
GENTEST	X		X	X	X	X
Huntingdon Life Sciences	X	X				
In Vitro Technologies	X		X	X	X	X
Marin Biologic	X					X
MetaXen			X		X	X
MRI	X			X	X	X
NaviCyte				X	X	X
MDS	X	X	X	X	X	X
Primedica		X		X		X
SRI–Serquest	X			X		X
SRA Life Sciences	X		X			X
SRI International	X	X	X			
TNO Pharma Institute	X	X	X	X	X	X

[a]In vitro and/or acute toxicology.
[b]Safety pharmacology.
[c]In vitro drug metabolism including enzyme induction, metabolic stability.
[d]In vitro and in vivo pharmacokinetics including protein binding and drug–drug interactions.
[e]Drug delivery including in vitro and in vivo absorption assessment.
[f]Bioanalytical chemistry method development and support.

OUTSOURCING OF NONCLINICAL DRUG DEVELOPMENT

Before entering into human clinical trials, a drug candidate undergoes various preclinical studies to define and characterize its safety and disposition profiles in animal models. After entering the clinic, information on the pharmacokinetics and toxicology of the drug candidate in the relevant species (human) finally becomes available. The results from earlier drug development experiments are usually re-evaluated in consideration of this new information to ascertain whether the animal models were predictive of the efficacy and safety observed in humans. If the animal results are extrapolative, the remaining nonclinical animal studies are fairly straightforward and are conducted to provide supportive information on the safety of the drug candidate. However, if the early animal data do not extrapolate to humans, additional animal experiments may be needed to more fully understand the observed pharmacology and/or toxicology in humans. The following discussion presents an overview of the research studies conducted during nonclinical drug development, which can divided into the broad categories of bioanalytical and analytical chemistry, formulation development, pharmacokinetics, drug metabolism, and toxicology. Some of the CSOs that offer services in a number of these disciplines are listed in Table 3.

A bioanalytical chemistry method is used to support definitive pharmacokinetic and toxicology studies after the assay has been appropriately validated. The validation experiments define acceptance and rejection criteria for the range of reliable results, the lower and upper limits of quantification, accuracy, precision, specificity, and recovery and should include appropriate stability studies (4, 5). The validated method needs to be documented in a test assay procedure, which lists the acceptance and rejection criteria for each parameter evaluated, and supported by appropriate SOPs.

Analytical chemistry and formulation development and characterization are aspects of manufacturing activities; however, these functions are critical for the successful completion of many nonclinical and clinical research studies. The section on outsourcing of manufacturing provides a summary discussion on analytical chemistry and formulation development.

Preclinical pharmacokinetic and bioavailability experiments are conducted to evaluate dose proportionality over the dose range used in toxicology studies and potential species-to-species differences in pharmacokinetic profiles. By incorporating one or two intravenous dose levels into the studies, absolute bioavailability can also be determined and information on the linearity of absorption, distribution, and disposition kinetics obtained. If more than one drug formulation is used in toxicology studies, relative

Table 3 CSOs providing various and multiple nonclinical services

CSO	Tox[a]	PK[b]	DM[c]	Bioan[d]	Form[e]
ABC Laboratories		X	X	X	
BIBRA International	X	X	X	X	
BioReliance	X		X	X	
Center de Recherches Biologiques	X	X	X	X	
ClinTrials Research	X		X	X	
Covance	X		X	X	X
Huntingdon Life Sciences	X	X	X	X	X
IIT Research Institute	X	X	X		
ILEX Oncology	X	X		X	X
Inveresk Research International Limited	X	X	X	X	X
ITR Laboratories Canada	X	X	X	X	X
LCG Bioscience	X	X	X	X	
Lovelace Respiratory Research Institute	X	X		X	X
MDS Pharmaceutical Services	X	X	X	X	
MRI	X	X	X	X	X
Northview Biosciences	X			X	X
Nucro-Technics	X			X	X
Oneida Research Services		X		X	X
Oread Inc.	X		X	X	X
PPD, Inc.		X	X	X	
Primedica	X	X	X	X	X
Quintiles Transnational	X	X	X	X	X
Ricerca	X	X	X	X	X
SGS Biopharma–Lab Simon	X	X		X	X
SRI–Serquest	X	X	X		X
SRI International	X	X	X	X	X
STS duoTEK	X		X	X	X
TNO Pharma Institute	X	X	X	X	X
WIL Research Laboratories	X	X	X	X	X

[a]Toxicology including subchronic and chronic, reproductive carcinogenicity.
[b]Pharmacokinetics including toxicokinetics.
[c]Drug metabolism including radiolabel synthesis.
[d]Bioanalytical chemistry.
[e]Formulation assessment, including solubility, stability, and delivery.

bioavailability experiments comparing the formulations can determine whether the extent of delivery is similar or different and thus can make extrapolation of pharmacology and toxicology results between animal species meaningful and useful in designing the later nonclinical studies and phase I safety and tolerance studies in humans. An important application of pharmacokinetics is determining the extent and duration of exposure, or toxicokinetics, in the test species. An ICH guideline (6) discusses the generation of toxicokinetic data to support the development of a drug candidate. Unless justified from pharmacokinetic results from humans or from toxicokinetic observations, additional animal pharmacokinetics are not usually conducted during nonclinical development. Types of animal pharmacokinetics that might be

performed include multiple-dose pharmacokinetics, bioavailability comparison when the formulation used in early toxicology studies is changed, newly identified drug candidate metabolites distribution and disposition evaluations, effect of food and time of feeding on the extent and duration of absorption, and drug–drug interactions if the animal model is considered predictive of humans.

Drug metabolism experiments in toxicology animal species are conducted to evaluate the protein binding, mass balance, and tissue distribution and to use an appropriately labeled compound. If the radiolabel is not nonmetabolically or metabolically stable, the results from the drug metabolism experiments or other studies using the labeled compound will have little if any meaning or usefulness in determining the metabolic fate of the drug candidate. The two most common preclinical drug metabolism studies are for mass balance, which includes metabolite profiling and identification, and for tissue distribution. A routine aspect of most tissue distribution studies is whole-body autoradiography. Nonclinical drug metabolism studies that may be conducted include multiple-dose tissue distribution [as addressed in an ICH guideline (7)], additional characterization and evaluation of metabolites, and studies such as fetal-placental transfer and lacteal secretion, which provide toxicokinetic support for developmental and reproductive toxicology evaluations.

A number of preclinical toxicology studies need to be completed and documented in a regulatory agency submission before initiating human clinical trials. The number and types of toxicology studies depend on the disease type, the duration of treatment, and the country(ies) in which clinical trials will be conducted. Preclinical toxicology studies include genetic toxicology, local tolerance, immunotoxicity, and acute and subchronic tests. After human clinical trials have been initiated, nonclinical toxicology is continued with chronic toxicology studies, developmental and reproduction studies, and carcinogenicity studies. One of the most troublesome problems in interpreting toxicology results is determining whether these data are predictive of toxicity in humans. Quite often, animal toxicology may not correlate with human safety because the observed toxicities are species-specific. Species specificity is sometimes discovered early in development and can be used to design the early human trials to ascertain whether humans also manifest the observed toxicity.

An ICH guideline (3) indicates that local tolerance evaluations are to be conducted in animals using the route of administration proposed for humans. The genotoxicity (8, 9) and immunotoxicity (3) potentials of a drug candidate are commonly studied shortly after a discovery lead has been selected for further development. The doses for definitive toxicology studies are defined in dose-range-finding studies, which have a primary goal of determining a maximum tolerated dose (MTD). The route of administration, frequency, and duration of dosing for this and other toxicology studies are determined from the expected clinical use of the drug candidate. When these parameters do not mimic those used in human clinical trials, unexpected findings surprises result, and the severity of the findings may be sufficient to stop development of an otherwise promising drug candidate. Most regulatory agencies require subchronic toxicity studies in two species, one of which must be a nonrodent, before the initiation of human clinical trials. ICH guidelines (3, 10) suggest the

minimum duration of toxicity studies needed to support phase I, II, and III clinical trials. Regulatory agencies (2, 3) require chronic toxicity studies in two species for drug candidates that are to be administered to humans for longer than 3 months. Both subchronic and chronic toxicology studies should include hematology, clinical chemistry, and histopathology evaluations. Developmental and reproduction toxicology studies are conducted to reveal any effect of a drug candidate or its metabolite on mammalian reproduction and to ascertain the potential risks to humans. These studies evaluate male and female fertility, embryo and fetal death, parturition and the newborn, the lactation process, care of the young, and the potential teratogenicity of the drug candidate. The combination of studies selected needs to allow exposure of mature adults and all stages of development from conception to sexual maturity to conception in the next generation (11, 12). Carcinogenicity studies encompass most of the life span of the test species and are conducted to measure tumor induction in animals and to assess the relevant risk in humans (13–16). These studies are normally conducted concurrently with phase III human clinical trials and are required by regulatory agencies when human exposure to a drug candidate is anticipated to be longer than 6 months.

OUTSOURCING OF CLINICAL DRUG DEVELOPMENT

Drug development is a long, complicated, highly regulated process, with the clinical trial aspect of the overall endeavor being both the most time-consuming and expensive. The clinical development stage requires approximately 75% of that time and over 50% of the money expended. Pharmaceutical companies are constantly searching for ways to shorten the clinical trial stage. However, with time and cost of drug discovery and development both still increasing, these efforts have not been overly successful to date. One approach, through the ICH process, is to harmonize many of the clinical trial tasks so that research studies conducted in one country are acceptable to the regulatory authorities in other countries. An ICH guideline (17) provides assistance on some general considerations for clinical trials. This section addresses clinical drug development, which is subdivided into four phases:

● *Phase I*: Safety and tolerance evaluation in human volunteers or in a small number of patients and pharmacokinetic and pharmacodynamic studies (human pharmacology)

- *Phase II*: Efficacy in patients and dose-response and dosing regimen definition (therapeutic exploration)
- *Phase III*: Definitive safety and efficacy in patients to define benefit-to-risk relationship and to confirm the dose-response relationship (therapeutic confirmation)
- *Phase IV*: Studies performed after marketing approval, related to the approved indication, and used to obtain a better understanding of the benefit-to-risk relationship and to identify less common adverse events (therapeutic use)

For each clinical trial study conducted to support the development of a drug candidate, certain features are necessary to ensure that the study is appropriately designed and conducted; that the data generated are collected, evaluated, and interpreted; and that the results are documented in a clinical trial study report. These features can be designated clinical trial design, investigator and clinical trial site selection, clinical trial site monitoring, clinical trial supply management, data collection and management, data evaluation and interpretation, report

Table 4   CSOs that conduct phase I–IV clinical trials

CSO	Phase I		Phase		
	Unit[a]	Spec[b]	II	III	IV
Advanced Biomedical Research	X	X			
Anapharm	X	X			
Applied Analytical Industries	X	X	X		
ASTER•CEPHAC	X	X	X		
BIBRA International	X	X			
Clinical Pharmacology Associates	X	X			
Clinical Research Services Turku	X	X	X	X	X
ICSL Clinical Studies	X		X	X	X
Colorado Medical Research Center	X	X	X	X	X
Covalent Group			X	X	X
Covance	X	X	X		
CroMedica Global	X	X			
Drug Research and Analysis Corporation	X	X			
FARMOVS	X	X	X	X	
Hill Top Research			X	X	X
Inveresk Research International Limited	X	X			
Kendle	X	X	X		
LCG Bioscience	X	X			
Lovelace Respiratory Research Institute	X		X	X	
MDS	X	X	X		
Medeval Limited	X	X	X		
Northwest Kinetics	X	X	X		
PAREXEL	X		X		
Pharma Bio-Research International	X	X			
PPD, Inc.	X	X			
PharmaKinetics Laboratories	X	X			
Premier Research Worldwide	X	X			
Quintiles Transnational	X	X			
Research Testing Laboratory			X	X	X
Simbec Research	X	X			
TNO Pharma Institute	X	X			
Valorum	X	X			
West Pharmaceutical Services	X	X	X	X	X

[a]Phase I unit with number of beds available listed, where known.
[b]Bioanalytical chemistry support and pharmacokinetic and special population studies conducted.

Table 5 CSOs providing multiple and various clinical trial support services

CSO	Phase	CTD[a]	SM[b]	DM/B[c]	RW[d]	CS[e]	A/RA[f]
Abt Associates Clinical Trials	I–IV	X	X	X	X		X
Advanced Biomedical Research	I–IV	X	X	X	X	X	
Analytical Sciences	I–IV		X	X	X		X
Anapharm	I–IV	X	X	X	X		X
Applied Analytical Industries	I–IV	X	X	X	X	X	X
Applied Logic Associates	I–IV	X	X	X	X		X
A.R. Kamm Associates	I–IV	X	X	X	X	X	X
Beardsworth Consult. Group	I–IV	X	X	X	X		X
Biomedical System	I–IV	X	X	X	X	X	
BZT	I–IV	X	X	X	X	X	X
Boston Biostatistics	II–IV	X	X	X	X		X
Cato Research	I–IV	X	X	X	X		X
Certus International	I–IV	X	X	X	X		X
Chiltern International	I–IV	X	X	X	X		X
Clinical Data Care	I–IV	X	X	X	X	X	X
Clinical Investigation Support	I–IV	X	X	X	X		X
Clinical R&D Services	I–IV	X	X	X	X		X
Clinical Research Services Turku	I–IV	X	X	X	X	X	
Clinimetrics Research Associates	I–IV	X	X	X	X		X
ClinPharm International	I–IV	X	X	X	X		X
ClinTrials Research	I–IV	X	X	X	X	X	X
Colorado Medical Research Center	I–IV	X	X	X	X		X
Covalent Group	II–IV	X	X	X			X
Covance	I–IV	X	X	X	X	X	X
CroMedica Global	I–IV	X	X	X	X	X	
Drug Research and Analysis Corporation	I–IV	X	X	X	X		X
FARMOVS	I–IV	X	X	X	X		X
Health Decisions	I–IV	X	X	X	X		X
IBAH	I–IV	X	X	X	X	X	X
ICON	II–IV		X	X	X	X	X
ILEX Oncology	I–IV	X	X	X	X		X
Innovus Research	II–IV	X	X	X	X		X
InSite Clinical Trials	II–IV	X	X	X	X		X
Integrated Research	II–IV	X	X	X	X		
Inveresk Research International Limited	I–III	X	X	X	X		X
IST Studien Therapeutica	II–IV	X	X	X	X	X	X
Kendle	I–IV	X	X	X	X	X	X
LCG Bioscience	I–IV	X	X	X	X	X	X
Lineberry Research Associates, L.L.C.	I–IV	X	X	X	X		X
MDS Pharmaceutical Services	I–IV	X	X	X	X	X	X
MEDDOC ApS	II–IV	X	X	X	X		X
Medical Industries Corporation	I–IV	X	X	X	X		X
MEDISEARCH International	I–IV	X	X	X	X		
MediTech International Company, Ltd.	I–III	X	X	X	X		X
METRONOMIA	I–IV	X	X	X	X		X
mimc-International Medical Consultants	II–IV	X	X	X	X	X	X
MTRA	II–IV	X	X	X	X		X
National Institute of Clinical Research	I–IV	X	X	X			X
OMEGA Contract Research Organization	III–IV	X	X	X	X		
Paragon Biomedical	II–IV	X	X	X	X	X	X
PAREXEL	I–IV	X	X	X	X	X	X

(Continued)

Table 5 CSOs providing multiple and various clinical trial support services (*Continued*)

CSO	Phase	CTD[a]	SM[b]	DM/B[c]	RW[d]	CS[e]	A/RA[f]
Pharma Bioresearch Int'l.	I–III	X	X	X	X		X
PPD, Inc.	I–IV	X	X	X	X	X	X
Pharmaceutical Research Associates	I–IV	X	X	X			X
PharmaKinetics Laboratories	I–IV	X	X	X	X		X
Pharmanet	II–IV	X	X	X	X		X
PharmaPart	I–IV	X	X	X	X	X	X
PharmaResearch	I–IV	X		X	X		X
Precision Research	I–IV	X	X	X	X	X	
Premier Research Worldwide	I–IV	X	X	X	X		X
ProTrials Research	I–IV	X	X	X	X	X	X
PSI Pharma Support	I–IV	X	X	X	X	X	X
Quintiles Transnational	I–IV	X	X	X	X	X	X
Research Services	I–IV	X	X	X	X	X	X
Research Testing Laboratories	II–IV	X	X	X	X		X
Schiff & Company	I–IV	X	X	X	X	X	X
SCIREX	I–IV	X	X	X	X	X	X
SGS Biopharm – Lab Simon	I–IV	X	X	X	X	X	X
Spadille ApS	I–IV	X	X	X	X	X	X
STATPROBE	I–IV	X	X	X	X		X
TOP Clinical Research	I–IV	X	X		X		X
Valorum	I–IV	X	X	X	X	X	X
Westat	I–IV	X	X	X	X	X	

[a]Clinical trial design and investigator and site selection.
[b]Clinical trial site monitoring.
[c]Data management and biostatistics.
[d]Report writing and other document preparation.
[e]Clinical trial supply management.
[f]Auditing and regulatory affairs.

writing, auditing, and regulatory affairs. CSOs have become major players in the clinical trial process. Their support ranges from designing and conducting a phase I clinical trial at a CSO's investigational site to coordinating a multinational, multisite phase III clinical trial. CSOs offering clinical trial services can be subdivided into two major classifications: those that actually conduct clinical trials and those that provide various clinical trial services. Table 4 lists a few CSOs that conduct clinical trials, and Table 5 lists some of the many CSOs that offer clinical trial support services in a variety of areas.

Phase I clinical trial studies include the initial administration of an investigational new drug to humans, usually healthy male volunteers, because the objectives of the study are nontherapeutic. However, women are now frequently included in these studies of first-time-use in humans Close attention is given to any adverse events (AEs) that occurs and to whether these events are related to the drug candidate and dose level, or are adverse drug reactions (ADRs). An ICH guideline (18) provides harmonized definitions for various terms including AE, ADR, serious adverse events (SAEs), and unexpected ADRs. A common practice in the first phase I clinical trial is to collect blood and urine specimens to obtain preliminary pharmacokinetic information in humans. Additional phase I clinical trials are frequently conducted later to address specific concerns such as relative bioavailability comparison when the formulation is changed; effect of food and time of feeding; potential for drug-drug interactions; pharmacokinetics in subpopulations such as the elderly, children, and ethnic groups; and possible change in clearance in renally or hepatically impaired patients.

Phase II clinical trial studies are designed primarily to explore the relationship between the dose level and frequency of administration and the efficacy and safety observed in patients with a particular therapeutic indication or disorder. Normally, a primary endpoint is selected to evaluate the efficacy; however, secondary endpoints are often included to establish criteria for monitoring patients in the more definitive phase III clinical trials. Phase II clinical trials are commonly placebo-controlled and blinded and may include a comparator drug. An ICH guideline (19) describes a number of possible study designs and also discusses the appropriateness of each design for the patient population and the disease indication and for obtaining the desired information. The study designs include parallel dose-response in which patients are randomized to several fixed dose groups, factorial parallel dose-response in which combination therapy is evaluated, cross-over dose-response in which each patient receives each dose level, forced titration in which all patients are administered a series of rising doses, and optional titration in which patients are titrated over a range of dose levels until they reach a predefined favorable or unfavorable response.

Phase III clinical trial studies are designed to confirm that the drug candidate is safe and effective in patients with the intended therapeutic indication and are conducted in a relatively large patient population and frequently at multiple sites. The size and duration of these studies make them, along with establishing the manufacturing facility, the most time-consuming and expensive aspects of drug development. Thus, phase III clinical trials need to be carefully planned and implemented so that the resulting database of generated safety and efficacy data is sufficient to demonstrate statistically that the drug candidate can effectively mediated the disease indication without causing substantial ADRs. For phase III clinical trial studies intended to show effective treatment for a chronic disorder, an ICH guideline (20) has been issued. Still another ICH guideline (21) discusses developmental approaches for drug candidates likely to be used in the elderly because the indication is a disease of aging, such as Alzheimer's disease, or the population with the disorder includes a significant number of geriatric patients. As with most pharmaceutical companies, CSOs do not have the necessary resources at their own facilities to actually conduct multisite, multinational phase III clinical trials.

Phase IV clinical trials start after a regulatory agency has granted a marketing authorization to a drug candidate, which is now a therapeutic product. These phase IV studies need to relate to the approved indication(s) and the dosage regimen(s) that were authorized and are intended to optimize the use of the drug. Phase IV clinical trials may include epidemiology, drug–drug interaction, and subpopulation studies.

Not all clinical trials, especially large, multisite, multinational phase III studies and phase IV postmarketing surveillance, pharmacoeconomic, and quality-of-life

studies, can be conducted at a CSO facility. These types of studies, and many phase II efficacy studies, are conducted in research- or university-based hospitals or other investigational sites where a sufficient patient population with the disease or disorder to be tested is available. A number of CSOs offer services to support clinical trial studies that are implemented at one or more clinical trial sites. These services can be broken down into relatively broad categories, which are summarized later.

CSOs assisting clients with clinical trial design need to be an extension of the client's project team and have access to all the data to assist in developing a realistic clinical trial package to determine the safety and efficacy of a drug candidate. In addition to assisting clients with clinical development plans and preparing clinical trial protocols, many of these CSOs also offer clients services for the preparation of CRFs, investigator brochures, IRB and IEC applications, and other clinical trial-related documents. Unless a clinical trial is being conducted at a predetermined site, selection of the clinical site(s) and the investigator(s) who will be responsible for the clinical trial is the next step. The pharmaceutical company is ultimately responsible for all research studies conducted during the development of a drug candidate. However, the clinical trial investigator is a key player (22) and has to have certain qualifications to assume a number of responsibilities. The next step is training of site personnel in the specific aspects and requirements of the study protocol. This training can be critical, especially when the study uses specialized or novel techniques for evaluating safety and/or efficacy. Clinical trial monitoring assists in ensuring that difficulties or problems are detected early and that their occurrence or recurrence is minimized. Overseeing the quality of a clinical trial involves checks of various aspects that may include ascertaining whether the study protocol and SOPs are being followed, whether GCP regulations and other regulatory agency regulations are being followed, the acceptability of data being generated and listed on CRFs and other clinical trial documents, the success in reaching planned patient accrual targets, success in keeping patients in the trial, and tracking clinical trial supplies. An ICH guideline (22) offers guidance on the various aspects of monitoring.

The proper management of the drug candidate and other products, such as comparator drugs and placebos, is in many respects as important to the success of a clinical trial as the care and management of the patients. The clinical trial supplies need to be appropriately characterized, manufactured in compliance with GMP regulations, and, if applicable, coded and labeled to protect the blinding of the clinical trial study (22). Outsourcing to CSOs or other companies of manufacturing and formulation development research is a common practice. This outsourcing does not relieve the clinical trial sponsor of responsibility for ensuring clinical trial supplies meet the requirements for the proper conduct of a clinical trial.

The primary focus of the data collection and management process is to provide a guaranteed, quality-assured, final database, which is accomplished by standardized strategies for handling data, verification of data, comparing and repairing data entries, and verifying the accuracy of the data. Inaccurate or incorrect clinical trial data can result in an otherwise successful clinical trial being erroneously interpreted for safety and/or efficacy parameters. Three ICH guidelines (18, 23, 24) address safety data management issues. The data collected from a well designed, well conducted clinical trial are evaluated to ascertain the benefit-to-risk relationship for the purposed therapy. When the patients who received a drug candidate have the disease manifestations completely eradicated and experience no other effects while patients treated with a placebo have a continuation of the disease process, the evaluation is not difficult. However, that is rarely, if ever, the case, and evaluation requires detailed statistical analysis of the collected data. An ICH guideline (25) covers statistical issues related to the scope of clinical trials, design techniques to minimize bias, types of clinical trial designs, conduct considerations, data analysis for efficacy, evaluation of safety and tolerance, and reporting.

Pharmaceutical companies are constantly bombarded with advertisements and brochures from CSOs and other groups that promise unrealistic speed in clinical trial design and management to expedite clinical development. What is missing from this picture? The compiling of the nonclinical and clinical findings in a detailed, well designed, believable story that results in the production of a high-quality regulatory agency submission for marketing authorization. This effort requires the expertise of scientific and medical writers who use clear, concise writing to share the science of drug development. All data and results, both positive and negative, generated during the development of a drug candidate need to be included. An ICH guideline (26) offers assistance in the generation and compilation of clinical trial study reports that are acceptable to all ICH region regulatory agencies. Many CSOs offer scientific and medical writing services, and some consider their medical writing capabilities to be more than just another service offered.

The audit of a clinical trial is independent and separate from routine clinical trial monitoring and quality-control functions. An audit is an aspect of quality assurance and evaluates clinical trial conduct and compliance with the study protocol; applicable SOPs; GCP, GLP, and GMP regulations; and applicable regulatory agency regulations (22). A clinical trial auditor is to be independent from the clinical trial. Because a clinical trial auditor(s) cannot have been involved in the study, clients who use a CSO to support the various aspects of clinical drug development and then contract with the same CSO to audit clinical trials need to ensure that the auditor(s) is truly independent. To achieve this goal, clients may contract with one CSO to support the clinical trial and another CSO or a qualified independent consultant(s) to conduct the audit. An estimated 80% of the regulatory agency approval process focuses on the clinical trial sections of a marketing application submission. To ensure that these, and other, sections are complete and meet the perceived specifications of the regulatory agency reviewers, most pharmaceutical companies have established regulatory affairs groups. These groups commonly assist drug development project teams and company management in defining and implementing regulatory strategies for the various aspects of drug candidate development, offer advice and recommendations on regulatory issues applicable to the countries where marketing approval is being sought, and serve as the primary contact between the company and regulatory agencies. Some CSOs offer regulatory affairs capabilities.

OUTSOURCING OF CONTROL, MANUFACTURING, AND CHEMISTRY

After clinical trials, the next most time-consuming and expensive aspect of the drug development process is the synthesis and characterization of the drug substance and drug product, i.e., the manufacturing process. A manufacturing process that is inappropriately designed, implemented, and controlled can kill a promising drug candidate or active pharmaceutical ingredient (API), which is the term used by most manufacturing groups, as easily as can life-threatening adverse effects or insufficient biological activity. A drug candidate that is costly to effectively produce results in high prices to patient, that, unless the drug is the best or the only therapy for a disease indication, lowers the market share and thus the revenue to the pharmaceutical company. Similarly, a complex manufacturing process that is difficult to control may result in API variations, in both amount and impurity profiles, that can hinder regulatory agency approval unless the manufacturer can prove that the production processes are being following and are producing the same material in each production batch.

The manufacturing process is frequently changed to improve yield or decease impurities. To ensure the drug substance is the same after processing changes, manufacturers develop and validate characterization procedures to demonstrate and document that the changes have not affected the material being produced and that no previously undetected impurities are present.

Many pharmaceutical companies outsource one or more of the control, manufacturing, and chemistry (CMC) processes, for which numerous regulatory agencies guidelines are available. Reasons for this outsourcing include but are not limited to:

• Avoiding capital investment in facilities, equipment, and personnel;
• Avoiding the need to establish and maintain a GMP manufacturing facility;
• Gaining access to additional capacity and technology;
• Accessing a contractor's expertise; and
• Expediting the time to market

Some CSOs that offer multiple CMC services to clients are listed in Table 6. These services have been subdivided into the major categories of manufacturing, raw materials, formulation development, method development, stability, packaging, and auditing.

The manufacturing process starts when the discovery scientists synthesizes a compound that has biological activity. The techniques used are usually sufficient to produce milligram to gram quantities for pharmacology studies but are rarely adaptable to the large-scale synthesis necessary for generating the much larger amounts of material needed for formulation development and preclinical and clinical studies. Shortly after a discovery lead is designated a preclinical drug candidate, the manufacturing group begins the research studies necessary to scale up the laboratory bench synthetic procedure to a larger, or manufacturing, process. Whether the drug substance is a small organic molecule or a macromolecule, the procedure may and usually does undergo substantial modification during scale up to commercial production. A few of the items that are evaluated during the establishment of a manufacturing process include:

• Identifying synthesis and formulation methods, including definition of equipment, processes, and scale of production;
• Defining and validating processes for fill, finish, and packaging;
• Determining procedures for waste disposal, including appropriate environmental assessments; and
• Determining the number of batches required to support development program and product launch.

One of the most important aspects of the manufacturing process is documentation and document control. Each step in the process, whether the results are positive or negative, needs to be evaluated and documented to show that the manufacturer understands what is happening and can control the synthesis, purification, formulation, and packaging of the drug product. Some of the documents needed include:

• Chemistry, manufacturing, and control documents;
• Appropriate standard operating procedures;
• Validation protocols for methods and processes;
• Progress and final reports for methods and processes; and
• Regulatory documents, such as IND, yearly updates, and NDA.

The raw materials used in the synthesis, purification, and formulation of an API are critical for the successful manufacture of a drug product. The supplier or vendor of each component and intermediate has to be identified and certified, commonly through a detailed site visit. The amount, timing, and cost of these supplies are negotiated so that the key ingredients are available when needed. Another important item is determining the shelf-life of each raw material to ensure that the ingredient has not deteriorated from the time of purchase to the time of use.

Once the drug candidate is available, formulation activities are initiated to develop a suitable dosage for administration to animals and, later, to humans. Depending on the route of administration, formulations may be solutions, suspensions, aerosols, creams, or solids. Because formulation ingredients can affect the delivery profile of a drug candidate, in some cases adversely, using a preclinical formulation that closely resembles and mimics the proposed clinical formulation is highly desirable. Thus, preformulation studies need to be conducted as early in the development process as possible. The formulation process usually continues throughout the development process, with changes made to improve stability, enhance delivery, or mask the taste or appearance of the drug product. Depending on the extent of the formulation change, additional nonclinical and clinical studies may be necessary to determine if the revised formulation has the same characteristics as the original formulation and, if not, what the extent and nature of the difference are.

Analytical chemistry methods are used for chemical characterization of the drug substance and drug product. This characterization includes qualitative tests for structural identification and for impurities, degradation products, and contaminants (27–29). Characterization relies on well characterized, validated, analytical

Table 6 CSOs that provide multiple and various CMC services

CSO	Manu[a]	RM[b]	Form[c]	MD[d]	Stab[e]	Pack[f]	Aud[g]
AAI	X		X	X	X		
Abbott Laboratories	X			X		X	
Alpharma USPD	X		X	X	X	X	
AMRESCO	X	X	X			X	X
Atlantic Pharmaceutical Services	X	X	X	X			
Ben Venue Laboratories	X		X	X	X		
BioAnalytika Laboratories				X	X		
Boston Analytics				X	X	X	
Catalytical Pharmaceutical	X	X	X	X	X	X	X
Charles River Laboratories				X	X		
Chesapeake Biological Labs	X		X	X		X	
Chromak Research		X	X	X	X		
Circa Pharmaceutical	X	X		X	X	X	
Collaborative BioAlliance, Inc.	X	X	X				
Covance, Inc.		X		X	X	X	X
Dow Chemical Manufacturing Services	X	X	X	X	X	X	
DPT Laboratories	X		X	X	X	X	
Elemental Research		X		X	X		
Gibraltar Laboratories		X	X	X	X		
Global Pharm Inc.	X	X		X	X	X	
Hauser, Inc.	X		X	X	X	X	X
IBAH Pharmaceutical Services	X	X		X	X	X	
IDEC Pharmaceutical Corporation	X	X		X			
International Processing Corporation	X		X	X	X	X	
J.B. Laboratories	X			X	X	X	
Kansas City Analytical Services		X		X	X		
Lancaster Laboratories		X		X	X		
Magellan Laboratories		X		X	X		
MDS Pharmaceutical Services	X	X	X	X	X	X	
Metrics, Inc.	X	X	X	X	X		
Metuchen Analytical		X		X	X		
Midwest Research Institute	X	X	X	X	X		
New Life Resources	X	X		X		X	X
Nycomed Amersham	X			X	X		
Oneida Research Services		X		X	X		
Oread	X		X	X	X	X	X
Patheon, Inc.	X	X	X	X	X	X	
Performance Solutions							X
Pharm-ECO Laboratories	X	X		X	X		X
Pharmaceutical Development Center	X	X	X	X	X	X	
Pharmaceutics International	X		X	X	X	X	
Pisgah Labs	X	X		X			
PPD, Inc.		X		X	X		
Proceutics				X	X		X
ProClinical Pharm. Services	X			X	X	X	
Quantitative Technologies		X		X	X		
Quality Chemical Laboratories		X		X	X		
Ricerca	X	X		X	X		
Schwarz Pharma	X			X		X	
SGS U.S. Testing		X		X	X	X	
Sharp		X			X	X	

(*Continued*)

Table 6   CSOs that provide multiple and various CMC services (*Continued*)

CSO	Manu[a]	RM[b]	Form[c]	MD[d]	Stab[e]	Pack[f]	Aud[g]
Shuster Laboratories		X	X	X	X		X
Southern Testing & Research Labs		X		X	X		
SP Pharmaceuticals	X		X		X	X	
SRI International	X	X	X	X	X		
STAT-A-MATRIX				X	X		X
Steifel Research Institute		X	X	X	X		
Taylor Pharmaceuticals	X	X		X	X	X	
Tetrionics, Inc.	X			X	X		
Tower Laboratories	X		X		X	X	
Vital Pharma, Inc.	X		X	X	X	X	
West Coast Analytical Services		X	X	X	X		
West Pharmaceutical Services	X			X	X	X	

[a]Manufacturing including process development and validation.
[b]Raw material including procurement and testing.
[c]Formulation development and characterization.
[d]Method development for drug substance and drug product characterization.
[e]Stability testing of drug substance and drug product.
[f]Packing services for drug product.
[g]GMP audit of chemistry, manufacturing, and control processes.

chemistry methods, which may include USP methods such as residual solvents, moisture content, residue on ignition, and thermal determinations and drug candidate-specific methods such as identification, concentration, impurity profiles, solubility profiles, and stability under various temperatures and conditions. For proteins and polypeptides, additional characterization is necessary. Several ICH guidelines (30–37) have been issued on characterization and discuss stability testing, including photostability, impurities, residual solvents, and test procedure and acceptance criteria specifications (33, 34). Quantitative analytical chemistry methods provide information on drug substance concentration, impurity profiles, and stability profiles. ICH guidelines (35, 36) for validation of analytical chemistry procedures address experiments to ascertain and set acceptance specifications for specificity, detection limit, quantification limit, linearity, range, precision, accuracy, and robustness. Analytical methods need to be validated for each sample type to be analyzed.

Stability testing determines how a drug substance or drug product may change with time under various conditions, such as temperature, humidity, and light and defines storage conditions and shelf-life. A number of ICH guidelines (30, 32, 37) describe and discuss stability issues and testing requirement for NCEs and macromolecules. These guidelines provide manufacturers and CSOs with acceptance specifications for

accelerated and long-term stability studies. In addition to the drug substance and drug product, stability assessment is frequently conducted on raw materials, key intermediates, formulation excipients, and packaging materials.

After the drug product is prepared, the next step is packaging and labeling the material. Packaging requirements depend on the final drug product (solid, suspension, liquid) and the clinical indication (hospital, physician office, or home use). For liquids to be dosed parenterally, sterility of the drug product is important and validated, and aseptic filling procedures are necessary. For other dosage forms, specialized equipment may be needed to place the drug product into the desired package. Compatibility of the drug product with any packaging material, such as vials, inner liners, and closure systems, with which the product comes into contact needs to evaluated. Proper labeling and package insert information is critical for the proper use of the drug product. The label and package insert provide physicians, pharmacists, and patients with information on:

- The drug substance, drug product, and formulation excipients;
- Clinical pharmacology and the biological action of the drug substance;
- Indications and usage for which the specific drug product has been approved;

- Contraindications for when the drug product should not be used;
- Warnings and precautions on the use of the drug product;
- Adverse reactions reported and attributable to the drug substance;
- Overdosage effects and treatment to counteract the effects;
- Dosage and administration specifications for the drug product; and
- How the drug product is supplied and appropriate storage conditions.

Audits are conducted to ensure that the manufacturer—either a pharmaceutical company or a CSO—has appropriately defined and documented the various processes and methods required to produce the drug substance and drug product and has the necessary personnel and facilities to conduct and control the manufacturing process and to determine whether GMP regulations are being followed. As with clinical trials, the pharmaceutical company developer is responsible for the manufacture of the drug substance and drug product, whether these activities take place at the company's facilities or are outsourced. Audits, whether conducted by regulatory agencies or by the developer, determine that the processes are under control and in compliance with GMP regulations. Problems discovered during audits can usually be resolved, and to prevent regulatory agencies from finding these areas of concern, pharmaceutical companies use their internal QA groups or their contract with the CSO or independent consultant to conduct GMP audits of the CMC aspects of drug development. As with its role in clinical trial auditing, the auditors have to be independent of the processes being audited, and at times, clients outsource auditing of a manufacturing CSO to another CSO that provides GMP auditing services.

VIRTUAL DRUG DEVELOPMENT ORGANIZATIONS AND CONSULTANTS

Another relatively new player in the drug discovery and development arena is the virtual drug development organization (VDO), which, like the CSO, offers pharmaceutical companies support in developing discovery ideas into therapeutic products. However, VDOs do not offer laboratory services, but provide clients with coordination of the various drug discovery and development activities necessary to characterize a drug candidate and produce the compound in sufficient quantity for nonclinical, clinical, and marketing efforts. This coordination is accomplished by designing and outsourcing the research studies to CSOs and then compiling the results generated into regulatory agency submissions. VDOs operate in one of two ways. One is to contract with the pharmaceutical client and serve as an extension of the client's program. The other is to out-license a drug candidate from a pharmaceutical company or university technology transfer group. In both cases, VDOs interact closely with CSOs. Pharmaceutical firms need to evaluate VDOs using the techniques and requirements used to select and monitor CSOs.

Consultants have supported the pharmaceutical industry for many years and provide expert advice on the many aspects of the drug discovery and development processes. This advice includes assisting in the selection and monitoring of CSOs and in the interpretation of results from outsourced studies. Pharmaceutical companies select consultants in a variety of ways, the most common being the "good-old-boy" network, in which a pharmaceutical company executive knows, or has a friend who knows, someone who is now a consultant, commonly a retired pharmaceutical executive, a former regulatory agency reviewer, or a pharmacology professor at a university. Is this the optimal means of identifying an expert? Probably not, if the company wants an expert with knowledge and experience in a particular area(s) research, such as drug metabolism or drug product stability. The techniques outlined above for selecting a CSO should also be used for evaluating consultants, with research area experience, integrity, and communication skills probably being the most important aspects. Choosing a toxicology or clinical pharmacology consultant to assist with evaluating human pharmacokinetic results may prevent the data from being used effectively to design additional nonclinical toxicology or clinical trial studies.

EMERGING TRENDS

Major changes have occurred, and are occurring, in the pharmaceutical industry and in the drug discovery and development processes. They have caused numerous changes in the way CSOs provide support services to drug developers. What can be expected in the future? Are more changes on the horizon, and, if so, what might they be and how will they affect pharmaceutical companies and their service providers? Although predicting the future is usually quite inaccurate and often misleading, some trends, based on recent events, may be extended into the near future.

For pharmaceutical companies, present trends indicate that:

- Mergers and acquisitions will result in formation of more mega-pharmaceutical companies. Reasons include the desire to have a more global presence, to enter into a therapeutic area with previously established research staff and drug development pipeline, and to obtain novel technology to assist in accelerating drug discovery and development. Whether these mega-firms have a better chance than midsized or small pharmaceutical houses in obtaining marketing approval for major therapeutic products is unknown.
- Numerous new companies, primarily biotechnology firms that hope to turn a discovery idea into a therapeutic product, will be formed. Funding for these firms will be difficult to obtain, will come primarily from venture capitalists and government grants, and will be insufficient to take a discovery lead through complete drug development. Most of these start-up companies will attempt to outlicense or sell for much-needed cash and future royalties their discoveries to pharmaceutical companies or VDOs. The further these small companies are along in the drug development process will determine how much they will receive for their discoveries. A number of companies, approximately the same number that are formed, will go out of business, merge, or be acquired when their discovery does not result in drug candidates with the necessary attributes to become therapeutic products.
- The ICH process will provide more standardization to the requirements for the worldwide development of drug candidates. A global marketing application package that meets the requirements of most regulatory agencies and that includes nonclinical, clinical, and manufacturing aspects will be defined and accepted.
- Even the best efforts of drug developers will not reduce the time and cost of drug discovery and development. However, as novel drug discovery and potential for development characterization techniques are put into place and the ICH process is more fully implemented, the time and cost will not increase as rapidly as in the past.

For CSOs and other support groups, the trends noted previously offer nothing but opportunities. The prospects for CSOs are very bright, and CSOs that capitalize on the present and future needs of their clients will be highly successful. Trends for the CSO industry include that:

- Pharmaceutical companies will increase their outsourcing efforts;
- Drug discovery and potential for development characterization services will be high-growth areas because these fields are presently bottlenecks, and the situation is not expected to get any better;
- CSOs offering primarily or exclusively nonclinical drug development services will have to broaden their capabilities to attract and maintain clients,
- Clinical CSOs will have more studies than they can support effectively and will most likely expand to meet the needs of their clients,
- Clinical CSOs that provide services in a number of aspects of clinical trials and have a worldwide presence will grow and prosper,
- More mega-CSOs, such as Quintiles and MDS, will emerge. Likely candidates are these mega-CSOs will offer clients many, but probably not all, services needed for drug discovery and development. Some of these large CSOs may attempt to become pharmaceutical houses and use their considerable expertise to discover and develop compounds obtained through their own efforts or by inlicensing,
- The CSO field will not be dominated by the mega-CSOs. The present and future bottlenecks experienced by pharmaceutical companies will result in more CSOs, not fewer. These new CSOs will offer clients specialized services in drug discovery and potential for development characterization to evaluate multiple discovery leads simultaneously,
- As pharmaceutical companies merge and continue to "right-size," CSOs will become more a true partner and less a pair of hands to complete tasks. The clients will have to share more scientific information, both positive and negative, to the service providers that, in turn, will need to learn more about the entire drug discovery and development process for these partnerships to be effective and beneficial for both parties.
- CSOs will be a primary source of employment for new graduates and for down-sized pharmaceutical company employees in various scientific disciplines. The new graduates will bring in the latest academic technology to assist in expanding or defining novel services to be offered to clients. These young, highly motivated employees will learn the more applied science of pharmaceutical development from the former pharmaceutical company employees.

Whether many or all of these potential trends will occur in the near future is not known. One thing is certain, change will happen. Those pharmaceutical companies and their CSO partners that embrace change and adapt to novel ideas and approaches to improve and possibly shorten the drug discovery and development processes will prosper. Companies that do not or are unwilling to embrace change will most likely become a memory. However, even a bad memory can offer guidance and be used to improve the process for finding novel therapeutic agents to treat one of the many human diseases or disorders that presently have only marginal or no effective treatment.

REFERENCES

1. *Drug Metabolism/Drug Interaction Studies in the Drug Development Process. Studies In Vitro*; US FDA: FDA Guidance for Industry: Washington, DC, 1997.
2. U.S. FDA's Proposed Implementation of ICH Safety Working Group Consensus Regarding New Drug Applications. Federal Register **1992**, *57* (73), 13105–13106.
3. *Non-Clinical Safety Studies for the Conduct of Human Clinical Trials for Pharmaceuticals*; ICH Harmonized Tripartite Guideline (M3); 1997.
4. Karnes, H.T.; Shiu, G.; Shah, V.P. Validation of Bioanalytical Methods, Pharm. Res. **1991**, *8* (4), 421–426.
5. Shah, V.P.; Midha, K.K.; Dighe, S.; McGilveray, I.J.; Skelly, J.P.; Yacobi, A.; Layloff, T.; Viswanathan, C.T.; Cook, C.E.; McDowall, R.D.; Pittman, K.A.; Spector, S. Analytical Methods Validation, Bioavailability, Bioequivalence and Pharmacokinetic Studies. Pharm. Res. **1992**, *9* (4), 588–592.
6. *Note for Guidance on Toxicokinetics: The Assessment of Systemic Exposure in Toxicity Studies*, ICH Harmonized Tripartite Guideline (S3A);1994.
7. *Pharmacokinetics: Guidance for Repeated Dose Tissue Distribution Studies*, ICH Harmonized Tripartite Guideline (S3B);1994.
8. *Guidance on Specific Aspects of Regulatory Genotoxicity Tests for Pharmaceuticals*, ICH Harmonized Tripartite Guideline (S2A); 1995.
9. *Genotoxicity: A Standard Battery for Genotoxicity Testing of Pharmaceuticals*, ICH Harmonized Tripartite Guideline (S2B); 1997.
10. *Duration of Chronic Toxicity Testing in Animals (Rodent and Non Rodent Toxicity Testing)*, ICH Harmonized Tripartite Guideline (S4A); 1998.
11. *Detection of Toxicity to Reproduction for Medicinal Products*, ICH Harmonized Tripartite Guideline (S5A); 1993.
12. *Toxicity to Male Fertility: An Addendum to the ICH Tripartite Guideline on Detection of Toxicity to Reproduction for Medicinal Products*, ICH Harmonized Tripartite Guideline (S5B); 1995.
13. *Guidelines on the Need for Carcinogenicity Studies of Pharmaceuticals*, ICH Harmonized Tripartite Guideline (S1A); 1995.
14. *Testing for Carcinogenicity of Pharmaceuticals*, ICH Harmonized Tripartite Guideline (S1B); 1997.
15. *Dose Selection for Carcinogenicity Studies of Pharmaceuticals*, ICH Harmonized Tripartite Guideline (S1C); 1994.
16. *Addendum to Dose Selection for Carcinogenicity Studies of Pharmaceuticals: Addition of a Limit Dose and Related Notes*, ICH Harmonized Tripartite Guideline (S1CR); 1997.
17. *General Considerations for Clinical Trials*, ICH Harmonized Tripartite Guideline (E8); 1997.
18. *Clinical Safety Data Management: Definitions and Standards for Expedited Reporting*, ICH Harmonized Tripartite Guideline (E2A); 1994.
19. *Dose-Response Information to Support Drug Registration*, ICH Harmonized Tripartite Guideline (E4); 1994.
20. *The Extent of Population Exposure to Assess Clinical Safety for Drug Intended for Long-Term Treatment of Non-Life-Threatening Conditions*, ICH Harmonized Tripartite Guideline (E1); 1994.
21. *Studies in Support of Special Populations: Geriatrics*, ICH Harmonized Tripartite Guideline (E7); 1993.
22. *Guideline for Good Clinical Practice*, ICH Harmonized Tripartite Guideline (E6); 1996.
23. *Data Elements for Transmission of Individual Case Safety Reports*, ICH Harmonized Tripartite Guideline (E2B); 1997.
24. *Clinical Safety Data Management: Periodic Safety Update Reports for Marketed Drugs*, ICH Harmonized Tripartite Guideline (E2C); 1996.
25. *Statistical Principles for Clinical Trials*, ICH Harmonized Tripartite Guideline (E9); 1998.
26. *Structure and Content of Clinical Study Reports*, ICH Harmonized Tripartite Guideline (E3); 1995.
27. *Impurities in New Drug Substances*, ICH Harmonized Tripartite Guideline (Q3A); 1995.
28. *Impurities in New Drug Products*, ICH Harmonized Tripartite Guideline (Q3B); 1996.
29. *Impurities: Guideline for Residual Solvents*, ICH Harmonized Tripartite Guideline (Q3C); 1997.
30. *Stability Testing of New Drug Substances and Products*, ICH Harmonized Tripartite Guideline (Q1A); 1993.
31. *Stability Testing: Photostability Testing of New Drug Substances and Products*, ICH Harmonized Tripartite Guideline (Q1B); 1996.
32. *Stability Testing: Requirements for New Dosage Forms, Annex to the ICH Harmonized Tripartite Guideline on Stability Testing for New Drugs and Products*, ICH Harmonized Tripartite Guideline (Q1C); 1996.
33. *Specifications: Test Procedures and Acceptance Criteria for New Drug Substances and New Drug Products: Chemical Substances*, ICH Harmonized Tripartite Guideline (Q6A); 1997.
34. *Specifications: Test Procedures and Acceptance Criteria for Biotechnology/Biological Products*, ICH Draft Consensus Guideline (Q6B); 1998.
35. *Text on Validation of Analytical Procedures*, ICH Harmonized Tripartite Guideline (Q2A); 1994.
36. *Validation of Analytical Procedures: Methodology*, ICH Harmonized Tripartite Guideline (Q2B); 1996.
37. *Quality of Biotechnological Products: Stability Testing of Biotechnological/Biological Products*, ICH Harmonized Tripartite Guideline (Q5C); 1995.
38. Corporate Capabilities. Bio. Pharm **1999**, *12* (12), 1–76.
39. The 2000 CSO Directory. Drug Information Association **2000**, *1–237*.
40. *2000 Corporate Capabilities*, LC-GC; North America 2000, 1–138.

41. GEN Directory to Contract Research Organizations, Genetic Engineering News Directory to Biotechnology Companies.

42. 1999/2000 Buying Guide. Pharm. Process. **1999**, *16* (6), 1–224.

43. *Larka Directory of Contract Pharmaceutical Manufacturers (CPMs) Europe*, Larka Directory of Contract Research Organization (CROs) Europe. Larka Pharmaceutical Publications.

44. *The Directory of Contract Services; Vol. I. Dosage Form Manufacturing, Formulation, Packaging and Analytical Services; Vol. II.*, Biologics API Manufacturing and Process Development; PharmSource Information Services, Inc.

45. *The Technomark Registers 2000; Vol. 1. CROs in Europe Offering Clinical Research Services, Data Management & Regulatory Affairs; Vol. 2. CROs in Europe Offering Preclinical, Toxicology & Analytical Services; Vol. 3. CPMs in Europe Offering Packaging & Manufacturing Services; Vol. 4. North American CROs & CPMs.*

46. Lakings, D.B. Biological CROs: Enhancing the Opportunity for a Successful Drug Discovery and Development Program. D&MD Reports, 1999; 1-1–10-348.

47. *New Drug Approval Process, The Global Challenge. Drugs and the Pharmaceutical Sciences,* 3rd Ed.; Guarino, R.A., Ed.; Marcel Dekker, Inc.: New York, 2000; 1–463.

PAPERLESS DOCUMENTATION SYSTEMS

Ellen M. Williams
Michael McKenna
Pfizer, Inc., New York, New York

INTRODUCTION

The fundamental purpose of documents is communication. Specifically, documents enhance the flexibility of communication. Documents improve the ability to transmit information in two ways. First, a document freezes a sender's message in time so that it may be accessed later. The wall of a cave marked with pictographs, a carved stone tablet, a photograph of the cave wall, a creased paper bag containing a shopping list, as well as a phonographic recording of a piano concerto all record information that persists through time beyond the act of its creation. The second way in which documents make our communications more versatile is by allowing the sender's message to travel through space independently of the sender. With the exception of the cave wall, each of the above examples is more or less portable. It is portability that gives documents the capacity to communicate across space as well as time.

By packaging a sender's message in such a way that it may be accessed by physically scattered recipients at any time after the original recording, documents enable marvelous things to happen. While proscribing real-time exchange between a message's sender and recipient, a physical record gives to ideas a life that they often would not have if merely spoken or performed once in time. Governments, religions, and much of society depend crucially on the existence of an ongoing exchange with certain key documents (1). On a smaller and more immediate scale, documents enable us to get things done in ways and on a scale that spoken words alone do not. Indeed, by allowing us to communicate across vast reaches of time and space, documents increase the coordination and scope of communication, thereby enabling tremendous feats of collaboration.

Perhaps more than other industries, pharmaceutical manufacturing and marketing depend on exquisite levels of collaboration among many different spheres of activity, ranging from analytical chemistry to clinical medicine, operations research, business, and the law. This complex coordination and a strict regulatory landscape, which ultimately dictates the viability of a pharmaceutical product, demand that all scientific and business decisions from discovery through postmarketing research be rigorously and thoroughly documented. The sheer volume of written procedures, forms, analyses, reports, and correspondence that must be managed across a single product's lifecycle is enormous. When one considers enterprise-wide management of documentation supporting a portfolio of dozens of drugs in various stages of development, the numbers are truly staggering. Although regulatory authorities have recently issued comprehensive regulations (2–4) and guidelines (5–7) on electronic records management, these standards and the predicate rules on which they are based could rapidly become outdated in the evolving world of computing and wireless data exchange (8).

Until recently, document management in an enterprise has been organized around distinct efforts involving the control of three kinds of paper document (forms, reports, and manuals) and the administration of the folders and archiving procedures used to manage them (9). A number of economic and technological forces over the last quarter century have changed business in such a way as to strain the traditional methods of document management, if not render them wholly obsolete. For one thing, improvements in organizational, manufacturing, and communications technology that have compressed production cycles and decreased the time from concept to market in nearly all industries have also yielded a corresponding acceleration in demand and consumption. With improvements in communications and techniques of distribution come unavoidable increases in the volume of business transactions (10). Speeded up markets beget more business, which necessitates more efficient management of ever more documentation. As computer technology has been introduced into business environments over the last 25 years to adapt to this quickening pace, the system designed to manage paper has met with great difficulty storing electronic documents as well (11). Computing and communications technology is changing the fundamental status of documents.

EVOLUTION OF DOCUMENTATION TECHNOLOGIES

Initially, the implementation of a paperless documentation system in an enterprise is driven by a need or mandate to eliminate paper, economize the use of physical space, improve the efficiency of document retrieval, or otherwise improve the storage of information assets. Paper document management has referred to the storage, modification, and retrieval of documents that distinguish themselves from each other in terms of content, purpose, or format. The emphasis is on the introduction of a system that provides a storage solution. The true strength of most electronic document management systems, however, lies beyond the simple capacity to warehouse digital representations of paper documents.

During the 19th and 20th centuries document technologies have followed an evolution that has repeatedly and alternately focused on document production, reproduction, and distribution. The first long wave of innovation was centered around the means of producing text. From as early as the fourteenth century, at least one hundred writing machines were invented before the Sholes and Glidden typewriter was produced by the gunmakers Remington and Sons some sixty miles west of Albany in 1874 (12). The second major development in the history of modern document technology sought to enable the rapid dissemination and reproduction of paper documentation and is marked by the Haloid (later Xerox) company's introduction of the photocopier around 1960 (13). In the mid-1960s, by way of the IBM Selectric typewriter, which had magnetic tape storage, and the text editor, which handily managed unformatted text for machine processing, the third evolutionary step brought the management of all aspects of the composition and formatting of individual documents in the form of the WYSIWYG word processor (14). By the mid-1990s, the word processor had effectively satisfied all needs surrounding the efficient production and stylistic control of single documents within a given operating system or platform. Concurrent with the improvement of word processing technology, much attention was paid to enhancing the distribution of textual information to disparate locations across computer networks. The shift in attention took place on two fronts, looking first to the distribution of formatted content across multiple platform-independent systems and then to managing the storage and retrieval of, as well as the complex relationships among, large volumes of documents. 1990 saw Tim Berners-Lee create the first web browser and a simple markup

language that would become HTML (hypertext markup language) at the European Laboratory for Particle Physics (CERN) to enable collaboration among disparately located scientists (15). This innovation is, in fact, not so new. It was actually presaged nearly half a century earlier by Vannevar Bush in an article written for the *Atlantic Monthly* that described his "memex" machine, which bears an eerily prescient resemblance to today's World Wide Web and the practice of hypertext linking (16). By the mid-1990s innovations in document warehousing and distribution were built atop mature relational database technologies and the ability to efficiently link document objects stored on a server platform with their associated indexing attributes in a database (17).

The evolution detailed above has alternately expanded and narrowed its focus, shifting from the domain of the document itself to the interstices between multiple documents and their authors and consumers. The development emphasis has cycled back and forth between the production of documents and the reproduction and distribution of documents. As we move into the 21st century, the prevailing trend in document technology appears to be moving in the direction of fusing the cycles of document production, reproduction, and distribution. As much as business allows, documents will soon be designed to allow their transmission, reuse, and machine processing in a simple fashion. Indeed, more and more, business models will be forced to adapt to a landscape that operates on such "documents." The need for immediate access to "decisionable data" in drug development, the need to control development costs, the need to shorten development times to protect patent life, the need to retrieve and analyze data for rapid response to regulatory and legal inquiries are but a few scenarios making the case for adapting to the new landscape in the pharmaceutical industry (18).

DOCUMENT MANAGEMENT PRINCIPLES

The traditional records management model is based on cabinets, folders, and files (9). This physical model was given its logical extension in the first electronic document management systems, where files were placed into virtual cabinets and folders.

File Room Model and Security

Security models for documents are all based on controlling who can see documents, who can create or edit documents, and who can delete documents. Securing these rights is implemented at numerous levels. It is illustrative to consider these in terms of a physical library or paper-based file room (9). First, you may need proper credentials simply to get in and browse the holdings. Second, once you've gained admittance to the filing area, your ability to view certain kinds of records may depend on your job title or departmental affiliation. Third, assuming you have rights to view a specific record, you may have permission only to view the final file (as opposed to a draft) under observation in the file room itself, and you may not be permitted to make a copy. Finally, if you are permitted to check the document out of the file room for a limited time, you will be required to sign your name to a dated logbook. Each of these constraints on your ability to interact with the holdings preserves the likelihood that files will remain unchanged for the next requestor and holds you accountable should they not.

Input–Output Model and Quality Control

Traditional document management rests on a very simple input–output model. An enterprise seeks to manage the storage of documents (input) in such a way that their retrieval (output) is simplified. The real goal is speedy retrieval of documents. Their intelligent storage is the means to achieve it. In most enterprises it will not do to sacrifice accuracy for speed, so the process must first attend to the security, integrity, and authenticity of the data being served. The enterprise must build in mechanisms to control and track input and output processes, which include versioning, searches, and collaborations or workflows. In the paperless environment, speed, intelligent storage, and accuracy of data and searching remain of paramount importance. As the paperless environment grows in volume and complexity, meeting these needs becomes increasingly difficult.

ELECTRONIC DOCUMENT MANAGEMENT SYSTEMS (EDMS)

Goals and Objectives

Electronic document management concepts have provided the bridge between traditional paper-based information management and the threshold of a new information age. The putative goals of moving from a paper-based to a paperless documentation system are to improve business processes and ultimately to enhance enterprise

performance and the bottom line by exploiting the numerous advantages of leaving paper behind (18). The core objectives that support the attainment of those goals include the following:

> Increase efficiency and effectiveness by stewarding the generation of paper and electronic documents within the individual's scope of control;
> Increase productivity by optimally using, reusing, and recycling enterprise documents where possible;
> Increase the consistency of classification, indexing, and retrieval of documents;
> Increase the sharing of documents within an organizational unit, and between and among organizational units, while maintaining necessary access controls;
> Preserve decision and accountability trails for documents;
> Automate the retention and disposal procedures for document review and retirement. Given these goals and objectives for paperless systems (19), it is perhaps helpful to look at the specific business and functional requirements that drive and enable them.

System Requirements

Before implementing any piece of technology in a business setting, it is necessary to define thoroughly both the business and functional requirements for the system. Business requirements describe, independently of technology, the high-level activities and processes that must be performed or enabled and the constraints that must be met by the system. Functional requirements outline in greater detail the lower level operations that must be performed and the constraints on the mechanisms for performing them.

Organization requirements: cabinet/folder structure

The most obvious business requirement for an EDMS is that it should enable the user to easily place and retrieve the items stored within. This means that files should be stored in the repository in an organized hierarchical file structure. Drug documents must be automatically stored in the appropriate location in the file structure based on their identifying information. Rather than having to manually place a file by navigating the entire hierarchy, which may be quite large in an enterprise with hundreds of compounds in various stages of development, a file could be placed following the entry of key content words or key file attributes (indexing information or metadata).

For a system managing documentation pertaining to the full life-cycle of drug development, including the conduct of clinical trials, a useful cabinet and folder hierarchy might resemble the following:

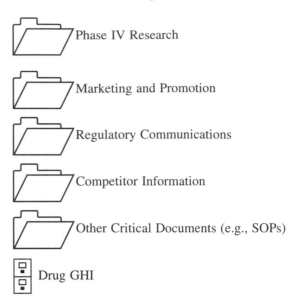

Drug ABC
Drug DEF

Patent Information

Chemical and Manufacturing Information

Nonclinical Research Information

Phase I Research

Phase II Research

Phase III Research

Study 123

Protocol

Case Report Forms

Data

Efficacy

Safety

Analysis Plan

Study Report

Study 456

Study 789

Phase IV Research

Marketing and Promotion

Regulatory Communications

Competitor Information

Other Critical Documents (e.g., SOPs)

Drug GHI

Input requirements: Creating and importing documents

The true business value of an EDMS is realized to the extent that it serves as more than just the terminus for document-related activities in an enterprise. To fully realize its goals, an enterprise paperless documentation system will perform functions across the entire document life-cycle. In addition to the storage of existing documents, users with appropriate system privileges must be able to create new electronic documents from within the electronic document management system. The system must explicitly support the file formats used by the business, which typically include word processing, spreadsheet, graphics, and database files.

An enterprise EDMS must be flexible enough to accommodate documents that do not originate within the system. It must be possible to import documents whether they are electronic or paper in format. Technologically speaking, there are no constraints on the files that can be stored in modern electronic document management systems. It should be noted, however, that certain file types (e.g., databases) cannot be rendered meaningfully to certain standard immutable display formats (e.g., PDF) and will often be viewed by default as read-only in the authoring application.

Modification requirements: Version control and document lifecycle

The ability to track changes in a fully rationalized manner is central to achieving enterprise objectives related to efficiency, data integrity, and accountability. To facilitate control over the full development lifecycle of documents, users with appropriate system privileges must be able to check out, modify, and check in documents.

In paper-based archives, questions about a document's authenticity or official status are usually answered by the surrounding policies and institutional mechanisms which dictate that only final and official documents are kept. In an EDMS environment, where document drafts are managed alongside their finalized counterparts, it is important to implement controls to ensure that the current version of a document is retrieved by default and that prior versions are retrieved only on explicit request. This is critical to both archiving and collaboration and workflow. The EDMS must implement a policy of nonreplication of documents and must also judiciously apply permissions to control changes in a document's life-cycle status. The system should distinguish between draft, review, approved, and final versions of a document and implement business rules defining security for the document based on its life-cycle status. For example, when a document is assigned a status of FINAL, users may view the document, but no one is permitted to modify it. The controls afforded by an EDMS should ensure confidence in answering questions about the official status or current version of a document.

Retrieving requirement: attributes and searching

In the digital age, ideas and information will be reprocessed and reused. Their portability and, consequently, their usefulness are dependent on the ability to find their particular data bit streams within a vast universe of binary number sequences. As the mass of documents in an enterprise EDMS grows and the filing structure that accommodates it both broadens and deepens, retrieving any specific item from the repository becomes more difficult. Speedy and accurate search and retrieval are achieved by allowing searches based on document content, attributes, or both. Users must also be able to save their queries for future reuse and store their queries in a centrally administered, single location. A simple FIND function must allow users to search either all versions of files or to restrict a search to only current versions of files. The system must validate and maintain a controlled list of category values and a controlled list of status values.

Searching for documents based on document content are "key word" searches using words or phrases. Document attributes, on the other hand, are summary information about the document, such as author's name, protocol number or drug name associated with the file, document title, modification date, business category, sponsoring business unit, document development milestones, project name, version status, version number, by which a document can be indexed. A document's attributes must uniquely identify it in the system. These

metadata allow for this intelligent searching through vast amounts of documentation. What metadata are captured at the time of document filing depends largely on the business requirements for searching through documents, though there are certain generic metadata that seem to apply across various settings.

As a company auditor, imagine we are confronted with the unwelcome but necessary chore of revisiting all approved contracts for the past five years undertaken by a particular division and involving a particular kind of endpoint analysis, "EP analysis," for compound XYZ. We need only briefly contemplate the prospect of searching through a paper-based archive for all occurrences of terms, say, "EP analysis" and "approved," to appreciate both immediately and fully the power of an electronic document management system. Even if we are able to physically separate all the paper contracts generated by the business unit in question, there is potentially still staggering work to be done in determining whether they involve the specified analysis or not. In a fully text-indexed EDMS with metadata indexing that anticipated the need for searching by business unit and the document type "contract," such a search would be trivial.

The richness of a business dialect probably varies directly with the specialization of the vertical market in which it competes. The ability to retrieve all relevant documents without having to specify every variant of equivalent terms can be of critical importance in performing effective and efficient searches. Such a method of searching through documents is the beginning of a movement away from the simple matching of string literals and towards the mining of data and meaning. The pharmaceutical industry is a striking example of an industry totally dependent on the ability to mine data and information for its economic viability.

In the end, EDMS systems allow for most effective searching when the filing hierarchy, indexing attributes, and some combination of full-text index, synonyms, or relevancy criteria are used in concert to specify the context around a particular search.

Output requirements: Viewing, printing, and exporting documents

Users with appropriate system privileges must be able to export documents in their native formats to any local or remote file systems to which they have access. Documents must be available for viewing in a standardized read-only format. Users must be able to view documents even if they do not have the native application. Users must also be able to match a printed or exported document to the original source file within the EDMS by means of unique system-generated identifiers referred to as watermarks.

Watermarks must not obscure any information on the document and must be in a standardized format. Watermarks must not be obscured when the document is bound.

Once a document is housed in an EDMS, it is very easy to publish it in many different places and still adhere to the principle of nonreplication. Enterprise intranets, local area networks (LANs) and wide area networks (WANs), make it possible to offer direct access to a document repository throughout an organization without requiring a physical replication of the database. Industrial strength document management systems are scalable and a single instance can support thousands of users. Also, even if the underlying filing hierarchy does not suit the needs of all customers, most EDMS packages allow for the repurposing of documents through a facility sometimes referred to as "virtual documents." This permits documents to be stored once in the repository but presented to various users in any number of ways. For instance, if both a clinical team and a biometrics team have their own standard document sets but each requires a copy of an investigator CV, two differently structured virtual documents can be created that each point to a single copy of the CV. Virtually all EDMS systems on the market today can serve as secure back-ends to web portals, enabling access to files stored in the system via ordinary HTML hyperlinks.

Electronic document management systems have the ability to distribute documents based on permissions or access control lists (ACLs). Document consumers can be notified automatically of a document's availability in the system. Once a file's status is updated to "final" or "approved," a message can be automatically sent to members of a distribution list alerting them that it has been published. Access to the document can be further streamlined by attaching to the email a pointer to the file in the EDMS.

Users with appropriate system privileges must be able to view documents. Typically, documents to be viewed in an EDMS are presented as read-only files, either in the authoring application or a standard immutable file format such as TIFF (Tagged Image File Format) or Adobe's portable document format (PDF). By virtue of its flexibility and platform-independence, PDF has become the storage standard in contemporary electronic document management systems (5). Most systems will automatically create PDF files and provide the PDF rendition in response to a user view request.

Workflow requirements: Collaboration and electronic approval

The pharmaceutical industry is a collaborative enterprise. An EDMS must provide the ability for users to electronically route documents with embedded messages to other users electronically for review and approval. The system must enable routing of multiple collaborative document types, such as SAS logs, lists, tables, graphics, datasets, and program files. The inclusion of routing features that enable files to be sent among users for review, annotation, and editing obviates the need for the handoff of multiple paper copies via interoffice mail. Moreover, the integration of such routing utilities with standard office email packages makes it possible to notify collaborators that an item is ready for review in the EDMS environment.

The capstone to fully electronic workflow and, indeed, the key to eliminating paper handoffs from the workplace is some kind of electronic approval facility. Electronic approval can be implemented in several ways, each of which is meant to substitute for a handwritten signature. Broadly construed, electronic signatures are linked to their owners in by verifying one of three things: (1) what the owner knows; (2) what the owner has; and, most secure, (3) what the owner is.

Encryption and certificate authorities

With the growth of electronic systems for creating, maintaining, and storing an organization's critical business documents, and with growing numbers of those documents existing only electronically, our electronic identities are forced to grow. Indeed, with increased mobility within and across job sectors, these electronic identities may span more than a single organization. In this light, encryption and digital certificates present an appropriate final issue to consider when confronting the security and validity of electronic approval. Certificate authorities (CAs) are the digital world's equivalent of passport offices. These businesses issue digital certificates and validate the holder's identity and authority. Public Key Infrastructures (PKIs) and digital certificates are most trustworthy when they are vouched for by a trusted certificate authority. CAs embed an individual's or an organization's public key along with other identifying information into each digital certificate and then cryptographically "sign" it as a tamper-proof seal, verifying the integrity of the data within it and validating its use (20).

What the signatory knows: This method of approval is the simplest to administer, because it relies on the assignment of unique ID and password combinations to every member of an enterprise, a practice that is already quite common as a result of the widespread application of networked computing.

What the signatory has: Here, approvals are issued by the use of a smart card or other object containing encoded identifying information.

What the signatory is: Arguably the most secure of the three approval methods, approval here relies on some sort of biometric identifier, some piece of physical and nonduplicable evidence of a person's identity. Such pieces of evidence include fingerprints, retinal vascular patterns, voice, and signature metrics, like speed, pressure, and stroke order (20).

Where electronic approval methods are implemented in the pharmaceutical industry, it will be of vital importance to comply with the FDA's Final Rule on Electronic Records and Electronic Signatures (21 CFR Part 11). In addition to broad guidance on the maintenance of the security and integrity of electronic records, the rule identifies specific requirements for the use of electronic signatures. First, signed records must indicate all of the following information: (1) the printed name of the signer; (2) the date and time of the signature; and (3) the meaning (e.g., review or approval). Second, the rule states that signatures executed to electronic records must be linked to the records in such a way that they cannot be excised, copied, or transferred to falsify an electronic record. Third, the rule establishes requirements around the uniqueness of electronic signatures to individuals within an organization and the controls that must be maintained to ensure that electronic signatures are used only by their genuine owners. Finally, and perhaps most importantly, 21 CFR Part 11 clarifies the necessity of notifying the users of electronic signatures that their electronic signatures are intended to be the legally binding equivalent of traditional handwritten signatures (2). The details of the rule surrounding electronic records and signatures are treated in greater detail later in this article

Security requirements: Protecting the corporate assets

Information and its knowledge base are the pharmaceutical company's most important asset after its people. The corporation's document management systems will either protect this asset or expose it to risk. Integrity of the information and assurance that the data were protected from fraudulent manipulation are at the heart of the new regulations (2) on controls for electronic records management systems. Technology has rationalized secure access to documents at each of the levels outlined in the schema of the paper-based file room. These levels range from broad to specific access privileges and are defined by (a) user login name (user security), (b) the user's affiliation with a group (group security), and (c) document status. The permissions associated with a given level of access entail those of all the more restrictive levels. For any user or group of users, the hierarchy of permissions is NONE, BROWSE, READ, WRITE, EDIT, DELETE, ALL.

Corporate network security: At the broadest level, access to the electronic file room must be monitored in the same way as access to the physical file room. A firewall is the equivalent of security guards at the entrance to the building. Corporate firewalls are barriers that exist between an enterprise's computer networks, or intranet, and any external network. Generally, firewalls filter inbound and outbound data, provide or manage public access to requested locations, deny all services except those explicitly permitted by the system administrator, log traffic and activity through the firewall, and activate alarms as prowlers are detected (21).

Database security: At the level of the EDMS application, access is governed by unique user ID and password combinations. Here, database security serves as the guard at the door who requests to see your badge before allowing entry. The system administrator maintains an updated register of valid IDs and passwords for gaining access to the system linked, typically, to the current list of employees maintained by human resources (9).

Folder security: As with our brick and mortar analog, entrance to the file room does not grant you free access to all the holdings. A folder may be accessible to a specific class of user. User permissions over folders are typically limited to NONE, BROWSE, or READ. The ability to CREATE folders is typically the restricted province of the EDMS administrators.

File security: While it may be that a specific class of user has access to the entire contents of a folder, it may just as well occur that members of that class have access to all documents in the folder with some exception. For example, Human Resources employees may have access to documents containing the terms of employment for all employees except those in Human Resources itself. Security must be applied to these particular documents in the EDMS such that they cannot be viewed by Human Resources personnel.

Version security: In the paper world, archival documents held in a file room are in some sense final drafts. Security for a product document must be determined by its status. The electronic document management environment in which documents are managed across their entire life cycle by its very nature allows for the inclusion of draft materials. So, in addition to permitting or disallowing the viewing of the final version of a file, the electronic world must consider and secure access to draft versions. Usually, only authors, editors, and reviewers of files have access to the drafts before they are finalized. Once files are promoted to final status, this version is then promulgated to a broader readership. The draft versions, by contrast, may continue to be accessible by the authors, or may be locked or purged from the system.

Disaster recovery

Any treatment of security in the context of document management would be remiss if it did not mention audit trails and disaster recovery.

The system must maintain a log of document creation, modification, or deletion. The automated log includes information about the document that was affected, the time at which the event occurred, and the user who caused the event (2).

Disasters include the full range of unplanned catastrophes, from internal or external sabotage to the extreme forces of nature, like fires, tornadoes, and earthquakes that do real damage to a corporation's physical assets. Each of these occurrences presents a serious risk to an enterprise's profitability and viability. It is, therefore, essential that disaster recovery plans be well-conceived and fully supported by management.

Retention requirements: Storage and deletion

In keeping with the dictum that an EDMS should enable management of files across the entire document lifecycle, the system should automate retention schedules. The system should calculate scheduled document expiry based on business rules that map to system file categories. The system should then be programmed to notify document owners, usually at some predefined interval prior to actual destruction, as a final check on extenuating business needs for extending retention. Business rules based on regulatory and statutory requirements can be built into the system's automatic monitoring and retention/deletion functionality. For a comprehensive discussion of storage media, see Pollnow (22).

Scheduled retirement of documents is especially critical in the pharmaceutical industry, where corporations are routinely subject to audits by the regulatory authorities or to discovery in litigation. In such cases, retention of draft documents and other aged files often unnecessarily increases the company's liability exposure. Although administered centrally, retention programs ideally devise a mechanism for notifying document owners prior to destruction, alienation, or transfer, as the document's owner may know of compelling business or legal reasons to delay the destruction of the document (23, 24). An EDMS allows an enterprise to automate and rationalize all aspects of the retention program, including scheduling, notification, and retirement.

The EDMS Toolbox

An electronic document management system is a configuration of design tools, data capture tools, messaging systems, repository databases, portals, and intra-/internetwork distribution and transfer options. There is no one magic bullet or single system that will provide solutions to the industry's document or knowledge management needs. With the almost daily introduction of new products, the best return on investment in technologies must be built on the principles of open architecture, best of breed products, and scalability. Designing, building, and constantly refining the corporate "digital nervous system" (18) is part of the cost of doing business in the paperless environment. In the next section we present an overview of key developments that undoubtedly will continue to redefine and reshape this complex and fluid corporate nervous system.

THE EMERGING PARADIGM

The transition from the paper environment to the early electronic environment was direct and intuitive. New computing models and technologies, however, are raising questions about the validity of this paradigm for complex information capture, access, and retention. In the current technology environment, forms, documents, data are not frozen, but dynamic and interactive. Communications and collaborations are as frequently machine to machine exchanges as direct human interactions.

It appears that in the rapidly evolving world of computing and communications (8, 25) the medium is indeed as important as the message. It is now possible to separate data and information from any document structure and technical platform. Whereas a document management system applies techniques of document locking, version control, and security to document objects, a component management system applies those same features to document fragments, or chunks, at a finer level of granularity. In other words, instead of checking out an entire document for editing, in a component management environment we may check out a single section, paragraph, or table. Much as the fundamental document objects that populate an EDMS can be combined in various ways as virtual documents, in a component management system document chunks form the basic elements and are "assembled" into whole documents. Component management is precisely the concept behind the regulatory search for a Common Technical Document (26).

The technology that enables both the creation of documents and the repurposing and redistribution of their content is XML, eXtensible Markup Language

(27). In terms of paperless documentation systems, XML signals a move from whole document management to component, or content, management. XML is a meta-language for describing languages that represent the content of a document. It is a subset of the Standard Generalized Markup Language (SGML), ISO Standard 8879, which has been around since 1986. SGML was devised as a means to create portable documents that are independent of any specific hardware or software.

HTML, which is also a subset of SGML, was developed as a means of transmitting hypertext documents over a network and specifies how a document should be displayed in a Web browser. HTML, however, describes neither the information content of a document nor its manner of organization. XML precisely fills this void by making use of tags and attributes to extend, validate, and unambiguously structure the content of a document.

Instead of viewing documents in an information system as passive objects to be served up to a human for reading, the SGML/XML paradigm regards them as active communications that can be parsed and manipulated by a computer. As such, they are data structures that can be used by computers rather than loose agglomerations of words, which can only be read by a human who comprehends the underlying grammar. XML's capacity to describe the content of a document as well as its organization makes it the ideal language for communication among both humans and machines. By encoding information in a format or tags that can be digested by both human and computational agents, XML is poised to become the true *lingua franca* of the Web in which both humans and silicon are initiators, brokers, and processors of transactions. To achieve this genuinely seamless communication, XML rethinks the very nature of documents themselves.

The usefulness of XML tags for structuring data presupposes the existence of a set of rules, or grammar, for their application. Such a grammar is embedded in either a Document Type Definition (DTD) or schema, both of which are defined by the XML author. A DTD is a set of syntax rules for tags. It establishes what tags may be used in a document, what attributes they have, and whether or not they can be nested inside other tags. Typically a DTD is maintained separately from a given XML document, though it can be part of it as well. Unlike HTML, which has a single DTD, XML supports as many user-defined DTDs as there are ways to structure information—thus, the extensibility. And also the danger. DTD's and, hence, XML are only as useful as the agreed upon standards that are used to implement them. The pharmaceutical industry stands to gain a great deal to the extent that it can establish and sustain extensive cross-corporation and FDA collab-

oration in the development of standard XML tags for its key documents. Should the industry fail to marshal a truly collaborative effort, it will have gained far less, being left instead with unique and peculiar DTDs and islands of XML that will exact a considerable cost to translate and maintain

Schemas are a newer development on the XML landscape. Like a DTD, a schema supplies the rules for building a document and indicates what tags may be used, what their attributes are, and how they relate to one another. Unlike a DTD, however, a schema has an additional level of specificity in that it can define data types. For example, a DTD might have a tag designated as <DOSE>, the content of which might be either numerical or a character string. A schema, by contrast, could ensure that the value entered was a number. This is clearly an appealing feature for the pharmaceutical industry, especially in the case of information exchange between databases or other applications making use of rigidly defined data types.

At the time of this writing, however, it still remains unclear whether schemas will overtake DTDs as the fundamental means of modeling XML documents.

XML structures document content but leaves presentation and formatting to other tools. The primary tool used for the job is now XSL, eXtensible Stylesheet Language. XSL consists of two parts: (1) a language for transforming XML documents and (2) an XML document for specifying formats. XSL allows users to process an XML document and dynamically render it to any number of formats. HTML, ASCII text, PDF, WML (wireless markup language) and XML itself are among the formats supported by the current technology.

XSL takes advantage of the intelligence built into the XML document to present its components in flexible ways. Thus, XSL does not merely apply style to the XML data; rather it evaluates, rearranges, and reassembles it. In fact, XSL permits multiple passes over an XML document so that information that appears once in the XML source can be presented multiple times in different formats within the same presentation. XSL, then, provides us with more than just an eye-catching rendition of XML data; it enables XML to realize its potential as flexible source information that can be created once but modified and presented infinitely many times. The application of this technology to the preparation and submission of information to multiple regulatory authorities is obvious.

Traditional paper models focused on discrete documents, file cabinets, and signature accountability. Setting aside the ability to commit fraud in any environment, the paper trail was clearly traceable from a physical file cabinet in the custody of a records manager responsible for a uniform indexing scheme to the data owner through the signature on the document. The computer network trail, on the contrary, runs through multiple virtual file cabinets under multiple ownership, custody, and indexing schema with multiple signatures or access authorities applied at both the data and systems levels. Added to this is the complex multilayered architecture supporting the exchange and communication of the information (28). All of these elements are the document. The medium can no longer be separated from the message.

THE REGULATORY ENVIRONMENT: EFFECT OF LEGISLATION ON TRADITIONAL AND EMERGING MODELS

Developments in paperless documentation systems for the pharmaceutical industry are intimately linked to regulatory developments.That "there is no alternative to moving towards complete electronic record keeping" is acknowledged by industry and regulators (29,30). The most documented environment in pharmaceutical industry is unquestionably the manufacturing segment. As early as 1983, FDA issued guidelines on the inspection of computerized systems used in drug manufacturing (31). In this environment, where there is no evidentiary trail to support either the compliance or integrity of claims and, where there is no documentation of data, messaging, transactions, actions, criteria applied, historical experience, audit experience, or staff experience and training, the event, action, collaboration, or data itself are considered nonexistent. Repeatedly and often, FDA officials have stated, "If it is not documented, it did not happen." FDA modeled the requirements and standards of the Final Rule on Electronic Records and Signatures (Part 11) on the GCMP regulations (32). The agency acknowledges that most predicate regulations, however, were written without contemplating the use of any technology other than paper (2). (Preamble Comment XVI.A, p.13462)

Basic differences between the manufacturing environment and other segments of the pharmaceutical industry, particularly the clinical research environment, pose additional special difficulties for industry and regulators in complying with and applying standards to the electronic management of data and documents. In the manufacturing environment, documentation of processes and results is fairly self-contained within a single location or plant. There is typically a single cohesive business culture focused on common deliverables where individual business units are relatively seamlessly integrated. At the other extreme, in the clinical research segment of the

industry, documentation of processes and results is spread across multiple locations (e.g., investigational sites, CRO facilities, laboratories, sponsor offices). There are multiple business cultures, each with distinct deliverables (e.g., research facilities, consultant services, data management groups, marketing departments, finance). These multiple cultures and business units are not typically well integrated by a paper or any other technology platform.

There have been four pivotal legislative developments between 1995 and 2000 impacting the pharmaceutical industry:

1. *FDA Final Rule on Electronic Records and Electronic Signatures* (effective August 20, 1997): This is a permissive regulation allowing any FDA-regulated industry to maintain paperless documentation systems that will be considered the legal equivalent of paper records and record keeping systems.
2. *ICH Recommendations for Electronic Standards for the Transfer of Regulatory Information (ESTRI)* (effective March and July 1997): This agreement by member states defines open nonproprietary international standards for electronic communications and the transfer of data and documents between industry and regulatory authorities.
3. *Government Paperwork Elimination Act, Title XVII of Pub.L. 105–277* (effective October 21, 1998): This is a U.S. law requiring federal agencies to be prepared to accept by 2003 electronic information from persons required to maintain, disclose, or submit information to the U.S. government.
4. *Electronic Signatures in Global and National Commerce Act* (effective October 1, 2000): Again, this is a U.S. law giving electronic signatures and electronically signed documents in commercial transactions the same legal status as handwritten signatures applied to paper documents.

The latter two laws, although specifically United States federal regulations, will impact all e-commerce transactions because of the importance of the U.S. economy in the world marketplace. U.S. industries will seek the competitive edge advantage provided by this legislation.

Regulatory authorities are fully aware of the complexities that the new, rapidly evolving computer environment poses for their oversight responsibilities. Both FDA and ICH wish to avoid rapid obsolescence by crafting regulations and guidelines based on open nonproprietary standards and generic tools such as Adobe Acrobat's free portable document format (PDF) codes and reader application. The ICH ESTRI Gateway agreement is the first step in attempting to define a platform independent environment.

Final Rule on Electronic Records and Electronic Signatures

FDA's Final Rule on Electronic Records and Electronic Signatures (the Final Rule, Part 11) requires special discussion since it is the most comprehensive regulation to date on applying computer technologies to regulated industry (33). The rule itself is contained on two Space consumption pages. The most important part of the rule for the pharmaceutical industry is, arguably, the Preamble, which comprises 34 pages of discussion on how and why the FDA made its decisions on the requirements it would enforce. The preambles to both the proposed rule making and the final rule making detail current regulatory thinking on and compliance concerns with paperless documentation systems (34).

Scope

The initial announcement of the proposed rule referred to the regulations as an electronic signature rule. By the time of publication of the Final Rule in the Federal Register (62 FR 13430, March 20, 1997) (2), the title had been expanded to "Electronic Records; Electronic Signatures." FDA rejected comments that would have limited the scope of the rule to signature authority and manifestation issues or to those records only that are required to be signed, witnessed, or initialed. The agency's rationale was that the "reliability and trustworthiness of the electronic signature depends in large measure on the reliability of the underlying electronic record" and that electronic records need to be reliable, trustworthy, and compatible with FDA's mandate to protect the public health "regardless of whether they are signed" (2). (Preamble Comment 26, p.13438) Therefore, regulation, in the agency's opinion, was required for electronic record keeping per se. By March of 1997, the regulatory authorities were fully aware of the power of the new computing and networking technologies and the communications explosions fostered by the internet and wireless possibilities.

Part 11 defines records management as the "creation, signing, modification, storage, access, and retrieval" of records and the software and hardware platforms used in these processes. This regulation applies to any documentation required by an FDA "predicate rule." The Authorities cited for the rule are Secs. 201–903 of the Federal Food, Drug, and Cosmetic Act (21U.S.C. 321–393); Sec. 351 of the Public Health Service Act (42 U.S.C. 262)]. For example, 21 CRF 820.70 requires documentation of process and production controls in quality systems for medical devices. This is a predicate rule. If any of this documentation is created, signed, modified, stored, accessed, or retrieved electronically, the requirements of Part 11 apply to the documentation and the hardware and software supporting it.

Applicability

There is a caveat to the application of Part 11. As noted, it is a permissive rule. Industry has the "option" of compliance. However, if a company currently uses any electronic systems to create, sign, modify, store, access, or retrieve records, it is presumed by the law that they have elected to follow the regulations and comply with the standards. Consequently, the company is subject to FDA enforcement of the rule under the food and drug regulations. If a company elects not to comply with the regulation, it must revert to all paper systems. No electronic systems are "grandfathered" under the Final Rule. Continued reliance on current electronic systems for any one of the electronic records management activities requires compliance with the requirements of Part 11 for security and controls (2). (Preamble Comment XVI.C.1, p. 13463)

Key issues

It is important for the industry to understand FDA's rationale in establishing these regulations, if appropriate and reasonable compliance policies and procedures are to be implemented. Any industry interpretation of the rule should be based on a thorough understanding of the preamble discussion of the final regulation (34). FDA's concern to protect the public health translates into four major issues addressed by the Final Rule: identification and authentication of data and source; system confidentiality and security; accountability for signing a document; and enforcement.

Identification and authentication of data and data source (audit trail): The ability to verify the integrity of records and to trace accountability for creation and modification of data are probably the most significant concerns of the FDA in relation to their ability to protect the public health and hold individuals and corporations accountable.

There must be a system-generated time-stamped audit trail, created independently of the operator of a system, for any access to, modification of, or deletion of records or the audit trail itself. This audit trail is intended to enable detection of record and signature falsifications and to provide an evidentiary trail in the event of falsification (2). (Preamble Comments 72–74)

Confidentiality and security (controls): FDA recognized that deliberate intent to commit fraud is very difficult to prevent (2). (Preamble Comment 7, p. 13433) Acknowledging this, the agency defined system control requirements at the operational, network, and device levels "to ensure that representations of database information have been generated in a manner that does not distort data or hide non-compliant or otherwise bad information, and that database elements themselves have not been altered so as to distort truth or falsify a record."

Requirements for controls are based on definition of "closed" or "open" system. Under these definitions there is no direct correlation between, for example, using a public phone line and an "open" system. Compliance with "closed" versus "open" standards is determined by how access rights to the data or documents are established and controlled by the owner(s) of this information. A system is defined as "closed" if access to the system containing the records or data is under the control of person(s) responsible for the content of the records or data in the system. A system is defined as "open" if access to the system is not under the control of the person(s) responsible for the content of the records therein. For example, dial-in retrieval over a public phone is "closed" where the records being accessed are under the control of the persons responsible for their content, whereas storage of records on a third party system is "open" because access to the records themselves is under the control of the third party. Sections 11.10 and 11.30 of the Final Rule list, respectively, the control measures required for establishing a "closed" or "open" system.

Access must be protected through use of unique biometric or digital identification technologies. Examples of biometric technologies include voice or fingerprint recognition. Nonbiometric or digital signatures must consist of two distinct identification codes such as a network user ID and password. All access rights and system supplied identification codes must be periodically reviewed, updated, and/or changed by the data/document owner(s) and all personal identification codes, such as passwords, periodically changed by the user to ensure that unauthorized parties do not gain access to the data/records. Open systems require an additional level of encryption on the data/records to prevent fraudulent access.

Accountability for signing (repudiation and links): Signatures can represent different intent and responsibility and the electronic signing must capture this metadata. Electronic signatures can be executed using biometric or digital technologies or a hybrid of these. Part 11 provides minimal standards and generic technical recommendations for ensuring that e-signatures can be unquestionably linked to their owners, cannot be repudiated, and are executed with clearly evident intent and understanding of the act of signing (35). Whatever final configuration of signature technologies is used, it must enable the FDA "to hold people (i.e., the individual) to the commitment they make under their electronic signature" (2). (Preamble Comment 19, p. 13456)

In fact, when it was suggested that FDA also hold business entities accountable as well as individuals, the agency rejected the idea because business entities do not sign records, individuals do (2). (Preamble Comment 90, p. 13450) (23)

Legal enforcement (authority, inspection, implementation): Part 11 cites the complete Federal Food, Drug, and Cosmetic Act as its authority for this regulation and for the scope of its enforcement jurisdiction. FDA wants "enforceable" baseline standards (2) (Preamble Comment 2, p. 13432) and intends to inspect any component of an electronic records and signature system that has bearing on the trustworthiness and reliability of the record or signature (2) (Preamble Comments 33, p. 13489). The agency reserves the right to conduct inspections, even of sensitive security systems, if deemed necessary "to enforce the provisions of the act and related statutes" (2). (Preamble Comments 32, p. 13439) Supplemental guidelines will provide additional detail on the standards against which FDA inspectors would judge compliance (7). FDA will consider the need for additional legislative initiatives or criminal law reform if their experience with the current rule warrants (2). (Preamble Comment 90 and 124, p. 13450 and p. 13458, respectively) The first FDA 483 inspection reports on compliance issues with Part 11 began to appear in 1999. Mr. Paul Motisse, widely considered FDA's architect of Part 11, was transferred to the inspection branch in the same year. As the agency gains experience and confidence with the new technologies, enforcement activities related to Part 11 will significantly increase.

Economic Impact

FDA asserts that the benefits of electronic record keeping in reduced review time and related business costs, such as space and rapid information access, will offset the costs of compliance with the rule (2). (Preamble Comment XVI.C.1, p. 13463) As industry and regulators enter the brave new paperless world, this remains to be verified.

It might be beneficial to discuss some of the current wisdom about the relative merits of paper-based and paperless documentation systems. Some of the claims about the outright superiority of electronic-based systems are perhaps overstated and highly context-dependent. Others probably have as much merit as their face value would seem to indicate. Table 1 provides a summary inventory of the pros and cons of the two models for document management.

Although a paper-based model for managing enterprise documentation appears to fall short of the promise for complex document management requirements, the

Table 1   Pros and cons of paper-based and electronic document management

Paradigm	Pros	Cons
Paper-based	Familiar Durable Transparent security model	Costly Inefficient searches Space consumption Inhibits leveraging of information assets Environmental impact Emphasis on separate repository function Audit management overhead
Digital	Space efficient Efficient searches Promotes leveraging of information assets Saves paper Integrates active file management and repository function Automates audit management	Durability of storage media Ever-changing technology standards High initial IT investment IT management overhead Environmental impact

paperless model is not without its own downside. Let us consider some of the issues in greater detail.

Cost

Paper-based systems are said to be costly. At roughly $0.10 per sheet of paper, printing and filing between 5 and 10 million pages—perhaps a conservative yearly estimate for an organization of 2,000 employees—would cost between $0.5 million and $1 million (19). Are digital documentation systems any less expensive given the costs of purchasing, servicing, and operating the component hardware and software systems? The answer depends on the level of digitization of the system. In a hybrid system, where some paper is printed and scanned into an electronic filing system, the average costs of implementing and maintaining a document indexing and scanning solution is $0.50 per page and ranges between $0.20 and $1.20 per page. It is difficult to assess the cost efficiencies of digitally based documentation systems for production and filing of documents. The full costs must include the initial investment in electronic systems and the outlays required to maintain them. It is no less incumbent on the pharmaceutical industry than any other e-commerce business to find a new measure, as precise as per page costs, for measuring its cost of doing business in the paperless environment (18).

Efficiency

Paper-based systems are increasingly considered inefficient. Relative to the file room scenario used to support the paper-based documentation model, it is hard to argue with the very real efficiencies afforded by the ability to search vast and disparately located document repositories electronically. In a paper-based environment, the effort required just to retrieve documents has been estimated to be on the order of 4–7 hours per week per person (19). This does not include the time required to travel physically from one's office to a file room, walk the aisles of the archives, peruse the shelves and folders, and finally to browse the file itself for the relevant passage. In a 2,000 person organization with 250 working days a year, this totals 50,000 to 87,500 person days per year across the organization.

By contrast, search and retrieval in an electronic environment is said to save 10 to 20 percent of the total individual work effort required, not just the effort required to retrieve documents. In one year, an electronic system would save this company 50,000 to 100,000 person-days of effort, potentially all the time spent searching in a paper-based system and more (19). If network downtime is equivalent to employee downtime, comparison between the two modes of search and retrieval appears absurd (36).

Space consumption

If the average enterprise professional creates approximately 500 documents a year, accumulates around 200–300 more from external sources, and an average document is from 5 to 10 pages in length, then an organization of 2,000 employees generates around 1 million documents containing some 5–10 million pages (19). Add the external documents and the organization contends with another 2 to 6 million pages. Continuing with the multiplication exercise, a ream of paper is about 2 inches thick, so given the above volumes an enterprise must find space to accommodate anywhere from 2,333 to 5,333 stacked feet of $8\frac{1}{2}$ by 11 inch paper, or between 1515 and 3463 cubic feet. In raw terms, the upper end of this volume will fit into a room measuring $35'$ by $10'$ by $10'$. When one considers that this does not take into account the folders, shelves, and aisle space required to intelligently store and navigate the documents, and that this is merely the volume of documentation encountered in a *single* year, entire floors of city-block-wide buildings can very rapidly disappear in an effort to retain it all.

Ten million pages requires about 500 gigabytes of disk storage space. The space occupied by the servers and disk drives for a decade worth of documents would probably not exceed the $35'$ by $10'$ room cited above as the minimum requirements for packing a year's worth of documents. Standard dimensions for 30-gigabyte hard drives on the market today are roughly $2.75''$ by $4''$ by less than half and inch in height. Simplifying somewhat, two hundred such drives, stacked one atop the other, would occupy less than 9 linear feet and only half a cubic foot. Even with the overhead required by server hardware, monitors, and the like, the space savings won by electronic storage of enterprise documentation are considerable. However, in the digital world, the cost of bandwidth is a major factor in "digitalizing" the workplace in both large and small corporate budgets (37).

Environmental impact

The high-tech digital alternative must be vastly more "green" by these measures. Yet, it is not immediately clear that the paperless documentation system is as environmentally friendly in practice. In general, the high-tech industry is pretty dirty. Chip manufacturing involves hundreds of chemicals (e.g., acids, cyanide compounds, silicon tetrachloride), many of them toxic or carcinogenic alone and, perhaps, more so in combination (39–42). The industry also wastes prodigious amounts of water, and pollutes both air and water (43). The reality of Moore's Law, which roughly states that the power of computer technology (i.e., the miniaturization and data density of transistors and microchips) doubles every 18 months, has landfills overflowing with obsolescent machines and components (44). Consider also the power required to operate electronic document management systems. The presumed environmental advantages, which prima facie seem obvious, are in fact not so clearcut.

Current wisdom maintains that paperless documentation systems are more environmentally friendly than paper-based systems. If an enterprise implements a system in which documents are generated, stored, and retrieved electronically, it can conceivably preserve the number of

trees corresponding to the number of sheets of paper it would otherwise generate. In a 2,000 person organization, which produces 10 million documents, that amounts to 850 trees a year (19). Typical offices produced 100 lbs of paper per head in 1975. In the still burgeoning paperless office, they produce more than 200 (1). One might argue that the paper industry exacts as in an even more terrible toll in terms of sulfur dioxide, resinous acid effluent (38).

Storage and durability

With respect to the most fundamental security issues (i.e., a document's persistence through time), it is rather easy to assume that digitized information, with its tight controls, rigid architecture and underlying ingenuity, must somehow offer greater long-term protection of stored document assets. To do so, however, is both to underestimate the durability of paper as a storage medium and overestimate that of digital media and the dominance of any single technology platform capable of reading digital media formats. Ineluctable technological obsolescence is perhaps the greatest threat to the preservation of electronic documents and data (45–48).

The above considerations have direct bearing on the presumed economic impact of regulations for the pharmaceutical industry on electronic record keeping systems. The pharmaceutical industry is, in fact, faced with a complex, costly development and implementation project once it heads down the road of electronic record management within the regulated parameters of Part 11. These costs and the attendant legal issues will increase within a fully digitalized, paperless environment. The key to a return on investment for the industry will be its ability to integrate and strategically plan technical implementations across multiple business divisions (49, 50).

CONCLUSIONS

Digital tools provide instantaneous distributed access to original experience. In a paperless world, one that is mobile, wireless, and extremely portable, customers seek data versus documents (37). Documents have become data embedded in inseparable multiple layered architectures (28). Technological and economic forces have essentially redefined document formats and purposes. The goal is more and more to preserve or re-create the immediacy of a communicative act, just-in-time delivery, real-time updates

"Document objects" have, in addition to text, come to include databases/spreadsheets, graphics, images, video, audio, web sites. What a document used to be is now a small part of documentation—audit trails, metadata, etc.—where documentation of immediate experience is immediately available to third parties. Documentation is now an environment of dynamic interactive support as opposed to the static support of imaged paper.

The pharmaceutical industry is traditionally document driven. The technology exists currently, however, for conducting research, manufacturing product, and promoting prescription drugs in a totally paperless environment. Several years ago the CEO of Boeing Corporation threw down a gauntlet to the aerospace industry. He asked what would happen if they designed and built a plane without any paper, and succeeded in doing it. In 1999, Bill Gates laid out the business case (18) for conducting any business as e-commerce. Both individuals were visionaries in understanding the possibilities of the new information technologies and translating them into a competitive edge for their industries.

Within the clinical research arena, the CRF, for example, will become a metaphor for a complex, multidimensional process of data collection providing an on-line interactive profile of the subject's experience and data. New technologies such as voice recognition, digital medical imaging, targeted drug discovery techniques, revolutions in computing design and power (8, 25) and the genome project (51, 52) are redefining for both industry and regulators how we capture and manage subject-specific data in a meaningful profile of an individual subject's experience. These same technologies, especially as they enable the discovery, mapping, and repeated use of genetic information, will redefine the execution and need to monitor informed consent rights for subjects. The protocol itself will be redefined as a set of "edit checks," access rights, system administration rules, and metadata structures controlling the on-line collection, verification, and analysis of data.

How should the pharmaceutical industry apply these possibilities to drug development and marketing? Fully "digitalizing" clinical research, for example, would revolutionize the industry's concepts of document, data, and regulatory review. It is no less impossible to apply Boeing's challenge to the manufacturing sector. Of all the areas in the industry, marketing, which is built on messaging and interactive communications, has innumerable models and other industry experience with e-commerce. Within the next five years, the industry needs to challenge its traditional thinking on pharmaceutical documentation and thoroughly explore the possibilities and issues involved in abandoning traditional paper paradigms for a fully digital environment (49, 53).

How can the regulatory agencies respond to this new environment in keeping with their legal mandate to protect the public health? The regulators have begun to tackle some of the issues in the Final Rule on Electronic Records (2) and the ICH ESTRI agreement (5). This legislation is merely the tip of a large, complex "iceberg" of law, public policy, and oversight techniques. Traditional documentation will become a metaphor for complex, integrated data capture and repository systems linked to enable dynamic "on-the-fly" profiling, analysis, and reporting of research and discovery results almost simultaneously with the direct research experience. The pharmaceutical industry, its regulators, and the consuming public have entered into a brand new collaborative world.

Glossary of Technical Terms

A comprehensive listing and definition of terms is available at http://www.webopedia.com

REFERENCES

1. Brown, J.S.; Duguid, P. *The Social Life of Information*; Harvard Business School Press: Boston, 2000.
2. *21 CFR Part 11: Electronic Records; Electronic Signatures; Final Rule*, Food and Drug Administration, 62 FR 13429, March 20, 1997.
3. *Government Paperwork Elimination Act*, Pub.L.105–277, Office of Management and Budget, Executive Office of the President, Proposed Implementation (64 FR 10895, March 5, 1999).
4. *Electronic Signatures in Global and National Commerce Act*, Pub.L.106–229, June 30, 2000.
5. *Electronic Standards for the Transfer of Regulatory Information (ESTRI)*, International Conference on Harmonization. M2 Recommendations, March 1997 (1.1–5.1) and July 1997 (5.2–5.3).
6. *Good Manufacturing Practice Guide for Active Pharmaceutical Ingredients*, International Conference on Harmonization, July 19, 2000; Draft Consensus Guideline.
7. Guidance for Industry: Computerized Systems Used in Clinical Trials, Food and Drug Administration, April 1999.
8. Mann, C.C.; Rotman, D.; Waldrop, M.M.; Garfinkel, S.L.; Regalado, A. Beyond Silicon: The future of computing. Technol. Rev. **2000**, *103* (3), 42–84.
9. Sutton, M.J.D. Chapter 8: Developing the Physical Model. *Document Management for the Enterprise: Principles, Techniques, and Applications*; John Wiley & Sons: New York, 1996; 223–244.
10. Harvey, D. *The Condition of Postmodernity: An Enquiry into the Origins of Cultural Change*; Blackwell: Cambridge, 1989.
11. Carlston, D. *Storing Knowledge*; www.longnow.com (accessed Oct 2000) Time & Bits.
12. Rehr, D. *The First Typewriter*; dcrehr@earthlink.net (accessed Oct 2000).
13. Carlson, C.F. *The Photocopier*; www.mit.edu (accessed Oct 2000).

14. *Word Processing; Information Processing*; www.britannica.com (accessed Oct 2000) Encylopaedia Britannica.

15. Connolly, D. *A Little. History of the World Wide Web*; www.w3.org (accessed Nov 2000), 1945–1995.

16. Bush, V. As We May Think. Atlantic Monthly **1945**, *176*, 101–108.

17. Sutton, M.J.D. Chapter 1: The Transition to Enterprise Document Management. *Document Management for the Enterprise: Principles, Techniques, and Applications*; John Wiley & Sons: New York, 1996; 1–22.

18. Gates, B. *Business @ The Speed of Thought, Using a Digital Nervous System*; Warner Books: New York, 1999.

19. Sutton, M.J.D. Chapter 3: Planning for Enterprise Document Engineering. *Document Management for the Enterprise: Principles, Techniques, and Applications*; John Wiley & Sons: New York, 1996; 53–92.

20. Yakal, K. Sign on the Digital Line. *PC Magazine*; Sept 19, 2000; 32–36.

21. Chapman, D.B.; Zwicky, E.D. *Building Internet Firewalls*; O'Reilly and Associates, Inc.: New York, 1995.

22. Pollnow, R.A. *Alphabet Soup, Acronyms Everywhere—Media Options in Data Storage*; Sept/Oct 2000; 44–47.

23. *Information Requirements Clearinghouse. Legal Responsibility for Records in a Corporation*; http://www.irch.com/irch_article2.htm (accessed Sept 2000).

24. *Information Requirements Clearinghouse. Legal Requirements for Filing Systems and Indexes*; http://www.irch.com/irch_article2.htm (accessed Sept 2000).

25. Williams, S. Computing After Silicon. Technology Review **2000**, *102* (5), 92–96.

26. *Organization of the Common Technical Document for the Registration of Pharmaceuticals for Human Use*, International Conference on Harmonization, July, Draft Consensus Guideline.

27. Bosak, J.; Bray, T. *XML and The Second-Generation WEB*; www.sciam.com (accessed Sept 2000): .

28. Horak, R.; Miller, M.A. Chapter 7: Fundamentals of Data Communications. *Communications Systems & Networks: Voice, Data, and Broadband Technologies*; M&Tbooks; Division of MIS: Press, Inc.; Subsidiary of Henry Holt and Company, Inc.: New York, 1997; 155–184.

29. *PhaRMA (Pharmaceutical Manufactuers' Association) Position Paper on 21CFR Part 11*, Docket No. 92N-0251Nov 30, 1999.

30. Raymond, R.; Galle, S.; Collom, W. Regulatory Submissions: From CANDA/CAPLA to 2002 and beyond. Drug Information Journal **2000**, *34* (3), 761–774.

31. Guide to Inspection of Computerized Systems Used in Drug Processing, U.S. Department of Health and Human Services, Public Health Service, Food and Drug Administration National Center for Drug and Biologics and Executive Director of Regional Operations, Feb 1983.

32. *Annual Report for 1999*; Food and Drug Administration, Office of Compliance.

33. Hoff, S. The Regulatory Environment for the New Millennium. Drug Information Journal **2000**, *34* (3), 659–672.

34. Woodrum, P. 21 CRF 11—more than meets the eye. Applied Clinical Trials **June 2000**, 86–94.

35. Bleicher, P. Sign Here, Please, Mr. Bondh. Applied Clinical Trials **August, 2000**,28–31.

36. Brin, S.; Page, L. *The Anatomy of a Large-Scale Hypertextual WEB Search Engine*; http://www7.scu.edu.au/programme/fullpapers/ 1921/com1921.htm (accessed Sept 2000).

37. Gingrande, A. *Wireless Applications For a Brave New World*; Sept/Oct 2000; 66.

38. http://www.greenpeace.org/toxics/reports/gopher-reports/papdam.txt (accessed Sept 2000).

39. Ayers, J. Controlling the Dangers of High-Tech Pollution. EPA Journal **1984**, *10*, 14–15.

40. Hayes, D. *Behind the Silicon Curtain: The Seductions of Work in a Lonely Era*; Black Rose Books: London, 1989.

41. Miller, M.W. Findings of Toxin Leakage in Silicon Valley Hurt Chip Makers' Reputation for Safety. Wall Street Journal **Aug 29, 1984**.

42. Seigel, L.; Markoff, J. *The High Cost of High Tech: The Dark Side of the Chip*; Harper & Row: New York, 1985.

43. Bills, B. *High Tech Toxins: Is the Computer Industry as Clean as it Seems*; www.canada.cnet.com (accessed Oct 2000).

44. Yang, D.J. *On Moore's Law and Fishing: Gordon Moore Speaks Out*; www.usnews.com (accessed Nov 2000).

45. Rothenberg, J. *Ensuring the Longevity of Digital Documents*; www.sciam.com (accessed Sept 2000).

46. Izarek, S. *Archiving Today's Digital Culture*; www.foxnews.com (accessed Oct 2000).

47. Lesk, M. Going Digital: Electronic Libraries will Make Today's Internet Pale by Comparison. But building them will not be easy. *Scientific American*; www.sciam.com (accessed Sept 2000).

48. Brand, S. Written on the Wind. *Civilization Magazine*; www.civmag.com (accessed Oct 2000).

49. Moore, G. *A Balanced Buy*; www.Darwinmag.com (accessed Nov 2000).

50. Heck, M. *Document Management Fuels e-Business*; www.infoworld.com (accessed Sept 2000).

51. Regalado, A. Mining the Genome Project. Technology Review **2000**, *102* (5), 57–63.

52. Philipkoski, K. *Genome Map Heralds Cheap Drugs*; www.wired.com (accessed Sept 2000).

53. Buderi, R. The Corporate Logic. Technology Review **2000**, *103* (3), 88–90.

PARTICLE-SIZE CHARACTERIZATION

Brian H. Kaye
Laurentian University, Sudbury, Ontario, Canada

SAMPLING PROCEDURES

The subject of powder sampling has been addressed extensively in standard reference books. Several companies sell sampling equipment for installation in industrial systems (1–7). Even when the sample received by the laboratory is a representative sample, the analyst still faces the difficult task of taking a small subsample from the powder supplied. It has been shown that one of the most efficient devices for taking a subsample of the powder is known as the spinning riffler, shown in Fig. 1a. It consists of a ring of containers that rotates under the powder supply. The total powder supply is processed using this instrument. It has been shown that to obtain a representative sample, the time of powder flow through the apparatus divided by the time of rotation of the ring of containers should be a large number (4, 7). Difficulties arise using such devices with very fine powders because air currents caused by the rotation of the system can blow the fines away. Furthermore, if the powder is cohesive (sticky), the powder flow through the funnel can be impeded. In some situations, the flow properties of the powder can be modified by adding a silica flow agent, provided this does not interfere with the size characterization procedures used subsequent to the sampling procedure (8).

Another approach to the sampling of powders has been developed by Kaye and coworkers. In this procedure, the powder is thoroughly mixed in such a way that any sample taken at random is a representative sample (9, 10). The equipment used in this technique is shown in Fig. 1c. The mixing chamber is placed in a rotating drum lined with dimpled foam. The foam serves two purposes: first, it promotes quiet tumbling of the chamber, and second, it accentuates the lifting power of the rotating drum so that it lifts the partially filled chamber up the wall of the drum until it tumbles chaotically to a new position of equilibrium before it is again lifted up for the next tumble. The chaotic tumbling of the mixing chamber creates ideal conditions for powder mixing, and short mixing times have proved to be efficient in mixing the ingredients (11). At the end of the tumbling procedure, a small sampling cup attached to the lid of the mixing chamber is used to retrieve a representative sample. The tumbling chamber can have various geometric shapes, and provided that dimpled foam is used, even a common laboratory jar can be tumbled. Efficiency of mixing is reduced if the jar is more than half-full, because this imposes restrictions on the free, random movement of the powder in the chamber. It is recommended that this type of device be used to homogenize any powder sample before using a subsample in an experimental investigation, if the sample has been kept for some time or has been poured in a laboratory environment. Powder segregation mechanisms are far more widespread in the laboratory than generally known (12, 13).

In Fig. 2, a new pneumatic sampler developed by Kaye and coworkers is shown. This instrument has the advantage that one can take a sample of any specified size by changing the position of the sintered frit in the central tube that is used when the sample is drawn into the equipment. Lubricating air provided through both concentric tubes enables the sampling device to be moved to a particular location within a powder. When the sampling location is reached, the airflow to the center tube is reversed to draw in the desired sample (14).

For sampling an aerosol system, a cascade impactor is used to fractionate the aerosol into various size ranges. A full discussion of these instruments has been reported by Kaye (1). Aerosols can also be sampled through various filter systems for subsequent examination by image analysis procedures. If the aim of the sampling process is to generate a deposit that can be examined through a microscope with an imaging system, surface filters, such as the Nucleopore filter and similar polycarbonate filters, are available in various pore sizes for filtering aerosols (15–17). The traditional paper filter is described technically as a depth filter. Although depth filters can sometimes be rendered transparent by using immersion oil, it is normally difficult to view the fine particles on depth filters because they penetrate into the pore structure of the filter (18).

The study of the size distributions of therapeutic aerosols creates a very difficult sampling task for the specialist. Wherever possible, size characterization of an aerosol system should be carried out in situ, using diffractometers as discussed later.

Encyclopedia of Pharmaceutical Technology

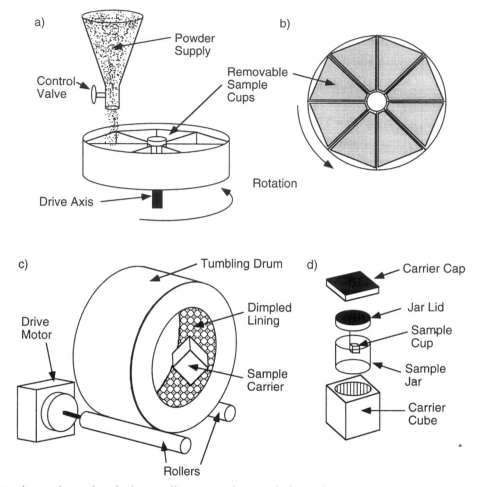

Fig. 1 Two devices that can be used to obtain a small representative sample from a larger supply. a) Systematic representative sampling of a powder can be achieved with the spinning riffler (7); b) the spinning riffler is composed of several removable sample cups; c) chaos-generating devices, such as the free-fall tumbling mixer, can be used for powder homogenization and sampling (11); d) exploded view of the sample carrier.

SAMPLE PREPARATION

In many situations, a powder sample to be characterized has to be prepared in a specified format for the characterization procedure. Thus, the powder may have to be spread out on a glass slide before microscopic examination, or a suspension of the material may have to be prepared in an appropriate liquid or gas. The act of dispersing the powder to be studied can change its size distribution radically, and the procedure used to prepare the sample for characterization should allow for what is known as the operational integrity of the fine particles. Thus, if the powder is to be dispersed in water, the use of ultrasonics to disperse it in the liquid can result in the shattering of agglomerates that would normally persist throughout the manufacturing and usage processes.

In general, the technology used to disperse a powder before a characterization study should match the severity of dispersion forces that the powder will experience in use. Alternatively, if ultrasonics is used to generate a well dispersed powder, the analytical procedure protocol should be defined rigorously to avoid variations from operator to operator. Dispersing agents are frequently used, and great caution should be exercised because they can alter the structure of the system in a fundamental manner (19).

SIZE CHARACTERIZATION OF FINE PARTICLES AND POWDERS

Direct Examination with Microscopes and Other Imagining Devices

Extensive pioneering fine particle characterization studies were carried out by Heywood and Hausner, respectively,

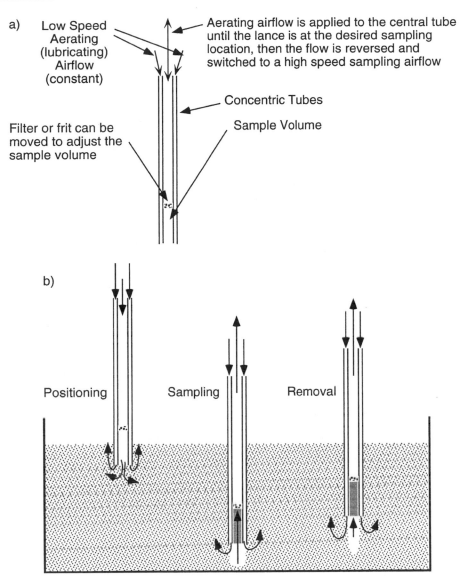

Fig. 2 The improved pneumatic lance is constructed from concentric tubes. Low-speed aeration from both tubes allows the lance to be inserted with minimum disturbance to the powder supply. Once the sampling location is reached, a high-speed flow is applied to the central tube to capture a sample below the filter or frit. a) Construction of the pneumatic sampler; b) process used to obtain a sample from a bulk of powder.

by examining images through microscopes and other imaging devices (20, 21). In these early works, the areas, or dimensions, of profiles were measured by direct comparison of the profile images with sets of reference circles engraved on what was known as an eye piece reticule (1). Recently, several sophisticated systems have been developed for computer-aided image analysis (1, 22).

The increased power of processing logic, available in modern computer-aided analysis systems, makes it possible to characterize the shape of fine particle profiles using Fourier analysis techniques and to describe

structures by means of fractal dimensions. The Fourier analysis techniques can be carried out in one or two dimensions (23). When exploring the structure of a profile in one-dimensional space by means of Fourier analysis, a reference point is located within the profile, and a geometric signature waveform is generated by rotating a vector at uniform angular velocity around the perimeter of the profile. The magnitude of the vector plotted against the angle of the vector generates the waveform. This waveform is subjected to Fourier analysis to generate a power spectrum of the various harmonics contributing to the structure of the waveform. This technique is useful for rounded objects but generates complex information if there are deep convolutions or sharp edges on the profile. For such profiles, two-dimensional Fourier transforms can be generated by computer (23, 24).

A different procedure for describing the structure of rugged profiles has been developed from the theorems of fractal geometry (24–29). The basic concept used in fractal geometry is to add a fractional number to the topological dimension of a system to describe the space-filling ability of the system being described. Thus, in Fig. 3a, all the lines have a topological dimension of one. The fractional number added to this dimension creates the boundary fractal dimension of the line, a parameter that describes the ruggedness of the line. In Fig. 3b, the basic logic used to evaluate the fractal dimension of a profile of a powder grain by the equipaced method is shown. Polygons are constructed on a digitized form of the profile, a sequential set of x,y coordinates representing the profile, by pacing out a given number of steps around the profile. Polygons constructed in this way become perimeter estimates at the inspection resolution represented by the number of steps paced out along the profile. The perimeter estimate and the resolution are normalized with respect to the maximum projected length of the profile. To estimate the magnitude of the fractal dimension of the profile, the normalized values of the perimeter estimates are plotted against the normalized resolution, as indicated in Fig. 3c. This plot is known as a Richardson plot after a pioneer of the detailed studies of convoluted profiles such as these of islands (25, 26). The slope of the data lines on the Richardson plot represents the fractional number that has to be added to the topological dimension to describe a structure of the boundary. As with the profile studied in Fig. 3b, some fine particle profiles exhibit different fractal dimensions at different levels of inspection. Thus, in this profile, what is known as the structural boundary fractal dimension is revealed by the course resolution data, and what is known as the textural boundary fractal dimension is revealed at high-resolution inspection. The structural fractal dimension probably governs the packing and flow properties of a powder, whereas the texture governs the dissolution rate, adsorptive capacity, and chemical activity.

Because of the large amount of visual information imparted by an image of a fine particle, there has been a tendency to regard image analysis inspection as a fundamental method against which all others should be measured. The principal problem involved in the inspection of a system by image analysis is the difficulty of deciding what constitutes a separate and operationally functional fine particle. A failure to record the density of coverage of the surface used in a microscopic study of a

powder is a major source of uncertainty in the value of the reported data, because random juxtaposition of fine particles on a surface can make them appear as preexisting agglomerates (30).

Sieve Fractionation

Sieving is a widely used method for characterizing the range of grain sizes present in a powder. In this technique, a quantity of powder is separated into two fractions on a surface containing holes of a specified uniform size. The two main problems associated with sieve characterization are the difficulty of determining the point at which the fractionation process is complete and coping with the variation in sieve apertures present in new and worn sieves. For a discussion of see Refs. 1 and 22. The photomicrograph of a woven wire sieve surface in Fig. 4a illustrates the problems associated with the variations in sieve apertures. In Fig. 4b the data on the variation of the sieve apertures as characterized by various studies are plotted (31). The midpoint diameter of the trapezium created by the projected image of the woven wire surface provides the operational diameter of the sieve, and the size distribution of the apertures can be measured with the help of image-analysis techniques. The size distribution determined in this way can then be normalized by the nominal aperture of the sieve. It can be demonstrated from the data in Fig. 4b that the aperture distribution is Gaussian.

In an alternative technique, spherical glass beads are separated on the sieve, and when the remaining oversize beads are poured off of the sieve, the near mesh-sized beads trapped in the mesh are removed by inverting the sieve and giving it a sharp rap on a surface. The beads collected in this way are then sized. If an irregularly shaped powder is used in such an experiment, a typical set of grains trapped in the openings of the sieve allows one to determine the shape distribution of the profiles, as illustrated in Fig. 5. Electroformed sieves have a much narrower distribution of aperture sizes but are more fragile and expensive than woven wire sieves (1).

Sedimentation Techniques

Sedimentation procedures to evaluate particle size in terms of the equivalent spheres, which have the same settling speed in laminar flow conditions, are the basis of many techniques used to characterize fine particles. A suspension of fine particles is prepared, and their falling speed is determined with an immersed balance pan or by monitoring the settlement of the fine particles with the help of light or X-ray beams. The measured falling speeds of the fine

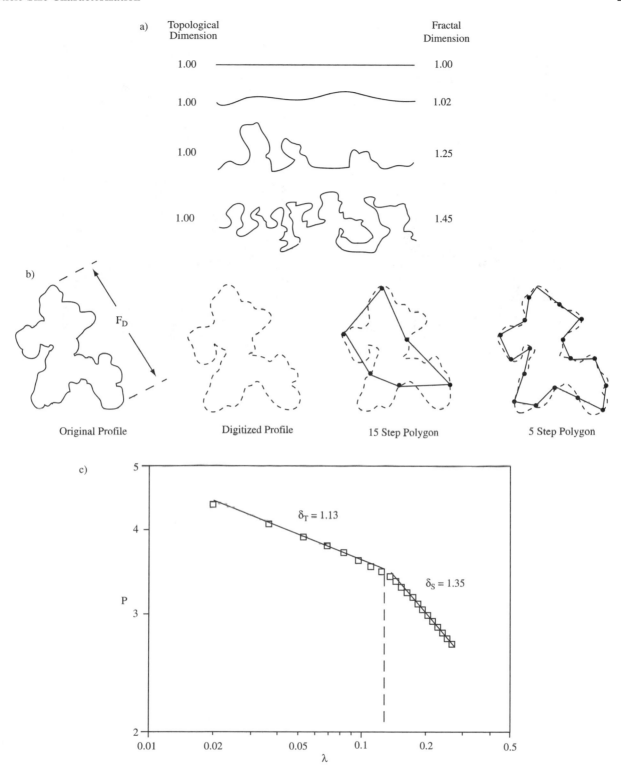

Fig. 3 Fractal dimensions can be used to evaluate the rugged structure of fine particles. a) Fractal dimensions used to describe the ruggedness of various lines; b) physical basis of the equipaced exploration technique for evaluating the fractal dimensions of rugged boundaries; c) data generated by the equipaced exploration technique for the profile of b; δ_S; structural boundary fractal dimension; δ_T; textural boundary fractal dimension.

a)

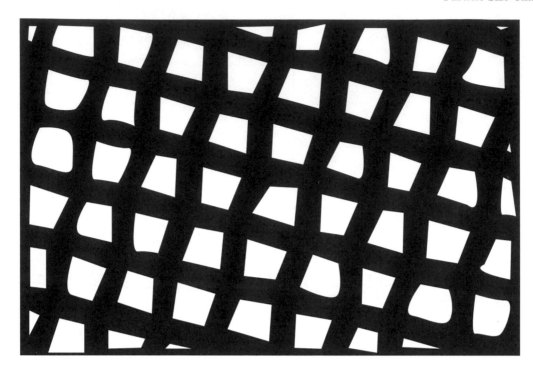

b)

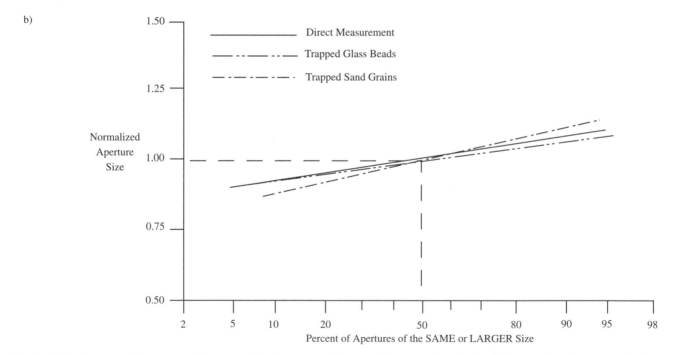

Fig. 4 Variations in mesh apertures of a woven wire sieve can be determined by several methods. a) Photograph of a woven wire sieve; b) the variations in sieve apertures can be determined either by direct inspection of the aperture or by examining near mesh size fine particles trapped in the apertures during the sieving process.

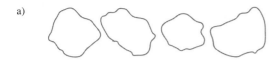

a)

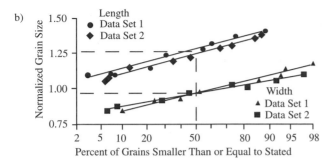

b)

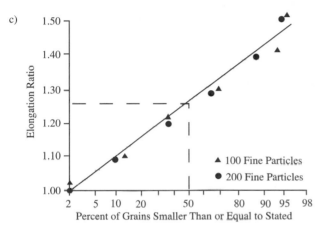

c)

Fig. 5 When calibrating a sieve mesh with trapped irregularly shaped grains, a subset of powder grains is obtained that can be used to generate a shape description of the powder grains (31). a) Profiles of typical sand grain trapped in a sieve mesh; b) length and width distributions of sand grains trapped in a sieve mesh; c) elongation ratio (shape) distribution for sand grains trapped in a sieve mesh.

particles are inserted, along with the other appropriate parameters of the suspension, into Stokes' equation

$$d_s = \sqrt{\frac{18\eta t}{(\rho_P - \rho_L)gh}}$$

where d_s = Stokes diameter of the fine particle; η = viscosity of the liquid; g = acceleration due to gravity; h = distance through which the fall is timed; t = time required to fall the distance h; ρ_P = density of the powder; and ρ_L = density of the liquid.

The configuration of the actual instrument used to measure the Stokes diameters of fine particles varies among instrument manufacturers (1, 22). Devices that

monitor the fine particle sedimentation with a light beam are known as photosedimentometers. Because of the difficulties of interpreting the concentration measurement of fine particles with diameters close to that of the wavelength of the light being used to monitor the dynamics of the suspension, some instruments use X-Ray beams to monitor the fine particle movements. Other instruments use centrifugal force to accelerate the settling dynamics of the suspended fine particles.

Sedimentation methods were the dominant size-characterization procedures in the 1950s and 1960s. In recent years, they have been replaced in the powder laboratory by the diffractometers. Diffractometers have the advantage of speed, but problems occur in the interpretation of the diffracted light signals. The X-ray-based sedimentometer manufactured by the Micromeretics Corporation, called the Sedigraph, is still widely used, partly because its use is written into some industrial standards governing size-characterization procedures (32, 33).

In recent years, disk centrifuges have been revived to characterize fine particles smaller than 1 μm, basically because of the work by Provder and coworkers in cooperation with Brookhaven Laboratories Ltd. (34).

Diffractometers

The advent of the laser has made the generation of diffraction patterns by a suspension of fine particles a relatively easy task. At the same time, the rapid development of computer-processing equipment and specialized photocells has made it possible to process the information in a group diffraction pattern to generate the particle size distribution of the fine particles in suspension. One of the first commercially available devices for generating size-distribution information from group diffraction patterns of a randomly dispersed array of fine particles was the CILAS device (Denver Autometrics, Inc., Boulder, CO) first developed in France to measure the size distribution of cement (35). Companies that have developed diffractometers do not divulge the structure of their software. The user of this equipment should be careful to obtain information on the data-processing protocol followed in any specific instrument to change the diffraction information into a size-distribution function. Some of the instruments assume a given distribution function and curve fit to accelerate the data processing. Sometimes such curve fitting can distort the data generated (36). Several manufacturers of these instruments provide extensive technical data on their performance, and the International Standard Organization is currently preparing a standard procedure for diffractometers. The laser diffractometers are particularly useful for studying the size distributions of sprays and aerosol clouds (37–43).

Time-of-Flight Instruments

Another type of instrument that has been made possible by the availability of lasers is known as the time-of-flight instrument. Here, a narrow focused beam of laser light explores an area of a suspension. The size of the particles in suspension is measured by the time it takes for a laser beam to pass across the profile of the fine particle. Sophisticated optical recording devices and electronic editors are used to generate the size distribution data from the information generated by the device.

An instrument developed and marketed by Galai Instruments (Haemek, Israel), sold in the United States for

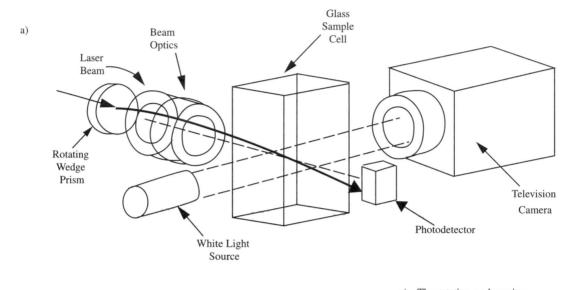

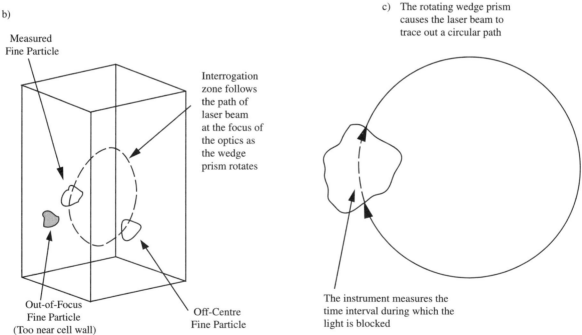

Fig. 6 The Galai particle-size analyzer uses a laser beam and a rotating wedge prism to measure the size of fine particles by the length of time the fine particle blocks the light reaching the photodetector. a) Basic layout of the Galai instrument; b) the laser beam traces a circular path within the sample cell, and the logic of the instrument rejects any particles that are off-center or out of focus; c) the length of time that the laser beam is blocked is related to the size of the fine particle. (From Ref. 44.)

several years by the Brinkmann organization but now marketed directly by Galai Instruments, is shown in Fig. 6. A useful feature of this instrument is that as the fine particles are being characterized by the scanning laser beam, they are also imaged on a television screen in such a way that any agglomeration can be detected during the analysis. The logic of the Galai system allows the fine particle shape to be measured concurrently with size (44).

Another time-of-flight size analyzer is known as the LASENTECH (Belleview, WA). This system is portable and has been suggested for use as an online monitor for fine particles moving in a system as well as in the laboratory (45). A different type of time-of-flight instrument is known as the Aerosizer (TSI, St. Paul, MN) (46). Here, the stream of aerosol fine particles is accelerated across a gap defined by two laser beams. The time of flight across this gap is measured from the light signals scattered from the two light beams, and an electronic editor ensures single occupancy for the measurement series. The larger fine particles are slow to accelerate across the gap, whereas the smallest move with the speed of the feed air jet. The system is calibrated using standard fine particles.

Another similar instrument is also manufactured by TSI. The basic system for measuring the aerodynamic

diameter of aerosol fine particles is shown in Fig. 7. Using this instrument, the velocity of a moving fine particle being accelerated across the inspection zone is measured with the Doppler shift in two beams that have a different directional reference to the moving airstream. From one perspective, the two lasers beams can be regarded as creating interference fringes, whereas the aerosol fine particle moving across the fringe system creates an oscillating signal that can be related to the fine particle size via calibration measurements. The fact that the instruments with which aerodynamic sizes are measured by the movement of the fine particles across crossed laser beams involves laser Doppler shifts is not immediately obvious from reading the trade literature of companies marketing this type of instrument. Indeed, in this class of instruments, the interpretive theory is complex, and the user is generally provided with a calibrated instrument to carry out the characterization studies of interest (46, 47).

Photon-Correlation Spectroscopy

Another instrument, in which the physics of the measurements are not immediately obvious to the outside observer, is part of a group of instruments variously referred to as photon correlation, dynamic light scattering,

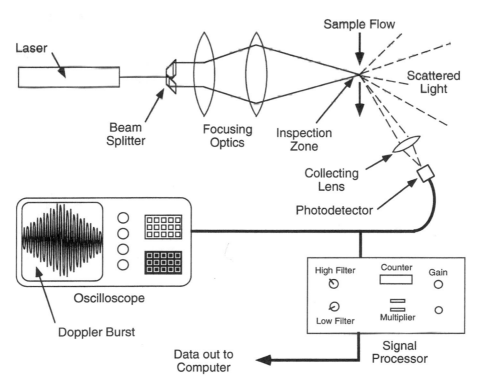

Fig. 7 A Doppler-shift procedure for measuring the aerodynamic size of aerosol fine particles is used by the TSI aerosol particle sizer. (Form Refs. 1 and 46.)

or quasielastic light scattering spectroscopes (often referred to as PCS, DLS, or QUELS). In this discussion, the term photon-correlation spectroscopy is used (48–51). Its physical basis is the monitoring of the Doppler shifts in reflected laser light created by the Brownian motion of submicron fine particles. In some cases, the technique can also be applied to fine particles of several microns in diameter. The equipment for actually measuring the Doppler shifts is relatively simple, but the overall expense is increased by the data-processing that is usually included. This instrument is useful for studying relatively simple size distributions such as latex suspensions. However, interpreting a wide range of sizes in suspension with this technique can involve complex data processing that, if carried out incorrectly, can generate confusing data (48, 50, 51).

Stream Counters

Another size characterization instrument group is known as stream counters, in which a stream of fine particles is passed through an inspection zone. The physical properties of the inspection zone are changed by the presence of the fine particles. The size of the fine particle is deduced from this change. In the Coulter counter, the fine particles to be characterized are placed in an electrolyte, and a stream of suspension is passed through an orifice between two electrodes as shown in Fig. 8 (52). The size of the fine particle is deduced from the measured resistance change between the electrodes.

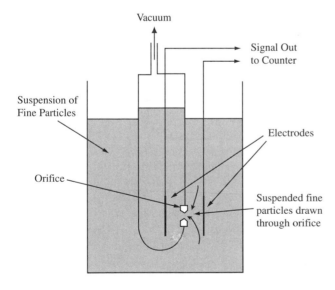

Fig. 8 Schematic representation of the operation of the Coulter counter. (Form Ref. 52.)

A major problem with stream counters is the single occupancy of the fine particles in the inspection zone. Should there inadvertently be two fine particles in the orifice, they register as one large fine particle, and the counting of the smaller particles has a deficit of two. This type of error is referred to as primary count loss (the undercounting of the smaller fine particles) and secondary count gain (the false registering of larger fine particles owing to multiple occupancy of the zone). Normally, the analysis with this type of instrument is carried out in a series of increasing dilutions until further dilution does not affect the measured size distribution. A difficulty sometimes encountered with this method is the availability of a conducting fluid that does not interact with the fine particles to be inspected. Over the years, various sophisticated data-processing techniques have been used to allow for problems associated with the Coulter counter, for example, when the fine particles are too close to the walls of the orifice or have extreme shape (1, 22).

In another group of stream counters, the fine particles in the inspection zone are monitored with a light beam. Various models of this type of instrument have been developed to count fine particles in liquids; others are specialized for the counting of dust fine particles in the air (1, 22, 53–55).

Elutriators for Size-Characterization Studies and Fine-Powder Fractionation

Elutriators are a class of instruments that fractionate fine particles according to their size by manipulating them in a moving fluid. They are among the first devices used for measuring size distributions of powders by fractionating them into various size groups and weighing the amount of powder in each group. The Roller elutriator was widely used in the powder metals industry (1). In recent years, elutriators have tended to be displaced from common use by diffractometers and other optically based instruments. They are still extremely useful, however, for fractionating powders into different sizes to study the physical variations of properties with size. Thus, a drug powder can be fractionated into various sizes to study the dependence of the bioavailability of a drug on its particle size. Fig. 9 shows three basic types of elutriators for fractionating powders and studying aerosol fine particles. In the gravity elutriator shown in Fig. 9a, air or another suitable fluid is passed upward through powder placed on a filter. As the air moves up through the column, the velocity of the moving fluid can be adjusted to move all fine particles below a certain size from the elutriator body to a fines collector, which may be a filter or a cyclone. The size limit, defining the size of the fine particles remaining

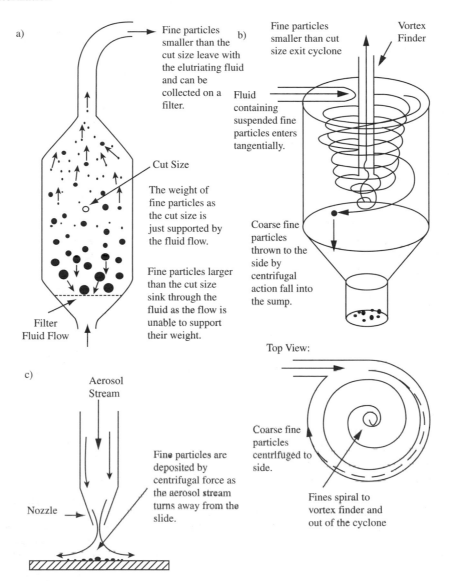

Fig. 9 Elutriators can use gravity or centrifugal force to separate fine particles into undersize and oversize fractions. a) Gravity elutriator; b) Cyclone (centrifugal elutriator); c) Impactor. (From Ref. 1.)

in the elutriator, is called the cut size of the elutriator. Because it is difficult to control the movement of the fluid and because of turbulence, the cut size and the fractionating power of an elutriator are not precise. A microscope or other suitable device is needed to investigate the actual fractionation of the powder in a given elutriator.

Cyclones are widely used in industry to fractionate powders. The operation of a cyclone, which is in fact a centrifugal elutriator, is shown in Fig. 9b (56). The stream of fluid suspension containing the fine particles to be fractionated enters the top of the cylindrical body tangentially. The fluid stream is made to spiral downward through the body of the cyclone until it can reverse its flow and leave through a pipe known as the vortex finder. As the feed stream spins around the body of the cyclone, the coarse particles in suspension are thrown to the wall by centrifugal force. At the wall, the coarser particles fall down into the conical bottom of the cyclone. The cut size of the cyclone, which determines how small the fine particles leaving through the vortex finder are, is determined by the dimensions of the cyclone and the velocity of the fluid stream. Small cyclones are widely used in occupational hygiene studies (56).

Another device for depositing fine particles from an airstream is the jet impactor, shown in Fig. 9c. The airstream containing the suspended particles is impinged onto a glass slide. As the airstream is forced to turn because of the slide under the jet, centrifugal force pushes the suspended fine particles onto the slide. The smallest fine particle, which is just deposited on the slide, is determined by the jet-slide configuration and the speed of the airstream moving through the equipment (1).

Giddings and coworkers have developed a series of cross-flow classifiers known as field-flow fractionation devices. The procedures, often referred to as FFF, are defined by Giddings (57) as: "a family of high resolution techniques capable of separating and characterizing materials in the macromolecular and colloidal range and beyond." Applications of FFF span a ten- to fifteen-fold mass range, extending from molecules under 1000 molecular weight to particles 100 microns in diameter. Particles as diverse as cells, subcellular particles, viruses, liposomes, protein aggregates, fly ash, waterborne colloids, and industrial latexes and pigments have been separated.

Characterization of Powder Surface Areas

In powder studies, the surface area of the powder is an important parameter. It can be measured directly by means of gas adsorption studies, in which the amount of gas or another molecular item, such as dye molecules adsorbed onto the powder to form a monolayer, is determined. Several books have been written describing the theory and procedures for gas adsorption studies. Before 1977, it was believed that one of the basic problems with surface area estimates by gas adsorption was that uncertainties in the knowledge of the cross-sectional area of the absorbed molecules made the estimates depend on the gas being used (58). In recent years, the gas adsorption studies of surface areas have been reinterpreted from the viewpoint of fractal geometry (59). It is now recognized that the surface area measured, using a given gas, depends on the accessibility of the rough surface to the adsorbed molecules, as illustrated in Fig. 10a. In a study of a series of adsorbent molecules of increasing size, Avnir and coworkers have shown that the surface area estimates can be plotted against the molecular size to obtain a Richardson plot from which the fractal roughness of the powder surface can be deduced (59, 60); a graph generated by Avnir and coworkers is shown in Fig. 10b. The slope of its data line can be used to deduce a fractal dimension of the rough surface. The fractal description of powder roughness is an important parameter for the bioavailability of a drug or the chemical reactivity of powder. Neimark has recently

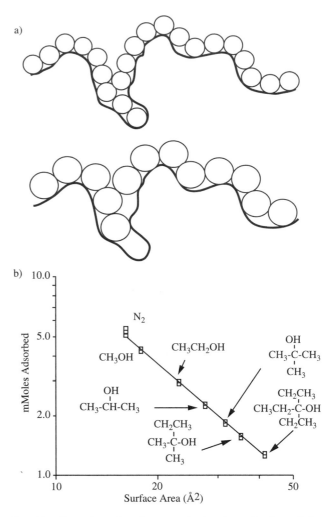

Fig. 10 Gas adsorption data permit the determination of the fractal dimension of a rough surface. a) The surface is estimated from the number of gas molecules that cover the surface. The estimate depends on the size of the gas molecule; b) the fractal dimension of a surface is derived from the results of gas adsorption studies with several different sized molecules (From Ref. 59.)

described a method for calculating the surface area and roughness of a powder by studying capillary condensation of a liquid on a powder (61).

The fineness of a powder can be studied with the help of permeability techniques, in which the resistance to fluid flow of a powder plug is measured and the fineness of the powder deduced from this measured resistance using various equations such as the Kozeny–Carmen equation. The interpretive equations used to calculate the surface area from permeability measurements make several assumptions concerning the pore structure of the packed powder bed, and the measured surface area from permeability studies should be regarded only as a measure of fineness and not as an absolute measure of surface. Instruments such as the Fisher Subsieve Sizer and the Blaine Fineness Tester are permeability-based methods that, in the past, have been widely used in industry and are still often used for quality control in industry. A major advantage of permeability methods is that they use large amounts of powder, which minimizes the problems of sampling (62, 63).

PORE-SIZE DISTRIBUTION MEASUREMENTS

When the pore size of a packed powder bed or of the structure of porous powder grains is of interest, mercury-intrusion studies can be used to investigate the pore structure. Fig. 11 shows data of a study using the mercury-intrusion technique to examine the structure of a powder bed of porous grains (64). The amount of mercury entering a bed at different pressures is used to generate the data. Using the known contact angle of mercury with the material of the powder, the applied pressure can be interpreted in terms of the capillary tube through which mercury moves at that pressure. However, there has always been some controversy as to the physical significance of mercury-intrusion data because it only measures access pore diameter, not the volume of the pore behind the neck. (Theories interpreting mercury-intrusion data in terms of pore diameter are often referred to as ink-bottle interpretive models, the idea being that it is the neck of the ink bottle that represents the penetration diameter, not the diameter of the bottle behind the neck.) For the data in Fig. 11a, at low pressures the mercury is entering the voids between the grains of the powder, but when a pressure of approximately 2000 psi (13.8 MPa) is reached, the mercury starts to intrude into pores within the powder grains having access diameters of the order of 0.1 μm. It has recently been shown that the traditional way of presenting mercury-intrusion data can be revised to generate a fractal dimension in data space. The revised data in Fig. 11a are shown in Fig. 11c. The slopes α and β of these diagrams are fractal dimensions in data space (65, 66).

STANDARD REFERENCE POWDERS

Some manufacturers of instruments for characterizing fine particles claim that their instruments do not need calibration. Such claims should be treated with skepticism. In practice, many sizing instruments have to be calibrated using standard powders available from several vendors (67, 68). Because the various methods of exploring the size

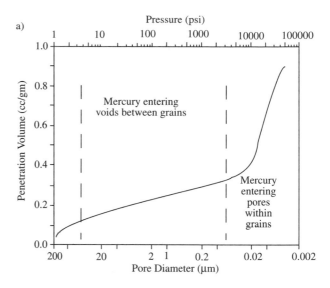

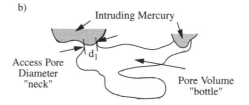

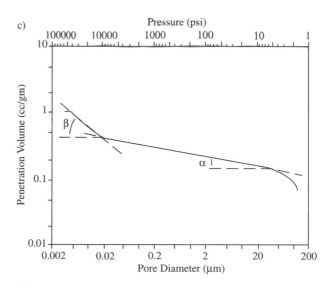

Fig. 11 Mercury intrusion porosimetry involves applying increasing pressure to a sample under study and noting the volume of mercury entering the pores within the sample. a) Traditional representation of mercury intrusion data; b) the physical significance of "ink bottle" theories of mercury intrusion have always been the subject of debate; c) a possible reinterpretation of the data in a) as fractal data. α and β are the slopes of particular regions of the resulting curve, which may be interpreted as fractal dimensions.

distribution of a powder evaluate different physical parameters, the size distributions of a powder generated by different methods do not always agree. The relationship between distribution functions, as evaluated by different methods, should be explored experimentally (69–72).

REFERENCES

1. Kaye, B.H. *Characterization of Powders and Aerosols*; Wiley-VCH: Weinheim, 1999.
2. Kaye, B.H. Efficient Sample Reduction of Powders by Means of a Riffler Sampler. Soc. Chem. Ind. Monogr. **1964**, 18, 159–163.
3. *British Standards Methods for the Determination of Particle Size Powders. Part I, Subdivision of Gross Sample Down to 0.2 ml*; BS3406, Part 1: London, 1961.
4. Kaye, B.H. An Investigation into the Relative Efficiency of Different Sampling Procedures. Powder Met. **1962**, 9, 213–234.
5. Sampling Equipment Literature is available from Gustafson, 6340 LBJ Freeway, Suite 180, Dallas, TX 75240.
6. Sampling Equipment Literature is available from Gilson Company Inc., P.O. Box 200, Lewis Center, OH 43035.
7. Information on the Spinning Riffler System is available from Microscal Ltd., 20 Mattock Lane, Ealing, London, W5 5BH.
8. Kaye, B.H. Powder Rheology. *Powder Mixing*; Chapman & Hall: London, 1997; 103–161, Ch.3, Now available through Kluwer Academic Publishers: Dordrecht, The Netherlands.
9. Kaye, B.H. *Chaos and Complexity*; VCH: Weinheim Germany, 1993; 148–154, See also Section 5.2, Poisson Tracking as a Technique for Studying Chaotic Conditions in a Mixer, in Ref. 8, 220–223.
10. Kaye, B.H.; Clark, G.G.; Bohan, Monitoring Mixer Performance using the Size Distribution Information on Samples taken from a Mixing Process. In *Proceedings of Fine Powder Processing 99*, The Pensylvania State University, University Park, PA, Sept, 20–22, 1999.
11. Kaye, B.H.; Clark, G.G. In Evaluating the Performance of Chaotic Powder and Aerosol Sampling Devices Using Tracker Fineparticles Proceedings of PARTEC, Nürnberg Conference on Particle Size, May, 1989; Nürnberg Messer Centrum, Nürnberg, 1989.
12. Kaye, B.H.; Turbitt-Daoust, C.; Clark, G.G. Segregation Dynamics of Powders Subjected to Vibration Proceedings of the Powder and Bulk Solids Conference, Rosemont, IL, May, 4–7, 1998; Reed Exhibition Companies, Norwalk, CT, 1998.
13. Kaye, B.H.; Fairburn, M.; Clark, G.G. Techniques for Monitoring and Combating Segregation in Powder Systems, Proceedings of the Powder and Bulk Solids Conference, Rosemont, IL, May, 10–13, 1999; Reed Exhibition Companies, Norwalk, CT, 1999.
14. Kaye, B.H.; Fairburn, M.; Hood, K.A. Efficient Sampling Protocols. In *Proceedings of the Powder and Bulk Solids Conference*, Rosemont, IL, May, 8–11, 2000; Proceeding published by Reed Exhibition Companies, Norwalk, CT.
15. Pall Gelman Laboratory, 600 South Wagner Road, Ann Arbor, MI 48103–9019 USA.
16. The Poretics Corporation, 151 Lindbergh Avenue, Livermore, CA.
17. Collimated Holes Incorporated, 460 Division St., Campbell, CA 95008.
18. Allen, T. Application of Precision Transparent Sieves to the Determination of Low Number Concentrations of Oversized Particles in Powders. *Part. Part. Syst. Characteristics*; Wiley-VCH: 1992; 9, 252–258.
19. Parfitt, G.D. *Dispersion of Powders in Liquids*, 2nd Ed.; Wiley: New York, 1973.
20. Heywood, H.H. Size and Shape Distribution of Lunar Fines, Sample, 12057, 72. In *Proceedings of Second Lunar Science Conference*, Vol. 13, 1971; 1989–2001.
21. Hausner, H.H. Characterization of the Powder Particle Shape, Proceedings of the Symposium on Particle Size Analysis, Loughborough, England, 1967, Society for Analytical Chemistry, London, 20–27 (See also Ref. 1, 205–232.)
22. Allen, T. *Particle Size Analysis*, 4th Ed.; Chapman and Hall: London, 1992.
23. Kaye, B.H. *Characterization of Powders and Aerosols*; Wiley-VCH: Weinheim, 1999, The Use of Fourier Techniques to Characterize the Shape of Profiles in Ch. 2, Direct Measurement of Larger Fineparticles and the Use of Image Analysis Systems to Characterize Fineparticles, 21–58, and Ch. 7, Light Scattering Methods for Characterizing Fineparticles, 205–232.
24. Kaye, B.H. Part I: Rugged Boundaries and Rough Surfaces Applied Fractal Geometry and the Fineparticle Specialist. Part. Part. Syst. Charact. **1993**, 10 (3), 99–110.
25. Kaye, B.H. *Chaos and Complexity, Discovering the Surprising Patterns of Science and Technology*; VCH: Weinheim Germany, 1993.
26. Kaye, B.H. *A Random Walk Through Fractal Dimensions*; VCH: Weinheim, Germany, 1989.
27. Mandelbrot, B.B. *Fractals: Form, Chance, and Dimension*; Freeman: San Francisco, 1977.
28. Schaeffer, D.W. Fractal Models and the Structure of Materials Matter. Res. Soc. Bull. **1988**, 13, 22–27.
29. Kaye, B.H. Multi-Fractal Description of a Rugged Fineparticle Profiles. Part. Part. Syst. Charact. **1984**, 1, 14–21.
30. *Coincidences, Clusters and Catastrophes*; Ch. 13, 483–534 in Ref. 25.
31. Kaye, B.H.; Yousufzai, M.A.K. Calibrating and Monitoring Woven Wire Sieving Surfaces. *Powder Bulk Eng.*, **1992**, (Jan.) , 29–34.
32. Sieves Sieving and Other Sizing Methods. *In Draft of Standard Determination of Particle Size Distribution, Laser Diffraction Methods*; International Organization for Standardization (ISO): Berlin, Germany.
33. Some of the Classical Sedimentation Equipment as well as other Sizing Equipment is Available from Gilson Company Inc., P.O. Box 200, Lewis Center, OH 43035.
34. Provder, T., Ed. *Particle Size Analysis*, ACS Symposium Series 332; American Chemical Society: Washington, DC, 1987.
35. CILAS U.S.A. available through Denver Autometrics, Inc., 6235 Lookout Road, Bolder, CO 80301. Company Headquarters in France, Osi 47, Rue de Javel, 75015 Paris.

36. Kaye B.H. Dangers of Curve Fitting in the Deduction of Size Distribution from Diffraction Data. Proceedings of the Powder and Bulk Solids Conference, Rosemont, IL, May 6–9, 1991.

37. Sympatec, Inc. Princeton Service Center, 34890 U.S. Route 1, Princeton, NJ 08540-5706.

38. See Trade Literature of Shimatzu Scientific Instruments Incorporated, 7102 Riverwood Drive, Columbia, MD 21046.

39. Holve, D.J. Using Ensemble Diffraction to Measure Particle Size Distribution. Powder Bulk Eng. **1991**, 5 June (6), 15–19, See also trade literature of INSITEC, 2110 Omega Road, Suite D, San Ramon, CA 94583.

40. See Trade Literature of Coulter Counter Electronics, 590 West 20th St., Hialeah, FL 33010.

41. Malvern Instruments Incorporated, 10 Southview Rd., Southborough, MA 01772.

42. MICROTRAC System Manufactured by Leeds and Northrop Instruments, 3000 Old Roosevelt Blvd., St. Petersburg, FL 33702.

43. Fritsch GmbH, Industriestrasse 8, D-55743, Idar-Oberstein, Germany.

44. Technical Literature Available from Galai Production Limited, Industrial Zone, 10500, Migdal, Haemek, Israel.

45. LASENTECH is available from Laser Sensor Technology Inc., P.O. Box 3912, Belleview, WA 98009.

46. TSI Particle Instruments/Amherst, 7 Pomeroy Lane, Amherst, MA 01002–2905, and TSI Inc., 2500 Cleveland Avenue, N, St. Paul, MN 55113.

47. Dantech Corporation, 777 Corporate Drive, Mahwah, NJ 07430.

48. Weiner, B.B. *Modern Methods of Particle Sizing*; Barth, H., Ed.; Wiley-Interscience: New York, 1984; Ch. 3.

49. See Technical Literature of Brookhaven Instruments Corporation, Brookhaven Corporate Park, 750 Bluepoint Road, Holtsville, NY 11742.

50. Nicoli, D.F.; Wu, J.S.; Chang, Y.J.; McKenzie, D.C.; Hasapidis, K.; Automatic High Resolution Particle Size Analysis by Single Particle Optical Sensing. Am. Lab. **1992**, July 24 (8), 39.

51. Mazumder, M.K.; E-Spart Analyzer: Its Performance and Applications to Powder and Particle Technology Processes. KONA **1993**, 11, 105–118, KONA is produced by the Hosokawa Micron International Inc., which Markets the E-SPART Analyzer; Literature is available from Micron Powder Systems (a member of the Hosokawa Micron group), 10 Chatham Rd., Summit, NJ 07901. (The term SPART Analyzer stands for: Single Particle Aerodynamic Relaxation Time analyzer).

52. Information on the Coulter Counter is available from Coulter Electronics, Inc., 590 West 20th St., Hialeah, FL 33010.

53. An Optical Stream Counter is available from the Climet Corporation, 1320 Colton Avenue, Redlands, CA 92373.

54. Royco Instruments for Studying Aerosols and Fineparticles in Liquids are available from Royco Instruments, Inc., 141 Jefferson Drive, Menlo Park, CA 94025.

55. The Widely used Stream Counter for Fineparticles in Fluid is the HIAC Counter, HIAC Instruments Division, P.O. Box 3007, 4719 West Brooke St., Monte Claire, CA 91763.

56. Humann, W.L. Cyclone Separators, a Family Affair. Chem. Eng. **1991**, June 8(6), 118–123.

57. Giddings, J.; Field Flow Fractionation. Chem. Eng. News **1988**, Oct. 95 (10), 34. (For Information on Field Flow Fractionation Research Development and Industrial Applications, Contact Field Flow Fractionation Research Center, Department of Chemistry, University of Utah, Salt Lake City, UT 84112.).

58. See Discussion of Gas Adsorption Methods in Ref. 22.

59. Avnir, D., Ed. *Fractal Approach to Heterogeneous Chemistry*; John Wiley & Sons: London, 1989.

60. Takayasu, H., Ed. *Fractals in the Physical Sciences*; John Wiley & Sons: New York, 1990.

61. Neimark, A.V. Percolation Theory of Capillary Hysteresis Phenomena and its Application for Characterization of Porous Solids. *Characterization of Solids II*; Rodrigues-Reinoso, F., et al. Eds.; Elsevier Science Publishers: Amsterdam, 1991; 67–75.

62. Kaye, B.H. Permeability Techniques for Characterizing Fine Powders. Powder Technol. **1967**, 1, 11–22.

63. Kaye, B.H.; Legault, P.E. Real-Time Permeability for the Monitoring of Fineparticle Systems. Powder Technol. **1973**, 23, 179–186.

64. Orr, C. Application of Mercury Penetration in Material Analysis. Powder Technol. **1969–1970**, 3, 117–123.

65. Kaye, B.H. Applied Fractal Geometry and the Fineparticle Specialist I. Rugged Boundaries and Rough Surfaces. Part. Part. Syst. Charact. **1993**, 10(3), 99–110.

66. Kaye, B.H. Fractal Dimensions in Data Space: New Descriptors for Fineparticle Systems. Part. Part. Syst. Charact. **1993**, 10, 191–200.

67. Standard powders are available from Duke Scientific Corporation, 135D San Antonio Rd. Palo Alto, CA 94303.

68. Calibration Fineparticles are available from Dyno Particles A. S., PO. Box 160N-2001, Lillestrom, Norway.

69. Merkus, H.G.; Bischof, O.; Drescher, S.; Scarlett, B. Precision and Accuracy in Particle Sizing. Round-Robin Results from Sedimentation, Laser Diffraction and Electrical Sensing Zone Using BCR 67 and 69. In Proceedings 6th European Symposium on Particle Characterization, *PARTEC*, Nurnberg, March 21–23, 1995.

70. Yamamoto, H.; Matsuyama, T. Comparative Study of Particle Size Analyses Using Common Samples. KONA **1995**, 13, 57–66.

71. Kaye, B.H.; Alliet, D.; Switzer, L.; Turbitt-Daoust, C. The Effect of Shape on Intermethod Correlation of Techniques for Characterizing the Size Distribution of a Powder I. Correlating the Size Distribution Measured by Sieving, Image Analysis, and Diffractometer Method. Part. Part. Syst. Charact. **1997**, 14, 219–224.

72. Kaye, B.H.; Alliet, D.; Switzer, L.; Turbitt-Daoust, C. The Effect of Shape on Intermethod Correlation of Techniques for Characterizing the Size Distribution of a Powder II. Correlating the Size Distribution as Measured by Diffractometer Methods, TSI-Amherst Aerosol Spectrometer, and Coulter Counter. Part. Part. Syst. Charact. **1999**, 16, 266–272.

P

PARTITION COEFFICIENTS

Eric J. Lien
Shijun Ren
University of Southern California, Los Angeles, California

INTRODUCTION

A thorough understanding of partition coefficients is important to all research scientists and product development staff in various branches of the pharmaceutical field. The principle and applications are involved in several different areas of current pharmaceutical interest. These include the techniques of extraction, preservation of oil–water systems, penetration through packaging materials, absorption and distribution of drugs in vivo, protein binding and hemodialysis, drug metabolism, enzyme inhibition, drug-receptor interactions, drug-delivery systems, and drug targeting. Because the partition coefficient is a measure of hydrophobic-bonding tendency, and all proteins (enzyme, membrane, plasma, and receptor proteins) contain 20 to 45% of amino acids with nonpolar groups (e.g., leucine, isoleucine, phenylalanine, tyrosine, tryptophan, etc.), continuing interest in using partition coefficients in correlating biological activity with molecular structure is expected. Other areas of interest in the application of partition coefficient fall beyond the scope of this article. These include analytical chemistry, toxicology, forensic medicine, ecology, and environmental protection.

HISTORICAL BACKGROUND

The first observation that the ratio of concentrations of a solute (e.g., I_2 or Br_2), when distributed between an organic solvent (e.g., CS_2 or ether) and water, remained constant even when the volume ratio of the immiscible solvents changed widely, was first reported by Berthelot and Jungfleisch in 1872, as illustrated by Eq. 1:

$$P = C_o/C_{aq} = \text{equilibrium constant } K \tag{1}$$

In 1921, Smith suggested that partition coefficient P can be converted from one solvent system to another.

Thirty years later, Collander presented the standard linear free-energy relationship, shown in Eq. 2, using water and different alkanols:

$$\log P_2 = a \log P_1 + b \tag{2}$$

where a is a coefficient, and b is a constant.

At the turn of the century, Meyer and Overton discovered that most organic compounds (except nutrients) penetrate tissue cells as a lipid barrier and that their narcotic action parallels the oil–water partition coefficients of the compounds. In the early 1950s, Collander demonstrated that the penetration rate of plant cell membranes by various organic compounds was related to their oil–water partition coefficients. Cohen and Edsal studied the ratios of alcohol solubility to water solubility to define the relative lipophilic character of amino acids. The limited additivity of the partition coefficients of organic compounds was observed by Collander, Cohen, and Edsal in their studies. In the early 1960s, Salame and Pinsky derived the permachor method, given in Eq. 3, for calculation of the P factor for the prediction of chemicals permeation through a plastic membrane:

$$\log P_f = 16.55 - 3700/T - 0.22\pi \tag{3}$$

where π is the permachor constant, and T is the absolute temperature. A general equation was presented by these investigators, as in Eq. 4:

$$\log P_f = K - R\pi \tag{4}$$

where K is a temperature correction constant, and R is a polymer (e.g., plastic) correction term. Interestingly, at about the same time Hansch, Fujita, and co-workers made the most significant contributions toward the understanding and application of partition coefficients ($\log P$ and π) and greatly extended the linear free-energy-related (LFER) approach from organic chemistry to medicinal chemistry and biology. This renewed interest in the application of partition coefficients has stimulated many excellent reviews, books, and monographs.

THEORY AND EXPERIMENTAL METHODS OF MEASUREMENTS

Because the partition coefficient is measured when an equilibrium is reached, it is characterized by the equality of the chemical potentials μ_o and μ_{aq} of the solute in the two phases (organic and aqueous), as shown by Eqs. 5, 6, and 7:

$$\mu_o = \mu_o^0 + RT \ln C_o \tag{5}$$

$$\mu_{aq} = \mu_{aq}^0 + RT \ln C_{aq} \tag{6}$$

If $\mu_o = \mu_{aq}$,

then:

$$P = C_o/C_{aq} = e^{-(\mu_{aq}^0 - \mu_o^0)/RT}$$
$$= e^{-\Delta\mu^0/RT} \tag{7}$$

where C_o and C_{aq} are the equilibrium concentrations of the solute in the organic and the aqueous phases, respectively; μ_o^0 and μ_{aq}^0 are the chemical potentials (in the organic and aqueous phases, respectively) at infinite dilution; and R is the gas constant, T the temperature, and P the partition coefficient. P is a constant for any compound in a given solvent system at a given temperature; this relationship is known as the Nernst law.

As with any equilibrium constant K, P is related linearly to the standard free-energy change when it is converted to the logarithmic scale, as in Eqs. 8, 9, and 10:

$$\Delta G^0 = -RT \ln K \tag{8}$$

For any equilibrium:

$$\Delta G^0 = -2.303\, RT \log K \tag{9}$$

For partition processes:

$$\Delta G^0 = -2.303\, RT \log P \tag{10}$$

Because of this linear free-energy relationship (LFER), log P is commonly used in most correlation studies instead of P.

In the past 35 years or so, 1-octanol-water has been the most commonly used solvent system. It has been shown that for correlation with biological activity, organic solvents (such as 1-octanol) capable of forming hydrogen bonds usually give better correlation than those not capable (e.g., CCl$_4$, cyclohexane, and other hydrocarbons). Extensive compilations on 1-octanol-water partition coefficient are available.

On the other hand, if one is interested in separating out thermodynamic properties such as enthalpy change (ΔH) and entropy change (ΔS), a solvent with minimum mutual solubility with water (such as cyclohexane or heptane) is preferable.

Apparent Versus True Partition Coefficient (log P' Versus log P)

If a solute is ionizable (either acidic or basic), two different species can exist in the aqueous phase, and therefore the apparent partition coefficient (P') or the true partition coefficients (P) can be measured, as shown below and in Eqs. 11, 12, 13, 14, 15:

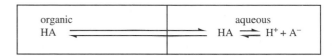

where

$$P = [HA]_o/[HA]_{aq} \tag{11}$$

$$P' = [HA]_o/([HA]_{aq} + [A^-]_{aq}) \tag{12}$$

and

$$P = P'/(1-\alpha) \tag{13}$$

where α is the degree of ionization: for acids:

$$\alpha = 1/[1 + \text{antilog}(\text{pKa} - \text{pH})] \tag{14}$$

for bases:

$$\alpha = 1/[1 + \text{antilog}(\text{pH} - \text{pKa})] \tag{15}$$

Because the degree of ionization is a function of the pH of the aqueous phase and the pKa of the solute, the apparent partition coefficient P' fluctuates as the pH of the aqueous phase (usually a buffer solution) is changed, whereas the true (or corrected) partition coefficient (P) should remain constant. However, in reality the different buffer species may not only affect P' but also P because of different degrees of ion-pair formation and the different polar nature of the counterions used. Among the different buffer species, 1-octanol-phosphate buffer appears to give the most consistent results compared with 1-octanol-water. In some publications, the apparent partition coefficient P' is also described as the distribution coefficient D.

Because the separation of immiscible phases takes place only in the presence of gravity, it would not be possible to measure partition coefficients in outer space where the gravity is zero.

Shake-Flask Method

The shake-flask method is used most commonly in the measurement of partition coefficients. It is also the standard procedure to validate other methods. A solute is simply shaken with two immiscible solvents (organic and aqueous), followed by analyzing the solute concentration in one or both phases. To avoid any volume changes in both phases, one phase is saturated with the other before the partitioning process. It is important to ensure that equilibrium is reached before the analysis. If a solute does not cause emulsification, vigorous shaking can reduce the time required to reach equilibrium, usually in a few minutes. However, if a solute with both polar and nonpolar groups present (such as saponin glycosides or surfactant-type compounds), a gentle and slow shaking procedure or even special devices such as a Doluisio and Swintosky Y-tube or a Schulman-type cell should be used.

Some true (undissociated, corrected) partition coefficients of representative drug molecules ranging from −2.26 to +15.69 are shown in Table 1.

For the quantitative analysis of the solute distributed in one or both phases, the most commonly used analytical methods include UV-visible spectrophotometric analysis for compounds with chromophore groups and gas-liquid chromatography (GLC). Colorimetric methods have also been used for specific compounds.

With the proper choice of solvent volume and sensitive analytical methods, log P values ranging from −5 to +5 can be measured. The temperature dependence of many partitioning systems is on the order of 0.01 log unit per degree in the 25°C range. Adequate temperature control is needed for high accuracy. This is more critical for volatile solvents like ether, choloroform, low-boiling hydrocarbons, and alcohols lower than 1-octanol.

Chromatographic Methods

In recent years, the availability of reproducible systems and precision instruments in high-performance liquid chromatography (HPLC) has prompted the application of chromatography in the rapid measurement of partition coefficients. In general, a linear relationship between log P and log K' from a set of compounds is required for the interpolation or extrapolation of log P values of additional compounds of congeneric nature, as shown in Eq. 16:

$$\log P = a \log K' + b \qquad (16)$$

where the capacity factor K' is determined from the net retention time t_R relative to the nonadsorbed time t_0, as defined by Eq. 17:

$$K' = (t_R - t_0)/t_0 \qquad (17)$$

This is similar to the linear relationship R_m measured by thin-layer chromatography (TLC), given in Eq. 18:

Table 1 Selected true (corrected) partition coefficients of representative drug molecules measured in 1-octanol-water or 1-octanol-phosphate buffer

Drug	log P
L-Tyrosine	−2.26
Hydroxyurea	−1.80
Citric acid	−1.72
Ascorbic acid (Vit. C)	−1.64
Phenol red	−1.45
Streptozotocin	−1.45
Sulfanilamide	−0.73
Theobromine	−0.72
Chlortetracycline	−0.62
Ethanol	−0.31
Ellagic acid	0.27[a]
Cimetidine	0.40
Atenolol	0.43
Metiamide	0.50
Procainamide	0.51
Morphine	0.76
Ephedrine	0.87
Aminopyrine	1.00
Colchicine	1.03
Chloramphenicol	1.14
Atropine	1.24
Digoxin	1.26
Nalidic acid	1.41
Phenobarbital	1.47
Daidzein	1.58[a]
Hydrocortisone	1.61
Benzoic acid	1.72
Salicyclic acid	1.73
Zileuton	1.81[a]
Benzylpenicillin	1.83
Chloroform	1.97
Dexamethasone	1.99
Podophyllotoxin	2.01
Metoprolol	2.04
Naloxone	2.09
Mathapyrilene	2.81
Phenformine	2.94
Labetalol	3.18
Benadryl	3.20
Propranolol	3.29
Clobetasol-17-butyrate	3.63
Progesterone	3.87
Estradiol	4.01
Tamoxifen	4.03
Propoxyphene	4.18
Mefepristone (Ru486)	5.48[b]
α-Tocopherol (vitamin E)	12.28[a]
β-Carotene	15.69[a]

[a]Calculated value using CQSAR program of BioByte.
[b]Calculated from the log P of progesterone and the π values of the substituents: log $P_{Ru\ 486}$ = log $P_{progesterone}$ − πCH_3 + $\pi_{double\ bond}$ + $\pi_{(CH_3)_2}N^+ \pi_{C_6H_4}$ − π_{COCH_3} + $\pi_{-O=C}$ + π_{CH_3} + π_{OH} = 3.87 − 0.5 − 0.2 + (−0.18) + 1.96 − (−0.71) + 0.48 + 0.5 + (−1.16) = 5.48.

$$R_m = \log K' = \log[(1 - R_f)/R_f] = \log(1/R_f - 1) \quad (18)$$

Because of the limits inherent in the mathematical formula, R_m ranges only from -1.996 to $+1.996$ for all possible compounds. This makes it less sensitive than the direct measurement of $\log P$. Nevertheless, for many compounds, it is much easier and more economical to measure $\log K'$ or R_m than $\log P$.

Countercurrent and Filter Probe Methods

A countercurrent-based device, known as AKUFVE, is useful when a large amount of information resulting from varying T or pH is required on one or only a few compounds. This method has the disadvantages of difficulties in cleaning and operation as well as in the need of large quantities of materials. Another method is Tomlinson's filter-probe method, which samples the phase with the larger volume (generally the aqueous phase) and pumps it through a UV detector to monitor the state of equilibrium. A heavy metal probe is attached to the circulating stainless steel tubing with a special filter that prevents entrapment of the unwanted phase. This method is related to the shake-flask method at high phase–volume ratio. It may be useful for unstable compounds and, as a closed system, may be used over a wide temperature range. Kaufman et al. have reported a microelectrometric titration method for the direct measurement of the pKa and partition and distribution coefficients of narcotics and narcotic antagonists and their pH and temperature dependence. Based on this principle, an automated instrument is now available for the simultaneous measurement of pKa and $\log P$ (pION Inc., Cambridge, MA).

Calculation of Partition Coefficients

Hansch-Fujita π constant

In 1964, Fujita et al. proposed that $\log P$ was an additive-constitutive property and can be calculated by taking the sum of the $\log P$ of the parent molecule and the π of the substituent, as in Eqs. 19, 20, 21:

$$\log P = \Sigma \pi \quad (19)$$

$$\pi_{substituent} = \log P_{substituted\ molecule} - \log P_{parent\ molecule} \quad (20)$$

For example:

$$\pi_{CH_3} = \log P_{CH_3C_6H_5} - \log P_{C_6H_6} = 2.69 - 2.13 = 0.56 \quad (21)$$

$$\log P_{Cl(C_6H_4)CH_3} = \log P_{C_6H_6} + \pi_{Cl} + \pi_{CH_3} = 2.13 + 0.71 + 0.56 = 3.40 \text{ (calculated), measured value} = 3.33.$$

By definition, the π of hydrogen is zero. A scale of the π values of various groups from very hydrophilic to very hydrophobic is shown in Table 2. Extensive compilations of the π constants of various functional groups are available in the literature.

Rekker's fragmental constant f

The fragmental (reductionist) approach of calculating $\log P$ was initiated by Rekker and coworkers. Based on a collection of measured $\log P$ values, they applied statistical analysis to determine the average contribution of simple fragments such as C, CH, CH_2, CH_3, OH, NH_2, $CONH_2$, OCH_3COOH, etc (see Table 2). It was found that it was necessary to introduce corrections if two polar groups were separated by only one or two aliphatic carbons. Their postulation is given in Eq. 22:

$$\log P = \Sigma a_m f_m + \Sigma b_m F_m \quad (22)$$

where a = the number of occurrences of fragment f of type n, and b = the number of occurrences of correction factor F of type m.

Leo-Hansch f constant

Hansch and Leo used a constructionist (synthetic) approach by starting with a few carefully measured values of $\log P$ of simple structures like H_2 and CH_4 and derived a separate set of fragment constants. The two columns in Table 2 show the slightly different values obtained by the two groups. Different π and f values should be used for an aliphatic system.

It is worth noting that although π_H is zero, f_H according to the Rekker's scale is 0.18 and according to the Hansch–Leo scale is 0.23. The calculation of $\log P$ using the fragment method has been computerized by the Hansch–Leo group. In this CLOGP program, all known correction factors have been incorporated. The structure of any compound can be entered by a linear notation called SMILES, and by going through a substructure search algorithm GENIE, the $\log P$ value can be calculated according to Eq. 22. The SMILES program includes all isomerisms.

Other methods

Other published methods of estimating partition coefficients include the use of molecular surface and volume in predicting solubilities and free energies of desolvation and the application of principal-component analysis based on partition coefficient data. Suzuki and Kudo's CHEMICAL (Combined Handling of Estimation Methods Intended for Completed Automated $\log P$ Calculation) as well as a

Table 2 The π and f constants for some functional groups

| Function x | π_x Aromatic system | π_x Aliphatic system | f_x Aromatic system | |
			Rekker	Leo–Hansch
H—	0	0	0.18	0.23
F—	0.13	−0.17	0.42	0.37
Cl—	0.76	0.39	0.93	0.94
Br—	0.94	0.60	1.18	1.09
I—	1.15	1.00	1.47	1.35
CH_3—	0.50	0.50	0.70	0.89
HC≡C—		0.48		
CH_2=CH—		0.70		
C_2H_5—	1.00	1.00		
H_2=C(CH_3)—		1.00		
CH_2=CHCH_2—		1.20		
n-C_3H_7—	1.50	1.50		
i-C_3H_7—	1.30	1.30		
n-C_4H_9—	2.00	2.00		
s-C_4H_9—	1.80	1.80		
t-C_4H_9—	1.68	1.68		
cyclo-C_3H_5—		1.21		
cyclo-C_5H_9—	2.14	2.14		
cyclo-C_6H_{11}—	2.51	2.51		
Adamantyl	3.30			
C_6H_5—	2.13	2.13	1.89	1.90
—$(CH_2)_3$	1.04			
—$(CH_2)_4$	1.39			
—$(CH)_4$—	1.24			
—CF_3	1.07		1.25	1.11
—CH_2OH	−1.03	−0.66		
—CH_2COOH	−0.72	−0.76		
—COOH	−0.32	−1.26	0.00	−0.03
—COO^-	−4.36			
—$CONH_2$	−1.49	−1.71	−1.13	−1.26
—$COOCH_3$	−0.01	−0.27		
—$COCH_3$	−0.55	−0.71		
—CN	−0.57	−0.84	−0.23	−0.34
—OH	−0.67	−1.16	−0.36	−0.44
—OCH_3	−0.02	−0.47		
—OCH_2COOH	−0.86			
—$OCOCH_3$	−0.64	−0.91		
—CH=NNHCONH_2	−0.85			
—CH= NNHCSNH_2	−0.27			
—O-β-Glucose	−2.84			
—NH_2	−1.23	−1.19	−0.90	−1.00
—N(CH_3)$_2$	−0.18	−0.32		
—NO	−0.12			
—NO_2	−0.28	−0.82	−0.09	−0.03
—NHCOCH_3	−0.97			
—NHCOC_6H_5	0.72			
—N=NC_6H_5	1.69			
—NHCONH_2	−1.01			
—N(CH_3)$_3^+$	−5.96			
—N_3	0.46			

(Continued)

Table 2 The π and f constants for some functional groups (*Continued*)

Function x	π_x Aromatic system	π_x Aliphatic system	f_x Aromatic system	
			Rekker	Leo–Hansch
—SH	0.39	0.28	0.62	0.62
—SCH$_3$	0.62			
—SCF$_3$	1.44			
—SCCl$_3$	1.65			
—SO$_2$				−2.17
—SO$_2$F				0.30
—SO$_2$CH$_3$	−1.26			
—SO$_2$CF$_3$	0.55			
—SF$_5$	1.55			
—SO$_2$NH$_2$	−1.82			−1.59

multidescriptor highly nonlinear regression model proposed by Bodor et al. were applied, in which a 10-parameter (15-term) equation was used to correlate with the log P values of 118 compounds of varying complexity. (All the descriptors were derived from AM1 calculation and were related to the surface area, dipole moment value, and charge densities of the molecule.) Some of the terms were raised to 10^4 and 10^2 powers to give the best fit. It is difficult to explain the physical meaning of the highly complex polynomial equation.

Several experts in the field suggest that the ultimate goal of flawless calculation of log P has not yet been fully realized, especially when dealing with a highly complex structure with de novo functional groups.

Physical Factors Contributing to Log P or π: Bulk and van der Waals Forces, Dipolar Interactions, and Hydrogen Bonding

Over the past 25 years, considerable efforts have been devoted to delineate the fundamental nature of partition coefficients (log P or π). As a result, many correlations between log P (or π) with other structural descriptors or physicochemical parameters have been reported by various investigators. For example, Moriguchi et al. dissected log P into two intrinsic components, namely, molecular volume and polar effect, and showed that the partition coefficient of a nonpolar molecule is a linear function of the volume. For polar molecules, a hydrophilic group effect has to be added as a correction term in the evaluation of log P. Kamlet et al. correlated log P with the solvatochromic parameters π^* and β, which were derived to measure dipolar and hydrogen bond acceptor strengths of pure bulk solvents as well as the corresponding properties of solutes.

Franke et al. examined the dependence of hydrophobicity on solvent and structure and showed that log P values depend on solute bulk and polar and hydrogen-bonding effects. Ou et al. examined the quantitative relationship of log P with molecular weight (log MW), dipole moment (μ), and hydrogen-bond capability (HB$_2$) of various compounds. For 222 of 282 compounds, log P values were correlated with these three parameters with a correlation coefficient of 0.938 and standard deviation of 0.492, as shown in Eq. (23):

$$\log P = 5.84 \log MW - 0.36\,\mu - 0.77\,HB_2 - 8.86 \quad (23)$$

$n = 222$, $r = 0.938$, $s = 0.492$ where HB$_2$ is the sum total of energy decrement in a hydrogen-bond group.

In a similar manner, Yang et al. reported the general Eq. (24) to be applicable to a wide range of nonpolar and polar substituents (with only a few notable exceptions):

$$\pi = +a\,MW\,(\text{or } vW) - b\,HB - c\mu + d \quad (24)$$

where vW is the van der Waals volume, and HB can be the number of atoms in a group capable of forming H bonds (HB$_1$), or HB$_1$ × energy (HB$_2$).

This general model has been extended to the log P of disubstituted aromatic compounds and the solubilities of tetracycline derivatives.

Applications

Extraction

In both organic and analytical chemistry laboratories, it is a common procedure to extract a compound from one solvent to another. It is also a common knowledge that it is more efficient to use small volumes and multiple extractions. This is shown by Eqs. 1 (given previously) and 25, 26, 27, assuming the two solvents are completely immiscible (e .g., H_2O–CCl_4).

$$P = (W_o/V_o)/[(W - W_o)V_{aq}] \qquad (25)$$

or

$$\text{or } W_o = WPV_o/(PV_o + V_{aq)} \qquad (26)$$

after n extractions:

$$W_n = W[PV_o/(PV_o + V_{aq})]^n \qquad (27)$$

where W is the water phase, and V is the volume.

If two solvents are partially miscible (e.g., ether-H_2O), the equation provides only approximate values, which may still be useful for practical purposes.

Preservation of oil–water systems

Many pharmaceutical preparations containing oil–water systems (creams, ointments, or suspensions) are subject to microbial contamination. Bacteria in these heterogenous systems are usually grown in the aqueous phase and at the oil–water interface. To preserve the shelf-life of these preparations, benzoic acid or other organic acids are added as preservatives. Because the microbial cell membrane is lipophilic in nature, the bacteriostatic actions of the acidic preservative are attributable almost entirely to the undissociated acid and not to the ionized form. A good understanding of the partition coefficient and the degree of ionization allows accurate calculation of the free un-ionized acid in the aqueous phase, which provides the bacteriostatic concentration.

Quantitative structure-activity relationships (QSAR)

Since the early work of Hansch et al., numerous examples of the quantitative correlation of biological activity with chemical structure have been reported. The success of QSAR relies heavily on the use of partition coefficients (log P or π) in extending the linear free-energy relationship (LFER) from homogenous organic chemical systems (i.e., the Hammett–Taft type approach) to compartmentalized heterogenous biological systems.

Further analysis of the physical nature of the partition coefficient reveals that it is a composite property depending on size, shape, dipole moment, and hydrogen-bonding ability. Although many researchers have attempted to replace log P with other simple parameters, only limited success has been achieved for some, but not all, molecules. It appears that for entirely new complex molecules, it still would be necessary to measure the partition coefficient, preferably validated by the conventional shake-flask method.

Partition coefficients of peptides and ampholytes

Since the publication of the first edition of the *Encyclopedia of Pharmaceutical Technology*, significant progress has been made in the experimental measurements and calculation of the log P' values of small peptides ranging from di- to pentapeptides with and without ionizable side chairs. Additional work will be needed to calculate the log P' values of large peptides and proteins. Testa's group has used a potential-pH representation to show ionic partition diagrams and analyzed the lipophilicity profiles of amphoteric compounds. They have also compiled a review on various computational approaches to lipophilicity, with 223 references cited.

Because an increasing number of new compounds are being synthesized every day, it is not feasible to have the partition coefficient of every new structure experimentally determined. According to the estimate of Leo and Hansch, the measured log P in octanol/water increases at the rate of approximately 1200/year. When a close congener with measured log P is available, it is easier to use the $\Sigma\pi$ method in calculating the log P of a structurally similar new derivative. On the other hand, for a large number of different structures, the CLOGP method based on the f constant of Hansch and Leo is suitable for obtaining calculated log P values fairly efficiently. An impressive correlation ($r^2 = 0.98$, $s = 0.21$) between the measured log P and calculated log P values of 9000 compounds has been obtained by this group. Regardless of the method used, it is necessary to measure the log P of a few model compounds for comparison. Many times, careful examination of the large deviation between the experimentally measured and the theoretically calculated values can uncover intra- or intermolecular interactions and thus lead to a better understanding of the phenomenon of partitioning of a solute between two immiscible phases saturated with each other.

The initial development of the fragmental constant f by Rekker has stimulated that of the systematic CLOGP method. Rekker has further compared the model of partition process with the passsage of a ball through a "brick wall" to account for a frequently observed "magic number." The model does not take into account the fact that neither 1-octanol nor the aqueous phase consists of homogeneous and ordered "bricks" as depicted in his diagram. At the present time, there is no rigorous theoretical method available for the calculation of log P of a complex de novo structure. Therefore, semiempirical methods and experimental methods will continue to be used.

For QSAR analysis, distribution coefficients (D) of ionizable compounds have been used by some investigators. From the mathematical formula of D, it can be demonstrated that it is the same as the apparent partition coefficient (P') and can be easily converted to a true (or corrected) partition coefficient P, as shown in Eqs. 28, 29, 30:

$$D = [HA]_o/([HA]_{aq} + [A^-]_{aq}) \tag{28}$$

$$P' = [HA]_o/([HA]_{aq} + [A^-]_{aq}) \tag{29}$$

$$D/(1 - \alpha) = [HA]_o/[HA]_{aq} = P \tag{30}$$

If limited data points are available in QSAR analysis, log P' (log D) can be used to account for different degrees of ionization as well as for different lipophilicities. If, on the other hand, a sufficient number of data points are available (more than 5 data points for each parameter being examined), it will be advantageous to use the log of the [undissociated] vs. [dissociated] ratio log U/D (= pKa − pH for acids, and pH − pKa for bases) as an independent variable as well as log P. This will separate the effect of ionization from that of relative lipophilicity.

Avdeef has recently reported the refinement of partition coefficients and ionization constants of multiprotic substances based on a generalized, weighted, nonlinear least-squares procedure and pH titration curve. This method allows for the determination of pKa and log P values of multiprotic substances with fairly close ionization constants.

A Prolog P program has been developed for the estimation of the distribution coefficients (log D) of ionizable compounds, based on LFER-derived microscopic dissociation constants. Several estimation methods for calculating octanol-water partition coefficients have been reported (e.g., Log KOW; X log P) using atom/fragment additive principles and correction factors. Clarke et al. have reported that for ionizable compounds, by using two different octanol volumes in a dual-phase potentiometric titration, both pKa and partition coefficient values can be obtained by curve fitting.

BIBLIOGRAPHY

Akamatsu, M.; Fujita, T. Quantitative Analyses of Hydrophobicity of Di- to Pentapeptides Having Unionizable Side Chains with Substituent and Structural Parameters. J. Pharm. Sci. **1992**, *81*, 164–174.

Akamatsu, M.; Katayama, T.; Kishimoto, D.; Kurokawa, Y.; Shibata, H.; Ueno, T.; Fujita, T. Quantitative Analysis of the Structure-Hydrophobicity Relationship for N-Acetyl Di- and Tripeptide Amides. J. Pharm. Sci. **1994**, *83*, 1026–1033.

Carrupt, P.A.; Testa, B.; Gaillard, P. Computational Approaches to Lipophilicity: Method and Applications. *Reviews in Computational Chemistry*; Lipkowitz, K.B., Boyd, D.B., Ed.; Wiley & Sons, Inc.: New York, 1997; 11, 241–315.

Clarke, F.H.; Cahoon, N.M. Partition Coefficients by Curve Fitting: The Use of Two Different Octanol Volumes in a Dual-Phase Potentiometric Titration. J. Pharm. Sci. **1996**, *85*, 178–183.

Csizmadia, F.; Tsantili-Kakoulidou, A.; Pander, I.; Darvas, F. Prediction of Distribution Coefficient from Structure. I. Estimation Method. J. Pharm. Sci. **1997**, *86*, 865–871.

Dearden, J.C.; Bresnen, G.M. The Measurement of Partition Coefficients. Quant. Struct.-Act. Relat. **1988**, *7*, 133–144.

Gao, H.; Wang, F.Z.; Lien, E.J. Hydrophobic Contribution Constants of Amino Acid Residues to the Hydrophobicities of Oligopeptides. Pharm. Res. **1995**, *12*, 1279–1283.

Gao, H.; Lien, E.J.; Wang, F.Z. Hydrophobicity of Oligopeptides Having Un-Ionizable Side Chains. J. Drug Target **1993**, *1*, 59–66.

Hansch, C.; Leo, A.; Hoekman, D. *Exploring QSAR: Hydrophobic, Electronic, and Steric Constants*; American Chemical Society: Washington, DC, 1995; 1–348.

Hansch, C.; Leo, A. *Exploring QSAR: Fundamentals and Applications in Chemistry and Biology*; American Chemical Society: Washington, DC, 1995; 1–557.

Lien, E.J.; Ren, S.J. QSAR and Molecular Modeling of Bioactive Phytophenolics. *Phytochemicals as Bioactive Agents*; Bidlack, W.R., Omaye, S.T., Meskin, M.S., Topham, D.K.W., Ed.; Chapter 2, Technomic Publishing Co.: Lancaster, PA, 2000; 21–41.

Lien, E.J. Partition Coefficients. *Encyclopedia of Pharmaceutical Technology*, 1st Ed. Swarbrick, J., Boylan, J.C., Ed.; Marcel Dekker, Inc.: New York, 1994; 11, 293–307.

Meylan, W.M.; Howard, P.H. Atom/Fragment Contribution Method for Estimating Octanol-Water Partition Coefficients. J. Pharm. Sci. **1995**, *84*, 83–92.

Pagliara, A.; Carrupt, P.A.; Caron, G.; Gaillard, P.; Testa, B. Lipophilicity Profiles of Ampholytes. Chem. Rev. **1997**, *97*, 3385–3400.

Palekar, D.; Shiue, M.; Lien, E.J. Correlation of Physicochemical Parameters to the Hydrophobic Contribution Constants of Amino Acid Residues in Small Peptides. Pharm. Res. **1996**, *13*, 1191–1195.

Reymond, F.; Steyaert, G.; Carrupt, P.A.; Testa, B.; Girault, H. Ionic Partition Diagrams: A Potential-pH Representation. J. Am. Chem. Soc. **1996**, *118*, 11951–11957.

Tsantili-Kakoulidou, A.; Panderi, I.; Csizmadia, F.; Darvas, F. Prediction of Distribution Coefficient from Structure, II. Validation of Prolog D, An Expert System. J. Pharm. Sci. **1997**, *86*, 1173–1179.

Wang, R.; Fu, Y.; Lai, L.A. A New Atom-Additive Method for Calculating Partition Coefficients. J. Chem. Inf. Comput. Sci. **1997**, *37*, 615–621.

Waterbeemd, H.V.D.; Mannhold, R. Programs and Methods for Calculation of Log P-Values. Quant. Struct.-Act. Relat. **1996**, *15*, 410–412.

PATENTS—INTERNATIONAL PERSPECTIVE

Stuart R. Suter
Suter Associates, Glenside, Pennsylvania

Peter J. Giddings
SmithKline Beecham plc, Brentford, United Kingdom

INTRODUCTION

A strong patent system is important to the research-based pharmaceutical industry. The success of the pharmaceutical industry has been based on the discovery of new products that treat human disease states in new and unique ways. The patent system has provided protection for these innovative products for a period of time, allowing the industry to use the revenues gained to search for the next generation of products that will improve the health of society. It is important that persons in R&D of the industry understand the basic principles of the patent system.

WHAT IS A PATENT?

A patent is a grant of exclusive rights from a government to inventors for their invention in exchange for the inventors disclosing their inventions to society. This quid pro quo is valuable to society because the disclosure stimulates additional innovation and development. The alternative for inventors is to keep their inventions secret and thus deprive society of the opportunity for further advancement.

Patent rights are limited in time and are also limited to the sole right of excluding others from making, using, and selling the invention. Because governments grant these rights, they are effective only in the area controlled by that government. Thus, a United States patent provides protection only in the United States and its territories such as Puerto Rico. If inventors desire protection in Japan, Canada, or any European country, they must apply for a patent in each of those countries as well.

It is important to understand that this right granted by the patent is solely a right to exclude others. It does not carry with it the right to practice the invention by the inventors themselves. This right to use by the inventor may be limited by the existence of other patents that would be needed to practice the invention or by laws or regulations having nothing to do with patents. An example of the latter is the health registration regulations in the countries where pharmaceutical products are being sold. An inventor not being free to use his invention because of other patents is also a common situation. For example, party X may have a patent claiming a broad genus of compounds useful to treat hypertension. Our inventor discovers a specific compound not disclosed specifically in the patent of party X, but through selection of the appropriate substituents in the defined genus this compound can be found. Its hypertensive properties are far superior to those of the compounds specifically disclosed in party X's patent, thus this inventor can obtain a patent for the compound but must obtain permission from party X before marketing the compound because of the patent rights of party X.

Patents belong to class of property that is referred to as "intellectual property." Intellectual property also includes trade secrets, trademarks, registered designs, and copyrights.

A trade secret is any information unknown to the public but gives the owner an economic or competitive advantage. Trade secrets have value only as long as they remain secret, which is difficult in this modern age. In the pharmaceutical industry, it is rare for any invention to be maintained as a trade secret because in the interests of public safety, the chemical composition of pharmaceutical products is always made public.

A trademark is a word, name, or symbol that identifies the source of the goods to which it applies. Two or more companies can sell the same product, but the public can identify each company's goods by the trademark. Pharmaceutical products available from multisources carry the same generic name and also the unique trademark of the specific seller; an example is the Tagamet brand of cimetidine.

A copyright protects the creations of artists and authors. In the pharmaceutical industry, copyrights are used to protect advertisements, product literature, and other copy used for product promotion.

A registered design right protects the aesthetic appearance of an article, i.e., features of a product's appearance rather than its technical features. In the pharmaceutical industry, a registered design right might be obtained, for example, in respect to a particular tablet shape or to the appearance of the product's packaging.

The patent system traces its history to early Venice, where patents were granted at least as early as 1460. The Anglo-American systems have their origins in Great Britain, where Parliament enacted the Statute of Monopolies in 1624. This law provided the basis for the British patent system for many years. The American colonies, before achieving independence, had no power to grant patents for inventions under the British system. The basic U.S. patent system is founded on the U.S. Constitution. Article I, Section 8, gives Congress the power "to promote the progress of science and useful arts by securing for limited times to authors and inventors the exclusive right to their respective writings and discoveries." The first Patent and Copyright Act in the United States was enacted on April 10, 1790.

PATENTS AND PHARMACEUTICALS

The patent system as applied to pharmaceuticals has been one of great controversy over the years. Many countries, especially those with few technology-based industries, have held that providing protection for drug products is against society's interests. Some countries include food in this category as well. Based on this theory, patents for pharmaceutical products have been limited or not allowed at all. The premise is usually that patents for chemical compounds can be claimed only for the process by which they are prepared. Thus, if someone develops a different process to make the compound, he or she can avoid the patent of the innovator.

Historically, as a country becomes more industrialized, it strengthens its patent system by providing protection for compounds per se, often referred to as "product protection." Examples are Germany and Japan, which had process protection for pharmaceutical products until 1968 and 1978, respectively, when they amended their laws to provide product protection. China had no patent law until June 1, 1985, when it introduced process-only protection for pharmaceuticals. Effective January 1, 1993, China amended its patent laws to allow product protection.

Since 1986, discussions have been ongoing at the governmental level to try to improve the standard of intellectual property laws around the world. These discussions, which have primarily been part of the General Agreement on Tariffs and Trade (GATT) negotiations among countries, culminated in 1994 with the signing of an agreement on Trade Related Aspects of Intellectual Property Rights (TRIPS). This agreement established comprehensive standards for the protection and enforcement of intellectual property rights and became effective in January 1995. The agreement is complex and covers a wide range of patent-related issues including, for example, the provision of patent protection for compounds per se and the provision of a patent term of 20 years from filing. As a general rule, the date of application of the agreement for countries classified as "developed" was January 1, 1996, and for "developing" countries January 1, 2000. The "least-developed" countries have the option to defer application of the agreement until January 1, 2006.

In summary, patent protection for pharmaceutical products has improved significantly in recent years and will continue to improve.

New compounds are not the only inventions important to the pharmaceutical industry. Many products have been developed from sources in nature, such as extracts from plants or compounds isolated from fermentation broths from various microorganisms. Protecting these inventions has been difficult at times in various countries because the materials were present in nature and thus were viewed as natural products, not new or novel. These difficulties can be overcome in certain cases by claiming the compounds in their pure form.

Patenting of "living matter" changed dramatically with the arrival of biotechnology methods and procedures. In 1980, the U.S. Supreme Court decided the famous Diamond vs. Chakrabarty case. In this case, a new strain of bacteria, produced by a reproducible artificial procedure, had the ability to digest oil and thus was useful in dispersing oil slicks. It was important to have patent protection on the bacteria per se because they were used themselves and not in a process to produce another product. Certain groups and individuals in the public sector expressed great concern that this decision would lead to patenting other higher forms of life. In 1988, U.S. Patent No. 4,736,866 was issued, claiming the "Harvard Mouse." This transgenic mouse has the special property of having an oncogene sequence in the germ and somatic cells that makes the mouse useful in testing for carcinogenic materials or for compounds that confer protection against neoplasms. Since then, many patents for higher life forms (but not humans) have been issued.

In Europe, the issues surrounding the patentability of biotechnological inventions are the subject of vigorous ongoing legal and political debate. In July 1998, the European Parliament approved Directive 98/44/EC aimed at harmonizing laws across Europe with respect to the patenting of biotechnological inventions. Member states had until July 2000 to bring their laws into conformity with the directive. However, the Dutch government has issued a challenge to the legality of the Directive at the European Court of Justice, and the decision of the court is awaited.

With respect to the specific case of the Harvard Mouse, an equivalent European patent has been allowed, but it is currently under opposition by a number of parties at the European Patent Office (EPO). Thus, the status of the patent is unclear at this time.

INTERNATIONAL TREATIES AND SYSTEMS

As noted above, patent protection is obtained on a country-by-country basis, and therefore patent applications must be filed in each country where protection is desired. International treaties and regional conventions have been set up to coordinate and make obtaining worldwide protection convenient and efficient. Several important treaties have been developed and are administered by the international organization known as the World Intellectual Property Organization (WIPO), centered in Geneva, Switzerland.

Paris Convention

This is the short title for the Paris Convention for the Protection of Industrial Property. This treaty was first signed in Paris in 1883 by 11 countries and has been revised several times over the years. Today 157 countries have ratified this treaty. A notable country of concern to the pharmaceutical industry that is not a member of the Paris Convention is Taiwan.

An important feature of the Paris Convention allows applicants to claim priority to their first-filed application in any member country, provided the applicant files a patent application in that country within 1 year. This is referred to as convention priority, and it is of great importance in the patent strategies developed in the pharmaceutical industry, as described below. If the first application meets the conditions of the Convention, the applications in all member countries are treated as if they were filed on the same day as the first application.

Budapest Treaty

When an invention involves a microorganism, most countries require the deposit of the biological material to complete the disclosure. WIPO established international uniformity under the Budapest Treaty of 1977, which became effective in 1980 and has been ratified by

48 countries. It provides for the establishment of a group of international deposit authorities. When a strain of microorganisms is deposited in any one of these authorities, this single deposit satisfies the necessary requirements for all signatory countries of this treaty. Under this convention, the formal requirements for making the deposit and maintaining the culture are set forth. Included in this is the possibility of a redeposit should the initial deposit become nonviable. The maintenance period of the deposit is a minimum of 30 years from the date of deposit.

Patent Cooperation Treaty (PCT)

The PCT first came into force in January 1978. It is in effect in 109 countries, including the United States, all the countries of the European Patent Convention, Japan, Canada, and China, as of January 1, 2001.

This treaty puts forth a process by which an applicant, through a simplified procedure, can file one application and designate that it be treated as an application in one or up to all of the PCT member countries. This application is filed in one of the official receiving offices in any of the official languages—English, German, French, Chinese, Japanese, Russian, and Spanish. The PCT has become a very important procedure in the pharmaceutical industry in providing an efficient means of obtaining maximum patent protection around the world in the most efficient and cost-effective manner.

The PCT application can be filed under the terms of the Paris Convention at the end of the 1-year period from the priority filing. The receiving office passes the application on to an International Searching Authority through which a search for the novelty of the invention is carried out. The application, together with the search report, is published 18 months from the priority date. After this publication, the applicant can choose two avenues for his application. First, if she or he wishes to proceed directly to each of the designated countries, the filing can be perfected in each of the designated countries within 20 months of the priority date. This is done by submitting the formal documents, translations, and fees required by each local patent office in each designated country. Alternatively, by the end of 19 months, a "demand" can be filed that the Preliminary Examining Authority of the PCT carry out a preliminary examination for patentability. This examination takes place between the 19th and 28th months of the priority date. During this period, the applicant receives the results of the examination and has the opportunity to present arguments in support of the patentability of his invention and/or amend his application. Again, the applicant must submit all formal documents, translations, and fees required by each designated country to perfect the individual national filings by the end of the 30th month.

The main advantage of the PCT process is that it allows the applicant time to determine more clearly the commercial viability and importance of the invention. In the pharmaceutical industry, patents are filed on new potential products very early in their development. Many of these fall by the wayside during the development process. The PCT allows for an application to be filed and maintained with minimum expense up to the 30th month before the significant expense of national filing fees and translations is required. Thus, under a strategy using the PCT, the pharmaceutical company can maintain patent applications for the major economically important countries at minimum cost while having 30 months in which to study the invention and determine its commercial potential.

This treaty has been gaining in popularity and use in recent years. In 1999, the PCT was used to file 74,023 applications, compared with 14,874 in 1989 and 2,625 in 1979.

European Patent Convention

A regional system is one that arises from a regional treaty entered into by a number of countries within a geographic area. The European Patent Convention (EPC) is the most important of several regional patent systems. It was negotiated by a number of European countries and entered into force on October 7, 1977. Eight countries ratified it by the time the European Patent Office (EPO) began accepting applications on June 1, 1978. As of January 2001, 20 countries have ratified the EPC. In addition, six other countries, including Slovenia and Romania, have indicated that granted European patents can be validated to have effect in their countries as an alternative to applying for national applications in those countries.

Under the EPC, applicants can file one application in the EPO and designate in which of the 20 countries they desire the application to have effect. The application is examined by the EPO, and if the invention is found patentable, the application is granted, not as a single patent, but as a national patent for each country designated by the applicant at the time of filing. Under the EPC, it is possible to challenge the grant of the patent, provided the challenge is made within 9 months of the patent grant. This provides the opportunity potentially to have the patent declared invalid in one set of proceedings. This procedure is referred to as an opposition and still takes places in the EPO. If there is no opposition filed to the grant of the patent, then challenges to validity of the patent and enforcement need to take place in each country under the national patent laws of that country.

This convention provides an efficient means of obtaining patent protection in up to 26 countries through the filing and prosecution of only one application. When the EPC first went into effect, there was concern that if the prosecution was unfavorable, the applicant would not have any patent protection, whereas if the national system had been used, he would. With the passage of time, this concern has been greatly diminished, and now the convention is used by most, if not all, in the pharmaceutical industry on a routine basis.

Other Regional Systems

There are a number of other regional patent application systems in operation. In Africa, two regional systems operate: the African Regional Industrial Property Organization (ARIPO), formed in 1976, and the African Intellectual Property Organization (OAPI), formed in 1962. These systems have 11 and 15 member states, respectively. In the Middle East, the Gulf Co-operation Treaty operate to provide protection in six countries (for example, Saudi Arabia and The United Arab Emirates), and the Eurasian Patent System operates to provide protection in nine countries of the former Soviet Union, including Russia.

CLAIMABLE INVENTIONS IN THE PHARMACEUTICAL AREA

Section 101 of the U.S. Patent Law defines inventions and discoveries for which a patent can be obtained in very broad terms. Specifically, these are processes, machines, articles of manufacture, and compositions of matter, or any new and useful improvements of these. Article 52 of the EPC provides that a patent will be granted for any inventions that meet the three requirements for patentability. It then lists exclusions, which include "scientific theories and mathematic methods" in addition to medical treatments, as noted below. Many different inventions arising from research in the pharmaceutical field can be protected under these broad definitions.

Chemical Inventions

In the pharmaceutical field, chemical inventions have become of primary importance. The traditional inventions for which the pharmaceutical industry has sought patents are set forth in Table 1.

Specifically, a new composition of matter (NCM) or new chemical compound prepared by synthetic methods is the primary area of interest. They may be made using

Table 1　Potential chemical inventions

Compound per se
Pharmaceutical compositions of new compounds
New pharmaceutical compositions of existing compounds
Method of treatment, mechanistically or by disease state or both
Compound for use (broad first use)
New medical use for existing compound (second use)
Analogy processes for new compounds
Process per se (when novel and inventive)
Intermediates
Processes for preparing compositions
Different salt forms, hydrates, or polymorphs

Table 2　Potential biotechnology inventions

Recombinant/genomics
　The protein perse
　Antibodies that react specifically with the protein and
　　antiidiotype antibodies
　rDNA that encodes the protein
　Expression systems
　Recombinant host cells containing the DNA
　Processes to make protein using recombinant host cells
　Processes for purifying the protein
　Processes to produce the antibody and antiidiotype antibodies
　Methods of using the DNA sequence
　Pharmaceutical compositions of the protein
　Method of treatment
　Vectors
　Promoters
　Single nucleotide polymorphisms (SNPs)
　Expressed sequence tags (ESTs)
　Genomic DNA
Monoclonal antibodies
　Monoclonal antibody (Mab)
　Hybridoma that produces Mab
　Process to prepare Mab
　Method to use Mab
　Pharmaceutical composition of the Mab
　Novel antigen and related processes and methods

synthetic methods or are isolated from natural sources such as plant or oceanic material or from fermentation broths. At times, a compound is known in an impure state that is unusable as a pharmaceutical product. If it is obtained in a purified state and meets the requirements of patentability, it can be claimed as a compound of a defined purity.

In addition to the compound per se, chemical processes for the preparation of the compound can be claimed. Analogous processes, which are a known chemical reactions that produce a new compound or use new starting materials, have various standards of patentability in different countries.

Pharmaceutical compositions of the new compound or new improved formulations of existing compounds are also patentable. For a new drug-delivery system, patent protection can be very important and useful, especially if developed for the delivery of an existing product.

A method of treating a particular disease or physiological condition is another important type of invention in the pharmaceutical field. It may be necessary to claim this type of invention by what is called "Swiss claims" to overcome the industrial applicability requirement in Europe. Such claims take the form of claiming the compound for use in the manufacture of a medicament for the treatment of a particular disease state. In the United States, the applicant may be required to provide proof to support the treatment claim. This is especially true if the invention is treating a disease that has been difficult or impossible to treat in the past, e.g., cancer or AIDS. A claim to "a method of treating cancer with compound X" will be challenged during examination. The most likely result will be amendment of the claim to a method of treating the specific cancer for which data can be provided to demonstrate utility.

Biotechnology Inventions

With the blossoming of biotechnology in the 1980s and, more recently, of genomics, a whole new specialty in

patent law has developed. In general, it is viewed that the principles of chemical patent practice apply equally to the biotechnology field. The Court of Appeals for the Federal Circuit (which is the U.S. Federal Court that hears all patent appeals from the Patent and Trademark Office and any Federal District Courts) has affirmed this in their decisions. Biotechnology inventions must satisfy the standard statutory requirements in the same manner as for any other invention. From the list of claimable inventions in Table 2, it is clear that biotechnology techniques have resulted in the production of inventions previously not obtainable by classic chemical methods.

REQUIREMENTS FOR PATENTABILITY

There are three basic requirements for patentability: novelty; nonobviousness or inventive step; and usefulness or industrial applicability. Each requirement may differ from country to country and is set forth by the statutes and regulations of each country.

Novelty

The first principle of patent law is that to obtain a patent, the invention must be new. The statutory requirements for novelty are set forth in Section 102 of the U.S. Patent Law and in Article 54 of the EPC.

In the United States, Section 102 has several stated requirements. One is that the invention must not have been known or used by others in the United States or patented or described in a printed publication in the United States or in any foreign country before the invention was made by the applicant. The second provision is that the invention must not have been patented or described in any printed publication anywhere in the world more than 1 year before the date of application in the United States. This is the 1-year grace period available in the United States but not in the rest of the world. These requirements are grouped under the term "anticipation" and mean that a single prior art reference must show the invention being claimed to nullify novelty. If an essential part of the invention is not present in a single publication, but is found in a second reference, anticipation does not exist (however, see the next section on obviousness).

Article 54 of the EPC defines an invention as "new if it does not form part of the state of the art." It goes on to specify that the state of the art comprises "… everything made available to the public by means of a written or oral description, by use or in any other way before the date of filing…."

Nonobvious or Inventive Step

In many cases, the requirement of nonobviousness or inventive step as it is referred to in Europe, is the one that presents the most difficulty during the examination process. It is governed by Section 103 of the U.S. Patent Law and by Article 56 of the EPC. The general principle is that even though an invention is novel, a patent cannot be granted unless the inventor has done something more than one would expect any given person to have done in the art or field to which the invention pertains. Two or more references can be used to make the case of what would have been obvious to the given person skilled in the art. In the pharmaceutical field, chemical compounds are often known that are very close structurally and/or have similar utilities to the compounds claimed in the application. In these situations, the issue of proving nonobvious is the of most concern during the examination process.

Usefulness or Industrial Applicability

This requirement is covered by Section 101 of the U.S. Patent Law and by Article 57 of the EPC.

In the United States, usefulness is a very broad concept and does not mean a commercial utility is in hand. In the pharmaceutical field, a showing of in vitro test results that have some nexus with treating a physiological condition is sufficient to meet this requirement. If, however, the invention is useful only as a scientific curiosity, this requirement is not met. Chemical intermediates may or may not have the required usefulness. If they are useful to prepare products that are themselves useful then they are patentable. However, intermediates that are only useful to prepare compounds with no utility are not patentable.

In Europe, industrial applicability is required. This means, for example, that methods of medical treatment or diagnosis performed on a human or an animal are not susceptible to industrial application. Nevertheless, substances that are useful in these methods are patentable.

OBTAINING A PATENT

When an invention is made, consideration must be given as to whether to obtain patent protection. Companies have a variety of internal procedures to determine when and where to seek patent protection.

After it has been decided to obtain patent protection, a patent application is prepared and filed. This first filing is referred to as a priority filing and the filing date as the priority date. This is the date against which the invention will be judged for purposes of determining whether a patent should be granted, as discussed above.

Filing Applications

This first patent application is usually filed in the home country of the inventors. In many countries, there are laws and/or regulations that require this, or, if the inventor wants to file in another country first, certain requirements must be met. In the United States, there are regulations against exporting technology to other countries without government approval. An invention made in the United States must be filed first in the United States and not in any foreign country for 6 months after this filing without obtaining an export license from the U.S. Patent Office. If the applicant wishes to file first in another country, he or she must submit the application to the U.S. Patent Office and obtain the export license before filing in that country.

After the priority application is filed, the applicant must decide in what additional countries the application should be filed during the 12-month convention period available under the Paris Convention. This is often referred to as the foreign filing decision. The cost of protecting the invention is directly proportional to the number of applications filed and the different language translations required by these filings. In times of cost consciousness, this foreign filing decision is not taken lightly.

Several options are available to applicants at this time. The first is to obtain a patent only in their home country and not pursue patent protection elsewhere. The second possibility is to proceed with a foreign filing in one or more foreign countries within the convention year. A final option is to abandon the home country application and not pursue patent protection.

The choice among these options depends on many factors. If the invention is completely or almost completely understood and its commercial potential known, then the decision as to in which countries to file can be made without much difficulty. Most pharmaceutical companies have listings of "filing groups" of countries that are used depending on the projected commercial potential for the invention. These filing groups may contain a few major countries up to a large number of countries, e.g., 50 to 100 countries or more. Each company develops its own set of filing groups based on numerous factors including costs, strength of protection in each country, the company's markets, etc. Likewise, the selection of the filing group for each particular invention depends on factors such as type of invention, perceived commercial potential, projected market areas, and the like.

Alternatively, if the invention and its commercial potential are not fully understood, the applicant could abandon or abandon and refile. This process carries with it the danger that someone else may have filed a patent application between applicant's priority date and the second priority date obtained through the refiling process. When this occurs, the applicant loses the rights to the invention in most countries. This can be especially dangerous in highly competitive areas in which many people are conducting research.

An alternate strategy is to file the foreign applications under the provisions of the PCT to obtain, an additional 18 months before the significant filing fees and cost of translations are incurred (see discussion under PCT, above).

Even after the 12-month priority period has passed, the applicant may still file patent applications, provided there has been no publication or public use of his invention. Applications filed in most countries including the EPO and PCT are published 18 months after the priority date. The United States will begin publishing applications filed on or after November 29, 2000. If the application has not been published and the applicant has not published in any scientific journals, he or she can still file in a country and obtain a patent. This is called a nonconvention filing because the applicant does not claim rights back to his first priority date. Therefore, if new information about the commercial potential of the invention becomes available between the 12th and 18th months, one should always review it carefully and decide whether nonconvention applications should be filed.

Examination of the Application

Once an application has been filed, each patent office will examine it before granting a patent. The completeness of this examination differs from country to country. In some countries, it is a matter of merely verifying that the application has all the proper formal papers required under the laws and regulations of that country. Other countries carry out a rigorous examination as to the patentability of the invention in addition to the formal matters of proper documents. The United States, Japanese, and European patent offices examine patent applications for all requirements of patentability. In the United States, applications filed on or after May 29, 2000, must be granted within 3 years. If it is not, a patent term adjustment is available, provided the applicant has followed all procedures in a timely manner. Currently, the EPO starts the examination process approximately 2 to 3 years after the application is filed. Japan uses a deferred examination process. An application filed in the Japanese Patent Office remains dormant until the applicant requests the patent office to examine it. It can be deferred up to 7 years from the filing date. Once requested, the examination process in Japan normally takes 2 to 3 years to complete. On occasion, this process can take significantly longer because Japan has a pregrant opposition system. This means that once the patent office makes a determination to grant an application, it is published, and within 90 days of that publication date, anyone may file an opposition to the grant. If this occurs, a lengthy proceeding can ensue, possibly deferring the patent grant for many years.

Content of a Patent Application

Each country sets forth the requirements for a patent application through its laws and regulations. The United States does this through Section 112 of the Patent Law. This section specifies that the application must contain two parts: the specification and the claims. The requirements of the specification are set forth in the first paragraph of Section 112, as follows:

> The specification shall contain a written description of the invention and the manner and process of

making and using it in such full, clear, concise and exact terms as to enable any person skilled in the art to which it pertains or with which it is most nearly connected to make and use the same and shall set forth the best mode contemplated by the inventor of carrying out his invention. To summarize, there are three requirements: a written description, an enabling disclosure, and the best mode. A written description and an enabling disclosure are universal requirements. However, the best mode requirement is distinctive to the U.S. patent system and is one that causes much debate among patent administrators. The requirement is based on the theory that applicants should not receive the privileges of patent protection if they have not disclosed the best methods of making and using the invention known to them at the time the patent application is filed. If applicants fail to disclose the best mode, even unintentionally, the patent can be held invalid.

Based on these disclosure requirements, the application normally contains the following:

1. Abstract
2. Summary of the background needed to understand the invention
3. Summary of the invention
4. Detailed description of how to practice the invention including appropriate examples and drawings.

The second paragraph of Section 112 requires that applicants point out and distinctly define the invention with a set of claims. Up to this point, a patent application has been a scientific article that teaches other people in the same field how to make and use the invention. This is no different than a scientific journal article. The claims, however, set forth what the applicant considers to be the invention for which patent protection is being sought. During the examination process, the claims may be modified to overcome objections. Therefore, one often finds, as a result of the examination process, the allowed claims of a granted patent often define less subject matter than is disclosed in the specification. Because the claims define the subject matter protected by the patent, when asked a question regarding infringement, a patent attorney will turn immediately to the claims to begin an analysis rather than to the description in the specification.

OWNERSHIP

Patents are property whose ownership may be governed law, contract, or by statutory provision. In many employer-

employee relationships, the employee has signed a contract of employment. This contract states that the employer owns all inventions made by the employee. In some countries, most notably Germany, there are elaborate statutory provisions for compensation of inventors by the employer. In all countries except the United States, the owner of the patent rights may file the patent application. Historically, the U.S. system has been based on rewarding the inventor and thus requires that the inventor apply for the patent. If the inventor is required by a contract of employment to assign the inventions to the employer, the U.S. application is made in the inventor's name, and an assignment noting the transfer of rights to the employer is recorded in the patent office.

INVENTORSHIP

In most of the world, inventorship of a patent may be relevant as to who owns the rights but it is not relevant to the validity of the patent. In fact, in some countries the inventor may never be mentioned or even appear on the patent. Again, the one important exception is the United States, where, as noted above, the inventor or inventors must file the patent application. If the wrong inventor or inventors intentionally apply for the patent, grounds for declaring the U.S. patent invalid are raised. Therefore, the proper inventors of the claimed invention are always determined according to the requirements of U.S. law.

It must be remembered that inventorship is different from authorship. Inventorship is based on legal requirements and must be strictly followed, whereas authorship is more arbitrary. The determination of inventorship is based on first inspecting the invention and determining what person or persons made an "inventive" contribution to the conception and reduction to practice of this invention. Conception is the mental steps taken to develop the invention. Reduction to practice is the physical process of taking the idea to the completed working invention. When two or more inventors (joint inventors) are involved, each must contribute to the claimed invention, but each is not required to have made a contribution to each claim of the patent.

Inventorship determination is not always straightforward and simple in today's research environment. However, to make these correct determinations, certain questions are asked. Did the person do only routine work or experiments as directed by another, or did he or she contribute something more? Was the invention completed because of the specific activity of this person? Did this person proceed beyond specific directions? In today's modern pharmaceutical research atmosphere, in which teams are involved in the discovery and development processes, the patent attorney may find the determination of the correct inventorship a very difficult aspect in the preparation of a patent application. In a 1972 decision, U.S. District Court Judge Newcomer made the following observation:

> The exact parameters of what constitutes joint inventorship are quite difficult to define. It is one of the muddiest concepts in the muddy metaphysics of patent law.

WHEN TWO OR MORE GROUPS MAKE THE SAME INVENTION

Sometimes two or more applicants make the same invention, but only one patent can be granted. The question is who receives the patent grant. In all countries except the United States, the first to file a patent application is granted the patent. In the United States, the patent is granted to the first to make the invention.

The first inventor is determined by a special administrative proceeding in the patent office called an interference. Evidence is presented by each applicant as to their earliest dates of conception and reduction to practice. Before January 1, 1996, only activities carried out in the United States could be used in these proofs. Now activities carried out in any country that is a member of the World Trade Organization can be used to prove when the invention was made.

In an interference, the proof requirements are very important. Activities or evidence given by the inventor must be collaborated in some manner. This is best accomplished through evidence from noninventors, although other forms of evidence have been used successfully in some cases. For this reason, research organizations have policies and procedures governing notebook recordkeeping in their laboratories.

Interferences are very complex and expensive proceedings that can delay the patent grant for many years. Fortunately, only less than 0.5% of all U.S. applications are involved in an interference.

LENGTH OF PATENT PROTECTION

The term of a patent grant is defined by the laws of each country, varying generally from 15 to 20 years. In some developing countries, patent terms are much shorter and

are of very little value to the pharmaceutical industry because the patent expires before the product can be marketed. Recently most countries, including the United States, have adopted a standard patent life of 20 years from the filing date. The United States, which until June, 1995, had a term of 17 years from the patent grant date, has recently enacted additional laws to restore any of the 20-year term lost because of delays in the patent office. Japanese patents have a 15-year term from the date of grant or 20 years from the date of filing, whichever is shorter.

In the pharmaceutical industry, the term of patent life is a very important factor. Because patents are filed very early in the life cycle of a new pharmaceutical product and much premarketing testing is needed before the health authorities will permit public sale of a product, a large portion of patent life is lost. Often, the term "effective patent life" for pharmaceutical products is used. Studies by the Pharmaceutical Research and Manufacturers of America have shown that effective patent life for pharmaceutical products averaged 15 years in the early 1960s and declined to 8 years in the early 1980s. Studies in Japan and Great Britain gave similar results. In recent years, the laws of many important countries have been changed to provide for the recapture of some of this lost patent life through patent term extension provisions.

Patent Term Extensions

Before 1980, in some countries, mainly those that were formerly part of the British Commonwealth, patent extensions were obtainable on petition at the end of the patent life. For a petition to be granted, the patent owner was required to show inability during the normal life of the patent to receive sufficient remuneration from the use of the patented invention. Under this system, patent extensions of 4 to 10 years could be obtained based on the evidence presented.

In 1984, the United States passed the first patent term restoration statute as part of the Drug Price Competition and Patent Term Restoration Act of 1984 (often referred to as the Waxman-Hatch Act). This was a significant law for the total pharmaceutical industry because it contained provisions important to both the research-based and the generic sections of the industry. Under this act, generic pharmaceutical companies were allowed to file abbreviated new drug applications (ANDA) and to do the testing required to submit an ANDA before the patent expired without being liable for patent infringement. The second part provided for the innovator of a new pharmaceutical product to receive up to 5 years of patent extension based on the time required to receive marketing approval from the Food and Drug Administration.

The extension can provide effective patent life for the product no longer than 14 years from the date of marketing approval.

Other countries have followed the U.S. lead regarding patent term extension. Japan enacted a provision effective January 1, 1986, whereby patents covering pharmaceutical products could be extended for up to 5 years. The Japanese provisions differ from the U.S. law in several ways. First, more than one patent can be extended for each product. Also, the Japanese law requires that the patent be granted 2 years before health authority approval of the product. Korea has enacted a patent term extension law very similar to that in the Japanese system. Australia has replaced its "lack of renumeration" system with a system based on regulatory delay.

Effective on January 1, 1993, Supplementary Protection Certificates (SPC), a system of providing extended protection for pharmaceutical products, was created by the European Community (EC). Such certificates do not actually extend the patent per se but confers protection for the product covered by the granted marketing approval (MA) and any use of the product as a pharmaceutical product for humans or animals. If more than one patent protects the product, the owner must select only one patent to be the basis for the SPC. SPCs are granted by individual national patent offices and come into effect only after the normal patent term expires. The duration of the SPC is equal to the time from the patent filing date to first MA in the EC, minus 5 years, subject to the limitations that the SPC cannot be effective for more than 5 years or provide protection for more than 15 years from the date of first MA in the EC.

The patent owner must request the SPC in the patent office of each country EC within 6 months of the first MA in that country or within 6 months of the patent grant date if it occurs after the first MA in that country. The SPC will be granted if, at the time the application is filed, 1) the patent has not expired; 2) an MA has been granted; 3) the product has not previously been the subject of an SPC; and 4) the MA is the first authorization to market the product.

The regulations allowed Spain and Greece to delay accepting the SPC system for 5 years. In addition, transitional provisions were adopted that allowed each country to choose to allow SPCs for products whose first MA was granted after January 1, 1982, June 1, 1985, or January 1, 1988.

MAINTAINING AND ENFORCING PATENTS

After a patent is granted, the owner must pay fees to keep it in force and may have to defend it from challenges to its validity and/or enforce it against infringers.

Maintenance Fees

In most countries, a patent does not automatically stay in force from the day it is granted until the end of its life. Most countries require payment of fees, referred to as renewal or maintenance fees, to keep the patent in force. In most countries, these fees are paid on an annual basis. Until 1980, the United States was a notable exception. However, in 1980 the United States modified its patent laws to require that fees be paid at three different time periods during the life of the patent. Specifically, renewal fees must be paid at 3.5, 7.5, and 11.5 years from the date the patent is granted. Although renewal fees vary from country to country, it is universal that the fees increase over the life of the patent. For example, the U.S. fees in 2000 are $930, $1870, and $2820 for the three periods, whereas in Germany fees begin at approximately 150 DM and increase to 3500 DM for the 20th year. If the owner of the patent knows that it has no value to himself or others, he or she will generally stop paying the fees and allow the patent to lapse. Maintenance fees on a portfolio of patents can become very expensive, therefore, most companies have a program of regular review of their patent portfolio. Patents, that are no longer of value to them are lapsed.

Invalidation

Once a patent is granted, the patent owner is not guaranteed that it is valid. Challenges to the validity of the patent again vary from country to country, depending on the specific patent law of each country.

In the United States, the patent law specifically provides that a granted patent carries with it a presumption of validity. Until 1980, the validity of a patent could be challenged only in a federal court as part of an infringement action or by suit for declaratory judgment of invalidity. This latter action could only be initiated by a party who was threatened by the patent owner so that the requisite legal dispute actually existed between the parties. In 1980, the patent law was amended to allow any person to file a request in the patent office for re-examination of a U.S. patent based on new prior art. The patent office studies the request and determines whether to grant reexamination. This procedure is not used very often because the third party requestor has little opportunity to fully present its views. On November 29, 1999, a new reexamination law was passed that applies to patents originally filed after that date, which allows for greater participation by the third party.

In Europe, challenges to the validity of patents must be made in each individual country unless a central opposition has been made to a European patent (see above).

PATENT INFRINGEMENT

A patent is infringed when someone makes uses or sells the claimed invention without the permission of the patent owner. When this occurs, the patent owner can take legal action against the party.

In the United States, this is a civil action brought in the federal courts. The specific federal district court in which a patent owner can sue an infringer is governed by federal law. Patent litigation is very expensive and time-consuming. For this reason, it is not entered into without careful consideration of the consequences and analysis of all options available. In recent years, various alternative dispute-resolution proceedings have been used more often.

Because patents are limited in their effect in a specific country, a company with a pioneering drug may find itself suing patent infringers in a number of other countries. Usually these actions are in countries where the patent system is not as strong as that in the United States and the major European countries. The direct costs of patent litigation are usually lower outside the United States, but the time requirements can be just as extensive.

Patents to compounds or pharmaceutical compositions are infringed by their sale or use in the country of issuance. Patents to processes for the preparation of a compound cause a different problem. There is no direct infringement if the compound is made by the process in a country without patent protection and then imported into the country where the process is patented. However, the laws of many countries specify that the sale or use of compounds made directly by a patented process is an infringement of the process patent. In most cases, "directly" means the final step to prepare the compound. Such protection was not available in the United States until 1986, when the patent laws were amended. The amendment also has a provision whereby a party can ask the producer of a compound for a list of any U.S. process patents that are owned or licensed.

REGULATORY EXCLUSIVITY AND ORPHAN DRUGS

Although patents are the main defense against generic copying in the pharmaceutical industry, another important form of protection that has developed in recent years relates to the data generated by the originator of a product in support of the marketing approval application. Specifically, valuable periods of so-called regulatory exclusivity have become available in the United States, Europe, and Japan. In addition, in the United States, the Orphan Drug Act has provided a special kind of regulatory exclusivity.

Regulatory Exclusivity

The interests of public safety and avoidance of unnecessary animal experimentation make it desirable that licensing authorities be able to cross-refer the originators file to establish safety and efficacy of generic versions of a product. Applications for marketing authorizations that rely on cross-referral to the originators full regulatory submission are generally known as abridged regulatory applications. Regulatory exclusivity is a temporary prohibition on cross-referral to the originator's data without the originator's consent. After a specified time, as detailed below, the originator cannot object to the cross-referral. Regulatory exclusivity is acquired rather than applied for by the originating drug manufacturer, and no certificate or other documentation is issued for the exclusivity period.

In 1980, Japan became the first country to have a regulatory exclusivity provision. The period is 6 years for new products, new combination products, or different routes of administration. For other modifications, such as a new indication or a new dosage regimen, the period of exclusivity is 4 years. If second applicants do their own complete safety and efficacy studies, these periods of exclusivity do not apply.

In the United States, these regulatory exclusivity rights are part of the Waxman-Hatch Act. The law provides that no abbreviated new drug application (ANDA) can be submitted for a generic equivalent for a new chemical entity (NCE) until 5 years after the approval date for the NCE. If the ANDA applicant certifies that the patent covering the NCE is invalid or not infringed, the period is 4 years. If a NCE is not involved or a pioneering supplemental NDA is approved,

Table 3   European regulatory exclusivity

10 Years	6 Years
United Kingdom	Denmark
Austria	Finland
France	Greece
Germany	Ireland
Belgium	Luxembourg
Holland	Portugal
Italy	Spain
Sweden	

a 3-year period exists before an ANDA can *become effective*. Thus, for non-NCEs, the regulatory period is reduced to 3 years. For a NCE the 5-year period is for *submission* of an ANDA, and so the FDA processing time would extend this exclusivity period.

Another interesting part of this law is that if a generic drug manufacturer challenges a patent and is successful, it is rewarded with a 6-month period during which no other generic products will be approved.

In Europe, regulatory exclusivity is more complex. More specifically, the countries may choose between a 10-year or 6-year period. According to European Community Directive 87/21, the national states can protect pharmaceutical products for 6 or 10 years from first marketing approval in the European Community. An exception to this is biotech products for which a 10-year period applies for all European countries. The countries that have chosen 10 or 6 years are presented in Table 3.

Orphan Drugs

Drugs that are used for treating rare diseases or conditions are called orphan drugs. The U.S. Orphan Drug Act provides that the FDA may not approve another application within 7 years of approval of the first unless the originator cannot assure availability to meet the needs of patients. This law was amended in 1985 to apply to patented as well as nonpatented drugs. The requirements to be recognized as an orphan drug that are 1) the disease affects fewer than 200,000 persons in the United States, or

2) recovery of the R&D costs from U.S. sales is unlikely. A request must be made to the FDA to obtain orphan drug status. The determination of eligibility is made as of the date of the request. This 7-year period of marketing exclusivity applies only to the individual uses of the compound or product and not to the compound itself.

In Japan, a law was introduced in October 1993 providing benefits for designated compounds including an accelerated examination, a 10-year rather than 5-year regulatory exclusivity period, and tax benefits. The conditions for orphan drug status are that the drug must be for the treatment of diseases with fewer than 50,000 patients in Japan and clinical trials essential to development for that use.

There are no specific orphan drug regulations in the EU. Other countries do not have exclusivity for orphan drugs at this time; however, provisions exist in some countries for speedier approval.

BIBLIOGRAPHY

Grubb, P.W. *Patents in Chemistry and Biotechnology*; Clarendon Press: Oxford, 1986.

Rosenstock, J. *The Law of Chemical and Pharmaceutical Invention: Patent and Nonpatent Protection*, 2nd Ed.; Aspen Law and Business: New York, 2000.

Wallerstein, M.B. Magee, M.E.; Schoen, R.A. *Global Dimensions of Intellectual Property Rights in Science and Technology*; National Academy Press: Washington, DC, 1993.

P

PATENTS—UNITED STATES PERSPECTIVE

Lorie Ann Morgan
GlaxoSmithKline, Research Triangle Park, North Carolina

Jeffrey Tidwell
University of North Carolina, Chapel Hill, North Carolina

INTRODUCTION

The importance of pharmaceutical patents has increased with the dramatic growth of the generic pharmaceutical industry in the United States and the resulting competition between the research-based pharmaceutical industry and the generic pharmaceutical industry. The research-based pharmaceutical industry provides a continuing supply of new and better pharmaceuticals to treat illness and improve lifestyle. The generic pharmaceutical industry, on the other hand, strives to provide lower-cost generic alternatives to already approved drugs. Patents provide the research-based pharmaceutical industry with an opportunity to recoup the extensive investment costs involved in providing new and better pharmaceuticals to the public. At the same time, patents restrict the generic pharmaceutical industry's ability to obtain approval for competing generic drugs. While a patent claiming the drug is in force, the generic pharmaceutical manufacturer is precluded from conducting infringing activities. The balance between the need for extensive Food and Drug Administration (FDA) review and approval of generic drugs and the need to preserve the enforceability of patents protecting newly developed drugs and provide incentives for further research and developement of new drugs prompted the Hatch–Waxman Amendments in 1984 (Drug Price Competition and Patent Term Restoration Act of 1984).

INNOVATOR PATENTS

Types of Patent Claims

Pharmaceutical companies spend billions of dollars on research and development programs each year in an effort to discover and develop innovative new medicines. As such, protection of these novel drugs and new technology developed during the research process from outside competitors is of paramount importance. The patent laws of the United States provide a mechanism by which research-based pharmaceutical companies can protect their inventions and commercialize them exclusively for a term of 20 years. When applying for a patent, an inventor sets forth the subject matter to be protected at the end of the patent specification in the claims. The claims of the patent determine the scope of protection during the 20-year exclusivity period.

Patentable subject matter is "... any new and useful process, machine, manufacture, or composition of matter, or any new and useful improvement thereof ..." (1). Patent laws provide that patents may be granted only for inventions that are deemed to be "new and useful." These requirements exclude pharmaceutical inventions that have not been shown to be reasonably safe and effective and chemical compounds that have no use except as intermediates for additional research. However, some special considerations have traditionally been applied in the case of chemical compounds, particularly those possessing therapeutic or pharmacological activity. A compound that is useful as an intermediate for the manufacture of a pharmacologically active compound may be claimed and afforded patent protection because it satisfies the utility requirement and is considered to be "useful." Further, a compound need not show therapeutic utility in humans to meet the utility requirement of patentability; pharmacological activity in animals or in vitro activity is considered sufficient in some cases. If the patent application purports to claim the use of a compound for the treatment of humans, the inventor must show that the compound is both safe and effective in humans.

Multiple patents may be issued that provide protection for the same new drug product because a single invention may be claimed in a number of different ways. For example, a patent may claim the compound itself, a novel use for the compound in treating disease, and a method for preparing and administering the compound.

Composition of matter

The most expansive protection is afforded by claims that present the particular novel product or drug compound

Encyclopedia of Pharmaceutical Technology

itself. Claims to specific chemical entities permit the innovator to exclude others from making, using, selling, offering for sale, or importing the drug compound into the United States regardless of the purpose for doing so and regardless of the formulation into which the drug is included.

Composition-of-matter claims can include claims to small organic compounds that may be useful as drug candidates as well as claims to more complex biomolecules. For example, a composition-of-matter claim may encompass claims to proteins, plasmids, pieces of DNA or RNA, and pharmacological receptors.

Another area of particular importance to the pharmaceutical industry of late is the patentability of living organisms. The last several years have seen a dramatic increase in the pace of biological research and technology. As a result, the courts have had to deal with the question of whether or not manmade living organisms qualify as patentable subject matter. Although the courts struggled with this issue, it is now fairly settled that manmade living organisms, such as genetically engineered animals, biologically pure cultures, and genetically engineered microorganisms, are patentable subject matter.

Natural products

An area of great importance to the pharmaceutical industry in particular relates to the patentability of natural products for use in treating disease. The last several decades have witnessed a dramatic increase in the search for compounds from natural sources, such as plants, for the treatment of human disease. It is established law that natural products are considered to exist in the "state of nature" and are not considered novel. Therefore, natural products generally cannot be claimed as a patentable composition of matter. This is true even if the natural product is isolated by novel means or is tested against novel drug targets. However, there are two ways in which natural products may be patentable. First, it is possible to obtain a method-of-use patent involving a natural product as it relates to novel biological or pharmacological activity. Second, it is possible to obtain composition-of-matter coverage for synthetic analogs of natural products because they are not considered to exist in the state of nature. This is of paramount importance because many new drugs are closely related, synthetic analogs of natural products.

Method claims

There are two types of method claims: method-of-making (or process) claims and method-of-using claims. An inventor may protect a new drug by claims directed toward the method of synthesizing the compound. Process claims provide the inventor with the right to exclude others

from using the claimed methods to prepare a chemical compound. In addition, the Process Patent Amendment Act (2), discussed below, provides the inventor with the power to prevent others from importing into the United States any compound or formulation thereof using the methods claimed in the patent. However, a process patent does not prevent others from making or using the compound or formulation when it is prepared by a method other than that claimed. Therefore, although method claims are valuable in serving to protect drug products, they are much more limited in scope than compound per se claims.

Another area of importance in terms of patenting methods of making relates to novel methods developed for the synthesis of chemical or biological target molecules. The last decade has witnessed an explosion of innovation in the areas of biochemistry and combinatorial chemistry, particularly as they apply to drug discovery and development. New methods of generating vast numbers of biological molecules, such as DNA and proteins, as well new technology used to prepare chemical "libraries" for use in screening new drug candidates have exponentially increased the number of patent applications directed toward these applications. It is generally established that these new types of technology are patentable subject matter and as such can be patented.

The second type of method-of-use claims relates to methods of using the invention. In terms of pharmaceuticals, method-of-use claims typically relate to the use of a particular drug in the treatment of specific diseases or conditions. FDA approval of a new drug is linked to specific therapeutic uses, and therefore these types of method claims provide important protection for the innovator. These claims are important because they provide patent protection that is in addition to any composition-of-matter claims that may be applicable. Method-of-treatment claims are particularly important for compounds that are already subject to composition-of-matter claims or for which composition-of-matter claims are not available. For example, an inventor may discover that a previously known compound possesses unreported and unexpected anti-inflammatory properties. The inventor may not obtain composition-of-matter protection for the compound itself because the compound is contained in the literature and therefore does not meet the novelty requirement for patentability. However, the inventor may instead obtain a method-of-use claim based on the unexpected anti-inflammatory properties because a compound's unexpected properties may be enough to support patentability.

Chemical intermediates

Generally, novel chemical compounds that are intermediates for the preparation of other chemical compounds of unknown utility are not considered patentable subject matter. However, if the intermediate is used to produce a compound that is known to be useful, then the utility requirement is satisfied, and a patent may be obtained for that intermediate. Claims directed toward chemical intermediates are particularly valuable when they cover stable intermediates that are critical to the only commercially feasible synthetic route to the drug.

Formulations

Still further protection may be afforded by claims that cite a specific formulation of a drug product. Formulation claims allow the inventor to exclude others from making, using, selling, offering for sale, or importing the claimed formulation into the United States. They represent an important opportunity for expanding the patent portfolio protecting a drug, in part because FDA approval for a drug is specific to the formulation containing the drug. Formulation claims may not provide exclusivity to the innovator, but formulation claims expiring after the expiry of compound claims may be a useful tool in maintaining maximum market share for as long as possible.

Reach-through claims

Another recent development in pharmaceutical patents involves so-called reach-through claims. Reach-through claims seek to cover, for example, drugs used for the treatment of conditions that are identified through a particular drug-screening assay without actually specifying the drugs that are covered. These claims, once granted, are exploited through licensing to seek royalties based on sales of products that are developed in part through use of the patented research tool assay. This particular strategy has become a favorite among smaller biotechnology companies that have expended a large portion of their capital in developing new technologies or materials. Several well known examples of reach-through claims are licenses under the Cohen-Boyer patent on basic recombinant DNA techniques and the patents on the Harvard recombinant onco-mouse and Roche polymerase chain reaction. The status of reach-through claims has yet to be determined in the courts.

Compound claims directed toward the drug compound generally afford the broadest scope of patent protection against competitors. However, no single type of claim can afford the best patent protection. The best protection against competitors includes a portfolio of patents, each of which is directed toward a different aspect of the drug. For example, an inventor may obtain a patent for composition of matter that covers the chemical compound itself, another for its method of synthesis, several relating to different formulations, and still others to different therapeutic uses

of the drug. Typically, one seeks to protect new drugs with a broad portfolio of patents to make it difficult for competitors to design around any one patent. As such, it is essential that generic drug manufacturers identify the full range of patents surrounding a particular product to avoid liability for patent infringement.

EXCLUSIVITY FOR THE INNOVATOR

Patent Exclusivity for the Innovator

Patent term

Before June 8, 1995, U.S. patents expired 17 years from the date the patent was issued. However, changes were made in the U.S. patent laws in 1994, in accordance with the Uruguay Round Agreements Act (URAA). The URAA governs the specific date on which a granted U.S. patent expires, which is 20 years from the filing date of the application (3). The changes enacted in response to the URAA were not made to extend patent terms, but to harmonize the term provisions of U.S. patent law with those of other, leading trading partners. In the case of applications filed as continuations or divisionals of previously filed applications, the filing date of the first U.S. priority application is the date from which the 20-year term is measured. For international applications filed under the Patent Cooperation Treaty (PCT), the 20-year term is measured from the filing date of the international application designating the U.S. Foreign national priority (under 35 U.S.C. §119) is not considered in the calculation of the 20-year term. For example, an application filed on June 10, 1995, that does not assert any claim priority to an earlier U.S. application would have an expiration date of June 10, 2015. However, an application filed on January 23, 1997, that is a continuation of an application filed on June 10, 1995, and that claims priority to that date, would have an expiration date of June 10, 2015. The expiration date is the same if the application claims a priority to a previous foreign application.

For those patents currently in force and those that will issue from applications filed before June 8, 1995, the patent term is the longer of either 17 years from the issue date or 20 years from the first U.S. filing date. It is possible for the terms of patents that have already been issued to be extended if they fall within the transition period. The expiration date of an issued patent is extended if the date that is 20 years from the first U.S. filing date is later than the date that is 17 years from the patent issue date. Consequently, any patent that required less than 3 years of prosecution from the first U.S. filing date receives an extension of term by virtue of the URAA 20-year term provisions.

A U.S. patent application filed on March 1, 1992, and issued on April 1, 1994, would have an expiration date calculated under the provisions for the transition period. The expiration date calculated 17 years from issue would be April 1, 2011. The expiration date calculated 20 years from the first U.S. filing would be March 1, 2012. Because the patent term as calculated 20 years from filing is longer, the expiration date of this patent would be extended to March 1, 2012; thus, the patent will receive an extension of term equal to 11 months. The extension is granted despite the fact that the patent was issued before the passage of the URAA provisions.

In addition to these term provisions, in 1999 Congress passed the Patent Term Guarantee Act as part of the American Inventors Protection Act. The Patent Term Guarantee Act, which will go into effect on May 29, 2000, provides that patent terms will be extended to compensate for certain processing delays in the U.S. Patent and Trademark Office and for delays in the prosecution of applications pending for more than three years. Also, extensions are available for delays in issuance of a patent attributable to interference proceedings, secrecy orders, and appellate review. Patent applicants that demonstrate due diligence in the prosecution of their application are guaranteed a minimum 17-year patent term. The act applies only to applications filed on or after the date of enactment, which is May 29, 2000.

Patent-term restoration

Patents claiming a pharmaceutical product, therapeutic uses for a pharmaceutical product, or methods of making a pharmaceutical product may also be eligible for an extension of patent term under the Patent Term Restoration Act (Hatch–Waxman Amendments) (4). Its purpose is to allow the innovator to recover valuable patent term lost during the regulatory review process. The innovator's patented product cannot be commercialized until regulatory approval is obtained. As a result, the innovator is not permitted to reap the benefits of its patent exclusivity until the lengthy approval process is complete. To be eligible for a patent term extension, the patent must claim a product or method of using or manufacturing the product, the patent must not have been previously extended, the application for patent term extension must be submitted within 60 days of approval, the product covered by the patent must have been subject to regulatory review before commercial marketing and use, the approved commercial marketing and use of the product must be the first commercial marketing or use under which the regulatory review period occurred, the patent must not have expired, and no other

patent term must have been extended based on the same regulatory review period (5). Although many patents may cover a single product, only one patent per product may be extended under these provisions, and the extension of the patent term applies to those claims that cover the product receiving regulatory approval.

The length of the patent term extension is directly related to the length of the regulatory review period. The period of extension is calculated by adding half of the length of the testing (IND) period to the length of the approval (NDA) period and subtracting any part of the period that occurred before the issuance of the patent and any part of the period in which the applicant did not act with due diligence (6). The maximum available term extension is 5 years (7). The total patent term, after the extension period, cannot exceed 14 years after the date of approval by the FDA (8). In other words, the patent expiry date, after the addition of the extension period, must be not later than 14 years after the date of FDA approval.

The passage of the URAA, adopting a 20-year patent term, raised questions in circumstances in which a single patent was eligible for a longer term under the URAA 20-year term provisions (hereinafter "URAA extension") and had also received an extension under the Patent Term Restoration Act (hereinafter "Section 156 extension"). The most important question was whether a patentee could reap the benefit of both extensions by adding the URAA extension and the Section 156 extension to prolong the period of patent exclusivity. The Federal Circuit Court of Appeal resolved this issue in *Merck & Co. v. Kessler* (9). In that case, the Court held that the expiration date of a patent having both a URAA and a Section 156 extension is 20 years from filing plus the Section 156 extension, unless the patent is in force on July 8, 1995, solely by virtue of the Section 156 extension. In other words, the foregoing rule applies, except when the patent's 17-year term had expired before June 8, 1995, and the patent is only enforceable by virtue of the Patent Term Restoration Act. Unfortunately, the Federal Circuit Court did not provide a calculation for the expiration date of patents that are in force on June 8, 1995, only because of the Patent Term Restoration Act. However, it would seem that few patents are affected by this omission.

FDA Exclusivity

In addition to patent exclusivity, an innovator may help preserve its market share for a new drug through FDA exclusivity. FDA exclusivity does not guarantee the innovator an exclusive right to market the drug, but it does operate to block approval of ANDAs for generic versions of the drug. FDA exclusivity does not prevent a manufacturer from developing and obtaining approval for a new formulation using the same active ingredient by filing a new drug application (NDA).

The length of the FDA exclusivity period depends on the nature of the new drug developed by the innovator. The statute provides that no ANDA may be submitted for a drug (i.e., new chemical entity) approved after September 24, 1984, until the expiration of 5 years from the date that the innovator received first approval, with one exception (10). An ANDA may be submitted before the expiration of 5 years if it contains a certification of patent invalidity or noninfringement (11). A new NDA for a previously approved drug, if supported by new clinical investigations, enjoys a 3-year exclusivity period during which no new ANDAs may be approved based on the new NDA (12). Supplemental NDAs supported by new clinical investigations also enjoy a 3-year period of exclusivity (13).

The Food and Drug Administration Modernization Act (FDAMA) was passed in 1998, providing for an additional period of exclusivity based on clinical trials conducted in pediatric patients (hereinafter "pediatric exclusivity"). The award of exclusivity is provided as an incentive to the industry to conduct pediatric studies that are requested, but not required, by the FDA. Pediatric exclusivity provides an additional 6 months of exclusivity at the end of any remaning exclusivity or patent life of any patents covering the approved product (14). To be eligible for pediatric exclusivity, the innovator must receive from the FDA a written request to conduct pediatric studies, submit study reports after receipt of the written request, and meet the conditions of the written request. The applicant may request that the FDA issue the necessary written request to qualify for pediatric exclusivity. The award of exclusivity attaches not only to the product tested in the pediatric studies but to any formulations, dosage forms, and indications for products having existing exclusivity or patent life that contain the same active ingredient.

Notice to Generic Manufacturers of Innovator's Exclusivity

The FDA provides notice of the innovator's FDA and patent exclusivity by publishing information regarding exclusivity in the FDA Approved Drugs Product List (the "Orange Book"). The Patent and Exclusivity Appendix to the list of approved products provides details regarding the expiry dates of all types of FDA exclusivity (including pediatric exclusivity) and the expiry dates of patents for each approved product.

The patent information provided in the Orange Book for an approved product is obtained from the innovator.

Innovators are charged with the duty to notify the FDA of the patent number and expiration date of any patent that claims the drug (i.e., the active ingredient or the formulation) or its approved therapeutic use (15). The innovator must update the patent information for an approved product in an appropriate and timely manner as new patents covering the approved product are granted. The innovator must also update the patent information to account for any patent term extension awarded. The submission of this patent information to the FDA ensures that generic drug manufacturers are on notice of the innovator's patent rights and invokes certain innovator rights, discussed below, with respect to notification of an ANDA filing by a generic drug manufacturer and infringement action based on ANDA filing. For these reasons, it is in the innovator's best interest to provide patent information in a timely manner, and, for purposes of competing with the innovator, it is in the generic drug manufacturer's best interest to be knowledgeable of the patent information provided in the Orange Book.

GENERIC COMPETITION

The ability of a generic pharmaceutical manufacturer to commercialize a generic version of an innovator's product centers around two closely related issues: FDA marketing approval and the innovator's patent portfolio. In addition to the requirements designed to establish that the generic drug is in fact equivalent to the approved innovator drug in terms of composition, manufacture, biological activity and labeling (16), the ANDA must also include a patent certification, also known as a paragraph i, ii, iii, or iv certification, regarding the nature of any patent exclusivity for the approved drug and its approved indications (17). The ANDA applicant must certify that in the opinion of the applicant and to the best of the applicant's knowledge with respect to each patent that claims the approved drug or its approved therapeutic use:

i. Patent information has not been filed;
ii. The patent(s) has expired;
iii. The date on which the patent(s) covering the approved drug will expire; or
iv. The patent(s) covering the drug is invalid or will not be infringed by the manufacture, use, or sale of the generic drug for which approval is sought.

The paragraph (i) certification states that patent information for the approved drug on which the ANDA is based has not been filed according to the requirements of the statute. This paragraph applies when there are no patents covering the approved product or its use or if the innovator has failed to properly list the patents covering the drug. It is very rare that no patents will exist for an approved drug, with the possible exception of very old drug products. This is because the investment required for an innovator to obtain marketing approval for a new drug is so great that it would not be feasible for an innovator to commercialize a new drug that lacked a significant period of patent exclusivity during which the innovator could recover the substantial costs of research and development. However, a paragraph (i) certification also applies when the innovator has failed to comply with the rules requiring the listing of all patents covering the approved drug. If the innovator failed to list the patents covering the approved product, and the ANDA applicant could establish that it was not aware of any unlisted patents that claimed the approved drug, the ANDA applicant would likely choose to include a paragraph (i) certification in the ANDA. An ANDA filed with a paragraph (i) certification may be approved effective immediately, barring any FDA exclusivity held by the innovator.

Under a paragraph (ii) certification, the generic drug manufacturer certifies that the patents covering the approved product have already expired. Typically, paragraph (ii) certifications are used only for older drug products because it is common for the ANDA to be filed before the actual expiry of the innovator's patents. An ANDA filed with a paragraph (ii) certification may be approved effective immediately, barring any FDA exclusivity held by the innovator.

Under a paragraph (iii) certification, the generic drug manufacturer certifies that the innovator patents will expire on a certain date and requests marketing approval as of that date. In this case, the FDA may grant tentative approval of the generic drug manufacturer's ANDA before the patent expires, but the generic drug manufacturer does not receive full approval and therefore cannot commercialize the generic product until after the patent expires.

Under a paragraph (iv) certification, the generic drug manufacturer certifies that the innovator patent(s) is either not infringed by the generic product or that the patent(s) is invalid or unenforceable. Paragraph (iv) certifications are discussed in more detail in the following section on infringement.

In this manner, the approval of an ANDA is, in part, dependent on the generic drug manufacturer avoiding infringement of the innovator's patents. The first step to avoiding infringement of the innovator's patents is to identify the particular patents that cover a particular approved product.

Identifying Patents Relating to a Drug

The Orange Book

There are several ways in which a generic pharmaceutical manufacturer can identify the extent of patent exclusivity on a product it wishes to produce. An innovator must submit to the FDA a list of patents that it believes covers the drug product, formulation, or specific therapeutic use of the new drug (18). The patents are subsequently published in the Orange Book. The patents to be listed must be submitted in a timely manner. Any patents directed toward the drug that might issue after the approval of the drug must be disclosed to the FDA within 60 days of issuance. This ensures that the FDA listing of patent exclusivity for a given approved drug is current. Although the FDA does not have the resources to police innovators to ensure compliance with the patent identification regulation, the courts have occasionally imposed a disincentive for failing to comply with the regulation. In particular, one court has determined that the innovator could not sue the ANDA applicant for infringement on the basis of filing the ANDA because the innovator did not list the patent in the Orange Book before filing the law suit (19). The rationale given by the court is that Congress intended that an ANDA applicant consult only the Orange Book to determine the existence of an applicable patent claiming the listed drug or a use of the listed drug.

The Orange Book is an appropriate starting place for the identification of patents claiming an approved drug, formulations of the approved drug, and therapeutic uses of the drug. However, innovators are not required to specify process patents in the Orange Book. As a result, the search for patents that may prohibit the commercialization of a generic form of the drug cannot be complete by merely referring to the Orange Book. For purposes of identifying relevant process patents relating to an approved drug, the Process Patent Amendment Act of 1988 requires the innovator to identify patents it considers relevant to a particular drug on receipt of a written request to do so.

Requests under the Process Patent Amendment Act

The Process Patent Amendment Act of 1988 encourages the generic pharmaceutical manufacturer to submit a request for disclosure of process patents relating to a particular drug to the innovator or patent holder (20). Making such a request is considered evidence of good faith on the part of the generic drug manufacturer in the event that litigation later ensues over the patent(s) (21). The request for disclosure must be in writing and be made to a person engaged in the manufacture of a product, asking for identification of all process patents owned by or licensed to that person as of the time of the request that the person reasonably believes could be asserted to be infringed if the product is imported into or sold, offered for sale, or used in the United States without prior authorization (22). The request for disclosure must be made by a person regularly engaged in the United States in the sale of the same type of products as those manufactured by the party to whom the request is submitted (23). It must also be made before the first importation, sale, or offer for sale of the product by the generic pharmaceutical manufacturer (24). Finally, it should include a statement that any patents identified by the innovator will be submitted to the party who will manufacture or supply the drug and that the generic drug manufacturer will request from the supplier a written statement that none of the processes claimed by the patents is used in the manufacture of the generic drug (25).

After the request for disclosure is received, the patent owner must reply within a reasonable period to be considered to have acted in good faith. However, no reply is required if the products are marked with the process patent numbers before the request is received by the innovator (26).

The Orange Book and the Process Patent Amendment Act are appropriate avenues for identifying the patent exclusivity of an innovator with respect to a specific drug. However, before proceeding with the investment required for the regulatory approval of a generic drug, the pharmaceutical manufacturer should conduct an independent search of the patent literature to identify additional relevant patents. For example, parties other than the innovator may hold patents that affect or even block the ability to commercialize a generic drug. Patent holders other than the innovator are not subject to the same statutory requirements and, furthermore, may not be readily identifiable without an independent search of the patent literature.

PATENT ENFORCEMENT BY THE INNOVATOR

General Principles of Patent Infringement

Infringement is defined as the making, using, selling, offering for sale, or importation into the United States of any patented invention without the authority of the patent owner (27).

Liability for patent infringement only extends throughout the life of the patent. Once the patent term expires, the invention is in the public domain and may be made, used, sold, and/or imported freely. Infringement liability attaches regardless of the quantity or amount of the patented invention that is made, used, sold, offered for sale, or imported. However, the quantity or amount of infringing products may be relevant in determining the damages to be awarded to the patent owner.

Infringement liability is limited territorially. Patent infringement of a U.S. patent arises only when the patented invention is practiced in the United States. The manufacture, use, or sale of the patented invention outside the United States cannot be prohibited by the patent owner, except to the extent that the patent owner also holds a patent in each of the countries where the invention is practiced.

One caveat to the foregoing is that anyone who, without the authority of the patent owner, imports a product into the United States that is prepared abroad by a process claimed in a U.S. patent infringes the U.S. process patent under the 1988 Process Patent Amendments Act (28). In other words, if an unlicensed party uses a process claimed in an unexpired U.S. patent to produce a product outside the United States and then imports that product, the party is liable for the infringement of the U.S. process patent. Thus, even though the patented process is being practiced outside the United States, the patent owner may recover damages for infringement of the process patent once the product produced by the claimed process is imported into the United States. However, the act also provides that a product will not be deemed to be made by the patented process if: 1) it is materially changed by subsequent processes; or 2) it becomes a trivial and nonessential component of another product. For example, see *Eli Lilly and Company v. American Cyanamid Company* (29) for a case concerning what constitutes a "material change" to a drug product under the applicable statute.

Standards for Proving Infringement

The issuance of a valid U.S. patent gives the patent holder the right to exclude others from making, using, selling, offering for sale, or importing the patented invention during the patent term (30). Anyone who makes, uses, sells, offers for sale, or imports the patented invention without the patent owner's consent infringes the claims of that patent. A product may infringe a patent literally or under the Doctrine of Equivalents.

Literal infringement

To define literal infringement, the plain language of the patent claims must first be properly interpreted. This is accomplished by consideration of the ordinary meaning of the language of the claim, the patent specification, the prosecution history of the patent, and the other claims in the patent. The individual claim elements are interpreted based on the ordinary meaning of the terms used, unless it is clear from the patent specification that the inventor intended to use a special meaning. The product or process in question is evaluated for infringement with respect to the properly interpreted claims, not the preferred embodiment set forth in the specification or any commercialized embodiment of the patented invention. Thus, with respect to claim interpretation, the words of the claims are interpreted without consideration of the product in question.

Literal infringement focuses on individual claim elements rather than on the invention as a whole. Whether a product infringes the claims of the patent depends on whether the product literally embodies each and every element of those claims (31). Each element of a claim is material and essential to the definition of the invention. If the product or process does not use even one element of the patent claim, it will not literally infringe the claims. However, the accused infringer usually cannot escape liability for literal infringement merely by adding elements that are not found in the patent claims if each element cited in the claims is found in the product or process under investigation.

Infringement under the Doctrine of Equivalents

Although the requirements of literal infringement may not be satisfied, infringement may still be found under the Doctrine of Equivalents. This doctrine is satisfied when the product in question contains elements identical or equivalent to each claimed element of the patented invention (32).

To determine whether this product possesses elements identical or equivalent to elements of the patented product, many factors may be considered. For example, if this product performs substantially the same overall function in substantially the same way, to obtain the same overall result as the claimed product, the conclusion that the element in question is equivalent is supported (33). However, this is not the only factor evaluated to analyze the doctrine of equivalents. In addition, known interchangeability of the elements used in the accused product compared with the elements of the claimed product by those skilled in the relevant art supports the conclusion that the element of the accused product is equivalent to the claimed product. On the other hand, evidence of lengthy efforts to design around the claims of the patent supports the conclusion that the accused product is not equivalent to the patented product.

The Doctrine of Equivalents has recently been severely restricted by the Court of Appeals for the Federal Circuit. In *Festo Corp. v. Shoketsu Kinzoku Kogyo Kabushiki Co., Ltd.* (33a) the Court held that amendments made to patent claims during prosecution of the patent application, for reasons related to patentability, foreclose the patent holder from subsequently proving infringement using the Doctrine

of Equivalents. Furthermore, patent applicants that amend claims during patent prosecution for unknown reasons are also precluded from relying on the Doctrine of Equivalents to prove infringement with respect to the amended claims.

Prosecution history estoppel

The basic effect of the doctrine of equivalents is to allow the patent owner to expand the scope of protection afforded by the literal language of the claims. However, the doctrine of equivalents does not allow the patent owner to expand the scope of the claims without restriction. The ability of the patent owner to expand the scope of the patent claims is restrained by the prior art and also by the doctrine of prosecution history estoppel.

The prior art limits the degree to which the claims may be interpreted because the claimed invention cannot be interpreted so broadly under the doctrine of equivalents as to encompass products that were known before the patent owner invented the claimed product. In other words, the claims may not be interpreted as broadly under the doctrine of equivalents as to read on the prior art.

The doctrine of prosecution history estoppel also limits the degree to which the claims may be interpreted under the doctrine of equivalents. The doctrine of prosecution history estoppel precludes the patent owner from interpreting the claims in a manner that would encompass, within the claim, subject matter that the patent owner surrendered during prosecution of the patent application to achieve issuance of the patent. Any subject matter that the patent owner surrendered during prosecution to obtain allowance of claims made in the application of the patent cannot be reclaimed under the doctrine of equivalents.

The fact that the accused infringer may have developed the accused product completely independently and without knowledge of the patent is irrelevant in the analysis of infringement liability. An accused infringer cannot escape liability by demonstrating that the accused product was developed wholly through independent research and development.

Invalidity as a Defense to Infringement

An important defense to infringement is that the patent in question is invalid. A patent, once issued, is presumed valid. However, occasionally patents are issued that are invalid for one or more reasons. The focus of the analysis of invalidity is on the mandates of 35 U.S.C. Sections 102 and 103, which set forth the conditions of patentability (although challenges under other sections can be raised as well). In particular, when a challenger presents evidence, such as a prior art reference, which is more pertinent than that considered by the patent examiner during the prosecution of the patent application, the burden of proving invalidity is more easily met (34).

Under Section 102(a), a patent claim is invalid if the claimed product was known or used by others in the United States, or was patented or described in a printed publication in the United States or a foreign country before the product was invented by the patentee (35). To anticipate a claim under Section 102(a), the challenger must show that the claimed product was publicly available before it was invented by the innovator, thus establishing that the patent owner was not the first to invent the claimed invention.

According to Section 102(b), a patent claim is anticipated, and therefore is invalid, if the claimed invention has been patented or described in a printed publication, or has been on sale, more than 1 year before the effective filing date of the application from which the patent was issued (36). To anticipate the claim, a single prior art reference must show each element of the claimed invention arranged as set forth in the claim. However, in the appropriate setting, a secondary reference may be used to explain or demonstrate that a primary reference anticipates a patent claim inherently.

A patent claim may also be invalidated if the challenger shows that the patent does not cite the true inventor(s) (37). A patent must list only the names of those individuals who contributed to at least one element of one or more claims. If the patent includes additional individuals who are not inventors or if the patent fails to include one or more true inventors, and the error in the naming of inventors occurred with deceptive intent, the claim(s) may be invalidated.

Section 103 can be used to invalidate patent claims even when the claimed invention is not identically disclosed or described for purposes of Section 102, if the differences between the claimed invention and prior art are such that the claimed subject matter as a whole would have been obvious at the time the invention was made (38). A determination regarding validity under Section 103 must address the following factors (39):

1. The scope and content of the prior art.
2. Differences between the prior art and the claimed invention.
3. The level of ordinary skill in the pertinent art, and
4. Secondary considerations evidencing nonobviousness.

The secondary considerations include commercial success, long-felt need, failure of others, copying, praise by persons in the industry, departure from accepted principles, and widespread recognition in the art of the invention's significance.

Remedies for Patent Infringement

Several remedies are available for patent infringement. The patent owner may obtain an injunction preventing the accused infringer from continuing the unauthorized practice of the claimed invention (40). The preliminary injunction is an important remedy because it enables the patent owner to immediately stop the activities of the infringer without the necessity of first obtaining a judgment of infringement through a lengthy litigation process.

The patent owner may also obtain monetary damages from the infringer (41), being entitled to adequate compensation for the infringement. Monetary damages may be measured in different ways to determine the amount that the patent owner can recover. For example, monetary damages may be based on the profits lost by the patent owner as a result of the infringement. In any event, the damages for the patent owner will not be less than a reasonable royalty for the practice of the invention (42).

When the infringement is shown to be willful or intentional, the patent owner may recover an increased monetary award of up to three times the amount of monetary damages shown, plus attorney's fees (43).

Infringement Exemptions for Generic Pharmaceutical Manufacturers under Hatch–Waxman Provisions

The Hatch–Waxman provisions were enacted to strike a balance between the competing interests of protecting the innovation of new drugs and providing an incentive for continued research and development of new drugs versus providing lower cost generic alternatives. To permit generic pharmaceutical manufacturers to begin the testing involved in obtaining FDA approval for a generic product, the Hatch–Waxman Act exempts the generic pharmaceutical manufacturer from patent infringement liability for certain activities. Under the Hatch–Waxman Act, it is not an act of infringement for a generic pharmaceutical manufacturer to make, use, sell, offer for sale, or import into the United States a patented drug if the act of doing so is reasonably related to the development and filing of an application for federal regulatory approval (e.g., FDA approval) (44). This exemption from the definition of infringement allows the generic pharmaceutical manufacturer to make or import and use the patented drug before the expiration of the patent, thus enabling the generic pharmaceutical manufacturer to initiate the FDA regulatory review process before the expiration of the patent. The ability to begin these activities before patent expiration is essential to obtaining FDA approval for commercialization as of the expiration date of the patent covering the drug. Without this provision, the patent owner would effectively receive the benefit of exclusivity not only during the patent term, but also during the regulatory review of the ANDA.

The purpose of the Hatch–Waxman Act is not, however, to insulate the generic pharmaceutical manufacturer from infringement liability to such an extent that the generic pharmaceutical manufacturer is permitted to start commercialization or even to obtain FDA approval before the expiration of the patent. As a corollary to the privileges granted to the generic pharmaceutical manufacturer, the Hatch–Waxman provision also specifies that the filing of an ANDA for the purpose of obtaining FDA approval for commercialization of a generic drug before the expiration of the patent covering the drug constitutes an act of infringement for which the generic pharmaceutical manufacturer may be liable (45).

The ANDAs that can be the subject of an infringement action under this provision include a paragraph (iv) patent certification, that is, a certification asserting either that the commercialization of the generic drug for which approval is being sought will not infringe the patent covering the innovator's drug or that the patent covering the drug is invalid. As noted above, an ANDA applicant including a paragraph (iv) certification is required by law to notify the patent owner that such an application has been filed. Thus, the patent owner is ensured of receiving notice of his right to commence an infringement action under Section 271(e). If after receiving such a notice the patent owner decides to file a lawsuit for infringement based on the filing of an ANDA including the paragraph (iv) certification, the owner must file the lawsuit within 45 days of receiving the notice of the ANDA filing (46). This action by the patent owner stops the FDA regulatory review of the ANDA, and approval would not be effective until 30 months after the date the patent owner received notification of the ANDA filing (47). The law does give some discretion to the court to shorten or lengthen the 30-month period, depending on the conduct of the parties during litigation (48). The act also provides exceptions to the 30-month period, depending on the outcome of litigation. For example, if the court finds that the patent is infringed and valid (contrary to the ANDA certification) before the expiration of the 30-month period, ANDA approval cannot become effective before the expiration date of the patent (49). This is true even if the 30-month period expires before the patent. If, on the other hand, the court finds that the patent is invalid or not infringed, the ANDA approval may be made effective as of the date of the court decision (50).

These provisions can be summarized as follows. A generic pharmaceutical manufacturer seeking to obtain FDA approval for a generic drug before the expiration of the patent covering the drug must file an ANDA including a paragraph (iv) certification asserting that the patent will not be infringed by the commercialization of the generic drug or that the patent is unenforceable or that the patent is invalid. The ANDA applicant making this certification must also notify the patent owner of the filing of the ANDA including this certification and provide the details regarding the rationale for the applicant's belief that the patent will not be infringed or is invalid. If the patent owner does not challenge the veracity of the ANDA certification, the ANDA may be approved effective immediately, and with this approval, the ANDA applicant may proceed with the commercialization of the generic drug. If, however, the patent owner does file an infringement action against the ANDA applicant within 45 days after receiving the notification of the ANDA filing, the ANDA may not be approved until 30 months from the date on which the patent owner received notification of the ANDA or the patent expires or the court determines that the patent is invalid or not infringed.

Remedies for the innovator for infringement based on an ANDA filing

If the court finds that an ANDA applicant has infringed a patent by filing the ANDA with a paragraph (iv) certification, the question remains as to what remedy is available to the patent owner. The law explicitly states that the patent owner may not obtain an injunction that would prevent the generic pharmaceutical manufacturer from making, using, selling, offering for sale, or importing the patented drug if the purpose of doing so is solely for the preparation and filing of an application for FDA approval (51). This provision prevents the patent owner from circumventing the provisions of the Hatch–Waxman Act that explicitly exclude these activities from the definition of infringement. However, an injunction can prevent the generic pharmaceutical manufacturer from commercializing the generic drug.

Monetary damages against the infringing ANDA applicant are also an available remedy. However, because the ANDA was not approved, commercial use or sales on which monetary damages could be based are highly unlikely. For the same reason, treble damages and attorney's fees based on willful infringement are, in reality, also unavailable. Perhaps the most important practical remedy for the patent owner is the fact that FDA approval of the ANDA is blocked by an infringement action. Without FDA approval, the generic drug cannot be commercialized, thus preserving the patent owner's exclusivity.

Case study: Bayer AG versus Elan Pharmaceutical Research Corporation

The Hatch–Waxman provisions are demonstrated by the case of *Bayer AG v. Elan Pharmaceutical Research Corporation* (52). Bayer AG and Bayer Corporation ("Bayer") filed an application and was granted U.S. Patent No. 5,264,446 (the '446 patent) in November 1993 covering nifedipine, a drug used for the treatment of hypertension. The '446 patent covered nifedipine itself as a composition-of-matter claim, a method for making the drug, as well as a method of treatment using the drug. The purpose of the patent was to provide patent coverage for a sustained-release version of the drug. The patent contained 12 independent claims, and each claim specified a specific surface area (SSA) for the nifedipine crystals used in making tablets of the drug. Specifically, the '446 patent covered nifedipine crystals with an SSA of 1.0 to 4 m^2/gram in admixture with a solid diluent to result in a sustained-release formulation of the compound.

In April 1997, Elan submitted an ANDA to the FDA seeking approval for a product they claimed was bioequivalent to Bayer's product containing nifedipine as the active ingredient. Elan's ANDA covered a once-daily formulation containing 30 mg of active ingredient with an SSA of no less than 5 m^2/gram. Pursuant to federal regulations (53), Elan sent notice of its ANDA filing and paragraph IV certification, noting that the nifedipine it intended to manufacture and market did not infringe the claims of Bayer's '446 patent. Bayer filed suit against Elan, claiming both literal infringement and infringement under the doctrine of equivalents. The District Court ruled in favor of Elan on both infringement issues, holding that Elan's proposed sale of a nifedipine product having an SSA greater than that claimed in the '446 patent did not constitute literal infringement and that prosecution history estoppel prevented Bayer from contending infringement under the doctrine of equivalents (54). Bayer appealed the decision of the District Court.

The United States Court of Appeals for the Federal Circuit subsequently upheld the decision of the District Court with respect to both issues of literal infringement and infringement under the doctrine of equivalents. With regard to the issue of literal infringement, the Court of Appeals reasoned that for a product to literally infringe a patent claim, the product in question must contain each limitation of the asserted claim. In other words, the accused product must contain each element of the patented composition to constitute direct infringement of the patent. If any claimed limitation is missing in the accused product, there is no literal infringement as a matter of law. Elan presented evidence at trial that the nifedipine crystals it intended to use in its product had an SSA equal to or greater than 5 m^2/gram. The Court of Appeals held that since the '446 patent covered only nifedipine crystals with an SSA between 1.0 and 4.0 m^2/gram, the manufacture and sale of Elan's nifedipine product did not constitute literal infringement.

Bayer alternatively argued that the manufacture and sale of Elan's nifedipine product constituted infringement under the doctrine of equivalents. As addressed previously, infringement under the doctrine of equivalents can occur if there is not a substantial difference between the limitations contained in the patent and the accused product. However, one caveat of the doctrine of equivalents is the theory of prosecution history estoppel under which a patentee is prevented from claiming infringment for subject matter that was clearly and unmistakably surrendered during prosecution of the patent application. In this case, there was clear evidence that the original application which eventually issued as the '446 patent contained claims for nifedipine with an SSA range of 0.5 to 6 m^2/gram. During prosecution of the application, the patent examiner rejected Bayer's claims as obvious over the prior art. In response to the examiner's rejection, Bayer amended its claims to restrict the scope to only nifedipine crystals with an SSA of 1.0 to 4 m^2/gram, claiming that crystals in this range provided unexpected and advantageous bioavailability and sustained-release properties. Elan argued that because Bayer had unequivocally surrendered any claims to nifedipine crystals having an SSA of greater than 4 m^2/gram, Elan's ANDA specifying crystals with an SSA of no less than 5 m^2/gram did not constitute infringement under the doctrine of equivalents. The Court of Appeals agreed with Elan's argument, reasoning that a competitor examining the entire prosecution history of the '446 patent would conclude that Bayer had surrendered any claim to a nifedipine drug product having an SSA greater than 4 m^2/gram. As a result, the Court of Appeal's held that Elan's ANDA for generic nifedipine did not infringe the claims of Bayer's '446 patent either literally or under the doctrine of equivalents. Consequently, the lawsuit instituted by Bayer was lost, and Elan's ANDA proceeded to approval by the FDA.

Process Patents and the Hatch–Waxman Act

Process patents (i.e., patents claiming processes for making a drug compound or formulation) are not listed by the FDA in connection with approved drug formulations. Thus, process patents are not subject to the patent certification requirements of ANDAs and do not invoke the Hatch–Waxman procedures relating to infringement outlined above. If the patent owner learns of the generic pharmaceutical manufacturer's use, sale, offer for sale, or importation of the drug or formulation prepared by the patented process, the patent owner has an action for infringement under the Patent Process Amendment Act, even if the process of making the drug or formulation is conducted outside the United States (55). The same is true if the generic pharmaceutical manufacturer uses, sells, offers for sale, or imports an intermediate useful for making the drug that is prepared by a process claimed in a U.S. patent. Thus, even though process patents do not invoke the important Hatch–Waxman provisions pertaining to infringement, the protection they provide may be invaluable particularly if the only commercially viable means of obtaining the drug is through the patented process. If this is the case, the patent owner may block the commercialization of the generic drug, not by blocking the FDA approval process, but by blocking the generic pharmaceutical manufacturer's ability to obtain the drug compound. Consequently, the protection afforded by the Patent Process Amendment Act, if used correctly, can be an important complement to the protection afforded by the Hatch–Waxman Act. As noted above, there are two important caveats to the Process Patent Amendment Act. A product imported into the United States will not be deemed to infringe on a valid process patent if: 1) the product is materially changed by subsequent processes, or 2) it becomes a trivial and nonessential component of another product. Of course, the terms "material change" and "trivial and nonessential" are vague and open to broad interpretation. The federal courts are still struggling with the meaning of this broad language and with what constitutes infringement.

MOTIVATIONS FOR CHALLENGING A PATENT

Irrespective of the potential liability for patent infringement, the motivation still remains for a generic pharmaceutical manufacturer to challenge the patent(s) covering a drug in an attempt to obtain FDA approval to market a generic version of the drug before the expiration of the innovator's patent(s). There are several incentives for challenging an innovator's patent. For example, although an issued patent is presumed to be valid, occasionally new evidence comes to light after grant that may invalidate one or more of the patent claims. If the generic pharmaceutical manufacturer obtains this evidence and discloses this to the patent owner in the notification required when filing an ANDA with a paragraph (iv) certification, the patent owner may prefer to negotiate a settlement with the generic

pharmaceutical manufacturer rather than risk the possibility of one or more of the claims being declared invalid by the court. Obviously, if the generic pharmaceutical manufacturer hopes to persuade the patent owner to accept such a compromise, the validity of the patent should be fully investigated before filing the ANDA.

If instead of reaching a settlement with the patent owner, the generic pharmaceutical manufacturer successfully challenges the patent, this company has the privilege of keeping the first generic drug on the market and has a head-start on would-be competitors. As a further incentive, the FDA regulations provide an exclusivity period for the first generic drug to enter the marketplace (56). The generic pharmaceutical manufacturer that successfully challenges the patent has an exclusivity period that extends for 180 days after either the first commercial marketing of the generic drug or the date of the first court decision holding the patent invalid or not infringed (57). During this period, no other ANDAs for the same drug may be approved. This period of exclusivity for the generic pharmaceutical manufacturer, coupled with the status of being the first generic drug on the market, can lead to the establishment of a strong market position and a return on the manufacturer's investment in challenging the patent.

CONCLUSION

Growth in the pharmaceutical industry has contributed significantly to the importance of pharmaceutical patents and the Hatch–Waxman Amendments in the United States. The importance of these issues will likely continue to increase as more and more foreign pharmaceutical companies reach toward the lucrative U.S. market for the sale of pharmaceutical products and formulations developed abroad. In the past, most small or midsize foreign pharmaceutical companies have avoided the U.S. markets because of stringent FDA regulations. As the demand for lower-cost pharmaceutical products increases, the profitable U.S. market can no longer be ignored. The balance between the rights of the patent owners and the desire for lower-cost generic alternatives to approved drugs will continue to elevate the importance of the Hatch–Waxman Amendments and will no doubt lead to significant debate as efforts begin for the revision of these provisions.

REFERENCES

1. 35 U.S.C. §101 and §100.
2. 35 U.S.C.§271(g).

3. 35 U.S.C. §154(a)(2).
4. 35 U.S.C. §156.
5. 37 C.F.R. §1.720.
6. 35 U.S.C. §156; 37 C.F.R. §1.775.
7. 35 U.S.C. §156(g)(6)(A).
8. 35 U.S.C. §156(c)(3).
9. 80F.3d 1543, 38 USPQ2d 1347 (Fed. Cir. 1996).
10. 21 U.S.C. §355(j)(5)(D)(ii). Other Time Periods Apply to Products Approved Before September 24, 1984. See 21 U.S.C. §355(j)(5)(D).
11. 21 U.S.C. §355(j)(5)(D)(ii).
12. 21 U.S.C. §355(j)(5)(D)(iii).
13. 21 U.S.C. §355(j)(5)(D)(iv).
14. 21 U.S.C. §355a.
15. 21 C.F.R. 314.53 and 21 U.S.C. §355(b)(1).
16. 21 U.S.C. §355(j)(2)(A).
17. 21 U.S.C. §355(j)(2)(A)(vii).
18. 21 C.F.R. 314.53 and 21 U.S.C. §355(b)(1).
19. *Abbott Labs r. Zenith Labs. Inc.*, 934 F.Supp 925, 36 USPQ2d 1801 (1995).
20. 35 U.S.C. §287(3).
21. 35 U.S.C. §287(3)(B)(i).
22. 35 U.S.C. §287(4).
23. 35 U.S.C. §287(4)(A)(i).
24. 35 U.S.C. §287(4)(A)(ii).
25. 35 U.S.C. §287(4)(A)(iii).
26. 35 U.S.C. §287(4)(C).
27. 35 U.S.C. §271(a).
28. 35 U.S.C. §271(g).
29. *Eli Lilly and Company v. American Cyanamid*, 82 F.3d 1568 (Fed. Cir. 1996).
30. 35 U.S.C. § 154(a)(1).
31. *Consolidated Aluminum Corp. v. Foseco Intl. Ltd.*, 716 F. Supp 316, 10 USPQ2d 1143 (N.D. Ill. 1988).
32. *Hilton Davis Chem. Co. v. Warner-Jenkinson Co., Inc.*, 62 F.3d 1512, 35 USPQ2d 1641 (Fed. Cir. 1995) (*En Banc*), *Revd. and Remanded*, No. 95–758 (U.S. March 3, 1997).
33. This Test was First Set Forth in *Pennwalt Corp. v. Durand-Wayland, Inc.*, 833 F.2d 931 (Fed. Cir. 1987).
33a. *Festo Corp. v. Shoketsu Kinzoku Kogyo Kabushiki Co., Ltd.*, 234 F.3d 558 (Fed. Cir. 2000).
34. *EWP Corp. v. Reliance Universal Inc.*, 755 F.2d 898, 225 USPQ2d 20 (Fed. Cir. 1985).
35. 35 U.S.C. §102(a).
36. 35 U.S.C. §102(b).
37. 35 U.S.C. §102(f).
38. 35 U.S.C. §103.
39. *Graham v. John Deere Co.*, 383 U.S. 1 (1966).
40. 35 U.S.C. §283.
41. 35 U.S.C. §284.
42. 35 U.S.C. §284.
43. 35 U.S.C. §285.
44. 35 U.S.C. §271(e)(1).
45. 35 U.S.C. §271(e)(2).
46. 21 U.S.C. §355(j)(4)(B)(iii).
47. 21 U.S.C. §355(j)(5)(B)(iii).
48. 21 U.S.C. §355(j)(5)(B)(iii).
49. 21 U.S.C. §355(j)(5)(B)(iii)(II).
50. 21 U.S.C. §355(j)(5)(B)(iii)(I).
51. 35 U.S.C. §271(e)(3).
52. *Bayer AG r. Elan Pharmaceutical Research Corp.*, 2000 WL 572705 (Fed. Cir. 2000).
53. 21 U.S.C. §505(j)(2)(B)(ii).
54. *Bayer AG v. Elan Pharmaceutical Research Corp.*, 64 F.Supp.2d 1295 (N.D. Ga. 1999).
55. 35 U.S.C. §271(g).
56. 21 U.S.C. §355(j)(5)(B)(iv).
57. 21 U.S.C. §355(j)(5)(B)(iv) and *Mylan Pharmaceuticals Inc. v. Shalala*, 53 USPQ2d 1449 (DC DC 2000).

Index

metered-dose inhaler, 2366-2367
nebulizer solutions, 2366
propellant-driven metered-dose
    inhalers, 2366-2367
radiolabeling, DPIs, 2367-2369
scatter correction, 2371-2372
single photon emission computed tomography,
    misconceptions of, 2370-2371
gamma-scintigraphic imaging
    data analysis, 2372
    lung deposition, 2369-2372
    scatter correction, 2371-2372
    single photon emission computed tomography,
        misconceptions of, 2370-2371
Radiopharmaceuticals, parenteral delivery
    drugs, 911
Randomization, clinical data management sys-
    tems, 443
Raoult's law, tonicity, 2812-2813
Rate of elimination, veterinary drugs, 2954-2955
Rate-preprogrammed delivery, 811-822
Rate theory, theoretical principles, 364-366
Raw materials
    analysis-gas chromatography, 375-400
    gelatin, 302-303
    hard capsules, 302-303
        gelatin, 302-303
R&D. *See* Research and developemnt
r-DNA technology, quality control tests in, 214
    biotechnology, 214
Reach-through claims, patents, 2034
Read-out devices, in ultraviolet spectropho-
    tometry, 2562
Reassembly, equipment cleaning, 1104
Receptors, 2375-2395
    adopted orphan receptors, 2388
    classification, 2375-2380
    cloned human receptors, 2386-2394
    combinatorial subunits, 2379
    conformational states, 2382-2383
    endogenous, surrogate ligands, screening
        for, 2391-2392
    human genome sequencing, 2392-2394
    interactions, real time, 2383-2384
    isoforms, 2380
    ligand-receptor interactions, 2380-2384
    molecular structure, 2375-2376
    multiligand/multireceptor families, 2379
    noncompetitive antagonists, 2383
    orphan, ligand fishing for, 2389
    orphan GPCR receptors, ligand
        identification, 2388-2389
    orphan receptors, 2380
    subtypes
        function, defining, 2385-2386
        functional roles, 2385-2386
    superfamilies, families, subtypes, 2376-2379
Recombinant DNA technology, 212-214
Recombinant human deoxyribonuclease, pulmon-
    ary absorption, 2121
Recombinant vaccines, 2897-2899
    anti-idiotypic vaccines, 2899
    bacterial vectors, 2897
    gene-deleted vaccines, 2898
    subunit vaccines, 2898-2899
        immunogenic antigen production, in
            plants, 2898-2899
    viral vectors, 2897
Recombivax, 219
Records, good manufacturing
    practices, 1412-1413
Recreational use of drugs, 24
Recruiting, in drug development, 1702
Rectal absorption, pediatric administration, 2050
Rectal administration, pediatric adminis-
    tration, 2063
Rectal delivery, peptides, proteins, 1887-1888

Rectal route, 932-944
    absorption, 11, 165, 939-942
    biochemistry of rectal tissues, 934-936
        advantages over oral systems, 937-938
        anatomy, 934-935
        biochemistry, 935-936
        model systems, 936-937
        in vitro models, 936-937
    constant environment, 938
    control, rectal drug absorption, 939-940
        charge, 940
        molecular size, 940
        nonspecific adsorption, 940
        pH partition, 939
        solubility, 940
        spreading, 940
    disadvantages, 938-939
    drug classes, 939
    enzymatic drug stability, 937
    hepatic first pass, avoidance of, 937
    higher drug load, 937-938
    limited fluid in, 939
    lymphatic delivery, 938
    market potential, 942
    nonspecific drug loss, 939
    optimizing absorption, 940-942
        enhancing agents, 940-941
        pH control, 941
        solubilizing agents, 941
        viscosity modifiers, 941-942
    overdosing, 938
    patient acceptance, compliance, 938
    physiologic issues, 934-939
    rectal formulations available, 932-934
        controlled-release formulations, 933-934
        gels/foams/ointments, 933
        marketed drugs, 934
        solid suppositories, 932
        solutions, 932-933
        worldwide market, 933
    rectum, limited fluid in, 939
    solutions, 932-933
    swallowing difficulty, 938
Red baneberry, toxicity, 2220
Reductions, 225-227
    biotransformation, 225-227
    carbon, 226
    expiration dating, 1217-1218
    nitrogen, 226
    sulfur, 226-227
Re-engineering, clinical data management sys-
    tems, 440
Reference CD spectra, chirotical analytical
    methods, 352-353
Reference diffraction patterns, x-ray powder
    diffractometry, 3006-3008
Reference electrodes, potentiometry, 2251-2253
Reference standards, 2190-2191
    harmonization, 1416-1417
Referrals from colleagues, contract manufactur-
    ing, 618
Refractive index detectors, chromatography, 421
Regranex, 217
Regulatory activity
    bacterial endotoxins test, 2347
    calorimetry, 299-300
    contract manufacturing, 623-624
        cooperation with regulatory agencies, 624
        dedicated equipment, 624
        inspections, 623
        international considerations, 623-624
        master files, 624
        pre-approval inspections, 623
        relations with regulatory agencies, 624
        requirements, biotechnology industry, 624
        status of contract manufacturer, 623
    cyclodextrins, 550-552

dry powder inhalation, 1538-1539
equipment cleaning, 1102
    validation, 1102
excipients, 1174-1180
expiration dating, 1211-1212
Food and Drug Administration, 1287-1298
generic drugs, 1345-1346
herbal medicine, 2216-2217
isolators, 1589
in process chemistry, 2302
protein binding, 2335-2336
in radiochemical analysis, 2363-2364
radiochemical analysis, 2363-2364
tablet evaluation, near-infrared spec-
    troscopy, 2691
topical drug delivery, 954-956
worldwide, coloring agents, 510-512
Regulatory agencies, electronic submission to,
    clinical data management systems, 447
Regulatory exclusivity, patents, 2030-2031
Rekker's fragmental constant f, 2015
Relative humidity
    control of, 2974-2976
    critical, measurement of, 2975
    measurement of, 2975
Releases
    excipients, 1152
    factors affecting, 141-142
    hard capsules, 312-314
Rembrandt mouth-refreshing rinse, 700
Remicade, 218
Removal of exudate, dressings, 787
Renal clearance, protein binding and, 2329
Renal disease
    adverse drug reaction and, 37
    protein binding and, 2333
Renal disorders, orphan drugs, 1943
Renal elimination, pediatric administration, 2052
Renal excretion, isomerism, 1612
Renal failure, hypoalbuminemia with, 37
Renal impairment, dosage adjusted for, 784
Renal system, cyclodextrins, 547-548, 548
ReoPro, 218
Reperfusion injury, free radicals, 108
Reporting
    clinical data management systems, 447
    derivations, clinical data management sys-
        tems, 447
    electronic submission to regulatory
        agencies, 447
    extracting data, 447
    reporting tools, 447
Reports
    good laboratory practice, 1401
    good manufacturing practices, 1412-1413
    validation, 2920-2921
Reproductive safety, cyclodextrins, 550
Reproductive toxicity
    drug safety evaluation, 1003-1005
        fertility studies, 1004
        perinatal toxicity, 1005
    perinatal toxicity, 1005
    in preservation, 2286
Reproductive toxicology, use of animals in
    testing, 75-76
Republic of South Africa, health care
    systems, 1429-1430
    organization, 1429-1430
    pharmaceuticals, 1430
Repulsion theory, super disintegrants, 2628
Research and development, 1693-1694
    economic characteristics, 1033-1036
        competition in pharmaceutical indus-
            try, 1034
        competitive process, 1033-1034
        internal organization, pharmaceutical
            firm, 1034-1035

Size exclusion chromatography, 420
Size reduction, classification, 2879-2882
    classification, size separation, 2881-2882
    grinding equipment, 2881
    mills, operation of, 2881
Skin, retention of compounds on, 949-950
Skin barrier function, 2125-2126
    stratum corneum, 2125-2126
Skin diffusivity, reduction of, 950
Skin graft product, 219
Skin irritation, with transdermal
    route, 951
Skin wound repair, absorbable gel-formers, 123
Slipping, two-dimensional mixing mechan-
    isms, 1797
Slits, in fluorescence spectroscopy, 2511-2512
Small intestinal absorption, oral drug deliv-
    ery, 2208
Small sample quantity analysis, nuclear magnetic
    resonance spectroscopy, 1912-1915
Small-volume injectables, parenteral
    route, 910-911
Small-volume probes, nuclear magnetic resonance
    spectroscopy, 1912-1915
Smectite clays, gels, 1341-1342
Smoking
    drug interactions, 992
    effects, pulmonary absorption, 2116
    oral drug delivery, 2208
    protein binding, 2333
Soap, cosmetic, 651
Social use of drugs, 24
Soda-lime-silica glasses, 1379
Sodium, 389, 391
    gels, 1338
    organic volatile impurities, 401
Sodium acetate, 408
Sodium acid phosphate, isotonicity, 2821
Sodium alginate
    as tablet binder, 2718
    as tablet disintegrating agent, 2722
Sodium ascorbate, 408
Sodium benzoate, 408
    isotonicity, 2821
    relative humidity value, 2978
Sodium bicarbonate, 408
    effervescent pharmaceuticals, 1039
    isotonicity, 2821
Sodium bisulfite, isotonicity, 2821
Sodium borate, 408
    isotonicity, 2821
Sodium butyrate, 408
Sodium caprate, oleic acid, 5
Sodium capsules, 381
Sodium carbonate, 390, 408
Sodium chloride
    isotonicity, 2821
    properties of, 2528
    relative humidity value, 2978
    as tablet diluent, 2716
Sodium chloride-potassium bromide, relative
    humidity value, 2979
Sodium cholate, 5
Sodium cromoglycate, for radiolabeling, 2368
Sodium dehydroacetate, 408
Sodium deoxycholate, 3, 5
Sodium fluoride, 408
    caries control, fluorides, 694
Sodium formaldehyde sulfoxylate, 408
Sodium fusidate, 3
Sodium glycine carbonate, as tablet disintegrating
    agent, 2722
Sodium glycocholate, 3
Sodium iodide, 408
    isotonicity, 2821
Sodium lauryl sulfate
    as tablet disintegrating agent, 2722

    as tablet lubricant, 2720
Sodium lauryl sulphate, 3, 5, 408
Sodium monofluorophosphate, 408
    caries control, fluorides, 694-695
Sodium nitrate, isotonicity, 2821
Sodium nitrite, titrations with, 2263
Sodium phosphate, 403
    isotonicity, 2821
Sodium propionate, 408
    isotonicity, 2821
Sodium salicylate, 408
    relative humidity value, 2978
Sodium starch glycolate, 2579
    as tablet disintegrating agent, 2722
Sodium stearate, 408
Sodium stearyl fumarate, 408
    as tablet lubricant, 2720
Sodium sulfite, isotonicity, 2821
Sodium taurodihydrofusidate, 3
Sodium valproate, veterinary drug, 2955
Soft capsules, 317-327
    description, 317
    fill formulation, 319
    formulation development, 317-319
    gelatin shell formulation, 318-319
        colorants/opacifiers, 318-319
        gelatin, 318
        plasticizers, 318
        water, 318
    gel compatibility, 320
    method of manufacture, 320-323
    new technology, 325
    patents, 325-326
    process development/trial manufacture, 320
    product development, 319-320
    product quality considerations, 324-325
        final product testing, 325
        ingredient specifications, 324-325
        in-process testing, 325
    therapeutic performance, 323-324
        decreased plasma variability, 324
        increased bioavailability, 324
        rate of absorption, 323-324
Soft contact lens cleaning, 1646-1648
    active components of, 1647-1648
        chelating agents, 1648
        deposit-shearing particles, 1648
        enzymes, 1647-1648
        oxidizing agents, 1648
        solvents, 1648
        surfactants, 1647
    active components of lens cleaners, 1647-1648
        chelating agents, 1648
        deposit-shearing particles, 1648
        enzymes, 1647-1648
        oxidizing agents, 1648
        solvents, 1648
        surfactants, 1647
    classification, lens cleaners, 1647
        consumer, *versus* professional use clea-
            ners, 1647
        consumer *versus* professional use clea-
            ners, 1647
        daily cleaners, *versus* weekly cleaners, 1647
        daily cleaners *versus* weekly cleaners, 1647
        in-the-eye, *versus* out-of-the-eye clea-
            ners, 1647
        in-the-eye *versus* out-of-the-eye clea-
            ners, 1647
    lens deposits, 1646-1647
        composition, 1646-1647
        problems associated with, 1647
Soft contact lenses, wear comfort, 1651-1652
    factors contributing to, 1651-1652
    lens comfort solutions, 1652
Soft gelatin capsules, 753-754
Software

computer-assisted drug design, 600-601
    medication error and, 1733
Sol-gel transition, 1331
Solid-crystalline suspensions, 1668-1670
    lipids, 1668-1670
Solid dispersions
    classification of, 642-644
        compound, complex formation, 644
        crystalline carrier, amorphous precipitations
            in, 644
        glass solutions, suspensions, 643-644
        simple eutectic mixtures, 642
        solid solutions, 642-643
    solubility of poorly water-soluble
        drugs, 635-636
Solid dosages, 749-754, 1132-1142
    absorption and, 17
    capsules, 753-754
    common excipients used in, 170
    controlled release, excipients, 1138-1139
    coprecipitates, 642-643
    hard gelatin capsules, 753
    lipids, 1670
    modified release dosage forms, 751-753
    orally administered, disposition of, 126
    powders, granules, 749
    soft gelatin capsules, 753-754
    specific types of tablets, 750-751
    sustained drug release, 850
    tablets, 749-750
    unit processes, 2890-2891
Solidification, tumbling blenders, 1808
Solid membranes, electrodes with, 2254
Solids
    compounding, 578-580
    flow properties, 1264-1285
        aerated bulk density, 1272-1273
        angle of repose, 1271-1272
        avalanche behavior, powder
            rheometers, 1280-1282
        bi, triaxial shear cells, 1279-1280
        classification systems, 1274-1275
        density, 1273
        factors influencing, 1264-1268
        flow enhancers (glidants), 1269-1270
        hopper flow models, 1268-1269
        Jenike shear cell, 1277
        measurement of, 1270-1274
        moisture, static charge, 1267
        orifice, flow through, 1270-1271
        packing properties, bulk
            densities, 1272-1274
        particle size, distribution, 1265
        plate-type shear cell, 1278
        powder
            cohesion, storage compaction, 1267
            granular properties, empirical measure-
                ments, 1271
            granulations, 1264-1265
        ring, annular shear cell, 1278-1279
        shape factors, 1265-1267
        shear cells, 1276-1280
        tapped, compressed bulk density, 1273
        temperature, 1268
    parenteral route, 913-914
        freeze-drying, 913
        powder-filled small volume
            injectables, 913-914
Solid-state detectors, in radiation detection, 2357
Solid-state nuclear magnetic resonance
    spectroscopy, 1917-1920
    anisotropy in solid state, 1918
    applications of solid state NMR, 1918-1920
    gel-phase NMR, 1918-1919
    magic angle spinning, 1918
    polymorph studies, 1919-1920
    solid-state structural studies, 1920

Brief Contents